LEUKEMIA

WILLIAM DAMESHEK and FREDERICK GUNZ'S

LEUKEMIA

THIRD EDITION—REVISED AND ENLARGED

Frederick Gunz, M.D., Ph.D.

Director of Medical Research,
Kanematsu Memorial Institute,
Sydney Hospital, Sydney, Australia

Albert G. Baikie, M.B.,
Ch.B. (Glasg.), F.R.C.P. (Edin.),
F.R.C.Path., F.R.A.C.P., F.R.C.P.A.

Professor of Medicine,
University of Tasmania;
Senior Physician, Royal Hobart Hospital,
Hobart, Tasmania, Australia

GRUNE & STRATTON
A Subsidiary of Harcourt Brace Jovanovich Publishers
New York   San Francisco   London

Library of Congress Cataloging in Publication Data

Gunz, Frederick.
    Leukemia.

    First-2d editions by W. Dameshek and F. Gunz.
    Includes bibliographies.
    1. Leukemia. I. Baikie, A. G., joint author.
II. Dameshek, William, 1900– Leukemia.
[DNLM: 1. Leukemia. WH250 G977L]
RC643.G94 1974   616.1'55   74-13366

Grune & Stratton, Inc.
111 Fifth Avenue
New York, New York 10003

Library of Congress Catalog Card Number 74-13366
International Standard Book Number 0-8089-0843-X
Printed in the United States of America

Contents

v

III   CLINICAL AND LABORATORY FEATURES

IV   TREATMENT

V   EPILOGUE

Preface to the Third Edition

This edition appears 10 years after its predecessor, a wide gap in an area where new developments are taking place with great rapidity. Unhappily, much of the delay was occasioned by the sudden death in 1969 of Dr. William Dameshek, the senior author of the first two editions, and a medical writer of such distinction that his loss was almost irreplaceable. In the preparation of this revision, we have attempted to adhere to the purpose set forth in the preface to the first edition, to present an account of those features of the leukemias in which practitioners such as internists, pediatricians, or clinical pathologists may be interested; an account which, without being encyclopedic, contains the most important information now available on human leukemia and related diseases. We have also tried to follow William Dameshek in making this a book to be read, rather than a catalog of facts and opinions. Since knowledge is still patchy in many areas of our subject, we have felt it important to pinpoint and to discuss deficiencies, as well as achievements, and, as in previous editions, to speculate on reasons for shortcomings and on likely lines of progress. No doubt some of our views will be found controversial by a number of readers.

Although the general structure of the work has been retained, we have rearranged some of the chapters in a more logical order, subdivided two of them, and, in place of the former Epilogue, added a brief account of very recent developments. To avoid duplications, the chapter on laboratory diagnosis has been amalgamated with that on the clinical features of the leukemias. Overall, a radical revision was found to be necessary, and much of the contents of the first two editions had to go, in order to make room for new material. Most importantly, we were fortunate in enlisting the help of a number of our colleagues who took over the rewriting of essential parts in their own specialized fields. We thank in this place Drs. M. A. McGrath, R. Penny, A. S. D. Spiers, P. C. Vincent, J. B. Ziegler, and the late Dr. Y. Rabinowitz for their most valuable contributions, without which we could not have completed our task. We are also grateful to many friends and their publishers for allowing us to reproduce illustrations or tables from their published work or for supplying us with original material for illustrations. Their generosity is acknowledged in the legends to the relevant figures.

In looking back over the years since the appearance of the second edition, we can discern solid progress on a wide front. The most spectacular advances have probably occurred in the therapy of the acute leukemias, with acute lymphocytic leukemia of childhood in the van. The extraordinary extension of survival of many such children is the first tangible reward for the enormous effort that has been made in so many fields of research, and gives hope for similar advances in the therapy of other forms of the disease. Yet it is sobering that, in spite of the steady widening and deepening of insights into the life history, the physical and chemical constitution, the kinetics, and immunology of normal hematopoietic cells and their pathologic counterparts; and despite the great improvements in pharmacology and therapeutic methods, we still lack basic information on the reasons why some leukemias—or certain patients with leukemia—respond to treatment, while others remain resistant. Nor are we as yet treating diseases whose causation is clearly understood. Much knowledge has been gained from the study of animal leukemias, their etiology and pathogenesis, but its application to the human disease still faces major obstacles. Progress here, as elsewhere in the leukemia field, is likely to come by means of multiple small steps, rather than by great breakthroughs which are so ardently hoped for by patients and their friends.

In completing this work, we should like to express our indebtedness to our publisher, Grune & Stratton, and to our wives and families for their tolerance and support over very many busy months.

F.G.
A.G.B.

Preface to the Second Edition

In the more than five years since this book was first published, enormous efforts by many different groups of workers have been made to advance the knowledge of leukemia and its treatment. In sifting through the great mass of publications, one may wonder if the progress that has been made can be equated with the quantity of work done. To be sure, neither the fundamental causative factors, nor the cure of the various disorders classified under the heading of leukemia have been elucidated, but perhaps a much clearer picture of a many-sided problem seems to be emerging. It is not too much to say that with the present logarithmic proliferation of basic knowledge, we may be on the verge of at least partial solutions.

Many of the advances have come from basic work on blood cells and their normal functions. In particular, the hitherto enigmatic lymphocyte has at length begun to shed some of its veils and something is now known of the history and purpose of its life. Connections between the recently "rediscovered" thymus, the growth of lymphocytes and immunologic phenomena have been found and the many analogies and relationships between immunologic and neoplastic lymphocytic and plasmocytic proliferations have emerged. Some forms of leukemia may, indeed, be perversions of normal reactions to foreign proteins, a possibility which constitutes a challenge to experimental investigation. Among other important advances is the unravelling of the minute structure of chromosomes from normal and leukemic blood cells. The Philadelphia chromosome, as noted in chronic granulocytic leukemia, the finding of trisomy for the G21 chromosome in Down's syndrome, the almost twenty-fold increase of acute leukemia in this condition—these correlations are fascinating developments. Information is very rapidly accumulating on the place of viruses in the causation of animal, but not yet of human, leukemias, although even here, there are hints of possibly important things to come. The Burkitt "lymphoma" with its relation to leukemia, the occurrence of acute leukemia in "clusters," the contention by some workers that immune bodies against leukemic tissue presumed to contain virus may be found in leukemic contacts—these are bits of evidence that must be seriously considered, especially in the light of future developments. The role in leukemogenesis of extraneous agents such as ionizing radiations has been more clearly assessed. Methods of therapy in both acute and chronic leukemia have been refined and several new and useful drugs have been introduced. The place of the corticosteroids in therapy, particularly with the use of large, "pharmacologic" doses of these materials in acute leukemia of adults and in the lymphoproliferative disorders has been a revelation.

In revising this monograph, we have tried to integrate an account of the newer knowledge with already established material and to present a balanced picture where this was possible. It must be confessed that not infrequently, we have resorted to speculation, particularly in relation to such things as abnormal or "forbidden" clones, matters of ecology and the closeness of autoimmune and certain leukemic disorders. This has seemed to us desirable in a field where so many uncertainties remain and where new work may conceivably be stimulated by, perhaps, unorthodox approaches. It has been our aim to include all relevant work, although omissions—some deliberate, others accidental—have been unavoidable. Some 1000 new references appear in this edition; a number of those previously cited have been deleted.

We have made more or less extensive additions and alterations in every chapter. The most complete reorganization has occurred in the clinical chapters, one of which has been subdivided. There is also a new chapter on lymphoproliferative diseases to balance that on the myeloproliferative disorders. Some illustrations have been changed and many new ones added. The index is new.

Without our many co-workers, and these include our Senior Associates: Drs. Mario Baldini, W. J. Mitus, Robert S. Schwartz and Joseph Sherman; our Clinical and Research Fellows in Hematology, our Trainees in Hematology, our technicians and our secretarial force, this book could not have got off the ground. We are particularly grateful to Dr. Brian MacMahon, Professor of Epidemiology, Harvard School of Public Health for his critique of the chapters devoted to Incidence and Etiology; to Dr. W. J. Mitus for his collaboration on the chapters devoted to the pathology of the leukemic cell and to the course and special pathology as related to symptomatology; to Dr. Anna Mitus for her help in writing the section on the treatment of childhood leukemia; to Lt. Commander Ross Moquin, USN, MC, for his close collaboration on the section devoted to the various chemotherapeutic agents; to Dr. Kosmas Kiossoglou for his studies on the chromosomes; to Mrs. Joan Gunz for her new index; and to Mrs. Virginia McKinney for her extraordinary secretarial efforts. To our friend, the publisher—Dr. Henry M. Stratton—we are, as ever, indebted for his excellent advice and sound judgment. To our patients with leukemia and particularly to parents of leukemic children, we extend the hope that some of the enormous research experience of today and tomorrow will be quickly channeled into practical accomplishment.

William Dameshek
Frederick Gunz

Contributors

Michael A. McGrath, M.B., M.R.A.C.P., Research Fellow in Medicine, St. Vincent's Hospital, Sydney, Australia.

Ronald Penny, M.D., F.R.A.C.P., F.R.C.P.A., Associate Professor of Medicine, University of New South Wales, Sydney, Australia.

Yale Rabinowitz, M.D. (deceased), Principal Investigator, Cell Research Section, Veterans Administration Hospital, Hines, Illinois.

Alexander S. D. Spiers, M.B., Ph.D., F.R.A.C.P., Lecturer in Haematology, Medical Research Council Leukaemia Unit and Department of Haematology, Royal Postgraduate Medical School, London, England.

Paul C. Vincent, M.B., B.Sc. (Med.), F.R.A.C.P., F.R.C.P.A., Clinical Haematologist, Kanematsu Memorial Institute, Sydney Hospital, Sydney, Australia.

John B. Ziegler, M.B., M.R.A.C.P., Research Fellow in Medicine, St. Vincent's Hospital, Sydney, Australia.

I

Introduction

1

Leukemia in the Past

Leukemia, since its recognition as a distinctive disease, has had a history of little more than 100 years, and it is therefore a comparative newcomer among the major known scourges of humanity. It was first described almost simultaneously by two brilliant young men who, after applying their great gifts to a meticulous exploration of its features in the living and the dead, engaged at once in an almost venomous wrangle over the honor of having been the first to identify this fatal disease. Progress in the knowledge of leukemia has been fitful since these beginnings. It should be realized that at the time of its discovery very little was known about the composition, the origins, and the functions of normal blood, nor were there any good methods available for investigating them. Each step forward had therefore to be preceded by an exploration of the normal. Where this lagged, speculation usurped the place of research, and theory that of fact. Much of the literature of the first hundred years echoes with the clash of controversy which, lacking a basis of substantial facts, could only be dialectic and unproductive. It is regrettable but true that even today we do not possess the answers to many of the fundamental questions about the mechanism of normal hematopoiesis or the regulation of the blood elements. In large measure, this fact explains our continuing ignorance of the causes of leukemia and of the means of subjugating it.

It seems likely that the first accurate description of a case of leukemia was given in 1827 by Velpeau.[37] His patient, a 63-year-old florist and seller of lemonade, "who had abandoned himself to the abuse of spirituous liquor and of women, without however, becoming syphilitic," fell ill in 1825 with a pronounced swelling of the abdomen, fever and weakness, and symptoms caused by urinary stones. He died soon after admission to the hospital and was at autopsy found to have an enormous liver and spleen, the latter weighing 10 pounds. The blood was thick, "like gruel . . . resembling in consistency and color the yeast of red wine. . . . One might have asked if it were not rather laudable pus, mixed with blackish coloring matter, than blood." It was, in fact, the peculiar character of the blood, as seen postmortem, which first attracted the attention of all the early observers of leukemia. Thus, Barth,[2] in 1839, was so interested in the autopsy findings in one of his patients that he submitted the blood to microscopic examination. This was carried out by Donné, who reported that more than half of the blood consisted of "mucous globules" which could not be distinguished from pus corpuscles. Thus, it appears that Donné[10] was the first to examine the blood of a leukemic patient during life; it was so full of colorless corpuscles that at first he thought it was pus.

In spite of these and other early observations, leukemia was not recognized as a definite entity until its description in 1845 by Bennett[4] in Scotland and by Virchow[38] in Germany. The independent publication, within 1 month of each other, of two cases of the same new disease, was less remarkable than the fact that each observation came from the pen of a man who was to become a leader in his own field, Bennett in physiology and Virchow in pathology. In each of the first two patients, it was the postmortem appearance of the blood which first gave the hint that an unusual condition was present. In Virchow's patient the blood vessels contained a "yellowish-white almost greenish mass." Microscopically, it contained "besides a very few red blood corpuscles . . . the same colorless or white bodies which also occur in normal blood, namely, small, not quite regular protein molecules, large, granular, fat-containing, non-nucleated corpuscles and granular cells with one rounded, horseshoe-shaped or trefoil-like or several hollowed-out distinct nuclei." The relationship between red and colorless corpuscles was the reverse of the normal, so that Virchow coined the term *white blood (weisses Blut)* to describe the condition. The spleen weighed 7 pounds, 12 ounces in Bennett's patient and measured nearly a foot in length in Virchow's patient. While thus the findings were similar, the two authors interpreted them in a different fashion: Bennett as "suppuration of the blood," Virchow, much more cautiously, as probably not "pyemic." A few months later in August 1846, having reconsidered, not only his own case, but also those published by Bennett,[4] Craigie,[8] and Fuller,[18] Virchow[39] took a much more definite attitude against the pyemic theory of leukemia, pointing out that there was no evidence of local suppuration which could have spread to the blood, that the "pus" corpuscles were identical with the colorless bodies normally occurring in the blood, and that in leukemia (still called white blood) there was merely an increase in the normal number of these latter cells. Such an increase was also shown by Fuller[18] who examined the blood three times during life in his patient and found on each occasion, "in addition to the natural blood-corpuscles, a very large proportion of abnormal, granular, colorless globules." (Craigie[8] observed his patient several years before those seen by Bennett and Virchow but did not realize the significance of his observations until he watched Bennett's autopsy of his own first patient. Both Craigie and Bennett thereupon reported their cases as instances of the same disease in the same number of the *Edinburgh Medical and Surgical Journal.* Fuller was apparently not cognizant of Bennett's and Virchow's papers when he presented his case at a meeting of the London Medico-Chirurgical Society in June, 1846).

Following these early publications, further cases were reported in rapid succession both by the two chief protagonists of the new disorder and by lesser figures, so that by 1852 Bennett[5] could publish a monograph on "leucocythaemia," in which he described 37 cases which were by then known; of these, 17 had been diagnosed during life by means of blood examinations, and at least one had been followed for 18 months, during which time the colorless corpuscles had been constantly increased. Meanwhile, Virchow introduced the term *leukemia* in 1847,[40] and published a series of brilliant studies on the nature of the disease, which he summarized in 1856 in a paper of great interest and importance.[41]

Virchow began by asserting that the colorless corpuscles are always present in normal blood and are increased after digestion, in pregnancy, and in most inflammatory conditions. Such an increase is not by itself a disease and must be distinguished from leukemia which is a definite pathologic state characterized not only by an increase in colorless cells, but also by a decrease in the number of red corpuscles, and is dependent on changes in certain organs. There are, in fact, two kinds of leukemia: the first, *splenic* or *lienal,* associated with a swelling of the spleen; the second, *lymphatic,* associated with tumefaction of the lymph nodes and the presence in the blood of colorless corpuscles resembling those which are ordinarily seen in the lymph nodes. Moreover, the changes in the organs precede those in the blood, for there are cases in which enlargement of the lymph nodes or spleen may be found months or years before changes develop in the blood. Pathologically, the lesions in both spleen and nodes are a hyperplasia of normal elements, and both the liver and kidney may be infiltrated with the cells present in the blood, although such foci are probably formed locally rather than from cells which have wandered out of the bloodstream. Virchow did not know the reason for these changes which he thought were not inflammatory, although they were sometimes accompanied by inflammatory lesions of the skin or mucous membranes; the latter were, however, likely to be a consequence rather than the cause of the blood and visceral changes.

This early paper of Virchow's contains in a rudimentary form many of the views on the pathology of leukemia which are still held today. It is all the more remarkable as there was extremely little knowledge at the time it was written concerning the sites and mechanisms of hematopoiesis, and the functions and fate of the blood cells. The general view on the origin of the red blood cell was still that put forward by Hewson in the eighteenth century, that is, that red cells are formed from the colorless corpuscles in the blood itself. Thus, in 1852 Bennett[5] suggested that the red cell was the "liberated nucleus of the colorless cell." Colorless corpuscles were thought to be formed in the "lymphatic glands," including the spleen, thymus, thyroid, suprarenals and pineal body, whence they entered the blood. They were probably produced "in an organic fluid by the production of molecules, the successive development and aggregation of which constitute the higher formations." Later the blood corpuscles are dissolved in the liquor sanguinis and "with the effete matter absorbed from the tissues constitute the blood fibrin." Virchow himself, like many others, had at first accepted the transformation of colorless into colored corpuscles in the circulating blood, and had explained leukemia as a retardation in this process, with the production of increased numbers of white and of decreased quantities of red cells. By 1856, however, he had abandoned this view and now regarded the white corpuscles as "simple, non-specific cells" which are not transformed into red corpuscles once they have left the sites at which they themselves are produced; they are rather "a relatively superfluous part of the blood, a sort of superfluous excess."[42] The transformation of lymph corpuscles into red cells does, however, take place in the spleen and lymph nodes; but once they have reached the bloodstream "their specific metamorphosis into colored corpuscles becomes impossible." They circulate for a brief while and then perish.

We may summarize this first phase of research on leukemia by saying that within 12 years of its recognition, the two chief varieties of chronic leukemia, as well as the acute form (Friedreich[17]) had been described, and the main clinical and pathologic features tabulated. Because of the exceedingly crude hematologic methods then available, it was possible to make only the most superficial examination of the leukocytes themselves, and though it was realized that there was more than one variety of these cells, they could not be characterized morphologically or traced back to the sites of their formation. It had, however, been acknowledged even by those who, like Bennett, had originally regarded leukemia as the result of a special kind of inflammation, that the changes in the blood were not caused by an admixture of pus, but probably by a proliferation of those white corpuscles which are a normal constituent of blood. The primary changes in the disease were now sought in the lymphatic organs rather than in the blood itself.

It is a significant sidelight on human vanity that in the face of the overwhelming evidence which pointed to leukemia as a distinct and, in many ways, remarkable disease, there were still loud voices which denied its very existence. At a discussion held in Paris in 1855, one physician[6] exclaimed: "Leukemia has no special causes, special symptoms, particular anatomic lesions or specific treatment, and I thus conclude that it does not exist as a distinct malady," while another[3] added: "There are enough diseases without inventing any new ones."

The 30 years which followed the publication of Virchow's great paper brought little significant progress. They were a time of consolidation of existing knowledge, although one notable addition to it was Neumann's demonstration that the bone marrow was an important site for the formation of blood corpuscles in health and disease.[24] His studies originated from the observation in 1870 of abnormal marrow appearances at the autopsy of a man who had died from obvious splenic leukemia. The marrow was not red like that of normal people, but "dirty yellow-greenish" like pus. Neumann thought that such changes might well be common in leukemia, and that they had probably not been previously described because nobody had looked for them. He surmised that there might, in fact, be a *myelogenous* leukemia, in addition to the splenic and lymphatic forms, and proceeded to prove this suspicion in a number of publications which he summarized in an extensive article, in 1878.[25] He was, by then, certain that the marrow normally formed colorless corpuscles and delivered them to the blood. Whether such corpuscles were transformed into colored ones, as had been generally assumed, appeared rather doubtful to Neumann, for he could show that the immediate precursors of the red cells were nucleated red cells which he found regularly in the marrow, and sometimes also in leukemic blood. If a transformation of white to red cells did occur, he reasoned, leukemia could be caused either by an overproduction of the former, or by a failure of their transformation to the latter; but if red cells were formed independently of the white ones, then there must also be a disturbance in their production in the marrow in order to account for their diminution in leukemic blood.

In 1879, Gowers,[19] in a masterly monograph on leukemia, took this argument a step farther by pointing out that the anemia in leukemia might theoretically be caused either by a diminished formation of red cells, or by their excessive destruction. He inclined to the view that the former mechanism was the main cause, although increased destruction might also play a part. It is of interest that this fundamental question has even now not been finally solved (see Chapter 14).

Although Gowers accepted Neumann's views on the role of the marrow in normal and leukemic hematopoiesis, he still regarded it as less important than that of the spleen and the lymph nodes, and subdivided leukemia into *splenic leukocythemia* and *lymphadenosis*. Very significantly he equated the latter term with *Hodgkin's disease* and thus foreshadowed an era of prolonged confusion about the diseases of the lymphatic tissues and their interrelations. Gowers believed that the increase in the number of white cells which occurred in splenic leukemia was only a symptom accompanying the primary changes in the blood-forming organs, and that it need not be present before the diagnosis of leukemia could be established. He thus anticipated the much later recognition of the subleukemic or aleukemic forms of leukemia which could only follow after new methods had permitted a separation of the various types of normal and abnormal leukocytes.

We now enter upon a period of uncertain groping for new truths during which efforts were made to define especially the features of the acute leukemias, and the position of all leukemias in the wider field of those diseases which affect the hematopoietic organs. Into this period, which extended well into the twentieth century, falls Ehrlich's discovery of staining methods which, for the first time, made it possible to see the cellular details of the various forms of leukocytes and to describe accurately the cytologic features of the leukemias. It required considerable time, however, before the new techniques could be assessed and assimilated and before it was feasible to trace securely the connections between the many different cell forms whose bewildering array now stood revealed. In the meantime, Ehrlich's stains probably added to, rather than relieved, the difficulties of classifying the leukemias.

During the late nineteenth and the early twentieth centuries, hematologists conjured with a host of new terms like *pseudoleukemia, leukosarcoma, chloroma, lymphosarcoma, myelosis, myeloma,* and various combinations. Many of these were ill-defined at the time of their first appearance, and definitions had to be altered in the light of accumulating clinical or pathologic experience, generally under the pressure of attacks by rival schools of physicians. Presently, the same term would be used in a variety of different ways by its proponents as well as its antagonists, until it might eventually become attached to conditions far removed from those to which it was originally intended to apply. Only a very brief account of this disturbed period need be given here and even this would be unnecessary but for the fact that faint echoes of these old battles are still heard today, and that some of the terms have survived to give useful descriptions of more precisely defined hematologic conditions.

A characteristic example of the metamorphosis and eventual disappearance of a hematologic neologism is *pseudoleukemia* which still appeared in official classifications of leukemias as late as 1938, although it had long since been discarded by serious students of the subject. This term was first used by Cohnheim[7] in 1865 to describe a disease which, to judge by its account, was undoubtedly an example of acute leukemia. The patient, who died 4 months after the onset of his illness, showed all the clinical and pathologic features of a rapidly progressive leukemia, but neither during life nor at autopsy was it possible to show an increase in the number of white blood corpuscles. It should be realized that at the time no actual blood counts could be made, and that only the relative proportions of red and white cells could be approximately determined, without attempts at "differential" counting. Hence, pseudoleukemia in effect described any condition associated with splenomegaly or lymphadenopathy in which there was no gross increase in the number of leukocytes, and which could not be otherwise diagnosed. The term was obviously a convenient one, and there is no doubt that many cases of tuberculosis and other infections, as well as of Hodgkin's disease, neoplasms and nonleukemic hematologic abnormalities were, at one time or another, included in the group of pseudoleukemias. Following the introduction of staining methods, attempts were made to define the condition more narrowly, a "relative" lymphocytosis becoming now an additional requirement.[27] By 1912, doubts about the existence of pseudoleukemia as a separate entity had grown so pronounced that even those who defended the usefulness of the term[16,33] appeared to be uncertain about the sense in which it was to be used. It was finally buried in 1918 by Symmers[35] who demanded that it "be discarded as a misleading and inappropriate designation" and suggested that "the lesion so named should be included among the lymphosarcomas"; a classification which would certainly be entirely inappropriate for Cohnheim's original case.

Of much greater importance than pseudoleukemia was the problem of the lymphosarcomas and their relation to leukemia. The name *lymphosarcoma* was first used by Kundrat[22] in 1893 for a primary affection of the lymph nodes or mucous membranes which sooner or later spread to neighboring structures in the fashion of some malignant diseases and, starting from one part of the lymphatic system, progressed by gradual stages to involve succeeding groups of lymph nodes. Kundrat thought it possible to distinguish this disease from leukemia by virtue of its greater local invasiveness, much less widespread generalized manifestations and absence of a leukemic blood picture. He believed that it was not a cancer and advanced chiefly, if not entirely, by lymphatic rather than by hematogenous channels.

The term *lymphosarcoma* as used by Kundrat soon became accepted as denoting the nodular and usually rapidly fatal affections of the lymph nodes, either regional or generalized, which occurred in the absence of a leukemic blood picture. It was not long, however, before Türk recognized that there were close connections between lymphosarcoma and leukemia, for many leukemias had little, if any, increase in the normal number of lymphocytes in the blood, and the clinical features of both conditions were very similar. In a remarkably farsighted paper published in 1903, Türk[36] grouped together the lymphatic leukemias, both chronic and acute, and the lymphosarcomata in one system of *lymphomatoses,* stating that this included benign (chronic lymphocytic leukemia), acute—either benign or malignant—(acute leukemia, chloroma), and chronic malignant (lymphosarcoma) forms, which differed from each other in only two ways: by the degree of proliferative activity and local invasiveness of the lymphoid cells; and by the presence or absence of blood invasion. Moreover, there might be transitions between the various lymphomatoses, although Türk thought that these were rare. Symmers,[35] some years later, went one step farther by actually including lymphocytic leukemia among the lymphosarcomas.

It is obvious that Türk's classification of the lymphomatoses, though differing from present-day views in some details, is fundamentally in harmony with all that is now known of the interrelationship of the various diseases of the lymphatic system. [We have used a somewhat similar term, the *lymphoproliferative disorders,* to describe the various proliferative lesions of the lymphoid tissue (see Chapter 12).] It is all the more regrettable that Türk's important theory became almost at once overshadowed by Sternberg's promotion of a new concept of what he called *leukosarcoma.* Because in earlier editions of this monograph we used this term as a generic one for leukocytic neoplasms, and in a sense that is quite different from Sternberg's and that of others, the development of the term is discussed rather fully here.

Sternberg[31,32] separated cases of lymphatic leukemia into two groups: the first showed the usual leukemic features and an infiltration with small lymphocytes of all those organs which normally contained lymphocytes; the second, which he termed *leukosarcoma,* also presented lesions of organs which were ordinarily free of lymphocytes. Many of the lesions were "tumorous," and showed large and often atypical lymphocytes, both in the tumors and in the blood. The most characteristic of such lesions, according to Sternberg, were mediastinal and arose either from the thymus or the mediastinal lymph nodes, spreading among the great vessels and sometimes enveloping the heart. Blood changes were always present but tended to be minimal, that is, seen only with careful study of a well-prepared and stained blood smear. In the second of his first two papers on the subject,[32] Sternberg discussed the relation of chloroma to the new syndrome, realizing that the two conditions might produce very similar appearances. He solved the problem by renaming chloroma as *chloromyelosarcoma,* inventing a corresponding *chlorolymphosarcoma,* and including both among his *leukosarcomas.*

The definition of Sternberg's new disease clearly cut across the lines of that of several of the leukemias, as well as of Kundrat's lymphosarcoma. His first group of cases certainly included some of acute granulocytic leukemia, as he later acknowledged.[34] It was, in fact, questionable from the first whether the condition leukosarcoma could actually be distinguished from either the leukemias or the lymphosarcomas, and such authors as Naegeli[13] and von Domarús[9] maintained very soon that this was merely a special type of leukemia. It was left to Sternberg's supporters, like Paltauf,[26] to attempt a more precise definition of leukosarcoma and especially its separation from acute leukemia. In spite of their efforts, the term began to assume a meaning practically synonymous with lymphosarcoma and to be applied especially to cases with pronounced mediastinal involvement.[43,44] The distinction from lymphocytic leukemia became gradually less and less clear-cut, so much so that Flashman and Leopold[14] in 1929 were able to return once more to a classification which was practically identical with that advanced by Türk more than 25 years earlier. These authors suggested a hierarchy of "lymphoid hyperplasias" extending from the most benign group of chronic lymphocytic leukemias to the most malignant lymphosarcomas, via an intermediate group of leukosarcomas which they considered as more or less localized primary and invasive lymphoid tumors accompanied by a leukemic blood picture. More recently, the term *leukosarcoma* has become a rather vague one, used by some authors[21a] synonymously with *lymphosarcoma* to designate certain cases of leukemia or lymphosarcoma in which the peripheral blood shows large, atypical, and definitely abnormal primitive lymphocytes, usually with indented or peculiarly shaped nuclei.

We may now return briefly to the developments in the knowledge of those leukemias which are not associated with primary changes in the lymph nodes. It will be recalled that since Virchow's time these were thought to follow primary changes in the spleen, and that Neumann added a myelogenous to the splenic form. Ehrlich[12] and his pupil Spilling,[30] by using the new panoptic staining method, showed that both splenic and myelogenous types were characterized by an overgrowth of the granular cells which form the greatest proportion among the normal leukocytes, and traced their origin back to a granular mononuclear precursor, the myelocyte, present in the normal and leukemic marrow and the leukemic spleen. As soon as this was realized, it became clear that Virchow's splenic and Neumann's myelogenous leukemias were actually the same disease, and terms like *splenomedullary* leukemia now came into use to describe this condition. Ehrlich regarded the eosinophils and basophils as the most characteristic cells in this form of leukemia, an assumption which was to delay considerably the recognition of the acute granulocytic leukemias in which these cells are usually absent from the blood.

It remained to find the source of the myelocytes themselves, and credit must be given to Hirschfeld[20] for identifying this in the nongranular mononuclear cells of the marrow and for describing their metamorphosis to granulocytes. Two years later, Naegeli[23] applied the term *myeloblast* to the same nongranular cells, but it is clear from his account that the name included all of the marrow cells which resembled "large lymphocytes," and that Naegeli was not yet able to distinguish genuine myeloblasts from lymphocytes. With the characterization of the complete granular cell series, the stage was set for evaluation of the acute leukemias.

Cases showing all the features which we now regard as typical of the acute forms of leukemia had been described by authors like Virchow since the earliest days, and Friedreich in 1857 had given a classic account of a woman dying from leukemia after a 6 weeks' illness with the prominent symptoms of weakness, hemorrhages, oral ulceration, and hepatosplenomegaly.[17] None of these early cases were however, designated specifically as "acute" by their chroniclers, and Gowers in 1879 defined leukemia as a chronic disease.[19] A type of leukemia which differed from the usual chronic forms was first recognized by Ebstein[11] who, in 1889, reported one case of his own and sixteen others collected from the literature as the distinct entity of "acute" leukemia. Apparently it needed only this single paper to release a whole flood of confirmatory reports, so that only 6 years after Ebstein's paper, Fraenkel[15] could claim that the acute was much commoner than the chronic form of leukemia. This author gave a good description of the clinical features of the disease as exemplified by nine personal cases, and stressed the point that in it, the blood shows an exclusive rise in mononuclear leukocytes which, in the days before the discovery of the early granulocytes, he regarded as lymphocytes. It is of interest that this author gave an early account of spontaneous remissions in two patients with acute leukemia.

The discovery of the myeloblast ushered in an era of dispute about the precise nature of the immature leukocytes of acute leukemia and also brought with it the distinct recognition of *aleukemic* leukemias in which (although the tissue changes were leukemic) the blood showed no leukocytosis but only the presence of abnormal leukocytes.[21,29] The lymphocytic form of aleukemic leukemia was seen to be similar to some of the pseudoleukemias, and it was now believed that there was also an aleukemic form of acute granulocytic leukemia (an "aleukemic myelosis") of which two types were described: one localized to the marrow and consisting of atypical myelocytes, the disease then known as *myelomatosis*; and the other generalized with involvement of the whole hematopoietic apparatus and the blood. Hirschfeld,[21] who must be regarded as one of the most astute investigators of his time (he described the first use of splenic punctures for the diagnosis of leukemia), also asserted categorically that in many cases of acute granulocytic leukemia the red cell precursors were involved in the leukemic process, owing to the "close genetic connection" between erythro- and myeloblasts. The time of *erythremia* and of *erythroleukemia* (see Chapter 11) was now fast approaching. Lastly, a short paper by Reschad and Schilling in 1913[28] reported a new form of acute leukemia in which the monocyte (or "splenocyte") was considered as the type-specific cell. Thus, there was now chronic lymphocytic and chronic granulocytic (myelogenous) leukemia, and acute lymphocytic, granulocytic (myeloblastic), and monocytic leukemia.

It would be unprofitable to linger over the prolonged polemics which were carried on in the medical press of the ensuing years concerning the identity, nature, and relationships of the various acute leukemias. Some of them now appear as mere exercises in semantics, and others are as yet unsettled. They will be referred to later (see Chapter 3). It is important, however, to stress that with the recognition of the acute and aleukemic forms of leukemia, the main phase of morphologic hematology as applied to leukemia was drawing to a close. Already the first "cytochemical" methods like the peroxidase stains were being used and the first tissue cultures of leukemic blood had been made.[1] Further research was to be focused progressively on the functional and dynamic aspects of the disease, and chemical, biochemical, biophysical, biological, cytogenetic, and immunologic techniques were to supplement more and more the classic methods of the histologist and cytologist. Although something of a renaissance of morphology has come about with the introduction of new techniques such as phase-contrast and electron microscopy, only a few significant discoveries have been made with these in the leukemia field. There can be no question that the simple act of looking at a cell still has considerable importance; but it is by the combined use of all the tools now available that progress is likely to come.

REFERENCES

1. Awrorow PP, Timofejewsky AD: Kultivierungsversuche von leukämischem Blute. Arch Pathol Anat 216:184, 1941.

2. Barth: Alteration du sang remarquable par la prédominance des globules blancs ou muqueux; hypertrophie considérable de la rate. Bull Soc Méd Hôp (Paris) 3:39, 1856.

3. Barthez F: Discussion. Bull Soc Méd Hôp (Paris) 3:55, 1856.

4. Bennett JH: Case of hypertrophy of the spleen and liver, in which death took place from suppuration of the blood. Edinburgh Med Surg J 64:413, 1845.

5. _____: Leucocythaemia or White Cell Blood. Edinburgh, Sutherland and Knox, 1852.

6. Cahen: Discussion. Bull Soc Méd Hôp (Paris) 3:55, 1856.

7. Cohnheim J: Ein Fall von Pseudoleukämie. Arch Pathol Anat 33:451, 1865.

8. Craigie D: Case of disease of the spleen, in which death took place in consequence of the presence of purulent matter in the blood. Edinburgh Med Surg J 64:400, 1845.

9. von Domarús: Der gegenwärtige Stand der Leukämiefrage. Folia Haematol 6:337, 1908.

10. Donné A: Cours de microscopie. Paris, Baillière, 1844, p 132ff.

11. Ebstein W: Ueber die acute Leukämie und Pseudoleukämie. Deutsches Arch Klin Med 44:343, 1889.

12. Ehrlich P: Farbenanalytische Untersuchungen zur Histologie und Klinik des Blutes. Berlin, Hirschwald, 1891.

13. Fabian E, Naegeli O, Schatiloff P: Beiträge zur Kenntnis der Leukämie. Arch Pathol Anat 190:436, 1907.

14. Flashman DH, Leopold SS: Leukosarcoma. With report of a case beginning with a primary retroperitoneal lymphosarcoma and terminating with leukemia. Amer J Med Sci 177:651, 1929.

15. Fraenkel A: Ueber acute Leukämie. Dtsch Med Wochenschr 21:639, 663, 676, 699, 712, 1895.

16. Fraenkel E: Ueber die sogenannte Pseudoleukämie. Zentralbl Allg Pathol 23 (suppl.):5, 1912.

17. Friedreich N: Ein neuer Fall von Leukämie. Arch Pathol Anat 12:37, 1857.

18. Fuller HW: Particulars of a case in which enormous enlargement of the spleen and liver, together with dilatation of all the blood vessels of the body, were found coincident with a peculiarly altered condition of the blood. Lancet 2:43, 1846.

19. Gowers WR: Splenic leucocythaemia, in Reynolds: System of Medicine, vol. 5. New York, Macmillan, 1879, p 216.

20. Hirschfeld H: Zur Kenntnis der Histogenese der granulirten Knochenmarkzellen. Arch Pathol Anat 153:335, 1898.

21. _____: Die generalisierte aleukämische Myelose and ihre Stellung im System der leukämischen Erkrankungen. Zentralbl Klin Med 80:126, 1914.

21a. Isaacs R: Lymphosarcoma cell leukemia. Ann Intern Med 11:657, 1937.

22. Kundrat H: Ueber Lympho-Sarkomatosis. Wien Klin Wochenschr 6:211, 234, 1893.

23. Naegeli O: Ueber rothes Knochenmark und Myeloblasten. Dtsch Med Wochenschr 26:287, 1900.

24. Neumann E: Ein Fall von Leukämie mit Erkrankung des Knochenmarkes. Arch Heilk 11:1, 1870.

25. _____: Ueber myelogene Leukämie. Ber Klin Wochenschr 15:69, 87, 115, 131, 1878.

26. Paltauf R: Leukosarkomatose und Myeloblasten Leukämie. Wien Klin Wochenschr 25:46, 1912.

27. Pinkus, R: Lymphatic leukemia, in Nothnagel CWH: Encyclopedia of Practical Medicine: Diseases of the Blood. Philadelphia, Saunders, 1905, p 539.

28. Reschad H, Schilling V: Ueber eine neue Leukämie durch echte Uebergangsformen (Splenozytenleukämie) und ihre Bedeutung für die Selbststandigkeit dieser Zellen. Münch Med Wochenschr 60:1981, 1913.

29. Schridde H: Die blutbereitenden Organe, in Aschoff L: Pathologische Anatomie, (ed. 2) vol. 2. Jena, Fischer, 1911, p 104.

30. Spilling E: Ueber Blutuntersuchungen bei Leukämie, in Ehrlich P: Farbenanalytische Untersuchungen zur Histologie und Klinik des Blutes. Berlin, Hirschwald, 1891, p 51.

31. Sternberg C: Ueber lymphatische Leukämie. Z Heilk 25:170, 201, 1904.

32. _____: Zur Kenntnis der Chlorome (Chloromyelosarkom). Beitr Pathol Anat 37:437, 1905.

33. _____: Ueber die sogenannte Pseudoleukämie. Zentralbl Allg Pathol 23 (suppl):22, 1912.

34. _____: Leukosarkomatose und Myeloblastenleukämie. Beitr Pathol Anat 61:75, 1916.

35. Symmers D: The relationship of the toxic lymphoid hyperplasias to lymphosarcoma and allied diseases. Arch Intern Med 21:237, 1918.

36. Türk W: Ein System der Lymphomatosen. Wien Klin Wochenschr 16:1073, 1903.

37. Velpeau A: Rev Med. 2: 218, 1827. Quoted by Virchow: Med Z 16:9, 15, 1847.

38. Virchow R: Weisses Blut. Froriep's Notizen 36:151, 1845.

39. _____: Weisses Blut und Milztumoren. 1. Med Z 15:157, 163, 1846.

40. _____: Weisses Blut und Milztumoren. 2. Med Z 16:9, 15, 1847.

41. _____: Die Leukämie, in: Gesammelte Abhandlungen zur wissenschaftlichen Medizin. Frankfurt, Meidinger, 1865, p 190.

42. _____: Die farblosen Blutkörperchen, in: Gesammelte Abhandlungen zur wissenschaftlichen Medizin. Frankfurt, Meidinger, 1865, p. 212.

43. Weber FP: Acute leukaemia and so-called mediastinal "leucosarcomatosis" (Sternberg). With the account of a case accompanied by myeloid substitution of the hilusfat of the kidneys. Q J Med 12:212, 1918–1919.

44. _____, Wolf F: Mediastinal leukosarcomatosis (Sternberg). Amer J Med Sci 152:231, 1916.

2

Definition

Although the term *leukemia* seems at first glance to be readily understood, its exact definition becomes rather difficult, as we will see below. Leukemia (white blood) implies a condition of the blood characterized by a greatly increased leukocyte count. Although this is frequently the case, it is by no means a constant phenomenon. Furthermore, what is fundamentally abnormal in leukemia is not in reality the *blood* but rather the tissues—the several tissues which produce the blood cells and, secondarily, the many tissues in which the leukemic cells may settle and accumulate. Indeed, the blood is of secondary importance in leukemia. In a measure, it may be considered only as a "traffic stream" through which cells pass from their site of origin in the blood-forming organs to tissues all over the body, and so to their eventual destruction.

As will be described in greater detail later (see Chapter 8), the quantity of leukocytes present in the blood is determined by three factors: their rate of entry from the blood-forming organs, the duration of their sojourn in the blood, and the rate of their disappearance into the tissues. Of these, the entry and disappearance rates are equal in the steady state. Rises in the leukocyte count may occur, theoretically, from an increased entry or decreased exit rate, or from a prolongation of the intravascular life span: the count may fall when there is decreased entry to or increased withdrawal from the blood, or when the intravascular life span is shortened. It should be emphasized that normally the movement of granulocytes is strictly in one direction, from the blood-forming organs, through the blood, to the tissues. There is no evidence that, having once left the blood, granulocytes can reenter it. In this they contrast with lymphocytes, many of which circulate from the blood through the lymph nodes and back into the blood, via the large lymphatic vessels. In certain forms of leukemia, however, granulocytes or their precursors may well return to the circulation after having passed through an organ such as the spleen.[2]

Although it has been the custom to consider leukemia as primarily and fundamentally a *proliferative disorder,* the rate of proliferation need not be faster than normal and is indeed often substantially slower. A basic defect of the leukemic leukocytes, especially in the acute forms, is a lack of normal *maturation*. So long as these cells remain immature, they retain the capacity for further proliferation, however slow this may be, and their lifetime may therefore be greatly increased. Indeed, many leukemic cells may be regarded as effectively immortal.

Because leukemic cells may have a prolonged total and reproductive life, they are likely to *accumulate* in the tissues, and this may be an essential element in the pathology of the disease. It is not the *rate* of cellular proliferation but the overall magnitude of the process which appears to be responsible for the distinctive character of leukemic cell growth.

Leukemia may thus be said to represent an *abnormal* form of proliferation of one of the white-cell–forming tissues, that is, the bone marrow, the lymphoid tissues, or the system of plasma cells. By "abnormal" in this context, we mean a new kind of white cell growth, in fact, the presence of a new "race" of leukocytes. Fortunately, not all leukocytic proliferations are leukemic; in fact *benign proliferations* of the white cells represent one of the commonest forms of normal bodily reactions. Thus polymorphonuclear leukocytosis occurs with trauma, exercise, or even with psychologic stress or excitement. The leukocytosis is not always the outcome of increased cellular growth, however, for a redistribution of granulocytes, with a shift of "marginated" cells into the circulating pool can lead to a rising granulocyte count (see Chapter 8). However, the leukocytosis of the many pyogenic bacterial infections (streptococci, staphylococci, etc.), in which there is a great increase in the polymorphonuclear cells of the blood, is a proliferation of the bone marrow granulocytes in response to a specific bacterial organism. The organism has invaded the body and lodged in a certain area such as the lung (pneumococcal pneumonia) or the meninges (meningitis) or the appendix (appendicitis). By obscure, though probably humoral mechanisms, the local infection evokes first a mobilization of existing bone marrow granulocyte reserves and then proliferation of the bone marrow granulocyte precursors. This proliferation is purposeful, and in direct relation to a well-defined etiologic agent; in this instance, a coccal bacterial organism. Once the invading organisms have been overwhelmed and there is no longer any need for excess numbers of granulocytes, the bone marrow reverts to its normal growth pattern, and the blood leukocytosis gives way to normal blood counts.

A similar mechanism, but one involving a different blood-cell forming system, is that found in the response to certain viral agents which can be seen most clearly in infectious mononucleosis. It is conceivable that the generalized proliferative reaction which takes place in this disorder is actually immunologic in nature, that is, that immunocytes of the lymphoid variety are proliferating with the eventual development of an immune response. In mononucleosis, the infective organism, which is probably the Epstein-Barr virus, induces an intense, perhaps purposeful proliferation of lymphoid tissues (lymph nodes, spleen, tonsils, Peyer's patches of the intestines, etc.). This results in generalized lymph node enlargement, both peripherally and centrally, in splenomegaly, and in many laboratory abnormalities, chiefly of the serum globulins. The leukocyte count is generally elevated to twice, three, or four times its normal value, with the presence of many abnormal lymphocytes. In a few weeks, however, certainly in a few months, the lymph nodes regress, the violent proliferation within them returns to normal, and the blood picture again reverts to its normal features, with perhaps a few abnormal lymphocytes present to indicate the previous disease. Similarly, other infections are characterized chiefly by a proliferation, at times quite intense, of the marrow cells (probably early members of the myeloid series) responsible for a monocytosis in the blood. This is noted in such conditions as tuberculosis, malaria, kala-azar, and in similar, rather indolent or chronic, disorders.

The polymorphonuclear responses of diverse origin, the lymphoid proliferative disorder known as infectious mononucleosis, the monocytic proliferation of tuberculosis, these are all generalized proliferations of one of the white-cell–forming tissues, but they are self-limited, that is, *reactive*. They are associated with the presence of a more or less well-defined etiologic agent to which there is a purposeful and self-limited response. Leukemia is not like this: it is not a normal self-limited reaction process, but an abnormal, generalized self-perpetuating proliferation of one of the leukopoietic tissues, in response to no well-defined, presently discernible agent; and apparently without purposeful or utilitarian value to the body.

This abnormal growth process appears to have an innate hardiness which gives it an ecologic advantage over the cells of the normal tissue: thus, it becomes a successful population. The principles of population dynamics have been applied by Burnet,[1] Gorman and Chandler,[3] and others to various types of cellular proliferative activities: immunologic, lymphoid, etc. They may have particular relevance in the case of leukemia, where the principle of "competitive exclusion," as stated by Hardin,[4] can also be invoked. Biological competition is most acute between the most similar populations, that is, between white cells which are almost, but not quite, similar, or perhaps even between the white and red cell precursors which are derived from a common stem cell (see Chapter 14). The most successful population tends to displace all others from a given ecologic niche, although a stable coexistence of two or more populations within a niche can occur. As Gorman and Chandler[3] wrote, "One population need have but an infinitesimally small advantage over another to displace it completely from the niche if enough time is allowed. The reasons for superiority of one population over another are often extremely subtle and are often not clear even after extensive study of a competitive situation." The inexorable course of leukemia is a demonstration of competitive population dynamics: its most graphic expression is seen in the clonal evolution which is featured in many cases of chronic granulocytic leukemia as they enter their terminal stage (see Chapters 6 and 10).

In brief, leukemia may be defined as an abnormal, neoplastic, generalized, self-perpetuating proliferation of one of the leukocytic tissues, often associated with abnormal white blood cell counts and an abnormal increase in leukocytic mass and leading to anemia, thrombocytopenia, and death.

This definition of leukemia has its limitations. Thus, there is no hint in it as to the *cause* of the proliferation; why should one of the leukocytic tissues suddenly develop this "obsessive" proliferation? In proliferations of infectious origin there is an inciting agent, usually a bacterium or a virus or an antigen. It is, of course, possible that a viral agent may be responsible for the proliferative process of leukemia, although in man there is so far no definitive evidence on this point (see Chapter 5). Moreover, it seems likely that a virus would constitute only one of a number of agents which must combine to cause leukemia in any given case, that is, to produce the self-perpetuating mechanism inherent in the leukemic disease. The abnormal cell proliferation in leukemia is, in fact, a "new way of life," or in the shorthand of language, "neoplastic." Thus, the self-perpetuating feature of the leukemic process, its tendency to recur even after reversal by a therapeutic agent, its relentless character terminating only with death of the individual—these features are synonymous with neoplastic disease. Leukemia may, therefore, be considered as generalized neoplasia of one of the white-cell–forming tissues or, more fundamental still, of the stem cells which are the progenitors of these tissues. The "why" of this apparently purposeless proliferation is by no means clear, and must be considered as the central investigative problem of leukemia, if not of hematology. The all-encompassing problem is that of *growth,* more particularly that of abnormal and successful neoplastic growth. Should the various complex mechanisms involved in growth be solved some day, one would be a long way toward solving the problems of abnormal or neoplastic growth and thus of leukemia itself.

REFERENCES

1. Burnet FM: The Clonal Selection Theory of Acquired Immunity. Nashville, Vanderbilt University Press, 1959.
2. Galbraith PR: The mechanism of action of splenic irradiation in chronic myelogenous leukemia. Can Med Assoc J 96:1636, 1967.
3. Gorman JG, Chandler JG: Is there an immunologically incompetent lymphocyte? Blood 23:117, 1963.
4. Hardin G: The competitive exclusion principle. Science 131:1292, 1960.

3

Classification

As stated in Chapter 2, leukemia may be considered as a generalized neoplastic proliferation of one of the leukocytic tissues. Since three lines of white cells may be distinguished—the granulocytes, the lymphocytes, and the monocytes—three main types of leukemia may be described: granulocytic, lymphocytic, and monocytic. To these main types may be added some others which occur occasionally as the result of invasion of the blood by cells not normally circulating in it, like those of lympho- and reticulosarcoma or perhaps the tissue mast cells. A special case may also be made for the inclusion of myelomatosis among the leukemias since its constituent plasma cells (mature or immature) can nearly always be found in the blood if sought for, and will occasionally produce a frankly leukemic picture (see Chapter 13).

Like other types of neoplastic proliferation, leukemia shows considerable variations in growth patterns. In some leukemic proliferations, this pattern may differ only slightly from the normal one. In such cases, examination of the tissue in question (whether bone marrow, lymph node, etc.) shows excessive numbers of the proliferating cell types, the proliferation appearing to take place in an orderly fashion, with eventual maturation to mature cells. The course of such cases is ordinarily protracted; this is *chronic* leukemia. There are, to be sure, varying degrees of chronicity, but all of them have these features in common: well-defined differentiation (maturation) to mature types of cells, a relatively indolent course, and a rather slow accumulation of the proliferating cells in various tissues. In contrast, the *acute* cases present histologically with large numbers of primitive cells, sometimes with many, sometimes with but few mitotic figures, but with little, if any, apparent tendency to differentiation or maturity. Again, there are many variations in the acute cases, some showing no apparent maturation of the proliferating cells, whereas others present with a clear tendency to maturation. Also variable is the clinical course, some cases having an acute onset, with anemia and thrombocytopenia developing rapidly, while others begin more insidiously and run a protracted course. Whether the term *subacute* should be reserved for the relatively slow acute cases is open to discussion. We prefer, however, to designate leukemia as either *acute* or *chronic,* realizing that many variations may occur in the two groupings and the *acute* and *chronic* are clinical and thus inexact terms for the fundamental histologic expression of undifferentiated or primitive cell leukemias as contrasted with well-differentiated, mature-cell leukemias.

The term *acute* is usually synonymous with the presence of large numbers of undifferentiated primitive cells in the bone marrow or blood. As already stated, this usually results from defective cellular maturation rather than from unduly rapid growth, although the total number of proliferating cells throughout the body is greatly increased. There are, furthermore, some cases of leukemia in which, although the course is chronic (i.e., lasting a few to several years), the blood and bone marrow show primitive leukocytes in greater or less degree, with apparently little tendency to differentiation. These cases are acute in the histopathologic sense, but chronic from the clinical or temporal standpoint. Certain cases of the so-called preleukemic state fall into this category. In addition, a variable number of primitive cells may be seen in some instances of generalized lymphosarcomatosis and in myelofibrosis with myeloid metaplasia (see Chapter 11); here myeloblasts and other primitive cells may form from 2–10 percent of the white cells in the blood for years without justifying a diagnosis of leukemia, let alone being an indication of acuteness.

In what has been rather ambiguously termed the *preleukemic status* there is generally a slow course with a relatively small proportion of apparently leukemic cells in the bone marrow. The chief feature is usually anemia with or without leukopenia and thrombocytopenia. Although unequivocal evidence of leukemia may be lacking, primitive leukocytes, usually myeloblasts, may be seen in small numbers in the blood, in association with similar, or somewhat higher, concentrations of the same cells in the bone marrow. The spleen may be normal or slightly enlarged. There may be a relatively static course of months or even several years. The term *preleukemic status* is probably misleading since this is actually leukemia. Chromosome studies[26] have shown that abnormal cell clones can coexist for long periods with the normal ones without expanding materially or overwhelming the host. It is even possible, though so far unproved, that at times a clone of abnormal leukocytes proliferates for a while and eventually dies off. There may be other cases in which a relatively small clone retains a foothold but does not gain a decisive ecologic advantage and fails to become generalized.[13] Perhaps if we knew what intrinsic or extrinsic forces in these cases kept the proliferative process relatively quiescent, we would have a useful tool in the management of more frank cases of acute leukemia which are far more formidable.

Theoretically, it should be possible to observe acute and chronic granulocytic, lymphocytic, and monocytic forms of leukemia. Of these, the monocytic forms are most difficult to define. Acute monocytic leukemia in the majority of cases resembles and behaves as a subtype of the acute granulocytic variety (myelomonocytic). Some authors have altogether denied the existence of a pure acute monocytic form (see below). Chronic monocytic leukemia is rare, perhaps nonexistent, though, especially among the elderly, there are cases of very long-continued monocytosis which eventually end in frank leukemia and can perhaps, therefore, lay claim to the title.[17]

The granulocytic leukemias merit special attention in view of their rather marked diversity. These are discussed in some detail in Chapter 11 which deals with the myeloproliferative syndromes. Chronic granulocytic leukemia (CGL), a relatively slow proliferative disorder of the bone marrow granulocytes, may be related to the more generalized chronic myeloproliferative disorders, that is, polycythemia vera and myelosclerosis-myeloid metaplasia. Acute granulocytic leukemia may be relatively *pure* or *myeloblastic,* showing an almost uniform proliferation of myeloblasts with a variable degree of maturation toward the myelocyte; *myelomonocytic,* with the blood showing a well-defined monocytosis, and the marrow showing, rather paradoxically, a marked degree of myeloblastic proliferation with a variable degree of monocytic proliferation and often also involvement of the erythrocytic series[3, 29]; *promyelocytic,* with predominance of very early myelocytes containing azurophil granulations, or a *mixed erythromyeloblastic* proliferation. This last we have called the DiGuglielmo syndrome. In this form, there appears to be a simultaneous proliferation not only of the myeloblasts but of erythroblasts as well, with the primary lesion in a common stem cell. This may rarely begin with what appears to be a pure red cell proliferation (*erythremic myelosis*), but gives way, as the case progresses, to mixed erythroblast-myeloblast proliferation and, eventually, to an almost complete leukemic status.

These different forms of granulocytic leukemia (and there are others as well) indicate that leukemia may not be as pure as it is customarily pictured. Thus, although it is the usual tendency to think of leukemia as purely a disease of one of the white cell systems, there are actually a number of cases in which simultaneous proliferation of both white cells and red cells and, indeed, of megakaryocytes and monocytes as well, may occur. Others may show pancytopenia, not only in the blood but in the marrow, thus resembling aplastic anemia rather closely; here the entire cellular content of the marrow may have been "insulted" by an unknown agent with the resultant simultaneous cessation in growth of red cells, white cells, and megakaryocytes. The bone marrow in such cases is hypocellular, but myeloblasts are usually found in small clusters. Later, these patients usually develop frank leukemia; before they do so, they might well be placed in the category of preleukemic status, for, in any given case characterized by pancytopenia with a low proportion of blasts, one could ask, with justification, *when* is leukemia?

Finally, mixed cell proliferations have been described consisting of monocytic cells with plasmocytosis or lymphocytosis of varying degrees and types.

Thirty years ago, the definition of leukemia was almost synonymous with a high leukocyte count. Now we realize that probably more than half of all patients with acute leukemia have normal or even low white cell counts. Such counts have often been called *aleukemic,* although strictly speaking, this is not only a paradoxical term (*aleukemic leukemia*), but in most cases, inaccurate as well. This is because almost all leukemia patients with normal or low leukocyte counts have abnormal or primitive cells in the blood. It is probably best to call these cases *subleukemic,* utilizing the designation of *aleukemic* for those in which the blood is totally devoid of any direct evidence of leukemia. Thus, cases of leukemia may be *leukemic,* that is, with high leukocyte counts; *subleukemic* with normal or low leukocyte counts, but with abnormal differential counts showing primitive leukocytes; and, very rarely *aleukemic,* with normal, usually low leukocyte counts but with no abnormal or primitive cells to be found in a careful study of the blood smear. According to this definition, multiple myeloma might be called aleukemic or subleukemic plasma cell leukemia. The occasional patients with high leukocyte counts and numerous blood plasma cells have usually been diagnosed as having "plasma cell leukemia," but it is doubtful if this distinction is justified.

Subleukemic and aleukemic forms are more common in the acute cases; chronic lymphocytic and chronic granulocytic leukemias are almost always leukemic. Why certain cases of leukemia should be associated with a high leukocyte count, and others with a low count, is indeed obscure. Do the subleukemic and aleukemic cases have a type of proliferation in which a high proportion of the primitive cells die before being released from the marrow, or are certain delivery mechanisms inhibited? Why do certain cases, aleukemic for months or years, eventually become leukemic, the bone marrow meanwhile showing but little change? Is the blood picture largely a fortuitous event in a given case of leukemia? Probably not, for the response to treatment and the prognosis may differ between the subleukemic and leukemic patients (see Chapters 18 and 19). It is apparent that in leukemia disturbed or abnormal delivery mechanisms or other equally obscure factors in the tissues may result in quite different pictures of the peripheral blood, though the bone marrow, lymph nodes, or other proliferating tissues appear identical. This indicates, not only that the blood is a more or less imperfect reflection of the status of the proliferating tissues, but also that a dynamic pathophysiology is present in leukemic proliferations, varying widely among patients and resulting thereby in differing blood pictures, or even in the same patient having different features at different times.

To summarize, leukemia may be

A	B	C
Granulocytic	Acute or chronic	Leukemic
Lymphocytic		Subleukemic
Monocytic		Aleukemic
Plasma cell		
Histiocytic		
Mast cell		

A given case of leukemia may be designated as follows: Acute subleukemic lymphocytic leukemia or chronic granulocytic leukemia. In the latter instance, the implication is present that the blood picture is leukemic, that is, having a high leukocyte count. The terms *aleukemic* or *subleukemic* are used only when the white count seems unusually low for leukemia.

Leukemia and the Solid Tumors of the Blood-forming Organs

Although leukemia, a *generalized* proliferation of the white cell tissues, is our principal topic, it should be recognized that localized forms of leukocytic proliferation occur whose histology and cytology closely resemble those of the generalized ones (Table 3-1). These conform more nearly to the usual conception of neoplastic disease than do the generalized proliferations we call leukemia. Localized forms, although they may occur in the course of the leukemic state, are ordinarily first seen as single or multiple tumors originating in various parts of the body, characteristically in the lymph nodes. As the disease progresses, it may spread from these localized foci and involve the bone marrow and bloodstream, thus becoming truly leukemic. Among the tumors in this group are some of the lymphomas, chloroma, and myeloma.

As pointed out more fully in the discussion of the lymphoproliferative disorders, the dividing line between lymphosarcomatosis and leukemia is often difficult, if

Table 3-1
Relationship Between Leukemias and
Solid Tumors of Blood-forming Organs

Generalized proliferation (Leukemia)	Initially localized proliferation (Solid tumors of blood-forming organs)
Acute and chronic forms	Acute and chronic forms
Leukemic, subleukemic, and aleukemic forms	Aleukemic and subleukemic forms almost invariably; leukemic forms may occur late in the disease, indistinguishable from typical leukemia
Granulocytic	Chloroma
Lymphocytic	Lymphosarcoma ⎫
Histiocytic	Reticulum cell sarcoma ⎬ Lymphomas
Plasma cell	Plasmacytoma; myeloma ⎭

not impossible, to define. Thus, certain cases of obvious chronic lymphocytic leukemia (CLL) may show gross lymph node or splenic enlargement which histologically cannot be distinguished from small-cell lymphosarcoma; conversely, what at one time appears to be an example of localized lymphosarcoma often becomes in the course of time a generalized proliferation of lymphoid tissues, that is, an example of leukemia, either of the classic small-celled type found in chronic lymphocytic leukemia or one showing the more immature cells characteristic of lymphosarcoma-cell leukemia. Between typical examples of chronic lymphocytic leukemia and lymphosarcoma, many transitional forms may be noted; in fact, they may be considered as closely related forms in a spectrum of neoplastic lymphoproliferative disorders. A very rare member of this group, the Sézary syndrome, is of particular interest. In this very chronic condition, large numbers of grossly abnormal lymphocytes with the cytogenetic characteristics of malignancy are present in the blood for many months or years without any obvious involvement of the marrow or lymph nodes (Fig. 3-1). This prelymphomatous condition may end in frank lymphoma or leukemia.[6]

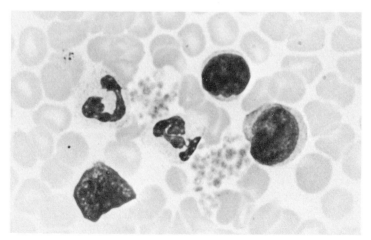

Fig. 3-1. Sézary cell, an abnormal lymphocyte. Such cells may circulate for years in large numbers in cases of the Sézary syndrome. Magnification × 1200.

In chloroma, a neoplasm of myeloblasts, which is probably rarer than was formerly thought, the blood picture is almost invariably myeloblastic at the time the diagnosis is made, the leukocyte count usually being high with a high proportion of myeloblasts (i.e., acute granulocytic or myeloblastic leukemia). However, we have seen one case in which a greenish utero-ovarian neoplasm was removed and diagnosed as "sarcoma, type undetermined," and in which the blood picture was at first stated to be normal; a few months later, the typical picture of the acute myeloblastic leukemia was present with striking involvement of the bone marrow. Postmortem examination in this case disclosed greenish tumors throughout the body, together with the typical features of acute leukemia. In solitary myeloma or plasmacytoma, which may arise anywhere in the body (we have seen it in the periepididymal area, in the tonsil, in a localized area of bone), the blood picture, the serum proteins, and the bone marrow examination may at first be completely normal. In the course of time, which may be 1–10 years later, and depending apparently upon the degree of malignancy of the proliferating cell, the entire bone marrow becomes involved with the plasma cell proliferation, and all the characteristic laboratory features of multiple myeloma are found, occasionally accompanied by frank leukemic changes (so-called plasma cell leukemia).

Reticulum cell sarcoma, a primary neoplasm of "reticulum cells," is at times associated with a leukemic picture in which the predominant cell is the histiocyte. This is exceptional. More often the bone marrow, lymph nodes, liver, spleen, etc. are extensively involved in a generalized reticulum cell proliferation, but the blood picture is relatively normal except perhaps for some degree of monocytosis (see below).

It would appear logical to include under single headings both the solid and the leukemic phases of the various leukocytic neoplastic proliferations. Thus, both chloroma and the many granulocytic leukemias would be included in the myeloproliferative, the lymphosarcomas and chronic lymphocytic leukemia in the lymphoproliferative group. Purists might add the rare reticuloproliferative and the plasma cell proliferative groups. As a further venture in classification, one may speculate that there are two broad groups of leukoproliferative disorders: the myeloproliferative, and the immunoproliferative. This admittedly speculative classification may possess some merit in contrasting the differing reactions of the granulocytic tissues as opposed to those of the reticulo-plasma-cell–lymphocytic tissues. The granulocytes represent the body's first and, in fact, chief protective mechanism against pyogenic organisms and nonspecific stimuli. On the other hand, the cells of the immunocyte complex react against antigenic substances of various types, either by cellular or humoral or combined immunologic means.

We believe there is some advantage in classifying leukemia in a dynamic rather than in a purely morphologic way. In particular, we should remember always that leukemia is by no means a single disease: it brings together under one heading a number of essentially different proliferative processes. Surely, there can be nothing more different than leukemia of the acute granulocytic and chronic lymphocytic varieties. To be sure, they both commonly have high white cell counts and both may lead eventually to the death of the patient, but they seem to be etiologically, physiologically, and in every other way entirely different diseases. They are classified together because they represent neoplastic proliferations of white blood cell-forming tissues but apparently of entirely different metabolic and pathogenic backgrounds.

The Reticuloses and Monocytic Leukemia

It is necessary at this point to consider briefly the so-called reticuloses and their relation to leukemia. The term *reticulosis* is probably one of the most confusing in medicine. It has been used in the most diverse senses by internists, pathologists, hematologists, and radiologists. To some, it means a collection of strictly defined and demarcated lesions of the lymph nodes; to others, a much wider group of conditions practically synonymous with the lymphomas; while in yet other hands, it has become a kind of procrustean bed on which such diverse diseases as tuberculosis, syphilis, the leukemias, and various lipoidoses have been stretched. The word, to quote Helen Russell,[28] "has appeared like a vague cloud." The original intention of those who introduced the term *reticulosis*[19,23] was to describe with it those diseases which arose from the multipotential cells lying in the connective tissue of the lymphoid and hematopoietic organs, as well as in other situations. In 1938, Robb-Smith[25] built an elaborate classification contrasting "reticulosis," which he conceived as "a progressive hyperplasia of reticular tissue" with the true blastomas. This author included the leukemias, Brill-Symmers' and Hodgkin's disease, as well as a number of rarer conditions in his portmanteau of "reticuloses," while leaving out the lympho- and reticulosarcomas and myeloma. Such a classification, while possibly satisfying to the histologic purist, seems of doubtful value in practice, since it describes static pictures, separates closely related clinical groups, gives no indication of prognosis, and ignores the not infrequent transitions from one condition to another.[7] Consequently, it is now mainly of historic interest.

It seems doubtful if much advantage accrues from the retention of the term *reticulosis* in its present multiple meanings. From the hematologist's point of view, the problem of the reticuloses is chiefly of interest because it impinges on that of the classification of monocytic leukemia. Monocytic leukemia has been recognized in numerous publications throughout the years[2,4,8,10,11,14,15,24,32,34] and treated extensively in a recent monograph by Leder.[18] It is generally agreed that there are many cases of the myelomonocytic variety[29] and that this is a subtype of acute granulocytic leukemia (see above). The question which has agitated hematologic minds for many years is whether a second "pure" monocytic variety[31] exists which is not basically derived from the granulocytic series. This question is tied up with that of the derivation of the monocyte itself. Is this cell, as has often been maintained, an offspring of Aschoff's "reticulo-endothelial system," arriving in the blood from its breeding grounds in the spleen, liver, lymph nodes, and perhaps other tissues? Does it have its own distinctive precursor, the monoblast, as stated by Sabin?[30] Or is it, as Naegeli believed, a member of the granulocytic family? We find it impossible to enter into the many arguments bedevilling this confused field. However, in our view the more recent evidence (especially cytochemical), as marshalled by Leder[18] and others,[16,33] is sufficiently strong to make it reasonably certain that monocytes originate not in the tissues but in the bone marrow from granulocytic precursors; and that the point at which the monocytic series diverges from the main granulocytic one is the promyelocyte stage. If this is so, there is little chance of a "pure" monocytic leukemia existing, and, indeed, since even grossly atypical monocytes can be distinguished from promyelocytes and later myeloid forms by cytochemical means, no cases of monocytic leukemia have yet been found, in which detailed studies did not disclose the simultaneous presence of both monocytes and myeloid

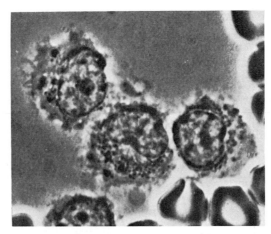

Fig. 3-2. Three reticulum cells observed in supravital films with the phase-contrast microscope. The mitochondria and a few cytoplasmic vacuoles are present. The lacelike outline of the membrane is prominent. The nucleus is eccentric. Nucleoli are prominent. Magnification approximately × 2260. (Bouroncle et al.,[5] courtesy of the authors and the publisher.)

cells.[18] Our own experience is similar, and we are, therefore, not convinced of the existence of a *pure* or *Schilling* type of monocytic leukemia.

On the other hand, there is no doubt that there are rare instances of so-called histiocytic leukemia arising from an invasion of the blood by the cells of certain reticulosarcomas. Although such cells may resemble monocytes morphologically, they differ from them cytochemically, especially in the absence of alpha-naphthyl acetate esterase.[18] Perhaps it is justified, as suggested in an earlier edition of this

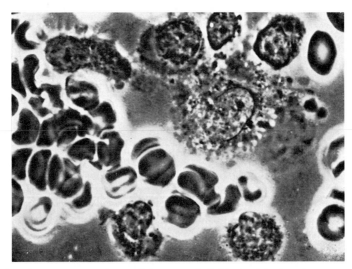

Fig. 3-3. Bone marrow observed in supravital films with the phase-contrast microscope. The elongated cell in the left upper corner has the morphologic characteristics of an endothelial cell as seen in leukemic reticuloendotheliosis. The larger cell is a phagocytic histiocyte. The others are reticulum cells. Magnification approximately × 1450. (Bouroncle et al.,[5] courtesy of the authors and the publisher.)

work, to include reticulum cell sarcomas and histiocytic leukemias in a group of reticuloproliferative neoplasms. Hodgkin's disease, often confused with reticulum cell sarcoma, would be excluded from this group, as there is no evidence to suggest a direct relationship between it and leukemia, although the two diseases may occasionally coexist.[12,22]

Bouroncle, Wiseman, and Doan[5] described, under the designation of "leukemic reticulo-endotheliosis," a group of cases characterized by hyperplasia of the reticulum tissue in the blood-forming organs with the appearance of reticuloendothelial cells in the blood. These free reticulum cells or histiocytes are identified in the blood by means of supravital studies, with or without phase microscopy, and present a characteristic lacelike outline to the cytoplasmic membrane. The nuclei contain prominent nucleoli (Figs. 3-2, 3-3). Mitus et al.[20] have described the cells seen in such patients as neoplastic lymphoid reticulum cells since many of them have the superficial appearance of lymphocytes. Rubin et al.[27] have more recently demonstrated that these neoplastic cells respond to stimulation with phytohemagglutinin (PHA): this is positive evidence that at least some of the cells first described by Bouroncle and her colleagues belong to the lymphocytic series. The condition is now often referred to as *hairy-cell leukemia* (see Chapter 21).

REFERENCES

1. Aschoff L: Das reticuloendotheliale System. Ergeb Inn Med Kinderheilk 26:1, 1924.

2. Belding HW, Daland GA, Parker F, Jr.: Histocytic and monocytic leukemia. A clinical, hematological and pathological differentiation. Cancer 8:237, 1955.

3. Bennett JM: Myelomonocytic leukemias: a historical review and perspective. Cancer 27:1218, 1971.

4. Berkheiser SW: Studies on the comparative morphology of monocytic leukemia, granulocytic leukemia and reticulum-cell sarcoma. Cancer 10:606, 1957.

5. Bouroncle BA, Wiseman BK, Doan CA: Leukemic reticulo-endotheliosis. Blood 13: 609, 1958.

6. Crossen PE, Mellor JEL, Finley AG, Ravich RBM, Vincent PC, Gunz FW: The Sézary syndrome. Amer J Med 50:24, 1971.

7. Custer RP, Bernhard WG: The inter-relationship of Hodgkin's disease and other lymphatic tumors. Amer J Med Sci 216:625, 1948.

8. Dameshek W: Acute monocytic (histiocytic) leukemia; review of literature and case reports. Arch Intern Med 46:718, 1930.

9. ———: Proliferative disease of the reticuloendothelial system. II. Aleukemic reticulosis. Folia Haematol (Leipz) 49:64, 1933.

10. Doan CA, Wiseman BK: Monocyte, monocytosis and monocytic leukosis: Clinical and pathologic study. Ann Intern Med 8:383, 1934.

11. Downey H: Monocytic leukemia and leukemic reticulo-endotheliosis, in, Downey's Handbook of Hematology. New York, Hoeber, 1938, p 1275.

12. Ezdinli EZ, Sokal JE, Aungst CW, Kim V, and Sandberg AA: Myeloid leukemia in Hodgkin's disease: Chromosomal abnormalities. Ann Intern Med 71:1097, 1969.

13. Finney R, McDonald GA, Baikie AG, Douglas AS: Chronic granulocytic leukemia with Ph¹-negative cells in bone marrow and a 10-year remission after busulphan hypoplasia. Br J Haematol 23:283, 1972.

14. Forkner CE: Clinical and pathological differentiations in acute leukemias with special reference to acute monocytic leukemia. Arch Intern Med 53:1,1934.

15. Herbut PA, Miller FR: Histopathology of monocytic leukemia. Amer J Pathol 23:93, 1947.

16. Huhn D, Schmalzl F, Demmler K: Monozytenleukämie. Licht-und Elektronenmikroskopische Morphologie und Zytochemie. Dtsch Med Wochenschr 96:1594, 1971.

17. Hurdle ADF, Garson OM, Buist DGP: Clinical and cytogenetic studies in chronic

myelomonocytic leukaemia. Br J Haematol 22:773, 1972.

18. Leder LD: Der Blutomonocyt. Berlin; Springer, 1967.

19. Letterer E: Aleukämische Retikulose. Frankf. Pathol 30:377, 1924.

20. Mitus WJ, Mednicoff IB, Wittels B, Dameshek W: Neoplastic lymphoid reticulum cells in the peripheral blood: A histochemical study. Blood 17:206, 1961.

21. Naegeli O: Lehrbuch der Blutkrankheiten und Blutdiagnostik. Berlin, Springer, 1931.

22. Osta S, Wells M, Viamonte M, Harkness D: Hodgkin's disease terminating in acute leukemia. Cancer 26:795, 1970.

23. Pullinger BD: Histology and histogenesis. Rose Research on Lymphadenoma. Bristol, Wright, 1932, p 115.

24. Rappaport AE, Kugel VH: Monocytic leukemia: A case report illustrating variations in clinical picture. Blood 2:332, 1947.

25. Robb-Smith AHT: Reticulosis and reticulosarcoma: A histological classification. J Pathol Bacteriol 47:457, 1938.

26. Rowley JD, Blaisdell RK, Jacobson LO: Chromosome studies in preleukemia. I. Aneuploidy of group C chromosomes in three patients. Blood 27:782, 1966.

27. Rubin AD, Douglas SD, Chessin LN, Glade PR, Dameshek W: Chronic reticulolymphocytic leukemia. Amer J Med 47:149, 1969.

28. Russell H: An essay on the reactions of the mesenchyme with especial reference to the "reticuloses." Edinburgh Med J 56:62, 1949.

29. Saarni MI, Linman JW: Myelomonocytic leukemia: Disorderly proliferation of all marrow cells. Cancer 27:1221, 1971.

30. Sabin FR: Studies on living human blood cells. Bull Johns Hopkins Hosp 34:277, 1923.

31. Schilling V: Der Monocyt in trialistischer Auffassung und seine Bedeutung im Krankheitsbilde. Med Klin 22:563, 1926.

32. Sinn CM, Dick FW: Monocytic leukemia. Amer J Med 20:588, 1956.

33. VanFurth R: Origin and kinetics of monocytes and macrophages. Semin Hematol 7:125, 1970.

34. Watkins CH, Hall BE: Monocytic leukemia of Naegeli and Schilling types. Amer J Clin Pathol 10:387, 1940.

4

Incidence

In this chapter two questions will be discussed: (1) How widespread is leukemia today; and (2) how much more widespread is leukemia today than formerly? Many statements have been, and are still being, published about the rapid increase in the incidence of leukemia and the menacing proportions which the total leukemia problem has assumed. Indeed, much of the available evidence shows that in many parts of the world both the number of cases and the rate of their notification have been rising for many years. It shows also that the increase has occurred at differing speeds in different areas; and that in some it has recently slowed down or even has been reversed. There are very large gaps in our knowledge concerning leukemia statistics which make it impossible to obtain a complete picture of the situation as it has developed or exists today. Much of the reported rise in leukemia incidence undoubtedly can be accounted for by progressive improvements in medical and diagnostic facilities. Whether, however, these factors alone are responsible is an unsolved question, although it can be said with some confidence that any increase in the *true* incidence of leukemia must have been of comparatively modest proportions.

Sources of Information

The *incidence* of leukemia, as used here, is the number of persons per 100,000 living in a given population who acquire the disease in any particular year. The *mortality* is the number of deaths from leukemia per 100,000 population per year. Both terms define rates or proportions rather than absolute figures. They may be presented as *crude* rates, that is, rates in a total unadjusted population, as *age-specific* rates, or as rates for a population whose age structure has been adjusted to resemble that of a given standard population (*age-adjusted* rate). Only the use of age-specific or age-adjusted rates makes comparisons between different populations meaningful, because crude rates are greatly influenced by the age structure of each given population. As will be seen later, leukemia occurs with varying frequencies at different ages, and because it is, for instance, less common in young than old people,

27

a relatively young population would automatically have a relatively low leukemia rate.

The terms *incidence* and *mortality* are often used loosely as though they were interchangeable. This is unjustified, despite the fact that the disease is almost universally fatal (in a few exceptional cases, especially in very chronic leukemias, patients may die from causes unconnected with their primary disease). In any event, incidence and mortality cannot be equal, for not every patient dies in the same year in which he acquires the disease. In 1947, for instance, the leukemia incidence in ten areas of the United States with a population of 14.6 million was 9.1 per 100,000 but the mortality was only 6.7 per 100,000, a ratio of 1.35:1 (Dorn and Cutler[22]: rates in this investigation were adjusted to the age distribution of the continental United States in 1950). In three other studies the ratios between incidence and mortality were 1.4, 1.1, and 1.2 respectively.[3,21,35]

The mortality of leukemia is easier to determine than its incidence because death certification is practised in nearly all countries whereas public health statistics of morbidity are obtainable only in a few countries in which either leukemia is notifiable or where special cancer registries exist. The most notable example of such a registry is in Denmark,[7-9] with others in New York State,[51,52] Connecticut,[33] Norway,[66] Eastern Germany,[91] Victoria, Australia,[44] and New Zealand.[24,28] The leukemia incidence has also been determined in some special surveys.[21,22,35,85] Figures obtained from registries and special surveys suffer from the defect that registrations do not usually come from the whole population, and that the reasons for incomplete reporting are not known. The populations investigated may not be fully representative, so that conclusions drawn cannot necessarily be applied to the whole population. An appraisal by Dorn and Cutler[22] of their results for a survey area as large as 10 percent of the United States suggested that the incidence found may have been 10 or 15 percent higher than that for the whole country. Because of the difficulties of obtaining statistics on the incidence of leukemia, estimates of the prevalence of the disease are usually based on its mortality.

Mortality figures, though readily obtainable, are not free from errors either, depending as they must on the accuracy of death certification. This is not likely to be uniform all over the world. Some leukemia patients are undoubtedly certified as dying from other diseases, and it has been stated that the recorded mortality may underestimate the true mortality by as much as 20 percent.[80] False positive diagnoses of leukemia, though rare, also occur. Special difficulties arise because of the different ways in which the leukemias and lymphomas have in the past been classified (see Chapters 1,3,12); consequently figures from different periods may not be comparable unless corrected with the use of factors which rest on somewhat uncertain assumptions.[73] Nevertheless, valuable information has been obtained from mortality statistics,[41,55,59,73,74] and much of present-day knowledge of the occurrence and distribution of leukemia still rests on them.

In former years, conclusions on leukemia statistics were often drawn on the basis of case series from single or groups of hospitals. This is not a safe procedure as such series can rarely be representative of the total population,[29,83] patients being selected for admission on a variety of criteria which are almost certain to bias the results. An even greater selectivity will be found among series of autopsy reports.

Geographic, Racial, and Social Distribution of Leukemia

The occurrence of leukemia appears to be worldwide, but there are considerable differences in its recorded incidence in different geographic areas. Figure 4-1 shows the incidence of leukemia in males, from data compiled by the International Union Against Cancer as a result of special surveys comprising the years 1950–1963.[85] Some of these data came only from small areas in the countries surveyed and may not be representative. The figures are, however, the best available, and as such suggest a fivefold higher incidence in some countries than in others. The differentials are particularly great in the youngest and oldest age groups, whereas in the middle years the incidence appears to be much more uniform. It seems likely

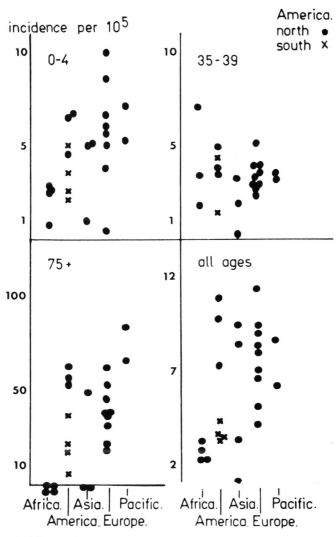

Fig. 4-1. Incidence of leukemia in males in five continents, based on figures compiled by the International Union Against Cancer. (Gunz,[36] courtesy of the authors and publisher.)

Table 4-1

Mortality Rates Per 100,000 from Leukemia 1962–1963:
Comparison Between Highest (H) and Lowest (L) in 24 Countries

Age and Sex	Highest	Lowest	Ratio H/L
All ages, M	8.00	3.44	2.32
All ages, F	6.32	2.76	2.30
Under 15, M	5.17	2.47	2.10
Under 15, F	4.68	1.02	4.64
15–55, M	4.10	2.78	1.47
15–55, F	4.19	2.05	2.02
Over 55, M	29.62	4.96	6.00
Over 55, F	22.53	3.33	6.74

Data from Segi and Kurihara.[72]

that medical services are most variable at the extremes of life, and especially at the oldest ages. This probably explains why the greatest variations in incidence and mortality are found in old people (Table 4-1).

In general, countries with non-European populations report low leukemia rates. In some (e.g., Samoa,[23] French Central Africa,[71] East Africa[19]), the disease was formerly said to be virtually absent. Where medical services were relatively good, however, as in areas served by medical schools, cases of leukemia were soon discovered where previously they were unknown,[1,20,86] and the incidence might even approach the European rates. This suggests that the real differences between geographic areas may be much less pronounced than those so far published.

It is debatable how many of the reported differences in leukemia incidence are due to genuine variations in racial susceptibility. Nearly everywhere environmental factors, as well as varying standards of case-finding, can be invoked in addition to the presumed genetic differences. The most striking example of a "racial" difference is the great rarity of the chronic lymphocytic type in Japanese and some other Oriental populations.[50,81,84,90] This cannot be explained simply on the basis of a non-European age distribution, with a relative shortage of old people. It may be a genuinely racial trait, although it has been reported[40,75] that in Japanese living in the United States the mortality from chronic lymphocytic leukemia is higher than among those living in Japan. The leukemia mortality in black Americans has been persistently lower than that among Caucasians,[29,30] but the difference has tended to diminish in recent years.[26] Here differences in access to medical facilities and in regional rates make an interpretation in terms of racial differences at present impossible. Similarly, the reportedly raised incidence among some Jewish groups in the United States,[55,63] and in those born in Russia, Poland, and Czechoslovakia[39] may be associated with social rather than racial factors.

It should be added that though different racial and social groups within some countries have been reported to have differing leukemia mortalities,[41,67,86] these relationships are inconstant and subject to rapid changes. Thus, in the United States, the mortality in 1950–1959 was higher in urban areas for white children but in rural areas for black children.[79] In England, leukemia used to be more common in the upper- than the lower-class social groups,[41] but this difference disappeared between 1931 and 1951.[21] Similarly, regional differences have not always been maintained.[11]

Table 4-2
Age-Adjusted Mortality from Leukemia in
24 Countries in 1962–1963

| | Mortality | |
Country	M	F
South Africa*	6.99	5.60
Canada	6.99	4.66
Chile	3.44	1.77
U.S.A., white	7.39	4.82
U.S.A., nonwhite	5.37	3.84
Israel	7.10	6.32
Japan	3.56	2.76
Germany, F.R.	5.84	4.36
Austria	6.21	4.16
Belgium	6.26	4.61
Denmark	8.00	5.41
Finland	6.74	5.28
France	6.56	4.74
Ireland	4.91	3.35
Italy	6.36	4.66
Norway	7.12	4.67
Netherlands	6.79	4.78
Portugal	4.22	3.73
England and Wales	5.46	4.05
Scotland	5.27	3.67
Northern Ireland	6.28	3.28
Sweden	7.26	5.06
Switzerland	5.92	4.64
Australia	6.03	4.23
New Zealand	7.29	4.62

*1962 only (white population)
From Segi and Kurihara[72]

Although some have been more constant than others the evidence suggests that they were not caused by purely geographic, but rather by social factors,[33,52,53,59] the most important of which may well be the quality and availability of medical care.

The leukemia mortality in 24 countries, most of them European or with Caucasian populations, is shown in Table 4–2, and in Figures 4–2 and 4–3. Although in general terms, there is a reasonably even distribution, some differences exist, and these are difficult to explain. Thus, the Scandinavian countries show rates which are consistently higher than the rest of Europe; the U.S. white population has had consistently higher rates than England and Wales (ratios between the two countries varied between 1.35 and 1.58:1 in males); and Portugal consistently has the lowest mortality in Europe. Japan's mortality is very low compared with that of all European countries but has been rising exceptionally fast, almost doubling between 1950–1951 and 1962–1963. The differences are much greater in the older age groups than the younger ones and the overall differences are largely accounted for by those among the old.[56,58]

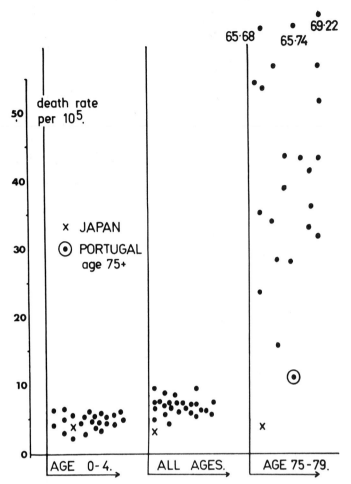

Fig. 4-2. Leukemia mortality in 24 countries for 1962–1963, based on the figures of Segi and Kurihara.[72] (Gunz,[36] courtesy of the authors and publisher.)

Total Prevalence of Leukemia

As has already been mentioned, figures for the incidence of leukemia are scanty and come only from countries or parts of countries in which voluntary or compulsory notification of malignant diseases is practiced. Figure 4-1 gives a résumé of the data collected by the International Union Against Cancer between 1950–1963. During this period, substantial changes in the recorded incidence took place. Table 4-3 shows the very wide variations observed in this material.

When mortality figures are examined, the size of the leukemia problem becomes most vividly illuminated. In the United States, there were 5,140 deaths from leukemia in 1940.[14] In 1950, there were 8,844; in 1951, 9,357; in 1952, 9,841; in 1953, 9,918; in 1954, 10,443; in 1955, 10,816; in 1956, 11,396; and in 1957, 11,718 deaths. Thus, in 8 years over 80,000 Americans died from leukemia. The number of new cases for 1968 was estimated at 19,000.[10] Figures given in Table 4-4 show that in one year, 1962, in 24 countries, 34,919 individuals died from leukemia. Since these countries had a population totaling about one-fifth that of the whole world, one

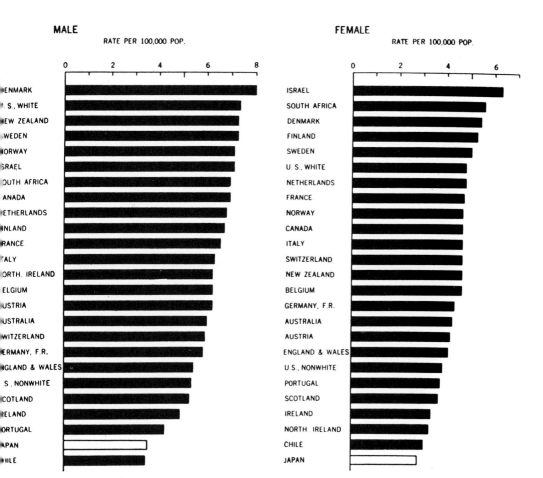

Fig. 4-3. Age-adjusted death rates for leukemia and aleukemia (all ages) for 1962–1963, in 24 countries. (Segi and Kurihara,[72] courtesy of the authors and publisher.)

Table 4-3
Range of Leukemia Incidence
Per 100,000 Living, 1950–1963

	Incidence per 100,000	
Ages	*Males*	*Females*
0– 5	0.8–10.2	0.5– 8.8
6–10	1.0– 6.0	0.7– 4.7
11–15	0.9– 6.3	0.6– 4.8
26–30	0.6– 4.0	0.5– 4.8
31–35	0.7– 5.8	0.3– 6.2
51–55	1.6–13.0	0.9–23.3
56–60	2.2–21.9	0.6–24.7
61–65	1.8–32.5	1.9–47.6
All ages	1.0–11.5	0.5– 8.4

From "Cancer incidence in five continents"[85]

Table 4-4

Total Deaths from Leukemia in 1962 and Leukemia Deaths as a
Percentage of All Cancer Deaths in 24 Countries

Country	M	F	Leukemia Deaths as % of All Cancer Deaths (1962–1963)	
			M	F
South Africa, white	99	89	4.2	4.7
Canada	682	444	5.0	4.1
Chile	126	121	3.3	2.9
U.S.A., white	6,757	4,881	5.2	4.4
U.S.A., nonwhite	491	402	3.7	3.5
Israel	69	63	6.4	5.2
Japan	1,606	1,306	3.0	2.9
Germany	1,807	1,703	3.0	2.7
Austria	243	205	2.7	2.5
Belgium	315	280	2.9	2.8
Denmark	224	163	4.3	3.3
Finland	142	136	3.6	4.4
France	1,751	1,434	3.4	3.3
Ireland	82	50	3.0	2.4
Italy	1.701	1,307	4.0	3.7
Norway	158	114	4.8	3.8
Netherlands	448	325	3.8	3.6
Portugal	192	174	3.9	3.8
England and Wales	1,392	1,315	2.6	2.8
Scotland	150	139	2.4	2.4
Northern Ireland	48	30	4.0	2.7
Sweden	370	261	4.7	3.8
Switzerland	177	161	3.3	3.2
Australia	358	265	4.3	3.9
New Zealand	88	75	4.8	4.0
	19,476	15,433		
	Total: 34,919		M:F=1.25:1	

Data from Segi and Kurihara.[72]

might expect about 180,000 leukemia deaths in the world in a single year. Although
this is probably an overestimate, because of the variability in the population structures, the figure gives a useful order of magnitude to show the extent of the global
leukemia problem. The years of potential life lost by death from leukemia in
England during 1953 (reckoning normal life to the age of 75) were estimated as
greater than those lost by death from peptic ulcer, nonrespiratory tuberculosis, or
all diseases conventionally attributed to viruses.[41]

Among the malignant neoplasms leukemia occupies a rather prominent
position which is, however, markedly age-dependent (Fig. 4-4). In children, nearly
half of all cancer deaths are due to leukemia, and in young adults about one in five,
whereas in the elderly the proportion falls to about 1:25. Internationally, the proportion varies from 2.4–6.4 percent in males and from 2.4–5.2 percent in females (Table
4-4). In the U.S. white population, in 1962–1963, deaths from leukemia were about
one-third those from cancer of the stomach and intestine, one-quarter those of the

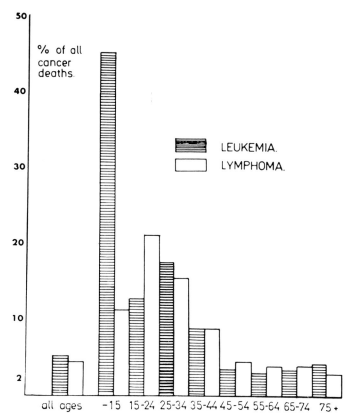

Fig. 4-4. Deaths from leukemia and lymphoma (males) as the percentage of all cancer deaths in New Zealand, 1964. (Gunz,[36] courtesy of the author and publisher.)

lung, bronchus, and trachea in males, and of the breast in females, but were equal to those of the buccal cavity, pharynx and esophagus, and of the pancreas. The probability of developing leukemia at any time during the individual's life drops from about 0.6 percent at birth to 0.14 percent at 80 years in males, and from 0.5 percent to 0.25 percent in females.[28,32]

Type Distribution

There are two main difficulties in assessing the prevalence of the various types of leukemia, as contrasted with that of leukemia as a whole. The first is that of obtaining adequate records. The classification of leukemia has been subject to continual changes, both among workers in the field and in the International List of Causes of Death which is used as the basis for certification in large parts of the world. Table 4-5 shows the current (eighth) revision of the list which came into use in 1968. Previously, the seventh revision permitted a division into "myeloid," "lymphatic," "monocytic," and "acute," the last embracing all types of acute leukemia. The sixth revision did not distinguish between acute and chronic types, except in a few cases. Earlier revisions had made distinctions between "leukemias" and "aleukemias," and from 1929–1938 the group of "pseudoleukemias" had included Hodgkin's disease as well as "aleukemia." It is clear that the fourth and fifth revi-

Table 4-5
International List of Causes of Death, Eighth Revision, 1967:
Neoplasms of Lymphatic and Hematopoietic Tissues (200–209)

200.	Lymphosarcoma and reticulum cell sarcoma
	200.0 Reticulum cell sarcoma
	200.1 Lymphosarcoma
201.	Hodgkin's disease
202.	Other neoplasms of lymphoid tissue
	202.0 Giant follicular lymphoma
	202.1 Mycosis fungoides
	202.2 Other primary malignant neoplasms of lymphoid tissue
	202.9 Other forms of lymphoma
203.	Multiple myeloma
204.	Lymphatic leukemia
	204.0 Acute
	204.1 Chronic
	204.9 Unspecified
205.	Myeloid leukemia
	205.0 Acute
	205.1 Chronic
	205.9 Unspecified
206.	Monocytic leukemia
	206.0 Acute
	206.1 Chronic
	206.9 Unspecified
207.	Other and unspecified leukemia
	207.0 Acute
	207.1 Chronic
	207.2 Acute erythremia (Di Guglielmo)
	207.9 Unspecified
208.	Polycythemia vera
209.	Myelofibrosis

sions are virtually useless for an analysis of type distribution, and that even the sixth cannot distinguish between the acute and chronic forms. Eventually, statistics compiled with the help of the seventh and eighth revisions may give a clearer picture, but this will depend on the widespread availability of first-class laboratory facilities.

The quality of vital statistics can only be as good as that of the diagnostic methods leading to their compilation, and diagnostic methods are still highly variable, even within individual countries and under favorable circumstances. Moreover, there is no consensus on some of the criteria used in classification. Observers may still differ on what constitutes acute and what chronic leukemia, to say nothing of the problems of subclassifying the acute leukemias, which are discussed in detail in Chapter 3. Mistakes even occur in the classification of the chronic leukemias.[47] For these reasons, the elaborate nomenclature of the eighth revision may not achieve the desired result of producing improved data on the type distribution among the leukemias.

Meanwhile, recourse must be had to alternative sources, either to hospital records or to the figures collected by cancer registries or in special surveys. The earliest series is that of Ward[88] who, in 1917, and "in such spare time as military

Table 4-6
Proportion of Acute Leukemias

Authors	Country	Years	Acute (%)	Remarks
Gauld et al.	Scotland	1938–1951	41.9	
MacMahon and Clark	U.S.A. (Brooklyn)	1943–1952	44.6	"Also 10.9 unknown and subacute"
Husabye and Gaustad	Norway (Oslo)	1946–1950	63.0	
Fischer	France (Montpellier)	1938–1954	61.0	
Keogh	Australia (Vic.)	1951–1955	68.0	
Pedersen and Magnus[66]	Norway	1953–1954	57.0	Also 23% "not specified"
Gunz and Hough	New Zealand	1950–1954	61.0	
Gunz[34]	New Zealand	1958–1961	60.0	
Court Brown and Doll	England	1955–1957	57.7	Adults only: males
Court Brown and Doll	England	1955–1957	60.0	Adults only: females
Court Brown et al.	England	1958–1961	63.5	Standardized for age

service provides," made a collection of 729 cases in the literature, finding 398 (54.5 percent) of acute, 247 (33.8 percent) of chronic granulocytic, and 84 (11.5 percent) of chronic lymphocytic leukemia. Probably by chance, Ward's proportion of 54.5 percent acute leukemias is almost precisely the same as that in a much larger American sample in 1960–1962.[18] As might be expected, the greatest divergencies in the literature concern the incidence of acute leukemia, with the figures ranging from 36–68 percent,[36,44] of all leukemias. In general, the more recent publications agree in assigning to the acute leukemias a dominant position, as indicated in Table 4-6. In one series totaling 10,148 patients of all ages,[18] the rising proportion of acute leukemia during a 23-year period can be clearly seen (Table 4-7). Different type distributions are found in non-European populations, notably in Japan, where well over 70 percent of all cases are acute.[84,87]

Considerable differences exist in the published rates for the chronic leukemias. In contrast to Ward's early figures, most Caucasian populations now show an excess of chronic lymphocytic over the chronic granulocytic forms (excess CL/CG in England and Wales, 1958–1961: 7 percent; Norway, 1957–1959: 20 percent; Finland, 1957–1961: 45 percent[17]; New Zealand, 1958–1961: 100 percent[34]). As a rough approximation, it may be concluded that in Western countries about 60 percent of all leukemias are acute, 25 percent chronic lymphocytic, and 15 percent chronic

Table 4-7
Proportion of Acute Leukemia in a Total of 10,148 Patients, 1940–1962

Sex	Percentage of Leukemias Classified as Acute				
	All Periods	1940–1949	1950–1954	1955–1959	1960–1962
Male	44	38	41	45	52
Female	49	41	46	49	56
Total	46	39	43	47	53

From Cutler, Axtell, and Heise.[18]

granulocytic. In Japan, only about 2.5 percent of all leukemias belong to the chronic lymphocytic type.

It is impossible to assess the incidence of monocytic leukemia from published statistics, since there is little common ground between different authors in their views of what constitutes this disease. In children, there is general agreement that the great majority of cases are acute. Opitz[65] found only 4.2 percent chronic forms in a total of 1357 cases; Oehme[64] 5.7 percent in 191; Cooke[13] 5 percent in 294, and

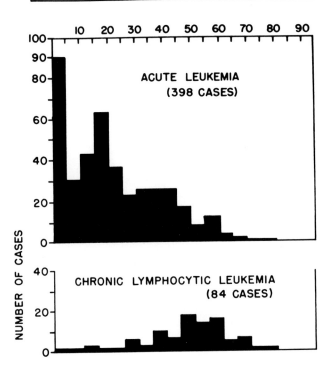
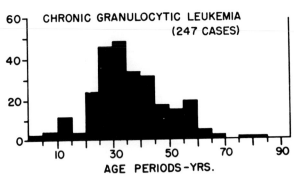

Fig. 4-5. Age distribution in 729 cases of leukemia, as given by Ward in 1917.[88] (Reproduced from Forkner CE, Leukemia and Allied Disorders. New York, Macmillan, 1938, courtesy of the publisher.)

Gunz and Spears[38] 2.7 percent in 288 cases. Almost all the chronic childhood leukemias are granulocytic.

Age Distribution

While there is much uncertainty about the type distribution of leukemia, we are
on firmer ground when its age incidence is examined. There is wide agreement on it
among reports originating during comparable periods of time, as well as good evidence of fairly uniform changes in the age incidence during the course of successive
periods. In Ward's[88] early series (Fig. 4-5), acute leukemia showed a peak incidence
below the age of 5, with a secondary peak between 15 and 20, and a fairly even level
up to 45, after which there were few cases. Most deaths from chronic granulocytic
leukemia occurred between 20 and 50 years, while the majority of chronic
lymphocytic leukemia clustered between 45 and 60. Other figures from this period
agree well with Ward's findings.[42,48,61,62,70,89] None of them established rates of incidence. Higher mean ages were recorded in more recent publications: Windeyer and
Scott,[92] for the years 1931–1949, found 38.8 years as the mean age for acute, 45.7
years for chronic granulocytic, and 55.0 years for chronic lymphocytic leukemia,
while for 1950–1954, Gunz and Hough[37] noted 46 percent of acute and 57.1 percent
of all leukemia deaths after the age of 50 (Fig. 4-6). Almost precisely the same
percentage (57) was found by Cooke[14] in an analysis of all leukemia deaths in the
United States in 1949 (Fig. 4-7). Throughout the years, chronic lymphocytic
leukemia has been shown to occur at significantly greater ages that any other type.

Over the years leukemia mortality rates have shown greater increases in the
older age groups than in the younger. An example from New Zealand is shown in
Figure 4-8.[36] In other countries a similarly disproportionate rise has occurred,[72]
but the actual rates are more variable in the elderly than for those of other ages

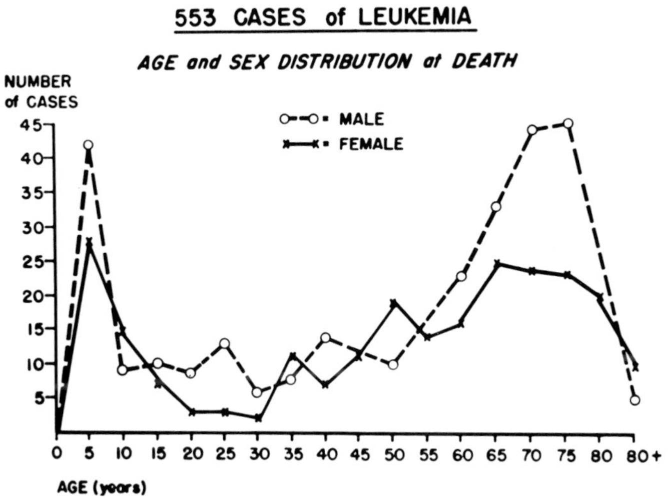

553 CASES of LEUKEMIA

AGE and SEX DISTRIBUTION at DEATH

Fig 4-6. Age and sex distribution of 553 cases of leukemia. Note the large number of
cases (57.1 percent) occurring after the age of 50. (Drawn from the figures of Gunz and
Hough,[37] courtesy of the publisher.)

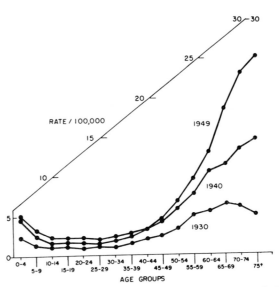

Fig. 4-7. Incidence of leukemia deaths by age for 1930, 1940, and 1949. Note increasing incidence of cases in older age groups in recent years. (Reproduced from Cooke,[14] courtesy of the publisher.)

(Fig. 4-2[36]). Even in Japan the increase above the age of 50 is greater than it is at younger ages (Fig. 4-9[87]).

The overall percentage of cases of leukemia at various ages in Western countries can be taken roughly as follows:[18,34]

	Percentage of Patients in Age Groups Shown		
Type	Age: 0–14	15–49	50+
All leukemias	20	20	60
Acute	35	23	42
Chronic	4	15	81

A peculiar age incidence is found in children in whom leukemia occurs more frequently in the first 5 years than at later ages. In Opitz' series,[65] which is typical, two-thirds of all cases occurred before the age of 6, and the rest between 6 and 14 years. A peak incidence between the ages of 3 and 5 began to appear in England from 1920 onward,[16] and in the United States after 1940.[5,12,69] Initially only white American children were affected during the earlier years, but recently a similar peak may have begun to appear in nonwhite American as well as in Japanese children.[26] The younger incidence, now a feature of leukemia statistics in most countries, is also reflected in malignant neoplasms of the kidneys and central nervous system.[25] Although its origin is obscure, it has been suggested that it might be at least partly caused by a decline in mortality for children of ages up to 2—possibly because these children survived longer with successful treatment.[76] Since in England the peak was present long before the introduction of effective chemotherapy for acute leukemia, this seems an unlikely explanation. It may be more rational to search for leuke-

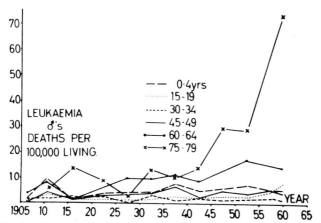

Fig. 4-8. Leukemia mortality by age groups in New Zealand males for 1907–1963. (Reproduced from Gunz,[36] courtesy of the publisher.)

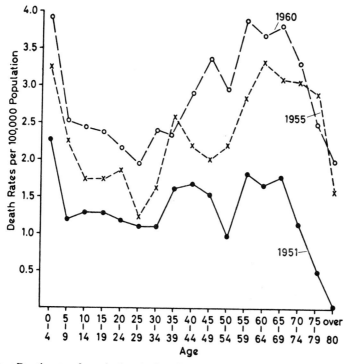

Fig. 4-9. Death rates from leukemia for all Japan in 1951, 1955, and 1960. (Reproduced from Wakisaka et al.,[87] courtesy of the authors and publisher.)

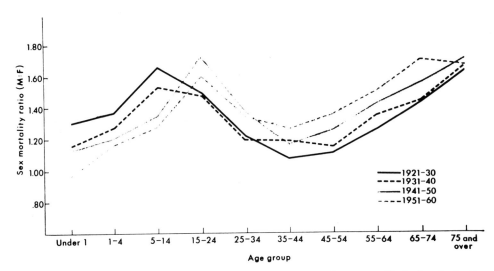

Fig. 4-10.   Trends in sex ratios (M:F) of average, annual, sex-specific leukemia death rates among the white population of the United States, 1921–1960. (Reproduced from Fraumeni and Wagoner,[27] courtesy of the authors and publisher.)

mogens which express themselves particularly at ages 3 and 4 and have only recently begun to affect nonwhite American and Japanese children. In many countries, a smaller but equally consistent peak occurs in male adolescents.[49,72]

Sex Distribution

Leukemia is more common in males than in females, the sex ratio in 1947 being 1.44:1 among the newly diagnosed cases in Dorn and Cutler's series.[22] There are, however, differences among the several types: In 1949, the ratio of males to females among all deaths attributed to granulocytic leukemia in the United States was 1.3:1, but it was 1.6:1 among the deaths attributed to lymphocytic leukemia.[29] In England, during 1955–1957, the sex ratios were 1.4:1 for acute, 1.2:1 for chronic granulocytic, and 2.0:1 for chronic lymphocytic leukemia.[15] In New Zealand[34] the corresponding ratios were 1.12, 1.30, and 2.02:1, respectively. The most consistent feature in these and other series were the high male:female ratios in chronic lymphocytic leukemia. Since this is predominantly a disease of old age, the highest sex ratios might be expected to be found in old people, and this is indeed the case (Table 4-8). By contrast, the sex ratios are lower at younger ages. Fraumeni and Wagoner have shown that in successive decades, in the U.S. white population, the sex ratio in children has become lower, while it has increased in old age (Fig. 4-10).[27] The sex ratio declines continuously from puberty to near the female climacteric, after which it increases rapidly, as the rising incidence of chronic lymphocytic leukemia begins to assert itself. International comparisons show that there have been no major or consistent changes in the sex ratio, except for the U.S. white population in which there has been a moderate rise (Table 4-8). The differences in the incidence of leukemia among the sexes make it appear possible that the sex hormones may, in some manner, be involved in the process of leukemogenesis.

Table 4-8
Sex Ratios in Age-Adjusted Populations, 1950–1963

Country	Years							1962–1963 (over 55)
	1950–1951	1952–1953	1954–1955	1956–1957	1958–1959	1960–1961	1962–1963	
South Africa*	1.26	1.23	1.45	1.67	1.43	1.52	1.25*	1.64*
Canada	1.19	1.44	1.35	1.39	1.38	1.43	1.50	1.79
Chile	1.22	1.48	1.42	1.31	1.40	1.10	1.12	1.22
U.S.A., white	1.41	1.43	1.45	1.44	1.51	1.55	1.54	1.75
U.S.A., nonwhite	1.43	1.35	1.65	1.57	1.53	1.40	1.40	1.62
Israel	1.16	1.21	1.04	1.12	1.07	1.73	1.12	1.24
Japan	1.47	1.33	1.52	1.40	1.29	1.30	1.29	1.49
Germany, F.R.	–	1.40	1.47	1.35	1.31	1.34	1.34	1.58
Austria	–	1.34	1.60	1.45	1.35	1.50	1.49	1.62
Belgium	–	–	1.21	1.17	1.43	1.59	1.36	1.49
Denmark	–	1.38	1.29	1.38	1.65	1.56	1.48	1.54
Finland	–	1.00	1.67	1.36	1.19	1.30	1.28	1.37
France	1.41	1.39	1.39	1.33	1.33	1.38	1.38	1.72
Ireland	1.69	1.23	1.08	1.54	1.19	1.74	1.47	1.72
Italy	–	1.32	1.35	1.38	1.37	1.38	1.37	1.67
Norway	–	1.39	1.18	1.38	1.58	1.36	1.52	1.67
Netherlands	1.31	1.25	1.28	1.39	1.30	1.32	1.42	1.62
Portugal	–	–	–	1.11	1.21	1.42	1.13	1.25
England and Wales	1.27	1.34	1.36	1.38	1.38	1.46	1.35	1.55
Scotland	1.28	1.47	1.64	1.49	1.30	1.45	1.44	1.60
Northern Ireland	1.32	1.48	1.50	1.76	1.40	1.36	1.91	2.11
Sweden	–	1.38	1.27	1.43	1.43	1.34	1.43	1.65
Switzerland	–	1.36	1.34	1.49	1.50	1.40	1.28	1.66
Australia	1.30	1.27	1.31	1.36	1.32	1.41	1.43	1.60
New Zealand	1.28	1.85	1.20	1.31	1.23	1.14	1.58	1.71

*1962 only (white population)
Data from Segi and Kurihara.[72]

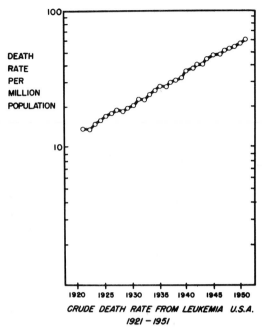

Fig. 4-11. Crude death rate from leukemia in the United States for 1921–1951. (Drawn after Shimkin,[73] courtesy of the publisher.)

Is There a Rising Incidence of Leukemia?

The mortality rate from leukemia rose steadily during the 30 years from 1920–1950. Figure 4-11 demonstrates this trend in the United States and can be taken as typical of what occurred in many other countries. Changes in the classification of the leukemias to which reference has already been made, were ineffective in modifying the upward trend by more than a minor degree. The striking rise of some 400 percent was widely assumed to mean that more people every year were acquiring and succumbing to leukemia. At the same time, however, it was apparent that a variety of changes were occurring in the practice of medicine which had the effect of greatly facilitating the early discovery of leukemia, a disease which depends on laboratory work for its diagnosis. Among these factors were the following:

1. Better and more widely available laboratory facilities.
2. Introduction of new laboratory methods, notably marrow biopsy.
3. Increased ease of access to physicians and hospitals.
4. Expansion of the specialty of hematology, with a great increase in the number of practicing hematologists.
5. Survival to the point of diagnosis of patients who would previously have died in the absence of ancillary methods of therapy such as antibiotics and blood transfusion.

An excellent account is given by Wood[93] of the effect which changing circumstances have had on the recorded leukemia mortality in a circumscribed part of England. While the factors listed above must have brought to light large numbers of

Table 4-9

Mortality from Leukemia in White Persons by Sex and Age. (Industrial Policyholders of Metropolitan Life Insurance Company, 1950–1954 and 1930–1934)

Age Period (yrs)	Death Rates per 100,000				% Increase 1950–1954 Since 1930–1934	
	Males		Females			
	1950–1954	1930–1934	1950–1954	1930–1934	Males	Females
1–74*	5.2	2.4	3.8	2.1	117	81
1–4	6.9	3.7	5.7	2.8	86	104
5–9	3.9	2.2	3.6	1.2	77	200
10–14	3.1	1.3	2.3	1.0	138	130
15–19	3.1	2.1	1.7	1.2	48	42
20–24	1.7	1.2	1.5	.9	42	67
25–34	2.3	1.2	1.8	1.4	92	29
35–44	3.2	2.0	2.7	1.8	60	50
45–54	6.7	3.6	5.1	3.5	86	46
55–64	14.1	5.9	9.6	5.4	139	78
65–74	28.0	6.6	17.0	6.5	324	162

*Adjusted on the basis of the standard million population of England and Wales, 1901.

patients with leukemia who would not otherwise have been diagnosed, the question remained whether they were enough to account for the whole of the rising mortality. Most workers in the field decided intuitively that they were not. This being so, it was logical to look for other causes responsible for the "genuine," as opposed to the "technical" rise in the incidence of leukemia. This could only be a new etiologic agent or group of agents, or the intensified action of previously existing ones. (The question of leukemogens is discussed in detail in Chapter 5.)

It is now necessary to point out that the simple line shown in Figure 4-11 is deceptive. In the first place, it conceals the fact that the leukemia mortality changes to very different degrees at different ages. Second, the steady rise until the early 1950s has been followed by a flattening-out and later by a down-turn of what is no longer a straight line.

Figures 4-8 and 4-9 show a disproportionally greater increase in leukemia for the age groups above 50 and especially for those above 60. This is also evident from Table 4-9 in which the leukemia mortality rates for 1950–1954 are compared with those for 1930–1934. Although there has been a marked overall increase, in the younger age groups it has been modest in comparison with that of the older ones. Table 4-10 gives the mortality figures for the entire U.S. white population in 1950–1951 and in 1962–1963. As will be noted, the picture has changed strikingly. While between 1930–1954 the average mortality for both sexes rose by an annual 5 percent, this had been reduced during the 1950–1963 period to a bare 1 percent. Moreover, in young children there had been a decline of over one-fifth, and lesser and variable decreases for most age groups up to 55 years in males and 65 in females. The small increase in the "all-ages" mortality was, in fact, entirely accounted for by progressively steeper rises in the groups from 55 upwards. It is noteworthy

Table 4-10

Mortality from Leukemia by Sex and Age, U.S.A. white population, 1950–1951 and 1962–1963

Age	Deaths per 100,000				% Increase or Decrease 1962–1963 Since 1950–1951	
	Male		*Female*		*Male*	*Female*
	1950–1951	1962–1963	1950–1951	1962–1963		
0– 4	6.45	5.01	5.32	4.16	− 22.0	− 21.8
5– 9	3.84	4.34	3.22	3.75	+ 13.0	+ 16.1
10–14	2.67	2.43	2.22	2.14	− 9.0	− 3.6
15–19	2.96	2.72	1.79	1.61	− 8.1	− 10.0
20–24	2.09	2.34	1.49	1.37	+ 12.0	− 8.0
25–29	2.49	2.15	2.08	1.42	− 13.7	− 31.7
30–34	2.81	2.40	2.18	1.90	− 14.6	− 12.7
35–39	2.91	2.86	2.80	2.21	− 1.7	− 21.0
40–44	4.14	3.71	3.86	3.20	− 10.2	− 17.1
45–49	5.61	5.47	4.31	4.06	− 2.5	− 5.7
50–54	8.52	7.68	6.10	4.87	− 9.5	− 20.2
55–59	12.14	12.43	9.08	7.57	+ 2.4	− 17.0
60–64	18.49	19.04	11.99	11.43	+ 3.0	− 4.7
65–69	25.82	29.97	14.93	16.96	+ 16.1	+ 13.6
70–74	34.39	43.10	18.50	23.18	+ 25.3	+ 25.3
75–79	40.25	57.14	25.85	31.00	+ 42.0	+ 20.0
80–84	39.34	72.03	23.71	44.38	+ 83.2	+ 87.2
85+	39.46	82.69	21.68	44.64	+109.4	+106.0
All ages	7.34	8.42	5.29	5.94	+ 14.7	+ 12.3

Data from Segi and Kurihara.[72]

that American blacks over 70 have a far lower leukemia mortality than do white Americans.[57]

The flattening-out of the leukemia mortality at younger ages began in the United States about 1940,[30] and a similar phenomenon was noted about the same period in England,[15] Australia,[44] Canada,[77] and Denmark.[9] An actual decline in childhood mortality began in England during the 1950s,[6] and the same leveling process occurred elsewhere. Examples from New Zealand and the United States are shown in Figures 4-12 and 4-13. Finally, in the period 1961–1965, an actual turning down of the "all-ages" mortality could be demonstrated in the U.S. white population but not in the U.S. nonwhite or the English populations (Fig. 4-14[26]).

It is too early to say what was responsible for the recent reversal in the mortality trends or how permanent they will prove to be. From an intuitive point of view, the reason seems less likely to be cessation of the activity of leukemogenic factors than the effect of changes in the processes of diagnosis and notification. In this context, one would like to know how the various types of leukemia have progressed. Because of difficulties in classification few data exist, but those from Britain[21] and New Zealand[35] suggest that all types of leukemia shared almost equally in the rise at ages above 50, possibly with a slightly greater proportional increase in the chronic lymphocytic type. Below 50, the changes were irregular, though the childhood decline was entirely accounted for by the change in the acute type.

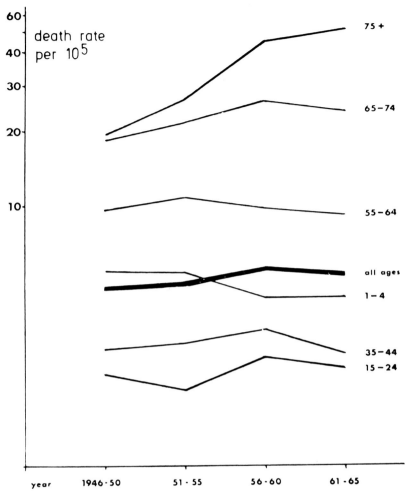

Fig. 4-12. Leukemia mortality by age groups in New Zealand for 1946–1965. (Reproduced from Gunz,[36] courtesy of the publisher.)

The diagnosis of leukemia, particularly the acute type, is more sophisticated than that of many other diseases, and this is especially so in older patients in whom its manifestations are often atypical. This being so, it is likely that its diagnosis will be missed relatively frequently, but that as knowledge of the disease and diagnostic facilities improve, recognition will be progressively more common, especially in the middle-aged and elderly. There must in many places be a backlog of leukemia which is gradually reduced as more cases can be recognized. Until it is completely abolished, one would therefore expect the increase in leukemia notifications to continue in general, and more rapidly (1) among the old and disadvantaged and (2) in countries with an initially low leukemia mortality. The process should then slow down, the flattening of the curve beginning in younger people and in countries with an initially high leukemia rate. This is precisely what is now happening. The age differences have already been discussed: Figure 4-15 shows the relationship between the 1950–1951 (or 1952–1953) mortality rates in twenty-one countries and the increases in mortality over a 10–12 year period. Clearly, there is a strong correlation,

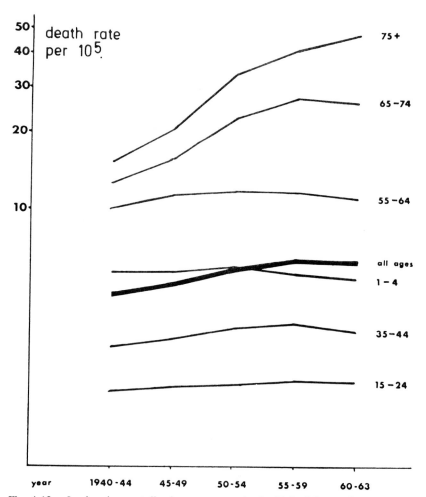

Fig. 4-13. Leukemia mortality by age groups in the United States for 1940–1963. (Reproduced from Gunz,[36] courtesy of the publisher.)

with countries with low initial mortalities having much greater increases than those with high ones. Moreover, in the low mortality countries, the rises extend through all age groups. Thus, in Japanese males the increase from 1950–1951 to 1962–1963 was 88.5 percent at ages 0–4; 91.5 percent at 20–24; 57.8 percent at 40–44; 130.5 percent at 60–64; and 415 percent at 80+. These figures are rather similar to those shown in Table 4-9 for the U.S. population between 1930–1934 and 1950–1954. All these findings suggest strongly that the low mortality groups are catching up with the high mortality groups, a phenomenon which could be explained by better case finding.

We are left to conclude that no decisive evidence exists as yet to prove that an actual, as opposed to an apparent, rise in the incidence of leukemia has occurred in past decades. There is a widespread impression that the rise in notifications indicates a truly increased prevalence of the disease. This is a personal view which cannot be disproved at this stage. However, the available evidence shows quite clearly that any

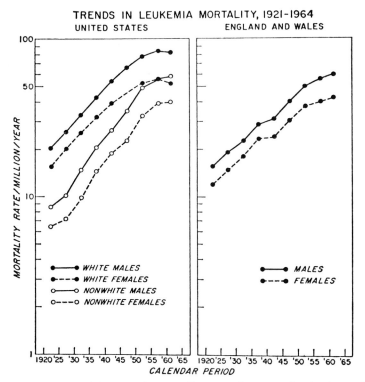

Fig. 4-14. Age-adjusted leukemia mortality rates by sex and calendar period in the United States white and nonwhite populations, and in England and Wales in 1921–1964 for all ages. (Reproduced from Fraumeni and Miller,[26] courtesy of the authors and publisher.)

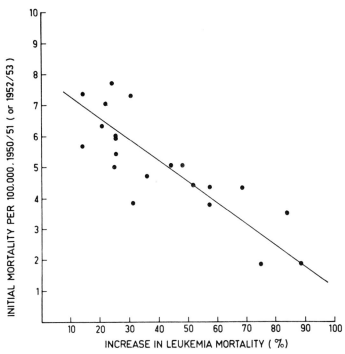

Fig. 4-15. Relationship between (a) increase in leukemia mortality between 1950–1951 (or 1952–1953) and 1962–1963, and (b) initial leukemia mortality per 100,000 in 1950–1951 (or 1952–1953): Age-adjusted rate for twenty-one countries. See text for detailed explanation. (Drawn from the figures of Segi and Kurihara,[72] courtesy of the publisher.)

real rise in leukemia mortality can have been only a moderate fraction of that recorded in public health statistics. It also shows that the rise may now have come to an end in some age groups and in some countries, suggesting that before many years it may do so everywhere and at all ages. There should then be a relatively stable situation which would give an opportunity for a more accurate assessment of the total size of the leukemia problem and of its background.

Leukemia Clustering

The term *clustering* signifies the occurrence, in a given space and during a circumscribed period of time, of a number of cases of a disease greater than that which is expected on the basis of its known incidence or mortality. Such time-space clusters of leukemia cases were described 35 years ago by Kellett,[43] and more recently by Heath and Hasterlik.[40a] Since then many further instances have come to light. One such example is shown in Figure 4-16. The sizes of reported clusters varied from two to ten or more cases, but all were relatively small. With few exceptions, the individuals within clusters were not related to or acquainted with each other.

The interpretation of the clustering phenomenon is difficult, for chance alone must produce some clusters. Many attempts have been made, by a variety of statistical techniques, to determine if clustering is more common than would be expected, and there is no consensus, although in at least three studies of large populations[31,45,82] a statistically significant degree of clustering was discovered in children under 6 with leukemia, but not in older children: nor was it present in adults with acute leukemia who were investigated by similar means.[38]

If the existence of clustering is accepted as a fact, it remains for us to inquire into its meaning. Small aggregations of cases may be caused by any number of agencies ranging, in the words of MacMahon, "from genes to lightning bolts."[54] Most investigators in this field have, however, assumed that clustering might provide support for an infectious—possibly viral—origin of leukemia. This possibility was first raised with regard to the cluster in Niles, Illinois,[40a] but evidence in its favor is exceedingly weak. Case-to-case infection seems most unlikely because of the absence of any known contacts, while infection from a common source would be expected to produce far larger numbers of cases than were found in any of the clusters, unless the degree of susceptibility to the common infectious agent should be extremely low. It is conceivable that the agent might act as a trigger in a few predisposed individuals (*see* Chapter 5), but there is no positive evidence to show the nature of any such agent, though it has been searched for many times. Another possibility, which is perhaps more likely, is that leukemia clusters are chance phenomena explained not by the presence of a leukemogenic agent in the area but by population movements during the study period, which made an accurate calculation of the expected number of cases impossible.[31] It seems at present unlikely that clustering, even if confirmed as more than a statistical artifact, will be found to yield many clues to the etiology of leukemia. These general conclusions on the evidence of time-space clustering in acute leukemia are not necessarily valid for other diseases of hematologic interest, notably Burkitt's lymphoma and Hodgkin's disease.[2]

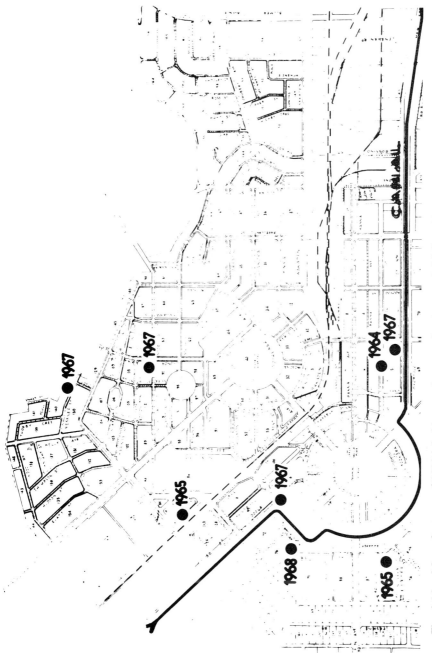

Fig. 4-16. Map of a town of 9500 inhabitants, the seat of a cluster of childhood leukemia and lymphoma cases which occurred between 1964–1968. The date and location of each case are marked on the map. Total of observed cases was eight, total expected 1.1 ($p < 0.0001$).

REFERENCES

1. Allan NC, Watson-Williams EJ: A study of leukaemia among Nigerians in Ibadan. Proceedings of the ninth Congress of the European Society Haematologists, New York, Karger, 1963, p. 906.

2. Baikie AG, Kinlen, LJ, Pike MC: Detection and assessment of case clustering in Burkitt's lymphoma and Hodgkin's disease, in Grundmann E and Tulinius H (eds): Current Problems in the Epidemiology of Cancer and Lymphomas. Berlin, Springer, 1972, pp 201–209.

3. Bailar JC III, Honeyman MS, Eisenberg H: Incidence and mortality rates for leukemia and lymphoma. Public Health Rep 77:281, 1962.

4. Bernhard WG, Gore I, Kilby RA: Congenital leukemia. Blood 6:990, 1951.

5. Bufkin JH, Davison WD: Childhood cancer (tumors, leukemia, and Hodgkin's disease). A review. J Pediatr 42:612, 1954.

6. Case RAM: Mortality from the cancers of childhood. Proc R Soc Med 58:607, 1965.

7. Clemmesen J: Statistical studies in the aetiology of malignant neoplasms. Copenhagen, Munksgaard, 1965.

8. Clemmesen J, Busk Th, Nielsen A: The topographical distribution of leukaemia and Hodgkin's disease in Denmark, 1942–46. Acta Radiol 37:223, 1952.

9. Clemmesen J, Sorensen J: Malignant neoplasia of haemopoietic and connective tissues in various countries. Danish Med Bull 5:73, 1958.

10. Statistics on Cancer. CA 18:16, 1968.

11. Cook PJ: The geography of human disease. Cited by Doll (Ref. 21).

12. Cooke JV: The incidence of acute leukemia in children. JAMA 119:547, 1942.

13. Cooke JV: Chronic myelogenous leukemia in children. J Pediatr 42:537, 1953.

14. Cooke JV: The occurrence of leukemia. Blood 9:340, 1954.

15. Court Brown WM, Doll R: Adult leukaemia. Trends in mortality in relation to aetiology. Br Med J 1:1063, 1959.

16. Court Brown WM, Doll R: Leukaemia in childhood and young adult life; trends in mortality in relation to aetiology. Br Med J 1:981, 1961.

17. Court Brown WM, Doll R, Hill ID: Leukaemia in Britain and Scandinavia. Pathol Microbiol 27:644, 1964.

18. Cutler SJ, Axtell L, Heise H: Ten thousand cases of leukemia: 1940–1962. J Natl Cancer Inst 39:993, 1967.

19. Davies JNP: Leukaemia in Trans-Saharan Africa. Acta Unio Internat Contra Cancrum 16:1618, 1960.

20. Davies JNP: Leukaemia in children in tropical Africa. Lancet 2:65, 1965.

21. Doll R: The epidemiological picture, in Hayhoe FGJ (ed): Current Research in Leukaemia. Cambridge, England, University Press, 1965, p 280.

22. Dorn HF, Cutler SJ: Morbidity from cancer in the United States. Washington, D.C., Public Health Monograph, 1955, no. 29.

23. Earle AM: Leukemia in American Samoa. J Pediatr 43:398, 1953.

24. Eastcott DF: Report of the B.E.C.C. (NZ) Branch Cancer Registration Scheme. Wellington, N.Z., Medical Statistics Branch, Department of Health, 1954.

25. Ederer F, Miller RW, Scotto J: U.S. childhood cancer mortality patterns, 1950–1959. JAMA 192:593, 1965.

26. Fraumeni JF Jr, Miller RW: Epidemiology of human leukemia. Recent observations. J Natl Cancer Inst 38:593, 1967.

27. Fraumeni JF Jr, Wagoner JK: Changing sex differentials in leukemia. Public Health Rep 79:1093, 1964.

28. Gardiner CE: Report of the Medical Statistician on Cancer Morbidity and Mortality in New Zealand. Wellington, N.Z., Department of Health, 1958.

29. Gilliam AG: Age, sex, and race selection at death from leukemia and the lymphomas. Blood 8:693, 1953.

30. Gilliam AG, Walter WA: Trends of mortality from leukemia in the United States, 1921–55. Public Health Rep 73:773, 1958.

31. Glass AG, Mantel N, Gunz FW, Spears GFS, Time-space clustering of childhood leukemia in New Zealand. J. Natl Cancer Inst 47:329, 1971.

32. Goldberg ID, Levin ML, Gerhardt PR, Handy VH, Cashman, RE: The probability of developing cancer. J Natl Cancer Inst 17:155, 1956.

33. Griswold MH, Wilder CS, Cutler SJ, Pollack ES, Cancer in Connecticut, 1935–1951. Hartford, Connecticut State Dept. of Health, 1955.

34. Gunz FW: Leukaemia in New Zealand and Australia. Pathol Microbiol 27:697, 1964.

35. Gunz FW: Studies on the incidence and aetiology of leukaemia in New Zealand. New Z Med J 65:857, 1966.

36. Gunz FW: The leukemia–lymphoma problem, in Zarafonetis CJD (ed): Proceedings of International Conference on Leukemia–Lymphoma. Philadelphia, Lea & Febiger, 1968, p 13.

37. Gunz FW, Hough RF: Acute leukemia over the age of fifty. A study of its incidence and history. Blood 11:882, 1956.

38. Gunz FW, Spears GFS: Distribution of acute leukaemia in time and space. Studies in New Zealand. Br Med J 4:604, 1968.

39. Haenszel W: Cancer mortality among the foreign-born in the United States. J Natl Cancer Inst 26:37, 1961.

40. Haenszel W, Kurihara M: Studies of Japanese migrants. I. Mortality from cancer and other diseases among Japanese in the United States. J Natl Cancer Inst 40:43, 1968.

40a Heath CW, Hasterlik RJ: Leukemia among children in a suburban community. Am J Med 34:796, 1963.

41. Hewitt D: Some features of leukaemia mortality. Br J Prev Soc Med 9:81, 1955.

42. Hoffman WJ, Craver, LF: Chronic myelogenous leukemia. Value of irradiation and its effect on the duration of life. JAMA 97:836, 1931.

43. Kellett CE: Acute myeloid leukaemia in one of identical twins. Arch Dis Child 12:239, 1937.

44. Keogh EV, McCall C, Rankin DW: Mortality from leukaemia in Victoria, 1946 to 1955: A report from the Central Cancer Registry, Melbourne. Med J Aust 2:632, 1958.

45. Knox G: Epidemiology of childhood leukaemia in Northumberland and Durham. Br J Prev Soc Med 18:17, 1964.

46. Latourette HB, Lampe I, Hodges FJ: Organized clinical investigation of cancer, ninth report. Univ Mich Med Cent J 20:283, 1954.

47. Lea AJ, Abbatt JD: The changing pattern of leukaemia. Lancet 1:389, 1957.

48. Leavell BS: Chronic leukemia. A study of the incidence and factors influencing the duration of life. Am J Med Sci 196:329, 1938.

49. Lee JAH: Acute myeloid leukaemia in adolescents. Br Med J 1:988, 1961.

50. Lee M, Lee JO, Seo HZ, Kim SI, Kim YI, Whang KS, Park HM, Song TS, Park HC: Clinical and statistical observations on malignant tumors. Korean J Hematol 2:23, 1967.

51. Levin ML: Cancer reporting in New York State. NY State J Med 44:880, 1944.

52. Levin ML, Haenszel W, Carroll BE, Gerhardt PR, Handy VH, Ingraham, SC, II: Cancer incidence in urban and rural areas of New York State. J Natl Cancer Inst 24:1243, 1960.

53. MacMahon B: Geographic variation in leukemia mortality in the United States. Public Health Rep 72:39, 1957.

54. MacMahon B: Epidemiologic aspects of acute leukemia and Burkitt's tumor. Cancer 21:558, 1968.

55. MacMahon B, Koller EK: Ethnic differences in the incidence of leukemia, in Jones AR (ed): Proceedings of the sixth International Congress of the Society of Hematology. New York, Grune & Stratton, 1957.

56. McCullough JJ, Rossow G, Hiller R: Leukemia deaths in Minnesota 1950–1964. Public Health Rep 82:946, 1967.

57. McPhedran P, Heath CW Jr, Garcia JS: Racial variations in leukemia incidence among the elderly. J Natl Cancer Inst 45:25, 1970.

58. Martin DC, Chin TDY, Larsen WE, Roth AE, Werder AA: Leukemia and lymphoma. J. Kans Med Soc 67:361, 1966.

59. Meadors GF: Epidemiology of leukemia. Public Health Rep 71:103, 1956.

60. Metropolitan Life Insurance Co., Recent trends in leukemia. Statistical Bull 36:3, 1955.

61. Minot GP, Buckman, TW, Isaacs R: Chronic myelogenous leukemia. Age incidence, duration, and benefit derived from irradiation. JAMA 82:1489, 1924.

62. Minot GP, Isaacs R: Lymphatic leukemia. Age incidence, duration, and benefit derived from irradiation. Boston Med Surg J 191:1, 1924.

63. Newill VA: Distribution of cancer mortality among ethnic subgroups of the white population of New York City, 1953–58. J Natl Cancer Inst 26:405, 1961.

64. Oehme J, Janssen W, Hagitte Ch: Leukämie im Kindesalter. Beiträge zur Morphologie, Klinik, Pathophysiologie und Therapie. Stuttgart, Thieme, 1958.

65. Opitz H: Das Leukämieproblem. Monatsschr. Kinderheilkd 102:120, 1954.

66. Pedersen, E, Magnus K: Cancer registration in Norway. The incidence of cancer in

Norway, 1953–1954. Oslo, The Norwegian Cancer Society, 1959.

67. Peltorven T, Pynnonen AL: Die Leukämie-sterblichkeit in Finnland im Zeitraum 1936–1956. Monatsschr. Kinderheilkd 108:469, 1960.

68. Pinkel D, Nefzger D: Some epidemiological features of childhood leukemia in the Buffalo, N.Y., area. Cancer 12:351, 1959.

69. Rodgers CL, Donohue, WL, Snelling CE: Leukaemia in children. Can Med Assoc J 65:548, 1951.

70. Rosenthal N, Harris W: Leukemia. Its diagnosis and treatment. JAMA 104:702, 1935.

71. Sankale M, LeViguelloux J, Oliveau–Lebreton G, Milhade J: Les tumeurs malignes des tissus hémopoïétiques en milieu africain au Soudan français. Sem Hôp Paris 34:2680, 1958.

72. Segi M, Kurihara M: Cancer mortality for selected sites in 24 countries, No. 4. (1962–1963). Sendai: Dept. Publ. Health, Tohoku University School of Medicine, 1966.

73. Shimkin MB: Hodgkin's disease. Mortality in the United States, 1921–1951; race, sex and age distribution; comparison with leukemia. Blood 10:1214, 1955.

74. Shimkin MB: Mortality from leukemia and lymphoma in the United States, in Jones AR (ed): Proceedings of the sixth International Congress of the Society of Hematology. New York, Grune & Stratton, 1957.

75. Shimkin MB, Loveland DB: A note on mortality from lymphatic leukemia in Oriental populations in the United States. Blood 17:763, 1961.

76. Slocumb JC, MacMahon B: Changes in mortality rates from leukemia in the first five years of life. N Engl J Med 268:922, 1963.

77. Sloman JG, Sellers AH: Trends in mortality from leukaemia in Ontario. Can J Public Health 50:518, 1959.

78. Söderhjelm L, Ranström S: Congenital leukemia with megakaryocytosis in extramedullary foci. Acta Soc Med Ups 56:233, 1952.

79. Stark CR, Oleinick A: Urban or rural residence and histologic type distribution in 21,000 childhood leukemia deaths in the United States, 1950–59. J Natl Cancer Inst 37:369, 1966.

80. Steiner PE: An evaluation of the cancer problem. Cancer Res 12:455, 1952.

81. Takeda K: Geographical pathology of leukaemia in Japan. Acta Unio Internat Contra Cancrum 16:1629, 1960.

82. Till MM, Hardisty RM, Pike MC, Doll R: Childhood leukaemia in Greater London: A search for evidence of clustering. Br Med J 3:755, 1967.

83. Tivey H: The prognosis for survival in chronic granulocytic and lymphocytic leukemia. Am J Roentgenol Radium Ther Nucl Med 72:68, 1954.

84. Tomonaga M: Statistical investigation of leukaemia in Japan. NZ Med J 65:863, 1966.

85. Cancer incidence in five continents, in Doll R, Payne P, and Waterhouse J, (eds): Unio Internationale Contra Cancrum. Berlin, Springer, 1966.

86. Vanier TM, Pike MC: Leukaemia incidence in tropical Africa. Lancet 1:512, 1967.

87. Wakisaka G, Uchino H, Yasunaga K, Nakamura T, Sakurai M, Miyamoto K, Yoshino T, Moriga M: Statistical investigations of leukaemia in Japan from 1956 to 1961. Pathol Microbiol 27:671, 1964.

88. Ward G: The infective theory of acute leukaemia. Br J Child Dis 14:10, 1917.

89. Warren SL: Acute leukemia: A review of the literature and of twenty-eight new cases. Am J Med Sci 178:490, 1929.

90. Wells R, Lau KS: Incidence of leukaemia in Singapore, and rarity of chronic lymphocytic leukaemia in Chinese. Br Med J 1:759, 1960.

91. Wildner GP: Zur Statistik der bösartigen Geschwulsterkrankungen in der DDR in den Jahren 1953 und 1954. Dtsch Gesundheitsw 14:494, 543, 1959.

92. Windeyer BW, Stewart JW: The leukaemias, in, Cade, S.: Malignant Disease and Its Treatment by Radium, vol. 4 (ed. 2). Bristol: Wright, 1952, p 347.

93. Wood EE: A survey of leukaemia in Cornwall, 1948–1959. Br Med J 1:1760, 1960.

II

Etiology, Pathogenesis, and Pathology

5

Etiology and Pathogenesis of Leukemia

In 1938, Forkner opened his chapter on the etiology of leukemia with the following words: "Almost nothing is known of the causes, either immediate or remote, of leukemia. In a minority of cases some disease or incident can be found in the patient's life to which the leukemia is sequential in time and to which, in some degree, it may be related. In the majority of cases no such antecedent is demonstrable. Those etiologic conditions which can be traced or suspected in some cases stand in a position with relation to the disease which is too uncertain to allow them to be considered as exciting or predisposing causes."[166] More than three decades after those lines were written, large parts of medicine have been revolutionized, but the causes of human leukemia still remain unknown. Yet, progress can be recognized in the understanding of its nature and of some of the factors concerned in its production. What is more, confidence can be placed in the continuance and acceleration of such progress. Thus, it is now almost generally accepted that human leukemia is essentially neoplastic in nature, and that a search for the factors and mechanisms involved in carcinogenesis in general has relevance to the special case of the cancers of the hematopoietic tissues.

Certainly, some of the more chronic forms of leukemia appear to be benign for long periods before passing into the malignant phase. Indeed, some never reach that phase, and here it may be difficult to distinguish neoplasia from other pathologic mechanisms. It has also become clear in recent years that the etiology of the various forms of human leukemia is not uniform and that the same agents may not be concerned in the causation of all of them. Probably what we designate as leukemia is actually a heterogeneous group of more or less closely related conditions whose origin is determined by the interaction of many different factors, some known, others as yet only surmised.

Among these factors are extrinsic agents, including the ionizing radiations, which have proved to be capable of inducing the disease, though in practice they may not often do so; and a galaxy of viruses or viruslike organisms whose role in human leukemogenesis is by no means established; and, underlying or associated with them is the genetic constitution which endows every individual with his own degree of susceptibility and response to the extrinsic agents. It is also likely that immunologic factors play an important part in at least some of the leukemias.

To set the stage for a detailed discussion of the leukemogenic factors, a rather brief historic description will be given of the manner in which present-day views on etiology have developed. Basic to these is the conviction that the leukemias are, in fact, neoplasms of the hematopoietic tissues, as shown by their classification in successive revisions of the International List of Causes of Death. Alternative and now largely discarded views on their nature will be mentioned in passing, to round off the picture, as will be the possible mechanisms by which the neoplastic transformation may be achieved.

Although this chapter is concerned with human leukemia and its etiology, a good deal of the discussion must be based on the results of extensive experimental work carried out on animals. Such studies are impossible in man, especially in the field of virology where positive findings have very largely come from fowl and rodent leukemias and related tumors. It is certainly pertinent to ask how far such findings can be extrapolated to the human disease. To this question there is as yet no conclusive answer, although at least some human leukemias behave very similarly to those found in animals, and may therefore have a related etiology.

THE NATURE OF LEUKEMIA

Historic Aspects

The nature of leukemia has been debated since the earliest papers of Bennett and Virchow in the late 1840s and 1850s (see Chapter 1), and something like a consensus of opinion has only emerged during the past 15 years. Previously, there was an abundance of theories which attributed leukemia to the whole range of agents known or suspected to be capable of initiating disease. Among these were infections of all kinds, toxic agents, trauma, deficiencies, hormonal imbalances, and a host of others, as discussed fully in Forkner's book.[166] The confusion was to be expected while diagnostic and statistical methods were inadequate. Lack of marrow biopsy data and autopsy findings, inadequate length of observation before and after diagnosis, ignorance of the etiology and pathology of other hematologic conditions such as the megaloblastic and hemolytic anemias all played their part. Even today, in spite of much stricter criteria, there is a borderland among the blood diseases where classification or determination of pathogenesis is difficult or impossible. The relationships between acute leukemia on the one hand and aplastic, refractory and sideroachrestic anemias on the other; or between chronic lymphocytic leukemia, the malignant lymphomas, and some of the autoimmune diseases are cases in point which are discussed in detail in other chapters.

INFECTION AND LEUKEMIA

Among the possible causes of leukemia, infection has held a high place ever since Bennett's first description of the new disease as a pyemia. Numerous organisms of all kinds were isolated from patients with leukemia and thought to be causative, but it became gradually clear that many of them were secondary invaders in a disease in which either cellular or immunologic defenses against infection were often depleted. Distinctions between leukemia and "leukemoid" reactions accompanying infections were difficult, especially in children with their more labile hematopoietic systems.[203] This led to many reports of cures of leukemia such as Gloor's[204] famous patient with "healed myeloblastic leukemia." Only recently a group of nonleukemic hyperleukocytoses in mongol infants was separated from genuine congenital leukemia.[490]

Among patients with leukopenia, the distinction between aleukemic acute leukemia and agranulocytosis due to infections or drugs was equally difficult. Sternberg, in 1911, claimed that there was no such disease as acute leukemia, and that the "blastic" blood picture was a peculiar response to infection.[525] It took another 30 years of painstaking work to establish clearly that two entities with superficial similarities existed.[110,305,492,539] Even today there can be doubts about the diagnosis in individual cases.

The precise relationship between agranulocytosis and leukemia is, in fact, often obscure; it is certainly not uniform in all cases. Both conditions may be preceded by infections, and both may show marrow hypoplasia.[40] This picture clears up in some patients, who then proceed to complete recovery; in others, it may appear to do so but leukemia later develops.[45,130,380,385,419] It is likely that often leukemia, or *preleukemia,* was present at the time the infection occurred[88,89,458] and that the latter merely revealed the underlying pathologic process. However, the possibility cannot be categorically excluded that the infection may at times be concerned in the pathogenesis of the leukemia. Some infections can certainly cause marrow hypoplasia, and it is conceivable that leukemogenic mutations may occur in the course of recovery. A similar mechanism has been postulated for some forms of radiation leukemogenesis.[68,529]

The infectious theory, in the form in which it was originally proposed, is certainly no longer tenable: no known organism *causes* leukemia. However, in a modified form it has experienced a remarkable renaissance, as will be seen in the section entitled, "Leukemia and Viruses."

IS LEUKEMIA A "METABOLIC" OR "DEFICIENCY" DISEASE?

Throughout the years numerous authors have been struck by the lack of normal maturation in leukemic cells and searched for factors which might remedy this defect.[286,588] The similarity of some leukemic marrows to those in the megaloblastic deficiency anemias encouraged hopes that, if only the missing maturation factors could be discovered, the marrow hyperplasia, organ infiltration, and other leukemic manifestations might disappear, just as the marrow and blood become normal in pernicious anemia treated with vitamin B_{12}.[491,502] Remissions, reported mainly in the French literature, and occurring in patients with acute leukemia after treatment with massive blood transfusions boosted these hopes briefly, while a lack of balance among various "leukopoietic" factors isolated from the urine were at times thought to be implicated in leukemogenesis.[167,264,403] No confirmation of these views has been forthcoming, and leukemia as a deficiency disease was, until quite recently, regarded as an unsubstantiated dream. Lately, there has been an unexpected renewal of interest in the possibility that a deficiency of a normal leukopoietic factor may be concerned in the genesis of some leukemias. Pluznick and Sachs,[460] and Bradley and Metcalf[56] almost simultaneously discovered a method of cultivating mouse marrow cells on agar plates. When certain stimulatory factors were present, colonies of granulocytes were obtained which were believed to be derived from "committed" granulocytic stem cells (see Chapter 8). The stimulatory factor (termed *CSF*, or colony-stimulating factor) was contained in murine and human urine and serum. It was believed that this factor might be a leukopoietin analogous to erythropoietin.[168] Extensive assays of CSF in patients with acute leukemia have shown that there is often an overproduction of CSF.[397]

Human marrow can be grown under similar conditions,[459] but the stimulation must be provided by *feeder layers* of living cells, either leukocytes or fetal kidney tubules.[60] In such a system marrow from patients with acute granulocytic leukemia will not proliferate normally,[60] but it has also been reported that in some cases of acute granulocytic leukemia *in relapse* normal granulocytic colonies were formed.[459] These challenging observations have revived speculations about a possible imbalance of leukopoietic factors in leukemia, and in a rapidly developing field there is promise of new discoveries of great basic importance.

MISCELLANEOUS THEORIES

Other authors attributed the genesis of leukemia partly or wholly to an excessive destruction of granulocytes, with compensatory hyperplasia,[5] to a fault in normal destruction or elimination of leukocytes,[42,298] or to a response to "stress factors."[449] While such theories have the merit of drawing attention to possible growth mechanisms in diseased cells, they cannot explain the basic processes leading to the disease itself. Other agents, including toxins, trauma, psychologic disturbances, etc., have been incriminated,[166] but such views are now only of historic interest.

Present Views

It is now believed by an overwhelming proportion of well-qualified observers that the leukemias should be included among the neoplasms, and that all of them are malignant, or potentially malignant.

As patients with leukemia are observed, the impression is strong that the inexorable progress, the lack of decisive response to treatment, and the invariably fatal outcome signify a neoplastic process. This impression is strengthened by the usual autopsy findings of widespread organ involvement, partly diffuse, but also at times in the form of local tumorous enlargement. Furthermore, there is an obvious close connection between those neoplasms of the leukopoietic tissues which are characterized by tumor formation without leukemic features, and those in which the bone marrow and blood are prominently affected. Transitions from solid, nonleukemic tumors to generalized dissemination and leukemia are commonly seen. The same experimental methods can cause true neoplasms and leukemia in animals, and the same therapeutic agents are capable of producing temporary regression in the growth of leukemic and frankly tumorous cells. At the same time there are some forms of human leukemia—especially the chronic variety—which in their comparatively slow rate of progress and lack of cellular abnormality resemble a benign rather than a malignant neoplasm.[20,140] These often show later transitions to a more malignant course. If the leukemias are to be regarded as neoplasms, it is probable that, as with other tumors, variations in degree of malignancy can occur, with some relatively benign and some highly malignant varieties, and with all manner of variations between. In the following paragraphs some of the evidence pointing to the neoplastic nature of leukemia will be marshalled in greater detail.

CYTOLOGY OF LEUKEMIC CELLS

Among the characteristics of malignant cells[377] are changes in the nucleocytoplasmic ratio; an unusually high number of mitotic figures, frequently in conjunction with mitotic abnormalities and the presence of double or multiple nuclei; and a lack of maturation or perfect differentiation of the cell. To this may be added other features such as abnormally large or numerous nucleoli, excessive nuclear segmentation or lobulation, and excessive basophilia of the cytoplasm, all signs of a disordered nucleic acid metabolism. Every one of these features is found in leukemia, as well as in malignant tumors, although their frequency differs greatly among different types of the disease, and in the same type at different stages of its evolution. A more detailed description of the cytology of leukemic cells will be given in Chapter 6. At this point, it should merely be noted that those cytologic signs which enable a pathologist to diagnose malignancy from sections or exfoliated tumor cells can be discovered in sections of leukemic tissues or in films of leukemic blood or marrow, particularly in the acute varieties.

CHROMOSOME CONSTITUTION

As will be discussed in greater detail later (see Chapter 6), clones of cells with chromosome abnormalities are found in a large proportion of leukemias,[282,444] and although there is no certainty whether these abnormalities are concerned in leukemogenesis or merely accompany the disease, the cells carrying them clearly have a growth advantage over those without them, a situation resembling that in the great bulk of other malignant tumors which have been examined.[596] Moreover, the abnormal karyotypes appear to be irreversible, although further and still more abnormal clones may arise during the course of the disease (clonal progression).[112,246] Clonal progression may be associated with an increased degree of malignancy as judged by the clinical picture.

RELATION OF LEUKEMIA TO TUMORS OF THE LYMPHATIC AND HEMATOPOIETIC SYSTEMS

The affections of the lymphatic and hematopoietic organs which Gall and Mallory[188] collectively termed *malignant lymphoma,* include the various forms of lymphosarcoma, follicular lymphoma, and reticulum cell sarcoma: all of these are now generally regarded as malignant neoplasms. They also include lymphocytic leukemia, for the simple reason that the histologic appearance in the frankly neoplastic group and in leukemia are identical. In fact, it is impossible, by merely examining tissue sections, to decide whether a given condition is chronic lymphocytic leukemia or lymphosarcoma. Histologically, the various types of lymphosarcoma can be distinguished on the basis of the type or types of cells which compose the abnormal tissues, and of the degree of invasiveness which these cells display. All forms, however, may become generally disseminated with the eventual development of abnormal blood pictures, that is, leukemia, and without an examination of the blood it is impossible to say if leukemia is present or not. Thus, it is possible to speak of leukemic and aleukemic phases of the lymphomatous processes.

The word *phase* indicates that a disease is capable of passing from one type of manifestation to another. Custer[100] has amply demonstrated the ease with which both follicular and other types of lymphosarcomas can pass over into lymphocytic leukemia. Gall and Mallory,[188] Berman,[36] and Israëls[299] have all put forward classifications of the *lymphomas* or *reticuloses* in which each type of tissue involvement is equated with a corresponding leukemic form. There is no need in this chapter to go into the complexities of nomenclature which have been a favorite battleground for morphologists for years; nor to adjudicate on the vexing question concerning the point at which an apparently fixed lymphoma becomes a leukemia. The one fact which we wish to emphasize is the impossibility of separating undoubted neoplasms of the lymphatic system from the various lymphocytic leukemias.

Another example of the same relationship is that which exists between plasmacytoma, myeloma, and plasma cell leukemia. There is no dispute that plasmacytoma is a genuine malignant neoplasm, which, when it disseminates, affects primarily the bone marrow, thus resulting in myeloma. It is also well recognized that in most, if not all, patients suffering from this disease, the more or less immature plasma cells of which the tumor is composed can be found in the blood, provided a careful search for them is made. In rare cases, however, these cells invade the blood in very much greater numbers so as to give rise to a truly leukemic picture (plasma cell leukemia). Again, no fundamental difference can be established between the myelomas with and without massive involvement of the bloodstream.

Even among the granulocytic leukemias, it is possible to find forms closely associated with tumor formation. The best-known example here is chloroma—a localized tumor, often multiple, and usually situated in the flat bones—which is almost invariably accompanied by acute granulocytic leukemia (AGL), otherwise indistinguishable from the nonchloromatous forms. That the chloroma is a genuinely malignant neoplasm is demonstrated by its tendency to invade and destroy bone and its neighboring structures. Nonchloromatous tumors have also been described in acute granulocytic leukemias,[415] although in some of these the precise classification is doubtful, and the possibility exists that they may have belonged to the lymphoproliferative group.

In Chapter 9, it will be shown that all forms of leukemia can give rise to tumor formation, especially in those organs which are not normally associated with hematopoiesis, such as the bones (excluding the marrow), the skin, and the central nervous system.[591] This is strong evidence in favor of the neoplastic nature of the leukemic process. It is probably best, as stated in Chapter 3, to consider the leukocytic neoplasms as leukosarcomas which, when generalized, are indistinguishable from and, in fact, are examples of leukemia. Our classification indicates that leukemia is a generalized neoplastic proliferation of the leukocyte precursors. Whether it arises *de novo* as a generalized process or becomes so from a previously isolated lesion is not clear; the result is the same in any event.

Leukemia in Animals and Its Relation to Human Neoplastic Disease

Leukemia is a widespread disease among animals, occurring spontaneously in birds, rodents, cattle, dogs, cats, primates and other species, and so much work has been done on it that even a concise description would demand a large separate volume; indeed, an early monograph by Engelbreth-Holm[139] fulfilled that function at the time it was written. A great many conclusions concerning the nature, causation, pathology, and treatment of human leukemia have been drawn on the basis of studies on animal leukemias. It must be recognized, however, that most of the latter were experimental varieties, nearly all in mice, and that these differ in many ways from the spontaneously occurring disease in rodents and other species, including man. For this reason there is room for doubt as to how far findings in artificially produced systems are applicable to the naturally occurring forms of leukemia. For extensive reviews of murine leukemias see Kirschbaum,[336] Kaplan,[322,325] and Furth and Metcalf.[186]

Morphologically, many spontaneous animal leukemias are remarkably similar to the types of the human disease, and in the mouse, for instance, all forms which occur in man can be found, with the exception of chronic lymphocytic leukemia.[183] The lymphocytic murine leukemias are far more common than the granulocytic ones. Most of them are subacute, rather than acute or chronic. The cells found in animal leukemias fulfill many of the morphologic and cytologic requirements of malignancy: an increased cell and nuclear size, the presence of large nucleoli, increased quantities of RNA, and often unusual and atypical mitotic activity. Obviously, these characteristics are akin to the human acute leukemias, especially those in childhood, rather than to the chronic forms, although types corresponding in appearance to chronic granulocytic leukemia have been seen in the mouse and the rat.

Mouse leukemia, like the human form, can be induced by ionizing radiations,[184,275,319,562,563] as well as by means of chemical[477] and hormonal carcinogens.[195] It is suppressed by the same therapeutic agents which are effective in man—x-rays, as well as many chemotherapeutic substances, a large proportion of which were first tried out in mice. These facts provide strong arguments in favor of the basic similarities between animal and human leukemias.

There are also dissimilarities. One of the more obvious is that in rodents, at any rate, the common lymphocytic forms start usually as localized tumors, especially in the thymus, and that a true leukemic picture occurs quite late in their course, if at all. The disease thus resembles lymphosarcoma rather than true leukemia.

Pure experimental lines of mice are established by brother and sister mating through many generations. Some of these lines are highly resistant to leukemia, with only 1 or 2 percent of animals developing the disease, usually at an advanced age. In other strains, as many as 90 percent of the members may manifest leukemia at 6-9 months. Purity of line can be demonstrated by means of grafting experiments, with hosts of the same inbred strains accepting grafts of skin or other organs, including tumors, without rejecting them at a later stage. Leukemia can be induced in normally low-leukemia strains by irradiation and other means, and the same agents may render animals in unrelated strains capable of accepting grafts of leukemic cells from each other.

Leukemia in pure strains of mice can be grafted by the transplantation of a single cell into an unaffected host.[185] From this, a new tumor will arise which ultimately enters the leukemic phase. This is certainly a malignant process, but one that cannot be copied in man. There is indeed much evidence that, far from spreading incontinently, the human disease may often lie dormant, giving rise to few or no symptoms, for considerable periods.[47,245] Possibly human leukemia may pass through a *dependent* phase—analogous to some endocrine tumors described by Furth[181] and others—during which the pathologic cells are still partly responsive to normal (and as yet undefined) regulatory factors.[396a,431] One would include in such a dependent category especially the chronic granulocytic leukemias whose cells are for long periods functionally indistinguishable from normal myeloid precursors.[570] With the onset of the acute blastic phase such cases come to resemble the mouse leukemias much more closely, and may then achieve the status of *autonomous* tumors, unrestrained by any regulators.

The genetic purity of experimental mouse strains constitutes a fundamental difference from the genetically heterogeneous human populations. Individual differences are minimal between members of inbred strains reared in the same environment, which explains the entirely predictable course of leukemia from its first appearance to the terminal stages, as well as the uniform responses to the various inducing and therapeutic agents. The only human parallel is found in uniovular twins.[375,410] Because of this essential difference between the animal and human leukemias there must always be some reservations about the degree to which experimental findings can be applied in the investigation of human disease.

To summarize: a large body of evidence exists which suggests that basically leukemia must be regarded as a neoplastic disease. This evidence stems partly from a consideration of the cytology and cytogenetics of leukemic cells, partly from the ability of many leukemias to form true tumorous growths, and from their close relationship with the undoubtedly neoplastic sarcomas; and largely from work with the mouse leukemias. Not all animal work may be directly applicable to the human disease. Marked differences exist in the cytology, pathologic and clinical behavior of various human leukemias, and it is possible that while some are true autonomous neoplasms from the moment of their inception, others may owe their initial development to alterations in the environment in which blood cells normally develop. Even these forms are likely to become eventually independent of their environment and will then fulfill all the requirements of malignant neoplasia.

MECHANISMS OF LEUKEMOGENESIS

If the neoplastic nature of the leukemias is acknowledged, as it is by the great majority of present-day students of the disease, then it becomes necessary to inquire in what way their precursors have become transformed into their neoplastic counterparts. This fundamental and so far unsolved question can only be touched on in this context, but a brief enumeration of the most important current views must be given in order to provide a background to the discussion of the various putative *leukemogenic* factors which is to follow in the next section. Many excellent reviews can be consulted by those interested in greater detail.[62–64,71,182,279,324,499,507,517,556]

In the words of Schultz, "it is a truism by now that the change from the normal to the neoplastic cell must involve a change in cellular heredity."[499] In the widest sense leukemogenesis involves a genetic problem, and the various alternative theories can be included in the overall picture of the genetic change. Among these are the theories attributing leukemia to somatic mutations, to gene deletions (with or without an immunologic element), to virus action, to metabolic alterations, or to endocrine imbalance. What is basically altered is the cellular genotype. Many of the theories, however, refer only to mechanisms of the phenotypic alterations and leave unspecified the underlying transformation of the genes controlling the phenotype. The reason for this is the comparative ease with which alterations in cellular structure and function can be described, and the almost insuperable difficulties opposed to an analysis of the underlying genetic changes in human material. We now proceed to a very brief consideration of the various theories of leukemogenesis.

The Theory of Somatic Mutation

This arose originally from early observations by Boveri[54] and others concerning the appearances of the chromosomes in malignant tumors. These investigators noted that grossly visible abnormalities such as nondisjunction and multiple mitoses were common and could lead to an asymmetrical distribution of the chromatin material. They argued that from this might follow an abnormal and unbalanced activity of the cellular metabolism controlled by the damaged chromosomes. According to this theory, mitotic abnormalities would generally lead to cell death, but in a few instances lead to the establishment of cell lines endowed with the capacity for excessive proliferation, the altered cells surviving and transmitting their progeny. Tumors, including leukemia, would thus arise.

This theory has been much altered during the course of time, and in particular the term *somatic mutation* has been understood in different ways by different workers. Whereas the earliest observers referred to gross structural alterations of the chromosomes, others have thought that point mutations invisible by optical and electron microscopy might give rise to the neoplastic changes. The somatic mutation theory has received much support from studies of the cellular changes induced by ionizing radiations and alkylating agents which are known to produce visible chromosome damage as well as being mutagenic in such material as *Drosophila*. In recent years the rapid developments in the field of cytogenetics have helped to bolster the somatic mutation hypothesis; this is particularly the case in chronic granulocytic leukemia where a consistent chromosomal abnormality has been found and clonal progression, with the development of new karyotypes, has been observed to run parallel with the acquisition of more obviously malignant characteristics.[358] By contrast, at least half of all acute leukemias show no chromosome abnormalities. It seems likely that when gross changes are found in any leukemia, they do not themselves represent the leukemogenic mutations required by the theory but are rather the result of submicroscopic changes in the genetic apparatus. Once genetic imbalance has occurred, it probably predisposes the affected cells to a sequence of further and progressively more detrimental changes, provided they survive the initial damage. Moreover, it may make them vulnerable to the activity of extrinsic leukemogenic agents. Very significantly, this initial imbalance need not be of mutagenic origin but may be congenital, as shown by the increased predisposition to leukemia of individuals with trisomy-21 and other rarer congenital abnormalities (see page 74).

An argument against the somatic mutation theory has been seen in those instances—now quite numerous—in which leukemia or other tumors have been induced by indirect means. One of the best-known examples is provided by Kaplan's original demonstration of the induction of lymphosarcoma in the thymus.[322] He irradiated thymectomized mice with x-rays and then transplanted thymus grafts from other unirradiated animals into them. Tumors arose in the grafted mice and could be shown to be derived from the nonirradiated donor cells. It appeared that the irradiated host environment was sufficient to induce leukemia in the nonirradiated cells, a truly indirect mechanism. More recent work[226,326,369] has shown that irradiation can activate a previously unobserved latent leukemogenic virus in such mice, and the indirect mechanism described is therefore virus-mediated. This is discussed below. Several other striking examples of indirect induction of neoplasms are quoted in Kaplan's earlier review.

In recent years the somatic mutation theory has been analyzed mathematically in detail by Burch who has proposed a series of mutations as being necessary for the initiation of leukemogenesis.[68-71] Some of these may be of prezygotic (inherited) and the rest of acquired origin. Before overt disease can arise, a final transformation of the potentially malignant cell is necessary, and this is brought about by an immunologic reaction such as that described below. Burch's theory is based on extensive analyses of the age and sex incidence and mortality of leukemia, as well as on dose relationships in its induction by radiations and other agents. It represents an attempt to account fully for the mechanism by which the leukemic genotype arises, as well as for the latent period between induction and development of the disease.

The Deletion Theory

This postulates the causation of neoplasia in the loss or deletion of specific enzyme systems concerned with cellular differentiation and normal function, with a consequent overactivity of those systems associated with cellular proliferation. Such deletions are thought to be produced by the combination of carcinogens with cellular proteins and especially nucleoproteins, and specific examples have been described by Miller and Miller,[402] and Wiest and Heidelberger.[589] The subject has been studied particularly in experimental hepatomas, in which very large and variable numbers of enzymatic changes are found, compared with normal liver cells.[470] The difficulty is to determine which, if any, of these changes are essential in the neoplastic transformation, and which merely accompany it or arise as its consequence.

It is suggested that what has undergone deletion are components of the enzyme system involved in cell maturation, with a strong possibility that their habitat within the endoplasmic reticulum may be specifically affected.[156] The actual deletion may be of immunologic origin.[219] This theory requires an initial combination between carcinogen and cellular protein which leads to a loss of normal *self-markers* and thus to the formation of a potentially autoantigenic protein. This, in turn, provokes the formation of autoantibodies, and the resulting antigen-antibody reaction is the basis of the eventual emergence of malignant cell clones which have lost the faculty of differentiation and are thereby enabled to proliferate freely. Burnet,[75,76] in his clonal selection theory, has provided the bridge spanning the gap between immunologic mechanisms and neoplasia, and Dameshek[104] has written persuasively about the loss of immunologic self-markers and its relationship to chronic lymphocytic leukemia (see Chapter 12).

The deletion theory of leukemogenesis has been particularly espoused by Haddow,[249] and by Osgood.[450-451] In Osgood's view, the deletion may affect the inhibitors of cell divisions which must normally check the proliferation of the stem (alpha) cells. Such inhibitors are postulated to be produced by the more mature members of a given cell series, and thus a reduction of the number of mature cells would automatically diminish the quantity of inhibitors available, thereby ensuring increased stem cell proliferation, the breakdown of a classic feedback mechanism. The inhibitors themselves have not been identified, but many enzymes are known to be diminished or absent in leukemic cells,[190] the best known of them, neutrophil alkaline phosphatase. Although it is not suggested that such enzymes are the deleted inhibitors of stem cell proliferation, their depression is evidence of profound alterations in the metabolism of the leukemic cell.

It should be observed that, instead of a *loss* of self-marker genes, carcinogenesis, in general, and leukemogenesis in particular, may involve a *gain* of tumor-specific antigens. Such antigens have been found in a variety of animal and human tumors.[208] In human leukemia, evidence for new antigens has been mainly obtained by means of the mixed lymphocyte reaction. A number of authors[19,174,471] have reported an immunologic reaction between leukemic blasts and lymphocytes from the same patients, and this has been interpreted as an indication of antigenic differences between leukemic and normal cells. An essential defect in neoplasia may be a failure of the body to recognize the new antigens as foreign and to dispose of the cells carrying them.[208] This lack of immunologic surveillance may be an important feature in leukemogenesis. It has, for instance, been suggested that the increased susceptibility to leukemia in trisomy-21 may be due to impaired cellular immunity.[539] The most significant examples of deletions in potentially malignant cells may be found in the lymphocytic and plasmacytic leukemias, in which loss of immunologic competency has been demonstrated both in vivo and in vitro. This is discussed in detail in Chapter 12.

The Virus Theory

For many years viruses have been thought to be carcinogens, although but little direct evidence has so far been produced in favor of their activity in human disease. The case is different with tumors of birds and some mammals, especially rodents, in which very detailed work has established their importance. Much is now known about the manifestations of viral activity in animal leukemogenesis, and its precise mechanism is gradually being clarified. Essentially, there are two different ways in which viruses could induce leukemia. They might act as one form of external carcinogen in the same way as ionizing radiations or alkylating chemicals, by causing one or more mutations and thus neoplasia in predisposed individuals. On the other hand, viruses—or, more likely, their genomes—might be resident in most or all individuals and transmitted through the generations as cells divide. Such *oncogenes*[291] might normally be repressed, giving rise to no disease and being difficult or impossible to demonstrate. If the oncogenes were derepressed or triggered they would then become *virogenes* or fully infectious viruses, with consequent development of neoplasia. It should be emphasized that the two theories mentioned are not mutually exclusive, for it could be envisaged that one strain of virus might trigger the oncogenes belonging to another. This whole subject is of such topical importance, especially where the etiology of leukemia is concerned, that it must be considered in some detail, and the discussion will be taken up in the section entitled "Leukemia and Viruses."

The Metabolic Theory

The father of the metabolic theory was Otto Warburg who discovered in 1923 that cancer cells have a lower rate of respiration and a higher fermentative metabolism than normal growing cells.[577] This appears to be a general property of malignant cells, and the ratio of aerobic glycolysis to respiration has been shown to vary in accordance with the degree of malignancy. Whether this alteration is basic in the causation of neoplasia or symptomatic of its occurrence is not, however, decided. There are a number of experimental tumors with only minimally raised glycolysis, and, again, some carcinogens do not depress respiration which had been thought by Warburg to be an essential first step in carcinogenesis. Possibly, therefore, the metabolic changes found in tumors result indirectly from the action of carcinogens whose primary effect is damage to cytoplasmic structures as well as to the enzymes normally produced by them.[156]

In leukemia there are special difficulties in that the metabolism of normal, as well as of leukemic, leukocytes differs in certain ways from that of other normal cells. This point is further considered in Chapters 6 and 7, where it will be seen that leukemic cells are deficient in some of the enzymes concerned in the glycolytic mechanism. Similar deficiencies have also been shown in other neoplastic cells. Since such alterations may well have been caused by gene deletions, the metabolic theory may thus be regarded as a special case in the general deletion theory of carcinogenesis and might be incorporated into it.

The Endocrine Theory

This has already been briefly mentioned during the discussion of dependence and autonomy in neoplasms. While it has its special application to tumors of the endocrine system, Furth has widened it so as to include leukemogenesis.[179–180] The concept, in this field, still lacks solid experimental support, but since it is consonant with much that is known about the clinical behavior of leukemias it should have great heuristic value for future research on the early stages of leukemogenesis.

In summary: the mechanism of leukemogenesis, as was pointed out above, is basically a genetic disturbance. It is obviously of great complexity, although it is likely that a certain simplification will be introduced into the subject as a result of what Furth[182] calls a "meeting of the ways" between workers in different fields. He continues, "One of the most salutary aspects of cancer research is that so many scholars in diverse disciplines are thinking about cancer, pursuing leads with their own techniques, and arriving at generalizations often contradictory to those of their peers. So arise one-sided theories."[182] None of the theories of carcinogenesis or leukemogenesis, which have been reviewed, can evidently claim to contain the whole truth, although probably each states some of the essence of the malignant transformation. Attempts at a synthesis have been most stimulating,[70, 450] but a great deal more experimental and statistical information is needed before any of the presently proposed schemes, even with modifications, can be accepted as a fully satisfactory explanation of the events leading to the development of leukemia.

ETIOLOGIC FACTORS

This section reviews some of the factors which, in the human, have been shown to be capable of causing leukemia or are suspected of doing so. In the former group—the agents which are definitely known to be leukemogenic—we still find only a solitary pair: the ionizing radiations and one chemical, benzol. Suspicions, on the other hand, have ranged widely but have lately tended to focus more and more on the viruses, mainly because of supposed analogies between human and animal leukemias. In addition, there has long been a feeling, amounting in some workers to a conviction, that genetic factors must somehow be concerned in leukemogenesis in man as they surely are in the mouse; this feeling has been strengthened by findings such as atypical palm prints (dermatoglyphs) in many patients with leukemia.[393,586]

Genetics and Leukemia

The clearest evidence pointing to the importance of gene action in leukemogenesis comes from the study of leukemic mice in which, as has been briefly described above, inbred strains have been established with a leukemia incidence varying from little more than zero to close on 100 per cent.[335] However, the genetic constitution, though crucial, is by no means the only variable, for, as has long been known,[337] the disease can be readily induced in normally low-leukemia strains by means of ionizing radiation[560–561] and other agents,[35] and prevented in high-leukemia strains by means of thymectomy.[373,396] Viruses are intimately concerned in the genesis of most, if not all, mouse leukemias, as will be discussed below, and factors such as age and sex and other hormones also enter the picture. Leukemogenesis in the mouse is thus an exceedingly complex phenomenon, where the genetic constitution appears to be the basis on which the various extrinsic and intrinsic factors operate. It is also very important to note that, in the mouse, leukemia is rarely inherited on a simple Mendelian (dominant-recessive) pattern which is determined by the action of single genes. Rather it develops as a threshold or quasi-continuous character whose expression is determined by the interaction of multiple genes, as well as of nongenetic factors.[279] Some of the loci, including the H2-histocompatibility locus, concerned in conferring resistance or susceptibility to leukemia, have recently been identified.[388,546] If the analogy between animal and human leukemogenesis is a valid one, it seems unlikely that the genetic aspects in man are less complicated than in the mouse. On the contrary, because of the impossibility of obtaining pure human strains, the demonstration of the genetic mechanisms, if any, must be peculiarly difficult.

It is not disputed that every case of human leukemia arises on a given genetic background, but considerable argument has arisen over the extent to which this background determines the occurrence of the disease and the way in which it does so.[32,600] The problem has been studied by means of surveys of the familial incidence of leukemia and of its occurrence in twins, and, more recently, also by analyses of the association between leukemia and other conditions with inherited or acquired chromosome abnormalities. Confusion has at times been due to terminology, since some authors have equated the terms *genetic* and *hereditary,* while others have accepted as *genetic* conditions those which, like mongolism (Down's syndrome), are clearly not heritable.

FAMILY SURVEYS

From the earliest days instances have been reported in which more than one case of leukemia occurred in the same family. Some of these did not stand up to critical analysis, but in a review in 1947 Videbaek accepted 26 as authentic up to that year, and mentioned a number of others as possibly acceptable. He himself reported a further 17 cases of familial leukemia, and a considerable number has been added since then.[12,55,236,278,315,360,482,484,568,578] Among our own earlier material, 6 of 45 leukemia patients had close relatives also dying from leukemia.[238] More recently, we have found 38 leukemia cases among the relatives of 680 leukemia patients (Gunz and Gunz, unpublished observations). These figures are much higher than those obtained, for example, by Guasch,[237] who procured from hematologists all over the world reports of 39 familial cases among a total of 8586 cases of leukemia—an incidence of only one in 220. The manner in which Guasch's figures were accumulated ensured an incomplete reporting of familial cases, since it relied entirely on the undocumented recollections of a multiplicity of physicians. Among more recent collections of familial leukemia are those of Miyata and Enomoto,[413] and of Kurita,[348] both from Japan, and of Rigby et al.[486]

That familial leukemia occurs is therefore not to be doubted. It is, however, equally certain that such cases are to be expected as the result of the operation of chance alone, and the only manner in which heredity can be indicated as an etiologic factor in human leukemia is by the demonstration that the incidence in the families of patients with leukemia is significantly higher than that in a control group. Controls may be obtained in two ways: either a series of nonleukemic patients, matched for sex, age, and other etiologic factors can be used, or a whole population can be employed as a control, provided the total incidence or mortality of leukemia is known. The selection of suitable matched controls is a matter of great difficulty, and for this reason some investigators[247,524] have dispensed with them entirely, preferring to check the incidence of familial leukemia against that expected on the basis of the incidence among the general population. Even this method is not fully satisfactory, because of the uncertainty of published statistics and of the information obtainable even from intelligent patients.

A number of controlled investigations have been made, of which the best known is that of Videbaek.[567] This author found among 209 patients with leukemia, 17 (8.1 percent) with a family history of other cases of leukemia. Among 200 controls there was only one case with a similar history, an incidence of 0.5 percent. Videbaek concluded that familial leukemia was therefore at least partially under hereditary control. Videbaek was unable to elucidate the precise mode of inheritance but suggested that what was inherited was a predisposition to leukemia in general, the gene or genes being dominant but with a low penetrance (failing dominance). At the same time, he discovered an increased incidence of cancer in the families of his patients compared with those of the controls, a fact which he interpreted as evidence in favor of leukemia being itself a neoplastic disease. It should be noted that Videbaek regarded the main types of human leukemia as constituting a single entity, "since the incidence of the various types among the familial cases corresponds exactly to their relative frequency among the nonfamilial cases. . . . The gene, or genes, which have the role in the production of leukemia are evidently not specific as regards the type of the disease."[567]

Videbaek's data and his conclusions, though partially supported by an earlier publication by Ardashnikov,[15] have been challenged by some statisticians, geneticists, and hematologists.[77,140,210,523–524] The chief criticism is based on the selection of his patients, and particularly of his controls, and on the methods by which cases of familial leukemia and cancer were inquired for. Busk[77] calculated from the cancer statistics in Denmark that in the families of Videbaek's leukemic patients there were approximately the numbers of relatives with cancer incidence which could be expected on the basis of the total cancer incidence; however, there was a marked deficiency of such cases among the families of the controls.

Videbaek's work illustrates the difficulties of finding adequate controls for a disease like leukemia.[479] Our own investigations[239–240] produced results similar to those of Videbaek, namely, an apparently significant excess of relatives with leukemia in leukemic patients compared with controls, but although a rough estimate showed that the mortality among the controls was probably not greatly deficient for leukemia compared with that in the general population, this could not be proved and the results were, therefore, equivocal. Similar or entirely negative findings were obtained by others.[8,317,430,498,523–524]

In the above-mentioned investigations all types of leukemia were included, and at times the types were not separated from each other. More recently, it was realized that this practice might dilute a familial clustering confined to only one or the other of the types, and since there was a suggestion that chronic lymphocytic leukemia might be the most likely to show such a pattern, we surveyed specifically the families of such patients,[247] using the expected mortality in the New Zealand population for comparison. A considerable excess was found in first-degree relatives of leukemia patients, especially brothers in whom the chance of developing leukemia was at least seven times that expected (Fig. 5-1). In children with acute leukemia, a small excess of siblings with leukemia has also been established.[24,408] This could have amounted to four times the expected rate. Familial chronic granulocytic leukemia is practically unknown, although Holton and Johnson[284] have reported a sibling pair with the juvenile form, and Weiner[583] an extraordinary family with three cases of chronic granulocytic, one of chronic lymphocytic leukemia, and several other members who were stated to have the Ph[1] chromosome but no leukemia. In another family, we found a mother and son with chronic granulocytic leukemia, and showed that the son had a Ph[1] chromosome in the marrow cells but not in the skin fibroblasts. Therefore, this was not a constitutional abnormality.[22] It is of interest that chronic granulocytic leukemia occurred in a number of the siblings of our patients with the CLL type.[247] Zuelzer and Cox believe that the most significant families from a genetic point of view are those in whom the disease is concordant as to type.[600]

From what has been said so far, it appears that the familial element in leukemogenesis may be real, at least in chronic lymphocytic leukemia of adults and acute lymphocytic leukemia of young children. However, the familial aggregation is certainly not pronounced. It is interesting that it does not appear to extend to other forms of cancer, although Videbaek thought so originally.[567] Neither Gunz and

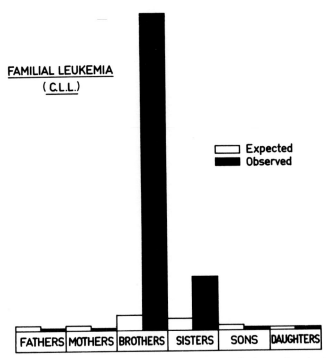

Fig. 5-1. Incidence of leukemia among first-degree relatives of patients with chronic lymphocytic leukemia.

Veale[247] nor Barber and Spiers[24] found an excess of cancer at other sites in their leukemic relatives. In this, the familial distribution resembles that found in other cancers, as of the breast[371] and lung,[550] in which concordant tumors were commonly observed but no excess of cancer of other sites was seen.

The presence of a hereditary factor in leukemia is certainly most likely in those instances in which multiple cases have occurred in close relatives. Such families have been reported by Reilly et al. (three brothers with chronic lymphocytic leukemia)[482]; Hornbaker (two sisters with chronic lymphocytic and a third with chronic granulocytic leukemia)[287]; Boggian (three siblings and one paternal cousin with chronic lymphocytic leukemia)[50]; Decastello (four, and possibly six cases in two generations)[111]; some of these were previously reported by Weiss[584]; Johnson and Peters (four of 12 siblings with acute leukemia)[315]; Anderson (lymphocytic leukemia in five of eight siblings)[12]; Gunz and Dameshek (identical twin brothers, previously published by Dameshek et al.[106], and one son, all with CLL)[243]; Campbell et al. (three siblings with acute leukemia)[78]; Heath and Moloney (five acute leukemias, among them three in siblings, in three generations)[260]; McPhedran et al. (six cases of chronic lymphocytic leukemia in two first-cousin sibships)[378]; Gunz et al. (four, and possibly five acute leukemias in siblings)[244]; Gunz and Veale (two siblings with chronic lymphocytic and one with chronic granulocytic leukemia)[247]; Fraumeni et al. (three siblings with chronic lymphocytic leukemia)[172]; Snyder et al. (three siblings and three other relatives with acute granulocytic leukemia)[516]; and Fitzgerald and Hamer (three siblings with the chronic lymphocytic type).[162] Steinberg mentioned two further families in which three of seven and four of twelve children, respectively, died of acute leukemia,[523] and Randall et al. published details of a "familial myeloproliferative disease," closely resembling acute granulocytic leukemia, occurring in nine children in a single family, among them four pairs of siblings.[476] It should be noted that once again the great majority of cases were chronic lymphocytic or acute leukemias. In several families multiple cases of leukemia were associated with other malignancies.[52,368]

Families such as those reported are of extreme rarity. Although there is a strong suggestion of a genetic, and, at times, a truly hereditary element in these reports, it must be remembered that close relatives are apt also to be exposed to closely similar environments, including possible leukemogens, and that familial clusters may therefore be at least partly due to extrinsic factors. Although case-to-case "infection," as suggested by Barbier et al.[25] and Debré et al.,[109] seems unlikely, there are reports of leukemia in husbands and their wives[9,82,401] which raises the question if such events may not perhaps be more than coincidences. The most likely interpretation of the high-leukemia familial clusters is that they result from interacting genetic and environmental factors, as discussed below.

TWIN STUDIES

It might be expected that an investigation of twins would throw some light on the genetics of leukemia, as it has done on that of other diseases. Leukemia in identical twins was first reported by Dameshek et al. in 1929.[106] By 1954, Guasch[237] had collected 14 pairs of identical and three pairs of nonidentical twins with concordant leukemia, but not necessarily identical types of the disease. In few of the identical twins was it possible to establish if the twins were indeed uniovular or fraternal. In a more recent survey of the literature, confined to cases in which the types of leukemia were known, there were 31 certainly or probably uniovular pairs, of whom 16 were discordant (only one member affected) and 15 concordant (both members affected).[344] Among nine fraternal pairs five were discordant and four concordant. It should be noted that concordance is much more likely to be reported than discordance, which is often regarded as comparatively uninteresting. Although isolated cases of discordance among twins have been published,[283,332,451,590] and larger groups have been noted by Steinberg[523] and Kosenow and Pfeiffer,[344] there must be a great discrepancy between numbers of cases occurring and those which reach the literature.[13] Of special interest are cases of chronic granulocytic leukemia in identical twins because of the presence of a marker chromosome (Ph[1]). Among six pairs reported in the literature, one had concordant disease with Ph[1] chromosome in both twins[551]; and five had discordant disease with the Ph[1] present only in the affected twin.[26,206-207,306,594] These findings provide confirmation of the generally held view that the Ph[1] chromosome is an acquired rather than inherited abnormality.

Some recent statistics have shown that there is an actual deficiency of twin-born children with leukemia, especially members of like-sex pairs, compared with those expected from the known numbers of twin births and the incidence of leukemia.[280,303] This deficiency, while relatively minor, is of importance, for it may indicate an increased intrauterine mortality among embryos predisposed to the later development of leukemia.

It has long been a tenet of genetics that concordant disease among uniovular twins is good evidence in favor of a hereditary mechanism and that discordant disease is against it. In leukemia the determination of rates of concordance is handicapped by its rarity and by the uncertain evidence of zygosity in many cases. Zuelzer and Cox[600] accept only 25 twin pairs with concordant leukemia, among them three with chronic lymphocytic and one with chronic granulocytic leukemia.[551] The rest were acute childhood leukemias. There is no question that concordant leukemia in twins is far more common than could be expected on the basis of chance.[453] Statistically, by means of comparatively extensive surveys, MacMahon and Levy,[375] Miller,[407,410] and Jackson et al.[303] established that concordance in presumably uniovular twins greatly exceeded expectation, amounting to about 25 percent of pairs, a figure subject to a large error because of the very few cases actually discovered. Characteristically, most of the children were very young and the onset of the disease in the members of the pairs occurred mostly in close succession, sometimes almost simultaneously (e.g., Joachim[314]). Whether the high concordance rate is necessarily a consequence solely of a genetic predisposition is, however, questionable. Zuelzer and Cox[600] point out that concordant leukemia in twin pairs (including those proved to be dizygous[244]) occurs substantially among infants, and calculations show that at that age the concordance rate may approach 100 percent while it becomes much lower in children over 4. This unusual age distribution—quite different from that in childhood leukemia as a whole—may indicate that the genetic factor is not of as much importance as had been thought, but that the disease in young twins could be due in part to intrauterine events of a postzygotic nature affecting both twins simultaneously.[331] Twins, more than other siblings, are exposed to similar environmental influences both in utero and postnatally. Therefore, the precise importance of genetic factors for leukemogenesis is still in question even in twins. At any event, it is unsafe to draw general conclusions as to the mechanism of childhood leukemogenesis from studies on a very small number of twins.

RELATIONSHIP OF LEUKEMIA TO CHROMOSOMAL ABNORMALITIES

One of the recently discovered associations, that between mongolian idiocy (Down's syndrome) and leukemia, constitutes perhaps a more direct piece of evidence in favor of the genetic background of some forms of leukemia than the surveys of familial and twin leukemia mentioned above. It has been repeatedly shown since 1956 that leukemia is far more common in mongols than in normal children,[346-347,394,534,540] the actual excess being rather variable in different series,[304] but probably at least 15 times the normal rate. There is a great predominance of very young children among mongols with acute leukemia, and a number of mongols with congenital leukemia have been reported.[39,285,473] Some of these cases may, in fact, not have been leukemias but atypical reactions to infections or other stimuli.[330,490] On the other hand, an increased incidence of leukemia of all types among older mongols has not been confirmed.[575]

Mongolism is now known to be a consequence of a congenital chromosome abnormality, trisomy 21, resulting from nondisjunction during meiosis.[307,359] The frequency of nondisjunction increases with maternal age, as does that of mongolism. Nondisjunction is not a random event but occurs preferentially in certain families.[261] In rare families there may even be an inherited tendency to nondisjunction.[21,334,404] It seems a reasonable assumption that leukemia in mongols is somehow determined by the existence of the chromosome abnormality, although the precise mechanism of the effect is by no means clear. Possibly any abnormality of the chromosome complement may lead to an overall instability during cell division and a tendency for further abnormalities to develop. Perhaps, on the other hand, chromosome defects make cells vulnerable to the action of extrinsic agents such as viruses. Miller and Todaro have shown that the oncogenic virus SV40 causes a malignant transformation in fibroblasts derived from mongols more readily than in those from normal persons.[412] Thus, there may be a collaboration between intrinsic and extrinsic agents in the mechanism of oncogenesis.

It has been found by most authors (though not all)[154] that the risk of leukemia in children—especially in those between 4–8 years—increases with maternal age, even in the absence of mongolism,[376,521–522,534] and it therefore seems that trisomy 21 is only one example of potentially leukemogenic disturbances in the genetic apparatus of aging parents. Many of these disturbances are too subtle for microscopic observation, the chromosomes appearing normal, just as they do in many trisomic mongols with leukemia,[86] and in about half the acute leukemias occurring in other patients (see Chapter 6). Point mutations may, of course, be present in many such cases, whether or not mongolism is an underlying abnormality.

A rare form of mongolism is due to a balanced and asymptomatic translocation of a 21-chromosome in one of the parents, and thereby to a functional rather than a structural trisomy-21. Since the parent carries the causative abnormality, there is a good chance of successive mongols being born in the resulting sibship. Interestingly enough, an early report described a family with three mongol sibs and one with acute leukemia, the mother being a translocation carrier.[66] In a sense, this is the clearest example of a truly inherited predisposition to leukemia.

In spite of the above example, and of a few other instances in which mongolism and leukemia occurred within the same family, mongolism has not been found to have a significantly increased incidence among the sibs of leukemic children,[24] although this had previously been suspected[405]; nor are other congenital defects unusually prevalent in such families.[408]

A number of cases of leukemia, mainly in children, have been described in which there were preexisting chromosome abnormalities other than trisomy 21.[51,171,554,601] Some of these affected the somatic and some the sex chromosomes. The rarity of such cases makes the significance of the associations problematic. Zuelzer and Cox found no significant preexisting karyotypic abnormalities, other than trisomy 21, in their large childhood material,[600] but Miller, in a detailed review of the literature, stressed the wealth of circumstantial evidence in favor of the predisposing activity of congenital chromosome abnormalities of all kinds in leukemogenesis.[408]

Two rare familial disorders associated with congenital abnormalities—Fanconi's and Bloom's syndromes—have both been shown to have an increased incidence of leukemia, as well as of chromosome abnormalities.[48,197,456,496,542] Both diseases are also regularly accompanied by cytogenetic alterations consisting in an unusual fragility of cultured lymphocyte chromosomes (Fig. 5-2) and sometimes in an increased tendency to endoreduplication. These in vitro phenomena probably do not indicate longstanding chromosome defects such as those which follow radiations (see below). As most of them affect chromatids rather than whole chromosomes they must have arisen while cells were preparing to divide in vitro,[97] and, therefore, a

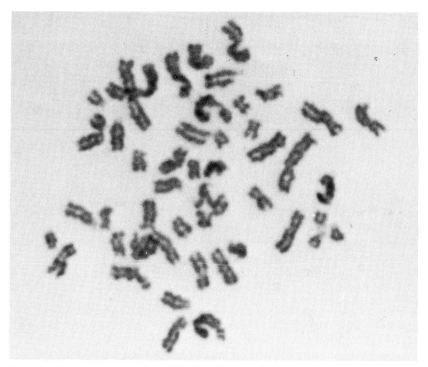

Fig. 5-2. Fanconi's anemia. Metaphase from cultured lymphocyte shows chromatid breaks and triradial figures.

mechanism regulating mitosis rather than the chromosomes themselves must be faulty. In the absence of adequate studies of bone marrow chromosomes, it is difficult to visualize a direct connection between the chromosome aberrations in cultured lymphocytes and the eventual development of leukemia, other than the above-mentioned predisposition of cells with unstable karyotypes to undergo further changes in their chromosome complement.

A variety of other congenital conditions (ataxia telangiectasia[262,353,457,481,513]; hereditary leukopenia[114]; phocomelia with hypoplastic thrombocytopenia[115]; Wiskott-Aldrich syndrome[454,545]) have been found to be associated with leukemia or lymphoma. Their precise significance is uncertain, though some, like ataxia telangiectasia, also show immunologic abnormalities and may therefore have a special significance (see Chapter 12).

The Fanconi and Bloom syndromes are examples of autosomal recessive conditions which can be recognized only in homozygotes. These are very rare but the heterozygotes carrying the mutant genes are rather common. Their frequency in the U.S. population is estimated as between 1 in 200 and 1 in 1000.[541] Preliminary evidence suggests that leukemia and other neoplasms may be unduly prevalent in heterozygotes, as well as in homozygotes, and if this should be confirmed, it can be calculated that the genes of one or the other of the rare neoplasia-prone syndromes may be present in as many as 5 or 10 percent of all leukemia patients.[541] This possibility throws an altogether new light on the role which genes may play in leukemogenesis. If there were a way of identifying the neoplasia-producing genes in carriers, the hypothesis might be tested directly. This may well become possible, for the oncogenic virus SV40 has already been shown to cause excessive malignant transformation in vitro of the cells of close relations of patients with Fanconi's anemia, as well as in those from the patients themselves.[124,412,548] Moreover, in a family with several leukemia cases, both patients and close relatives showed a greatly increased rate of in vitro transformation with SV40.[516] If such studies could be more widely extended, an increased susceptibility to virus action might well be found in a proportion of apparently healthy persons, and this might be an indication of their liability to leukemia. This work has opened a highly promising line of investigation into the genetics of leukemogenesis.

INTERPRETATION OF GENETIC STUDIES

The genetic basis of human leukemia is still uncertain, although to the extent that each patient is an individual, his genetic constitution must be concerned in the development of the disease. Surveys of families and of twin pairs have indicated a greater than expected incidence of cases among relatives, especially of patients with chronic lymphocytic leukemia and of children with the acute type, many of them very young. No excess of familial cases has yet been found in chronic granulocytic leukemia. The existence of a small number of families with multiple cases among close relatives, particularly sibs, has raised the question if these may fall into a separate group; and the same possibility exists in the exceedingly small group of uniovular infant twins in whom a very high concordance rate has been established.

No reliable evidence has been produced to show that leukemia in man is inherited in a Mendelian fashion, either by means of a dominant or recessive mechanism. It is much more likely that, as in mice, there is a polygenic background of the threshold or quasi-continuous type.[95] This theory postulates that there is an underlying variable, "liability to develop leukemia," that this is widespread in the population, and that all individuals in whom this genetically determined variable exceeds a certain threshold develop the disease. It has been shown that a quasi-continuous variation of genetic characters is difficult to distinguish from a dominant inheritance with a very low penetrance.[136] This may explain certain of the reports in which the latter mechanism was postulated.[567]

It must be presumed that environmental factors of all kinds act on the stage set by the genetic constitution. The same factors which would not produce disease in most individuals will cause the leukemogenic threshold to be exceeded in persons or families with a naturally high polygenic setting for leukemia. This would suffice to account for the cases of familial leukemia—possibly even the exceptionally large family clusters—as well as the cases of concordant disease in young twins who share the same environment more intimately than any other blood relations. The possible nature of the environmental factors concerned will be discussed below.

Some individuals have congenital chromosome abnormalities and a greatly increased susceptibility to leukemia. Chief among these are mongols, together with rarer groups with autosomal and, possibly, with sex chromosome abnormalities. Here the connection between the genetic background and the occurrence of leukemia is particularly evident, though the leukemogenic mechanism itself is obscure. Possibly the chromosomal defect makes these people more susceptible than normal to the leukemogenic action of extrinsic factors. This is suggested by studies such as those of Miller and Todaro,[412] in which a virus was shown to be unduly carcinogenic in vitro when acting on cells from congenitally defective individuals.

In summary, evidence is beginning to accumulate that gene action, in conjunction with the activity of extrinsic factors, may be of importance in the genesis of at least certain forms of leukemia. As yet there is no precise knowledge of its mechanism. Nor is it known whether, as suggested by Zuelzer and Cox,[600] it is significant only in a small minority of cases or plays a part, albeit often a subordinate one, in a sizable proportion. Work now in progress may help to decide this important question.

Hormones

Whereas there is evidence in some strains of mice that estrogenic hormones are leukemogenic,[195] that the incidence of spontaneous leukemia is higher in females than in males,[432] and that it can be reduced by ovariectomy,[179] there is nothing to suggest that the female sex hormones may play a similar part in human leukemia. Indeed, such data as are available all point in the opposite direction, for all forms of leukemia are commoner in human males than females, and in chronic lymphocytic leukemia this sex difference is particularly apparent (see Chapter 4). This fact suggests that the sex hormones may play a part in the etiology of human leukemia, but there are no data to elucidate the mechanism of any such effect. A strange irregularity in the sex incidence is found in chronic granulocytic leukemia. In the middle-

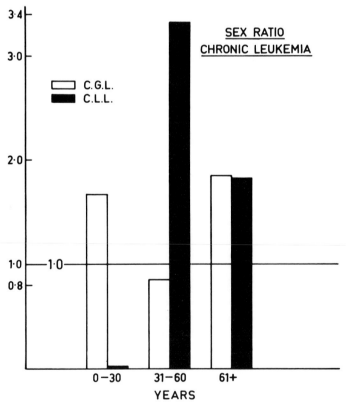

Fig. 5-3. Sex ratios at various ages in chronic granulocytic and chronic lymphocytic leukemia. (Ratios in excess of 1.0 denote predominance of males.)

aged groups, this type is almost equally common in the two sexes, whereas males predominate in younger and older persons (Fig. 5-3).

No other hormones are recognized as being leukemogenic in man.

Leukemia and Viruses

The relationship between tumor viruses and leukemia has become a burning question since Ludwik Gross showed, in 1951, that some forms of leukemia in inbred strains of mice are transmissible by means of cell-free filtrates of leukemic tissues.[222] A long series of investigations by Gross and by others has proved that the agents involved in such transmissions are viruses; that they are widely, if not universally, present in laboratory mice, often without giving rise to overt disease, and that they have many of the same basic characteristics as the fowl leukosis viruses which have been much longer known. More recently, leukemia in cats has been shown to be associated with similar viruses which are transmissible to newborn kittens and grow in vitro, not only in feline, but also in canine and in human tissues. There are strong suspicions that leukemia in dogs, cattle, and perhaps in pigs is also virus induced. Many argue that, with this growing wealth of evidence from the animal field, man, too, must eventually come into line, and that human leukemia will be found to be a virus disease.

So far this argument has not been backed by any incontrovertible evidence. Although viruses have been discovered in patients with leukemia and human leukemic tissues have been seen to harbor viruslike particles resembling those in leukemic mice or birds, it has not been demonstrated that these were causally related to the disease. The case for a viral etiology of human leukemia still rests on indirect and circumstantial evidence.

FOWL LEUKEMIA

As long ago as 1908, Ellerman and Bang[137] proved that leukosis of domestic fowls could be transmitted by means of the inoculation of cell-free extracts and thus propagated through several generations of birds. These observations were confirmed and extended by a number of later workers, especially Furth,[177–178] Engelbreth-Holm,[138] and the Beards and their coworkers.[28–30] Their studies indicated that the disease was caused by self-propagating, filter-passing agents with all the characteristics of viruses. Fowl leukosis occurs in several forms characterized by the predominance of erythroblasts, myeloblasts, or lymphocytes. It may spread either horizontally from chicken to chicken, or vertically through infected eggs. Its economic importance is enormous as it often affects and destroys whole flocks.

The viruses of avian erythroblastosis and myeloblastosis have been isolated and characterized in detail.[29,30,46,131,134,135,248,343] They belong to the group of RNA viruses which have a central spherical nucleoid surrounded by an outer envelope (Fig. 5-4), the total diameter being some 70–120 mμ. In ultrathin sections, under the electron microscope, they can be recognized as so-called *C-type* particles,[102,103] which are characteristically situated in the cellular cytoplasm or between cells and arise by budding from the cell membrane or some internal membrane such as the endoplasmic reticulum (Fig. 5-5). With one exception, all the known avian, murine, and feline leukemogenic viruses belong to the RNA group resembling myxoviruses,

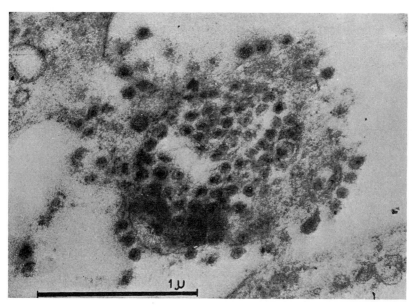

Fig. 5-4.   Chicken leukemia. Detail of viruslike particles. Electron micrograph, × 450,-000. (Courtesy of Dr. Marcel Bessis, Paris.)

as does the closely related Rous sarcoma virus (RSV) which produces solid tumors in birds. This last virus can be readily obtained from many experimental leukemias and tumors, but in others it disappears once a tumor has been induced. This is now known to be due to the fact that the RSV is defective and requires the help of a second virus, that of chicken lymphomatosis, to produce infective particles. The addition of such a helper virus to apparently virus-free tumor cells can rescue the RSV, which thereupon becomes evident in its original infective form.[251] Similar defective strains have more recently been found among the murine leukemia viruses (see below), and if defectiveness should be a general phenomenon in the leukemia field, it might have obvious relevance to the etiology of the human disease.

The single exception to the rule that all leukemogenic viruses in birds are of the RNA type is formed by the newly discovered virus of Marek's disease (neural lymphomatosis) in chickens.[83] This is a DNA virus of the herpes group, and the possible significance of this fact is discussed on page 94.

MURINE LEUKEMIA

Whereas the leukosis of fowls was clearly demonstrated to be virus-induced early in the century, attempts to transmit mammalian leukemia by means of cell-free extracts remained unsuccessful for many years, until 1951 when Gross showed that transmission is possible, provided newborn animals are used as hosts.[222] This discovery has since been repeatedly confirmed and has led to a great upsurge of interest in this field.

The Gross Virus.   The early experiments of Gross were carried out with two inbred strains of mice, Ak and C3H. The former of these has a very high incidence of spontaneous leukemia, no fewer than 85 percent of all animals succumbing in middle age to a rapidly growing lymphocytic leukemia which shows its most pronounced le-

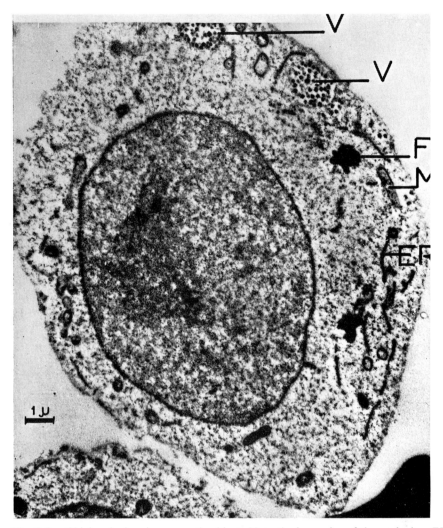

Fig. 5-5.   Chicken leukemia, proerythroblast. Note the large size of the nucleolus. ER: endoplasmic reticulum; F: fat granules; M: mitochondria; V: vacuoles, full of viruslike particles. Electron micrograph, × 13,500. (Courtesy of Dr. Marcel Bessis, Paris.)

sions in the thymus. Like many other murine leukemias it has the characteristics of a lymphosarcoma whose cells may eventually invade the bloodstream. The C3H strain has a spontaneous leukemia rate of only 0.5 percent. Gross succeeded in transmitting leukemia from Ak donors to C3H recipients. In his early work he used newborn (less than 16 hours old) C3H mice and inoculated them with suspensions of leukemic Ak cells. Tumors appeared at the site of inoculation within 2–3 weeks, and were usually followed within another week or two by a generalized leukemia. These tumors could be transplanted back to normal Ak but not to adult C3H mice; they were therefore merely grafts, the very young C3H mice serving as a medium for the growth of the implanted Ak leukemic cells (immunological tolerance of the newborn mouse.)

The next step in Gross's experiments was the inoculation of cell-free extracts of leukemic Ak organs into newborn C3H mice.[223] No immediate tumors occurred at

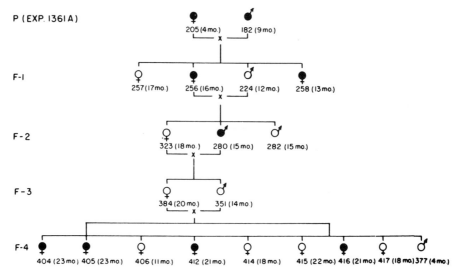

Fig. 5-6. Vertical transmission, that is, from one generation to another, of leukemia in the C3H strain of mice. Only female 205 and her brother 182 had been injected (within a few hours after birth) with Ak leukemic extracts. Their offspring were untreated. Black color indicates the development of leukemia. It is evident that leukemia developed in several descendants of successive generations (this strain of mice is essentially free from spontaneous leukemia). The inoculation of the parent couple 205 and 182 with the leukemic agent apparently initiated vertical transmission of this disease in this particular family of mice. (Reproduced from Gross,[225] courtesy of the publisher.)

the inoculation site, but after an interval averaging 10 months, 28 percent of the C3H mice developed leukemia, which could be transplanted to further C3H mice. It therefore appeared that this was not merely a graft of leukemic cells but a newly induced form of leukemia in a previously low-leukemia strain of mice. Later, Gross prepared a uniformly pathogenic filtrate by passing a particularly active extract serially through newborn mice.[227] This "Passage A" agent had all the properties of an oncogenic virus and was intensely and uniformly leukemogenic to many strains of mice, as well as to suckling rats.[232] It is now known as the Gross leukemia virus (GLV). Although usually this produces the lymphocytic form of the disease, with thymic tumors and splenic, hepatic, and lymph node involvement but few blood changes, the GLV is capable also of causing typical acute lymphocytic, myelocytic, monocytic, chloroleukemic, and erythroblastic forms.[232] A similar polymorphic picture can be produced by the Graffi strain of murine leukemia viruses after prolonged cell-free passage.[215]

C-type particles of the GLV are contained in high concentration in the plasma of leukemic mice and in their leukemic organs, as shown by transmission experiments and in electron photomicrographs. Spherical particles resembling the GLV have been seen in ovaries of a high-leukemia strain[506]; leukemia has been transmitted through cell-free extracts of ground-up, apparently normal embryos,[225] and GLV has been demonstrated by electron microscopy in such embryos.[122] C-type particles have been found in the genital organs of both males and females.[155] All these findings suggest that the GLV is transmitted "vertically" from generation to generation through both the male and female gametes, at least in the high-leukemia strains such as Ak and C58. In low-leukemia strains, vertical transmission cannot usually be demonstrated, but in some strains the GLV appears in the mammary glands and can be transmitted to sucklings through the mother's milk.[234] Horizontal transmission among litter mates or unrelated animals is never found.

In high-leukemia strains, the disease is thus transmitted mainly through embryos (Fig. 5-6). The virus remains latent for long periods in any given mouse, sometimes throughout its whole lifetime, and during this period the host remains in perfect health. The disease becomes obvious only at later ages, but its onset can be accelerated through the injection of a potent viral preparation such as the Passage A agent. The etiology of mouse leukemia is determined by the genetic background and such factors as age and hormonal balance, as well as the quantity of virus present.

There are, however, also other factors involved in leukemogenesis, as is most clearly seen in the usually low-leukemia strains. Animals belonging to such strains can be induced to develop leukemia by means of exposure to x-rays[226,255,369,573] or to chemical carcinogens[253,294] (see also page 000), and the leukemias so induced are fully transmissible. Budding C-type particles can be seen in the organs within a few days of irradiation, and long before leukemia appears (Figs. 5-7–5-10).[235] These findings provide strong evidence for the presence of virus in *unirradiated* mice of low-leukemia strains, and it must be assumed that the x-rays and carcinogens act by triggering or releasing this virus. In addition, the state of the host's immunologic defences appears to be crucial in its resistance to virus leukemia.[254,392] In fact, Gross's original discovery was possible only because newborn mice happen to be tolerant to virus infections. By means of irradiation experiments, leukemia virus has been demonstrated to be present even in germ-free mice.[316]

The work of Gross and of many others may now be summarized. There is a strong genetic background—that of strain specificity—against which other agents, both intrinsic and extrinsic, can be seen to act. Among intrinsic agents are sex and other hormones, immunologic factors and the tissue changes caused by ageing. Viruses are ubiquitously present and vertically transmitted through several generations. Extrinsic agents such as ionizing radiations or chemical carcinogens, can release or trigger the virus and lead to the onset of the disease. In addition, the expression of leukemia can be manipulated by such means as thymectomy or thymic grafting.

As has been noted above (page 69), the genetic element in murine leukemia is of a quasi-continuous nature in which multiple genes are concerned, as well as nongenetic factors. The mechanism of leukemogenesis may be graphically shown as in Figure 5-27. There is a threshold of leukemogenic factors which must be exceeded before the disease develops. Genetic factors, quantity of virus, and activity of triggering mechanisms are all concerned in determining whether the threshold is to be crossed in any individual.

Other leukemogenic agents in mice. Besides the mouse leukemia agent described by Gross, many others have been discovered in the past 20 years. These include:

1. An agent obtained by Graffi from a variety of spontaneous mouse tumors (not

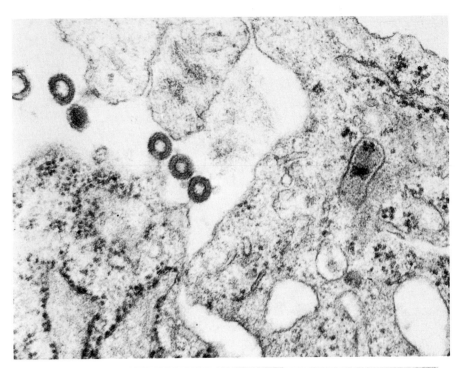

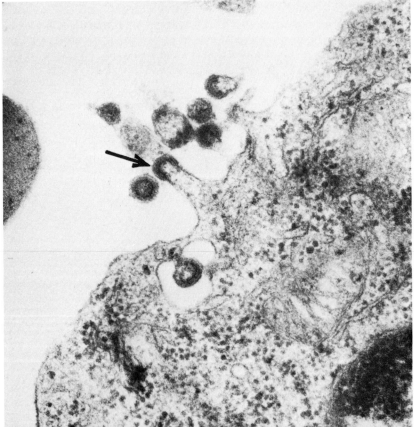

Figs. 5-7 and 5-8. Spleen sections from mice with radiation-induced leukemia showing the presence of virus particles, including a budding particle (*arrow*). Electron micrographs, × 62,000. (Reproduced from Gross and Feldman,[235] courtesy of the authors and publisher.)

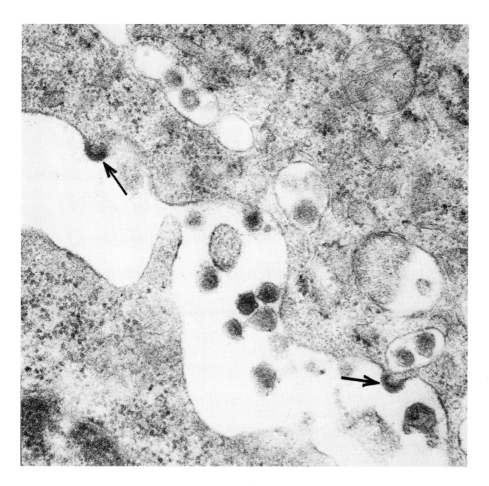

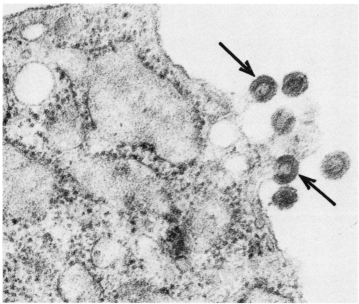

Figs. 5-9 and 5-10. Lymph node sections from a mouse with radiation-induced leukemia showing budding (*arrows*) and other virus particles. Electron micrographs, × 62,000. (Reproduced from Gross and Feldman,[235] courtesy of the authors and publisher.)

   leukemia), especially the Ehrlich carcinoma.[213-214] This produces not the customary lymphocytic (lymphosarcoma) type of leukemia but an unusual form of
   myeloid (chloro-) leukemia which can be transmitted by cell-free filtrates to
   several strains of mice, as well as to rats.[216]

2.   An agent similarly derived from the Ehrlich carcinoma of Swiss mice by
     Friend[175] and causing in the same strain a leukemia, interpreted as being of re-
     ticulum cell origin with an erythroblastosis.[398]
3.   An agent derived by Moloney from mouse sarcoma 37 and causing a
     lymphocytic leukemia in a wide variety of inbred as well as in Swiss mice,[420] and
     in rats.[421] This agent has been propagated serially in vitro.[381]
4.   A virus isolated by Rauscher[478] in 1962, capable of causing both erythroblastic
     and lymphoid leukemia.
5.   A virus described by Rich in Swiss mice.[483]
6.   The "radiation leukemia virus" of Lieberman and Kaplan[369] (see page 99).

   All these organisms have been characterized as RNA viruses, and ultra-
structurally the various viruses are indistinguishable from each other.
   Antigenically, there are differences: although common antigens have been
found in all by means of immunodiffusion[199] and complement fixation tests,[257] other
work has shown that serologically the mouse leukemia viruses fall into two broad
groups, the first with the GVL as prototype, the second containing the Friend, Moloney, and Rauscher viruses.[447] It is of great interest that there are group-specific
(gs) antigens common to the leukemias of the mouse, rat, hamster, and cat, but that
these differ from the antigens of the avian leukoses.[198] Group-specific antigens can
be detected even when no infectious virus is present, and in infected animals they are
demonstrable in normal hematopoietic as well as in tumor tissues. They are also
contained in young mouse embryos in strains which normally reveal little or no expression of the RNA virus postnatally,[290] as well as in seemingly uninfected "wild"
house mice.[194] This evidence has become the foundation of the new oncogene-
virogene theory of Huebner and Todaro.[291,548a] This postulates that RNA tumor
virus genomes are ubiquitous in all strains of mice, and possibly in all mammals.
These *virogenes* are vertically transmitted through the generations and incorporated
in the host genomes. They contain a special portion, the *oncogene,* which carries the
information for transforming normal cells into tumor cells. Normally the virogene-
oncogene is repressed until some further event, either endogenous or exogenous,
causes derepression of the whole virogene or of portions of it; accordingly, cells will
either produce infectious virus without transformation or become transformed, with
or without the production of infectious virus.
   Gross[230,232-233] has suggested that the GLV is the organism which gives rise to
naturally occurring mouse leukemia, and its wide distribution in many strains
provides evidence in favor of this view. The other viruses are not normally pathogenic and do not cause murine leukemia except under artificial (i.e. experimental)
conditions.

VIRUSES IN THE LEUKEMIAS OF HIGHER ANIMALS

   Leukemia is a common disease in many higher animals. In cattle it occurs as a
lymphosarcoma which is accompanied by a lymphocytosis and affects animals in
certain herds, particularly in the countries of northern Europe.[32] Although in such

herds it has many of the features of an infectious disease, and although C-type particles have been isolated from the milk of leukemic cows,[132] the disease has not been
transmitted, and the evidence for a virus etiology is still circumstantial.

C-type particles have been seen in canine[81] and feline leukemias, but only in the
cat has a virus been isolated and positively shown to be concerned in leukemogenesis
(Figs. 5-11–5-18).[310–311,350–351] The feline leukemia virus (FeLV) has been isolated
from a number of leukemic cats, transmitted to healthy newborn kittens with causation of the disease, and grown in tissue culture. C-type particles have been seen in
the spleen, marrow, platelets, and salivary glands of affected and, even of normal,
animals. Cultures of human embryonic cells, as well as those of canine and feline
tissues support the growth of FeLV[311,495] FeLV shares group-specific antigens with
the viral genomes of mouse, rat, and hamster, but so far no similar homology has
been found with canine and human antigens.[193] Indeed, in the dog, RNA viruses have
not been definitely identified in any naturally occurring tumors, though FeLV can be
cultured in canine tissues.

Because cats—and to a lesser extent dogs—develop leukemia quite frequently,
it has often been thought that contact with infected animals might be responsible for
some cases of human leukemia. These suspicions became acute with the discovery in
1964 of the FeLV in cats with sporadic leukemia,[312] and especially of the capacity of
the FeLV to multiply in cultures of tissues from several species, including man.

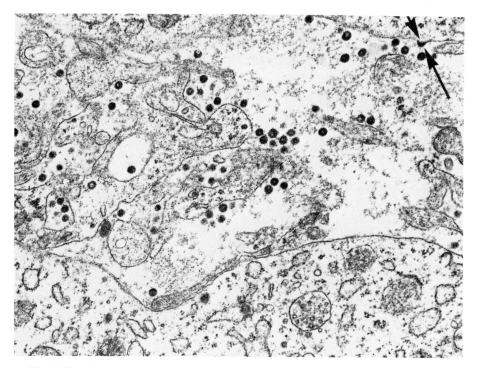

Fig. 5-11.   Bone marrow section from kitten infected with FeLV. Numerous virus particles are seen near the surface of a macrophage; one budding virus is marked by *arrows*. × 20,-
000. (Courtesy of Dr. Helen Laird, Department of Veterinary Pathology, University of
Glasgow.)

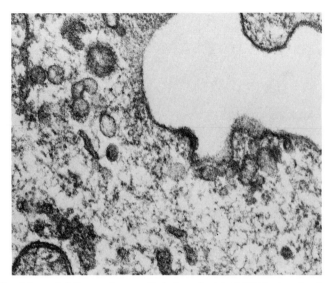

Fig. 5-12.   Normal feline embryo cells infected with FeLV leukemia virus. Early stage of virus budding from a cell membrane. × 80,000. (Courtesy of Dr. Helen Laird, Department of Veterinary Pathology, University of Glasgow.)

Moreover, the fact that FeLV could be found in cat salivary glands,[193] seemed to explain how the disease could be transmitted.

When it is, however, remembered that, so far as is known, all mammalian leukemias are transmitted vertically rather than horizontally, a transmission from pet to owner seems rather unlikely, and the evidence is, in fact, negative up to the present. No human antigens capable of reacting with antibodies against FeLV have been found,[256] and laboratory personnel working with FeLV failed to develop anti-

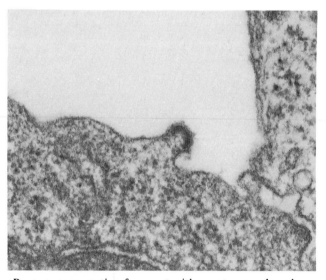

Fig. 5-13.   Bone marrow section from cat with spontaneous lymphosarcoma. A virus bud protrudes from the cell membrane; the formation of the virus internal membranes is demonstrated. × 80,000. (Courtesy of Dr. Helen Laird, Department of Veterinary Pathology, University of Glasgow.)

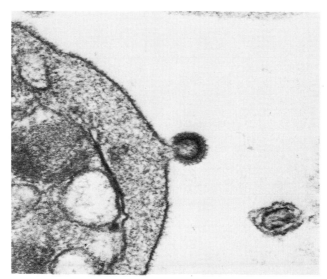

Fig. 5-14. Blood platelet from kitten infected with FeLV. An almost complete virus particle is attached to the cell surface by a narrow neck of membrane. × 80,000. (Courtesy of Dr. Helen Laird, Department of Veterinary Pathology, University of Glasgow.)

bodies against it[193]; nor could epidemiologic surveys show any increased exposure to cats in the households of leukemia patients.[252] Similarly negative findings were obtained when excessive contacts with dogs, either healthy or diseased, were sought.[443,497,564] Finally, the leukemia death rate is not raised in veterinarians.[154] It has also been pointed out that because FeLV can be propagated in canine and human tissues in vitro, this should not be taken to imply that either species will support infections with the virus in vivo.[193]

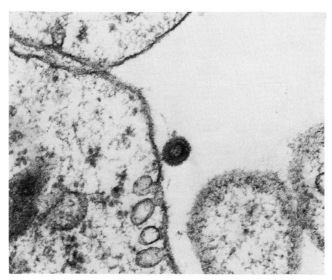

Fig. 5-15. Normal feline embryo cells infected with FeLV. A fully formed particle is seen near the cell surface; the two internal membranes and the spiked layer on the outer surface of the virus are shown. × 80,000. (Courtesy of Dr. Helen Laird, Department of Veterinary Pathology, University of Glasgow.)

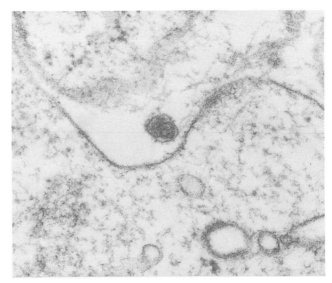

Fig. 5-16. Normal feline embryo tissue culture infected with FeLV. A complete virus particle with the electron-dense nucleoid form is seen in an intercellular space. × 90,000. (Courtesy of Dr. Helen Laird, Department of Veterinary Pathology, University of Glasgow.)

VIRUSES IN HUMAN LEUKEMIA

There is as yet no direct evidence that viruses are concerned in the etiology of human leukemia. This negative conclusion has to be drawn in spite of an enormous quantity of research on this subject, some of which will now be briefly reviewed.

Attempts have been made for many years to transmit human leukemia to animals or other human beings. These have been uniformly unsuccessful, although a

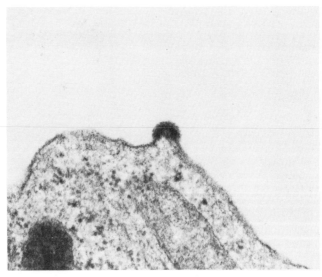

Fig. 5-17. Bone marrow section from kitten infected with FeLV. A virus particle is seen budding from the cell membrane. × 60,000. (Courtesy of Dr. Helen Laird, Department of Veterinary Pathology, University of Glasgow.)

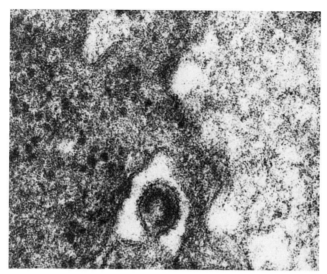

Fig. 5-18. Detail of the final stage of virus budding. Section of spleen megakaryocyte from kitten infected with FeLV. × 120,000. (Courtesy of Dr. Helen Laird, Department of Veterinary Pathology, University of Glasgow.)

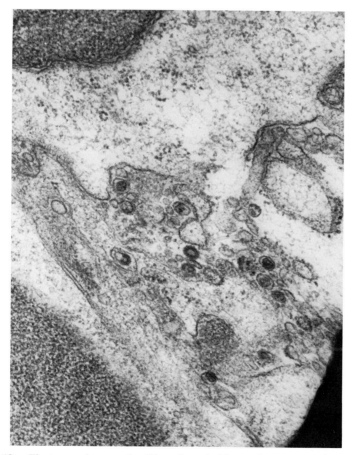

Fig. 5-19. Electron micrograph of lymph node biopsy from human lymphosarcoma showing extracellular mature and immature C-type particles and a budding particle in a cell vacuole. (Courtesy of Dr. Leon Dmochowski, M.D. Anderson Hospital, Houston, Texas.)

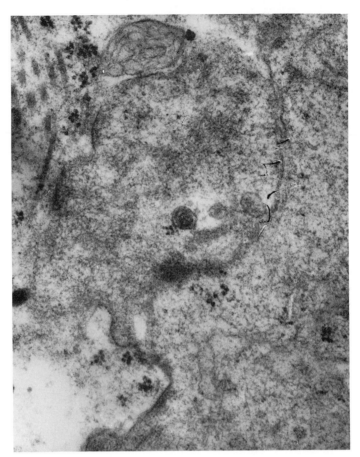

Fig. 5-20. Electron micrograph of section of human osteosarcoma biopsy showing a mature extracellular C-type particle. (Courtesy of Dr. Leon Dmochowski, M.D. Anderson Hospital, Houston, Texas.)

variety of other lesions have been produced in the course of such experiments. To prove an etiologic relationship between injected human material and leukemia subsequently developing in animals, a minimum requirement would be the demonstration that leukemic material from a diseased animal reacts immunologically with the serum of the donor patients.[508] This proof does not appear to have been brought in any one instance. Indeed, in at least one case in which it was claimed that the inoculation of cell-free splenic extracts from a patient with leukemia had caused leukemia in mice,[277] it was later shown by serologic techniques that this leukemia was of murine and not of human origin.[158]

RNA viruses. Electron micrographic methods have been used for a number of years in attempts to demonstrate viruses in human leukemic tissues. The greatest success in this field has been attained by Dmochowski and his colleagues.[116–120,123] By means of ultrathin sectioning, C-type particles, some of them showing the budding phenomenon, were found in a proportion of lymph node biopsies, plasma and bone marrow pellets, and tissue cultures derived from leukemic patients (Figs. 5-19 and 5-20). These particles were exceedingly few in number in any one patient, so that prolonged efforts had to be made to locate them, a procedure sometimes referred to as the "needle-in-the-haystack" method.[64]

Some years ago a spate of reports appeared on the visualization or isolation of viruses and viruslike particles in centrifuged plasma or marrow of patients with leukemia[7,72,297,433,437]; some of these turned out to be contaminants or cellular debris; others were not viruses but mycoplasmas whose relationship to human leukemia is highly problematic.[151–152,202,221,259] A major difficulty in studies of this nature is the fact that RNA viruses have no specific surface structure so that they cannot be positively identified by optical means but are easily confused with other particulate matter arising from normal cell organelles—mitochondrial debris, vesicles, and other small granules—or degenerating cells, especially when the material is treated by means of negative staining, rather than by thin-sectioning.[16,440,489] Reports on a positive correlation between the presence of viruslike particles in the plasma and the clinical status of patients with leukemia have not been confirmed.[361]

In 1965 a committee of the World Health Organization[595] suggested two principal criteria on which the relationship between viruslike particles and leukemia should be judged in any given case. There was likely to be a causative relationship if large numbers of uniform particles were found, and especially if an origin of the particles by budding could be observed. As pointed out by Dalton,[103] neither of these criteria is likely to be helpful when human plasma preparations are studied; first, to go by the experience gained with murine and other animal leukemias, large numbers of particles are never found in cases of spontaneous disease (as opposed to those induced by deliberate injection of a potent virus preparation); second, budding will be seen only when cells are present, and not in pellets from cell-free plasma centrifugates. For these reasons, the most suggestive—but so far inconclusive—evidence in favor of RNA viruses in human leukemia comes not from the examination of body fluids but from the careful tissue studies carried out by Dmochowski[116–120] and some other groups.[103,467]

Attempts have been made to demonstrate the presence of virus in human leukemic cells by immunologic methods. Rabbits were immunized with plasma which had been shown to contain viruslike particles, and the resultant antibodies, absorbed with various normal human blood components, were tested against leukemic cells by means of an immunofluorescent technique.[159–161,597] Positive results were interpreted as showing the presence of virus material in fluorescent cells. Later work, however, cast doubts on this interpretation when it was shown that positive fluorescence could be abolished when antisera were absorbed with normal human bone marrow powder.[598]

Recently, much interest was created by the discovery of a new test which, it was hoped, might reveal the presence of RNA viruses in human tissues. It had long been a mystery how RNA viruses could induce a heritable change in cells destined to become neoplastic without contributing genetic information in the form of DNA to the cellular genome. An explanation was eventually found in the form of an enzyme, viral RNA-dependent DNA polymerase (reverse transcriptase), which is capable of using viral RNA as a template for the formation of new DNA.[23,544] The DNA becomes polymerized through the action of other enzymes, including a DNA-directed polymerase,[414,518] and thus can be incorporated into the host genome. Reverse transcriptase has been found in all known oncogenic RNA viruses including those of avian, murine, and feline leukemias, but not in nononcogenic viruses, with the exception of the foamy viruses of monkeys, cats and cattle—a widely distributed group of viruses of uncertain pathologic significance.[189] It seemed likely that possession of reverse transcriptase might be found to characterize a given RNA virus as oncogenic, and, furthermore, that the discovery of the enzyme in a strain of cells would denote the presence of oncogenic viruses in them. Reverse transcriptase was, in fact, discovered in human leukemic cells[192] and later found also in a number of apparently normal tissues.[503] It has, however, become clear that these cellular enzymes are not identical with the viral enzyme,[99] and that therefore they cannot be regarded as a sign of viral infection. Antibodies prepared against reverse transcriptases from various sources have shown that, like the group-specific antigen (see page 86), the enzyme has both species-specific and interspecies antigenic characteristics.[547] Thus, the source of the reverse transcriptase can be identified by immunologic means, and this fact was used for the first time to show that a reverse transcriptase in a C-type virus isolated from a cultured Burkitt tumor[191,472] was not of human but of murine origin.[504] The discovery of reverse transcriptase is obviously of the greatest importance, both from a theoretical and a practical point of view, but, to date, its full significance in relation to human leukemia remains problematic.

DNA viruses.   As stated above, with the exception of the recently discovered virus of Marek's disease, all the known leukemogenic viruses belong to the RNA group. However, a group of DNA viruses are now known which can induce neoplastic changes, but not leukemia, in experimental conditions. To this group belongs Gross's original mouse *parotid tumor virus*[223-224] which was later rechristened the *polyoma virus*[535-537]; the Simian virus SV40, isolated from monkey kidneys which had been used for making poliomyelitis vaccine; and the human adenoviruses of which the 12-type in particular has been shown to be potentially oncogenic. These organisms cause tumors in suitable experimental animals and tranformation in tissue cultures, SV 40 being the only virus which transforms cultures of human cells. Reference has already been made to the increased ease of transformation by SV 40 of cultures derived from patients with Down's syndrome and Fanconi's anemia, and from their close relatives; and of the association between vulnerability to SV 40 and leukemia incidence[412,516] (see page 77).

A possible connection between a DNA virus and human leukemia has been explored in recent years in consequence of the discovery of a new organism of the herpesvirus group, the Epstein-Barr virus or EBV.[143,145-146] As a result of extensive studies by workers in several countries, it has been found that infection with the EBV is extremely widespread; that the virus has a propensity for growing in lymphoid cells and in no other type of cell; that it has a clear association with Burkitt's lymphoma; and that it is almost certainly the cause of infectious mononucleosis. However, there is little evidence as yet to indicate a special role of the EBV in leukemogenesis.

The EBV (Fig. 5-21), like other DNA and unlike RNA viruses, has a distinctive surface structure which allows it to be positively identified as a member of the herpes group of viruses. Serologically, it is distinct from others in the same group such as herpes simplex, cytomegalovirus, and varicella.[211-212,270] The first isolations were made from suspension cultures of Burkitt tumor cells originating in African patients.[145] The Burkitt tumor or African lymphoma is discussed in Chapter 12. Cultures of tumors from the United States[446] as well as from New Guinea,[144,146] yielded the same organism as those from Africa, and this could be shown, by means

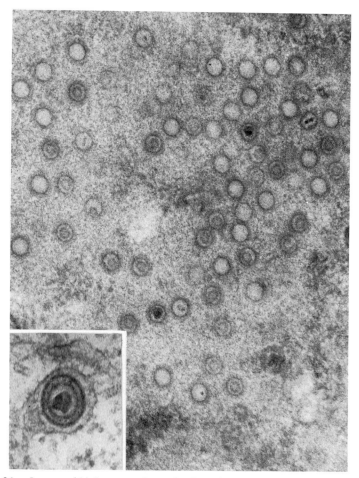

Fig. 5-21. Low- and high-power views of cultured EBV stained negatively. Electron micrographs. (Courtesy of Professor M. A. Epstein, University of Bristol.)

of electron microscopy and immunofluorescent studies, to be contained in a small minority of the cultured cells (0.3–10 percent).[141,142] The virus was at first thought to be peculiar to Burkitt's tumor, especially as it was found that, by growing normal leukocytes together with x-irradiated, nonproliferating Burkitt cells, the normal cells too could be transformed so as to become capable of indefinite growth in vitro.[269] Cultures of leukemic cells were next established, and also found at times to contain the EBV,[300,428,464] which again could transform normal cells in culture.[465,466] Finally, it was discovered that leukocytes from normal donors could be made to grow in otherwise untreated suspension cultures[211,427]; and that such cultures also contained the virus.[211,313,364] The morphology of the cells growing in all long-term cultures was similar, whether they were derived from Burkitt, leukemic or normal sources.[429,480] They were lymphoblastoid cells resembling those transformed by phytohemagglutinin (PHA),[474] with a varying proportion of more mature lymphoid cells among them. Several chromosomal abnormalities were noted, including what was at first thought to be a constant marker in a C-group chromosome[341–342,538,555]; later this was found to be inconstant and nonspecific.[289,587]

The proportion of successful long-term cultures established from the several sources was variable. Significantly, the very great majority of such cultures contained EBV, and it could be concluded that this organism has a special relationship with lymphoid cells from human sources, preferring them as a habitat, and possibly causing their multiplication in the conditions obtaining in culture. It should be noted that the EBV has not been found in monolayer cultures from hematopoietic tissues which consist mainly of fibroblasts.[117,118] However, lymphoblastoid lines could be developed from some monolayer cultures and propagated in suspensions.[34] Herpeslike virus particles were found in some such lines.[512]

Antibodies against the EBV can be detected by several techniques,[271,339–340] and at least four types have been identified in association with the presumed or definite presence of the EBV.[338] One or more of them are present in high proportions of the population in many parts of the world, their incidence rising with age. Infection with the EBV must therefore be a very common occurrence, and probably many such infections are subclinical or completely asymptomatic. Most antibody titers in random subjects are low or moderate, but in infectious mononucleosis they reach high levels. It has also been shown that infectious mononucleosis occurs only in people with no antibodies[147] or in those with very low titers.[526] When clinical symptoms develop, antibody titers rise spectacularly[273,441] and remain at an elevated level for years. Not only infectious mononucleosis patients but some of their family contacts develop EBV antibodies. These findings are extremely strong evidence in favor of a specific causal relationship of the EBV to infectious mononucleosis, although for final proof, transmission experiments may be necessary.

The exact relationship between the EBV and the Burkitt lymphoma is less clear than that between it and infectious mononucleosis. Many strains of virus have been isolated from tumor cells in culture, but not all tumors contain infectious virus. Antibodies are however present in much higher proportions of patients with Burkitt's lymphoma than of controls, both normal and those with various lymphoproliferative diseases, and the titers are much higher.[272] The only other disease with similar EBV titers is anaplastic nasopharyngeal carcinoma which contains a high proportion of lymphoid cells,[274] and in which antigens indistinguishable from those of Burkitt's lymphoma cells have been demonstrated.[113] In both Burkitt's lymphoma and nasopharyngeal carcinoma antibodies against EBV develop, with mean titers about eight times higher than those in controls, but the types and titers of antibodies vary among the cases from various sources.[338] Recently EBV DNA has been isolated from Burkitt's lymphoma which lacked infectious virus, and this provided direct evidence that even apparently virus-free Burkitt's lymphoma and nasopharyngeal cells contained masked EBV.[602,603] Thus, it is now established that EBV, either free or masked, exists in most, if not all, Burkitt lymphomas and nasopharyngeal carcinomas, but it is still not certain whether the organism is actually capable of causing the tumors: its role in vivo might still be that of a passenger rather than of an oncogen, in spite of all that is known about its "transforming" activity in vitro.

In any event, it is at present difficult to visualize the mechanism which could make the virus pathogenic in a population already heavily infected from an early age. It has been suggested that for the tumor to arise there must be previous overstimulation of the reticuloendothelial system, as by chronic malaria which is holoendemic in all tropical areas where the tumor flourishes.[73,101,445] Another possibility is a synergism between EBV and other organisms such as reovirus, type 3.[31,363–364,520]

Prolonged longitudinal observation of many children in areas with a high tumor prevalence will be needed to settle these questions.

Because several of the earliest isolations of the EBV came from patients with leukemia, a relationship between the virus and leukemia seemed possible despite the fact that the known leukemogenic viruses were all of the RNA type. Further support was lent to this theory when the organism of Marek's disease (a condition closely similar to chicken lymphomatosis) was discovered to belong to the herpes group of viruses.[83] The recently reported induction of malignant lymphoma in owl monkeys by *herpesvirus saimiri*[3] was obviously of still greater significance. It must, however, be stated that little fresh evidence has been produced in favor of a leukemogenic activity of the EBV virus. In particular, the proportion and titer of antibodies in patients with most forms of leukemia are not higher than those among normal individuals[211] though in one study the sera of patients with chronic lymphocytic leukemia were found to have a higher anti-EBV titer than those of CGL patients.[362] Such longitudinal studies as have been carried out have shown no consistent movements of antibody titers in the course of the leukemia. Our own studies on a group of 44 patients with acute leukemia have shown no unduly high titers and no consistent changes in the titers in the course of the disease (Pope, Speden, and Gunz, unpublished observations) but children with acute lymphocytic leukemia are said often to have a *lower* than normal titer.[187] Whether there could be a synergism between vertically transmitted RNA virus genomes (oncogenes) and EBV, acting as a trigger, is a question which cannot as yet be answered.

Several patients have been reported who contracted infectious mononucleosis during the course of acute leukemia and in whom antibody studies were made.[108,173,475,527] It was found in some that anti-EBV titers were absent or low during leukemia and before the onset of infectious mononucleosis, but rose sharply as symptoms and hematologic findings of infectious mononucleosis developed, and remained high thereafter. This would suggest a lack of association between the causes of acute leukemia and infectious mononucleosis, but curiously enough the supervention of infectious mononucleosis appeared to have a favorable effect on the course of the leukemia in several of the patients.[527] Taylor[543] nearly 20 years ago claimed to have produced remissions in acute leukemia by the injection of serum from patients convalescing from infectious mononucleosis, and it seems possible that some unsuspected connections between leukemia, infectious mononucleosis, and the EBV may yet be uncovered.

It must be said in summary that the role of viruses in human leukemogenesis is still conjectural. This is perhaps not surprising when it is recalled that the mouse leukemia viruses were discovered only as a result of persistent search in strains bred artificially for an extremely high-leukemia incidence. Such strains carry virus in much higher concentrations than are found in the spontaneous disease. Human leukemia occurs sporadically, and if virus is present at all, its concentration must be expected to be very low. Furthermore, some avian and murine oncogenic viruses are known to be defective and cannot be demonstrated unless rescued by helper viruses. Defectiveness has been shown in some strains of the EBV[268]; hence, possibly, oncogenic viruses in man may also need rescue. Lastly, as recently suggested by Huebner and Todaro,[291] RNA virus material could be carried in an inactive or repressed form (oncogenes) and only become evident when derepressed by one or more intrinsic or extrinsic agents. Proof of such an association would pose formidable technical problems. However, techniques in this field are advancing so fast that a solution of the virus problem, even in human leukemia, may not be very distant. Conceivably, viruses other than those currently regarded as oncogenic may be involved in human leukemogenesis. Thus, it was recently found that the leukemia and lymphoma incidence in children whose mother had had influenza during pregnancy was nine times higher than that in children without such a maternal history.[154a] Other instances of an increased leukemia incidence after exposure to nononcogenic viruses may well be discovered.

Ionizing Radiations

The ionizing radiations constitute the only group of agents which has been unequivocally shown to be able to cause leukemia in man as well as in experimental animals. Although it has been known for over 40 years that x-rays can induce leukemia,[345] it was only the development of nuclear energy which suddenly thrust this fact into the focus of medical and even of popular interest. The spectacular rise in leukemia incidence in the survivors of the atomic bombing of Hiroshima and Nagasaki gave rise to a reexamination of the effects of medically applied radiations, and soon there were reports of leukemia following in the wake of therapeutic and even of diagnostic x-irradiation. Some of these have been confirmed, while the significance of others remains doubtful. However, little light has so far been shed on a question of particular importance in the present context, namely, the role which should be attributed to radiation in the etiology of sporadic human leukemia. It is obviously not enough to say that ionizing radiations *can* cause leukemia; we need to know *under what circumstances* they do so. Unfortunately, few definitive answers are available. So long as there is doubt about the relationship between the dose of radiation administered and the response in terms of leukemia induced, we can only guess what proportion of the cases of leukemia may be radiogenic in populations which have not been exposed to any exceptional rate of irradiation.

Though the position is still in need of clarification, the trend of recent work has been to suggest that radiations do not play a major part in the causation of human leukemia. In particular, they are not alone responsible for the rise in leukemia notifications which has occurred in so many countries. From the point of view of its practical importance, it would, in fact, be permissible to deal rather briefly with the leukemogenic activity of the ionizing radiations. However, a more detailed account appears necessary in view of the great interest, if not passion, which has been aroused by this question, and of the many misleading statements which have been made and need correction. Also, the hope exists that though today the radiations constitute the only proved leukemogen, but a minor one, in man, a close study of their mode of action may lead to the prevention of at least some cases of leukemia, as well as to give us a clearer understanding of leukemogenesis as a whole.

LEUKEMIA IN ANIMALS

In 1930, Krebs, Rask-Nielsen, and Wagner[345] showed that, whereas lymphocytic leukemia occurred spontaneously in only 0.29 per 1000 white mice, after irradiation of either the whole animal or its posterior part, the incidence rose to 3.6 per 1000. Furth and Furth[184] used three strains of mice and showed an eightfold increase in the incidence of myelosis and a sevenfold increase in that of lymphosarcoma following the application of x-rays. A total body dose of 200 rad given up to six times in 20 weeks to C57 mice increased the incidence of leukemia from 7 to 30 percent.[275] The effect was more marked the younger the mice.[319] Single doses of 112 rad of x-rays or their equivalent as slow neutrons were effective in raising significantly the incidence of leukemia, both lymphocytic and granulocytic, in mice of the RF strain.[562]

In the past 20 years, radiation leukemogenesis in the mouse has been found to be an exceedingly complex process.[322,325,372,416] In addition to the size of the dose given, the rate of its administration and degree of fractionation are of importance.[418] The strain, age, and sex of the irradiated animals influence the response,[320-321,399,417] as does the presence or absence of the thymus in lymphoma,[395,396,561] and that of the spleen in granulocytic leukemia.[563] Shielding of part of the marrow during irradiation, or injections of unirradiated marrow into irradiated animals[328] reduces the number of lymphomas induced and so does the injection of cortisone.[329] On the other hand, transplantation of unirradiated thymus into thymectomized irradiated hosts causes lymphoma to arise in the graft. Factors other than the direct action of the ionizing radiations must therefore be concerned in the induction of mouse leukemia.

At least three such factors are now thought to be involved. One is the activity of leukemogenic viruses which appear to be present in all strains of laboratory mice, including those with a low spontaneous leukemia rate,[121,235] and even in germ-free lines.[316,463] Irradiation activates or triggers viruses in some lines, so that the leukemia becomes transmissible by means of cell-free extracts,[355,369] but the mechanism of this effect is still uncertain.

A second factor of importance in the mouse is the quantity of cells susceptible to the leukemogenic action of the radiation or of the virus activated by it.[129] This may be the essential variable in the experiments in which lymphoma induction was altered by removal or grafting of the thymus.

Third, radiation may interfere with the immunologic defenses and thus conceivably disturb the equilibrium between the animal host and clones of potentially malignant cells. The mode of interaction between these various factors will be considered below.

Much effort has been spent in attempts to establish a relationship between the dose of radiation administered and the size of the leukemogenic response. In view of what has been said, it would be surprising if a constant simple relationship (such as a linear one) had been found.[418] One of the chief aims of this animal work has been to find the effect of comparatively small doses, in order to obtain evidence for or against the proposition that human leukemia can be caused by low-grade irradiation. Unfortunately, this evidence is likely to be slow in forthcoming since, as pointed out by Brues[61] and by Lamerton,[352] prohibitively large numbers of animals would have to be used to obtain statistically significant results at the low levels of radiation in which interest centers.

HUMAN LEUKEMIA FOLLOWING CHRONIC EXPOSURE TO SMALL DOSES OF X-RAYS

Sixty years ago the first cases of leukemia were reported in persons who had been professionally exposed to x-rays over a number of years.[309] Since then there has been a steady procession of similar cases, with reviews, at intervals by Evans and

Roberts,[148] Rolleston,[488] Aubertin,[17] Nielson,[442] and many others. At the same time, it had been known since the early days of radiology that x-rays and radium have a destructive action on blood cells or their precursors,[263-265] though much work was required before the order of sensitivity of the various cell types could be established.[18,33,49,79,308,400] This field was reviewed by Dunlap.[128] Changes were found in the blood of early radium and x-ray workers by Amundsen,[10] Rolleston,[488] and Goodfellow,[209] and it was shown by these authors that whereas such changes were reversible in their earlier stages, they became permanent if the degree of exposure exceeded a certain level. More recently, as a result of improved working conditions, gross changes in the blood after radiation have become extremely uncommon, but subtle alterations in the morphology, chiefly of lymphocytes, are still being found where workers are carefully supervised.[267,295-296]

It has been generally assumed that radiations which damage hematopoietic tissues are capable, if long continued, of causing leukemia. Although this intuitive assumption seems reasonable, there is little evidence to back it. For instance, Martland investigated a famous group of women workers who, in the course of their occupation as painters of watch dials, had ingested huge quantities of radium and were subject to a very high rate of osteogenic sarcoma.[387] Although postmortem studies performed by Martland found bone marrow changes in which he thought "a myeloid leukemia could easily develop," there was no excess of leukemia when the whole group of 400 was followed up to 40 years later.[258] Another group of nearly 1000 individuals was given large "therapeutic" injections of radium during the postwar years. Again osteogenic sarcomas developed in a large proportion of subjects, but the leukemia incidence was not higher than expected.[519] In mice chronically irradiated with doses corresponding to those received by radiologists in the course of their work, leukemia failed to develop.[371]

Thus, there is no *direct* evidence as yet to show that those cases of leukemia which have been found in radiation workers are actually the result of the radiation received by them. By virtue of the fact that such workers usually have numerous blood counts in the course of their professional lives, a number of leukemias have been followed in them from the earliest stages to their termination.[357,379,442,585] It is, however, impossible to assert that these cases would not have developed in the absence of radiation: as in the case of heredity, the influence of chance must be excluded. In this field, as a result of large-scale statistical investigations, this has been done conclusively, and it is in this *indirect* way that the leukemogenic action of frequent small doses of ionizing radiations has been established.

By means of the analysis of large numbers of death certificates and of death notices in a medical journal, Henshaw and Hawkins found the incidence of leukemia in physicians to be 1.7 times as high as that in the general population.[276] Almost exactly the same ratio was obtained in a later analysis by Dublin and Spiegelman.[127] When these figures were further examined, it was found that this raised incidence could be almost entirely accounted for by a much higher leukemia rate among radiologists which exceeded that among nonradiological physicians nine times and was statistically highly significant.[382-384,557] Even without radiologists being included in the total, the leukemia rate among physicians was still somewhat higher than that in the general population. The reason was thought to be that many physicians other than radiologists (e.g., dermatologists), were in the habit of using and receiving considerable doses of radiation. It is interesting that in physicians the mortality from leukemia was found to be excessive within the first 5 years of their exposure to radiation,[455] a fact which strengthens the likelihood of radiation being a significant leukemogenic agent.

In recent years, the leukemia incidence among radiologists has been falling[582] (Fig. 5–22) and that among nonradiologic physicians rising, probably because the former used greater safety precautions but the latter more radiologic apparatus.[500] Even as late as 1935–1958, however, American radiologists still had 2.5 times as much leukemia as did opthalmologists.[505] It appears significant that among British radiologists there was no excess mortality from leukemia except in the group entering practice before 1921.[92] The reason for the discrepancy between the British and American experience seems to lie in the fact that adequate safety regulations were introduced in England much earlier than across the Atlantic, and only the earliest pioneers were probably working without any effective protection, and they died from leukemia more frequently than other practitioners. Between them, the reports dealing with leukemia among radiologists provide suggestive evidence in favor of the leukemogenic action of x-rays in small doses over prolonged periods. The actual

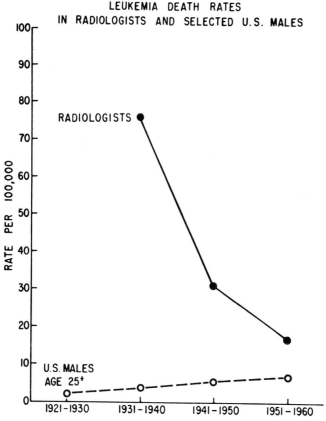

Fig. 5-22. The incidence of leukemia in radiologists compared with that of the population of the United States. Note the marked decrease in incidence among radiologists as greater precautions against overexposure have been taken. (Reproduced from Warren,[582] courtesy of the author and the publisher.)

Table 5-1

Incidence of Leukemia in the Population of the City of Hiroshima (Per 100,000 Per Year)

| Year | All City | | | A-Bomb Survivors | | | | | | | | | Nonexposed | | |
| | | | | 0–1,499 m | | | 1,500–9,999 m | | | All Exposed | | | | | |
	Cases	Population	Incidence	Cases	Population	Incidence	Cases	Population	Incidence	Cases	Population	Incidence	Cases	Population	Incidence
1946	0	171,902	0	0	11,546	0	0	79,808	0	0	91,354	0	0	80,548	0
1947	3	224,100	1.34	1	11,546	8.66	1	79,808	1.25	2	91,354	2.19	1	132,746	0.75
1948	12	246,134	4.88	6	11,546	52.00	3	79,808	3.76	9	91,354	9.85	3	154,780	1.94
1949	12	270,863	4.43	4	11,546	34.64	3	79,808	3.76	7	91,354	7.66	5	179,509	2.79
1950	8	285,712	2.80	5	11,546	43.31	1	79,808	1.25	6	91,354	6.57	2	194,358	1.03
1951	21	299,839	7.00	13	11,306	114.98	3	78,258	3.83	16	89,564	14.86	5	210,275	2.38
1952	18	311,042	5.79	10	11,095	90.13	2	77,113	2.59	12	88,208	13.60	6	222,834	2.69
1953	21	334,864	6.27	11	10,853	101.35	6	75,440	7.95	17	86,293	19.70	4	248,571	1.61
1954	15	352,648	4.25	4	10,577	37.82	6	73,929	8.12	10	84,506	11.83	5	268,142	1.86
1955	19	366,205	5.19	7	10,312	67.88	2	72,266	2.77	9	82,578	10.78	10	283,627	3.53
1956	16	378,197	4.23	2	10,072	19.86	5	70,624	7.08	7	80,696	8.67	9	297,501	3.03
1957	18	400,368	4.50	5	9,851	50.76	7	68,651	10.20	12	78,502	15.29	6	321,866	1.86
1958	22	416,840	5.28	6	9,627	62.39	2	67,027	2.98	8	76,654	10.44	14	340,186	4.12
1959	19	431,254	4.41	3	9,399	31.92	8	65,274	10.63	11	74,673	14.73	8	356,581	2.24
1960	12	443,285	2.71	1	9,170	10.80	1	63,534	1.57	2	72,704	2.75	10	370,581	2.70
1961	19	459,301	4.14	2	9,170	21.59	5	63,534	7.87	7	72,704	9.63	12	386,597	3.10
1962	15	474,357	3.16	4	9,170	43.18	5	63,534	7.87	9	72,704	1.24	6	401,653	1.49
1963	14	491,889	2.64	3	9,170	32.39	2	63,534	3.15	5	72,704	6.88	9	419,185	2.17
1964	16	507,363	3.15	1	9,170	10.80	2	63,534	3.15	3	72,704	4.13	13	434,659	2.99
1965	2	522,685	0.38	0	9,170	0	0	63,534	0	0	72,704	0	2	449,981	4.44
Total	282	7,388,858*	5.32	88	205,844*	42.75	64	1,428,825*	4.48	152	1,634,669*	9.30	130	5,754,179*	2.26

*Person—years at risk.

Based on data from the late Dr. M. Tomonaga.

doses received are discussed below. It is reassuring to know that the leukemia incidence was found to be normal in over 6000 x-ray technologists who served in the U.S. Army during World War II.[411]

LEUKEMIA IN HIROSHIMA AND NAGASAKI SINCE WORLD WAR II

The delivery of two atomic bombs at Hiroshima and Nagasaki in 1945 may be said to have constituted an experiment on an almost cosmic scale by which the leukemogenic effect of a single dose of ionizing radiation could be investigated. The results have been examined with great care and published in a series of papers from the Atomic Bomb Casualty Commission.[43-44,59,163,281,354,422,424-426,574] These clearly indicated a remarkable increase in the incidence of leukemia in the years following the bombing of the two cities. Details are shown in Tables 5-1–5-3 and in Figure 5-23.

It can be seen that an excess of leukemia was first detectable in 1948, that a peak was reached between 1950 and 1955, and that by 1965 the rate had returned to somewhere near that in Japan as a whole. There is also a clear correlation between the dose of radiation received (as shown by the subjects' distance from the hypocenter of the explosion) and the leukemia rate. In Hiroshima, those within 1000 meters at the time of the detonation had a leukemia risk over sixty times higher than those unexposed. The ratio at Nagasaki was somewhat lower, as was the dose of radiation yielded by the bomb. In neither city was the rate among those beyond 2000 meters from the hypocenter significantly higher than among the unexposed.

The radiation-induced leukemias were either of the acute or chronic granulocytic but not the chronic lymphocytic types. There was a relatively greater rise in chronic granulocytic leukemia than in acute leukemia, and the former type had a shorter induction time or latent period.[43] All forms had a shorter induction time in those most heavily irradiated than in the lightly irradiated survivors. Moreover, the youngest and oldest subjects had higher rates than the middle-aged, and it seems clear that radiation caused "a constant multiple of the natural incidence at the particular age in question, rather than a constant number of additional cases."[561]

It is of interest that preleukemic changes could be found in the blood for many months before the onset of symptoms in patients who had been under regular supervision (Figs. 5-24 and 5-25).[425] Twenty years after the detonation, on the other hand, the marrows of apparently healthy survivors were normal and showed no chromosomal changes.[318] Besides leukemia, an increase in myelofibrosis and possibly some lymphomas occurred in the atom bomb survivors,[14] and in recent years a probable rise in some solid cancers has been noted.[301] It was of great interest that the leukemia rate was not significantly increased in children who had been irradiated while in utero,[302] for this finding conflicted with that of Stewart and her collaborators in children receiving intrauterine diagnostic radiation (see below).

DEVELOPMENT OF LEUKEMIA FOLLOWING EXPOSURE TO MEDICAL RADIATIONS

In 1955, it was reported[90,566] that among patients with ankylosing spondylitis treated by radiotherapy there were numbers of cases of leukemia almost certainly in excess of those in the general population. Ankylosing spondylitis, a relatively common condition in Europe, was treated in many centers by large-field application of x-

Table 5-2

Incidence of Leukemia in the Population of the City of Nagasaki (Per 100,000 Per Year)

| | All City | | | A-Bomb Survivors | | | | | | | | | Nonexposed | | |
| | | | | 0-1,499 m | | | 1,500-9,999 m | | | All Exposed | | | | | |
Year	Cases	Popula-tion	Inci-dence	Cases	Popula-tion	Inci-dence	Cases	Popula-tion	Inci-dence	Cases	Popula-tion	Inci-dence	Cases	Popula-tion	Inci-dence
1946	2	186,119	1.13	0	4,100	0	2	88,000	2.27	2	92,100	2.22	0	94,109	0
1947	6	195,174	3.03	2	4,100	48.78	3	87,000	3.45	5	91,100	5.49	1	104,074	0.96
1948	4	213,698	1.88	2	4,000	50.00	0	87,000	0	2	91,000	2.20	2	122,698	1.63
1949	4	229,823	1.75	1	3,904	25.61	1	86,036	1.16	2	89,940	2.22	2	139,883	1.43
1950	13	241,805	5.38	4	3,904	102.46	5	86,036	5.81	9	89,940	10.01	4	151,865	2.63
1951	9	258,392	3.48	3	3,763	79.72	4	84,293	4.75	7	88,056	7.95	2	170,336	1.17
1952	10	266,374	3.74	4	3,664	109.17	4	82,695	4.84	8	86,359	9.26	2	180,015	1.11
1953	5	274,809	1.83	2	3,586	55.78	2	80,612	2.48	4	84,198	4.75	1	190,611	0.52
1954	9	281,192	3.20	1	3,490	28.66	6	79,272	7.57	7	82,762	8.46	2	198,430	1.01
1955	12	305,891	3.93	1	3,408	29.34	7	77,607	9.02	8	81,015	9.87	4	224,876	1.78
1956	9	312,886	2.88	1	2,968	33.69	3	75,960	3.95	4	78,928	5.07	5	233,958	2.14
1957	12	321,827	3.73	1	2,718	36.79	7	75,000	9.33	8	77,718	10.29	4	244,109	1.64
1958	13	331,080	3.92	3	2,600	115.38	3	74,000	4.05	6	76,600	7.83	7	254,480	2.75
1959	9	336,741	2.67	1	2,500	40.00	4	73,000	5.48	5	75,500	6.62	4	261,241	1.53
1960	14	345,335	4.05	1	2,400	41.67	4	72,000	5.56	5	74,400	6.72	9	270,935	3.32
1961	18	350,230	5.14	0	2,300	0	6	72,000	8.33	6	74,300	8.08	12	275,930	4.35
1962	7	376,048	1.86	0	2,200	0	1	71,000	1.41	1	73,200	1.37	6	302,848	1.98
1963	15	395,652	3.79	1	2,100	47.62	1	70,000	1.43	2	72,100	2.77	13	323,552	4.02
1964	15	399,258	3.77	0	2,000	0	2	69,000	2.90	2	71,000	2.84	13	328,258	3.96
1965	18	407,686	4.42	1	1,900	52.63	4	68,000	5.88	5	69,900	7.15	13	337,786	3.85
Total	204	6,030,020*	3.38	29	61,605*	47.04	69	1,558,511*	4.43	98	1,620,116*	6.05	106	4,409,904*	2.40

*Person—years at risk.

Based on data from the late Dr. M. Tomonaga.

Table 5-3

Summary of Incidence of Leukemia in Residents of Hiroshima and Nagasaki, by Distance from Hypocenter (1945-1965)

Exposure Distance (m)	Hiroshima			Nagasaki		
	Person Years at Risk	*Cases*	*Incidence**	*Person Years at Risk*	*Cases*	*Incidence**
0– 999	21,475	28	130.4	8,309	6	72.2
1000–1499	184,369	60	32.5	57,603	23	39.9
1500–1999	319,208	20	6.3	69,380	6	8.6
2000 and over	1,109,615	44	4.0	1,485,669	63	4.2
Total						
Exposed	1,634,669	152	9.3	1,620,961	98	6.0
Nonexposed	5,754,179	131	2.3	4,409,904	106	2.4

*Incidence per 100,000 population per year.
Based on data from the late Dr. M. Tomonaga.

rays to the back and joints, the total dose amounting in individuals up to 12,000 R or more, given over periods of months or years.[566] The findings with respect to leukemia were so arresting that a large-scale investigation was set in train by the Medical Research Council in England. An extensive report of its results was published in 1957.[91] This report recorded that among 13,352 patients presumed to have ankylosing spondylitis who were given x-rays for this condition, there were 37 with leukemia or probable leukemia. In these, the disease followed the irradiation within a period of some years, the average being six. Most of the cases were chronic

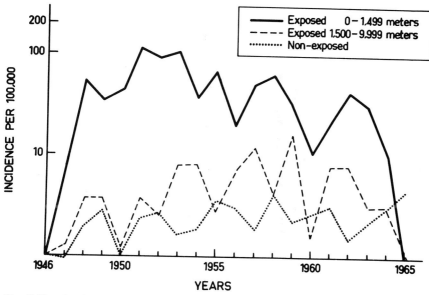

Fig. 5-23. Leukemia incidence in Hiroshima 1946–1965. Comparative incidence among exposed and nonexposed population. (Drawn from figures kindly supplied by the late Dr. M. Tomonaga.)

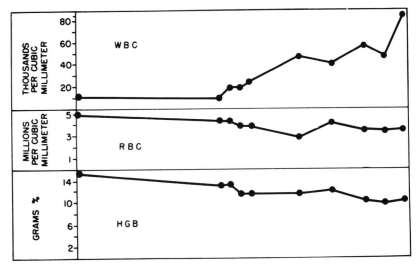

Fig. 5-24. Changes in white blood cell count, red blood cell count, and hemoglobin levels over a period of 32 months in a case of chronic granulocytic leukemia. (Reproduced from Moloney and Lange,[426] courtesy of the publisher.)

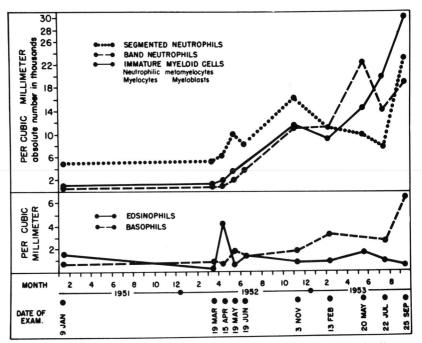

Fig. 5-25. Same patient as in Figure 5-24. Absolute numbers of myeloid cells over a period of 32 months. (Reproduced from Moloney and Lange,[426] courtesy of the publisher.)

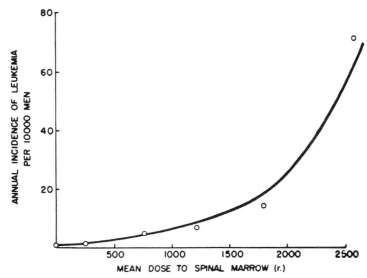

Fig. 5-26. The incidence of leukemia standardized for age, in relation to the mean dose of radiation to the spinal marrow. (Reproduced from Court Brown and Doll,[91] courtesy of the Controller of H. M. Stationery Office.)

granulocytic or acute in type; only one was chronic lymphocytic, and in this the diagnosis was later queried.[93] The expected number of leukemias in a group of the general population of similar size and age distribution was 2.9, so that there was a highly significant rise in the leukemia incidence in the irradiated group.

A further report included some additional patients and extended the total time of follow-up to 5–25 years.[93] There were then 52 cases of leukemia, against an expected number of 5.48, a ratio of 9.5:1. In addition, several aplastic anemias were probably leukemias. Although there may be a mildly increased leukemia rate in patients with spondylitis who have not been irradiated,[2] it seems clear that all, or nearly all the "excess" cases of leukemia occurring in the treated spondylitics were induced by radiation. A clearcut dose-relationship (Fig. 5-26) makes this conclusion inescapable. As in Japan, the risk of leukemia being caused depended on the patient's age. For a given exposure, at least five times as many cases were induced among the elderly than within the younger groups.

The British work on the role of irradiation in spoldylitis has been confirmed by a number of other authors[217,509] and constitutes the best documented pointer to the leukemogenic activity of therapeutic radiations. Other investigations have produced confirmatory results. Thus, excessive numbers of leukemia cases were found in children whose thymus was irradiated during infancy.[434,511] In such material it obviously is difficult to exclude from the analysis children irradiated for thymic enlargement, which might itself have been due to early leukemia, and Simpson's results have, in fact, not been fully confirmed by others.[87,356,493,515,553] The development of leukemia following other forms of radiotherapy has been reported in a few cases,[241,423,469] but leukemia incidence was probably not excessive in several large groups of women irradiated for the treatment of cancer of the cervix.[293,510,599] In Israel, large numbers of immigrant children from Afro-Asian countries were, during 1949–1958, treated for ringworm of the scalp by means of epilating doses of x-rays averaging 450 r in divided doses. A disproportionate rise in the leukemia mortality of Israeli children originating in Afro-Asian countries during 9 years has been thought to be connected with this large-scale radiotherapy.[107]

Although a number of cases of leukemia have followed the administration of ^{131}I for the treatment of hyperthyroidism,[96] statistical evidence does not suggest that they were excessive compared with the number expected.[461,494] However, there may be an association between the disease, thyrotoxicosis itself, and an increased incidence of leukemia.[494]

There is no good statistical evidence to show that diagnostic x-irradiation, except when given in gross excess,[193a,241] is leukemogenic in adults.[53,149,150,438-439,571] Theoretical considerations suggest that doses received by average members of a population, such as that in England, could at worst increase the risk of contracting leukemia by some two chances per million per year over that of 50-60 per million experienced by those who have no x-ray examinations, if, in fact, such irradiation has any leukemogenic effect.[391]

The situation may be different in children under 10, for the work of Stewart[530-531,533-534] has shown an increased risk of leukemia in the offspring of women undergoing diagnostic irradiation of the abdomen during pregnancy, most commonly in the third trimester. The leukemia incidence increases with the size of the dose, as measured by the number of films used.[532] There has been some debate on the absolute size of the risk,[94,165,218,302,323,366,434,462] but in the most extensive study reported[374] it was calculated to be about 40 percent in excess of the expected rate. Reductions in the dosage used during diagnostic radiation could decrease the risk considerably,[532] but for the time being it must be accepted that diagnostic radiations during pregnancy carry a definite chance of causing leukemia in the child, probably because of increased radiosensitivity of the fetal tissues.[559] Whether irradiation of the mother before conception increases the likelihood of leukemia in subsequently born children is still controversial.[200,288,409]

THE RISK OF PRODUCING LEUKEMIA BY IONIZING RADIATIONS

During the past 25 years enough evidence has been produced to establish the fact that ionizing radiations can cause leukemia in human beings. We must now discuss the practical meaning of this statement. We need to ask how many sporadic cases of leukemia are caused by radiations and how far the action of radiations can account for the almost universal rise in the recorded leukemia incidence. These questions have been the subject of a spirited and, so far, inconclusive debate. No final answers have yet been forthcoming because there is an unsolved fundamental problem at the bottom of the controversy: namely, the minimum size of the dose of radiation which may be expected to be leukemogenic. In those instances in which radiation had most clearly caused the disease, the doses received by the victims were obviously quite large—that is, they were almost without exception in the range of several hundred rads. There are also probably large numbers of unrecorded, albeit rather poorly documented cases of leukemia in which there is a strong history of x-ray therapy, usually for neoplastic disease.[96] The question is whether doses below 100 rads can still cause leukemia, and if, in fact, there is a threshold dose of radiation below which there is no danger.

Little information is available on this point. Estimates of the life-time doses received by American radiologists, before the adoption of present-day precautions, vary from 1000 R[580] to 2000 R.[57] The doses received by those exposed to the atomic bombs are even now not precisely known in spite of a huge effort; they range from about 100 r upward according to the victim's position in relation to the hypocenter and to other factors.[281,574] Only one of the British spondylitics developing leukemia had been given less than 450 R to the spinal marrow, while most of the doses were much higher (Fig. 5-26).[91] The single exception, in which there was a possibility that leukemia might have been caused by low doses of x-rays, was Stewart's series of children who had been given intrauterine irradiation. Even here, it has been calculated that at least in some cases, doses in the known leukemogenic range must have been received by the fetuses.[242] Patients treated for hyperthyroidism with multiple courses of ^{131}I may receive blood doses up to 160 rads with an estimated marrow dose of 80 percent of that in the blood,[220] but so far have shown no excess of leukemia.[494]

The results of Court Brown and Doll,[91] as well as the figures from Hiroshima[59] suggested that at dose levels above 100 rads there is a linear relationship between the dose of radiation administered and the response in terms of numbers developing leukemia. Over at least the range of 100–900 rads the rate of increase with dose, as determined from the Japanese and British experiences, is of the order of one to two cases per year per rad per million exposed individuals. Below the level of 100 rads there is insufficient knowledge to be certain about the shape of the dose-response curve[96,281,560] although Lewis,[366] among others, claimed that there was an overall linear dose response and an absence of a threshold of radiation leukemogenesis. This conclusion has been strongly attacked[61,333,352] as being unjustified on the strength of present-day knowledge about the effect of low doses of radiation, and as being, in fact, unlikely. Animal experiments[417,418] have not yet produced a clear answer to the low dosage problem, except for showing that, not only the dose of radiation, but also the mode of its administration is important in influencing the degree of response (see above). Nothing like the number of human beings necessary for statistically valid results have been or are likely to be examined.[65] The question concerning the leukemogenic effect of small doses of radiation thus remains open, although Stewart's work suggests that the risk of leukemia per unit dose may be several times higher in the fetus in utero than in adults. Many competent observers still consider that a threshold may exist at a dose level of 50–100 rads for adults,[581] and that smaller doses are unlikely to be leukemogenic. It is, moreover, becoming clear that the risk of developing leukemia following radiation does not persist indefinitely through the subject's remaining lifespan. It declines perceptibly after about 6 years, becomes much diminished after 10 years, and is probably quite low after about 15 years.[84,96]

Clearly, it is impossible at this stage to say what proportion of sporadic leukemias may be radiation-induced. An upper limit may be set by adopting Lewis's pessimistic assumptions on the mode of action of radiation, namely, that there is full linearity and no threshold, that the dose alone determines the response, and that the effect of any given dose continues indefinitely.[366] With these assumptions, 10 percent of all leukemias might be caused by natural background and another 10 percent by man-made radiation. On the other hand, other types of dose-response relationships might be envisaged, such as the quadratic one proposed by Burch. This would yield fewer than 1 percent of radiation-induced leukemias. Even the higher figure would be quite insufficient to account by itself for the rise in leukemia mortality during the first half of the century.[75,386,592] Much of what is now known about the complexities of radiation leukemogenesis in laboratory animals (see above) would tend to speak against a simple linear dose response.

We may now summarize what is known about the relationship of human leukemia to ionizing radiation. That radiation can cause and has caused leukemia is unquestionable. Some hundreds of reasonably well-authenticated cases were known to have followed the administration of moderately large or large quantities of radiation given either as single or fractionated doses to the whole body, or to large parts of the body. The evidence for these statements is contained in a number of official publications,[389-391, 435-436, 558-559] as well as in numerous research papers. Whether small doses of radiation can cause leukemia is, however, doubtful, and no definite answer can be given so long as it is unknown if there is a threshold to radiation leukemogenesis. In ordinary peacetime circumstances, medical radiations represent the only form of ionizing radiation which is capable of being leukemogenic. Of these, the relatively heavy doses used in radiotherapy have the greatest chance of producing leukemia, but the risk is small when compared to the great capacity of this form of treatment for relieving the symptoms of grave disease and for prolonging life. No firm evidence exists to show that diagnostic radiology, except when applied during fetal life, has caused leukemia, although in exceptional conditions, patients have received doses of diagnostic radiation comparable to those used in radiotherapy. There is nothing to indicate that the extremely small quantities of radiation so far provided by nonmedical sources (fallout) are leukemogenic.[85]

In the etiology of leukemia, radiation undoubtedly plays a part, but it is likely to be a small one. Even the most pessimistic estimates have produced no support for the suggestion that a rise in the population exposure to radiation can account for the rise in leukemia incidence which has taken place in large parts of the world in past years. Direct investigations of case histories have made it seem likely that not more than one leukemia patient in 20 has ever been exposed to significant doses of radiation in the past.[241]

Chemical Leukemogens

Chemicals have for long been suspected of being leukemogenic. Because so many substances are known to be myelotoxic, it was natural to assume that anything which is capable of injuring the marrow might also produce a neoplastic change in it. From this standpoint, an almost limitless list of candidates could be established, beginning with the early agents used for leukemia therapy (arsenic, benzene, etc.) and proceeding via the sulphonamides and antibiotics to practically any of the multitude of chemotherapeutic drugs introduced during the past 20 years. Results in the exploration of this vast field of potential leukemogens have been meager, the very multiplicity of substances forming a serious obstacle to their statistical evaluation.

Even now benzene is the only serious contender for the status of an accepted leukemogen. There is little question that cases of leukemia—mainly acute—have occurred more frequently in persons with a history of heavy occupational exposure to benzene or its congener toluol than among the general population.[37,201,292,448,565] The occupations chiefly affected are leather and shoe manufacture which use glues containing benzene,[44] drycleaning, rotogravure printing in which some inks might contain up to 40 percent benzene, and spray-painting where benzene-containing solvents are employed.[569]

Exposure in all known cases was prolonged and heavy, few precautions having been employed—the victims usually came from small workshops or home industries. Nearly always the leukemia was preceded by some years during which various blood abnormalities were noted (preleukemia).[205] Marrow depression is a much more common sequel of benzene poisoning than leukemia (five to six times),[569] and it seems likely that leukemia arises in a small proportion of damaged marrows, perhaps in the presence of other leukemogenic factors.

The other putative leukemogens, which have made their appearance in the literature, have generally reflected the therapeutic fashions of the day. Because of their ubiquity, the sulphonamides and antibiotics have often been suspected, but the few statistically acceptable studies[2,534] have failed to provide confirmation. Two substances, chloramphenicol and phenylbutazone, have been most frequently incriminated because of the ease with which they can cause marrow damage, and a number of well-documented cases are known in which leukemia followed the administration of one or the other of the two.[27,58,125,593] In a few of these the leukemia was preceded by a period of marrow depression, with or without an apparent temporary recovery,[58,250,593] and it is here that the strongest evidence for the causal relationship between the drug and the disease is found, analogous to that in the case of benzol or radiation leukemia. Statistical evaluation of the incidence of leukemia among patients having adverse drug reactions has so far produced only equivocal results.[170]

Very recently a new kind of association between chemotherapeutic agents and leukemogenesis has moved into the center of interest. It was noted that since Waldenström introduced melphalan as a treatment for myelomatosis in 1964,[576] acute leukemia had occurred in a number of patients so treated. Andersen and Videbaek,[11] and Kyle et al.[349] have each reported four cases, and we have seen another ourselves. Similarly, acute leukemia has followed the use of triethylenethiophosphoramide (thio-TEPA) in carcinoma,[6,196,514] and of chlorambucil in lymphomas.[80,164] These drugs are known to be immunosuppressive and carcinogenic in experimental animals, and the sudden spate of cases raised a strong suspicion that they may be leukemogenic in man. Although the risk may be small, it should be considered when alkylating agents are used in the therapy of nonmalignant conditions.

Other chemical agents—whether of pharmaceutic, industrial, or other origin—should certainly not be regarded as above suspicion, for among the many varieties capable of damaging the bone marrow there may well be several which could cause leukemia. However, their investigation, in the presence of many other pollutants of the environment, is bound to be an extremely complex undertaking, and no quick results can be expected.

Summary

Although much remains to be learned about the etiology of human leukemia—some would say nearly everything—progress has been made in the past few years. In spite of profound biologic differences, the laboratory mouse has become a useful

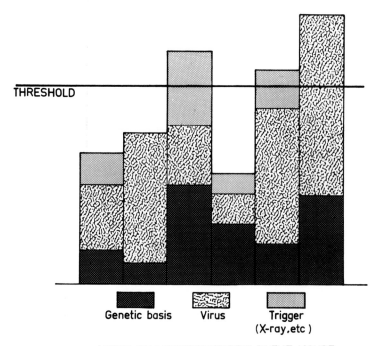

THRESHOLD

Genetic basis   Virus   Trigger
(X-ray,etc)

MODEL OF LEUKEMOGENESIS IN THE MOUSE

Fig. 5–27. Model of leukemogenesis in the mouse with genetic factors and extrinsic leukemogens interacting. Each column represents a hypothetic strain of mice. When the combined factors exceed the threshold, leukemia develops.

model for the human situation, for it demonstrates clearly the interplay between genetic, intrinsic, and extrinsic factors in the causation of leukemia (see Fig. 5-27). Most of the leukemogenic factors now known to be active in the experimental model have been recognized as significant in the etiology of human leukemia. In particular, the influence of the genetic predisposition has become more clearly understood, and that of the individual's immunologic reactivity can at last be investigated. The possible role of viruses remains to be elucidated.

Mathematical models of leukemogenesis have been constructed, and provide at least glimpses of theoretical possibilities. There are few doubts left that this is a multistage process, basically a series of damaging encounters between leukemogenic agents and genetic material which is in varying degree predisposed toward oncogenesis. A wise choice of ancestors may perhaps be as important in the prophylaxis of leukemia as it is in that of coronary disease.

The nature of leukemogens and the ways in which they act are likely to differ in the different types of leukemia. Thus, radiation is important (we do not know how important) in chronic granulocytic and in acute leukemias but not in the chronic lymphocytic variety in which the activity of genetic factors can be most clearly recognized. Chronic lymphocytic leukemia is also closely associated with immunologic factors, as observed both in vivo and in vitro. This will be discussed in greater detail in Chapter 12. The interaction of the immunologic constitution and of leukemia viruses is an exciting new experimental concept.[392,501] This may conceivably be of practical importance, as in two cases of acute leukemia treated by marrow transplantation in which the transplanted cells assumed leukemic properties.[156a,546a]

Many factors must be concerned in human leukemogenesis, besides the main groups which have been discussed. Some are known, but their mode of action is uncertain. It has been established, for instance, that women who have had stillbirths or abortions (fetal wastage) have an increased expectation of producing children who will get leukemia,[200] but the relationship between these two statistics must be complex. Similarly, children with leukemia often have histories of severe infections some time before the onset of the disease. Do such infections assist in the causation of leukemia or are they a consequence of the blood disease? Are the antibiotics used in the treatment of infections perhaps themselves leukemogenic in suitable hosts? More widely, is the virtual conquest of fatal infectious disease in childhood partly responsible for increased numbers of leukemias by permitting those to survive, and to get leukemia, who would have formerly died from pneumonia?[528]

Progress in research on the etiology of human leukemia appears to be accelerating. Further epidemiologic and statistical studies are likely to produce results which will supplement those now coming from the experimental laboratory. Although problems are still plentiful, the right questions may by now have been asked, and this surely encourages the expectation that solutions will eventually be found in man, as they have been in the mouse.

REFERENCES

1. Abbatt JD, Lea AJ: The incidence of leukaemia in ankylosing spondylitis treated with x-rays. Lancet 2:1317, 1956.

2. _____, Lea AJ: Leukaemogens. Lancet 2:880, 1958.

3. Ablashi DV, Loeb WF, Valerio MG, Adamson RH, Armstrong GR, Bennett DG, Heine U: Malignant lymphomas with lymphocytic leukaemia induced in owl monkeys by "herpesvirus saimiri." J Natl Cancer Inst 47:837, 1971.

4. Aksoy M, Dincol K, Erdem SA, Dincol G: Acute leukemia due to chronic exposure to benzene. Am J Med 52:160, 1972.

5. Aleksandrowicz J: Considérations sur la pathogénèse de la leucémie myéloblastique à la lumière des recherches sur la granulocytolise. Proceedings of the Third International Congress of the International Society of Hematology. New York, Grune & Stratton, 1950, p 245.

6. Allan WS: Acute myeloid leukaemia after treatment with cytostatic agents. Lancet 2:775, 1970.

7. Almeida JD, Hasselback, RC, Harn AW: Virus-like particles in blood of two acute leukemia patients. Science 142:1487, 1963.

8. Amiotti, PL: Sulla incidenza sei tumori nei familiari di bambini leucemici. Minerva Pediatr 5:449, 1953.

9. Amos DA, Wellman WE, Bowie, EJW, Linman JW: Acute leukemia in a husband and wife. Mayo Clin Proc 42:468, 1967.

10. Amundsen P: Blood anomalies in radiologists and in persons employed in radiological service. Acta Radiol 3:1, 1924.

11. Andersen E, Videbaek A: Stem cell leukaemia in myelomatosis. Scand J Haematol 7:201, 1970.

12. Anderson RC: Familial leukemia. A report of leukemia in five siblings with a brief review of the genetic aspects of this disease. Am J Dis Child 81:313, 1951.

13. _____, Herrmann HW: Leukemia in twin children. JAMA 158:652, 1955.

14. Anderson RE, Ishida K: Malignant lymphoma in survivors of the atomic bomb in Hiroshima. Ann Intern Med 61:853, 1964.

15. Ardashnikov, SN: The genetics of leukaemia in man. J Hyg 37:286, 1937.

16. Arnoult J, Haguenau F: Problems raised by the search for virus particles in human leukemia. A study with the electron microscope of blood plasma, cerebrospinal fluid and megakaryocytes from bone marrow. J Natl Cancer Inst 36:1089, 1966.

17. Aubertin C: Leucémie myéloide chez les radiologistes. Bull Off Soc F Electrothér Radiol 40:218, 1931.

18. _____, Beaujard E: Action des rayons X sur le sang et les organes hématopoiétiques. C R Soc Biol 58:217, 1905.

19. Bach ML, Bach FH, Joo P: Leukemia-associated antigens in the mixed leukocyte culture test. Science 166:1520, 1969.

20. Baikie AG: Chromosomes and leukaemia. Acta Haematol 36:157, 1966.

21. _____, Buckton KE, Court Brown WM, Harnden DG: Two cases of leukaemia and a case of sex-chromosome abnormality in the same sibship. Lancet 2:1003, 1961.

22. _____, Garson OM, Spiers ASD, Ferguson J: Cytogenetic studies in familial leukaemias. Aust Ann Med 18:7, 1969.

23. Baltimore D: RNA-dependent DNA polymerase in virions of RNA tumour viruses. Nature 226:1209, 1970.

24. Barber R, Spiers P: Oxford survey of childhood cancers; progress report 11. Monthly Bull Ministry of Health 23:46, 1964.

25. Barbier J, Guillermet J, Morel P: Deux leucémies aiguës successives dans la même famille. Lyon Med 182:379, 1949.

26. Bauke J: Chronic myelocytic leukemia. Chromosome studies of a patient and his nonleukemic identical twin. Cancer 24:643, 1969.

27. Bean RHD: Phenylbutazone and leukaemia. A possible association. Br Med J 2:1552, 1960.

28. Beard JW: Etiology of avian leukosis. Ann NY Acad Sci 68:473, 1957.

29. _____: Isolation and identification of tumor viruses. Tex Rep Biol Med 15:627, 1957.

30. _____: Physical methods for the analysis of cells. Ann NY Acad Sci 69:530, 1957.

31. Bell TM, Massie A, Ross MGR, Williams MC: Isolation of reovirus from a case of Burkitt's lymphoma. Br Med J 1:1212, 1964.

32. Bendixen HJ: Epidemiological studies of bovine leukosis in Denmark. Proc Roy Soc Med 59:657, 1966.

33. Benjamin E, Von Reuss A, Sluka E, Schwartz G: Beiträge zur Frage der Einwirkung der Röntgenstrahlen auf das Blut. Wien Klin Wochenschr 19:788, 1906.

34. Benyesh-Melnik M, Fernbach DJ, Dessy S, Lewis RT: Studies on acute leukemia and infectious mononucleosis of childhood. III. Incidence of spontaneous lymphoblastoid transformation in bone marrow cultures. J Natl Cancer Inst 40:111, 1968.

35. Berenblum I, Trainin M: Possible two-stage mechanism in experimental leukemogenesis. Science 132:40, 1960.

36. Berman L: Malignant lymphomas. Their classification and relation to leukemia. Blood 8:195, 1953.

37. Bernard J, Braïer L: Les leucoses benzéniques. Proceedings of the Third International Congress of the International Society Hematology. New York, Grune & Stratton, 1951, p 251.

38. _____, Jacquillat Cl, Chavelet F, Boiron M, Stoitchkov Y, Tanzer J: Leucémie aiguë d'une enfant de 5 mois née d'une mère atteinte de leucémie aiguë au moment de l'accouchement. Nouv Rev Fr Hématol 4:140, 1964.

39. Bernhard WG, Gore I, Kilby RA: Congenital leukemia. Blood 6:990, 1951.

40. Beyers MR, Meyer LM, Lowenthal M, Oehrig RJ, Sawitsky A: Hypocellular marrow in acute leukemia. Report of two cases. Arch Intern Med 88:803, 1951.

41. Bieber A: Sopra un caso di emopatia (leucemia linfatica) in una coppia di gemelli bicori (falsi gemelli). Riv Clin Pediatr 49:161, 1951.

42. Bierman HR, Byron RL, Kelly KH, Dod KS, Black PM: Studies on cross circulation in man. I. Methods and clinical changes. Blood 6:487, 1957.

43. Bizzozzero OJ Jr, Johnson KG, Ciocco A: Radiation-related leukemia in Hiroshima and Nagasaki, 1946–64. I. Distribution, incidence and appearance time. N Engl J Med 274:1095, 1966.

44. _____, Johnson KG, Ciocco A, Kawasaki S, Toyoda S: Radiation-related leukemia in Hiroshima and Nagasaki, 1946–64. II. Observations on type-specific leukemia, survivorship and clinical behavior. Ann Intern Med 66:522, 1967.

45. Black AB, Meynell MJ: Aleukaemic myeloid leukaemia presenting as aplastic anaemia. Br Med J 1:1430, 1951.

46. Black PH: Recent advances in the study of oncogenic viruses. N Engl J Med 275:377, 1966.

47. Block M, Jacobson LO, Bethard WF: Preleukemic acute human leukemia. JAMA 152:1018, 1953.

48. Bloom GE, Warner S, Gerald PS, Diamond LK: Chromosome abnormalities in constitutional aplastic anemia. N Engl J Med 274:8, 1966.

49. Bloom MA, Bloom W: The radiosensitivity of erythroblasts. J Lab Clin Med 32:654, 1947.

50. Boggian B: Considerazioni sopra due case di leucemia familiare. Policlinico (Prat) 45:472, 1938.

51. Borges WH, Nicklas JW, Hamm CW: Prezygotic determinants in acute leukemia. J Pediatr 70:180, 1967.

52. Bottomley RH, Trainer AL, Condit PT: Chromosome studies in a "cancer family." Cancer 28:519, 1971.

53. Bousser J, Brousseau C, Christol D: Les antécédents d'exposition aux radiations ionisantes chez les sujets atteints de leucose. Sang 30:154, 1959.

54. Boveri T: The Origin of Malignant Tumors. Baltimore, Williams & Wilkins, 1929.

55. Bowie W: Report of leukaemia occurring in father and daughter. Can Med Assoc J 78:259, 1958.

56. Bradley TR, Metcalf D: The growth of mouse bone marrow cells *in vitro*. Aust J Exp Biol Med Sci 44:287, 1966.

57. Braestrup CB: Past and present radiation exposure to radiologists from the point of view of life expectancy. Am J Roentgenol Radium Therap Nucl Med 78:998, 1957.

58. Brauer MJ, Dameshek W: Hypoplastic anemia and myeloblastic leukemia following chloramphenicol therapy. N Engl J Med 277:1003, 1967.

59. Brill AB, Tomonaga M, Heyssel RM: Leukemia in man following exposure to ionising radiation. Ann Intern Med 56:590, 1962.

60. Brown CH, Carbone PP: In vitro growth of normal and leukemic human bone marrow. J Natl Cancer Inst 46:989, 1971.

61. Brues AM: Critique of the linear theory of carcinogenesis. Science 128:693, 1958.

62. Bryan WR: A reconsideration of the nature of the neoplastic reaction in the light of recent advances in cancer research. J Natl Cancer Inst 24:221, 1960.

63. ———: The viral study of leukemia and related neoplastic diseases: a problem apart, in Dameshek W and Dutcher RM (eds): Perspectives in Leukemia. New York, Grune & Stratton, 1968, p 94.

64. ———: Rationale for virus research in human leukemia, in Zarafonetis CJD (ed): Proceedings of the International Conference on Leukemia-Lymphoma. Philadelphia, Lea & Febiger, 1968, p 73.

65. Buck C: Population size required for investigating threshold doses in radiation-induced leukemia. Science 129:1357, 1959.

66. Buckton KE, Harnden DG, Baikie AG, Woods GE: Mongolism and leukaemia in the same sibship. Lancet 1:171, 1961.

67. Burch PRJ: Radiation carcinogenesis: A new hypothesis. Nature 185:135, 1960.

68. ———: A biological principle and its converse: some implications for carcinogenesis. Nature 195:241, 1962.

69. ———: Carcinogenesis and cancer prevention. Nature 197:1145, 1963.

70. ———: Human cancer: Mendelian inheritance or vertical transmission? Nature 197:1042, 1963.

71. ———: Leukemogenesis in man. Ann NY Acad Sci 114:213, 1964.

72. Burger CL, Harris WW, Anderson NG, Bartlett TW, Knisely RM: Virus-like particles in human leukemic plasma. Proc Soc Exp Biol Med 115:151, 1964.

73. Burkitt DP: Etiology of Burkitt's lymphoma—an alternative hypothesis to a vectored virus. J Natl Cancer Inst 42:19, 1969.

74. Burnet FM: Leukemia as a problem in preventive medicine. N Engl J Med 259:423, 1958.

75. ———: The clonal selection theory of acquired immunity. Nashville, Vanderbilt University Press, 1959.

76. ———: Somatic mutation and chronic disease. Br Med J: 1:338, 1965.

77. Busk Th: Some observations on heredity in breast cancer and leukaemia. Ann Eugenics 14:213, 1948.

78. Campbell WAB, Macafee AL, Wade WG: Familial neonatal leukaemia. Arch Dis Child 37:93, 1962.

79. Casati A: Experimentelle Untersuchungen über die Röntgenwirkung auf das Knochenmark. Strahlentherapie 32:721, 1929.

80. Catovsky D, Galton DAG: Myelomonocytic leukaemia supervening on chronic lymphocytic leukaemia. Lancet 1:478, 1971.

81. Chapman AL, Bopp WJ, Brightwell AS, Cohen H, Nidsen AH, Gravelle CR, Werder AA: Preliminary report on virus-like particles in canine leukemia-derived cell cultures. Cancer Res 27:18, 1967.

82. Chen WY, Crittenden LB, Mantel N, Cameron WR: Site distribution of cancer deaths in husband-wife and sibling pairs. J Nat Cancer Inst 27:875, 1961.

83. Churchill AE, Biggs PM: Agent of Marek's disease in tissue culture. Nature 215:528, 1967.

84. Cobb S, Miller M, Wald N: On the estimation of the incubation period in malignant disease. J Chron Dis 9:385, 1959.

85. Conard RA, Hicking A: Medical findings in Marshallese people exposed to fallout radiation. JAMA 192: 457, 1965.

86. Conen PE, Erkman B: Combined

mongolism and leukemia. Report of eight cases with chromosome studies. Am J Dis Child 112:429, 1966.

87. Conti EA, Patton GD, Conti JE, Hempelmann LH: Present health of children given x-ray treatment of the anterior mediastinum in infancy. Radiology 74:386, 1960.

88. Cooke JV: Acute leukemia in children. JAMA 101:432, 1933.

89. _____: The incidence of acute leukemia in children. JAMA 119:547, 1942.

90. Court Brown WM, Abbatt JD: The incidence of leukaemia in ankylosing spondylitis treated with x-rays. A preliminary report. Lancet 1:1283, 1955.

91. _____, Doll R: Leukaemia and Aplastic Anaemia in Patients Irradiated for Ankylosing Spondylitis. London, Her Majesty's Stationery Office, 1957.

92. _____, _____: Expectation of life and mortality from cancer among British radiologists. Br Med J 2:181, 1958.

93. _____, _____: Mortality from cancer and other causes after radiotherapy for ankylosing spondylitis. Br Med J 2:1327, 1965.

94. _____, _____, Hill AB: Incidence of leukaemia after exposure to diagnostic radiation in utero. Br Med J 2:1539, 1960.

95. Crittenden LB: An interpretation of familial aggregation based on multiple genetic and environmental factors. Ann NY Acad Sci 91:764, 1961.

96. Cronkite EP, Moloney W, Bond VP: Radiation leukemogenesis. An analysis of the problem. Am J Med 28:673, 1960.

97. Crossen PE, Mellor JEL, Adams AC, Gunz FW: Chromosome studies in Fanconi's anaemia before and after treatment with oxymetholone. Pathology 4:27, 1972.

98. _____, Mellor JEL, Vincent PC, Gunz FW: Clonal evolution in human leukaemia. Cytobios 4:29, 1971.

99. Culliton BJ: Reverse transcription: One year later. Science 172:926, 1971.

100. Custer RP: Borderlands dim in malignant disease of the bloodforming organs. Radiology 61:764, 1953.

101. Dalldorf, G, Linsell CA, Barnhart FE: An epidemiologic approach to the lymphomas of African children and Burkitt's sarcoma of the jaws. Perspect Biol Med 7:435, 1964.

102. Dalton AJ, Moloney JB, Porter GH, Frei E, Mitchell EZ: Studies on murine and human leukemia. Trans Assoc Amer Physicians 77:52, 1964.

103. _____, Rowe WP, Mitchell EZ, Pugh WE: Detection of virus particles in leukemia-lymphoma by electron microscopy, in: Zarafonetis CJD (ed), Proceedings of the International Conference on Leukemia-Lymphoma. Philadelphia, Lea & Febiger, 1968, p 87.

104. Dameshek W: Chronic lymphocytic leukemia—an accumulative disease of immunologically incompetent lymphocytes. Blood 29:566, 1967.

105. _____, Gunz FW: Diagnostic and therapeutic x-ray exposure and leukemia. JAMA 163:838, 1957.

106. _____, Savitz HA, Arbor B: Chronic lymphatic leukemia in twin brothers aged fifty-six. JAMA 92:1348, 1929.

107. Davies AM, Modan B, Djaldetti M, De Vries A: Epidemiological observations on leukemia in Israel. Arch Intern Med 108:86, 1961.

108. Deardorff FW, Gerber P, Vogler WR: Infectious mononucleosis in acute leukemia with rising Epstein-Barr virus antibody titers. Ann Intern Med 72:235, 1970.

109. Debré R, Bernard J, Buhot S: Leucose aiguë familiale. Evolution rapprochee d'une leucose aiguë du même type chez une enfante et chez son père. Bull Mém Soc Méd Hôp. Paris 67:183, 1951.

110. Decastello A: Akute Leukämie und Sepsis. Wien Arch Inn Med 11:217, 1925.

111. _____: Beitrag zur Kenntnis der familiären Leukämie. Med Klin 35:1255, 1939.

112. De Grouchy YJ, De Nava C, Cantu JM, Bilski-Pasquier G, Bousser J: Models for clonal evolution: A study of myelogenous leukemia. Am J Hum Genet 18:485, 1966.

113. De Schryver A, Friberg S Jr, Klein G, Henle W, Henle G, De Thé G, Clifford P, Ho HC: Epstein-Barr virus-associated antibody patterns in carcinoma of the postnasal space. Clin Exp Immunol 5:443, 1969.

114. De Vries A, Peketh L, Joshua H: Leukaemia and agranulocytosis in a member of a family with hereditary leukopenia. Acta Med Orient 17:26, 1958.

115. Dignan P St J, Mauer AM, Frantz C: Phocomelia with congenital hypoplastic thrombocytopenia and myeloid leukemoid reactions. J Pediatr 70:561, 1967.

116. Dmochowski L: Electron microscope studies of leukemia in animals, and man, in: ITO Subviral Carcinogenesis. Monograph of the First International Symposium on Tumor Viruses, Nagoya, Japan, 1966, pp 362–407; Kyoto, NISSHA Co., 1967.

117. _____: Viral studies in human leukemia and lymphoma, in Zarafonetis CJD (ed): Proceedings of the International

Conference on Leukemia-Lymphoma. Philadelphia: Lea & Febiger, 1968, p 97.

118. _____: Ultrastructural studies in leukemia, in Dameshek W and Dutcher RM (eds): Perspectives in Leukemia. New York, Grune & Stratton, 1968, p 34.

119. _____: Recent studies on leukemia and solid tumors in mice and man. Bibl Haematol 31:285, 1968.

120. _____, Grey CE: Subcellular structures of possible viral origin in some mammalian tumors. Ann NY Acad Sci 68:599, 1957.

121. _____, _____, Gross L: The role of viruses in x-ray induced leukemia, in: Radiation Biology and Cancer. Austin: University of Texas Press, 1958, p 382.

122. _____, _____, Padgett F, Sykes JA: Studies on the structure of the mammary tumor-inducing virus (Bittner) and of leukemia virus (Gross) in: Viruses, Nucleic Acids and Cancer. Baltimore, Williams & Wilkins, 1963, p 85.

123. _____, Yumoto T, Grey CE, Hales RL, Langford PL, Taylor HG, Freireich EJ, Shullenberger CC, Shively JA, Howe CD: Electron microscopic studies of human leukemia and lymphoma. Cancer 20:760, 1967.

124. Dosik H, Hsu, LY, Todaro, GJ, Lee SL, Hirschhorn K, Selirio E, Alter AA: Leukemia in Fanconi's anemia: Cytogenetic tumor virus susceptibility studies. Blood 36:341, 1970.

125. Dougan L, Woodliff HJ: Acute leukaemia associated with phenylbutazone treatment: A review of the literature and report of a further case. Med J Aust 1:217, 1965.

126. Dougherty TF, White A: Effect of pituitary adrenotropic hormone on lymphoid tissue. Proc Soc Exper Biol Med 53:132, 1943.

127. Dublin LI, Spiegelman M: The longevity and mortality of American physicians, 1938–1942; preliminary report. JAMA 134:1211, 1947.

128. Dunlap CE: Effects of radiation on the blood and the hemopoietic tissues, including the spleen, the thymus and the lymph nodes. Arch Pathol 34:562, 1942.

129. Duplan JF, Latarjet R: Studies on the mechanism of radiation-induced leukemogenesis in C57BL mice. Cancer Res 26:395, 1966.

130. Dustin P Jr: Myélose aplasique récidivante chez un enfant. Crise leucémoïde aiguë terminale. Sang 16:394, 1944.

131. Dutcher RM: Viruses as etiological factors in leukemia-comparative studies, in Dameshek, W and Dutcher RM: Perspectives in Leukemia. New York, Grune & Stratton, 1968, p 13.

132. _____, Larkin EP, Tumilowicz JJ, Nazerian K, Eusebio CP, Stock ND, Guest GB, Marshak RR: Evidence in support of a virus etiology for bovine leukemia. Cancer 20:851, 1967.

133. Ebbin AJ, Heath CW Jr, Moldow RE, Lee J: Down's syndrome and leukemia in a family. J Pedriatr 73:917, 1968.

134. Eckert EA, Beard D, Beard JW: Dose-response relations in experimental transmission of avian erythromyeloblastic leukosis. III. Titration of the virus. J Natl Cancer Inst 14:1044, 1954.

135. _____, _____, _____: Virus of avian erythroblastosis. I. Titration of infectivity. J Natl Cancer Inst 16:1099, 1956.

136. Edwards JH: Familial predisposition in man. Br Med Bull 25:58, 1969.

137. Ellermann V, Bang O: Experimentelle Leukämie bei Hühnern. Vorläufige Mitteilung. Zentralbl. Bakteriol 46:595, 1908.

138. Engelbreth-Holm J: Bericht über einen neuen Stamm Hühnerleukose. (Vorläufige Mitteilung). Z Immunitaetsforsch Allerg Klin Immunol 73:126, 1931.

139. _____: Spontaneous and Experimental Leukaemia in Animals. London, Oliver & Boyd, 1942.

140. _____: On leukaemia research, in: Ciba Foundation Symposium on Leukaemia Research. Boston, Little, Brown, 1954, p 5.

141. Epstein MA, Achong BG: Specific immunofluorescence test for the herpes-type EB virus of Burkitt lymphoblasts, authenticated by electron microscopy. J Natl Cancer Inst 40:593, 1968.

142. _____, _____: Observations on the herpes-type EB virus in cultured Burkitt lymphoblasts, using a specific immunofluorescence test. J Natl Cancer Inst 40:609, 1968.

143. _____, _____, Barr YM: Virus particles in cultured lymphoblasts from Burkitt's lymphoma. Lancet 1:702, 1964.

144. _____, _____, Pope JH: Virus in cultured lymphoblasts from a New Guinea Burkitt lymphoma. Br Med J 2:290, 1967.

145. _____, Barr YM, Achong BG: A second virus-carrying tissue culture strain (EB2) of lymphoblasts from Burkitt's lymphoma. Pathol Biol (Paris) 12:1233, 1964.

146. _____, Henle G, Achong BG, Barr YM: Morphological and biological studies on a virus in cultured lymphoblasts from Burkitt lymphoma. J Exp Med 121:761, 1965.

147. Evans AS, Niederman JC, McCollum RW:

Seroepidemiologic studies of infectious mononucleosis with EB virus. N Engl J Med 279:1121, 1968.

148. Evans WH, Roberts RE: Splenomedullary leukaemia in an x-ray worker, with discussion of previously reported cases. Lancet 2:748, 1928.

149. Faber, M: Radiation-induced leukaemia in Denmark, in: Advances in Radiobiology. Edinburgh, Oliver & Boyd, 1957, p 397.

150. ———: Ioniserende Stråling som pathogenetisk Faktor ved Leukaemi. Nord Med 59:839, 1958.

151. Fallon RJ, Grist NR, Inman DR, Lemcke RM, Negroni G, Woods DM: Further study of agents isolated from tissue cultures inoculated with human leukaemic bone marrow. Br Med J 2:388, 1965.

152. ———, Jackson DK: Relation between mycoplasmas and leukaemia and related diseases. Br Med J 4:225, 1968.

153. Fasal E, Jackson EW, Klauber MR: Mortality in California veterinarians. J Chron Dis 19:293, 1966.

154. ———, ———, ———: Birth characteristics of leukemia in childhood. J Natl Cancer Inst 47:501, 1971.

154a. Fedrick J, Alberman ED: Reported influenza in pregnancy and subsequent cancer in the child. Br Med J 2:485, 1972.

155. Feldman DG, Gross L: Electron microscopic study of vertical transmission of the mouse leukemia virus (Gross) through genital organs of male and female C3H(f) and Ak mice. Cancer Res 27:1513, 1967.

156. Fiala S: The cancer cell as a stem cell unable to differentiate. A theory of carcinogenesis. Neoplasma 15:607, 1968.

156a. Fialkow PJ, Thomas ED, Bryant JI, Neiman PE: Leukaemia transformation of engrafted human marrow cells in vivo. Lancet 1:251, 1971.

157. Finch CS, Hoshino T, Ichimaru M, Ingram RH Jr: Chronic lymphocytic leukemia in Hiroshima and Nagasaki, Japan. Blood 33:79, 1969.

158. Fink MA, Herbut PA, Sibal LR, Wivel NA: Probable murine origin of a virus (HHLV-2) recovered from leukemic mice after inoculation of human leukemic material. J Natl Cancer Inst 39:1253, 1967.

159. ———, Karon M, Rauscher FJ, Malmgren RA, Orr HC: Further observations on the immunofluorescence of cells in human leukemia. Cancer 18:1317, 1965.

160. ———, Malmgren RA, Rauscher FJ, Orr HC, Karon M: Application of immunofluorescence to the study of human leukemia. J Natl Cancer Inst 23:581, 1964.

161. ———, Manaker RA, Dalton AJ, Cranford VL: Immunofluorescence of tissue cultured cells derived from human lymphoid tissues, in Winquist, (ed): Symposium on Comparative Leukaemia Research. Oxford, Pergamon Press, 1966, p 45.

162. Fitzgerald PH, Hamer JW: Third case of chronic lymphocytic leukaemia in a carrier of the inherited Ch¹ chromosome. Br Med J 3:752, 1969.

163. Folley JH, Borges W, Yamawaki T: Incidence of leukemia in survivors of the atomic bomb in Hiroshima and Nagasaki, Japan. Am J Med 13:311, 1952.

164. Forbes IJ: Development of acute leukaemia in Waldenstrom's macroglobulinaemia after prolonged treatment with chlorambucil. Med J Aust 1:918, 1972.

165. Ford DD, Paterson JCS, Treuting WL: Fetal exposure to diagnostic x-rays and leukemia and other malignant diseases in childhood. J Natl Cancer Inst 22:1093, 1959.

166. Forkner CE: Leukemia and Allied Disorders. New York, Macmillan, 1938.

167. Foster CG, Miller FR: Presence of myelokentric and lymphokentric acid in sera of patients with lymphomatoid diseases. Proc Soc Exp Biol Med 75:633, 1950.

168. Foster R, Metcalf D, Robinson WA, Bradley TR: Bone marrow colony stimulating activity in human sera. Br J Haematol 15:147, 1968.

169. Fraumeni JF Jr: Sex ratio of children of leukemic mothers. Pediatrics 33:587, 1964.

170. ———: Bone marrow depression induced by chloramphenicol or phenylbutazone. JAMA 201:828, 1967.

171. ———, Miller RW: Epidemiology of human leukemia: Recent observations. J Natl Cancer Inst 38:593, 1967.

172. ———, Vogel CL, De Vita VT: Familial chronic lymphocytic leukemia. Ann Intern Med 71:279, 1969.

173. Freedman MH, Gilchrist GS, Hammond GD: Concurrent infectious mononucleosis and acute leukemia. JAMA 214:1677, 1970.

174. Fridman WH, Kourilsky FM: Stimulation of lymphocytes by autologous leukaemic cells in acute leukaemia. Nature 224:277, 1969.

175. Friend C: Cell-free transmission in adult Swiss mice of a disease having the character of leukemia. J Exp Med 105:307, 1957.

176. Furth J: Nature of agent transmitting leucosis of the fowl. Proc Soc Exp Biol Med 28:449, 1930.

177. ———: On the resistance and filterability

of the agent transmitting leucosis. Proc Soc Exp Biol Med 28:985, 1931.

178. _____: Immunity phenomena in transmissible leucosis of fowls. Proc Soc Exp Biol Med 29:1236, 1932.

179. _____: Recent experimental studies on leukemia. Physiol Rev 26:47, 1946.

180. _____: Conditioned and autonomous neoplasms: A review. Cancer Res 13:477, 1953.

181. _____: The concept of conditioned and autonomous neoplasms, in: Ciba Foundation Symposium on Leukemia Research. Boston, Little, Brown, 1954, p 38.

182. _____: A meeting of ways in cancer research: thoughts on the evolution and nature of neoplasms. Cancer Res 19:244, 1959.

183. _____, Ferris, HW, Reznikoff P: Relation of leukemia of animals to leukemia of man. JAMA 105:1824, 1935.

184. _____, Furth OB: Neoplastic diseases produced in mice by general irradiation with x-rays. I. Incidence and type of neoplasm. Am J Cancer 28:54, 1936.

185. _____, Kahn MC: The transmission of leukemia of mice with a single cell. Am J Cancer 31:276, 1937.

186. _____, Metcalf D: An appraisal of tumor-virus problems. J Chron Dis 8:88, 1958.

187. Gahrton G, Wahren B, Killander D, Foley GE: Epstein-Barr and other herpesvirus antibodies in children with acute leukemia. Int J Cancer 8:242, 1971.

188. Gall EA, Mallory TB: Malignant lymphoma. A clinicopathologic survey of 618 cases. Am J Pathol 18:381, 1942.

189. Gallo, RC: RNA-dependent DNA polymerase in viruses and cells: Views on the current state. Blood 39:117, 1972.

190. _____, Perry S: Enzyme abnormality in human leukemia. Nature 218:465, 1968.

191. _____, Sarin PS, Allen PT, Newtown WA, Prior ES, Bowen JM, Dmochowski L: Reverse transcriptase in type C virus particles of human origin. Nature 232:140, 1971.

192. _____, Yang SS, Ting RC: RNA dependent DNA polymerase of human acute leukaemic cells. Nature 228:927, 1970.

193. Gardner MB: Current information on feline and canine cancers and relationship or lack of relationship to human cancer. J Natl Cancer Inst 46:281, 1971.

194. _____, Officer, JE, Rongey RW, Ester JD, Turner HC, Huebner RJ: C-type RNA tumour virus genome expression in wild house mice. Nature 232:617, 1971.

195. Gardner WU, Dougherty TF, Williams WL: Lymphoid tumors in mice receiving steroid hormones. Cancer Res 4:73, 1944.

196. Garfield DH: Acute erythromegakaryocytic leukaemia after treatment with cytostatic agents. Lancet 2:1037, 1970.

197. Garriga S, Crosby WH: The incidence of leukemia in families of patients with hypoplasia of the marrow. Blood 14:1008, 1959.

198. Geering G, Aoki T, Old LJ: Shared viral antigen of mammalian leukaemia viruses. Nature 226:265, 1970.

199. _____, Old LJ, Boyse EA: Antigens of leukemias induced by naturally occurring leukemia virus: their relation to the antigens of Gross virus and other murine leukemia viruses. J Exp Med 124:753, 1966.

200. Gibson RW, Bross IDJ, Graham S, Lilienfeld AM, Schuman LM, Levin ML, Dowd, JE: Leukemia in children exposed to multiple risk factors. N Engl J Med 279:906, 1968.

200a. _____, Graham S, Lilienfeld A, Schuman L, Dowd JE, Levin ML: Irradiation in the epidemiology of leukemia among adults. J Natl Cancer Inst 48:301, 1972.

201. Girard R, Revol L: La fréquence d'une exposition benzénique au cours des hémopathies graves. Nouv Rev Fr Hématol 10:477, 1970.

202. Girardi AJ, Hayflick L, Lewis AM, Sommerson ML: Recovery of mycoplasmas in the study of human leukaemia and other malignancies. Nature 205:188, 1965.

203. Gittins R: Studies in anaemias of infancy and early childhood. Leukaemia (leucosis) in children. Arch Dis Child 8:291, 1933.

204. Gloor W: Ein Fall von geheilter Myeloblastenleukämie. Münch Med. Wochenschr 77:1096, 1930.

205. Goguel A, Cavigneaux A, Bernard J: Les leucémies benzéniques. Bull Inst Natl Santé Rech Méd 22:421, 1967.

206. Goh KO, Swisher SN: Identical twins and chronic myelocytic leukemia. Arch Intern Med 115:475, 1965.

207. _____, Herman EC: Chronic myelocytic leukemia and identical twins. Additional evidence of the Philadelphia chromosome as postzygotic abnormality. Arch Intern Med 120:214, 1967.

208. Good, RH, Finstad J: Essential relationship between the lymphoid system, immunity, and malignancy. Natl Cancer Inst Monogr 31:41, 1969.

209. Goodfellow DR: Leucocytic variations in radium workers. Br J Radiol 8:669, 752, 1935.

210. Gorer, PA: Videbaek A: Heredity in human leukaemia and its relation to cancer (a review). Ann Eugenics 14:346, 1949.

211. Grace, JT Jr: Studies of a herpes-type virus

in human lymphoma and leukemia, in Za-rafonetis CJD (ed): Proceedings of the International Conference on Leukemia-Lymphoma. Philadelphia, Lea & Febiger, 1968, p 115.

212. _____: Studies of Epstein-Barr virus. Ann NY Acad Sci 174:946, 1970.

213. Graffi A: Chloroleukemia of mice. Ann NY Acad Sci 68:540, 1957.

214. _____: Experimentelle Untersuchungen zur Ätiologie der Leukämien. Z Gesamte Inn Med 13:961, 1958.

215. _____, Fey F, Schramm T: Experiments on the hematologic diversification of viral mouse leukemias. Natl Cancer Inst Monogr 22:21, 1966.

216. _____, Gimmy J: Über die Wirkung des Virus der myeloischen Leukämie der Maus bei der Ratte. Z Gesamte Inn Med 13:881, 1958.

217. Graham DC: Leukemia following x-ray therapy for ankylosing spondylitis. Arch Intern Med 105:51, 1960.

218. Graham S, Levin ML, Lilienfeld AM, Schuman LM, Gibson R, Dowd JE, Hempelmann L: Preconception, intrauterine and postnatal irradiation as related to leukemia. Natl Cancer Inst Monogr 19:347, 1966.

219. Green HN: The immunologic theory of cancer. Some implications in human pathology. J Chron Dis 8:123, 1958.

220. Green M, Fisher M, Miller H, Wilson GM: Blood radiation dose after I^{131} therapy of thyrotoxicosis. Calculations with reference to leukaemia. Br Med J 2:215, 1961.

221. Grist NR, Fallon RJ: Isolation of viruses from leukaemia patients. Br Med J 2:1263, 1964.

222. Gross L: "Spontaneous" leukemia developing in C3H mice following inoculation in infancy with AK leukemic extracts of AK embryos. Proc Soc Exp Biol Med 76:27, 1951.

223. _____: A filterable agent recovered from AK leukemic extracts causing salivary gland carcinomas in C3H mice. Proc Soc Exp Biol Med 83:414, 1953.

224. _____: Induction of parotid carcinomas and/or subcutaneous sarcomas in C3H mice with normal C3H organ extracts. Proc Soc Exp Biol Med 88:362, 1955.

225. _____: Mouse leukemia: An egg-born virus disease. Acta Haematol 13:13, 1955.

226. _____: Attempt to recover filterable agent from x-ray induced leukemia. Acta Haematol 19:353, 1958.

227. _____: Biological and pathogenic properties of a mouse leukemia virus. Acta Haematol 23:259, 1960.

228. _____: Induction of leukemia in rats with mouse leukemia (passage A) virus. Proc Soc Exp Biol Med 106:890, 1961.

229. _____: Serial cell-free passage in rats of the mouse leukemia virus. Effect of thymectomy. Proc Soc Exp Biol Med 112:939, 1963.

230. _____: Attempt at classification of mouse leukemia viruses. Mouse leukemia virus type A and the Friend virus. Acta Haematol 32:81, 1964.

231. _____: How many different viruses causing leukemia in mice? Acta Haematol 32:44, 1964.

232. _____: Are the common forms of spontaneous and induced leukemia and lymphomas in mice caused by a single virus? Natl Cancer Inst Monogr 22:407, 1966.

233. _____: The Rauscher virus: A mixture of the Friend virus and of the mouse leukemia virus (Gross). Acta Haematol 35:200, 1966.

234. _____, Dreyfuss Y: How is the mouse leukemia virus transmitted from host to host under natural life conditions?, in: Carcinogenesis: A Broad Critique. Baltimore, Williams & Wilkins, 1967, p 9.

235. _____, Feldman DG: Electron microscopic studies of radiation-induced leukemia in mice: virus release following total-body-x-ray irradiation. Cancer Res 28:1677, 1968.

236. _____, Matte ML: The occurrence of tumors and leukemia in members of families of patients suffering from leukemia. NY State J Med 48:1283, 1948.

237. Guasch J: Hérédité des leucémies. Sang 25:384, 1954.

238. Gunz FW: The etiology of leukemia: Review and pilot investigation. Bull. Tufts-N.E. Med. Center 3:121, 1957.

239. _____: Incidence of some aetiological factors in human leukaemia. Br Med J 1:326, 1961.

240. _____: Leukaemia in New Zealand and Australia. Pathol Microbiol (Basel) 27:697, 1964.

241. _____, Atkinson HR: Medical radiations and leukaemia: A retrospective survey. Br Med J 1:389, 1964.

242. _____, Borthwick RA, Rolleston GL: Acute leukaemia in an infant following excessive intrauterine irradiation. Lancet 2:190, 1958.

243. _____, Dameshek W: Chronic lymphocytic leukemia in a family, including twin brothers and a son. JAMA 164:1323, 1956.

244. _____, Fitzgerald PH, Crossen PE, Mackenzie IS, Powles CP, Jensen GR: Multiple cases of leukemia in a sibship. Blood 27:482, 1966.

245. _____, Hough, RF: Acute leukemia over the age of 50. A study of its incidence and natural history. Blood 11:882, 1956.

246. _____, Ravich RBM, Vincent PC, Stewart JH, Crossen PE, Mellor J: A case of acute leukemia with a rapidly changing chromosome constitution. Ann Génét 13:79, 1970.

247. _____, Veale AMO: Leukemia in close relatives—accident or predisposition? J Natl Cancer Inst 42:517, 1969.

248. Haddad MN, Weinstein D, Bonar RA, Beaudreau GS, Becker C, Beard D, Beard JW: Virus of avian myeloblastosis. XV. Structural loci of virus synthesis and adenosine triphosphatase activity by electron and light microscopy of myeloblasts from tissue culture. J Natl Cancer Inst 24:971, 1960.

249. Haddow A: Experimental and clinical aspects of the action of various carbonylic acid derivatives in the aromatic nitrogen mustard series, in: Ciba Foundation Symposium on Leukaemia Research. London, Churchill, 1956, p 196.

250. Hamer JW, Gunz FW: Multiple aetiological factors in a case of acute leukaemia. NZ Med J 71:141, 1970.

251. Hanafusa H, Hanafusa T, Rubin H: The defectiveness of Rous sarcoma virus. Proc Natl Acad Sci 49:572, 1963.

252. Hanes B, Gardner MB, Loosli CG, Heidbreder G, Kogan B, Marylander H, Huebner RJ: Pet association with selected human cancers: A household questionnaire study. J Natl Cancer Inst 45:1155, 1970.

253. Haran-Ghera N: A leukemogenic filtrable agent from chemically induced lymphoid leukemia in C57BL mice. Proc Soc Exp Biol Med 124:697, 1967.

254. _____: The mechanism of radiation action in leukaemogenesis. The role of radiation in leukaemia development. Br J Cancer 21:739, 1967.

255. _____, Peled, A: The mechanism of radiation action in leukaemogenesis. Isolation of a leukaemogenic filtrable agent from tissues of irradiated and normal C57BL mice. Br J Cancer 21:730, 1968.

256. Hardy WD Jr, Geering G, Old LJ, De Harven E, Brodey RS, McDonough S: Feline leukemia virus: occurrence of viral antigen in the tissues of cats with lymphosarcoma and other diseases. Science 166:1019, 1969.

257. Hartley JW, Rowe WP, Capps WI, Huebner RJ: Complement fixation and tissue culture assays for mouse leukemia viruses. Proc Natl Acad Sci 53:931, 1965.

258. Hasterlik RJ, Finkel AJ, Miller CE: The cancer hazards of industrial and accidental exposure to radioactive isotopes. Ann NY Acad Sci 114:832, 1964.

259. Hayflick L: The mycoplasma (PPLO) specter of man. Trans NY Acad Sci 27:817, 1965.

260. Heath CW Jr, Moloney WC: Familial leukemia. Five cases of acute leukemia in three generations. N Engl J Med 272:882, 1965.

261. Hecht F, Bryant JS, Gruber D, Townes PL: The nonrandomness of chromosome abnormalities. N Engl J Med 271:1081, 1964.

262. _____, Koler RD, Dahnke GS, Case MP, Tisdale V, Miller RW: Leukaemia and lymphocytes in ataxia-telangiectasia. Lancet 2:1193, 1966.

263. Heineke H: Über die Einwirkung der Röntgenstrahlen auf innere Organe. Münch Med. Wochenschr 51:785, 1904.

264. _____: Experimentelle Untersuchungen über die Einwirkung der Röntgenstrahlen auf innere Organe. Mitt Grenzgeb Med Chir 14:21, 1904–1905.

265. _____: Experimentelle Untersuchungen über die Einwirkung der Röntgenstrahlen auf das Knochenmark, nebst einigen Bemerkungen über die Röntgentherapie der Leukämie und Pseudoleukämie und des Sarkoms. Dtsch Z Chir 78:196, 1905.

266. Heinle RW, Wearn JT, Weir DR, Rose FA: Myeloid hyperplasia and metaplasia induced by extracts of urine from patients with myelogenous leukemia. Ann Intern Med 17:902, 1942.

267. Hempelmann LH, Lisco H, Hoffman JG: The acute radiation syndrome: A study of nine cases and a review of the problem. Ann Intern Med 36:279, 1952.

268. Henle W: Evidence for viruses in acute leukemia and Burkitt's tumor. Cancer 21:580, 1968.

269. _____, Diehl V, Kohn G, Zur Hausen H, Henle G: Herpes-type virus and chromosome marker in normal leukocytes after growth with irradiated Burkitt cells. Science 157:1064, 1967.

270. Henle G and Henle W: Studies on cell lines derived from Burkitt's lymphoma. Trans NY Acad Sci 29:71, 1966.

271. _____, _____: Present status of the herpes-group virus associated with cultures of the hematopoietic system, in Pollard, M (ed): Perspectives in Virology, vol. 6, New York, Academic Press, 1968.

272. _____, _____, Clifford P, Diehl V, Kafuko GW, Kirya BG, Klein G, Morrow RH, Munube GMR, Pike P, Tukei PM, Zie-

gler JL: Antibodies to Epstein-Barr virus in Burkitt's lymphoma and control group. J Natl Cancer Inst 43:1147, 1969.

273. _____, _____, Diehl V: Relation of Burkitt tumor-associated herpes-type virus to infectious mononucleosis. Proc Natl Acad Sci 59:94, 1968.

274. _____, _____, Burtin P, Cachin Y, Clifford P, De Schryver A, De Thé G, Diehl V, Ho HC, Klein G: Antibodies to Epstein-Barr virus in nasopharyngeal carcinoma, other head and neck neoplasms, and control groups. J Natl Cancer Inst 44:225, 1970.

275. Henshaw PS: Leukemia in mice following exposure to x-rays. Radiology 43:279, 1944.

276. _____, Hawkins JW: Incidence of leukemia in physicians. J Natl Cancer Inst 4:339, 1944.

277. Herbut PA: Human leukemia virus in mice. Arch Pathol 83:123, 1967.

278. Herrell WE, Ruff JD, Bayrd ED: Multiple myeloma in siblings. JAMA 167:1485, 1958.

279. Heston WE: Genetic factors in the etiology of cancer. Cancer Res 25:1320, 1965.

280. Hewitt D, Lashof JC, Stewart AM: Childhood cancer in twins. Cancer 19:157, 1966.

281. Heyssel R, Brill AB, Woodbury LA, Nishimura ET, Ghose T, Hoshino T, Yamasaki M: Leukemia in Hiroshima atomic bomb survivors. Blood 15:313, 1960.

282. Hirschhorn K: Cytogenetic alterations in leukemia, in Dameshek W, and Dutcher RM (eds): Perspectives in Leukemia. New York, Grune & Stratton, 1968, p 113.

283. Hitzig WH, Rampini S: Leukämie bei Zwillingen. Helvet paediatr Acta 14:67, 1959.

284. Holton CP, Johnson WW: Chronic myelocytic leukemia in infant siblings. J Pediatr 72:377, 1968.

285. Honda F, Punnett HH, Charney E, Miller G, Thiele HA: Serial cytogenetic and hematologic studies on a mongol with trisomy-21 and acute congenital leukemia. J Pediatr 65:880, 1964.

286. Hoogstraten J: The nature of leukemia, in Proceedings of the Third International Congress of the International Society of Hematology. New York, Grune & Stratton, 1951, p 244.

287. Hornbaker JH: Chronic leukemia in three sisters. Am J Med Sci 203: 322, 1942.

288. Hoshino T, Kato H, Friech SC, Hrubec Z: Leukemia in offspring of atomic bomb survivors. Blood 30:719, 1967.

289. Huang CC, Minowada J, Smith RT, Osunkoya BO: Reevaluation of relationship between chromosome marker and Epstein-Barr virus: Chromosome and immunofluorescence analyses of 16 human hematopoietic cell lines. J Natl Cancer Inst 45:815, 1970.

290. Huebner RJ, Kelloff GJ, Sarma PS, Lane WT, Turner HC, Gilden RV, Oroszlan S, Meier H, Myers DD, Peters RL: Group-specific antigen expression during embryogenesis of the genome of the C-type RNA tumor virus. Implication for ontogenesis and oncogenesis. Proc Natl Acad Sci 67:366, 1970.

291. _____, Todaro GJ: Oncogenics of RNA tumor viruses as determinants of cancer. Proc Natl Acad Sci 64:1087, 1969.

292. Hunter FT: Chronic exposure to benzene (benzol). II. The clinical effects. J Indust Hyg Toxicol 21:331, 1939.

293. Hutchinson GB: Leukemia in patients with cancer of the cervix uteri treated with radiation. A report covering the first five years of an international study. J Natl Cancer Inst 40:951, 1968.

294. Igel HJ, Huebner RJ, Turner HC, Kotin P, Falk HL: Mouse leukemia virus activation by chemical carcinogens. Science 166:1624, 1969.

295. Ingram M, Adams M, Coonan L, Jespersen J, Nielsen G, Piatt D, Yettewich G: The occurrence of lymphocytes with bilobed nuclei in cyclotron personnel. Science 116:706, 1952.

296. _____, Barnes SW: Experimental confirmation of a previously reported unusual finding in the blood of cyclotron workers. Science 113:32, 1951.

297. Inman DR, Woods DA, Negroni G: Electron microscopy of virus particles in cell cultures inoculated with passage fluid from human leukaemic bone marrow. Br Med J 1:929, 1964.

298. Isaacs R, Danielian AC: Maintenance of leukocyte level and changes during irradiation; study of white blood corpuscles appearing in saliva and their relations to those in blood. Am J Med Sci 174:70, 1927.

299. Israels MCG: The reticuloses. A clinicopathological study. Lancet 2:525, 1953.

300. Iwakata S, Grace JT: Cultivation in vitro of myeloblasts from human leukemia. NY State J Med 64:2279, 1964.

301. Jablon S: Radiation-induced cancer in atomic bomb survivors. Proceedings of the Tenth International Cancer Congress, Houston, 1972.

302. _____, Kato H: Childhood cancer in relation to prenatal exposure to atomic bomb radiation. Lancet 2:1000, 1970.

303. Jackson EW, Morris FD, Klauber MR: Childhood leukemia in California-born twins. Cancer 23:913, 1969.

304. _____, Turner JH, Klauber MR, Norris FD: Down's syndrome: Variation of leukemia occurrence in institutionalized populations. J Chron Dis 21:247, 1968.

305. Jackson H Jr: The differential diagnosis of agranulocytic angina from acute leukemia. Am J Med Sci 188:604, 1934.

306. Jacobs EM, Luce JK, Cailleau R: Chromosome abnormalities in human cancer. Report of a patient with chronic myelocytic leukemia and his nonleukemic monozygotic twin. Cancer 19:869, 1966.

307. Jacobs PA, Court Brown WM, Baikie AG, Strong JA: The somatic chromosomes in mongolism. Lancet 1:710, 1959.

308. Jacobson LO, Marks EK, Gaston EO, Simmons EL, Block MH: Studies on radiosensitivity of cells. Science 107:248, 1948.

309. Jagié N, Schwartz G, Von Siebenrock L: Blutbefunde bei Röntgenologen. Klin Wochenschr 48:1220, 1911.

310. Jarrett O, Laird HM, Hay D: Growth of feline leukaemia virus in human cells. Nature 224: 1208, 1969.

311. _____, _____, _____, Crighton GW: Replication of cat leukaemia virus in cell cultures. Nature 219:54, 1968.

312. Jarrett WF, Crawford EM, Martin WB, Davie F: Virus-like particle associated with leukaemia (lymphosarcoma). Nature 202:567, 1964.

313. Jensen EM, Korol W, Dittmar SL, Medrek TJ: Virus-containing lymphocyte cultures from cancer patients. J Natl Cancer Inst 39:745, 1967.

314. Joachim H: Acute leukemia in uniovular twins: Review of genetic aspects of human leukemia. Cancer 15:539, 1962.

315. Johnson MSE, Peters CH: Lymphoma in four siblings. JAMA 163:20, 1957.

316. Kajima M, Pollard M: Wide distribution of leukaemia in strains of laboratory mice. Nature 218:188, 1968.

317. Kaliampetsos G: Kommen Blutkrankheiten und Karzinome unter den Verwandten von Leukämie-Kranken gehäuft vor? Dtsch Med Wochenschr 79:1783, 1954.

318. Kamada N: Studies on bone marrow chromosomes in atomic bomb survivors in Hiroshima. Acta Haematol Jap 32:236, 1969.

319. Kaplan HS: Observations on radiation-induced lymphoid tumors of mice. Cancer Res. 7:141, 1947.

320. _____: Preliminary studies of the effectiveness of local irradiation in the induction of lymphoid tumors in mice. Cancer Res 10:267, 1949.

321. _____: Influence of thymectomy, splenectomy and gonadectomy on incidence of radiation-induced lymphoid tumors in strain C57 black mice. Cancer Res 11:83, 1950.

322. _____: On the etiology and pathogenesis of the leukemias: A review. Cancer Res 14:535, 1954.

323. _____: An evaluation of the somatic and genetic hazards of the medical uses of radiation. Am J Roentgenol Radium Therap Nucl Med 80:696, 1958.

324. _____: Some implications of indirect induction mechanisms in carcinogenesis. A review. Cancer Res 18:791, 1959.

325. _____: The role of radiation in experimental leukemogenesis. Natl Cancer Inst Monogr 14:207, 1964.

326. _____: On the natural history of the murine leukemias. Cancer Res 28:1325, 1967.

327. _____: Induction of murine leukemia: Interaction of viruses, target cells, host factors, and exogenous agents, in Vincent, P. (ed): The Nature of Leukaemia. Sydney: N.S.W. Government Printer, 1972, p 13.

328. _____, Brown, MB, Paule J: Influence of bone marrow injections on involution and neoplasia of mouse thymus after systemic irradiation. J Natl Cancer Inst 14:303, 1953.

329. _____, Marder SN, Brown MB: Adrenal cortical function and radiation-induced lymphoid tumors of mice. Cancer Res 11:629, 1951.

330. Kaufman HJ, Hess R: Does congenital leukaemia exist? Br Med J 1:867, 1962.

331. Keith L, Brown E: Epidemiologic study of leukemia in twins (1928–1969). Acta Genet Med Gemellol 20:9, 1971.

332. Kellett CE: Acute myeloid leukaemia in one of identical twins. Arch Dis Child 12:239, 1937.

333. Kimball AW: Evaluation of data relating human leukemia and ionizing radiation. J Natl Cancer Inst 21:383, 1958.

334. Kiossoglou, KA, Rosenbaum ER, Mitus WJ, Dameshek W: Multiple chromosome aberrations in Down's syndrome associated with twinning and acute granulocytic leukaemia. Lancet 2:944, 1963.

335. Kirschbaum A: Rodent leukemia: Recent biological studies. A review. Cancer Res 11:741, 1951.

336. _____: Etiology of leukemia, in: Etiology and Treatment of Leukemia. Proceedings of

the First Louisiana Cancer Conference St. Louis: Mosby, 1958, p 29.

337. _____, Mixer H: Induction of leukemia in eight inbred stocks of mice varying in susceptibility to the spontaneous disease. J Lab Clin Med 32:720, 1947.

338. Klein G: Immunological studies on Burkitt's lymphoma. Postgrad Med J 47:141, 1971.

339. _____, Klein E, Clifford P: Host defences in leukemia and Burkitt tumor. Cancer 21:587, 1968.

340. _____, Pearson G, Nadkarni JS, Nadkarni JJ, Klein E, Henle G, Henle W, Clifford P: Relation between Epstein-Barr viral and cell membrane immunofluorescence of Burkitt tumor cells. J Exp Med 128:1011, 1021, 1968.

341. Kohn G, Diehl V, Mellman WJ, Henle W, Henle G: C-group chromosome marker in long-term leukocyte cultures. J Natl Cancer Inst 41:795, 1968.

342. _____, Mellman WJ, Moorhead PS, Loftus J, Henle G: Involvement of C-group chromosomes in five Burkitt lymphoma cell lines. J Natl Cancer Inst 38:209, 1967.

343. Koprowski H: Virus-induced tumors and leukemias. Am J Med 38:716, 1965.

344. Kosenow W, Pfeiffer RA: Chronisch myeloische Leukämie bei eineiigen Zwillingen. Dtsch Med Wochenschr 94:1170, 1969.

345. Krebs C, Rask-Nielsen HC, Wagner A: The origin of lymphosarcomatosis and its relation to other forms of leucosis in white mice. Acta Radiol (suppl 10), 1930.

346. Krivit W, Good RA: The simultaneous occurrence of leukemia and mongolism. J Dis Child 91:218, 1956.

347. _____, _____: Simultaneous occurrence of mongolism and leukemia. Am J Dis Child 94:289, 1957.

348. Kurita S: Familial leukemia. Acta Haematol Jap 31:748, 1968.

349. Kyle RH, Pierre RV, Bayrd ED: Multiple myeloma and acute myelomonocytic leukemia. N Engl J Med 283:1121, 1970.

350. Laird H, Jarrett O, Crighton GW, Jarrett WFH: An electron microscopic study of virus particles in spontaneous leukemia in the cat. J Natl Cancer Inst 41:867, 1968.

351. _____, _____, _____, _____, Hay D: Replication of leukemogenic-type virus in cats inoculated with feline lymphosarcoma extracts. J Natl Cancer Inst 41:879, 1968.

352. Lamerton LF: An examination of the clinical and experimental data relating to the possible hazard to the individual of small doses of radiation. Br J Radiol 31:229, 1958.

353. Lampert F: Akute lymphoblastische Leukämie bei Geschwistern mit progressiver Kleinhirnataxie (Louis-Barr-Syndrom). Dtsch Med Wochenschr 94:217, 1969.

354. Lange RD, Moloney WC, Yamawaki R: Leukemia in atomic bomb survivors. I. General observations. Blood 9:574, 1954.

355. Latarjet R, Duplan JF: Experiments and discussion on leukemogenesis by cell-free extracts of radiation-induced leukemia in mice. Int J Radiat Biol 5:339, 1962.

356. Latourette HB, Hodges FJ: Incidence of neoplasia after irradiation of thymic region. Am J Roentgenol Radium Therap Nucl Med 82:667, 1959.

357. Leibetseder F: Monocytenleukose als Folge chronischer Röntgen-Radium Schädigung. Med Klin 47:46, 1952.

358. Lejeune J: Aberrations chromosomiques et cancer, in Harris RJC (ed): UICC Monograph Series., Ninth International Cancer Congress, vol. 9. Berlin: Springer, 1967, p 71.

359. _____, Gautier M, Turpin R: Etude des chromosomes de neuf enfants mongoliens. CR Acad Sci (Paris) 248:1721, 1959.

360. Lentz O: Gehören Leukämie und perniciöse Anämie zu den bösartigen Geschwülsten? Folia Haematol 69:5, 1949.

361. Levine PH, Horoszewicz JS, Grace JT Jr, Chai LS, Ellison RR, Holland JF: Relationship between clinical status of leukemic patients and viruslike particles in their plasma. Cancer 20:1563, 1967.

362. _____, Merrill DA, Bethlenfalvay NC, Dabich L, Stevens DA, Waggoner DE: A longitudinal comparison of antibodies to Epstein-Barr virus and clinical parameters in chronic lymphocytic leukemia and chronic myelocytic leukemia. Blood 38:479, 1971.

363. Levy JA, Henle G, Henle W, Zajac BA: Effect of reovirus 3 on cultured Burkitt's tumour cells. Nature 220:607, 1968.

364. _____, Tanabe E, Curnen EC: Occurrence of reovirus antibodies in healthy African children and in children with Burkitt's lymphoma. Cancer 21:53, 1968.

365. _____, Virolainen M, Defendi V: Human lymphoblastoid lines from lymph node and spleen. Cancer 22:517, 1968.

366. Lewis EB: Leukemia and ionizing radiation. Science 125:965, 1957.

367. _____: Leukemia, multiple myeloma, and aplastic anemia in American radiologists. Science 142:1492, 1963.

368. Li FP, Fraumeni JF: Soft-tissue sarcomas, breast cancer, and other neoplasms. A fa-

milial syndrome. Ann Intern Med 71:747, 1969.

369. Lieberman M, Kaplan HS: Leukemogenic activity of filtrates from radiation-induced lymphoid tumors of mice. Science 130:387, 1959.

370. Lilienfeld AM: Formal discussion of: Genetic factors in the etiology of cancer: an epidemiologic view. Cancer Res 25:1330, 1965.

371. Lorenz E: Some biologic effects of long-continued irradiation. Am J Roentgenol Radium Therap Nucl Med 63:176, 1950.

372. Ludwig FC, Elashoff RM, Wellington JS: Murine radiation leukemia and the preleukemic state. Lab Invest 19:240, 1968.

373. McEndy DP, Boon MC, Furth J: On the role of the thymus, spleen and gonads in the development of leukemia in a high leukemia stock of mice. Cancer Res 4:377, 1944.

374. MacMahon B: Prenatal x-ray exposure and childhood cancer. J Natl Cancer Inst 28:1173, 1962.

375. _____, Levy MA: Prenatal origin of childhood leukemia: Evidence from twins. N Engl J Med 270:1082, 1964.

376. _____, Newill VA: Birth characteristics of children dying of malignant neoplasms. J Natl Cancer Inst 28:231, 1962.

377. MacMahon HE: The pathology of malignancy, in: Cancer: A manual for Practitioners (3 ed.). Boston: American Cancer Society (Massachusetts Division, Inc.), 1956, p 15.

378. McPhedran P, Heath CW Jr, Lee J: Patterns of familial leukemia. Ten cases of leukemia in two interrelated families. Cancer 24:403, 1969.

379. Maingot G, Girard L, Bousser J: Poussées leucocytaires transitoires suivies de leucocytose durable et de leucémie myélogène chez un radiologiste. Contribution à la pathogenie et à la prophylaxie de la leucémie myélogène des radiologistes. Sang 12:569, 1938.

380. Mallarmé J: Les débuts hématologiques des leucoses malignes. Sang 20:429, 1949.

381. Manaker RA, Strother PC, Miller AA, Piczak CV: Behavior in vitro of a mouse lymphoid leukemia virus. J Natl Cancer Inst 25:1411, 1960.

382. March HC: Leukemia in radiologists. Radiology 43:275, 1944.

383. _____: Leukemia in radiologists in a 20-year period. Am J Med Sci 220:282, 1950.

384. _____: Leukemia in radiologists, ten years later. Am J Med Sci 242:137, 1961.

385. Marchal G, Deprez V, Blanc G: Syndrome agranulocytaire par chimiothérapie, transformé en cryptoleucémie aiguë à evolution lente. Sang 16:133, 1944.

386. Martin JH: An estimate of the potential leukaemogenic factor in the diagnostic use of x-rays. Med J Aust 2:157, 1958.

387. Martland HS: The occurrence of malignancy in radioactive persons. A general review of data gathered in the study of radium dial painters, with special reference to the occurrence of osteogenic sarcoma and the inter-relationship of certain blood diseases. Am J Cancer 15:2435, 1931.

388. Meier H, Myers DD, Huebner RJ: Genetic control by the hr-locus of susceptibility and resistance to leukemia. Proc Natl Acad Sci 63:759, 1969.

389. Medical Research Council: The Hazards to Man of Nuclear and Allied Radiations. London, Her Majesty's Stationery Office, 1956.

390. _____: The Hazards to Man of Nuclear and Allied Radiations. A Second Report to the Medical Research Council. London, Her Majesty's Stationery Office, 1960.

391. _____: Committee on radiological hazards to patients. Final report of the Committee. London, Her Majesty's Stationery Office, 1965.

392. Mellors RC, Aoki T, Huebner RJ: Further implication of murine leukemia-like virus in the disorders of NZB mice. J Exp Med 129:1045, 1969.

393. Menser MA, Purvis-Smith SG: Dermatoglyphic defects in children with leukaemia. Lancet 1:1076, 1969.

394. Merrit DH, Harris JS: Mongolism and acute leukemia. J Dis Child 92:41, 1956.

395. Metcalf D: Adrenal cortical function in preleukemic AKR mice. Proceedings of the Eighth International Congress of the International Society of Hematology. Tokyo, Pan-Pacific Press, 1960.

396. _____: The Thymus. Berlin, Springer, 1966.

396a. _____: The nature of leukaemia: Neoplasm or disorder of haemopoietic regulation? Med J Aust 2:739, 1971.

397. _____, Chan SH, Gunz FW, Vincent PC, Ravich RBM: Stimulation and inhibition of bone marrow colony formation in vitro by serum and urine from patients with acute granulocytic leukemia. Blood 38:143, 1971.

398. _____, Furth, J, Buffett RF: Pathogenesis of mouse leukemia caused by Friend virus. Cancer Res 19:52, 1959.

399. Mewissen DJ: Dose-response relationship in radiation leukaemia. Nature 184:1669, 1959.

400. Milchner R, Mosse M: Zur Frage der Behandlung der Blutkrankheiten mit Röntgenstrahlen. Berl Klin Wochenschr 41:1267, 1904.

401. Milham S Jr: Leukemia in husbands and wives. Science 148:98, 1967.

402. Miller EC, Miller JA: In vivo combinations between carcinogens and tissue constituents and their possible role in carcinogenesis. Cancer Res 12:547, 1952.

403. Miller FR, Turner DL: The action of specific stimulators on the hematopoietic system. Am J Med Sci 206:146, 1943.

404. Miller OJ, Breg WR, Schmickel RD, Tretter W: A family with an XXXXY male, a leukaemic male, and two 21-trisomic mongoloid females. Lancet 2:78, 1961.

405. Miller RW: Down's syndrome (mongolism), other congenital malformations and cancers among the sibs of leukemic children. N Engl J Med 268:393, 1963.

406. _____: Relation between cancer and congenital defects in man. N Engl J Med 275:87, 1966.

407. _____: Deaths from childhood cancer in sibs. N Engl J Med 279:122, 1968.

408. _____: Relation between cancer and congenital defects: An epidemiological evaluation. J Natl Cancer Inst 40:1079, 1968.

409. _____: Delayed radiation effects in atomic bomb survivors. Science 166:569, 1969.

410. _____: Deaths from childhood leukemia and solid tumors among twins and other sibs in the United States, 1960–1967. J Natl Cancer Inst 46:203, 1971.

411. _____, Jablon S: A search for late radiation effects among men who served as x-ray technologists in the U.S. Army during World War II. Radiology 96:269, 1970.

412. _____, Todaro GJ: Viral transformation of cells from persons at high risk of cancer. Lancet 1:81, 1969.

413. Miyata H, Enomoto H: Familial leukemia. Jap J Clin Hematol 5 (suppl): 15, 1964.

414. Mizutani S, Boettiger D, Temin HM: A DNA-dependent DNA polymerase and a DNA endonuclease in virions of Rous sarcoma virus. Nature 228:424, 1970.

415. Moeschlin S, Rohr K: Klinische und morphologische Gesichtspunkte zur Auffassung der Myelose als Neoplasma. Ergeb Inn Med Kinderheilkd 57:723, 1939.

416. Mole RH: The development of leukaemia in irradiated animals. Br Med Bull 14:174, 1958.

417. _____: The dose-response relationship in radiation carcinogenesis. Br Med Bull 14:184, 1958.

418. _____: The leukaemogenic effect of whole-body irradiation of the mouse: Experimental work at the Radiobiological Research Unit, in: The Hazards to Man of Nuclear and Allied Radiations. London, Her Majesty's Stationery Office, 1960.

419. Moller B: Myeloblastic leukaemia. Acta Paediatr 37:492, 1949.

420. Moloney JB: Biological studies on a lymphoid-leukemia virus extracted from sarcoma 37. I. Origin and introductory investigations. J Natl Cancer Inst 24:933, 1960.

421. _____: Properties of a leukemia virus, in: Symposium on Phenomena of the Tumor Viruses. Nat Cancer Inst Monogr 4:7, 1960.

422. Moloney WC: Leukemia in survivors of atomic bombing. N Engl J Med 253:88, 1955.

423. _____: Leukemia and exposure to x-ray: A report of six cases. Blood 14:1137, 1959.

424. _____, Kastenbaum MA: Leukemogenic effects of ionizing radiation on atomic bomb survivors in Hiroshima City. Science 121:308, 1955.

425. _____, Lange RD: Cytologic and biochemical studies on the granulocytes in early leukemia among atomic bomb survivors. Texas Rep Biol Med 12:887, 1954.

426. _____, _____: Leukemia in atomic bomb survivors. II. Observations on early phases of leukemia. Blood 9:663, 1954.

427. Moore GE, Gerner RE, Franklin HA: Culture of normal human leukocytes. JAMA 199:519, 1967.

428. _____, Grace JT, Citron P, Gerner R, Burns A: Leukocyte cultures of patients with leukemia and lymphomas. NY State J Med 66: 2757, 1966.

429. _____, Kitamura H, Hoshima S: Morphology of cultured hematopoietic cells. Cancer 22:245, 1968.

430. Morganti G, Cresseri A: Nouvelles recherches génétiques sur les leucémies. Sang 25:421, 1954.

431. Morley A, Baikie AG, Galton DAG: Cyclical leucocytosis as evidence for retention of normal homeostatic control in chronic granulocytic leukaemia. Lancet 2:1320, 1967.

432. Murphy JB: The effect of castration, theelin and testosterone on the incidence of leukemia in a Rockefeller Institute strain of mice. Cancer Res 4:622, 1944.

433. Murphy WH, Ertel IJ, Zarafonetis CJD: Virus studies of human leukemia. Cancer 18:1329, 1965.

434. Murray R, Heckel P, Hempelmann LH: Leukemia in children exposed to ionizing radiation. N Engl J Med 261:585, 1959.

435. National Academy of Sciences: Biological Effects of Atomic Radiation. Washington, D.C.: National Research Council, 1956.

436. ———: Implications to man of irradiation by internally deposited strontium-90 and cesium-137. Washington, D.C., National Research Council, 1964.

437. Negroni G: Isolation of viruses from leukemia patients. Br Med J 1:927, 1964.

438. Neumann G: Leukämie und Tuberkulose. Beitr Klin Erforsch Tuberk Lungenkr 118:348, 1958.

439. ———: The mortality from leukaemia in Western Germany from 1948 to 1956. Ger Med Mon 4:86, 1959.

440. Newell GR, Harris WW, Bowman KO, Boone CW, Anderson NG: Evaluation of "virus-like" particles in the plasmas of 255 patients with leukemia and related diseases. N Engl J Med 278:1185, 1968.

441. Niederman JC, McCollum RW, Henle G, Henle W: Infectious mononucleosis: clinical manifestations in relation to the EB virus. JAMA 203:205, 1968.

442. Nielson J: Chronic occupational ray poisoning; a discussion based on a case of leukemia in a radium worker. Acta Radiol 13:385, 1932.

443. Norris FD, Jackson EW, Aaron E: Prospective study of dog bites and childhood cancer. Cancer Res 31:383, 1971.

444. Nowell PC: Chromosome abnormalities in human leukemia and lymphoma, in Zarafonetis CJD (ed): Proceedings of the International Conference on Leukemia-Lymphoma. Philadelphia, Lea & Febiger, 1968, p 47.

445. O'Conor GT: Persistent immunologic stimulation as a factor in oncogenesis with special reference to Burkitt's tumor. Am J Med 48:279, 1970.

446. O'Conor GT, Rabson AS: Herpes-like particles in an American lymphoma: preliminary note. J Natl Cancer Inst 35:899, 1965.

447. Old, LJ, Boyse EA, Stockert E: The G (Gross) leukemia antigen. Cancer Res 25:813, 1965.

448. Oldfelt CO, Knutson D: Chronic benzene poisoning. Acta Med Scandinav (suppl 206):331, 1948.

449. Olmer J, Gascard E: Essai d'interprétation des leucoses aiguës. Sem Hôp Paris 27:3771, 1951.

450. Osgood EE: A unifying concept of the etiology of the leukemias, lymphomas and cancers. J Natl Cancer Inst 18:155, 1957.

451. ———: Ross Conference on Pediatric Research, Nov., 1959. In Hammond D (ed): 34th Report: Current Concepts in Leukemia. Columbus, Ohio, Ross Laboratories, 1960, p. 90.

452. ———: The etiology of leukemia, lymphomas and cancers. Geriatrics 19:208, 1964.

453. Pearson HA, Grello FW, Cone TE Jr: Leukemia in identical twins. N Engl J Med 268:1151, 1963.

454. ———, Shulman NR, Oski FA, Eitzman DV: Platelet survival in Wiskott-Aldrich syndrome. J Pediatr 68:754, 1966.

455. Peller S, Pick, P: Leukemia and other malignant disease in physicians. JAMA 147:893, 1951.

456. Perkins J, Timson J, Emery AEH: Clinical and chromosome studies in Fanconi's aplastic anaemia. J Med Genet 6:28, 1969.

457. Peterson RDA, Kelly WD, Good RA: Ataxia telangiectasia. Its association with a defective thymus, immunological deficiency disease and malignancy. Lancet 1:1189, 1964.

458. Pierce M: Childhood leukemia. J. Pediatr 8:66, 1936.

459. Pike BL, Robinson WA: Human bone marrow colony growth in agar-gel. J Cell Physiol 76:77, 1970.

460. Pluznick DH, Sachs L: The cloning of normal "mast" cells in tissue culture. J Cell Comp Physiol 66:319, 1965.

461. Pochin EE: Leukaemia following radioiodine treatment of thyrotoxicosis. Br Med J 2:1545, 1960.

462. Polhemus DW, Koch R: Leukemia and medical radiation. Pediatrics 23:453, 1959.

463. Pollard M, Matsuzawa T: Radiation-induced leukemia in germ-free mice. Proc Soc Exp Biol Med 116:967, 1964.

464. Pope JH: Establishment of cell lines from Australian leukaemic patients: presence of a herpes-like virus. Aust J Exp Biol Med Sci 46:643, 1968.

465. ———, Horne MK, Scott W: Transformation of foetal human leucocytes in vitro by filtrates of a human leukaemic cell line containing herpes-like virus. Int J Cancer 3:857, 1968.

466. ———, ———, ———: Identification of the filtrates leukocyte-transforming factor of QIMR-WIL cells as herpes-like virus. Int J Cancer 4:255, 1969.

467. Porter GH III, Dalton AJ, Moloney JB, Mitchell EZ: Association of electron dense particles with human leukemia. J Nat Cancer Inst 33:547, 1964.

468. Portmann UV, Robinson WH: Lymphatic leukemia occurring simultaneously in

Negro brother and sister. Cleve Clin Q 18:33, 1951.

469. Poth JL, George RC Jr, Creger WP, Schrier SL: Acute myelogenous leukemia following localized radiotherapy. Arch Intern Med 128:802, 1971.

470. Potter VR, Watanabe M: Some biochemical essentials of malignancy: the challenge of diversity, in Zarafonetis CJD (ed): Proceedings of the International Conference on Leukemia-Lymphoma. Philadelphia, Lea & Febiger, 1968, p 33.

471. Powles RL, Balchin LA, Fairley GH, Alexander P: Recognition of leukaemia cells as foreign before and after autoimmunization. Br Med J 1:486, 1971.

472. Priori ES, Dmochowski L, Myers B, Wilbur JR: Constant production of type C virus particles in a continuous tissue culture derived from pleural effusion cells of a lymphoma patient. Nature 232:61, 1971.

473. Propp S, Brown CD, Tartaglia AP: Down's syndrome and congenital leukemia. NY State J Med 66:3067, 1966.

474. Pulvertaft RJV: Phytohaemagglutinin in relation to Burkitt's tumour. Lancet 2:552, 1964.

475. Ragab AH, Vietti TJ: Infectious mononucleosis, lymphoblastic leukemia, and the EB virus. Cancer 24:261, 1969.

476. Randall DL, Reiquam CW, Githens JH, Robinson A: Familial myeloproliferative disease. A new syndrome closely simulating myelogenous leukemia in childhood. Am J Dis Child 110:479, 1965.

477. Rask-Nielsen R: Investigations into varying manifestations of leukaemic lesions following injection of 9:10-dimethyl-1:2 benzanthracene into different subcutaneous sites in street mice. Br J Cancer 3:549, 1949.

478. Rauscher FJ: A virus-induced disease of mice characterized by erythrocytopoiesis and lymphoid leukemia. J Natl Cancer Inst 29:515, 1962.

479. Razis DV, Diamond HD, Craver LF: Familial Hodgkin's disease: Its significance and implications. Ann Intern Med 51:933

480. Recher L, Sinkovics JG, Sykes JA, Whitescarver J: Electron microscopic studies of suspension cultures derived from human leukemic and nonleukemic sources. Cancer Res 29:271, 1969.

481. Reed WB, Epstein HL, Boder E, Sedgwick R: Cutaneous manifestations of ataxia telangiectasia. JAMA 195:746, 1966.

482. Reilly EB, Rapaport SI, Karr NW, Mills H, Carpenter GE: Familial chronic lymphatic leukemia. Arch Intern Med 90:87, 1952.

483. Rich MA, Johns LW Jr: Morphology of an agent associated with a murine leukemia. Virology 20:373, 1963.

484. Riel L: Akute lymphatische Leukämie bei eineiigen Zwillingen. Kinderärztl Prax 16:148, 1948.

485. Rigby PG, Hanson TA, Smith RS: Passage of leukemic cells across the placenta. N Engl J Med 271:124, 1964.

486. _____, Pratt PT, Rosenlof RC, Lemon HM: Genetic relationships in familial leukemia and lymphoma. Arch Intern Med 121:67, 1968.

487. Robinson WA, Pike BL: Colony growth of human bone marrow cells in vitro, in: Stohlman F Jr (ed): Hematopoietic Cellular Differentiation. New York, Grune & Stratton, 1970, p 249.

488. Rolleston H: Critical review. The harmful effects of irradiation (x-rays and radium). Q J Med 23:101, 1930.

489. Ross A, Harnden D: Ultrastructural studies on normal and leukaemic human haematopoietic cells. Eur J Cancer 5:349, 1969.

490. Ross JD, Moloney WC, Desforges JF: Ineffective regulation of granulopoiesis masquerading as congenital leukemia in a mongoloid child. J Pediatr 63:1, 1963.

491. Sabin FR, Austrian CR, Cunningham RS, Doan CA: Studies on the maturation of myeloblasts into myelocytes and on amitotic cell division in the peripheral blood in subacute myeloblastic leukemia. J Exp Med 40:845, 1924.

492. Sabrazès J, Saric R: Angines Lympho-Monocytaires, Agranulocytoses, Leucémies Leucopéniques. Paris: Masson, 1935.

493. Saenger EL, Silverman FN, Sterling TD, Turner ME: Neoplasia following therapeutic irradiation for benign conditions in childhood. Radiology 74:889, 1960.

494. _____, Thoma GE, Tomkins EA: Incidence of leukemia following treatment of hyperthyroidism. JAMA 205:855, 1968.

495. Sarma PS, Huebner RJ, Basker JF, Vernon L, Gilden RV: Feline leukemia and sarcoma viruses: susceptibility of human cells to infection. Science 168:1098, 1970.

496. Sawitsky A, Bloom D, German J: Chromosomal breakage and acute leukemia in congenital telangiectatic erythema and stunted growth. Ann Intern Med 65:487, 1966.

497. Schneider R, Dorn CR, Klauber MR: Cancer in households: A human canine retrospective study. J Natl Cancer Inst 41:1285, 1968.

498. Schönbauer L: Karzinom und Blutkrankheiten. Wien Med Wochenschr 103:113, 1953.

499. Schultz J: Malignancy and the genetics of the somatic cell. Ann NY Acad Sci 71:994, 1958.

500. Schwartz EE, Upton AC: Factors influencing the incidence of leukemia; special consideration of the role of ionizing radiation. Blood 13:845, 1958.

501. Schwartz RS, André-Schwartz J, Armstrong MYK, Beldotti L: Neoplastic sequelae of allogeneic disease. I. Theoretical considerations and experimental designs. Ann NY Acad Sci 129:804, 1966.

502. Schwind JL: Partial maturation of leukemic myeloblasts following fresh plasma transfusions. Am J Med Sci 213:170, 1947.

503. Scolnick EM, Aaronson SA, Todaro GJ, Parks WP: RNA dependent DNA polymerase activity in mammalian cells. Nature 229:318, 1971.

504. _____, Parks WP, Todaro GJ, Aaronson SA: Immunological characterization of primate C-type virus reverse transcriptases. Nature 235:35, 1972.

505. Seltser R, Sartwell PE: The influence of occupational exposure to radiation on the mortality of American radiologists and other medical specialists. Am J Epidemiol 81:2, 1965.

506. Seman G, Dmochowski L: Studies on the possible transmission of virus and mycoplasma in leukemia. Med Record Ann 58:400, 1965.

507. Shimkin MB: On the etiology of cancer. J Chron Dis 8:38, 1958.

508. Shope RE: Koch's postulates and a viral cause of human cancer. Cancer Res 20:1119, 1960.

509. Silberberg DH, Frohman LA, Duff IF: The incidence of leukemia and related diseases in patients with rheumatoid (ankylosing) spondylitis treated with x-ray therapy. Arth Rheumat 3:64, 1960.

510. Simon N, Brucer M, Hayes R: Radiation and leukemia in carcinoma of the cervix. Radiology 74:905, 1960.

511. Simpson CL, Hempelmann LH, Fuller LM: Neoplasia in children treated with x-rays in infancy for thymic enlargement. Radiology 64:840, 1955.

512. Sincovics JG, Sykes JA, Shullenberger CC, Howe CD: Patterns of growth in cultures derived from human leukemic sources. Tex Rep Biol Med 25:446, 1967.

513. Smeby B: Ataxia telangiectasia. Acta Paed Scand 55:239, 1966.

514. Smit CG, Meyler L: Acute myeloid leukaemia after treatment with cytostatic agents. Lancet 2:671, 1970.

515. Snegireff LS: The elusiveness of neoplasia following roentgen therapy for thymic enlargement in childhood. Radiology 72:508, 1959.

516. Snyder AL, Henderson ES, Li FP, Todaro GJ: Possible inherited leukaemogenic factors in familial acute myelogenous leukaemia. Lancet 1:586, 1970.

517. Southam CM: Relationships of immunology to cancer: A review. Cancer Res 20:271, 1960.

518. Spiegelman S, Burny A, Das MR, Keydar J, Schlom J, Traunicek M, Watson K: DNA-directed DNA polymerase activity in oncogenic RNA viruses. Nature 227:1027, 1970.

519. Spiess H: Carcinogenesis by bone seeking ^{224}Ra, in: Proceedings of the Tenth International Cancer Congress, (1970) Houston, 1972.

520. Stanley NF: The aetiology and pathogenesis of Burkitt's African lymphoma. Lancet 1:961, 1966.

521. Stark CR, Mantel N: Effects of maternal age and birth order on the risk of mongolism and leukemia. J Natl Cancer Inst 37:687, 1966.

522. _____, _____: Maternal-age and birth-order effects in childhood leukemia: Age of child and type of leukemia. J Natl Cancer Inst 42:857, 1969.

523. Steinberg AG: A genetic and statistical study of acute leukemia in children, in: Proceedings of Third National Cancer Conference. Philadelphia, Lippincott, 1957, p 353.

524. _____: Genetics of acute leukemia in children, in Hammond D (ed): Proceedings of Ross Conference on Pediatric Research, Nov., 1959. 34th Report: Current Concepts in Leukemia. Columbus, Ohio, Ross Laboratories, 1960, p 85.

525. Sternberg C: Ueber die akute myeloische Leukämie. Wien Klin Wochenschr 24:1623, 1911.

526. Stevens DA, Pry TW, Manaker RA: Infectious mononucleosis—always a primary infection with herpes-type virus? J Natl Cancer Inst 44:533, 1970.

527. _____, Levine PH, Lee SK, Sonley MJ, Waggoner DE: Concurrent infectious mononucleosis and acute leukemia. Am J Med 50:208, 1971.

528. Stewart A: Aetiology of childhood ma-

lignancies. Congenitally determined leukaemia. Br Med J 1:452, 1961.

529. _____, Barber R: Survey of childhood malignancies. Progress report and new ideas: Fieldwork carried out by county and county borough health departments. Med Officer 107:3, 1962.

530. _____, Draper GJ: X-rays and childhood cancer (letter). Lancet 2:829, 1968.

531. _____, Hewitt D: Leukaemia incidence in children in relation to radiation exposure in early life, in Ebert M, Howard A (eds): Current Topics in Radiation Research. Amsterdam, North-Holland, 1965.

532. _____, Kneale GW: Radiation dose effects in relation to obstetric x-rays in childhood cancers. Lancet 1:1185, 1970.

533. _____, Webb J, Giles D, Hewitt D: Malignant disease in childhood and diagnostic irradiation in utero. Lancet 2:447, 1956.

534. _____, _____, Hewitt D: A survey of childhood malignancies. Br Med J 1:1495, 1958.

535. Stewart SE: Leukemia in mice produced by a filterable agent present in AKR leukemic tissues with notes on a sarcoma produced by the same agent. Anat Rec 117:532, 1953.

536. _____: Neoplasms in mice inoculated with cell-free extracts or filtrates of leukemic mouse tissues. I. Neoplasms of the parotid and adrenal glands. J Natl Cancer Inst 15:1391, 1955.

537. _____: Neoplasms in mice inoculated with cell-free extracts or filtrates of leukemic mouse tissues. II. Leukemia in hybrid mice produced by cell-free filtrates. J Natl Cancer Inst 16:41, 1955.

538. _____, Lovelace E, Whang JJ, Ngu VA: Burkitt tumor: Tissue culture, cytogenetic and virus studies. J Natl Cancer Inst 34:319, 1965.

539. Stodmeister R, Büchmann P: Die funktionell-pathologischen Beziehungen zwischen aplastischer Anämie und akuten Leukämien. Ergebn Inn Med Kinderheilkd 60:367, 1941.

539a. Sutnick AI, London WT, Blumberg BS, Gerstley BJS: Susceptibility to leukemia: Immunologic factors in Down's syndrome. J Natl Cancer Inst 47:923, 1971.

540. Sutow WW, Welsh VC: Acute leukemia and mongolism. J Pediatr 52:176, 1958.

541. Swift M: Fanconi's anaemia in the genetics of neoplasia. Nature 230:370, 1971.

542. Swift MR, Hirschhorn K: Fanconi's anemia. Inherited susceptibility to chromosome breakage in various tissues. Ann Intern Med 65:496, 1966.

543. Taylor AW: Effects of glandular fever infection in acute leukaemia. Br Med J 1:589, 1953.

544. Temin HM, Mizutani S: RNA-dependent DNA polymerase in virions of Rous sarcoma virus. Nature 226:1211, 1970.

545. Ten-Bensel RW, Stadlan EM, Krivit W: The development of malignancy in the course of the Aldrich syndrome. J Pediatr 68:761, 1966.

546. Tennant JR, Snell GD: The H-2 locus and viral leukemogenesis as studied in congenic strains of mice. J Natl Cancer Inst 41:597, 1968.

546a. Thomas ED, Bryant JI, Buckner CD, Cliff RA, Fefer A, Johnson FL, Neiman P, Ramberg RE, Storb R: Leukaemic transformation of human marrow cells in vivo. Lancet 1:1310, 1972.

547. Todaro GJ: Reverse transcriptases of RNA tumour viruses, in Vincent, PC (ed): The Nature of Leukaemia. Sydney, N.S.W. Government Printer, 1972, p 79.

548. _____, Green H, Swift MR: Susceptibility of leukemic diploid fibroblast strains to transformation by SV40 virus. Science 153:1252, 1966.

548a. _____, Huebner RJ: The viral oncogene hypothesis: New concepts. Proc Natl Acad Sci USA 69:1009, 1972.

549. _____, Zeve V, Aaronson, SA: Virus in cell culture derived from human tumour patients. Nature 226:1047, 1970.

550. Tokuhata GK, Lilienfeld AM: Familial aggregation of lung cancer in humans. J Natl Cancer Inst 30:289, 1963.

551. _____, Neely CL, Williams DL: Chronic myelocytic leukemia in identical twins and siblings. Blood 31:216, 1968.

552. Tomonaga M: Statistical investigation of leukaemia in Japan. NZ Med J 65:863, 1966.

553. Tooyoka ET, Pifer JW, Crump SL, Dutton AM, Hempelmann LH: Neoplasms in children treated with x-rays for thymic enlargement. II. Tumor incidence as a function of radiation factors. J Natl Cancer Inst 31:1357, 1963.

554. Tough IM, Baikie AG, Harnden DG, King MJ, Brown WMC, Buckton KE, Jacobs PA, McBride JA: Cytogenetic studies in chronic myeloid leukaemia and acute leukaemia associated with mongolism. Lancet 1:411, 1961.

555. _____, Harnden DG, Epstein MA: Chromosome markers in cultured cells from Burkitt's lymphoma. Eur J Cancer 4:637, 1968.

556. Tyler A: Clues to the etiology, pathology and therapy of cancer provided by analogies with transplantation disease. J Natl Cancer Inst 25:1197, 1960.

557. Ulrich H: The incidence of leukemia in radiologists. N Engl J Med 234:45, 1946.

558. United Nations: Report of the Scientific Committee on the effects of atomic radiation. New York, 1958.

559. United Nations: Report of the United Nations Scientific Committee on the effects of atomic radiation. New York, 1964.

560. Upton AC: The dose-response relation in radiation-induced cancer. Cancer Res 21:717, 1961.

561. ———: The role of radiation in the etiology of leukemia, in Zarafonetis CJD (ed.): Proceedings of the International Conference on Leukemia-Lymphoma. Philadelphia, Lea & Febiger, 1968, p 55.

562. ———, Furth J, Christenberry KW: Late effects of thermal neutron irradiation in mice. Cancer Res 14:682, 1954.

563. ———, Wolff FF, Furth J, Kimball AW: A comparison of the induction of myeloid and lymphoid leukemias in x-radiated RF mice. Cancer Res 18:842, 1958.

564. Van Hoosier GL Jr, Stenback WA, Mumford DM, Hill WA, Dunn SC, MacDonald EJ, MacDonald MC, Taylor HG, Trentin JJ: Epidemiological findings and electron microscopy observations in human leukemia and canine contacts. Int J Cancer 3:7, 1968.

565. Vannucchi V: Mielosi acute da benzolismo cronico con aspetto iniziale di aplasia e aspetto successivo di leucemia o di eritroleucemia. Riv Crit Clin Med 57:51, 1957.

566. Van Swaay H: Aplastic anaemia and myeloid leukaemia after irradiation of the vertebral column. Lancet 2:225, 1955.

567. Videbaek A: Heredity in Human Leukemia and Its Relation to Cancer. Copenhagen, Ejnar Munksgaard, 1947.

568. ———: Familial leukaemia. Acta Pathol Microbiol Scand 44:372, 1958.

569. Vigliani EC, Saita G: Benzene and leukemia. N Engl J Med 271:872, 1964.

570. Vincent PC, Cronkite EP, Greenberg ML, Kirsten C, Schiffer LM, Stryckmans PA: Leukocyte kinetics in chronic myeloid leukemia. I. DNA synthesis time in blood and marrow myelocytes. Blood 33:843, 1969.

571. Voll A, Tveit J: Leukemi hos tidligere roentgen/radiumbehandlete pasienter. Nord Med 58:1114, 1957.

572. Wahren B, Lantorp K, Sterner G, Espmark A: EBV antibodies in family contacts of patients with infectious mononucleosis. Proc Soc Exp Biol Med 133:934, 1970.

573. Walburg HE Jr, Upton AC, Tyndale RC, Harris WW, Grove GE: Preliminary observations on spontaneous and radiation-induced leukemia in germ-free mice. Proc Soc Exp Biol Med 118:11, 1965.

574. Wald N: Leukemia in Hiroshima City atomic bomb survivors. Science 127:699, 1958.

575. ———, Borges WH, Li CC, Turner JH, Harnois MC: Leukaemia associated with mongolism. Lancet 1:1228, 1961.

576. Waldenström J: Melphalan therapy in myelomatosis. Br Med J 1:859, 1964.

577. Warburg O: On the origin of cancer cells. Science 123:309, 1956.

578. Ward JE, Galinsky I, Newton BL: Familial leukemia: a report of three cases of leukemia and one leukemoid reaction in one family. Am J Hum Genet 4:90, 1952.

579. Warkany J, Schubert WK, Thompson JN: Chromosome analysis in mongolism (Langdon-Down Syndrome) associated with leukemia. N Engl J Med 268:1, 1963.

580. Warren S: Longevity and causes of death from irradiation in physicians. JAMA 162:464, 1956.

581. ———: The pathological effects of small doses of radiation. Bull. NY Acad Med 34:633, 1958.

582. ———: Radiation carcinogensis. Bull NY Acad Med 46:131, 1970.

583. Weiner L: A family with high incidence leukemia and unique Ph[1] chromosome findings. Blood 26:871, 1965.

584. Weiss J: Über die gegenseitigen Beziehungen zwischen Schulzschem Symptomenkomplex (Mucositis necroticans agranulocytica), akuter Leukämie und septischem Infekt. Wien Arch Inn Med 14:303, 1927.

585. Weitz W: Über einen von Anfang an beobachteten Fall von myeloischer Leukämie bei einer Röntgenlaborantin. Klin Wochenschr 17:1579, 1938.

586. Wertelecki W, Plato CC, Fraumeni JF Jr: Dermatoglyphics in leukaemia. Lancet 2:806, 1969.

587. Whang-Peng J, Gerber P, Knutsen T: So-called C-marker chromosome and Epstein-Barr virus. J Natl Cancer Inst 45:831, 1970.

588. Whitby L: Whither clinical pathology? Trends and opportunities. J Clin Pathol 4:129, 1951.

589. Wiest WG, Heidelberger C: The interaction of carcinogenic hydrocarbons with tissue

constituents. Cancer Res 13:246, 250, 255, 1953.

590. Willi H: Die Leukosen im Kindesalter, Abh. Kinderheilk, no. 43. Berlin, Karger, 1936.

591. Wintrobe MM, Mitchell DM: Atypical manifestations of leukaemia. Q J Med 9:67, 1940.

592. Witts LJ: Recent work on leukaemia in man. Br Med J 1:1197, 1957.

593. Woodliff HJ, Dougan L: Acute leukaemia associated with phenylbutazone treatment. Br Med J 1:744, 1964.

594. _____, _____, Onesti P: Cytogenetic studies in twins, one with chronic granulocytic leukaemia. Nature 211:533, 1966.

595. World Health Organization: Statement on the detection of viruses by electron microscopy in human leukaemia tissues and extracts and in similar material from domestic animals. Bull WHO 34:953, 1966.

596. Yamada K, Takagi N, Sandberg AA: Chromosomes and causation of human cancer and leukemia. II. Karyotypes of human solid tumors. Cancer 19:1879, 1966.

597. Yohn DS, Grace JT Jr: Immunofluorescent studies in human leukemia. Proc Am Assoc Cancer Res 7:78, 1967.

598. _____, Horoszewics JS, Ellison RR, Mittelman A, Chai LS, Grace JT Jr: Immunofluorescent studies in human leukemia. Cancer Res 28:1692, 1968.

599. Zippin C, Bailar JC III, Kohn HI, Lum D, Eisenberg H: Radiation therapy for cervical cancer: Late effects on life span and on leukemia incidence. Cancer 28:937, 1971.

600. Zuelzer WW, Cox DE: Genetic aspects of leukemia. Sem Hematol 6:228, 1968.

601. _____, Thompson RI, Mastrangelo R: Evidence for a genetic factor related to leukemogenesis and congenital anomalies: Chromosomal aberrations in pedigree of an infant with partial D trisomy and leukemia. J Pediatr 72:367, 1968.

602. Zur Hausen H, Schulte-Holthausen H: Presence of EB virus nucleic acid homology in a "virus-free" line of Burkitt tumour cells. Nature 227:245, 1970.

603. _____, _____, Klein G, Henle W, Henle G, Clifford P, Santesson L: EBV DNA in biopsies of Burkitt tumours and anaplastic carcinomas of the nasopharynx. Nature 228:1056, 1970.

6

The Pathology and Pathophysiology
of the Leukemic Cell

The fundamental nature of the leukemic process is unknown, as has been repeatedly noted in previous chapters. Toward its illumination, many approaches have been made, some of which will be considered here. The purpose of this chapter is the description and analysis of leukemic cells and their activities, including studies of cell morphology as well as of the chemical constitution and metabolic activity of leukocytes, both at the cellular and tissue levels.

DEVELOPMENT

It is impossible to understand the morphologic and physiologic alterations found in leukemic cells without appreciating the fundamentals of normal hematopoiesis. These consist, as does the development of all other somatic cells, in a nicely balanced combination of the two separate functions of proliferation and maturation (as is described in greater detail in Chapter 8). Whereas proliferation comprises the processes of DNA synthesis and cell division, maturation includes the sum total of those events which take place while cells alter their features from complete immaturity devoid of individual characteristics to the adult stage when they can be recognized and separated from other types of cells and become capable of subserving their specific functions.

The morphology of the leukocytes as seen in conventionally (Romanowsky) stained films is largely determined by their nucleic acid constitution, chiefly DNA in the nucleus, RNA in the cytoplasm. While in fully mature granulocytes or lymphocytes the DNA content per nucleus is constant, it undergoes cyclical changes in immature proliferating cells, doubling before mitosis and returning to the normal diploid quantity after that. If nuclear DNA is thus measured in a series of normal immature cells such as myelocytes, values ranging from diploid (2n) to tetraploid (4n) will be obtained for individual cells according to the stage of DNA synthesis in which they are found. Resting or fully mature cells, by contrast, will show a sharp DNA peak around the 2n value (Fig. 6-1).

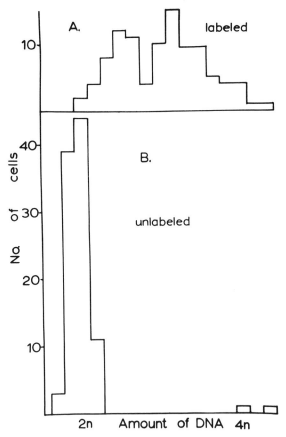

Fig. 6-1. DNA contents (in arbitrary units) of normal, immature marrow cells, measured by microdensitometry. Top, cells labeled with radioactive thymidine which synthesize DNA. Values of DNA range from 2n–4n. Bottom, cells unlabeled by radioactive thymidine and, therefore, in the resting phase. Most have a DNA value of 2n.

In many leukemic cells, especially in the acute forms, and in the metamorphosis of chronic granulocytic leukemia (CGL), the nuclear pattern in Romanowsky films is disturbed in comparison with that of normal cells in the same stage of development. Increases in nuclear size, folding, and lobulation are commonly seen and raise the suspicion that the nuclear DNA content may be abnormally high, a condition which might arise either because the cell contained excessive numbers of chromosomes or abnormally large quantities of DNA per chromosome. Direct measurements have, in fact, shown that the nuclear content of DNA is not raised in most leukemic cells,[90] the increased nuclear size being chiefly explained by a raised protein content.[159] Although direct chromosome counts (described below) have shown the presence of additional chromosomes (hyperdiploidy) in a number of leukemias, the increase in DNA thus produced is nearly always too small to be measurable by optical methods, except in a few instances in which the cells are tetraploid or of even higher degrees of ploidy. Abnormally high quantities of DNA have, on the other hand, been found in the presence of normal chromosome counts. These findings are attributable to cells which have begun the synthesis of DNA prior to division but are

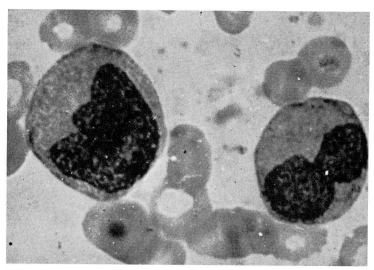

Fig. 6-2. Chronic granulocytic leukemia showing late granulocytes, with grossly deficient granulation as well as nuclear abnormalities.

blocked from entering mitosis either because of metabolic abnormalities inherent in the disease process or, more often, by therapeutic agents[16,50] (see chapter 17).

Many of the most characteristic morphologic abnormalities of leukemic cells do not result from disturbances in proliferation but rather occur in the process of cellular *maturation*. Normal leukocytes, like other cells, proliferate while they are young, ceasing to do so when they have reached a level of maturation which enables them to carry out their specific functions; this change occurs at the myelocyte stage in the granulocytic series and at the prolymphocyte stage in the lymphocytic series. This is probably the consequence of a radical and progressive alteration in cellular metabolism. The primitive type is directed largely toward the synthesis of nucleoproteins needed for the formation of new cells. This is altered later to a form capable of supplying the energy for the defensive and other functions of the mature leukocytes. (See Rebuck for a review of leukocytic functions.[209]) Cytologically, the change is seen in an alteration of the nuclear chromatin pattern from a fine and almost uniform network to an irregular arrangement of variously condensed blocks. There is a decrease in the nuclear-cytoplasmic ratio, usually with a change in nuclear outline from a circular to a less regular oval or indented configuration, a disappearance of the nucleoli and the chromatin condensations associated with them (perinucleolar crown),[202] and a gradual decline in the intensity of the cytoplasmic basophilia with a concurrent appearance of the specific granulations. Biochemically, profound changes in the nucleic acid constitution of the cell occur.

The basophilia of the cytoplasm is a reflection of its content of RNA. In the normal cell, the cytoplasmic RNA diminishes from a concentration in excess of 5 percent in the immature phases to one of zero percent during maturity.[212,253] Simultaneously, the nucleolus, which is also largely composed of RNA, disappears. In the maturing cell nuclear changes are closely coordinated with the gradual loss of cytoplasmic RNA. In leukemia, by contrast, there is often an apparent lack of such coordination, with cytoplasmic maturation lagging behind that in the nucleus, or occasionally the reverse. This applies particularly to the acute forms as well as to the later stages of chronic granulocytic leukemia, in which, as noted by Bessis[32] and many others, there is a progressive lack of maturation as the disease advances. In chronic lymphocytic and chronic granulocytic leukemia in its chronic phase, on the other hand, we see none of the cytologic signs pointing to a fundamentally disordered protein metabolism.

The most frequent morphologic abnormalities seen in leukemic cells in acute leukemia are the following: an abnormally long retention of the fine, immature, nuclear chromatin pattern, often, as has already been mentioned, associated with an increase in nuclear size which may lead to convolution or actual reduplication of the nucleus; an overdevelopment of the nucleolar apparatus, either in number or size of the nucleoli or both; and an unusually late persistence of cytoplasmic basophilia, frequently with poor development of the signs of cytoplasmic maturity like the specific granulations (Fig. 6-2). Optical and chemical estimations of the cellular nucleic acids have shown that in many leukemias the cytoplasmic RNA is much higher than in normal leukocytes of the same stage of development.[253] This may lead to an increased ratio of the RNA to the DNA content of the cells.[62, 101, 171]

MORPHOLOGY

In the preceding section an attempt was made to show the differences in the nucleoprotein of normal and leukemic leukocytes, and the disturbances in proliferation and maturation resulting from them. We must now state these differences in the more conventional terms of hematologic morphology, and describe those cytologic features which characterize the various types of leukemic cells.

In this connection, we can deal very briefly with the cells found in the earlier stages of the chronic leukemias, since they do not differ significantly from the normal cells at the same stage of development. Thus, we find apparently normal mature lymphocytes in chronic lymphocytic leukemia—even though they may differ profoundly from the functional point of view (Chapters 10 and 12)—and normal polymorphonuclears, metamyelocytes, myelocytes, and occasionally younger cells in chronic granulocytic leukemia. Moreover, these cells appear identical with their normal counterparts whether they are examined in Romanowsky-stained blood films, by supravital stains, phase-contrast or electron microscopy. The nucleus and cytoplasm show their usual structures and complements of organelles such as granules, mitochondria, and Golgi apparatus. On the other hand, the mature granulocytes of chronic granulocytic leukemia commonly have an enzyme abnormality (page 145) and invariably a specific chromosomal anomaly (page 157).

We are on much more uncertain ground when we examine the cells found in the acute or the later phases of the chronic leukemias, one of the chief difficulties being the classification of the leukocytes which characterize these conditions. In the granulocytic series, for instance, there is normally an unbroken line of development from very immature to completely mature cells, and any desire to separate the various stages from each other must of necessity result in arbitrary divisions. There is no unanimity about the positions at which the dividing lines are drawn, and different authors use identical terms for obviously different developmental stages. Terminological differences complicate in particular the distinction between promyelocytes and myelocytes, and between myelocytes and metamyelocytes.

Where such difficulties exist in the nomenclature of the normal cell series, they become much greater in the acute leukemias in which there is an infinite variety of atypical cells characterized, not only by nuclear and cytoplasmic abnormalities, but also by an often striking asynchronism between the maturation of nucleus and cytoplasm. A cell with an undoubtedly primitive nucleus may, for instance, show quite numerous azurophil cytoplasmic granules; or conversely, a convoluted or hypersegmented nucleus may be surrounded by a basophilic and nongranulated cytoplasm. Such abnormal cells, although they have been dignified with an astonishing variety of names (paramyeloblasts, paralymphoblasts, parapromyelocytes, monocytoid paramyeloblasts, monocytoid cells, and many more) are often extremely difficult to classify, or even to identify clearly as members of any one cell line. It is here that cytochemistry has come into its own since it affords an additional and very precise means of studying the characteristics of individual leukemic cells. However, when the prevalent cell type is very primitive, even the most searching investigations may fail to yield definite information on its origin and classification. Wherever cytochemical methods are used in the leukemias, the interpretation of results calls for a careful and critical approach, eschewing all unwarranted presumptions.[126]

It is usual to distinguish acute granulocytic, lymphocytic, and monocytic leukemias. A further type has been given a great many more or less descriptive names in various countries, ranging from acute *stem cell* to *hemocytoblastic* leukemia, but we prefer to refer to it as the *acute undifferentiated type,* inasmuch as it is impossible, by present means, to classify its very primitive cells. The diagnosis of the cellular type is in the first instance attempted by an analysis of its morphology in Romanowsky-stained films, including cell size, nuclear shape, chromatin pattern, nuclear-cytoplasmic ratio, cytoplasmic staining characteristics, and the presence of granules and other intracytoplasmic structures. Further hints as to the nature of the type-specific cells may at times be found in the more mature cells present together with them. Thus, there may be a clearly defined line of maturation leading from the dominant blasts, through promyelocytes to myelocytes and beyond, in which case there is little doubt about the granulocytic nature of the case, even though the blasts themselves show few or no distinctive features.

More often than not, however, there is no such obvious maturation line, and, indeed, arrest or abnormality of cellular maturation is probably the most characteristic feature in the acute leukemias. When this happens, primitive cells are accompanied by few, if any, intermediate forms. Mature forms may be present in some numbers: the so-called hiatus leukaemicus of Naegeli is conceived to be the simultaneous presence of primitive and mature cells, with a lack of intermediate forms. In such cases the mature cells are usually derived from surviving *normal* precursors which are in the process of final extinction, and therefore they convey no diagnostic message. Thus, the type of acute leukemia can only rarely be diagnosed from the "company kept" by the blasts. On the contrary, it would seem more rational to assume that *absence* of mature cells of a certain line gives a clue as to the nature of the primitive cells: a blast cell leukemia associated with a severe neutropenia, for instance, is nearly always granulocytic in type.

Even when maturation does occur in the acute leukemias, it is often pathologic. Nucleocytoplasmic asynchronism, abnormal nuclear development with atypical lobulation, segmentation, and imperfect maturation of the cytoplasmic granulations conspire to produce appearances far removed from those of normal cells. In par-

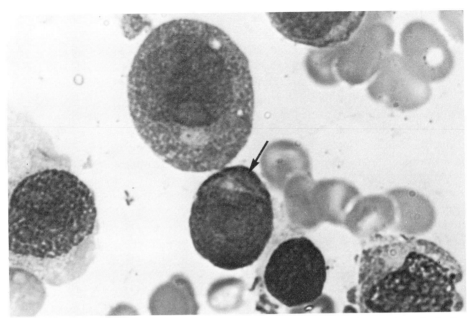

Fig. 6-3. Acute granulocytic leukemia. Myeloblasts, one showing an Auer body (*arrow*).

ticular, distinctions between the neutrophil and monocyte series become difficult (see Chapter 3), and this is responsible for the enormously confusing literature on acute monocytic leukemia.

Thus, it is evident that in a proportion of cases of acute leukemia neither the morphology of the leukemic cells nor the general character of the blood picture is capable of providing a firm diagnosis of the type. Conventional examination of Romanowsky-stained films proves insufficient, for whether a given cell is a myeloblast, lymphoblast, or monoblast, it will be large, with a primitive nucleus, one or more nucleoli, and a strongly basophilic nongranular cytoplasm. Therefore, we must examine the special diagnostic criteria which have been advocated as useful in this predicament.

Presence of Auer bodies.   These azurophil rods (Fig. 6-3) whose nature has been extensively investigated by Bessis,[33] Bessis and Breton-Gorius,[36] Ackerman,[2] Freeman,[94] Huhn and Borchers,[131] and McDuffie[167] give all the staining reactions of azurophil granules, particularly the oxidase, peroxidase, and acid phosphatase reactions, and are crystalline coacervates of granules which occur only at the acid pH prevailing in young cells. Almost all authors agree that they are characteristic of granulocytic leukemia and are found in from 0.1–30 percent of leukemic myeloblasts,[61] but never in lymphoblasts. If Auer bodies are seen, it appears justifiable to label the case as one of acute granulocytic leukemia.

The pseudo-Pelger phenomenon.   The congenital leukocytic anomaly named after Pelger[197] and Huët[132] is characterized by lack of segmentation and by abnormal chromatin condensations in the granulocytic series, most obvious in its maturest members whose nuclei are rod- or dumbbell-shaped, but recognizable also in

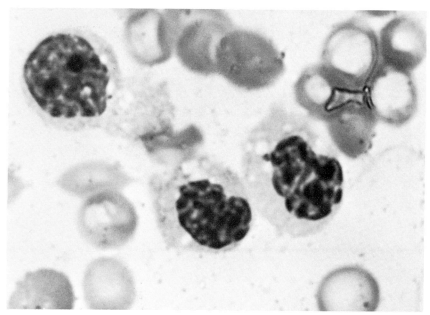

Fig. 6-4.   Acute granulocytic leukemia. Three leukocytes showing the pseudo-Pelger anomaly.

the immature granulocytes as early as the myelocyte stage (Fig. 6-4). Inherited as a dominant, it inflicts no clinical handicaps on its carriers. An acquired form closely resembling the congenital variety is frequently found in cases of acute leukemia[60,70,232] in which there is no indication of a familial incidence of the anomaly (Fig. 6-4). The importance of this anomaly lies in the fact that it is an acquired and not a congenital aberration and clearly stigmatizes the affected granulocytes as the derivatives of abnormal and, hence, presumably leukemic precursors. The discovery of pseudo-Pelger cells provides an additional diagnostic criterion in favor of the granulocytic type of acute leukemia.[114]

The nucleolar formula.   Normal myeloblasts are stated to have usually two or more nucleoli, but lymphoblasts have only one. If this difference were constant, and if it were found in leukemic as well as in normal cells, this would, of course, be a valuable diagnostic criterion. Unfortunately, there is a large range of nucleolar counts among the cells of either series, and although the means may differ, the ranges overlap, particularly in the often grossly abnormal leukemic blasts. Moreover, specialized staining methods have shown that nucleoli can often be shown where the traditional Romanowsky stains fail to do so.[103,224] Those authors[99,156,157] who rely on nucleolar counts do not appear aware of these difficulties, and though we believe that the discovery of unequivocal single nucleoli may add a rather weak argument in favor of a diagnosis of the lymphocytic type in a given case of acute leukemia, the usefulnes of the nucleolar formula as a diagnostic tool appears limited.

Supravital staining and phase-contrast microscopy.   These methods permit an observation of the cells in the unfixed living state and reveal intracellular structures

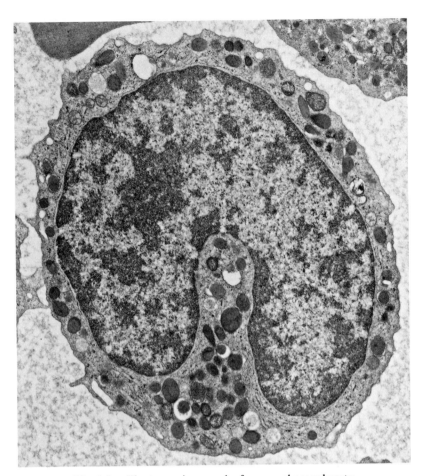

Fig. 6-5. Electron micrograph of a normal granulocyte.

which remain invisible in most conventionally stained films.[229] According to some older authors,[214] both myeloblasts and lymphoblasts are motile in supravital preparations, but their mode of locomotion differs. More recent investigations[61] have revealed little if any motility in either class of cells, but a rather characteristic spreading of the living myeloblast, which is not observed in lymphoblasts. Mitochondria are stained by the supravital technique and can be easily observed under phase-contrast microscopy, with or without vital staining. In the myeloblast, they tend to be numerous, fine, and spread throughout the cells; in the lymphoblasts, few, coarse, and usually in a juxtanuclear position.[45,61] This may be a useful distinguishing feature, provided the cells are typical; but difficulties at once arise in atypical leukocytes[229] and it is here that the need for reliable diagnostic criteria is most marked.

Electron microscopy. The development of electron microscopy of ultrathin sections of blood cells, notably by Bessis and his group, has added a new dimension

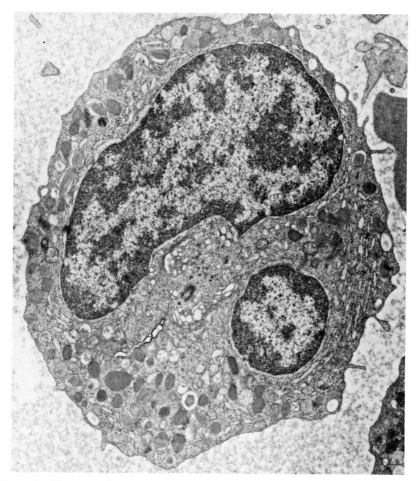

Fig. 6-6.   Electron micrograph of a normal granulocyte showing nuclear condensation and lobulation, and well developed cytoplasmic granules. × 16,000.

to the morphologic study of leukemic cells. Many alterations have been found in comparison with the appearances of normal cells (Figs. 6-5–6-8), but from the point of view of the type diagnosis of acute leukemias, electron microscopy has proved to be of little help.

Among the electron microscopic features peculiar to leukemic cells are *fibrillar* bodies in the cytoplasm (Fig. 6-9).[33,35,94] Often there is "anarchy" of the cellular organelles, resulting in a loss of their normal sequential and interdependent development.[34] This is seen in unusual nuclear projections, abnormalities of the granulations, both azurophil and specific (diminution in number of the granules, vacuolization, lack of the normal paracrystalline structure), and deficiencies and abnormalities of ribosomes, mitochondria, and ergastoplasmic profiles; above all, the same asynchronism prevails between nuclear and cytoplasmic development which is also found in conventional blood and marrow films.[36] The striking development of crystalline Auer rods from azurophil granules has already been mentioned (Fig. 6-

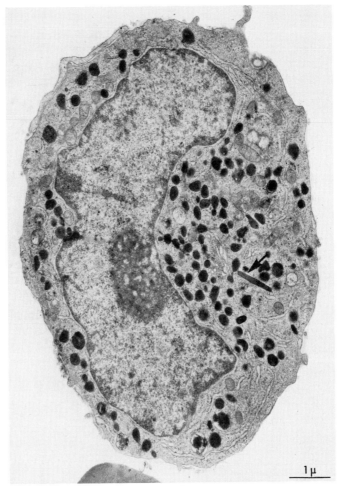

Fig. 6-7. Electron micrograph of an AGL granulocyte. Note the nuclear cytoplasmic asynchrony. A large number of azurophil and specific granules are present, one of them, rod-shaped, an early Auer body (*arrow*). The nucleus lacks condensations and contains a large nucleolus. Ribosomes and ergastoplasmic profiles are abundant in the cytoplasm. (Reproduced from M. Bessis: Cellules du Sang Normal et Pathologique. Paris, Masson et Cie, 1972, courtesy of the author and publisher.)

10). In many instances of acute leukemia the variety of structural abnormalities is such that it "can render cytologic diagnosis impossible to establish, even with the electron microscope."[36]

The preceding paragraphs may be summarized by stating that, when all possible diagnostic methods have been employed, there remains a sizeable group of acute leukemias in which a decision as to type cannot be made by objective criteria. This group forms such a large proportion of all cases that it must seriously affect the statistics of type distribution, and there seems no doubt that this accounts for the extraordinarily variable percentages which have been reported from different

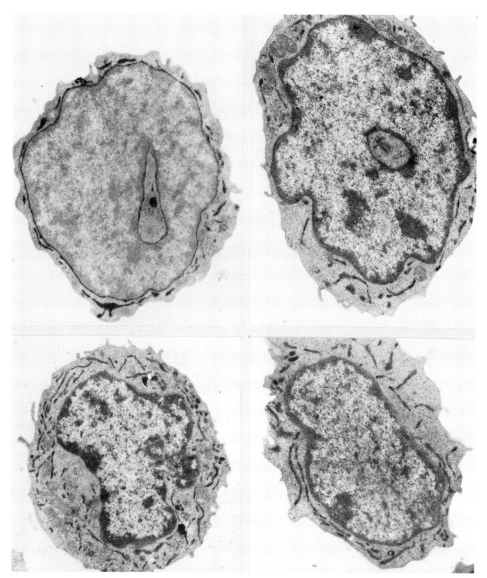

Fig. 6-8. Electron micrographs of four AGL granulocytes. All lack specific granulations. The dark streaks are caused by the peroxidase reaction which has produced staining of the nuclear membranes and ergastoplasmic profiles, as well as a few tiny cytoplasmic granules. (Reproduced from M. Bessis: Cellules du Sang Normal et Pathologique. Paris, Masson et Cie, 1972, courtesy of the author and publisher.)

centers.[116] In relation to both treatment and prognosis—especially in acute leukemia of childhood—the most important differentiation to be made is whether the leukemia is lymphocytic or nonlymphocytic. The differentiation of the acute myelomonocytic (often called monocytic) variety from the more common acute granulocytic form is of much less significance.

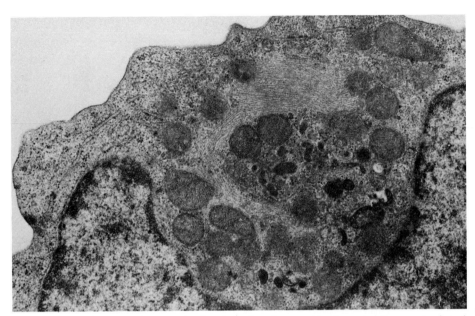

Fig. 6-9. Electron micrograph of early leukemic granulocyte containing a cytoplasmic fibrillar body. These bodies are often crescentic or cylindrical and may contain cytoplasm, granulations, or mitochondria. (Reproduced from M. Bessis: Cellules du Sang Normal et Pathologique. Paris, Masson et Cie, 1972, of the author and publisher.)

CHROMOSOMES

Proliferation in hematopoietic cells takes place, as in other somatic cells, by means of mitotic divisions in the immature members of all series: myeloblasts, promyelocytes and myelocytes, proerythroblasts and early erythroblasts, and megakaryocytes. As will be seen, there is evidence that these three series are derived from a common ancestor. In the lymphocytic series, mitosis occurs in lympho-blasts: mature lymphocytes, in contrast to mature granulocytes, will also divide when stimulated by phytohemagglutinin (PHA) or other mitogens (see Chapter 12).

The kinetics of cellular division are discussed in Chapter 8. In this section we are concerned with the number and structure of the chromosomes in leukemic cells, their comparison with those of their normal equivalents, and the part which chro-mosomal abnormalities may play in the leukemic process. Studies in this field have become feasible as the result of new techniques[92, 181] which permit the even and un-distorted spreading of chromosomes following metaphase arrest of mitosis. Cells from both marrow and peripheral blood are routinely examined, and less frequently those from the spleen[238] and the lymph nodes.[239] Marrow cells are usually studied in *direct* preparations, without previous culture,[160] whereas peripheral blood cells are examined after incubation lasting 1–7 days in various culture media. Under these conditions normal blood cells will show very few divisions unless stimulated by PHA. In cultures to which PHA has been added, the lymphocytes become transformed to blastlike cells which divide. When leukemic blood is cultured, im-mature cells such as blasts or myelocytes often divide without stimulation, and when mitoses are found in such cultures, they may reasonably be taken to be derived from leukemic cells, unless PHA has been added. In PHA cultures of leukemic blood the

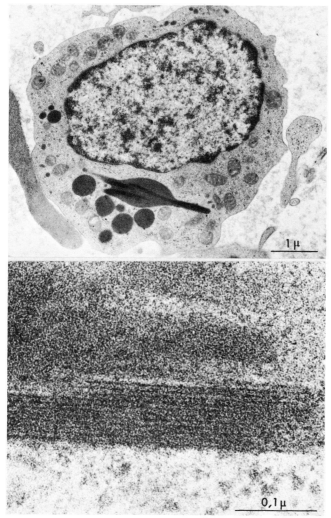

Fig. 6-10. Electron micrographs of Auer bodies. Top, a leukemic myeloblast whose cytoplasm contains mitochondria and azurophil granules of various sizes. The Auer body arises from the fusion of some large azurophil granules. Bottom, high-power magnification of an Auer body showing its periodic structure. (Reproduced from M. Bessis: Cellules du Sang Normal et Pathologique. Paris, Masson et Cie, 1972, courtesy of the author and publisher.)

mitoses are likely to be mixed, some coming from leukemic cells and some from normal lymphocytes.

Chronic Granulocytic Leukemia

In this disease a constant chromosomal abnormality has been found. Studies by many workers have shown the presence of an abnormally small acrocentric chromosome, the Philadelphia or Ph[1] chromosome, in a very high proportion of patients (Fig. 6-11).[12,85,187–189,255] The Ph[1] replaces one of the small acrocentric chromosomes originally thought to be number 21 but now identified by fluorescence microscopy as 22.[190] In the marrow, it occurs in all dividing cells during relapse and,

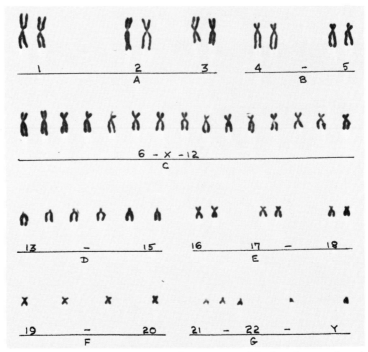

Fig. 6-11. Karyogram of a metaphase from a man with chronic granulocytic leukemia in the chronic phase. The Philadelphia chromosome (Ph[1]) is shown replacing a number 22 chromosome of the G group.

surprisingly, also during full remission.[254,256,259,278]* This is so because, not only granulocyte precursors, but also erythroblasts[54,208] and megakaryocytes contain the Ph[1]. This is strong evidence in favor of a stem cell common to all three series, for an identical mutation occurring separately in all three of them is a highly unlikely event.

While the Ph[1] is carried by hematopoietic cells wherever they may be found— marrow, blood, or spleen[238]—it is not carried by other tissues such as skin fibroblasts, or by lymphocytes. In the blood, therefore, the Ph[1] can be seen only so long as leukemic cells capable of division are present, that is, in relapse. During remission PHA-stimulated blood cultures are usually Ph[1]-negative because all mitoses are derived from lymphocytes; without PHA there are few or no mitoses in chronic granulocytic leukemia during remission.

The Ph[1] is clearly an acquired and not an inherited abnormality (in a single family described by Weiner,[273] the Ph[1], or a predisposition to its acquisition, was apparently inherited). Its origin is almost certainly clonal, that is, all cells carrying it are derived from a single mutant cell. Strong support for this theory was discovered when it was found that women with chronic granulocytic leukemia, who were heterozygous for the enzyme glucose-6-phosphate-dehydrogenase, had red and white cells which carried only one of the two types of the enzyme.[81] Normally, all cells including erythrocytes and leukocytes should have carried a mixture of the two

*There are few but important exceptions to this rule, generally in cases of marrow hypoplasia induced by busulfan.[83]

enzyme types, and this was indeed the case in the skin fibroblasts. Hence, all the hematopoietic cells in these individuals must have formed a single clone; a clone which carried the Ph[1] chromosome. Evidence in favor of a clonal origin of Ph[1] also came from a patient with chronic granulocytic leukemia who also had a mosaic Klinefelter syndrome. In this patient the normal (XY) cells were Ph[1]-positive but the XXY cells were negative.[88]

The mechanism by which the Ph[1] arises is not clear. It may be either the result of a deletion or of a translocation to another chromosome. The defect represents about 39 percent of the affected small acrocentric chromosome or 0.5 percent of the total diploid complement.[223] This is such a small proportion that present cytogenetic methods are not sensitive enough to distinguish between translocation of the missing segment or its outright loss (see, however, Chapter 21).

In the majority of cases of chronic granulocytic leukemia the Ph[1] is the only chromosome abnormality during the chronic phase. However, in a small subgroup of men there is an associated absence of the Y chromosome in the hematopoietic but not in other cells. These men often have a peculiarly benign form of the disease with a prolonged course.[8, 18, 100, 193, 237, 256] A similar XO condition of the marrow cells has been found in three cases of chronic myelomonocytic leukemia, but without the Ph[1] chromosome.[134]

Abnormalities in addition to the Ph[1] arise in at least half the cases of chronic granulocytic leukemia as they approach or enter the acute (blastic) phase, the so-called metamorphosis.[10] At that stage, the previously stable karyotype changes by a process which has been termed *clonal evolution*,[63, 164] which is closely associated with the more malignant phase of the disease. Clinically, lymphadenopathy may now be prominent, while it is generally absent during the chronic phase.[72, 148] Among the most common of the additional abnormalities is a second Ph[1] chromosome,[3, 58, 119, 136, 194, 240, 243, 246] but many other chromosomal duplications or, less commonly, deletions have been described as well (Figs. 6-12 and 6-13).[75, 142, 192, 195–196] The most extensive studies in this field have been conducted by de Grouchy,[63–65] and by Spiers and Baikie.[240, 243] De Grouchy and his colleagues have described seven different models for clonal evolution. The chromosomal changes in the acute phase of chronic granulocytic leukemia resemble closely those of the acute leukemias (see below), as do, of course, the clinical and hematologic features, and it is often possible in serial studies to analyze the cytogenetic mechanisms which have produced these changes by means of clonal evolution. Both in chronic granulocytic and in acute leukemias (where it is rare), clonal evolution seems to be an orderly process which appears at a late stage and leads to increasing acuteness of the disease.[58] Clonal changes during metamorphosis may be reversible if a remission is induced. In such patients, the marrow picture returns to simple Ph[1]-positivity without other abnormalities.[49]

The specificity and significance of the Ph[1] have been much debated. Apart from chronic granulocytic leukemia, the abnormality has been described in a few cases of the eosinophilic variety,[74, 111] and in a small number of patients with other myeloproliferative disorders, especially acute granulocytic leukemia.[52, 130, 141, 148, 169, 280] Some of these cases were probably atypical chronic granulocytic leukemia, and others may have been discovered in the acute phase of CGL, the chronic phase having been unusually brief. There appears to be no incontrovertible evidence to show that the Ph[1] chromosome occurs in any condition other than chronic granulocytic leukemia.

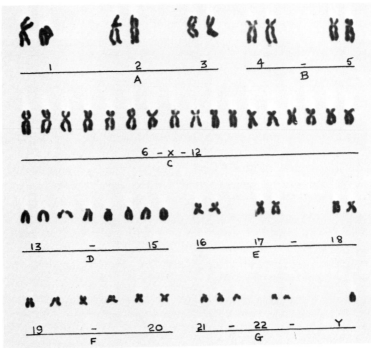

Fig. 6-12. Karyogram from a man with chronic granulocytic leukemia in metamorphosis. There are 53 chromosomes, including two Ph[1] and additional members of the C, D, and F groups.

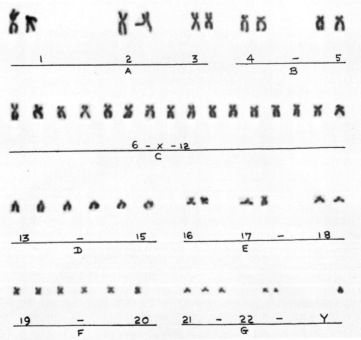

Fig. 6-13. Karyogram from a man with chronic granulocytic leukemia in metamorphosis. There are 50 chromosomes including two Ph[1], one additional C-group and two additional F-group chromosomes.

The opposite situation—chronic granulocytic leukemia without a Ph[1] chromosome—is more controversial. Both in adults[152,254] and in children,[121] cases have been described which clinically and hematologically resemble chronic granulocytic leukemia but cannot be shown to have any consistent chromosome abnormality. In childhood, the Ph[1]-negative (juvenile) type of the disease differs clearly from the typical Ph[1]-positive type, which although rare in children, certainly occurs. The "juvenile" type is found almost entirely in young infants and is characterized by an acute course resistant to therapy, as well as by some unusual hematologic features, especially a very high fetal hemoglobin content of the erythrocytes.[40] In adults, the proportion of Ph[1]-negative cases of chronic granulocytic leukemia varies greatly according to the source of the report, but in one series it was as high as 15 percent of all cases of chronic granulocytic leukemia.[79] The same authors, however, as well as earlier ones,[152] made the point that the Ph[1]-negative cases differed clinically and hematologically from the classic Ph[1]-positive type: the course in the former was more acute, they were resistant to therapy, the blastic crisis appeared earlier, and the overall prognosis was worse. In our view, the distinction between the two types is a fairly clear one, and we prefer, therefore, to regard them as different members of the myeloproliferative group. Semantically, it appears more logical to restrict the name chronic granulocytic leukemia to cases which show the Ph[1] chromosome and form a rather homogeneous group from the clinical point of view. We reserve the term *atypical myeloproliferative syndrome* for the Ph[1]-negative cases. This has been our practice for some time, and in our terminology, therefore, chronic granulocytic leukemia is synonymous with 100 percent Ph[1]-positivity.

The relationship of the Ph[1] to the leukemic process has long been a matter of the greatest interest. Theoretically, the abnormality could either be causally related to the disease, or again, it could arise in its course but promote its progression; or it could be an unimportant by-product of its activity. The very consistency of the presence of the Ph[1] would indicate a special relationship to chronic granulocytic leukemia, or perhaps, more fundamentally, to the regulation of granulocytic proliferation, and this feature probably excludes the third possibility mentioned above. That the Ph[1] occurs early in the disease, and sometimes in its preclinical stages, is also evident.[140] However, apart from a few instances in which chromosomes said to resemble the Ph[1] were found in individuals exposed to intensive irradiation[104] the Ph[1] has not yet been unequivocally found in people without chronic granulocytic leukemia who later developed the disease. Therefore, it cannot be asserted that the abnormality precedes the leukemic process or leads to its onset. However, whether it does so is perhaps less important than the undoubted fact that the Ph[1] chromosome occurs in all cases of chronic granulocytic leukemia. We believe that this signifies an intimate connection with the nature and progress of the disease and, furthermore, that the possession of the Ph[1] predisposes the carrier eventually to further clonal changes associated with increasing malignancy. Enough is now known to make this interpretation of the course of events in chronic granulocytic leukemia and in its metamorphosis a matter of overwhelming probability.

Acute Leukemia

In this type it was realized from an early stage that no uniform chromosomal abnormality is present, but that changes, when they occur, are manifold and variable among patients.[13-14,86,93,133,147,225] In substantial numbers of patients, no ab-

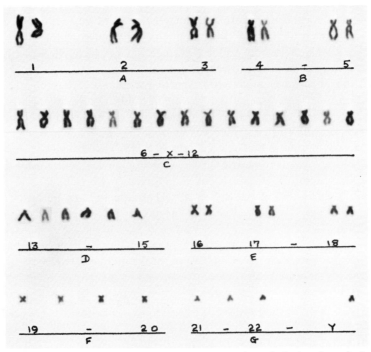

Fig. 6-14. Karyogram from a man with acute lymphocytic leukemia and a hypodiploid karyotype. There are 45 chromosomes. One G-group chromosome is missing.

normalities whatever are found. The proportion of those showing abnormalities has been variously estimated, most commonly at about 50 percent. Among 45 patients with acute lymphocytic leukemia, Whang-Peng et al.[279] found only 29 percent with significant cytogenetic abnormalities, among 73 with acute granulocytic leukemia there were 29.1 percent,[280] and our own results in 79 adults with acute leukemia, mainly granulocytic, were almost exactly the same.[113]

The abnormalities in acute leukemia are both numerical and structural. Hypo-, hyper-, and pseudodiploid mitoses occur (Figs. 6-14 and 6-15), generally in distinct clones, although in some patients there is a wide range of abnormalities. Marker chromosomes (Fig. 6-16) often characterize individual clones of cells. As a rule, once an abnormal clone is found in a patient, it remains with him throughout the course of his illness. In complete remission, the abnormal clone frequently disappears, and only normal mitoses are found, but as relapse occurs, the clone reappears, sometimes in a modified state. Clonal progression—the acquisition of fresh abnormalities in the course of the disease—is rarer in acute than in chronic granulocytic leukemia, but it is demonstrable in some patients.[31,58,92,117,135,153,165,211] Its frequency has probably been underestimated.

In acute lymphocytic leukemia the abnormal clones are most often hyperdiploid,[226] but in the granulocytic forms, including erythroleukemia, all varieties of abnormalities—hyper-, pseudo-, and hypodiploidy—may be seen.[127,183,280] Members of any of the chromosome groups may be either duplicated, deleted, or structurally altered; statistically, the incidence of abnormalities is higher than expected in the G group,[113,243,279,280] but in no other.

It has been stated that chromosomal abnormalities are more common in the late than in the earlier stages of acute leukemia.[279] If true, this would imply a poorer

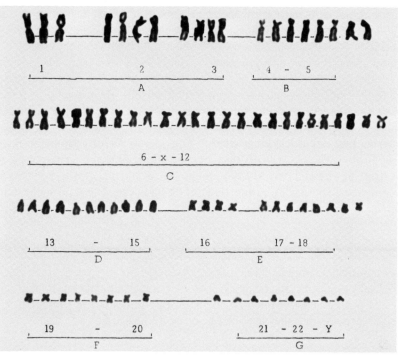

Fig. 6-15. Karyogram from a man with acute granulocytic leukemia and a hyperdiploid (polyploid) karyotype. There are 84 chromosomes with additional chromosomes in all groups.

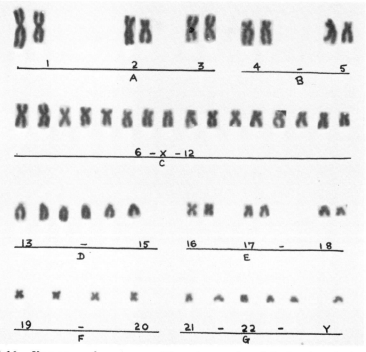

Fig. 6-16. Karyogram from a man with acute granulocytic leukemia and a hyperdiploid karyotype. There are 48 chromosomes with additional members of the C- and G-groups, and a large marker chromosome in the A group.

prognosis for patients with cytogenetic abnormalities, and this has not generally been found,[11,113] although an association between various specific abnormalities and the clinical outlook has been claimed.[123] It must be remembered that therapy—both radio- and chemotherapy—can produce chromosomal abnormalities, though these are not clonal in nature. Making allowance for such iatrogenic appearances, there is no conclusive evidence to show any correlation between the presence or absence of chromosomal abnormalities and the prognosis of acute leukemia.

On the other hand, it is evident that, when changes are discovered, these characterize the actual leukemic clones. This clearly follows from the fashion in which abnormalities are seen to disappear in remission and reemerge as relapse asserts itself. In the majority of cases, moreover, abnormal clones, when first seen, are accompanied by varying proportions of diploid cells. These probably represent the remaining nucleus of normal cells which can displace the abnormal clones during remission.[113] Why abnormal clones are not always found in acute leukemia is not certain, but it may be presumed that when there are only diploid complements during relapse, submicroscopic changes are actually present in some or all of them. Perhaps new techniques will reveal these. Again, the persistence of abnormal clones in individual cases suggests strongly that they are intimately associated with the pathogenic process itself. However, as in chronic granulocytic leukemia, it is still impossible to assert that they precede the onset of the disease.

Preleukemia

The relationship between chromosomal changes and leukemia has been investigated by studies on preleukemic conditions of which the refractory anemias and myeloproliferative conditions are the most common. This subject has recently been fully reviewed,[30,112] and the following are the salient points emerging from this analysis.

The presence of an abnormal clone in a marrow, thought to be preleukemic but not as yet definitely leukemic, signifies a high chance of an early conversion to full leukemia, especially if the clone is unstable.[30,184-186] However, the change to overt leukemia is not invariable, for some patients have been followed for many months or even years without it occurring, in spite of the undoubted presence of clonal abnormalities.[30,222]

In the myeloproliferative conditions such as polycythemia vera the situation is somewhat similar, for though clonal changes are fairly common, they do not always indicate the early onset of leukemia.[138-139,166,174] Conversely, absence of chromosomal abnormalities does not exclude the possibility of leukemia developing, even in the imminent future, which is not surprising since at least half of all cases of definite acute leukemia lack any recognizable chromosomal lesions.

Chronic Lymphocytic Leukemia and the Lymphomas

The study of the chromosomes in this form of leukemia is handicapped by the fact that, unlike the normal lymphocyte which divides upon stimulation by PHA or other mitogens, its leukemic counterpart does so only to a very slight extent or not at all. Mitoses are not found in bone marrow lymphocytes, while there are few in PHA blood cultures from patients with chronic lymphocytic leukemia: it is not even

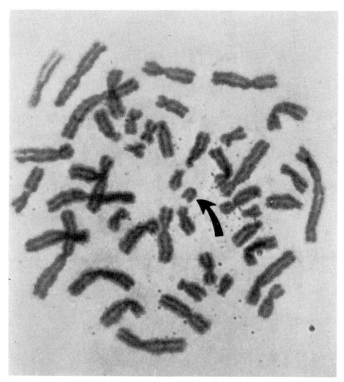

Fig. 6-17. Metaphase plate from a leukocyte, cultured from the blood of a patient with chronic lymphocytic leukemia, showing the Ch¹ chromosome (*arrow*). × 1900

certain whether those in the blood are derived from normal or leukemic lymphocytes (see Chapter 10). Significantly, no chromosomal abnormality was found in mitoses from lymph nodes in chronic lymphocytic leukemia.[241] Very few chromosomal abnormalities have thus far been described in this type, and those which have were inconstant and of doubtful significance.[9,29,84] In one exceptional family described by the authors, three siblings with chronic lymphocytic leukemia, as well as some unaffected members, carried a constitutional abnormality of one of the G-group chromosomes, termed the *Christchurch* or *Ch¹ chromosome* (Fig. 6-17).[87,115] While its possession may well have predisposed members of this family to chronic lymphocytic leukemia, it does not appear to have any wider significance.

Many abnormalities have been found in the solid lymphomas by means of studies of the chromosomes in the lymph nodes, marrow, or serous effusions.[162,173,241] These resemble the changes found in many other solid tumors[227] in being polymorphic, with changes in all chromosome groups. An occasional case of clonal evolution has been described.[241] Spiers and Baikie[242] have drawn attention to the frequency with which abnormalities occur in the 17 and 18 chromosomes of the E group and have made a case for a special role of this group in the lymphomas and, possibly, some of the leukemias.[76] The appearance of lymphomatous cells in the blood may lead to the finding of abnormal clones in cultures with or without PHA.[57]

It should be noted that until now the study of chromosomes and their structure has been carried out by relatively unsophisticated methods. Thus, it has been possible to identify the majority of the chromosomes only as members of groups and not as individual units. Hopes based on the introduction of autoradiographic labeling have only been partially realized.[273] As a result of these difficulties, some lesions of individual chromosomes have probably been overlooked and others misinterpreted. The recent development of new technical methods—the staining of chromosomes with fluorescent dyes or with Romanowsky dyes at high pH, and their examination after pretreatment with enzymes—gives promise of a more precise identification of most, if not all, of the 46 human chromosomes and with it of a much more precise analysis of their defects and the mechanism of their production.[51, 118, 190–191, 230]

CYTOCHEMISTRY

Although the chemical composition of the leukocytes has been investigated for a considerable period of time, reliable results have been obtained only in recent years. Work has proceeded along two distinct lines: the analysis of large quantities of leukocytes before or after their separation from the other blood constituents, and that of individual cells by cytochemical methods. Both of these have their own advantages and difficulties.

The examination of sizable volumes of leukocytes is capable of yielding quantitative results with the comparatively small errors inherent in chemical as opposed to biologic methods. It requires rather large quantities of blood and an efficient means of separating leukocytes from the red cells, platelets, and plasma, and, in many instances, the separation of the various types of leukocytes from each other. Such techniques have been developed during the past few years, and it is now possible, by means of differential centrifugation, flotation methods, and the use of filtration through glass beads, cotton-wool, or nylon fibers, to obtain pure or greatly enriched preparations of the lymphocytes or granulocytes of normal blood or of the type-specific cells in various forms of leukemia.[78] The methods are particularly suitable for the determination of leukocyte metabolism and its aberrations in the leukemias, but can provide relatively little information on the changes in individual cells. Cytochemical methods, by contrast, can give only qualitative or at best semiquantitative results, but they permit the identification of specific substances and of their intracellular location by direct inspection. The cytochemical analysis of cell constituents is made by indirect tinctorial means, which may involve an element of initial ambiguity and often the need for batteries of tests. Such combinations of techniques have come into use in the years since 1964[126] and constitute valuable tools for the identification of leukemic cell types. This work rests on foundations laid by many earlier workers[82, 105, 213, 269, 283] and is still in a period of rapid progress.

The Peroxidase Reaction

The peroxidase contents of granulocytes and the absence of the enzyme from cells of the lymphocytic series has been known for many years, and as early as 1947, Cazal suggested that the reaction could be used to differentiate the granulocytic and lymphocytic types of acute leukemia (Fig. 6-18).[53] Peroxidase is contained in the azurophilic granules which can first be demonstrated in promyelocytes, but there is none in the secondary specific granules which are developed at later stages of matu-

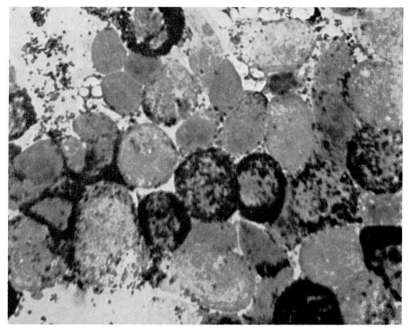

Fig. 6-18. Acute granulocytic leukemia. Marrow. Peroxidase reaction. × 2000

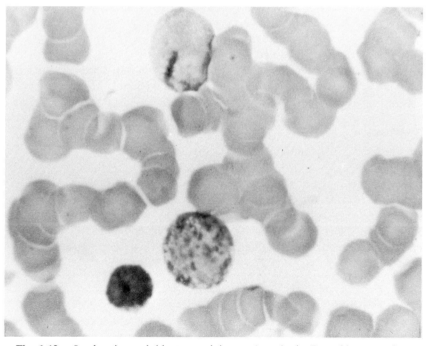

Fig. 6-19. Leukemic myeloblast containing an Auer body. Peroxidase reaction.

ration.[71] Before its distinctive localization in the azurophil granules, the enzyme can be shown to be present in the perinuclear space, the endoplasmic reticulum, and the Golgi apparatus which is the source of at least part of the azurophil granules.[46] Such granules are also found in early and later monocytes though occurring in smaller numbers than in promyelocytes, and, hence, promonocytes and monocytes are also peroxidase-positive. The granules themselves conform in their enzyme contents and structure to that of lysosomes.[95,268] In the acute leukemias, they may form the abnormal crystalline coacervates known as Auer bodies which are thus also peroxidase-positive (Fig. 6-19).

From the diagnostic point of view, the peroxidase reaction has a limited usefulness. If positive, it characterizes a given class of cells as belonging either to the granulocytic or monocytic series, but it cannot distinguish definitively between the two. A negative peroxidase reaction is against a diagnosis of acute granulocytic leukemia, with certain reservations: first, to give a reaction, azurophil granules must be present; hence, myeloblasts are themselves peroxidase-negative. Second, as has already been stated, the pathologic leukemic cells may have abnormal granulations, and these may be difficult to see in Romanowsky or electron microscopic preparations and give doubtful peroxidase reactions. In our experience, the peroxidase reaction is only occasionally valuable as a diagnostic aid.

Sudan Black

The use of Sudan black B, a lipophilic stain, has become popular mainly as a result of the studies of Hayhoe and his collaborators.[126] Previously, studies by Rheingold and Wislocki,[213] and by Wislocki et al.[283] had shown that lipids are contained almost exclusively in the cytoplasmic granules of the granulocytic series, from the earliest promyelocytes onward, and Storti had used the Sudan black B stain for the differential diagnosis of the acute leukemias.[201,245] In the normal granulocyte series, Sudan black-positivity is localized in the azurophil granules.[228] It is first seen as a rather faint brownish black stain in the promyelocytes: myelocytes and more mature granulocytes show a much more vigorous reaction which may be granular or occupy the cytoplasm as an unbroken mass. Monocytes and their precursors are also Sudan black-positive, with delicate discrete granules. Whether the lipids stained by Sudan black are neutral lipids is doubtful; they may be phospholipids.[27]

In the acute leukemias, Sudan black-positivity excludes a diagnosis of the lymphocytic type. However, the characteristics of the granulation are generally not distinctive enough to make possible a separation between granulocytic and monocytic leukemias. In our experience, the Sudan black reaction tends to be positive in peroxidase-positive cases, as well as in occasional peroxidase-negative ones. It is a more sensitive test than the peroxidase reaction, but a diagnosis of acute granulocytic leukemia is not finally excluded, even when the cells are Sudan black-negative.

Esterases

Among the many nonspecific esterases present in leukocytes, those of prime cytochemical interest are α-naphthyl acetate esterase (NA), naphthol-AS-D-acetate esterase (NADA), and napththol-AS-D-chloroacetate esterase (NACA). Small

Table 6-1

Cytochemical Differentiation Between Granulocytes
and Monocytes by Means of Esterase Reactions

Reaction	Granulocytes	Monocytes
α–Naphthyl acetate esterase (NA)	+	++
Naphthol–AS–D–acetate esterase (NADA)	+	++
NADA + sodium flouride	+	±
Naphthol–AS–D–chloroacetate esterase (NACA)	++	+

quantities of NA are present in most blood and marrow cells, including granulocytes, lymphocytes, erythroblasts, and megakaryocytes,[158,163] but by far the most
obvious cytochemical reactions for both NA and NADA are given by monocytes,
both mature and immature. The reaction in the monocytic series is inhibited by previous incubation with sodium fluoride.[228] In the granulocytic series, the reaction with
NA and NADA is weaker than in monocytes and is not inhibited by sodium fluoride.
NACA is present only in the granulocytic series and can be demonstrated from the
promyelocytic state onward.[129,180] This enzyme, like peroxidase and acid phosphatase, is lysosomal in type and is contained in the azurophil granules. Between
them, the esterase reactions provide helpful evidence enabling cells of the granulocytic and monocytic series to be separated (Table 6-1).

In the acute leukemias, the use of the esterase reactions has been found of some
assistance in differentiating the various types of granulocytic leukemia, and, in particular, to make distinctions between promyelocytes and monocytoid cells. The
former tend to be strongly NACA-positive, whereas the latter show much weaker
staining for NACA but prominent NA- and NADA-positivity, inhibited by sodium
fluoride.[59,89,129,163,220] Unfortunately, like other cytochemical tests, the esterase
reactions depend greatly on the normal maturation of the cellular organelles, and
equivocal results are obtained when this is disturbed, as in many acute leukemias.

Phosphatases

Many studies have shown striking and consistent differences in the concentration of neutrophil alkaline phosphatase (NAP) in normal as compared with abnormal leukocytes, both by chemical and cytochemical methods. NAP is contained
in the secondary specific granules of the mature neutrophils and is believed to participate in both their protein and carbohydrate metabolism. Wachstein, who showed
in 1946 that considerable quantities of NAP occur in the cytoplasm of mature
granulocytes,[269] worked with the original qualitative cytochemical method of
Gomori,[105] but semiquantitative results are now usually reported with the use of
diazo methods.[125,137,150] Normally, about 20 percent of mature granulocytes are
positive with either of these reactions.[176] Wachstein[269] showed that in infections both
the number of NAP-positive cells and the strength of the reaction is greatly increased, but that in chronic granulocytic leukemia, in striking contrast, there is a
decrease in the NAP-positivity of the cells. Only two of Wachstein's thirteen cases
of chronic granulocytic leukemia showed an activity comparable to that of normal
blood. One case of nonleukemic myelosis showed a large number of strongly positive
granulocytes.

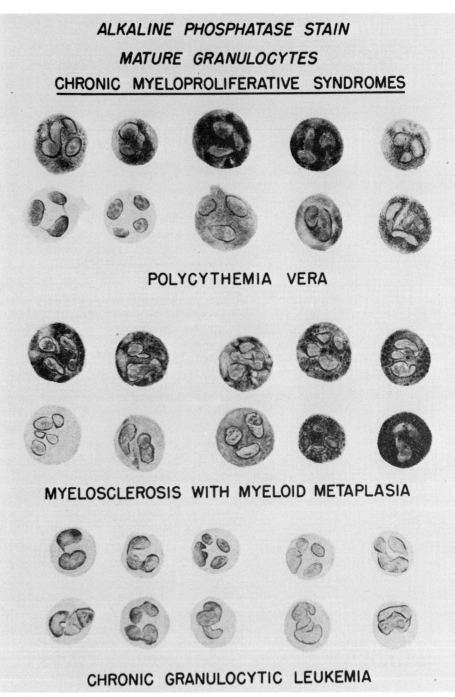

ALKALINE PHOSPHATASE STAIN

MATURE GRANULOCYTES

CHRONIC MYELOPROLIFERATIVE SYNDROMES

POLYCYTHEMIA VERA

MYELOSCLEROSIS WITH MYELOID METAPLASIA

CHRONIC GRANULOCYTIC LEUKEMIA

Fig. 6-20. Alkaline phosphatase stains of mature granulocytes in chronic myeloproliferative syndromes: polycythemia vera, myelosclerosis with myeloid metaplasia, and chronic granulocytic leukemia. × 1430.

Wachstein's findings have been confirmed and extended by Valentine who, with his associates, has done a great deal of work on this subject.[23,260,261,262,263] With the use of biochemical methods, they found that leukocyte NAP is greatly reduced in chronic granulocytic leukemia, but that it is much higher than normal in polycythemia vera and in many cases of myelosclerosis with myeloid metaplasia of the spleen. Extensive cytochemical studies by Mitus and his colleagues[176,178] have shown that high, normal, and low NAP values can be found in individual cases of myelosclerosis (Fig. 6-20). Similar findings have come from Koler et al.,[150] Meislin et al.,[170] and Merker and Heilmeyer.[172] The low NAP concentrations found in chronic granulocytic leukemia are quite striking and serve as an empirical diagnostic criterion, in that patients having a normal or high NAP content are unlikely to belong in this group of leukemias. However, a low NAP content does not by itself mean a diagnosis of chronic granulocytic leukemia. Thus, some cases of myelosclerosis have low values; furthermore, occasional instances of low NAP concentrations have been found in other blood dyscrasias, the most striking being in paroxysmal nocturnal hemoglobinuria and pernicious anemia.[172,248] It is interesting that low NAP figures were discovered in the granulocytes of some of the Japanese victims of atomic bombings years before they developed the overt signs of granulocytic leukemia.[179]

Although NAP is very low or absent in nearly all cases of chronic granulocytic leukemia, the enzyme score may rise to normal or even to elevated levels in certain circumstances, notably, in some remissions[155,285] and when the disease enters the acute phase. Very occasionally, there is a rise of NAP in infections, following the administration of pyrogens,[198] and when additional tumors are present.[282] The mechanism of this effect is not clear. Originally it was believed that a double population of cells—one leukemic, the other normal—might be present, but the persistence of the Ph[1] chromosome in all metaphases in such cases has invalidated this hypothesis. Although there have been reports to the effect that the NAP in chronic granulocytic leukemia and polycythemia vera differed in its electrophoretic pattern from that in normal granulocytes,[217,258] this has been denied.[110] It now appears that though chemically and immunologically there are no differences between the NAP in normal and leukemic subjects, the enzymes differ in their specific activity.[41] In the acute leukemias, the NAP tends to be normal in the lymphocytic but diminished in the granulocytic form.[126]

The studies on NAP provided the earliest clear evidence showing that morphologically indistinguishable cells can show definite chemical differences. Much effort has been expended in a search for the mechanism controlling cellular NAP contents. The coexistence in the same patient of abnormally low NAP values with the Ph[1] chromosome gave rise to the speculation that genes controlling NAP metabolism might be situated on chromosome 21; and this was strengthened when abnormally high NAP values were discovered in patients with Down's syndrome who were trisomic for the 21 chromosome.[4,257] As was soon pointed out, however, the presence on the 21 chromosome of structural genes concerned with NAP synthesis was difficult to reconcile with the fluctuations of NAP in certain CGL patients.[146] Since then, several more elaborate theories have been put forward which would put regulator or modifier genes for NAP synthesis, rather than structural genes, on this chromosome.[219,250] Much of this work has been invalidated since new banding techniques indicated that the Ph[1] abnormality does not arise in the same pair of small acrocentric chromosomes as that which becomes trisomic in Down's syndrome.[190]

It appears that in NAP estimations we have a useful means of obtaining guidance on the nature of the granulocytes in the granulocytic leukemias, as well as in the other myeloproliferative disorders. However, these are so far empirical findings whose significance is by no means clear. NAP activity appears to be closely connected with the presence of zinc ions.[266] This may provide an explanation for the low zinc concentrations found in cases of untreated chronic granulocytic leukemia (see below). The fact that in normal individuals—but not usually in those with chronic granulocytic leukemia—the unit cellular NAP is significantly increased by the administration of corticosteroids,[260,264] a phenomenon which can be reproduced in vitro,[281] may indicate that the NAP level is under endocrine control.

In contrast with the studies of alkaline phosphatase, those on the distribution of leukocyte acid phosphatase have provided fewer significant data.[207] This is one of the lysosomal enzymes contained in the azurophil granules of the granulocytic series, as well as in monocytes, reticulum cells, lymphocytes, megakaryocytes, platelets, and erythroblasts. Unusually strong positivity for acid phosphatase may be found in some of the granulocytic leukemias, both acute and chronic, and especially in the immature cells of the myelomonocytic type,[163,175,218,228] as well as in some myeloma cells.[1] In some of the lymphoproliferative disorders the acid phosphatase content of the lymphocytes is unusually low.[286]

Glycogen

Chemical methods have suggested that the glycogen in whole blood is contained exclusively in the leukocytes.[263,272] With cytochemical investigations, it was found that platelets also contain small amounts of glycogen.[102,270] The results of glycogen determinations are somewhat contradictory, perhaps due to the diversity of analytical methods and of the methods for expressing results. Thus, some chemists have measured glycogen per unit wet weight of leukocytes [272] and others per unit number of cells.[263] Histochemists have used a variety of stains; in some, enzymatic digestion (diastase, saliva) is employed to identify the substance. It is generally accepted that a large proportion of the leukocytic glycogen is contained in the granulocytes, small quantities being identifiable as early as the promyelocyte stage, larger quantities in the more mature cells. This being so, it is not surprising that increased amounts are found in the blood cells of chronic granulocytic leukemia. However, Valentine et al. stated that the glycogen content per unit number of leukemic granulocytes, exclusive of blasts (which are devoid of glycogen), is only one-half that of normal granulocytes.[263] This has more recently been confirmed by means of cytophotometry of individual cells stained with periodic acid-Schiff (PAS). By this method, mature neutrophils from acute granulocytic leukemia in relapse contain 25–50 percent less PAS-positive material—almost certainly glycogen—than do normal neutrophils,[97] while in untreated chronic granulocytic leukemia there is a similar considerable reduction.[98] In both conditions the onset of a remission is accompanied by a return of the PAS levels toward normal.

The PAS method stains cells of the granulocytic series, beginning with a faint pinkish tinge in the promyelocytes which increases in depth with increasing maturation. Mature neutrophils are usually packed with small cherry-red granules.

Myeloblasts are PAS-negative and this distinguishes them from lymphoblasts which generally contain small-to-coarse PAS-positive granules. Both the number of granules per cell and the proportion of cells giving a positive reaction are highly variable, however, so that the PAS reaction alone, or even in combination with other cytochemical methods, is often unable to distinguish between primitive blasts of the various series.[27,126]

Normally, about 20 percent of lymphocytes contain some PAS-positive granules; their number is markedly increased in the lymphocytes of chronic lymphocytic leukemia and in the abnormal lymphoid cells of lymphosarcoma cell leukemia.[6,7,177] Successful treatment of the former leads to a return to normal of the lymphocytic glycogen.[205] The content of PAS-positive material increases in normal lymphocytes cultured in the presence of PHA, but falls in those from chronic lymphocytic leukemia in relapse.[204]

Some of the abnormal erythroblasts found in the DiGuglielmo syndrome are strongly PAS-positive,[15,206] and this feature has been used in distinguishing the syndrome from other forms of acute leukemia[126] and from some of the refractory anemias.

Histamine

As early as 1941, it was found that the blood histamine is mainly contained in the leukocytes,[55] and that bone marrow contains more of this substance than does peripheral blood. The blood histamine remains normal in infections, leukocytosis, and in chronic lymphocytic, monocytic, and other acute leukemias, but tends to be increased in chronic granulocytic leukemia and in polycythemia vera.[233,251-252] The reason is that the basophils are the most important carriers of histamine in the blood, containing fifty times as much of it as any other blood cell,[108,215-216] and that basophils are constantly augmented in chronic granulocytic leukemia from the earliest to the late stages, except in pure blastic metamorphosis. Good correlations between the percentage of basophils and the histamine contents were obtained in chronic granulocytic leukemia by Valentine and his colleagues.[265] The elevated histamine contents of basophils and neutrophils in chronic granulocytic leukemia and other myeloproliferative disorders is probably a consequence of large concentrations of the enzyme histidine decarboxylase.[151] The urinary excretion of histamine and histamine metabolites in chronic granulocytic leukemia rises up to twenty times over that in normal individuals.[28]

Nonprotein Sulfhydryls and Sulfatases

This group of substances includes glutathione (GSH), cystine, and cysteine and is of obvious physiologic importance since it is known to be necessary for cell division. In leukocyte metabolism, cystine and cysteine appear to play an almost unique role as has been demonstrated by the important studies of Weisberger and his colleagues.[274-276] If radioactive L-cystine is given orally, its presence can be demonstrated within 10 minutes in the circulating leukocytes, the concentration rising gradually to reach a peak within 5 days in normal blood. Inorganic sulfur, on the other hand, is hardly incorporated by the leukocytes. Leukocytes in both acute and chronic leukemia incorporate L-cystine more rapidly than do normal leukocytes, probably because of the increased proportions of immature cells. In acute granulocytic leukemia there is a lower and in the chronic variety a higher peak level of radioactive sulfur than in normal leukocytes. Conversely, in chronic lymphocytic leukemia the cells show a very slow incorporation with a low and long-continued plateaulike level in the leukocytes. These varying peak levels are probably associated with the varying life span of the different classes of leukocytes.

The blood GSH is contained in both the red cells[39] and the leukocytes, but the content is four to seven times higher, cell for cell, in the latter.[109,120] There is some disagreement as to the changes which occur in leukemic leukocytes. Thus, Contopoulos and Anderson report a raised GSH content in most leukemic cells and a return to normal levels under treatment,[56] whereas Hardin et al. note no consistent changes in chronic granulocytic leukemia, but a low concentration in the chronic lymphocytic and the acute blastic leukemias. Other authors found varying concentrations of GSH in leukemia.[37-38] No abnormalities have been found in the enzymes synthesizing and degrading GSH in leukemic cells.[122]

Sulfatases are widely distributed in the body. The aryl sulfatases occur in three main types—A, B, and C—which hydrolyse various organic sulfates. Most leukocytes contain cytoplasmic C-type aryl sulfatase which can be demonstrated cytochemically as brownish granules and whose physiologic role is unknown. *Nuclear* aryl sulfatase, by contrast, is stated to be present only in lymphoblasts and lymphocytes but not in the granulocytic series.[73] If this were an absolute distinction, such tests could provide valuable diagnostic help in the differentiation of the acute leukemias, but, unfortunately, nuclear aryl sulfatase-positivity has occasionally also been found in nonlymphocytic leukemias,[43,235,249] so that the value of this reaction is somewhat uncertain.

Other Substances

The content of a variety of enzymes and trace metals has been determined in normal and leukemic cells. Among the enzymes is β-glucuronidase, a lysosomal enzyme, which may be concerned with detoxication processes. It is evenly distributed among the various leukocytes,[221] and shows irregular changes in the leukemias, though it is generally low in chronic lymphocytic leukemia and other lymphomas.[5,91,286] Xanthine oxidase and uricase are involved in purine catabolism and show a lower than normal concentration, at least in mouse leukemia cells.[80] A good deal of work has been done on the nucleic acid depolymerases of human leukocytes (deoxyribonuclease and ribonuclease) and their naturally occurring inhibitors.[168] The latter may be present in excess in leukemic cells[128,154] while the lysosomal deoxyribonuclease is decreased in acute leukemia during relapse, returning to normal in remission.[77] The enzymes concerned in intracellular hydrogen transport systems have been investigated by Stuart et al.[247] In leukemic lymphoblasts there was an increase of extramitochondrial dehydrogenases but not of the intramitochondrial variety. This may signify that leukemic blasts show diminished hydrogen transport to the intramitochondrial respiratory pathway. The well-known increase in lactic acid dehydrogenase concentration in such blasts (see pages 68 and 164) may be compensatory for this defect.

The most important trace metals appear to be zinc and magnesium, both of which are enzyme activators. The zinc content of the leukocytes in chronic granulocytic, chronic lymphocytic, and monocytic leukemia is markedly decreased compared with that of normal leukocytes and tends to rise as the leukocyte count falls after treatment.[66,267] As mentioned above, zinc is concerned with activation of alkaline phosphatase,[266] and the fluctuations of the zinc content of leukemic cells may be associated with changes in their NAP content.

Leukocyte lipids have already been referred to in the section dealing with Sudan black. Not all of the cellular lipid is, of course, contained in the granules, for much of it is in the cell membrane, and there may be some in the nucleus.[203] Differences in the total cellular lipid of some leukemic cells compared with their normal counterparts have been described,[107] but do not at present add up to a clearly recognizable pattern.

LEUKOCYTE METABOLISM

The metabolism of proteins, carbohydrates, and lipids has been studied in leukocytes, both normal and leukemic, for many years, and from this work has arisen a literature which is "highly contradictory and dissentient."[25] The aim was initially to discover differences between normal and leukemic cells and when found, to use them for the purposes of diagnosis or, on a more fundamental plane, in attempts to explain the mechanism of leukemogenesis. More recently, biochemical research has become orientated toward the possible exploitation of any existing metabolic differences.

Protein metabolism. An early example of such endeavors was the use of a selenium analog of the amino acid cystine for the treatment of acute leukemia.[277] In the past few years, attention in this field shifted to some of the ordinarily nonessential amino acids, especially serine and aspartic acid with its amide asparagine. Serine, though not required for protein synthesis by all tissues, was found to be essential in normal and leukemic granulocytes,[210] with the earlier, and particularly the blast forms having particularly high requirements.[68] Similarly, aspartic acid is incorporated with unusual avidity into the leukocytes of acute granulocytic leukemia and especially chronic granulocytic leukemia in the blastic phase.[68] The most immediately exploitable feature of leukocyte metabolism, however, is the requirement of some lymphomatous and leukemic cells for asparagine, and the consequent antineoplastic activity of L-asparaginase.[17,48,69,124,236] This important subject is fully discussed elsewhere (see Chapters 17 and 18).

Carbohydrate metabolism. Studies of the leukocyte carbohydrate metabolism have been repeatedly reviewed,[21–22,25,199,271] and the emerging picture has been confused because of the difficulties—many of them only recently recognized—peculiar to work in this area. Among these were the wide metabolic differences among leukocytes from different sources, the obstacles to efficient separation of the various cell types, the ease with which leukocytes were injured during experiments, and the many different ways in which results were expressed.[21,161] Now that these sources of confusion have been partly clarified, it may be expected that results will become more consistent and perhaps more meaningful.

The chief aim of most early investigators in this field was to establish if leukemic leukocytes had a "malignant" metabolism in the sense of Warburg, that is, a metabolism characterized by a relatively high aerobic glycolysis and a relatively low respiratory rate. (It has long been realized that a number of normal tissues share this type of malignant metabolism.) After initial controversy, it has now become reasonably certain that mature granulocytes, both normal and leukemic, have a high aerobic glycolytic rate, relative to respiration, and that this is not merely a sign of cell injury as had been suspected.[21–22,161,231] Immature granulocytes from acute granulocytic leukemia also have a high aerobic glycolytic rate but, in contrast to normal granulocytes, they respond to lack of glucose by greatly raising their respiratory rate. There are quantitative differences between the glycolytic rates of normal leukocytes and those from chronic granulocytic and chronic lymphocytic leukemias, as shown some years ago by Beck and Valentine.[24,26] The lower rates for the chronic leukemias are accompanied and possibly accounted for by lower concentrations of several of the enzymes of the Embden-Meyerhof cycle, notably hexosekinase, and by a deficiency of ADP-generating systems in leukemic cells.[19,20] Since these results were all obtained with mixed cell populations, they are in need of confirmation. Somewhat less than 10 percent of glucose utilized by normal leukocytes traverses the hexose-monophosphate shunt pathway, but the proportion is higher in leukemic leukocytes.[20]

Evidence is beginning to accumulate that lymphocytes, both normal and leukemic, have relatively high respiratory rates but little aerobic glycolysis as compared to granulocytes. Moreover, similar ratios have been found in the blasts from about 38 percent of acute leukemias, which have been identified as lymphocytic.[161,231] CLL lymphocytes show even less glycolysis than normal lymphocytes, both through the Embden-Meyerhof and the hexose-monophosphate pathways.[47]

If these findings are confirmed, a new means of classifying the acute leukemias on the basis of their carbohydrate metabolism will be available. Further, it will then be clear that undoubtedly normal cells—those of the granulocyte series—may have a high ratio of aerobic glycolysis to respiration while undoubtedly malignant cells—those from some acute leukemias—may have a low ratio. "In the light of these facts, the conception of a so-called cancerous metabolism, based on the recognition of aerobic glycolysis as a specific sign of neoplasia, is deprived of experimental basis." [231]

Lipid metabolism. As might be expected from the cytochemical studies already discussed (page 156), the lipid content of granulocytes is far higher than that of lymphocytes, and this has been confirmed by chemical studies.[42] Among the various lipid fractions, phospholipids—especially phosphatidyl choline and phosphatidyl ethanolamine—predominate; cholesterol is mainly present in the free rather than the esterified form; and there are varying quantities of triglycerides.[106,145] The ratios between the fractions show minor differences between normal leukocytes and those of chronic granulocytic and chronic lymphocytic leukemias, but normal leukocytes have a higher absolute lipid content and more cholesterol than do their leukemic counterparts. The absolute quantities of lipids present in normal and CLL lymphocytes are only about half those in normal neutrophils, probably because of their smaller size and fewer lipid-containing organelles.

Lipid synthesis, as measured by the incorporation of ^{14}C-acetate into lipids, is high in AGL and CGL leukocytes but low in ALL and CLL leukocytes.[143-144] Here may be yet another means of classifying the various types of acute leukemia, though whether this adds much to the cytochemical evidence provided by lipophilic stains is doubtful.

REFERENCES

1. Abbrederis K, Schmalzl F, Braunsteiner H: Zur Differentialdiagnose akuter Leukämien mittels zytochemischer Methoden. Schweiz Med Wochenschr 99:1425, 1969.

2. Ackerman GA: Microscopic and histochemical studies on the Auer bodies in leukemic cells. Blood 5:847, 1950.

3. Adams A, Fitzgerald PH, Gunz FW: A new chromosome abnormality in chronic granulocytic leukaemia. Br Med J 2:1474, 1961.

4. Alter AA, Lee SL, Pourfar M, Dobkin M: Leukocyte alkaline phosphatase in mongolism: a possible chromosome marker. J Clin Invest 41:1341, 1962.

5. Anlyan AJ, Gamble J, Hoster HA: Beta-glucuronidase activity of white blood cells in human leukemias and Hodgkin's disease. Cancer 3:116, 1950.

6. Astaldi G: The behaviour of the glycogen content in normal leukaemic leukocytes during survival and after x-ray irradiation. Transactions of the Sixth Congress of the European Society of Haematology, 1957, p 324.

7. Astaldi G, Verga L: Ricerche citochimiche sul contenuto in glicogeno dei linfociti della leucemia linfatica in rapporto al loro grado di maturazione. Bull Soc Ital Biol Sper 33:247, 1957.

8. Atkin NB, Taylor MC: A case of chronic myeloid leukaemia with a 45-chromosome cell-line in the blood. Cytogenetics 1:97, 1962.

9. Baikie AG: Chromosomal aspects of leukaemia. Proceedings of the Eleventh Congress of the International Society of Hematology, Plenary Sessions. Sydney, N.S.W., Government Printer, 1966, p 202.

10. _____: Chromosomes and leukaemia. Acta Haematol 36:157, 1966.

11. _____: What is a leukaemic remission? The evidence from cytogenetic studies, in Vincent PC (ed): Proceedings of the International Cancer Conference, Sydney. Sydney, N.S.W., Government Printer, 1972, p 231.

12. _____, Court Brown WM, Buckton KE, Harnden DG, Jacobs PA, Tough IM: A possible specific chromosome abnormality in human chronic myeloid leukaemia. Nature 188:1165, 1960.

13. _____, _____, Jacobs PA, and Milne JS: Chromosome studies in human leukaemia. Lancet 2:425, 1959.

14. _____, Jacobs PA, McBride JA, Tough IM: Cytogenetic studies in acute leukaemia. Br Med J 1:1564, 1961.

15. Baldini M, Fudenberg HH, Dameshek W: The anemia of the Di Guglielmo syndrome. Blood 14:334, 1959.

16. Ball CR, Connors TA, Cooper EH, Topping NE: Cytochemical observations on the nucleolus-ribosome system. Effect of Actinomycin D and nitrogen mustard. Neoplasma 14:253, 1967.

17. Banerjee SP, Gallmeier WM, Schmidt CG: Bestimmung der Asparagin—Synthetase in Leukämie—Zellen als Indikator für die Enzymtherapie von Hämoblastosen. Dtsch Med Wochenschr 95:994, 1970.

18. Bauters F, Croquette MF, Delmas-Marsalet Y, Deminatti M, Goudemand M: Une forme particulière de leucémie myéloïde chez l'homme: évolution prolongée et présence du chromosome philadelphie avec perte du chromosome Y dans les cellules myéloïdes. Nouv Rev Fr Hématol 10:697, 1970.

19. Beck WS: The control of leukocyte glycolysis. J Biol Chem 232:251, 1958.

20. _____: Occurrence and control of the phosphogluconate oxidation pathway in normal and leukemic leukocytes. J Biol Chem 232:271, 1958.

21. _____: Leukocyte metabolism. Ser Haematol I:69, 1968.

22. _____: Biochemical properties of normal and leukemic leukocytes, in Zarafonetis CJD (ed): Proceedings of the International Conference on Leukemia-Lymphoma. Philadelphia: Lea & Febiger, 1968, p 245.

23. _____, Valentine WN: Biochemical studies

on leukocytes. II. Phosphatase activity in chronic lymphatic leukemia, acute leukemia and miscellaneous hematologic conditions. J Lab Clin Med 38:245, 1951.

24. _____, _____: The aerobic carbohydrate metabolism of leukocytes in health and leukemia. I. Glycolysis and respiration. Cancer Res 12:818, 1952.

25. _____, _____: The carbohydrate metabolism of leukocytes: a review. Cancer Res 13:309, 1953.

26. _____, _____: The aerobic carbohydrate metabolism of leukocytes in health and leukemia. II. The effect of various substances and coenzymes on glycolysis and respiration. Cancer Res 12:823, 1962.

27. Bennett JM, Dutcher TF: The cytochemistry of acute leukemia: Observations on glycogen and natural fat in bone marrow aspirates. Blood 33:341, 1969.

28. Berg B, Granerus G, Westling H, White T: Urinary excretion of histamine and histamine metabolites in leukaemia. Scand J Haematol 8:63, 1971.

29. Berger R, Parmentier C: Leucémie lymphoïde chronique et chromosomes. Nouv Rev Fr Hematol 11:261, 1971.

30. Berry EW: Cytogenetic studies in myeloproliferative disorders and other potentially leukaemic states. M.D. thesis, University of Otago.

31. _____, Desforges JF: Changing cytogenetic factors in an acute myeloproliferative disorder. Am J Med 47:229, 1969.

32. Bessis M: La différenciation et la maturation des cellules leucémiques. Considérations cytologiques et cliniques. Rev Hématol 9:745, 1954.

33. _____: Cytology of the blood and the blood-forming organs. New York, Grune & Stratton, 1956.

34. _____: Ultrastructure of normal and leukemic granulocytes, In Zarafonetis CJD (ed): Proceedings of the International Conference on Leukemia-Lymphoma. Philadelphia, Lea & Febiger, 1968, p 281.

35. _____, Breton-Gorius J: Examen des cellules leucémiques au microscope électronique par la méthode des coupes. Presse Méd 63:189, 1955.

36. _____, _____: Pathologie et asynchronisme de développement des organelles cellulaires au cours des leucémies aiguës granulocytaires. Etude au microscope electronique. Nouv Rev Fr Hématol 9:245, 1969.

37. Bichel J: Le glutathione reduit dans le sang des cancéreaux. Acta Pathol Microbiol Scand 22:248, 1945.

38. Bichel J: Blood glutathione in leucoses. Acta Med Scand 124:160, 1946.

39. Binet L, Bernard J, Wellers G, Mathé G: La glutathionémie au cours des leucoses aiguës. Presse Med 60:961, 1952.

40. Bloom GE, Gerald PS, Diamond LK: Chronic myelogenous leukemia in an infant: Serial cytogenetic and fetal hemoglobin studies. Pediatrics 38:295, 1966.

41. Bottomley RH, Lovig CA, Holt R, Griffin MJ: Comparison of alkaline phosphatase from human normal and leukemic leukocytes. Cancer Res 29:1866, 1969.

42. Boyd EM: The lipid composition of the white blood cells in leukemia. Arch Pathol 21:739, 1936.

43. Boysen G: An evaluation of aryl sulphatase activity in leukaemic cells. Scand J Haematol 6:246, 1969.

44. Böyum A: Separation of leucocytes from blood and bone marrow. Scand J Clin Lab Invest 21 (suppl. 97):31, 1968.

45. Brausil B: Diagnostic differences between atypical myeloblasts and lymphoblasts in the phase contrast microscope. A morphological study of 32 cases. Acta Haematol 12:276, 1954.

46. Breton-Gorius J, Guichard J: Etude au microscope électronique de la localisation des peroxydases dans les cellules de la moelle osseuse humaine. Nouv Rev Fr Hématol 9:678, 1969.

47. Brody JI, Oski FA, Singer DE: Impaired pentose phosphate shunt and decreased glycolytic activity in lymphocytes of chronic lymphocytic leukemia. Metabolic pathway? Blood 34:421, 1969.

48. Broome JD: L-asparaginase: The evolution of a new tumor inhibiting agent. Trans NY Acad Sci (ser. II) 30:690, 1968.

49. Canellos GP, DeVita VT, Whang-Peng J, Carbone PP: Hematologic and cytogenetic remission of blastic transformation in chronic granulocytic leukemia. Blood 38:671, 1971.

50. Caspersson T, Farber S, Foley GE, Killander D: Comparison of nitrogen mustard-sensitive and -resistant Yoshida sarcomas. II. Effect of treatment on cell kinetics. Exp Cell Res 32:529, 1963.

51. Caspersson T, Zech L, Johansson C, Modest EJ: Identification of human chromosomes by DNA-binding fluorescent agents. Chromosoma 30:215, 1970.

52. Castoldi G, Yam LT, Mitus WJ, Crosby

WH: Chromosomal studies in erythro-leukemia and chronic erythremic myelosis. Blood 31:202, 1968.

53. Cazal P: Analyze cytologique des leucémies à cellules atypiques. Utilité de la formule peroxydasique. Rev Hématol 2:507, 1947.

54. Clein GP, Flemans RJ: Involvement of the erythroid series in blastic crisis of chronic myeloid leukaemia. Br J Haematol 12:754, 1966.

55. Code CF, Jensen JL: A comparison of the histamine content of blood and bone marrow. Am J Physiol 131:768, 1941.

56. Contopoulos AN, Anderson HH: Sulf-hydryl content of blood cells in dyscrasias. J Lab Clin Med 36:929, 1950.

57. Crossen PE, Mellor JEL, Finley AG, Ravich RBM, Vincent PC, Gunz FW: The Sézary syndrome. Am J Med 50:24, 1971.

58. _____, _____, Vincent PC, Gunz FW: Clonal evolution in human leukaemia. Cytobios 4:29, 1971.

59. Daniel M-Th, Flandrin G, Lejeune F, Liso P, Lortholary P: I. Les estérases spécifiques monocytaires. Utilisation dans la classification des leucémies aiguës. Nouv Rev Fr Hématol 11:233, 1971.

60. Darte JM, Dacie JV, and McSorley JGA: Pelger-like leucocytes in chronic myeloid leukemia. Acta Haematol 12:117, 1954.

61. Dausset J: Essai de différentiation des diverses variétés des leucémies aiguës par l'examen du sang et de la moelle à l'état frais. Sang 21:610, 1950.

62. Davidson JN, Leslie I, White JC: Quantitative studies on the content of nucleic acid in normal and leukaemic cells from blood and bone marrow. J Pathol Bacteriol 63:471, 1951.

63. De Grouchy J, De Nava C: A chromosomal theory of carcinogenesis. Ann Intern Med 69:381, 1968.

64. _____, Cantu JM, Bilski-Pasquier G, Bousser J: Models for clonal evolutions: A study of chronic myeloid leukemia. Am J Hum Genet 18:485, 1966.

65. _____, _____, Feingold J, Bilski-Pasquier G, Bousser J: Onze observations d'un modèle précis d'évolution caryotypique au cours de la leucémie myéloide chronique. Eur J Cancer 4:481, 1968.

66. Dennes E, Tupper R, Wormall A: Zinc content of erythrocytes and leucocytes of normal and leukaemic subjects. Nature 187:302, 1960.

67. Dienard AS, Page AR: An improved method for performing neutrophil survival studies. Blood 36:98, 1970.

68. Dimitrov NV, Hansz J, Toth MA, Bartolotta B: Serine and aspartic acid metabolism in leukemic leukocytes: correlation to effectiveness of therapy. Blood 38:638, 1971.

69. Dolowy WC, Henson D, Cornet J, Sellin H: Toxic and antineoplastic effects of L-asparaginase. Cancer 19:1813, 1966.

70. Dorr AD, Moloney WC: Acquired pseudo-Pelger anomaly of granulocytic leukocytes. N Engl J Med 261:742, 1959.

71. Dunn WB, Hardin JH, Spicer SS: Ultrastructural localization of myeloperoxidase in human neutrophil and rabbit heterophil and eosinophil leukocytes. Blood 32:935, 1968.

72. Duvall CP, Carbone PP, Bell WR, Whang J, Tjio JH, Perry S: Chronic myelocytic leukemia with two Philadelphia chromosomes and prominent peripheral lymphadenopathy. Blood 29:652, 1967.

73. Ekert H, Denett X: An evaluation of nuclear aryl sulphatase activity as an aid to the cytological diagnosis of acute leukaemia. Australas Ann Med 15:152, 1966.

74. Elves MW, Israëls MCG: Cytogenetic studies in unusual forms of chronic myeloid leukaemia. Acta Haematol 38:129, 1967.

75. Engel E, Flexner JM, Engel-De Montmollin ML, Frank HE: Blood and skin chromosomal alterations of a clonal type in a leukemic man previously irradiated for a lung carcinoma. Cytogenetics 3:228, 1964.

76. _____, McKee LC, Bunting KW: Chromosomes 17-18 in leukaemias. Lancet 2:42, 1967.

77. Eschenbach C: Cytochemischer Nachweis von saurer Desoxyribonuclease im Cytoplasma von Blutzellen. III. Aktivität der sauren Desoxyribonuclease im Cytoplasma von Leukocyten akuter Leukosen im Kindesalters. Klin Wochenschr 49:958, 1971.

78. Evans CA, Middleton VL: Evaluation of methods for preparing pure lymphocyte suspensions from peripheral blood. J Clin Pathol 23:822, 1970.

79. Ezdinli EZ, Sokal JE, Crosswhite L, Sandberg AA: Philadelphia-chromosome-positive and -negative chronic myelocytic leukemia. Ann Intern Med 72:175, 1970.

80. Feigelson P, Ultmann JE, Harris S, Dashman T: Cellular xanthine oxidase and uricase levels in leukemic and normal

mouse leukocytes. Cancer Res 19:1230, 1959.

81. Fialkow PJ, Gartler SM, Yoshida A: Clonal origin of chronic myelocytic leukemia in man. Proc Natl Acad Sci USA 58:1468, 1967.

82. Fieschi A: Semeiologia del midollo osseo: Studio di morfologia clinica (ed. 2). Milan, Garzanti, 1946.

83. Finney R, McDonald GA, Baikie AG, Douglas AS: Chronic granulocytic leukaemia with Ph[1]-negative cells in bone marrow and a ten-year remission after busulphan hypoplasia. Br J Haematol 23:283, 1972.

84. Fitzgerald PH, Adams A: Chromosome studies in chronic lymphocytic leukemia and lymphosarcoma. J Natl Cancer Inst 34:827, 1965.

85. ———, ———, Gunz FW: Chronic granulocytic leukemia and the Philadelphia chromosome. Blood 21:183, 1963.

86. ———, ———, ———: Chromosome studies in adult acute leukemia. J Natl Cancer Inst 32:395, 1964.

87. ———, Hamer JW: Third case of chronic lymphocytic leukaemia in a carrier of the inherited Ch[1] chromosome. Br Med J 3:752, 1969.

88. ———, Pickering AF, Eiby JR: Clonal origin of the Philadelphia chromosome and chronic myeloid leukaemia: Evidence from a sex chromosome mosaic. Br J Haematol 21:473, 1971.

89. Flandrin G, Daniel M-Th, Blanchet Ph, Brière J, Bernard J: La leucémie aiguë monocytaire. Situation clinique et pronostique actuelle à la lumière des techniques de détermination des esterases spécifiques. Nouv Rev Fr Hématol 11:241, 1971.

90. Foadi MD, Cooper EH, Hardisty RM: DNA synthesis and DNA content of leucocytes in acute leukaemia. Nature 216:134, 1967.

91. Follette JH, Valentine WN, Lawrence JS: The beta glucuronidase content of human leukocytes in health and disease. J Lab Clin Med 40:825, 1952.

92. Ford CE, Clarke CM: Cytogenetic evidence of clonal proliferation in primary reticular neoplasms. Can Cancer Conf 5:129, 1963.

93. ———, Jacobs PA, Lajtha LG: Human somatic chromosomes. Nature 181:1565, 1958.

94. Freeman JA: The ultrastructure and genesis of Auer bodies. Blood 15:449, 1960.

95. ———: Origin of Auer bodies. Blood 27:499, 1966.

96. ———, Samuels MR: The ultrastructure of a fibrillar formation of leukemic human blood. Blood 13:725, 1958.

97. Gahrton G: The periodic acid-Schiff reaction in neutrophil leukocytes in untreated and myleran-treated chronic myelocytic leukemias. A quantitative microspectrophotometric study. Blood 28:544, 1968.

98. ———, Brandt L, Franzen S, Norden A: Cytochemical variants of neutrophil leukocyte populations in chronic myelocytic leukaemia. Scand J Haematol 6:365, 1969.

99. Gardikas C, Israëls MCG: The Feulgen reaction applied to clinical haematology. J Clin Pathol 1:226, 1948.

100. Garson OM, Milligan WJ: The 45, XO, Ph[1] subgroup of chronic granulocytic leukaemia. Scand J Haematol 9:186, 1972.

101. Gavosto F, Maraini G, Pileri A: Nucleic acid and protein metabolism in acute leukemia cells. Blood 16:1555, 1960.

102. Gibb RP, Stowell RE: Glycogen in human blood cells. Blood 4:569, 1949.

103. Gillis EM, Baikie AG: Method for the demonstration of nucleoli in lymphocytes and other blood and marrow cells. J Clin Pathol 17:573, 1964.

104. Goh KO: Smaller G chromosome in irradiated man. Lancet 1:659, 1966.

105. Gomori G: Microtechnical demonstration of phosphatase in tissue sections. Proc Soc Exp Biol Med 42:23, 1939.

106. Gottfried EL: Lipids of human leukocytes: Relation to cell type. J Lipid Res 8:321, 1967.

107. ———: Lipid patterns in health and disease. Sem Hematol 9:241, 1972.

108. Graham HT, Wheelwright F, Parish HH Jr, Marks AR, Lowry OH: Distribution of histamine among blood elements. Fed Proc 11:350, 1952.

109. Green R, Martin SP: The nonprotein soluble sulfhydryl content of human leukocytes and erythrocytes in infection and leukemia. J Lab Clin Med 45:119, 1955.

110. Griffin MJ, Lovig CA, Bottomley RH: Alkaline phosphatase of human normal and leukemic granulocytes. Proc Am Assoc Cancer Res 8:23, 1967.

111. Gruenwald H, Kiossoglou KA, Mitus WJ, Dameshek W: Philadelphia chromosome in eosinophilic leukemia. Am J Med 39:1003, 1965.

112. Gunz FW: Preleukemic conditions. In Mandelli F (ed): Trattato di Ematologia. Liechtenstein, Enciclopedia dei Trattati Internazionali Medico-Chirurgici. In press.

113. ———, Bach BI, Crossen PE, Mellor JEL,

Singh S, Vincent P: The relevance of the cytogenetic status in acute leukemia in adults. J Natl Cancer Inst 50:55, 1973.

114. _____, Burry AF: Cellular types in acute leukaemia: Diagnosis and significance. Br J Haematol 16:325, 1963.

115. _____, Fitzgerald PH, Adams A: An abnormal chromosome in chronic lymphocytic leukaemia. Br Med J 2:1097, 1962.

116. _____, Hough RF: Acute leukemia over the age of fifty. A study of its incidence and natural history. Blood 11:882, 1956.

117. _____, Ravich RBM, Vincent PC, Stewart JH, Crossen PE, Mellor J: A case of acute leukemia with a rapidly changing chromosome constitution. Ann Génét 13:79, 1970.

118. Hamerton JL: Banding patterns of metaphase chromosomes in Down's syndrome. Nature 230:167, 1971.

119. Hammouda F, Quaglino D, Hayhoe FGJ: Blastic crisis in chronic granulocytic leukaemia. Cytochemical, cytogenetic and autoradiographic studies in four cases. Br Med J 1:1275, 1964.

120. Hardin B, Valentine WN, Follette JH, Lawrence JS: Studies on the sulfhydryl content of human leukocytes and erythrocytes. Am J Med Sci 228:73, 1954.

121. Hardisty RM, Speed DE, Till M: Granulocytic leukaemia in childhood. Br J Haematol 10:551, 1964.

122. Harrap KR, Jackson RC: Some biochemical aspects of leukaemias: leucocyte glutathione metabolism in chronic granulocytic leukaemia. Eur J Cancer 5:61, 1969.

123. Hart JS, Trujillo JM, Freireich EJ, George SL, Frei E III: Cytogenetic studies and their clinical correlates in adults with acute leukemia. Ann Intern Med 75:353, 1971.

124. Haskell CM, Canellos GP, Cooney DA: Biochemical and pharmacologic effects of L-asparaginase in man. J Lab Clin Med 75:763, 1970.

125. Hayhoe FGJ, Quaglino D: Cytochemical demonstration and measurement of leucocyte alkaline phosphatase activity in normal and pathological states by a modified azo-dye coupling technique. Br J Haematol 4:375, 1958.

126. _____, _____, Doll R: The cytology and cytochemistry of acute leukaemias. A study of 140 cases. London; Her Majesty's Stationery Office, 1964.

127. Heath CW Jr, Bennett JM, Whang-Peng J, Berry EW, Wiernick PH: Cytogenetic findings in erythroleukemia. Blood 33:453, 1969.

128. Henstell HH, Freedman RI, Ginzburg B: An inhibitor of desoxyribonuclease in human white blood and bone marrow cells and its relationship to cellular maturity. Cancer Res 12:346, 1952.

129. Hermansky F, Lodrova V, Pössnerova V: Significance of cytochemical methods for the diagnosis and classification of immature leukemias of myeloid origin. Neoplasma 15:203, 1968.

130. Hossfeld DK, Han T, Holdsworth RN, Sandberg AA: Chromosomes and causation of human cancer and leukemia. VII. The significance of the Ph[1] in conditions other than CML. Cancer 27:186, 1971.

131. Huët GJ: Familial anomaly of leukocytes. Ned Tijdschr Geneeskd 75:5956, 1931.

132. Huhn D, Borchers H: Elektronenmikroskopisch-zytochemische Untersuchungen der Auer-Stäbchen bei akuter Paramyeloblasten-Leukämie. Blut 17:70, 1968.

133. Hungerford DA: Chromosome studies in human leukemia. I. Acute leukemia in children. J Natl Cancer Inst 27:983, 1961.

134. Hurdle ADF, Garson OM, Buist DGP: Clinical and cytogenetic studies in chronic myelomonocytic leukaemia. Br J Haematol 22:773, 1972.

135. Jensen MK: Cytogenetic studies in acute myeloid leukaemia. Acta Med Scand 190:429, 1971.

136. Kamada N, Uchino H: Double Ph[1] chromosome in leukaemia. Lancet 1:1107, 1967.

137. Kaplow LS: A histochemical procedure for localizing and evaluating leukocyte alkaline phosphatase activity in smears of blood and marrow. Blood 10:1025, 1955.

138. Kay HEM, Lawler SE, Millard RE: The chromosomes in polycythaemia vera. Br J Haematol 12:507, 1966.

139. _____, Millard RE, Lawler SD: Aneuploidy of C-group chromosomes in chronic myeloproliferative disorders. Haematol Rev 2:19, 1970.

140. Kemp NH, Stafford JL, Tanner R: Chromosome studies during early and terminal chronic myeloid leukaemia. Br Med J 1:1010, 1964.

141. Khan MH, Martin H: Myeloblastenleukämie mit Philadelphia-Chromosom. Klin Wochenschr 45:821, 1967.

142. Khouri FP, Shahid MJ, Kronfol N: Chromosomal pattern in the progression of chronic granulocytic leukemia. Cancer 24:807, 1969.

143. Kidson C: Lipid synthesis in human leu-

cocytes in acute leukaemia. Australas Ann Med 10:282, 1961.

144. _____: Leucocyte lipid metabolism in myeloproliferative states. Australas Ann Med 11:50, 1962.

145. Kim H, Suzuki M, O'Neal RM: Leukocyte lipids of human blood. Am J Clin Pathol 48:314, 1967.

146. King MJ, Gillis EM, Baikie AG: Alkaline-phosphatase activity of polymorphs in mongolism. Lancet 2:1302, 1962.

147. Kinlough MA, Robson HN: Study of chromosomes in human leukaemia by a direct method. Br Med J 2:1052, 1961.

148. Kiossoglou KA, Mitus WJ, Dameshek W: Two Ph¹ chromosomes in acute granulocytic leukaemia. A study of two cases. Lancet 2:665, 1965.

149. _____, _____, _____: Chromosomal aberrations in acute leukemia. Blood 26:610, 1965.

150. Koler RD, Seaman AJ, Osgood EE, and Vanbellinghen P: Myeloproliferative diseases. Diagnostic value of the leukocyte alkaline phosphatase test. Am J Clin Pathol 30:295, 1958.

151. Krauss S, Gilbert HS, Wasserman LR: Leukocyte histidine decarboxylase: properties and activity in myeloproliferative disorders. Blood 31:699, 1968.

152. _____, Sokal JE, Sandberg AA: Comparison of Philadelphia chromosome-positive and -negative patients with chronic myelocytic leukemia. Ann Intern Med 61:625, 1964.

153. Krompotic E, Silberman S, Einhorn M, Uy ES, Cherray PR: Clonal evolution in Di Guglielmo syndrome. Ann Génet 11:225, 1968.

154. Kurnick NB, Schwartz LI, Praiser S, Lee SL: A specific inhibitor for human desoxyribonuclease and an inhibitor of the lupus erythematosus cell phenomenon from leukocytes. J Clin Invest 32:193, 1953.

155. Lambers K: Die alkalische Phosphataseaktivität bei Leukosen und anderen pathologischen Zuständen. Z. Klin Med 155:176, 1958.

156. Lambin P: Recherches hématologiques sur la leucémie aiguë. Bull Acad R Med Belg 2:224, 1937.

157. _____: La formule nucléolaire dans les leucémies aiguës. Sang 12:901, 1938.

158. Lambrecht J: Cytochemische Untersuchungen über die unspezifische Esterasereaktion kernhaltiger Zellen im Blutausstrich bei Leukämien. Blut 17:129, 1968.

159. Lampert F, Deckelnik KH: Das Kern-

trockengewicht von menschlichen Leukämie—und Lymphosarkomzellen im Vergleich zu normalen Lymphozyten. Z Gesamte Exp Med 48:28, 1968.

160. Lam-Po-Tang, PRLC: An improved method of processing bone marrow for chromosomes. Scand J Haematol 5:158, 1968.

161. Laszlo J: Energy metabolism of human leukemic lymphocytes and granulocytes. Blood 30:151, 1967.

162. Lawler SD, Pentycross CR, Reeves BR: Chromosomes and transformation of lymphocytes in lymphoproliferative diseases. Br Med J 4:213, 1968.

163. Leder L-D: Der Blutmonocyt. Heidelberg, Springer, 1967.

164. Lejeune J: Leucémies et cancers, in: Les chromosomes humains. Paris, Gauthiers Villard, 1965.

165. _____, Berger R, Haines M, Lafourcade J, Vialatte J, Satge P, Turpin R: Constitution d'un clone à 54 chromosomes au cours d'une leucoblastose congénitale chez une enfant mongolienne. CR Acad Sci (Paris) 256:1195, 1963.

166. Levan A, Nichols WW, Hall B, Löw B, Nilsson SB, Norden A: Mixture of Rh-positive and Rh-negative erythrocytes and chromosomal abnormalities in a case of polycythaemia. Hereditas 52:89, 1964.

167. McDuffie NG: Crystalline patterns in Auer bodies and specific granules of human leukocytes. J Microscopie 6:321, 1967.

168. Maney BE, Moloney WC, Taylor FHL: Nucleic acid depolymerases of human leukocytes. Lab Invest 9:466, 1960.

169. Mastrangelo R, Zuelzer WW, Thompson RI: The significance of the Ph¹ chromosome in acute myeloblastic leukemia: serial cytogenetic studies in a critical case. Pediatrics 40:834, 1967.

170. Meislin AG, Lee SL, Wasserman LR: Leukocyte alkaline phosphatase activity in hematopoietic disorders. Cancer 12:760, 1959.

171. Menten ML, Willms M: Nucleic acid content of cells of bone marrow aspirated from patients with leukemia. Cancer Res 13:733, 1953.

172. Merker H, Heilmeyer L: Die alkalische Phosphatase neutrophiler Leukozyten. Dtsch Med Wochenschr 85:253, 1960.

173. Millard RE: Chromosome abnormalities in the malignant lymphomas. Eur J Cancer 4:97, 1968.

174. _____, Lawler SD, Kay HEM, Cameron CB: Further observations on patients with a

chromosomal abnormality associated with polycythaemia vera. Br J Haematol 14:363, 1968.

175. Mitus WJ, Bergna LJ, Mednicoff IB, Dameshek W: Atypical myeloblasts in acute leukemia. Clin Res Proc 5:149, 1957.

176. _____, _____, _____, _____: Alkaline phosphatase of mature neutrophils in chronic forms of the myeloproliferative syndrome. Am J Clin Pathol 30:285, 1958.

177. _____, _____, _____, _____: Cytochemical studies of glycogen content of lymphocytes in lymphocytic proliferations. Blood 13:748, 1958.

178. _____, Gherardi GJ, Mednicoff IB, Dameshek W: Cytochemistry of myelofibrosis with myeloid metaplasia in relation to spleen changes. Arch Pathol 67:188, 1959.

179. Moloney WC, Lange RD: Leukemia in atomic bomb survivors. II. Observations on early phases of leukemia. Blood 9:663, 1954.

180. _____, McPherson K, Fliegelman L: Esterase activity in leukocytes demonstrated by the use of naphthol AS-D chloroacetate substrate. J Histochem 8:200, 1960.

181. Moorhead PS, Nowell PC, Mellman WJ, Battips DM, Hungerford DA: Chromosome preparation of leukocytes cultivated from human peripheral blood. Exp Cell Res 20:613, 1960.

182. Naegeli O: Blutkrankheiten und Blutdiagnostik. Leipzig, von Veit, 1908.

183. Naman R, Cadotte M, Long LA: Les chromosomes dans les érythro-leucemies. Nouv Rev Fr Hématol 11:211, 1971.

184. Nowell PC: Prognostic value of marrow chromosome studies in human "preleukemia." Arch Pathol 80:205, 1965.

185. _____: Chromosome abnormalities in human leukemia and lymphoma, in Zarofonetis CJD (ed): Proceedings of the International Conference on Leukemia-Lymphoma. Philadelphia, Lea & Febiger, 1968, p 47.

186. _____: Marrow chromosome studies in "preleukemia." Further correlation with clinical course. Cancer 28:513, 1971.

187. _____, Hungerford DA: A minute chromosome in human chronic granulocytic leukemia. Science 132:1497, 1960.

188. _____, _____: Chromosome studies on normal and leukemic human leukocytes. J Natl Cancer Inst 25:85, 1960.

189. _____, _____: Chromosome studies on human leukemia. II. Chronic granulocytic leukemia. J Natl Cancer Inst 27:1013, 1961.

190. O'Riordan ML, Robinson JA, Buckton KE, Evans HJ: Distinguishing between the chromosomes involved in Down's syndrome (trisomy 21) and chronic myeloid leukaemia (Ph¹) by fluorescence. Nature 230:167, 1971.

191. Patil SR, Merrick S, Lubs HA: Identification of each human chromosome with a modified Giemsa stain. Science 173:821, 1971.

192. Pedersen B: Three cases of chronic myeloid leukaemia with presumably identical 47-chromosome cell-lines in the blood. Acta Pathol Microbiol Scand 61:497, 1964.

193. _____: Males with XO Ph¹-positive cells: A cytogenetic and clinical subgroup of chronic myelogenous leukaemia? Acta Pathol Microbiol Scand 72:360, 1968.

194. _____: Ph¹-disomy and prognosis in chronic myelogenous leukaemia. Acta Haematol 39:102, 1968.

195. _____: Relation between karyotype and cytology in chronic myelogenous leukaemia. Scand J Haematol 8:494, 1971.

196. _____, Videbaek A: Several cell-lines with abnormal karyotypes in a patient with chronic myelogenous leukaemia. Scand J Haematol 1:129, 1964.

197. Pelger K: Demonstratie van een paar zeldzaam voorkommende typen van vloedlichchampjex en gesprefing der patiëntin. Ned Tijdschr Geneeskd 72:1178, 1928.

198. Perillie PE: Studies of the changes in leukocyte alkaline phosphatase following pyrogen stimulation in chronic granulocytic leukemia. Blood 29:401, 1967.

199. Perry S: Biochemistry of the white blood cell. JAMA 190:918, 1964.

200. Perry VP, Kerby CC, Gresham RB: Further observations on the collection, storage and transfusion of peripheral blood leukocytes. Ann NY Acad Sci 114:651, 1964.

201. Perugini S: Morfochimica della leucopoiesi e della piastrinopoiesi normali e patologiche. Haematol Lat 2:235, 1959.

202. Pittaluga G, Bessis M: The structure and function of the nucleoli in normal and pathologic cells. Puerto Rico J Publ Health 19:180, 1943.

203. Polli E, Ratti G: Studien über Leukocyten; die Fettfraktionen in intakten Zellen und in isolierten Zellkernen bei normalen und pathologischen Zuständen. Biochem Z 323:546, 1953.

204. Quaglino D, Cowling DC: Cytochemical studies on cells from chronic lymphocytic leukaemia and lymphosarcoma cultured

with phytohaemagglutinin. Br J Haematol 10:358, 1964.

205. _____, Hayhoe FGJ: Observations of the periodic acid-Schiff reaction in lymphoproliferative diseases. J Pathol Bacteriol 78:521, 1959.

206. _____, _____: Periodic acid-Schiff positivity in erythroblasts with special reference to DiGuglielmo's disease. Br J Haematol 6:26, 1959.

207. Rabinovitch M, Junqueira LCU, Mendes FT: Cytochemical demonstration of "acid" phosphatase in bone marrow smears. Science 107:322, 1948.

208. Rastrick JM, Fitzgerald PH, Gunz FW: Direct evidence for presence of Ph¹ chromosome in erythroid cells. Br Med J 1:69, 1968.

209. Rebuck JW: The functions of the white blood cells. Am J Clin Pathol 17:614, 1947.

210. Regan JD, Vodopick H, Takeda S, Lee WH, Faulcon FM: Serine requirement in leukemic and normal blood cells. Science 163:1452, 1969.

211. Reisman LE, Zuelzer WW, Thompson RI: Further observations on the role of aneuploidy in acute leukemia. Cancer Res 24:1448, 1964.

212. Reisner EJ Jr, Korson R: Microspectrophotometric determination of desoxyribosenucleic acid in megaloblasts of pernicious anemia. Blood 6:244, 1951.

213. Rheingold JJ, Wislocki GB: Histochemical methods applied to hematology. Blood 3:641, 1948.

214. Rich AR, Wintrobe MM, Lewis MR: The differentiation of myeloblasts from lymphoblasts by their manner of locomotion, a motion picture study of the cells of normal bone marrow and lymph nodes, and of leukemic blood. Johns Hopkins Med J 65:291, 1939.

215. Riley JF: Heparin, histamine and mast cells. Blood 9:1123, 1954.

216. _____: The Mast Cells. Edinburgh, Livingstone, 1959.

217. Robinson JC, Pierce JE, Goldstein DP: Leukocyte alkaline phosphatase: electrophoretic variants associated with chronic myelogenous leukemia. Science 150:58, 1965.

218. Rosales CL, Bennett JM, Rutenberg AM: Histochemical demonstration of leukocyte acid phosphatase in health and disease. Br J Haematol 12:172, 1966.

219. Rosen RB, Teplitz RL: Chronic granulocytic leukemia complicated by ulcerative colitis: elevated leukocyte alkaline phosphatase and possible modifier gene deletion. Blood 26:148, 1965.

220. Rosenszajn L, Leibovich M, Shoham D, Epstein J: The esterase activity in megaloblasts, leukaemic and normal haemopoietic cells. Br J Haematol 14:605, 1962.

221. Rossiter RJ, Wong E: Beta-glucuronidase of human white blood cells. Blood 5:864, 1950.

222. Rowley JD, Blaisdell RK, Jacobson LO: Chromosome studies in preleukemia. I. Aneuploidy of Group C chromosomes in three patients. Blood 27:782, 1966.

223. Rudkin GT, Hungerford DA, Nowell PC: DNA contents of chromosome Ph¹ and chromosome 21 in human chronic granulocytic leukemia. Science 144:1229, 1964.

224. Salsbury AJ: Nucleolar staining in the differentiation of acute leukaemias. Br J Haematol 13:768, 1967.

225. Sandberg AA, Ishihara T, Miwa T, Hauschka TS: The in vivo chromosome constitution of marrow from 34 human leukemias plus 60 non-leukemic controls. Cancer 21:678, 1961.

226. _____, _____, Kikuchi Y, Crosswhite LH: Chromosome differences among the acute leukemias. Ann NY Acad Sci 113:663, 1964.

227. _____, Yamada K: Chromosomes and causation of human cancer and leukemia. I. Karyotypic diversity in a single cancer. Cancer 19:1869, 1966.

228. Schmalzl F, Braunsteiner H: The application of cytochemical methods to the study of acute leukaemia. Acta Haematol 45:209, 1971.

229. Schwind JL: The supravital method in the study of the cytology of blood and marrow cells. Blood 5:597, 1950.

230. Seabright M: A rapid banding technique for human chromosomes. Lancet 2:971, 1971.

231. Seitz JF, Luganova IS: The biochemical identification of blood and bone marrow cells of patients with acute leukemia. Cancer Res 28:2548, 1968.

232. Shanbrom E, Collins Z, Miller S: "Acquired" Pelger-Huët cells in blood dyscrasias. Am J Med Sci 240:732, 1960.

233. Shimkin MB, Sapirstein L, Goetzl FR, Wheeler PM, Berlin NI: Blood histamine in leukemia and erythremia. J Natl Cancer Inst 9:379, 1949.

234. Shortman, K., 1969. The separation of T lymphocyte populations on glass bead columns, in Gerritsen T (ed): Progress in Separation and Purification, vol 2. New York, Wiley, 1969, p 91.

235. Smutka P, Brunning RD: An evaluation of nuclear aryl-sulfatase activity in acute leukaemias. Acta Haematol 41:290, 1969.

236. Sobin LH, Kidd JG: A metabolic difference between two lines of lymphoma 6C3HED cells in relation to asparagine. Proc Soc Exp Biol Med 119:325, 1965.

237. Speed DE, Lawler SD: Chronic granulocytic leukaemia. The chromosome and the disease. Lancet 1:403, 1964.

238. Spiers ASD, Baikie AG: Chronic granulocytic leukaemia: Demonstration of the Philadelphia chromosome in cultures of spleen cells. Nature 208:497, 1965.

239. _____, _____: Cytogenetic studies in the malignant lymphomas. Lancet 1:506, 1966.

240. _____, _____: Cytogenetic evolution and clonal proliferation in acute transformation of chronic granulocytic leukaemia. Br J Cancer 22:192, 1968.

241. _____, _____: Cytogenetic studies in the malignant lymphomas and related neoplasms. Results in twenty-seven cases. Cancer 22:193, 1968.

242. _____, _____: A special role of the group 17, 18 chromosomes in reticuloendothelial neoplasia. Br J Cancer 24:77, 1970.

243. _____, _____: Anomalies of the small acrocentric chromosomes in human tumour cells. Aust NZ J Med 2:188, 1972.

244. Steele MW: Autoradiography may be unreliable for identifying human chromosomes. Nature 221:1114, 1969.

245. Storti E, Perugini S: Cytochemical researches on the lipids of the hematic cells with particular attention to those of acute leukosis. Acta Haematol 5:321, 1951.

246. Strieff F, Peters A, Gilgenkrantz S: Anomalies chromosomiques au cours de la transformation blastique terminale d'une leucémie myéloide chronique: prédominance d'un clone à 48 chromosomes avec deux chromosomes Ph¹. Nouv Rev Fr Hématol 6:417, 1966.

247. Stuart J, Simpson JS, Mann JR: Intracellular hydrogen transport systems in acute leukaemia. Br J Haematol 19:739, 1970.

248. Tanaka KR, Valentine WN, Fredricks RE: Diseases or clinical conditions associated with low leukocyte alkaline phosphatase. N Engl J Med 262:912, 1960.

249. Tanzer J, Dallapiccola B, Philippe N, Lanoe R, Seban C, Boiron M, Bernard J: Intérêt diagnostique possible de la coloration cytochimique de l'arylsulfatase en hématologie. Données préliminaires. Nouv Rev Fr Hématol 9:706, 1969.

250. Teplitz RL: Regulation of leucocyte alkaline phosphatase and the Philadelphia chromosome. Nature 209:821, 1966.

251. Thiersch JB: Histamine and histaminase in chronic myeloid leukaemia of man. I. Histamine in the blood of chronic myeloid leukaemia. Aust J Exp Biol Med Sci 25:73, 1947.

252. _____: II. Histamine and histaminase in the blood of cases of myeloid leukaemia under and after deep x-ray treatment. Aust J Exp Biol Med Sci 25:75, 1947.

253. Thorell B: Studies on the formation of cellular substances during blood cell production. Acta Med Scand (suppl 200), 1947.

254. Tjio JH, Carbone PP, Whang J, Frei E III: The Philadelphia chromosome and chronic myelogenous leukemia. J Natl Cancer Inst 36:567, 1966.

255. Tough IM, Baikie AG, Harnden DG, King MJ, Court Brown WM, Buckton KE, Jacobs PA, McBride JA: Cytogenetic studies in chronic myeloid leukaemia and acute leukaemia associated with mongolism. Lancet 1:411, 1961.

256. _____, Jacobs PA, Court Brown WM, Baikie AG, Williamson ERD: Cytogenetic studies on bone marrow in chronic myeloid leukaemia. Lancet 1:844, 1963.

257. Trubowitz S, Kirman D, Masek B: The leucocyte alkaline phosphatase in mongolism. Lancet 2:486, 1962.

258. _____, Miller WL: Electrophoretic heterogeneity of leucocyte alkaline phosphatase in normal man and in patients with polycythemia vera. Proc Soc Exp Biol Med 123:187, 1966.

259. Trujillo JM, Ohno S: Chromosomal alteration of erythropoietic cells in chronic myeloid leukemia. Proceedings of the Ninth Congress of the International Society of Hematology, Mexico City, 1962.

260. Valentine WN: The biochemistry and enzymatic activities of leukocytes in health and disease, in Tocantins L (ed): Progress in Hematology, vol. I. New York, Grune & Stratton, 1956, p 293.

261. _____: The metabolism of the leukemic leukocyte. Am J Med 28:699, 1960.

262. _____, Beck WS: Biochemical studies on leucocytes. I. Phosphatase activity in health, leucocytosis and myelocytic leucemia. J Lab Clin Med 38:39, 1951.

263. _____, _____, Follette JH, Mills H, Lawrence JS: Biochemical studies in chronic myelocytic leukemia, polycythemia

vera and other idiopathic myeloproliferative disorders. Blood 7:959, 1952.

264. ———, Follette JH, Solomon DH, Reynolds J: Biochemical and enzymatic characteristics of normal and leukemic leukocytes with particular reference to leukocyte alkaline phosphatase, in: The Leukemias. New York, Academic Press, 1957, p 457.

265. ———, Lawrence JS, Pearce ML, Beck WS: The relationship of the basophil to blood histamine in man. Blood 10:154, 1955.

266. ———, Tanaka KR, Fredricks RE: Studies on leukocyte alkaline phosphatase: Role of zinc and magnesium. J Lab Clin Med 55:303, 1960.

267. Vallee BL, Altschule MD: "Trace" metals in blood with particular reference to zinc and carbonic anhydrase. Editorial. Blood 4:398, 1949.

268. Van Furth R, Hirsch JG, Fedorko ME: Morphology and peroxidase cytochemistry of mouse promonocytes, monocytes and macrophages. J Exp Med 132:794, 1970.

269. Wachstein M: Alkaline phosphatase activity in normal and abnormal human blood and bone marrow cells. J Lab Clin Med 31:1, 1946.

270. ———: The distribution of histochemically demonstrable glycogen in human blood and bone marrow cells. Blood 4:54, 1949.

271. ———: Histochemistry of leukocytes. Ann NY Acad Sci 59:1052, 1955.

272. Wagner R: Studies on the physiology of the white blood cell. The glycogen content of leukocytes in leukemia and polycythemia. Blood 2:235, 1947.

273. Weiner L: A family with high incidence leukemia and unique Ph[1] chromosome findings. Blood 26:871, 1965.

274. Weisberger AS, Heinle RW: The protective effect of cysteine on leucopenia induced by nitrogen mustard. J Lab Clin Med 36:872, 1950.

275. ———, Levine B: Incorporation of radioactive L-cystine by normal and leukemic leukocytes in vivo. Blood 9:1082, 1954.

276. ———, Suhrland LG: Comparative incorporation of S35-L-cystine + S35 sodium sulfate by normal and leukemic leukocytes. Blood 10:458, 1955.

277. ———, ———: Studies on analogues of L-cysteine and L-cystine. II. The effect of selenium cysteine on leukemia. Blood 11:19, 1956.

278. Whang J, Frei E, III, Tjio JH, Carbone PP, Brecher G: The distribution of the Philadelphia chromosome in patients with chronic myelogenous leukemia. Blood 22:664, 1963.

279. Whang-Peng J, Freireich EJ, Oppenheim JJ, Frei E, III, Tjio JH: Cytogenetic studies in 45 patients with acute lymphocytic leukemia. J Natl Cancer Inst 42:881, 1969.

280. ———, Henderson ES, Knutsen T, Freireich EJ, Gart JJ: Cytogenetic studies in acute myelocytic leukemia with special emphasis on the occurrence of Ph[1] chromosome. Blood 36:448, 1970.

281. Wiltshaw E, Moloney WC: Studies on various factors influencing leukocyte alkaline phosphatase activity. J Lab Clin Med 47:691, 1958.

282. Winkelstein A, Goldberg LS, Tishkoff GH: Leukocyte alkaline phosphatase and the Philadelphia chromosome. Arch Intern Med 119:291, 1967.

283. Wislocki GB, Dempsey EW: Observations on the chemical cytology of normal blood and hemopoietic tissues. Anat Rec 96:249, 1946.

284. ———, Rheingold JJ, Dempsey EW: The occurrence of the periodic acid-Schiff reaction in various normal cells of blood and connective tissue. Blood 4:562, 1949.

285. Xefteris E, Mitus WJ, Mednicoff IB, Dameshek W: Leukocytic alkaline phosphatase in busulfan-induced remissions of chronic granulocytic leukemia. Blood 18:202, 1961.

286. Yam LT, Mitus WJ: The lymphocyte β-glucuronidase activity in lymphoproliferative disorders. Blood 31:480, 1968.

Yale Rabinowitz, *deceased*

7

RNA and DNA Metabolism in Normal and Leukemic Leukocytes

Recent reviews relevant to various aspects of the metabolism of RNA, DNA, and their nucleotide precursors in normal and leukemic leukocytes include those by Cline,[15,17] Beck,[4] Gallo,[32–33] Perry and Gallo,[55] and Perry.[54]

The fundamental features of nucleic acid metabolism in mammalian cells are to be found in normal leukocytes. There are differences in enzyme content between differentiated and immature cells. In general, these are quantitative rather than qualitative. Some precursor enzymes are missing, perhaps because the liver manufactures and supplies intermediate metabolites such as purines. This applies particularly to the early enzymes of purine synthesis. Synthesis of DNA is chiefly by means of a DNA-directed DNA polymerase which requires all four 5'-triphosphate deoxyribonucleotides. Synthesis of DNA on RNA templates by an RNA-directed DNA polymerase has been found to occur with animal RNA leukemia viruses and may be important in human leukemia (see below). RNA synthesis by RNA polymerase on DNA templates requires all four ribonucleotide 5'-triphosphates. Pathways for the production of the nucleotide precursors (Figs. 7-1–7-3) have received considerable attention in the hope of finding exploitable differences between normal and leukemic cells. Some of the most effective therapeutic agents against leukemia interfere with nucleic acid synthesis by blocking specific enzymes involved in the synthesis of purine or pyrimidine nucleotides (see chapter 17, and the review by Wilmanns.[82])

Studies of partially to completely separated normal and leukemic leukocytes[58–64] showed that there were differences in the content of the enzymes of nucleotide and nucleic acid metabolism among cell types and between normal and leukemic cells. Immature cells retaining a capacity for cell division were characterized by high activity of anabolic enzymes, while mature cells showed high activity of catabolic enzymes. Myeloblasts thus showed high levels of activity of such enzymes as thymidine (TdR) kinase, dihydrofolate reductase, thymidine-5'-monophosphate (TMP) synthetase, and DNA polymerase, while more mature granulocytes had high activities of nucleases, phosphatases, and phosphorylases. Most studies of the enzymes of nucleic acid metabolism in both normal and

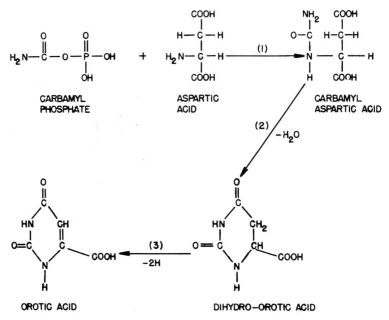

Fig. 7-1. Enzymes found in leukocytes for *de novo* synthesis of the pyrimidine ring: 1. aspartate carbamyl transferase, 2. dihydro-orotase, 3. dihydro-orotic dehydrogenase.

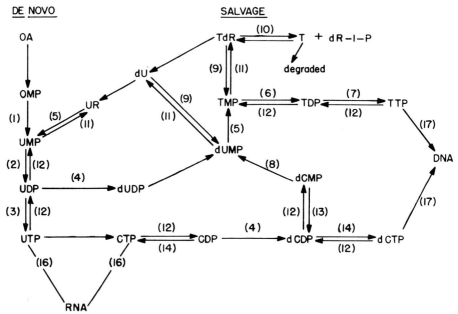

Fig. 7-2. Enzymes of pyrimidine nucleotide synthesis: completion of *de novo* synthetic pathways (see Fig. 7-1 for initial enzymes) and enzymes of salvage. 1. orotidylate decarboxylase, 2. uridine 5′ monophosphate (UMP) kinase, 3. uridine diphosphate (UDP) kinase, 4. ribonucleotide reductase, 5. thymidine synthetase, 6. TMP kinase, 7. TDP kinase, 8. deoxycytidylate deaminase, 9. thymidine (deoxyuridine) kinase, 10. thymidine phosphorylase, 11. 5′-nucleotidase, 12. pyrophosphatase, 13. dCMP kinase, 14. dCDP kinase, 15. uridine kinase, 16. RNA polymerase, 17. DNA polymerase.

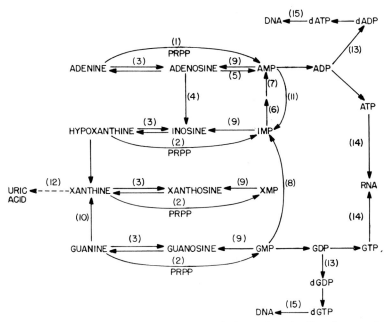

Fig. 7-3. Purine salvage enzymes: 1. adenine phosphoribosyl transferase, 2. hypoxanthine—guanine phosphoribosyl transferase, 3. purine nucleoside phosphorylase, 4. adenosine deaminase, 5. adenosine kinase, 6. adenylosuccinate synthetase, 7. adenylosuccinate lyase, 8. GMP reductase, 9. 5'-nucleotidase, 10. guanine deaminase, 11. AMP deaminase, 12. xanthine oxidase (not present in blood cells), 13. ribonucleotide reductase, 14. RNA polymerase, 15. DNA polymerase.

leukemic leukocytes have been done with crude cell extracts containing a mixture of enzymes which may be in competition with each other. Unfortunately, limitations in the number of cells available have usually prevented separation and purification of the individual enzymes. The results obtained represent a balance of the activities of the enzymes present, as well as the effects of such factors as end-product inhibition, substrate concentration, pH, etc. Under these conditions, the absence of activity of a given enzyme may merely indicate that it is inhibited, or its substances are being removed, or that its product is being used as a substrate by another enzyme. It would thus be possible in some instances for the presence of an anabolic enzyme, such as DNA polymerase, to be obscured because a high level of 5'-phosphatase activity has removed its nucleotide triphosphate substrates. Separation of the individual cell types, of course, helps to yield more meaningful results. Removal of granulocytes with their high levels of catabolic enzymes from a mixture of cell types, permits the anabolic enzymes of the less differentiated cells to become more evident. In any case, valuable information is obtainable from such studies, but one must remain cognizant of the fact that the absence of the product of an enzyme's activity does not necessarily indicate that the enzyme itself is absent.

FEEDBACK INHIBITION

Feedback inhibition of an initial, and usually rate-limiting, enzyme of a pathway of nucleotide synthesis by the end-product of the pathway appears to be an important mechanism in the control of the production of the four deoxy- or ribonucleotides needed for the synthesis of DNA or RNA, respectively. Inhibition may result from attachment of the end-product of a synthetic sequence at an allosteric site[48] on the initial or allosteric enzyme of the pathway. This alters the enzyme so that it is prevented from combining with the substrate at its normal attachment site. The potential complexity of this control mechanism is suggested by the fact that thymidine-5'-triphosphate (TTP), one of the four nucleotide substrates for DNA polymerase, exerts a powerful inhibitory effect on several enzymes leading to its synthesis from different directions. Some of these enzymes also are inhibited by other small molecules, such as adenosine triphosphate (ATP).[34,62] Inhibition by TTP of thymidine kinase[11] and deoxycytidylate deaminase[74] has been demonstrated in leukocytes. TTP inhibition of ribonucleotide reductase was found in leukemic mouse spleen,[29,30] and that of aspartic transcarbamylase in mammalian cells,[38] but not as yet in leukocytes. Although changes in nucleotide synthesis perhaps provide only a coarse adjustment[32] in the control of nucleic acid synthesis, it seems, nevertheless, to operate effectively.

PYRIMIDINE NUCLEOTIDE SYNTHESIS

Leukocytes can synthesize pyrimidines *de novo* from simple compounds (Fig. 7-1). Enzymes of salvage pathways for reutilization of the pyrimidine bases (thymine, uracil, and cytosine) are also found in the leukocytes (Fig. 7-2). The synthesis of TTP has received special attention because of the specificity of the thymine base for DNA. TTP may be the end-product of either *de novo* synthesis or the thymidine salvage pathway.[14] The relative importance of these two pathways is not completely clear. Rate-limiting enzymes in both pathways show increased activities in cells which are dividing. The increases are, however, greater in the salvage pathway.[22]

The activities of aspartate carbamyl transferase,[77] thymidylate synthetase,[67,75] dihydrofolate reductase,[6,66-67,80] thymidine kinase,[8,11,50] and ribonucleotide reductase[30] are increased in leukocytes from patients with acute leukemia or chronic granulocytic leukemia. The level of enzyme activity was found to correlate with the number of blasts present and to diminish with cell maturity.[30,50,61-62,67] Levels of these enzymes were low in lymphocytes from patients with chronic lymphocytic leukemia, as well as in normal lymphocytes unless stimulated by phytohemagglutinin (PHA).[61,64] Silber et al.[75] and Bertino et al.[7] were unable to demonstrate thymidylate synthetase activity in CLL lymphocytes, although low levels were found by Roberts and Hall.[67]

Smith et al.[77] studied the activities of a sequence of three enzymes which produce the pyrimidine, orotic acid, from carbamyl phosphate and L-aspartic acid (Fig. 7-1). They found that in CGL cells the activities of the enzymes aspartate carbamyltransferase, dihydro-orotase, and dihydro-orotic dehydrogenase were increased severalfold above normal values for mature polymorphonuclear leukocytes. The increased enzyme activity of dihydro-orotic dehydrogenase was particularly marked, being as much as fourteen times elevated in acute leukemia. Generally, they found, as they anticipated, that in leukemic leukocytes increased enzyme activity tended to parallel cytological evidence of immaturity of the cells. Leukocytes from patients with infection or with myeloproliferative disorders showed similar but less marked alterations of their enzyme patterns. In comparison with normal polymorphonuclear leukocytes, lymphocytes from patients with chronic lymphocytic leukemia had similar activities of aspartate carbamyltransferase and dihydro-orotase, but dihydro-orotic dehydrogenase was increased four- to sevenfold. Unfortunately, normal lymphocytes were not available for comparison. Dihydro-orotic dehydrogenase, absent from mature erythrocytes, was found to be present in the nucleated erythrocytes in the Di Guglielmo syndrome. The point where the *de novo* and salvage pathways of TTP synthesis join is TMP (see Fig. 7-2). TMP is synthesized in the *de novo* pathway by methylation of deoxyuridine 5'-monophosphate (dUMP) by TMP synthetase. This occurs in the presence of tetrahydrofolate which is reduced in the following process: N^5, N^{10} – methylene tetrahydrofolate + dUMP → TMP + dihydrofolate. Dihydrofolate reductase is needed to reoxidize the dihydrofolate to tetrahydrofolate.[6-7] The dUMP may come also from the deamination of deoxycytidine 5'-monophosphate (dCMP),[74] or from salvage of uridine.[44] In the TdR salvage pathway the synthesis of TMP from TdR has been extensively studied because TdR kinase activity was found to be increased in actively dividing cells.[9,26] As already noted, both TMP synthetase and TdR kinase are subject to inhibition by TTP, the end-product in common of both pathways.

Bianchi demonstrated that leukocytes could phosphorylate TdR to TTP.[8] Leukocytes from chronic granulocytic leukemia patients were more active than those from normal cells. Nakai et al., also using mixed cell suspensions and supernatant fractions of cell homogenates, thought that some generalizations could be made.[50] They recognized the difficulties present in interpretation of results complicated by competing reactions and negative feedback inhibitions. They found that chronic granulocytic leukemia increased TdR kinase activity, decreasing with therapy, which correlated with a shift in differential count. Chronic lymphocytic leukemia had relatively low TdR kinase activity and high TMP phosphatase activity. Acute granulocytic leukemia, however, inexplicably appeared to have low TdR kinase activity, but a relatively normal deoxythymidine-5'-monophosphate (dTMP) phosphatase activity. Perhaps the low phosphatase activity of the CGL cells permitted greater accumulation of the product. In contrast, Roberts and Hall[67] did find TdR kinase activity high in both acute and chronic granulocytic leukemias.

When enzymes of the TdR salvage pathway were studied[62,64] in glass-column-separated normal and leukemic leukocytes,[58,59] differences in enzyme content of the individual cell types became apparent. Most of the cells studied were able to phosphorylate TMP to TTP. TdR kinase activity was negligible in mature granulocytes, low in normal and CLL lymphocytes, but was high in all types of blast cells. TdR phosphorylase and 5'-nucleotidase activities were high in granulocytes and in both normal and CLL lymphocytes. Blast cells, on the other hand, showed low levels of TdR phosphorylase and 5'-nucleotidase activity. In cultures of normal and CLL lymphocytes,[64] response to PHA stimulation with blast-cell formation was accompanied by large increases in TdR kinase activity.

Evaluation of results, even when separated cells were studied, presented some difficulties, since the cells still contained a mixture of enzymes. Rabinowitz et al.[62] found that phosphatase and TdR phosphorylase activity was high in granulocytes and in normal and leukemic lymphocytes, even at optimal ATP concentrations but the activities of these enzymes only became apparent in blasts in the absence of ATP. It was evident that with mixed enzyme preparations the assay conditions might be crucial in determining the end-products. With TdR or TMP as the substrate, the end-products obtained varied greatly with the concentration of ATP and Mg^{++} in the reaction mixture, undoubtedly by affecting the various enzymes in different ways. ATP may function in these reactions to supply energy, as a coenzyme, as a phosphate donor, as an enzyme activator, or as an enzyme inhibitor. Changes in ATP levels in cell loci may contribute to the control of TdR metabolism and thus serve in regulating DNA synthesis.

Studies in leukocytes of pyrimidine pathways other than those of TTP production have been limited. Although dCMP deaminase is one of the enzymes which has been associated with cell growth,[45] Silber et al.[75] found the levels of this enzyme's activity to be similar in normal and leukemic leukocytes of all types. Silber[74] did show that the dCMP deaminase of leukocytes was subject to inhibition by TTP, a potential end-product of the pathway. The activity of uridine kinase, which is subject to end-product inhibition, increases in PHA-stimulated lymphocytes.[44] Its activity is high in leukemic myeloblasts.[67] In studies of glass-column-separated cells,[61] it was found that cellular maturity, as represented by normal granulocytes and lymphocytes, was associated with a balance of enzyme activities leading to the breakdown of deoxycytidine to deoxyuridine and uracil, while showing minimal production of dCTP and TTP. A balance, on the other hand, in favor of anabolic enzymes was associated with cellular immaturity as was shown with myeloblasts, monoblasts, as well as with lymphocytes which had responded to PHA stimulation. Lymphocytes from patients with chronic lymphocytic leukemia showed a wide range of enzyme activities which seemed to correlate with their ability to respond to PHA.

PURINE NUCLEOTIDE SYNTHESIS

The *de novo* pathway of purine synthesis is incomplete in leukocytes.[40] Scott showed that leukocytes could incorporate formate-C^{14} into nucleic acid purine if supplied with 5-amino-4-imidazolecarboxamide (AIC) or its ribotide (AICR).[73] The formate only served to close the purine ring of the otherwise complete precursor. *De novo* purine synthesis from formate-C^{14} without the addition of AIC was found only with acute leukemic cells and, even in these, its addition produced a great increase in purine production. Recently, Reem demonstrated two alternative pathways for synthesis of phosphoribosyl-1-amine in human spleen and in Burkitt lymphoma cells.[65] This may indicate that the subject of *de novo* synthesis in leukocytes is not closed, but the chief source of purines for the blood cells appears to be exogenous. Available evidence indicates that the liver is the primary source of bone marrow purines.[41,57] The compounds transported from the liver have not been rigidly determined, but are probably adenine, hypoxanthine, and guanine. The bone marrow is also a potential major source of purine bases for salvage, but dietary purines are probably unimportant. Enzymes (Fig. 7-3) of the purine salvage pathway (hypoxanthine-guanine phosphoribosyl transferase and adenine phosphoribosyl transferase) convert the bases to inosine 5'-monophosphate (IMP), 5'-guanylic acid (GMP), and 5'-adenylic acid (AMP).[49] The blood cells do not contain xanthine oxidase and cannot complete the catabolism of purines to uric acid.

The phosphoribosyl transferases have become notorious because of their involvement in Lesch-Nyhan disease.[42] Interest in hypoxanthine-guanine phosphoribosyl transferase has also been stimulated by the enzyme's function in converting 6-mercaptopurine to its ribonucleotide—a step which appears to be the site of the drug's blocking action. Resistance by bacteria to 6-mercaptopurine is associated with loss of the enzyme.[2] Davidson and Winter found that all except one of their acute leukemic patients had activities of hypoxanthine-guanine phosphoribosyl transferase equal to that of normal leukocytes; thus, they could not attribute drug resistance, when it occurred, to loss of this enzyme.[25] The leukemic cells did show a two- to threefold higher activity of adenine phosphoribosyl transferase than did normal leukocytes. Smith et al. obtained essentially similar results.[76] None of their drug-resistant patients showed reduced enzyme activities. They found that the level of hypoxanthine transferase activity was significantly increased in AGL leukocytes compared with normal ones. In both AGL and ALL patients the activities of the adenine and hypoxanthine transferases were more variable than normal. They thought the cause of these findings was "obscure."

SYNTHESIS OF DEOXYRIBONUCLEOTIDES

Ribonucleotide reductase catalyzes the reduction of ribonucleotides (chiefly the diphosphates) to deoxyribonucleotides needed for DNA synthesis. This enzyme was shown by Fujioka and Silber to be most active in cells from patients with acute lymphocytic leukemia, chronic granulocytic leukemia, or from normal marrow.[30] Much lower levels of activity were found in lymphocytes from chronic lymphocytic leukemia, and the lowest levels occurred in normal mature leukocytes.

Alternative means for production of deoxynucleotides without conversion to ribonucleotides is provided by salvage enzymes which have been studied extensively by Gallo, Perry, and their associates.[55] They showed that leukocytes could synthesize thymidine from thymine by two different enzyme reactions:

$$\text{TdR phosphorylase}$$
$$T + dR\text{-}I\text{-}P \leftrightarrow TdR + Pi$$

and

$$\text{pyrimidine deoxyribosyl transferase}$$
$$T + dU \leftrightarrow TdR + U$$

The first enzyme also synthesized deoxy-uridine (UdR). The same investigators also studied a deoxynucleoside phosphorylase which in the presence of deoxyribose-1-P converted hypoxanthine to deoxyinosine and guanine to deoxyguanosine, but did not react directly with adenine. Deoxyadenosine must be produced by the amination of deoxyinosine 5'-monophosphate (dIMP) to deoxy 5'-adenylic acid (dAMP). This is a step which it may be difficult for leukocytes to make. It does not occur in human erythrocytes. Our own initial efforts to demonstrate its occurrence in normal and leukemic cells have thus far been unsuccessful. The phosphorylases may function chiefly to break down nucleotides to their bases for salvage.[46] Leukocytes do make greater use of exogenous thymidine than thymine for DNA synthesis.[10, 22]

DNA-DIRECTED DNA POLYMERASE

DNA polymerase activity in mature granulocytes was virtually absent, while in lymphocytes it was comparatively high.[60] In chronic lymphocytic leukemia, DNA polymerase levels were moderately elevated above normal, perhaps because of the presence of some lymphoblasts. In chronic granulocytic leukemia, in studies of partially or completely separated cells, enzyme activity was very high in immature forms, but fell sharply with increasing maturity, approaching zero in segmented cells. Levels of DNA polymerase activity appeared to parallel the cells' potential for cell division. With cell maturity, granulocytes lose the capacity to divide and to synthesize DNA. With remission in chronic granulocytic leukemia, there was a fall in DNA polymerase activity which was attributed to the change from immature to mature cells. With an acute blastic crisis on the other hand, a large increase in DNA polymerase activity occurred.

Ove et al., while agreeing that DNA polymerase activity was high in mixed cell suspensions from patients with chronic granulocytic leukemia, reported that DNA polymerase content was a function of leukemia rather than of cellular immaturity.[52] This judgment was based on their finding of relatively low DNA polymerase activity in cells with similar differential counts from patients with leukemoid reactions. This discrepancy may be due to differences in alkaline phosphatase content. The low alkaline phosphatase activity of CGL granulocytes, even in remission, may permit persistence of the 5'-triphosphate nucleotides needed for DNA synthesis. Any preparation containing normal mature granulocytes, on the other hand, has high phosphatase activity which may destroy the nucleotide substrates of DNA polymerase. It has been our experience that a mixed cell preparation, which contains mature normal granulocytes in any significant number, may show an apparent absence of DNA polymerase activity, even though enzyme activity is demonstrable in separated immature cells from the same blood sample. Some variation in enzyme content may also be the result of differences in size of cells from patients with chronic granulocytic leukemia.[67]

Loeb et al. found that normal human lymphocytes which responded to PHA in cultures with blast-cell formation showed a significant increase in DNA polymerase activity.[43] It was also shown that only those CLL lymphocytes which could respond to PHA with blast-cell production, showed increased DNA polymerase activity.[62] Again, ability to divide was associated with high DNA polymerase activity in both normal and CLL lymphocytes.

RNA-DEPENDENT DNA POLYMERASE

Temin and Mizutani[79] and Baltimore[3] demonstrated that oncogenic RNA viruses contained a DNA polymerase which could synthesize DNA on a viral RNA template. Gallo et al. reported an RNA-dependent DNA polymerase in acute leukemic lymphoblasts, but not in PHA-stimulated normal lymphocytes.[37] They considered the latter to be the best available normal cell for comparison with the leukemic blast. Later studies reopened the question of the presence of RNA-dependent RNA polymerase in normal cells.[33] Synthetic RNA-DNA and RNA-RNA have proved to be most effective templates for RNA-dependent DNA polymerase. With a synthetic RNA-DNA template (rA · dT), Scolnick et al.[72] found RNA-dependent DNA polymerase activity in nonleukemic mammalian cells in tissue cultures. Gallo,[33] while noting that his laboratory did find DNA polymerase activity in PHA-stimulated lymphocytes with a synthetic rA · dT, had reservations concerning the specificity of the synthetic DNA-RNA complex for RNA-dependent DNA polymerase. He noted that there was little or no evidence of such polymerase activity in normal cells using natural templates. Ross et al. reported that they were able to identify the RNA-dependent DNA polymerase of murine leukemic virus-transformed cells as physically and antigenically different from that of normal cells.[68] They purified RNA-dependent DNA polymerase from normal and virus-transformed mouse BALB/3T3 cells and compared the properties with the polymerase from murine leukemia virus. They found the viral and cellular enzymes to be chromatographically and antigenically different, and virus-specific DNA polymerase could be identified in virus-transformed cells. Since the RNA-dependent DNA polymerases of the known mammalian leukemia viruses are antigenically related[1] it seemed relevant to search for virus-specific polymerase activity in human leukemia cells. If a unique peak were found, it should be possible to ascertain if it were a mammalian virus enzyme, with obvious implications.

MITOCHONDRIAL DNA

A circular dimer of mitochondrial DNA was found by Clayton and Vinograd[12,13] in CGL leukocytes, but not in normal cells. It was thought that this might be important in the leukemic process. Gallo,[32] in view of the subsequent finding that these circular dimers could be produced in cultured mouse fibroblasts, known as L-cells, under special conditions, implied that the importance of this finding was doubtful.[51] Polli,[56] on the other hand, did not think that these findings detracted from the relevance of the observation of Clayton and Vinograd.[12,13] He noted that this was the first time since the discovery of the Philadelphia chromosome that a correlation had been established between the leukemic process and a specific modification of the DNA of a leukemic cell.

SATELLITE DNA

Corneo et al. demonstrated that human leukemic DNA contains a fraction of nuclear satellite DNA, demonstrable as distinct bands in equilibrium density gradients in the analytical ultracentrifuge.[23,24] These contain highly repeated nucleotide sequences, which constitute about 3–4 percent of the DNA. An intermediate fraction with less frequently repeated nucleotide sequences was about 16–17 percent, while the remaining 80 percent was made up of heterogenous DNA without the repeated nucleotide sequences. So far no differences have been found between normal and leukemic cells.

METABOLISM OF RNA

The enzymes of RNA synthesis and the classes of RNA found in leukocytes[17] are essentially the same as in the other mammalian cells.[53] RNA polymerase in the presence of all four 5'-ribonucleotide triphosphates and a DNA template produces a polyribonucleotide strand which is a transcription of one of the twin strands of the DNA. The principal site of RNA synthesis appears to be the nucleolus, from which it is transferred to the cytoplasm. Cytoplasmic RNA consists chiefly of low molecular weight, 4S RNA which is chiefly transfer RNA (tRNA) and two ribosomal RNA species, 18S and 28S, which are formed from newly synthesized 45S RNA.[16,21] Messenger RNA (mRNA) appears to be included in newly synthesized polydisperse higher molecular weight RNA, but has not been well characterized in leukocytes.[17] The mRNA is incorporated with ribosomes into polysomes to provide the genetic information for coding protein synthesis. Small fractions of several other RNA species are identifiable, but their function is obscure. These include 5S RNA and high molecular weight polydisperse RNA.

The tRNA is involved in reading the genetic code, and its function in the control of protein synthesis is becoming increasingly apparent.[55] Gallo and Pestka,[36] noting that a considerable body of evidence had already been presented that changes in aminoacyl-tRNA accompany differentiation, studied differences in tRNA species in PHA-stimulated normal lymphocytes and leukemic lymphoblasts as a possible site of translational control. They found:

1. At least 56 species of tRNA fractionated from both normal and leukemic cells on reverse-phase partition chromatography columns.
2. For the most part, the profiles of double-labeled co-chromatographed aminoacyl-tRNA samples were similar in normal and leukemic cells.
3. Small but reproducible differences were found for leucyl-, seryl-, threonyl-, and pronyl-tRNA.
4. The most pronounced differences were found with tyrosyl-tRNA and glutaminyl-tRNA.

The latter feature, however, was thought to be caused by differences in the enzyme preparation rather than the tRNA itself. Fujioka et al. demonstrated some additional differences in the profiles of low molecular weight (4S and 5S) RNA from normal and leukemic cells.[28] It would appear that a mechanism for altered protein synthesis[55] is present in these findings, especially if they are consistent and reproducible.

Synthesis of 45S ribosomal RNA precursor with production and conservation of 28S and 18S ribosomal RNA results from the stimulation of normal lymphocytes by PHA.[18,19,39,47,69,70] Wasting of 18S RNA occurred in cultures of unstimulated lymphocytes, or in those reverting to the resting state.[20] Conservation of 18S RNA was considered by Rubin to be an important factor in the control of ribosomal assembly.[69,70] The poor responses of CLL lymphocytes to PHA stimulation were attributed by Rubin to failure to conserve ribosomal RNA,[71] even though synthesis increased initially in some cases. Rabinowitz et al. found that unstimulated CLL lymphocytes may show higher rates of RNA synthesis than normal lymphocytes during the initial hours of culture.[62] With PHA stimulation of normal lymphocytes, on the other hand, RNA synthesis doubled during the first 1–2 hours, while CLL lymphocytes showed little or no change. Rubin found that CLL lymphocytes, in some cases at least, did show increased incorporation of ^{3}H-uridine into 28S and 18S ribosomal RNA to a degree comparable with normal lymphocytes during the first hours of culture with PHA, but that after 6 hours, wasting of 18S RNA began.

In summary, despite difficulties arising from the study of mixed cell populations, a large number of differences has been described in the RNA and DNA metabolism of normal and leukemic leukocytes. Not surprisingly, the abnormalities differ from one type of leukemia to another, and none has yet emerged as a specific abnormality inherently related to leukemogenesis. Indeed, many of the apparent abnormalities of leukemic cells seem to be mere concomitants of their immaturity. These are all the more difficult to assess because comparable samples of normal cells of the same degree of immaturity are not readily obtained. Certain morphologic and tinctorial resemblances between leukemic blasts and PHA-stimulated normal lymphocytes have led to the use of the latter in various comparative studies. It appears that response to PHA is associated with several detectable changes in the metabolism of lymphocytes, but these do not necessarily correspond with the abnormalities found in leukemic blast cells.

REFERENCES

1. Aaronson S, Parks WP, Scolnick EM, Todaro GJ: Antibody to the RNA dependent DNA polymerase of mammalian C-type RNA tumor viruses. Proc Natl Acad Sci (USA) 68:920, 1971.

2. Balis ME: Antagonists and Nucleic Acids. Amsterdam, North Holland, 1968.

3. Baltimore D: RNA-dependent DNA polymerase in virions of RNA tumor viruses. Nature 226:1209, 1970.

4. Beck WS: Biochemical properties of normal and leukemic leukocytes, in Zarafonetis CJD (ed): Proceedings of the International Conference on Leukemia–Lymphoma, Philadelphia, Lea & Febiger, 1968, p 245.

5. Beltz RE: Comparison of the content of thymidylate synthetase, deoxycytidylate deaminase and deoxyribonucleoside kinases in normal and regenerating rat liver. Arch Biochem Biophys 99:304, 1962.

6. Bertino JR: The mechanism of action of the folate antagonists in man. Cancer Res 23:1286, 1963.

7. _____, Silber R, Freeman M, Alenty A, Albrecht M, Grabicio BW, Huennekens FM: Studies on normal and leukemic leukocytes. IV. Tetrahydrofolate-dependent enzyme systems and dihydrofolic reductase. J Clin Invest 42:1899, 1963.

8. Bianchi PA: Thymidine phosphorylation and deoxyribonucleic acid synthesis in human leukaemic cells. Biochim Biophys Acta 55:547, 1962.

9. Bollum FJ, Potter VR: Nucleic acid metabolism in regenerating rat liver. VI. Soluble enzymes which convert thymidine to thymidine phosphates and DNA. Cancer Res 19:561, 1959.

10. Breitman TR, Perry S, Cooper RA: Pyrimidine metabolism in human leukocytes. III. The utilization of thymine for DNA-thymine synthesis by leukemic leukocytes. Cancer Res 26:2282, 1966.

11. Bresnick E, Karjala RJ: End-product inhibition of thymidine kinase activity in normal and leukemic human leukocytes. Cancer Res 24:841, 1964.

12. Clayton DA, Vinograd J: Circular dimer and catenate forms of mitochondrial DNA in human leukaemic leucocytes. Nature 216:652, 1967.

13. _____, _____: Complex mitochondrial DNA in leukemic and normal human myeloid cells. Proc Natl Acad Sci (USA) 62:1077, 1969.

14. Cleaver JE: Thymidine metabolism: Pathways of incorporation and degradation, in Neuberger A and Tatum EL (ed): Frontiers of Biology, vol. 6. Amsterdam, North Holland, 1967, p 43.

15. Cline MJ: Metabolism of the circulating leukocyte. Physiol Rev 45:674, 1965.

16. _____: Ribonucleic acid biosynthesis in human leukocytes: The fate of rapidly labeled RNA in normal and abnormal leukocytes. Blood 28:650, 1966.

17. _____: Leukocyte metabolism, in Gordon AS (ed): Regulation of Hematopoiesis, vol. 2. New York, Appleton-Century-Crofts, 1970, p 1045.

18. Cooper HL: Ribonucleic acid metabolism in lymphocytes stimulated by phytohemagglutinin. J Biol Chem 243:34, 1968.

19. _____: Ribosomal ribonucleic acid production and growth regulation in human lymphocytes. J Biol Chem 244:1946, 1969.

20. _____: Ribosomal ribonucleic acid wastage in resting and growing lymphocytes. J Biol Chem 244:5590, 1969.

21. _____, Rubin AD: RNA metabolism in lymphocytes stimulated by phytohemagglutinin: Initial responses to phytohemagglutinin. Blood 25:1014, 1965.

22. Cooper RA, Perry S, Breitman TR: Pyrimidine metabolism in human leukocytes. I. Contribution of exogenous thymidine to DNA thymine and its effect on thymine nucleotide synthesis in leukemic leukocytes. Cancer Res 26:2267, 1966.

23. Corneo G, Ginelli E, Polli E: Repeated sequences in DNA. J Mol Biol 48:319, 1970.

24. _____, _____, _____: Repeated sequences in human leukemic DNA. Acta Haematol 45:167, 1971.

25. Davidson JP, Winter TS: Purine nucleotide pyrophosphorylases in 6-mercaptopurine-sensitive and -resistant human leukemias. Cancer Res 24:261, 1964.

26. Fausto N, Van Laucher JL: Molecular mechanisms of liver regeneration. IV. Thymidylic kinase and deoxyribonucleic acid polymerase activities in normal and regenerating liver. J Biol Chem 240:1247, 1961.

27. Feinendegen LE, Bond VP, Hughes WL: Physiological thymidine reutilization in rat bone marrow. Proc Soc Exp Biol Med 122:448, 1966.

28. Fujioka S, O'Hopp S, Gerber P, Gallo RC: Comparison of chromatographic patterns of

low molecular weight RNA from Burkitt lymphoma, infectious mononucleosis, EB-virus transformed and normal human lymphoblasts. Blood 39:60, 1972.

29. _____, Silber R: Purification and properties of ribonucleotide reductase from leukemic mouse spleen. J Biol Chem 245:1688, 1970.

30. _____, _____: Leukocyte ribonucleotide reductase: Studies in normal subjects and in subjects with leukemia or pernicious anemia. J Lab Clin Med 77:59, 1971.

31. Gallo RC: RNA dependent DNA polymerase of human acute leukaemic cells. Nature 228:927, 1970.

32. _____: Synthesis and metabolism of DNA and DNA precursors by human normal and leukemic leukocytes. Acta Haematol 45:136, 1971.

33. _____: RNA-dependent DNA polymerase in viruses and cells: Views on the current status. Blood 39:117, 1972.

34. _____, Breitman TR: The enzymatic mechanisms for deoxythymidine synthesis in human leukocytes. III. Inhibition of deoxythymidine phosphorylase by purines. J Biol Chem 243:4943, 1968.

35. _____, Perry S: The enzymatic mechanisms for deoxythymidine synthesis in human leukocytes. IV. Comparisons between normal and leukemic leukocytes. J Clin Invest 48:105, 1969.

36. _____, Pestka S: Transfer RNA species in normal and leukemic human lymphoblasts. J Mol Biol 52:195, 1970.

37. _____, Yang SS, Ting RC: RNA-dependent DNA polymerase of human acute leukaemic cells. Nature 228:927, 1970.

38. Gerhart JC, Schachman HK: Distinct subunits for the regulation and catalytic activity of aspartate transcarbamylase. Biochemistry 4:1054, 1965.

39. Kay JE, Cooper HL: Rapidly labelled cytoplasmic RNA in normal and phytohemagglutinin-stimulated human lymphocytes. Biochim Biophys Acta 186:62, 1969.

40. Lajtha LG: Utilization of formate-C^{14} for synthesis of deoxyribonucleic acid by human bone marrow cells in vitro. Nature 174:1013, 1954.

41. _____, Vane JR: Dependence of bone marrow cells on the liver for purine supply. Nature 182:191, 1958.

42. Lesch M, Nyhan WL: A familial disorder of uric acid metabolism and central nervous system function. Am J Med 36:561, 1964.

43. Loeb LA, Agarwal SS, Woodside AM: Induction of DNA polymerase in human

lymphocytes by phytohemagglutinin. Proc Natl Acad Sci (USA) 61:827, 1968.

44. Lucas ZJ: Pyrimidine nucleotide synthesis: Regulatory control during transformation of lymphocytes in vitro. Science 156:1237, 1967.

45. Maley F, Maley GF: Nucleotide interconversions. II. Elevation of deoxycytidylate deaminase and thymidylate synthetase in regenerating rat liver. J Biol Chem 235:2968, 1960.

46. Marsh JC, Perry S: Thymidine catabolism by normal and leukemic human leukocytes. J Clin Invest 43:267, 1964.

47. Monjardino JPPV, MacGillivray AJ: RNA and histone metabolism in small lymphocytes stimulated by phytohemagglutinin. Exp Cell Res 60:1, 1970.

48. Monod J, Changeux JP, Jacob I: Allosteric proteins and cellular control systems. J Mol Biol 238:1467, 1963.

49. Murray AW: The biological significance of purine synthesis. Ann Rev Biochem 40:811, 1971.

50. Nakai GS, Michael E, Peterson M, Craddock CG: Thymidine and thymidylate kinase, and thymidylate phosphatase in human leukemic leukocytes. Clin Chim Acta 14:422, 1966.

51. Nass MMK: Reversible generation of circular dimer and higher multiple forms of mitochondrial DNA. Nature 233:1124, 1969.

52. Ove P, Kremer WB, Laszlo J: Increased DNA polymerase activity in human leukaemic cells. Nature 220:713, 1968.

53. Penman S: Ribonucleic acid metabolism in mammalian cells. N Engl J Med 276:502, 1967.

54. Perry S: Proliferation of myeloid cells. Ann Rev Med 22:171, 1971.

55. _____, Gallo RC: Physiology of human leukemic leukocytes: Kinetic and biochemical considerations, in Gordon AS (ed): Regulation of Hematopoiesis, vol. 2. New York, Appleton-Century-Crofts, 1970, p 1221.

56. Polli E: Introduction to: Nucleic acid metabolism in normal and leukemic cells. Acta Haematol 45:133, 1971.

57. Pritchard JB, Chavez-Peon F, Berlin RD: Purines: Supply by liver to tissues. Am J Physiol 219:1263, 1970.

58. Rabinowitz Y: Separation of lymphocytes, polymorphonuclear leukocytes and monocytes on glass columns, including tissue culture observations. Blood 23:811, 1964.

59. _____: Adherence and separation of

leukemic cells on glass bead columns. Blood 26:100, 1965.

60. _____: DNA polymerase and carbohydrate metabolizing enzyme content of normal and leukemic glass column-separated leukocytes. Blood 27:470, 1966.

61. _____, Farmer R, Czebotar V: Deoxycytidine pathway in separated normal and leukemic leukocytes with effects of culture. Blood 38:312, 1971.

62. _____, McCluskey IS, Wong P, Wilhite BA: DNA polymerase activity of cultured normal and leukemic lymphocytes: Response to phytohemagglutinin. Exp Cell Res 57:257, 1969.

63. _____, Wilhite BA: Thymidine salvage pathway in normal and leukemic leukocytes with effects of ATP on enzyme control. Blood 33:759, 1969.

64. _____, Wong P, Wilhite BA: Effect of phytohemagglutinin on enzymes of thymidine salvage pathway of cultured chronic lymphatic leukemic lymphocytes. Blood 35:326, 1970.

65. Reem GH: De novo purine biosynthesis by two pathways in Burkitt lymphoma cells and in human spleen. J Clin Invest 51:1058, 1972.

66. Roberts D, Hall TC: Dihydrofolate reductase activity and deoxynucleoside incorporation into DNA of human leukocytes. Relation to Methotrexate administration. Cancer 20:905, 1967.

67. _____, _____: Enzyme activities and deoxynucleoside utilization of leukemic leukocytes in relation to drug therapy and resistance. Cancer Res 29:166, 1969.

68. Ross J, Scolnick EM, Todaro GJ, Aaronson SA: Separation of murine cellular and murine leukaemia virus DNA polymerases. Nature 231:163, 1971.

69. Rubin AD: Possible control of lymphocyte growth at the level of ribosome assembly. Nature 220:196, 1968.

70. _____: Ribosome biosynthesis in cultured lymphocytes. III. The role of ribosomal RNA production in the initiation and maintenance of lymphocyte growth. Blood 35:708, 1970.

71. _____: Defective control of ribosomal RNA processing in stimulated leukemic lymphocytes. J Clin Invest 50:2485, 1971.

72. Scolnick EM, Aaronson SA, Todaro GJ, Parks WP: RNA dependent DNA polymerase activity in mammalian cells. Nature 229:318, 1971.

73. Scott JL: Human leukocyte metabolism in vitro. Incorporation of adenine 8-C^{14} and formate-C^{14} into the nucleic acids of leukemic leukocytes. J Clin Invest 41:67, 1962.

74. Silber R: Regulatory mechanisms in the human leukocyte. I. The feedback control of deoxycytidylate deaminase. Blood 29:896, 1967.

75. _____, Gabrio BW, Huennekens FM: Studies on normal and leukemic leukocytes. VI. Thymidylate synthetase and deoxycytidylate deaminase. J Clin Invest 43:1913, 1963.

76. Smith JL, Omura GA, Krakoff IH, Balis ME: IMP and AMP: pyrophosphate phosphoribosyltransferase in leukemic and normal human leukocytes. Proc Soc Exp Biol Med 136:1299, 1971.

77. Smith, LH, Barker FA, Sullivan M: Pyrimidine metabolism in man. II. Studies of leukemic cells. Blood 15:360, 1960.

78. Spiegelman S, Burny A, Das MR, Keydar J, Schlom J, Travnicek M, Watson K: Synthetic DNA-RNA hybrids and RNA-RNA duplexes as templates for the polymerases of the oncogenic viruses. Nature 228:430, 1970.

79. Temin HM, Mizutani S: RNA-dependent DNA polymerase in virions of Rous sarcoma virus. Nature 226:1211, 1970.

80. Wilmanns W: Bestimmung, Eigenschaften und Bedeutung der Dihydrofolsaure-Reduktase in den weissen Blutzellen bei Leukamien. Klin Wochenschr 40:533, 1962.

81. _____: Thymidin-Kinase in normalen und leukämischen myeloischen Zellen. Klin Wochenschr 45:505, 1967.

82. _____: DNA synthesis in leukemic cells under the action of cytotoxic agents in vitro and in vivo. Natl Cancer Inst Monograph 34:153, 1971.

P. C. Vincent

8

Cell Kinetics of the Leukemias

Hematopoietic cells are normally produced in the bone marrow by an orderly, controlled proliferation in which cells mature progressively as they divide. Proliferation is fed by an input of cells from a pluripotential stem cell compartment, via intermediate stem cells committed to either erythropoiesis, granulopoiesis, or thrombopoiesis, and it is terminated when a critical stage of cell maturity is reached. The process is irreversible; proliferating cells do not give rise to less differentiated forms and the mature cells do not regain the capacity to divide. Mature cells remain in the marrow for some time before release into the blood, which again is an orderly process with the delivery of the oldest cells first. Cells leave the blood after a given time and either enter the tissues (in the case of neutrophils) or are removed by the reticuloendothelial system (in the case of erythrocytes and platelets).

For each cell type, the system of proliferation, maturation, and release into and disappearance from the blood is normally in a steady state. This means that in the long run the rates of production, release, and turnover are all equal and the population as a whole remains constant in size.

The characteristics of normal hematopoietic cell production by the bone marrow are summarized below:

1. It originates from normal stem cells.
2. It is orderly and irreversible.
3. It is controlled by feedback mechanisms.
4. In the long run it is in a steady state.
5. Maturation occurs with, and ultimately terminates, proliferation.
6. The cells produced cannot resume division.*

---

*This is true for granulocyte, erythrocyte, and megakaryocyte proliferation. Lymphocytes and monocytes, however, can resume division when suitably stimulated.

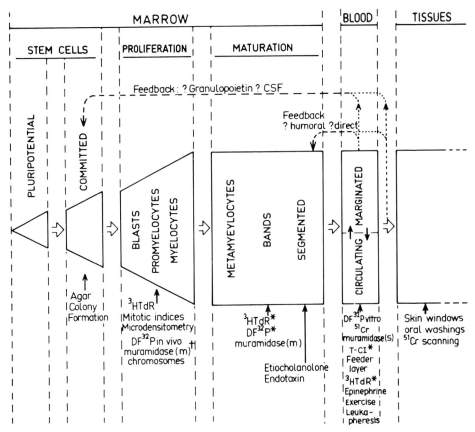

Fig. 8-1. Schematic representation of neutrophil granulocyte production showing methods of analysis, and known feedback loops. Note that it is not known whether the feedback loop acting on the stem cell is activated by a change in the neutrophil concentration in the blood or by the rate of neutrophil migration into the tissues. The loop acting on neutrophil release is probably triggered by a change in blood neutrophil levels. *Flow of cells labeled in vivo with ^{3}HTdR or DF^{32}P; T-C1: transcobalamin 1; †, (m): Marrow concentration, (s): Serum concentration.

NORMAL GRANULOCYTE KINETICS

This subject has been extensively reviewed elsewhere[11,39,55,62,65,66,184,232] and will only be summarized briefly here. Neutrophil granulocyte production can be analyzed in terms of stem cell, proliferative, maturative, blood, and tissue compartments, each of which is amenable to study (Fig. 8-1). In addition, techniques for measuring factors which might exert feedback control are becoming available.

Stem Cell Compartments

Neutrophil granulocyte precursors are believed to arise from a pluripotential stem cell—the common ancestor of granulocytes, erythrocytes, and platelets—probably via an intermediate stem cell committed to granulopoiesis.[109,151,194,196,232]

Pluripotential stem cells can be assayed in animals by their ability to form colonies in the spleen of irradiated recipients,[151,227] but techniques for their detection in man have not yet been developed. The intermediate granulopoietic-committed stem cell is thought by most workers to be identical with the cell which forms colonies in semisolid cultures of marrow from mouse,[25,189] or man,[32,109,200] although others believe that the cells which grow under these conditions are more likely to be pluripotential stem cells.[71] The great majority of pluripotential stem cells are in a resting or G_0 phase; this means that they are not actively dividing under normal circumstances, but can reenter division if necessary.[138-140,151] By contrast, most of the committed stem cells are actively dividing.[195,196]

The morphology of marrow stem cells is not known with certainty, but Fliedner and his colleagues have produced compelling evidence to suggest that they are indistinguishable in appearance from bone marrow lymphocytes.[22,86,111,112] Stem cells capable of forming spleen colonies have been shown to differ from those which grow in culture, by their adherence to glass beads; the latter adhere, while the former do not.[168] The two types of cells also differ in their density distributions, but the differences are not great enough to allow their separation by this technique.[116,168,246]

Feedback Control

The rates at which neutrophils are produced by the bone marrow, and released into the blood, are controlled by negative feedback mechanisms.[176] One such mechanism, which appears to be humorally mediated, acts at the committed stem cell level, while the other causes the release of stored mature granulocytes from the marrow (Fig. 8-1). The latter mechanism is triggered by a decrease in the neutrophil concentration of blood perfusing the marrow,[72,73] which is associated with the presence of a leukocytosis-inducing factor in the serum,[106] but it may also be mediated by intramedullary nerve pathways.[86]

The nature of the humoral substance controlling stem cell proliferation (granulopoietin) is not known. Growth of bone marrow colonies in semisolid cultures requires the presence of a stimulatory substance, and it is widely assumed that this is a granulopoietin. In the case of human marrow, this substance can be provided if nondividing peripheral blood leukocytes are present as a feeder layer,[109,200] or if a supernatant from incubated blood leukocytes[44] or incubated human spleen[182] is used. Human urine and serum which contain colony-stimulating factor (CSF), a substance capable of stimulating murine bone marrow growth in culture, are either ineffective or markedly inferior as stimuli for the growth of human bone marrow. Thus, while CSF levels in human urine and serum (assayed by mouse marrow culture) do fluctuate with changes in granulopoiesis,[167,243] the precise significance of these fluctuations on feedback control is not yet clear. The most likely reason for the failure of CSF to stimulate human marrow is that CSF is a partial degradation product of a human granulopoietin, which is still capable of stimulating murine bone marrow cells in culture. The presence of substances in human serum which inhibit the growth of mouse bone marrow cells has been extensively investigated,[41,42,167] but their significance in the control of human granulopoiesis has yet to be defined.

Substances in murine sera which stimulate mouse bone marrow growth in culture seem to fulfil most of the requirements of a mouse granulopoietin.[177,193,215] Their level fluctuates with demand, rising at the time of radiation-induced neutropenia,[177,193] although changes in serum inhibitor levels may also be important.[41]

Recognizable Granulocyte Precursors in the Marrow

Proliferation and maturation occur at the myeloblast, promyelocyte, and myelocyte stages. The transition from myelocyte to metamyelocyte marks the end of the proliferative capacity of the cell; thereafter cells continue to mature, but do not divide again.

The synthesis of tritiated thymidine (^{3}HTdR) at Brookhaven opened the way to a study of the kinetics of proliferating cell populations.[24,61,63,121] Parenterally administered ^{3}HTdR is available only for a brief period (30 minutes), during which time it is incorporated via a salvage pathway (see Chapter 7) only into those cells synthesizing DNA; these then retain the intranuclear label for the rest of their life.[82] Labeled cells can be detected autoradiographically; the short track length of the low-energy beta particle from tritium is ideal for this purpose. Autoradiography also has the advantage of allowing the identification of the type and the number of cells labeled. Liquid scintillation counting, although much less tedious, does not permit the identification of the labeled cells.[144]

Various parameters can be calculated following the intravenous administration of ^{3}HTdR. Marrow samples obtained after about 30–60 minutes show what is known as the flash labeling index, that is, the ratio of the number of cells synthesizing DNA to the total number of cells in the population. The labeling index is *not* a direct measure of the rapidity of cell division, although this is often assumed incorrectly to be the case.

Following administration of ^{3}HTdR, labeled cells move through G_2 into mitosis, which produces two daughter cells, each labeled with approximately half the activity of the parent. If the daughter cells are capable of dividing further, labeled cells then move through G_1, the next S phase, and the next mitosis. Nondividing daughter cells remain labeled with ^{3}HTdR and can be followed during subsequent maturation and migration. Time parameters (T_S, T_M, and T_G) appropriate to these phases of the cycle can be calculated by various methods, including analysis of labeled mitoses,[126,224] by double-labeling with ^{3}HTdR and ^{14}CTdR,[235] and by grain-count halving techniques.[52,181] The time parameters of normal granulopoietic proliferation have been estimated as follows: T_S, 12–14 hours; T_M, 1–1.5 hours; and T_{G2}, 2–3 hours.[224] The generation time (T_G) appears to be longer (52 hours) in myelocytes than in myeloblasts, where it is of the order of 24 hours.[126]

As will be seen later, these values are greater in most cases of acute leukemia— that is, normal cells have a shorter T_G and T_S than are found in acute leukemia. As a result, the fractional rate at which cells are produced (cells produced per 100 per hour) is *less* in acute leukemia than in normal granulopoiesis.

^{3}HTdR-labeled cells flow through the nondividing compartments in a sequential orderly progression from metamyelocytes to band forms and mature granulocytes.[62,65,66] Labeled metamyelocytes are first seen about 3 hours after ^{3}HTdR injection and then increase at a linear rate, determined by the transit time of cells through the compartment. Labeled granulocytes appear in the blood between 4–6 days after giving ^{3}HTdR.[87] This represents the minimum transit time through the maturing cell compartments in the marrow. Labeled granulocytes appear in extravascular sites at the same time.[88]

Intravenous diisopropyl fluorophosphate-^{32}P (DF^{32}P) has also been used to study the proliferation of granulocyte precursors.[39,157] The proliferative characteris-

Table 8–1

Normal Values for Blood Granulocyte Kinetics

Total blood granulocyte pool	70×10^7 cells/kg
Circulating granulocyte pool	31×10^7 cells/kg
Marginated granulocyte pool	39×10^7 cells/kg
Granulocyte blood half-time	6.7 hr
Granulocyte turnover rate	6.8×10^7 cells/kg/hr
Ratio marginated to circulating cells	1.26:1

Data from Cartwright et al.[39]

tics of myelocytes, labeled at the time of injection, are reflected in blood radioactivity curves obtained when granulocytes derived from these cells enter the blood.

Blood Granulocytes

The kinetics of peripheral blood granulocytes can be studied readily using cells labeled in vitro with $DF^{32}P$[5,39,67,156] or with ^{51}Cr[74,152] and reinfused. Using these techniques, granulocytes have been shown to disappear randomly from the blood, and the size of the blood granulocyte pool has been calculated.[3] Blood granulocytes are partitioned between marginated and circulating pools of cells which, however, behave kinetically as a single entity. The granulocyte turnover rate can be calculated from the total blood granulocyte pool and the half time of the blood granulocyte disappearance curve. Normal values are given in Table 8-1.

CELL KINETICS IN ACUTE LEUKEMIA

Before methods were available for the study of cell kinetics, it was assumed as an article of faith that acute leukemia was a disease caused by rapid cellular proliferation. The opposite has nearly always been shown to be the case; leukemic cells take longer to synthesize DNA and divide more slowly than do normal hematopoietic precursors.[48,58,97,107,127–130,132,238,240] Despite this apparently subdued behavior, leukemic cells accumulate relentlessly in most cases, and compete more than successfully with normal hematopoietic cellular proliferation. Recent studies which are reviewed below have shed light on the reasons for these apparent paradoxes. The characteristics of normal hematopoietic cellular proliferation have been described (page 189). Leukemic cells behave abnormally in respect of each of these characteristics (Table 8-2).

Stem Cells in Acute Leukemia

The extent to which input from a stem cell compartment serves to maintain a leukemic cell population, once the disease is established, is not known with certainty, but evidence to be reviewed later suggests that its contribution is small. It is unlikely that the stem cell compartment is as large relative to the recognizable cell population in acute leukemia as it is in normal granulopoiesis.

Despite the quantitively small contribution made by a stem cell pool toward

Table 8–2
Abnormalities of Cellular Proliferation in Acute Leukemia

Process	Normal	Leukemic
Stem cells	Normal	Abnormal
Maturation	Synchronous with Proliferation	Asynchronous
	Terminates division	Does not terminate division
Feedback	Controls Production	Absent or ineffective
Steady state	Yes	No
Release	Orderly	Random
End-product	Mature cells—	Immature cells—
	cannot resume division	can resume division

maintaining the leukemic process, however, there is quite good indirect evidence that leukemogenesis involves a primary somatic mutation occurring in a stem cell. The best evidence for this has been obtained by the finding of the Philadelphia (Ph[1]) chromosome in chronic granulocytic leukemia (see section, "Cell Kinetics in Chronic Granulocytic Leukemia"). Chromosomal abnormalities are less common in the acute leukemias, being found in fewer than half the cases reported. In these, however, the abnormalities may be shown to be clonal, suggesting again that the leukemic cells originate from a single ancestor. Chromosomal studies have also suggested that erythroid cells in AGL marrows arise from abnormal (i.e., leukemic) stem cells.[130,134,135]

Clinical reports of leukemia arising in a marrow recovering from induced or even idiopathic aplasia[68] offer further evidence that an abnormal stem cell is responsible for leukemogenesis. Another disease assumed to result from somatic mutation—paroxysmal nocturnal hemoglobinuria—is also known to have occurred in similar circumstances,[145,190] and it has also been reported as preceding acute leukemia[119,124,125] (see Chapter 14).

Killmann has reviewed available data concerning the stem cell in leukemia.[127–130] He has proposed two functional states for normal stem cells, either *sleepers* or *feeders,* the former being equivalent to resting (G_0) cells which have completed relatively few divisions and which have consequently been exposed to fewer of the risks of genetic error in replication and division. He postulates, however, that an error occurring in one of these sleeper stem cells would have far-reaching (i.e., leukemic) effects if it gave rise to a feeder clone, and further that the possibility of recruiting a defective sleeper stem cell would be greater in individuals whose marrow was recovering from aplasia.

In Vitro Study of Agar Colony-forming Cells in Leukemia

The in vitro agar-culture technique for the study of normal granulopoiesis has been described previously (page 60). The same technique has been used in the study of human leukemia, with interesting results.

Reports have been conflicting regarding colony growth of AGL marrow in relapse, ranging from a finding of no colonies at all[32,109,172,214] through small numbers of colonies,[32,122,214] to numerous colonies.[182,200] Some of these differences have been due to technical reasons, such as the use of suboptimal stimuli,[114] and different definitions of what constitutes a colony (e.g., more than 10 cells,[214] 20 cells,[122] 30 cells,[114] 40 cells,[172] 50 cells,[32,182] 100 cells,[200] or 150 cells[109]). However, a pattern is emerging in which it appears that there is considerable variation among patients.[53,109,200] In addition, it is not uncommon for leukemic marrows, when grown in agar, to give rise to numerous cell clusters which are smaller than colonies.[32,109,172] These are also seen in normal marrow cultures, but in much smaller numbers.

Marrows from patients with acute lymphocytic leukemia and acute undifferentiated leukemias usually show little or no colony growth in agar.[32,172,200] Patients in remission, regardless of the type of leukemia, have normal numbers of marrow colony-forming cells.[32,53,109,214]

Leukemic peripheral blood samples have also been cultured on agar. Normal peripheral blood contains a small number of cells capable of forming colonies.[45,136,150] In some cases of acute granulocytic leukemia, large numbers of such cells are present,[172,182,197,198] although this has not been a universal finding.[32] Bloods from patients with acute lymphocytic or acute undifferentiated leukemias have no more of these cells than normal.[198]

The nature of these cells in acute leukemia is of considerable interest. Maturation has been reported in colonies grown in vitro from marrow and blood of some patients in frank relapse,[109,182,197,198] and it has been suggested that leukemia is due to defective regulation in vivo rather than to an intrinsic defect in the cell's ability to respond.[197] The maturation which does occur, however, is frequently abortive, and its products are reminiscent of the monocytoid cells not uncommonly seen in the marrow in acute granulocytic leukemia. Cultures grown in agar cannot be stained by Romanowsky dyes, and morphology has to be interpreted using aceto-orcein. This obstacle can be overcome by culturing marrow on methylcellulose.[32]

Activity of Leukemic Cells in Stimulating in vitro Colony Growth of Marrow

Normal peripheral blood leukocytes, prepared as feeder layers, will stimulate the growth of normal human marrow.[200] When leukemic peripheral blood leukocytes are tested in the same system, they are found to be either ineffective or suboptimal as a stimulus.[109,198,200] Nonleukemic murine bone marrow will grow on leukemic cell feeder layers[45,147,172] which will not support the growth of human marrow.[148] The ability to stimulate human marrow colony growth is related to the number of granulocytes in the feeder layer,[109] and the failure of leukemic cell feeder layers to stimulate human marrow might be because of the small number of normal granulocytes present in most leukemic blood samples.* In this case, the ability of murine bone marrow to respond to leukemic feeder layers could be in response to the release of a substance from leukemic cells which is ineffective for normal human marrow growth. There is evidence that human and murine bone marrow cells in vitro respond to different substances, both of which are released by normal, human leukocyte feeder layers.[147]

---

*More recent evidence suggests that monocytes, rather than granulocytes, are responsible for stimulation (see chapter 21).

CSF in Serum and Urine from Leukemic Patients

The CSF present in human urine and serum, which stimulates the growth of murine but not human bone marrow in culture, has been discussed above (page 000). Elevated levels of CSF have been reported in serum and urine from a proportion of patients with acute granulocytic leukemia[166,167,197,199] as well as decreased levels of serum inhibitors of CSF.[41,166]

Kinetics of Recognizable Leukemic Cells

PROLIFERATING AND NONPROLIFERATING POOLS

The ^{3}HTdR-labeling index of leukemic cells obtained at the time of first diagnosis is almost always low, and much lower than that of normal myeloblasts.[48,50,96,98,102,107,126,127,132,159,170,212] In turn, the labeling index of blasts in the blood is lower than it is in the marrow.[46,50,126,127,159,160,212] Possible reasons for a low labeling index are as follows:

1. Thymidine incorporation may be defective:
2. T_s may be abnormally short relative to T_G:
3. T_G may be abnormally long relative to T_s:
4. There may be separate compartments of blasts, one proliferating and the other nonproliferating.

Defective thymidine incorporation is unlikely in view of the fact that all the mitoses which are seen after in vivo ^{3}HTdR are labeled.[107,159] Evidence to be reviewed later shows clearly that T_s in blasts is usually prolonged and never shorter than normal, and although T_G is also prolonged this is not sufficient to account for a low labeling index. This leaves the fourth possibility, namely, that at any one time some blasts belong to a proliferating population, while others are nonproliferating. There is now considerable evidence to show that this is indeed the case.

When autoradiographs of acute leukemic marrow exposed to ^{3}HTdR either in vivo or in vitro were examined closely, it was obvious that the vast majority of labeled blasts were large, and, conversely, that the labeling index of large blasts was similar to that of normal myeloblasts. By contrast, very few, if any, small blasts were labeled.[98-100,107,159] It was also found that labeled cells tended to be "typical" blasts, while those with a low labeling index were blasts which were morphologically atypical.[126] In vivo studies then showed that large blasts gave rise to small blasts,[91,97,99,100,146,159] and that marrow blasts gave rise to blasts which entered the blood.[132] Even more importantly, it was shown that small blasts were capable of reentering the cell cycle either spontaneously[49,206,240] or following depletion of the proliferating pool by chemotherapy.[91] Further evidence of the proliferative ability of resting leukemic cells was provided by studies showing the capacity of these cells, but not of normal cells, to repair DNA.[222,225]

The relationship of proliferating and nonproliferating leukemic cell compartments can be summarized as shown in Figs 8-2 and 8-3. On the average, between 10 and 25 percent of marrow blasts are proliferating[107,202]; this is similar to the proportion of proliferating granulopoietic cells (20 percent) in normal marrow.[65] Morphologically, proliferating leukemic cells are mostly large typical blasts, while the nonproliferating population is made up particularly of small blasts. Nonpro-

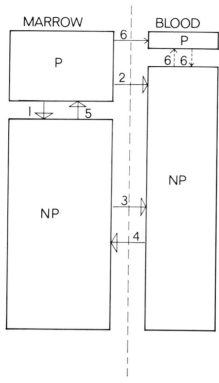

Fig. 8-2. Model of the likely relationships between proliferating (P) and nonproliferating (NP) leukemic cells in marrow and blood in acute granulocytic leukemia. The proportion of proliferating cells (predominantly large blasts) is greater in the marrow than in the blood. Proliferating cells give rise to NP cells within the marrow (1) and to NP cells in the blood (2). Cells also enter the blood directly from the marrow NP compartment (3). Leukemic cells in the blood can return to the marrow (4), and NP cells in the marrow can transform to proliferating cells (5). The relationship of P cells to NP cells in the blood and P cells in the marrow has not been defined, but interchanges probably occur (6).

liferating cells are more numerous in the blood than in the marrow, from which they are released preferentially (Fig. 8-2).[132,159]

Proliferating cells, when they divide, usually give rise to small nonproliferating cells,[99,100,159] so that the proliferating compartment—unlike a stem cell compartment—is not strictly self-maintaining.[100] However, the numbers of large proliferating cells are continually replenished by transformation of small nonproliferating blasts, and the system as a whole moves in a circle (Fig. 8-3). Even allowing for considerable death of cells, it is apparent that such a system is not only self-maintaining,[49] but would, in fact, relentlessly increase in size. The rate at which the increase would occur has been shown, using computer simulation techniques, to depend on the number of cells entering the resting phase, and the extent of cell death.[81,158,163]

Nonproliferating leukemic cells are generally regarded as being in a G_0 state, that is, they are not in cycle at the time, but are capable of resuming division,[48,49,206,240] although the possibility that some might be in a very long G_1 phase cannot be excluded.[48,107] Many other G_0 cells require a stimulus before

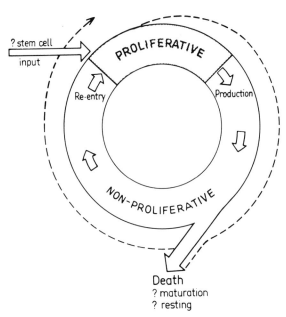

Fig. 8-3. Relationship of proliferative and nonproliferative leukemic cells. Proliferative leukemic cells feed into the nonproliferative pool, from which some are lost by death, possibly by maturation and possibly by entry into a resting pool. Nonproliferative cells reenter the proliferative pool, leading to a progressive increase in cell numbers (*broken line*). The magnitude and importance of a continued stem cell input are unknown.

resuming division—for example, antigen binding for lymphocytes, and critical cell mass for renal cells—and it would be important to know whether G_0 leukemic cells also need a trigger to cause them to divide again. Such a trigger might be an increase in cell size, or it might be a leukemogenic agent serving to maintain the disease. Leukemia appears to have developed in apparently normal marrow cells transplanted into two leukemic recipients.[83, 226]

Time Parameters of Leukemic Cell Division and Rates of Cell Production

In most published series, the duration of the cell cycle and of its divisions in leukemic cells have been longer than in normal myeloblasts or erythroblasts,[2, 62, 65, 113, 224] although Greenberg et al. have pointed out that proliferating leukemic cells are perhaps not so unlike normal myeloblasts as had been thought.[107] Estimates of the generation time of large blasts from T_S and the labeling index (of large blasts) $\left[T_G = \dfrac{T_S}{LI} \right]$ have to be accepted with caution, however, since many patients fail to show a second division of blasts within a time period longer than that expected from such calculations.[70, 107] This is hardly surprising, since the majority of large blasts give rise to small (nonproliferating) blasts following division.[100, 159, 206] A more realistic interpretation of the generation time—the time from one division to the next—would thus be much longer than that computed from the value of T_s, and would vary considerably, depending on the time small blasts spent in a resting phase before resuming division.[49] The number of cells produced per hour per thousand cells is similar in leukemic and normal marrows,[107] the production rate in each case being of the order of about five cells per thousand per hour if related to the whole population, or about 25 cells per thousand per hour if related only to the proliferating fraction. In the case of normal granulopoiesis, these cells mature and ultimately migrate out of the bloodstream; in the case of acute leukemia, a fraction of this production—its size depending on the frequency of cell death—returns to augment the proliferating pool.

Kinetics of Peripheral Blood Cells in Acute Leukemia

In acute granulocytic leukemia, and in many cases of acute lymphocytic leukemia, the ³HTdR labeling index of leukemic cells is lower in the blood than in the bone marrow.[46,126,159,160,212] However, some cases of acute lymphocytic leukemia show the opposite,[46,101,103] and Gavosto et al. have postulated that these have a predominantly extramedullary site of leukemic cell production.[101]

Following injection of ³HTdR in vivo, labeled leukemic cells appear in the blood.[50,101,103,132,159,229] The rate of appearance, calculated from published data, has ranged from approximately 0.04 percent per hour (Patient TM,[229]) to between 0.51 percent per hour (Patient JS,[132]) and approximately 0.6 percent per hour (Patient YN,[229]). These figures would correspond to blood transit times in the range of 104 to 7 days if only labeled cells entered the blood. However, where transit times have been calculated by following the disappearance of heavily labeled cells only,[50,132] transit times in the range of 33–36 hours have been obtained. The most likely explanation for this difference is that unlabeled as well as labeled cells leave the marrow.[132] Autologous leukemic cells, labeled in vitro with ³H-cytidine and reinfused, disappear from the blood in a double exponential fashion. The slow component (half-time 2.5–6 days)[118] would correspond to a transit time of the order of 4–9 days for these cells. ³H-cytidine studies have also shown that leukemic cells return from the blood to the marrow in acute granulocytic leukemia.[133]

Liquid scintillation studies of peripheral blood radioactivity, following injection of ³HTdR in acute lymphocytic leukemia and acute granulocytic leukemia at first presentation show two peaks of activity, the first between 25–50 hours, and the second between 65–120 hours.[104] With remission, a normal pattern returns, with the appearance of labeled neutrophils at 8–10 days.

Autologous leukocytes labeled with DF³²P and reinfused in patients with acute leukemia show delayed, complex disappearance patterns.[93,220]

Kinetics of Leukemic Blasts at Different Stages of Disease

If a patient with acute leukemia is followed, the percentage of proliferating blasts is almost always higher when relapse occurs following remission than it was at the time the disease was first diagnosed.[48,49,205] The smaller fraction of proliferating cells at the time of first diagnosis is thought to be because of a crowding effect similar to that seen in the late phases of experimental tumor growth,[9,10,115,141] whereas close surveillance of the patient allows detection of relapse at an earlier stage of cell population growth. At first diagnosis, patients with symptoms of longer duration tend also to have a smaller proportion of proliferating cells than those with symptoms of recent onset.[205]

Understanding the regrowth of leukemic cells following induced remission is a problem. The duration of unmaintained remissions is commonly much longer than would be predicted from the unfettered doubling of surviving cells, even if only one cell had survived the original therapy.[48,58] The same question may be relevant to the long latent period in the development of leukemia in atomic bomb survivors.[58,64] Factors to be considered in this regard include the extent of cell death suffered by regenerating leukemic cells, the possible requirement for leukemic cell-cell interaction for growth to occur, the dormancy of leukemic cells, the possibility that established normal hemopoiesis might inhibit leukemic cell growth, and the possibility that leukemia might be reinduced in normal cells.[83,226]

Relationship of Normal and Leukemic Cells

Failure of normal hemopoiesis is a major problem in acute leukemia, and attempts have been made to interpret this in kinetic terms. There is evidence to suggest, in acute granulocytic leukemia at least, that morphologically normal neutrophils and erythrocytes arise from abnormal (leukemic) stem cells, and that normal stem cells have either disappeared or been completely suppressed.[97,128,130,134,135] Suppression is compatible with available data, particularly with the occurrence of remissions after profound, drug-induced marrow hypoplasia.[97,128,130] Comparison of the proliferative rates of erythropoietic and leukemic cells in acute granulocytic leukemia,[48,50,52] and study of erythropoiesis in a transplanted rat leukemia[89] also lead to the conclusion that normal stem cells may be suppressed in acute granulocytic leukemia. Studies of the in vitro colony-forming ability of leukemic marrow (see above) have also been interpreted as showing the presence of suppressed stem cells with the capacity for normal differentiation, but the evidence for this is not convincing.

Decreased red cell production in acute leukemia is caused by a combination of decreased stem cell input and ineffective erythropoiesis. There is also evidence to suggest that erythroid cells seen in acute granulocytic leukemia arise from leukemic stem cells.[130,134,135] In most studies,[48,50,52,95] the ^{3}HTdR-labeling indices of erythroblasts were similar to normal, although in one series they were found to be significantly lower,[120] and, in some cases, impaired incorporation of ^{3}HTdR has been demonstrated.[80] In erythroleukemia, anemia occurs as a result of markedly ineffective erythropoiesis.[89]

In the small number of patients with leukemia in whom studies of recognizable (?normal) granulocyte precursors have been possible, the proliferative and emergence patterns of these cells have been close to normal.[48,50,52]

Leukemic Cell Kinetics and Chemotherapy

While most chemotherapeutic agents used in the treatment of leukemia were developed on the assumption that leukemic cells were proliferating more rapidly than normal, they appear paradoxically to be effective despite the error of this assumption. Cytokinetic studies in leukemia have led to a reappraisal of the mode of action of these drugs, and to exploration of ways in which the proliferative abnormalities of leukemia might be exploited to enhance drug effectiveness.[59,70,94,102,127,144,153,155,164,192,222,239] Models utilizing the L1210 mouse leukemia

have been developed in an attempt to relate kinetic behavior of leukemic cells to chemotherapy.[12,192,218,219] Unfortunately, the proliferative characteristics of human
leukemia differ from those of mouse leukemia,[94] and these models are of limited application to the human situation.

Some chemotherapeutic agents act on particular segments of the cell cycle
(cycle-active drugs) while others exert a general effect on cells, regardless of the
stage of the cell cycle. Drug effects may be further complicated by the possibility
that drug uptake occurs in one phase of the cycle, and drug action in another. The
known sites of action of various drugs are listed in Table 8-3. In addition, ^{3}HTdR in
large doses has been shown to have a cytocidal effect in two cases of acute
leukemia.[108]

Attempts have been made to manipulate the proliferative pattern of leukemic
cells, either by synchronizing cell division,[48,49,78–80,142–144,155,236] or by recruiting cells
into the proliferative pool.[36,40,77,144] Evidence of synchronization has been found
using cytosine arabinoside,[142–144,166] vincristine,[142,143] methotrexate,[78,80,144,164] and
hydroxyurea,[236] and after stopping antimetabolite therapy.[48,49] In each case the particular drug was given with the intention of killing or inhibiting cells in a particular
phase of the cycle. During the period of drug availability, cells in the rest of the cycle
move forward and accumulate at the site of the block, to be released as a
synchronous wave when inhibition wears off. This synchronous wave should then be
more susceptible to a second drug. These studies have also pointed to the necessity,
when using cycle-active drugs, to combine them in such a way that their effects do
not cancel each other.[80,142]

Prednisone has a cycle-specific effect on leukemic lymphoblasts, inhibiting the
influx of cells from G_1 into S[78,79,142] and is potentially capable also of producing
synchronization. The capacity of daunorubicin to block G_2 cells in vitro[28] has not
been tested as a synchronizing maneuver in vivo. Recruitment of cells from the
nonproliferating into the proliferating pool has been attempted using extracorporeal

Table 8–3
Relationship of Cytotoxic Drug Effects to Cell Cycle

Drug	Cycle-phase Independent Effect	Cycle-specific Effect
Prednisone (in acute lymphocytic leukemia)	Cell destruction	Blocks $G_1 \longrightarrow S$
Vincristine		Blocks mitosis
		? Blocks cells $G_0 \longrightarrow G_1$
Cytosine arabinoside*		Inhibits DNA synthesis
Hydroxyurea		Inhibits DNA synthesis
Methotrexate*	Inhibits RNA synthesis	Inhibits DNA synthesis
6-mercaptopurine	Inhibits RNA synthesis	Inhibits DNA synthesis
Daunorubicin	General DNA complexing	Blocks $G_2 \longrightarrow M$[28]
Cyclophosphamide	General DNA complexing	Inhibits DNA synthesis
		Blocks $G_1 \longrightarrow S$
		Blocks mitosis
L-asparaginase		Blocks $G_1 \longrightarrow S$

*Recruitment of cells from G_0 to G_1 has been reported with methotrexate[91] and cytosine ara-
binoside followed by administration of vincristine or methotrexate.[144]

Data from Lampkin et al.,[142,144] and Mauer.[155]

irradiation of the blood[40,77] and drug therapy.[36,91,144] Following irradiation of the blood, the labeling index of leukemic cells in the marrow increased, suggesting an increase in the proliferating pool, mediated possibly by feedback from the depleted blood pool.[40,77] One drug regimen which utilized cyclophosphamide in an attempt to deplete the proliferating pool did not produce recruitment.[36] On the other hand, return of nonproliferating blasts to the proliferating pool has been reported following methotrexate[91] and cytosine arabinoside plus vincristine or cytosine arabinoside plus methotrexate.[144]

Cytokinetic parameters which might predict the likelihood of response to treatment have yet to be fully explored. In one series, patients with high ^{3}HTdR and ^{3}H cytosine arabinoside labeling indices were more likely to respond,[36] while in another study, patients who ultimately responded showed a rise in ^{3}HTdR labeling indices after 3 weeks' treatment, before any morphologic evidence of remission was seen.[46] There have been few reports of leukemic cell kinetics during chemotherapy. Those that have appeared have shown prolongation of the generation time during treatment with cytosine arabinoside,[48] or thioguanine,[49] which was reversed when treatment was stopped. The possibility of delayed effects of chemotherapy on cell proliferation must also be considered.[48]

The relationship of proliferating and nonproliferating pools is clearly of the greatest significance in planning chemotherapy. Most efforts have been directed to increasing the size of the proliferating pool in order to offer a larger target to subsequent chemotherapy. The alternative approach—that of putting as many cells as possible into the nonproliferating pool and keeping them there—could give acceptable control of the disease.

The effect of chemotherapy on the kinetics of normal hematopoietic cells has also to be considered.[60] Cytotoxic therapy will produce a cyclical neutropenia in experimental animals[178] and, when given intermittently, cyclical neutropenia and thrombocytopenia in patients with AGL in remission (personal observations).[37]

CELL KINETICS IN CHRONIC GRANULOCYTIC LEUKEMIA

Cell Traffic

Hematologists had long suspected that immature granulocytes in chronic granulocytic leukemia were capable of migrating between the bone marrow and the spleen via the blood, and recent studies utilizing ^{3}HTdR, DF^{32}P, or ^{51}Cr as labels have demonstrated the existence of cellular traffic of this type.[47,76,92,179,181,187] The picture is complicated, however, by the possibility that cells might either leave the marrow, the blood or the spleen while they are immature, or remain in situ to mature further before migrating to other tissues. For example, a myelocyte in the spleen could either stay where it is and mature to a metamyelocyte, or enter the blood as a myelocyte. Once in the blood, the same cell could either mature, enter the marrow, or return to the spleen. The theoretical pathways open to granulocytic precursors in chronic granulocytic leukemia are represented in Figure 8-4.

The migrations of immature granulocytes in chronic granulocytic leukemia from blood to marrow,[47,179] from blood to spleen,[76] and from spleen to marrow[181]

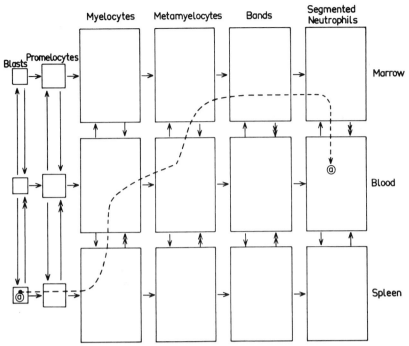

Fig. 8-4. Schematic representation of the pathways of migration and maturation in chronic granulocytic leukemia. *Horizontal arrows* represent maturation. *Vertical arrows* represent migration, the principal pathways of which are shown by *double-headed arrows*. Immature.cells in the blood originate chiefly in the spleen, while the marrow contributes the bulk of the mature cells. The hypothetical pathways followed by one descendant of a blast "a" is shown by a *dotted line*. This cell originated in the spleen, matured to a myelocyte there, entered the blood, matured to a metamyelocyte, entered the marrow, and matured to a segmented form before being released again into the blood. Kinetic studies have shown that pathways like this, or even more complex ones, are common in chronic granulocytic leukemia.

are well documented. In addition, the immature blood cells label readily with [3]HTdR—that is, many of them are synthesizing DNA prior to division. Despite this, mitoses are rarely seen in the blood in chronic granulocytic leukemia in relapse (in contrast to the blood in myelofibrosis),[131,181,235] so these cells clearly leave the blood before dividing.

Data obtained by infusion of [3]HTdR into the splenic artery show that the majority of immature granulocytes in the blood originate in the spleen.[51,181] It thus seems possible that most of the *marrow* cells in chronic granulocytic leukemia mature in situ, and are released in a reasonably normal fashion into the blood as polymorphonuclears. It has been shown that cells which return to the marrow are located in the marrow parenchyma and are not simply present in marrow sinusoids.[47] Under these conditions, continued delivery of immature cells from blood to marrow would cause a progressive expansion of the immature cell compartments which could only be relieved by maturation of the cells. It is, however, difficult to visualize the mechanism by which immature cells can enter the marrow but not leave it, and further investigation of this point is needed.

Proliferative Characteristics of Recognizable Granulocytic Precursors in Chronic Granulocytic Leukemia

Cell proliferation has been studied using injections or infusions of ³HTdR followed by autoradiographic analysis of marrow,[132,171,181,234,235] blood,[126,131,132,171,181,201,234,235] by splenic aspirates,[181] or by liquid scintillation counting of blood[75,104,179,186,187,231] or marrow[179,187], and in vivo DF³²P followed by determination of total blood radioactivity.[43,231] In vitro studies have also been reported, both to determine the in vivo labeling index after incubation with ³HTdR[23,26,56,126,201] and to study the behavior of cells in culture.[11,110,245]

Studies Utilizing ³HTdR

Myeloblasts. The ³HTdR labeling index of myeloblasts is lower in CGL marrow than in normal marrow, both in vivo[7,132,181,234] and in vitro[181,201], and it is lower in the blood than in the marrow.[132,181,234] The generation time of CGL myeloblasts has been estimated to be in the range of 40–88 hours in both blood and marrow,[132,181,234] with an average of about 60 hours. This is very much longer than the generation time of about 24 hours estimated for normal myeloblasts.[62,65,66] From the average generation time of 60 hours and an average labeling index of about 20 percent in CGL marrow myeloblasts[181] the DNA synthesis time in these cells can be calculated to be about 12 hours—similar to that found in normal[62,65,66,224] and CGL myelocytes[235]—if all the cells are in cycle. Indirect estimates of T_s in CGL myeloblasts have ranged from 7–21 hours.[7,132] If some CGL myeloblasts, like blasts in acute leukemia, are not in cycle, the estimate of T_s would be longer than this.* However, data obtained by continuous infusion of ³HTdR[51,181] make it unlikely that there are significant numbers of nonproliferating myeloblasts in CGL. The great majority of those which do not flash label with ³HTdR but are in cycle must therefore be in G_1, which is probably of the order of 45 hours in these cells.

Promyelocytes. These cells tend to have a higher labeling index and a similar[234] or longer[181] generation time than CGL myeloblasts, and a lower labeling index and longer generation time than normal promyelocytes. Their DNA synthesis time has not been measured directly but it has been estimated as 20 hours. Again, it is unlikely that significant numbers of these cells are nonproliferating because more than 70 percent of blood promyelocytes are labeled following continuous infusion of ³HTdR into the splenic artery.[181]

Myelocytes. The DNA synthesis time of CGL myelocytes has been measured directly in vivo by a double-labeling technique,[235] and has been found to be about 14 hours in both blood and bone marrow. Generation times computed from the DNA synthesis time and labeling indices are in the range of 43–74 hours (averaging 52 hours), which are similar to those measured by grain count-halving techniques (68 hours[181] and 75 hours[234]). The initial ³HTdR-labeling index of CGL myelocytes is be-

---

*$T_S = \dfrac{N_S}{N_G} \times T_G$. If some cells were not in cycle, so that $N_G < N$, T_S would be: $\dfrac{N_S}{N} \times T_G \times \dfrac{N}{N_G}$ and would be greater than these estimates.

tween 9 and 26 percent.[7,181,234] A few of the cells which do not flash label are in G_2 and in mitosis, but the majority are in G_1. The duration of G_1 is in the order of 36–60 hours. It is probable that the small myelocytes which can be distinguished morphologically from large myelocytes, and which form a distinct subpopulation as distinguished by nuclear area, represent G_1 cells.[65,66]

SPLENIC GRANULOPOIESIS IN CHRONIC GRANULOCYTIC LEUKEMIA

Clarkson and his colleagues have provided considerable insight into the kinetics of splenic granulopoiesis in chronic granulocytic leukemia, using infusions of ^{3}HTdR into the splenic artery[51,181] and autoradiographs of splenic aspiration biopsies following systemic ^{3}HTdR injection.[181] Their data show a striking similarity of kinetic patterns in the marrow and the spleen. Even more striking, however, is their finding that the great majority of the immature granulocytes (myeloblasts through metamyelocytes) in the blood originate in the spleen. The implication of this finding for cell traffic in chronic granulocytic leukemia has already been discussed.

Leukocyte kinetics have also been studied following splenectomy. No difference was detected in the pattern of labeling in blood and marrow in one patient studied before and 1 year after splenectomy.[181] Another patient, studied by means of liquid scintillation counting 6 weeks after (but not before) splenectomy, failed to show a delayed peak of activity seen in other CGL patients.[187] It is possible that, in the short term, the removal of splenic hematopoiesis interrupts the flow of immature cells into the blood, while in the long-term extrasplenic extramedullary hematopoiesis is responsible for a return to a kinetic state similar to that found preoperatively.

PROLIFERATIVE CELLS IN THE BLOOD
IN CHRONIC GRANULOCYTIC LEUKEMIA

Autoradiographic study of blood samples obtained immediately after a single injection of ^{3}HTdR in CGL patients shows labeled myeloblasts, promyelocytes, and myelocytes. As mentioned earlier, the flash-labeling indices of myeloblasts and promyelocytes are lower in the blood than in the marrow, while labeling indices of myelocytes are comparable in the two sites.[7,181,234] Very few, if any, small myelocytes label initially with ^{3}HTdR. The labeling indices of myeloblasts and promyelocytes in the blood rise significantly between 24 and 48 hours after ^{3}HTdR injection, to levels higher than the initial labeling index in the marrow in the case of myeloblasts, and to levels comparable with the marrow in the case of promyelocytes.[132,234] In the case of myeloblasts, this rise suggests the inflow of cells from a precursor compartment, other than myeloblasts in the marrow, with a high labeling index.

Serial blood studies show secondary peaks in the labeling indices of myeloblasts[132,234] and promyelocytes[234] 48 to 60 hours after the first peaks. These time intervals are close to the generation times for these cells.[132] Sequential blood samples show considerable differences between the labeling patterns of large as compared with small myelocytes.[234] In the case of large myelocytes, the labeling index falls initially and then rises again after 48 hours; in some, but not all patients, a further peak is seen at about 5 days. By contrast, the labeling index of small myelocytes rises progressively, from virtually zero to over 50 percent in the first 36–48 hours following ^{3}HTdR injection.[234] This pattern is consistent with the concept that small myelocytes are G_1 cells.[65,66]

Nondividing Granulocytic Precursors

In chronic granulocytic leukemia, labeled metamyelocytes, bands, and segmented granulocytes appear in the blood and marrow in an orderly sequential fashion following ³HTdR injection.[181,234] Qualitatively, the sequence of events is similar to that seen in normal marrow.[62,65,66] The emergence time—the time from injection of ³HTdR to the first appearance of labeled cells—is about 1–2 hours for metamyelocytes, about 1–3 days for bands, and about 4–5 days for segmented cells.[87,181,234] Labeled bands and segmented granulocytes tend to appear a little sooner in the marrow and the spleen than in the blood. Estimation of transit times through the nondividing compartments (as the reciprocal of the rate of appearance of labeled cells; see p. 192) is complicated by the fact that cells can enter and leave a compartment by migration as well as by maturation.

The appearance of ³HTdR-labeled cells at an extravascular site (the oral cavity) has also been studied. Labeled, segmented granulocytes appeared simultaneously in the mouth and in the blood in CGL patients,[234] in the same way as they do in normals.[88] Immature cells were not seen in the mouth, suggesting that they are unable to migrate out of blood vessels. A similar predominance of mature granulocytes is seen in induced inflammatory exudates in patients with chronic granulocytic leukemia.[8,21,183]

Liquid Scintillation Blood Studies Following ³HTdR

Perry and his colleagues have used liquid scintillation counting to study the emergence into the blood of cells labeled in vivo by ³HTdR. This technique has the advantages of speed and simplicity over autoradiography, but it has disadvantages as well. The activities of different cell types cannot be distinguished, and the measured activity does not correlate directly with the labeling index.* In normal individuals a single peak of blood radioactivity is seen 7 days after ³HTdR injection, and this is due almost exclusively to labeled, segmented granulocytes.[186,187] The situation is more complex in patients with chronic granulocytic leukemia. In relapse, significant radioactivity is found in blood samples obtained within the first few hours, because of the presence of proliferating cells. Thereafter, major peaks of radioactivity are seen at 30–40 hours and 120–144 hours.[186,187,231] Similar peaks are seen if the total activity of samples analyzed by autoradiography is calculated.[234] The first peak consists chiefly of labeled myelocytes, while the peak seen at 120–144 hours is predominantly due to labeled bands and segmented granulocytes[234] and not, as was previously suggested,[187] to labeled myelocytes. As mentioned earlier, one patient studied after splenectomy failed to show this secondary peak of leukocyte radioactivity. Liquid scintillation counting has also been used to show that CGL leukocytes, labeled in vitro with ³HTdR and reinfused, return to the bone marrow.[179]

Studies Utilizing Diisopropyl Fluorophosphate (DFP) in Chronic Granulocytic Leukemia

In vitro labeling with DF³²P. The use of diisopropyl fluorophosphate-³²P (DF³²P) in the study of normal granulocyte kinetics has been described earlier. Myelocytes, metamyelocytes, and bands, as well as segmented granulocytes, label

---

*The total activity measured is related to the number of cells labeled *and* the intensity of their labeling. It can be approximated as being equal to the labeling index multiplied by the mean grain count.

with DF^{32}P.[137] Leukocyte radioactivity measured after reinfusion of CGL blood labeled with DF^{32}P in vitro thus reflects the rate of disappearance of all these cell types. Not surprisingly, many patients show biphasic, exponential, or even more complex curves, although approximately half show a single exponential disappearance pattern.[6,92,231]

In all cases, however, the rate of disappearance of DF^{32}P-labeled autologous leukocytes is much slower in chronic granulocytic leukemia patients than in normals.[6,43,92,162,231] The reason for this is not clear.[43] Some workers believe that it is partly (but not entirely) due to the presence of immature cells in the blood,[6,38] and they point to similarly prolonged disappearance times in cases of myelofibrosis and polycythemia with significant numbers of immature cells in the blood.[4] This view is also strengthened by autoradiographic analyses of CGL blood labeled with ^{3}HDFP which show a slower disappearance of immature cells.[231] The scarcity of immature cells in inflammatory sites[8,19,123,183] and in the oral cavity[234] suggests that immature cells do not migrate readily from the blood into the tissues. On the other hand, other studies with both DF^{32}P[92,212] and with ^{51}Cr[212] suggest that mature granulocytes in chronic granulocytic leukemia have an intrinsic defect which causes them to disappear more slowly from the blood than do normal mature granulocytes.

In addition to their restricted capacity for emigration from the blood, immature cells may also cause an apparent prolongation of leukocyte survival by leaving the blood and dividing to give rise to labeled progeny which later return to the blood.[212] Cell traffic of this type between marrow, blood, and spleen in chronic granulocytic leukemia has already been described. Early disappearance of significant numbers of labeled cells from the blood of some patients is thought to be due to equilibration of cells between the blood and extravascular pools.[92]

The grossly expanded total blood granulocyte pool (TBGP) in chronic granulocytic leukemia has also been considered as a possible cause of the slow disappearance of blood leukocytes.[6,38,43] However, cross-circulation experiments make this unlikely, since isologous normal leukocytes infused into CGL patients disappear at a normal rate.[6,92] Any effect due to an expanded TBGP would be expected to delay the disappearance of these cells as well as of autologous cells.[6]

The circulating granulocyte pool (CGP), marginated granulocyte pool (MGP), and granulocyte turnover rate, as well as the TBGP, are all grossly expanded in chronic granulocytic leukemia.[6,162] The ratio of the MGP to the CGP is, however, normal[6] by contrast with other conditions associated with a leukocytosis such as myelofibrosis and polycythemia vera in which this ratio is increased.[4] The MGP in chronic granulocytic leukemia consists of immature as well as mature cells, and can be mobilized by epinephrine.[6]

Comparison with results obtained using ^{51}*Cr-labeled cells.* Blood radioactivity curves, similar in most respects to those obtained with DF^{32}P, are found when blood is labeled with ^{51}Cr in vitro and reinfused in chronic granulocytic leukemia.[76,213] Surface counting reveals significant uptake of radioactivity by the spleen, some of which is probably caused by the migration of cells into extravascular spaces.[76,213] However, this activity decreases during epinephrine infusion, and it seems likely that a significant proportion of the marginated blood pool is also located in the spleen.[213]

Cross-transfusion studies with DF^{32}P-labeled cells. Isologous normal leukocytes infused into CGL patients disappear normally, while CGL leukocytes infused into patients with carcinoma disappear from the blood in a slower but more complex fashion, presumably because of the presence of immature cells and mature, leukemic granulocytes.[6,38,92] DF[32]P-labeled marrow cells infused intravenously show a similar pattern.[6] Cross-transfusion studies between two CGL patients have been interpreted as showing an extravascular abnormality in CGL patients which alters the disappearance of intrinsically abnormal (CGL) cells.[92]

Chronic granulocytic leukemia in remission. It is generally agreed that granulokinetics measured by DF[32]P tend toward normal in patients in remission, although in a number of cases the disappearance curves are still complex.[6,92,231] Galbraith believes there is evidence to show that CGL leukocytes are still intrinsically abnormal in remission, even when their apparent survival has returned to within the normal range.[92]

In vitro labeling with tritiated DFP. Tritiated DFP ([3]HDFP) has the advantage that the type of cell labeled can be detected by autoradiography.[137,231] With its use in chronic granulocytic leukemia, immature cells have been shown to disappear more slowly from the blood than do mature granulocytes.[231] [3]HDFP tends to underestimate granulocyte survival compared with DF[32]P,[33] but it can produce a valid comparison of the survival of different cell types in chronic granulocytic leukemia provided that there is no great difference in the rate at which the [3]HDFP is degraded by each.

In vivo studies with DF[32]P. Normal individuals show a plateau of blood activity following injection of DF[32]P, which corresponds to the average time taken for labeled nondividing cells in the marrow to complete their maturation and emerge into the blood.[39,157] However, in patients with chronic granulocytic leukemia, in vivo labeling with DF[32]P is followed by a steady decline in blood activity[43] caused by the breakdown of the orderly maturation of cells before their release into the blood.

Leukapheresis Studies in Chronic Granulocytic Leukemia

In hematologically normal subjects, the selective removal of leukocytes from the blood (leukapheresis) is followed by a prompt granulocytosis.[15,16] By contrast, studies in chronic granulocytic leukemia show a fall in leukocyte count either during or after leukapheresis, with a subsequent slow rise toward pretreatment values.[17,34] The failure to produce a prompt leukocytosis is thought to be caused by relatively small reserves of mature granulocytes in chronic granulocytic leukemia,[17] although it has been pointed out that the degree of leukopenia produced might not be sufficient to trigger their release.[43] The subsequent delayed rise probably represents a slow replenishment of blood pools in chronic granulocytic leukemia.

Other Studies of Granulocyte Kinetics in Chronic Granulocytic Leukemia

The response of most CGL patients to injections of endotoxin is subnormal, indicating either that their marrow reserves are relatively inadequate or that the release mechanism is abnormal.[154] Patients with chronic granulocytic leukemia in remission show a normal response. Similar studies with etiocholanolone have not been reported.

Differential counts and relative in vitro ³HTdR-labeling indices in spleen and marrow have also been used in the study of CGL kinetics.[26,27] An increase in the proportion of granulopoietic precursors, but a decrease in the rate of ³HTdR incorporation, were seen in the marrow in patients with the highest white cell counts. In the spleen, the proportion of precursors was unaltered, but the rate of ³HTdR incorporation was increased.[27]

Feedback Control of Granulopoiesis in Chronic Granulocytic Leukemia

Morley and his colleagues have concluded that cyclical fluctuations seen in blood granulocyte levels in normal individuals are the result of feedback mechanisms,[173,176] which are exaggerated in cyclical neutropenia[175] and in drug-induced marrow depression.[178] Similar fluctuations have been observed in a few cases of chronic granulocytic leukemia,[174,216] suggesting that feedback mechanisms may have been sufficiently active to produce discernible changes in the leukocyte count. The existence of feedback control in chronic granulocytic leukemia would favor the concept that this disease is a "conditioned" neoplasm.[174] The possibility must also be considered that feedback from the excessive number of cells in chronic granulocytic leukemia prevents the development of normal stem cells.[43]

Elevated levels of CSF are usually found in the urine and sera of CGL patients,[167,199] but the relationship of this activity to feedback control is not yet established. CGL leukocytes used as feeder layers will stimulate the growth of normal numbers of murine bone marrow colonies in the agar colony system,[172] but they have very little stimulatory activity for the growth of normal human marrow.[148] As discussed above, mouse and normal human bone marrow probably respond to different substances in peripheral blood feeder layers. CGL granulocytes may be deficient in the substance capable of stimulating *human* marrow. CGL sera also contain a substance which stimulates granulopoiesis in explant cultures of normal marrow,[191] while sera from patients following splenic irradiation have been reported to contain an inhibitor.[217]

Studies of CGL Kinetics Utilizing In Vitro Cultures

Peripheral blood in the chronic phase of chronic granulocytic leukemia contains more agar colony-forming cells (CFC) than normal.[172,182] The colonies grown from these cells in vitro have been reported to consist of Ph¹-positive cells,[151,172] and evidence has been presented to suggest that these cells differ in their physical and biological characteristics from normal blood CFC.[172] If, as many workers believe, CFC are stem cells committed to granulopoiesis, their increased number in CGL blood would suggest that there is a considerable stem cell traffic within the blood in this disease. By contrast with the situation in the chronic phase, CFC are virtually absent from the blood in the acute phase of chronic granulocytic leukemia.[172,182]

The behavior of recognizable granulocytic precursors from CGL patients has been extensively studied by in vitro culture.[110,149,188,207,244,245] In most cases the cells die after 7–10 days, but occasionally they survive longer[110] and a few long-term cultures (with persistence of the Ph¹ chromosome) have been established.[149] Maturation of immature CGL cells in vitro has been demonstrated and mitoses are readily found, in contrast with their rarity in the blood in vivo.[110,188,207,244,245] The proliferative and maturation kinetics of CGL cultures in vitro have been studied following the addition of [3]HTdR.[245] The DNA synthesis time of immature leukocytes (blasts through myelocytes) was in the range of 20–26 hours in cultures from patients in the chronic phase, compared with the time of 14 hours observed in vivo.[235] Estimates of the generation time were similar in vitro to those found in vivo, but maturation was slower.[181,234,235,245]

Kinetic Studies in the Acute Phase of Chronic Granulocytic Leukemia

Kinetic studies in the acute phase of this form of leukemia are broadly similar to those seen in acute leukemia. The [3]HTdR-labeling index of myeloblasts in the acute phase is greater than in the chronic phase.[131,132] However, their generation times are similar.[132,181,234] Liquid scintillation studies following [3]HTdR injection have shown an absence or modification of the late secondary peaks of blood activity seen in the chronic phase.[75,104] The virtual absence of CFC from the blood in the acute phase has been mentioned above. Migration of leukocytes into inflammatory sites is severely curtailed in the acute phase of chronic granulocytic leukemia.[8]

KINETICS IN CHRONIC LYMPHOCYTIC LEUKEMIA

Normal Lymphocyte Kinetics

Lymphocyte kinetics have been extensively studied in experimental animals, but there have been relatively few studies in man.[54] In animals, the existence of a large pool of small, long-lived lymphocytes, recirculating from blood to lymph to blood,[90,105] which behaves as a single kinetic entity,[230] has been well established. These cells are in G_0, and are able to resume division when exposed to antigens to which they are specifically committed. They are responsible for cell-mediated immunity and are known as T (or thymus-derived) lymphocytes.[169] Other small lymphocytes (B, or bone marrow-derived lymphocytes) do not recirculate, are shorter-lived, and are responsible for humoral immunity.[90,169] In addition to these two pools of small blood lymphocytes, a lesser pool of dividing cells with a high proliferative rate,[203,233,241] and pools of fixed lymphocytes, are found in lymphoid tissues.[208]

The existence of long-lived lymphocytes[35,180] and recirculation of lymphocytes from blood to lymph[31,185] have both been demonstrated in man. Transfusion of autologous, isotopically labeled lymphocytes[29,30,85,117,153,211,221,223,228] has shown an initial rapid equilibration with a pool of cells larger than the circulating pool, followed by the disappearance of the remaining cells in a complex pattern consistent with interchange with at least two extravascular pools. The pool in which rapid equilibration occurs has been called the readily exchangeable, or marginated, lymphocyte pool, and is similar in many respects to the MGP (see page 193). Its size is approximately two to six times that of the circulating pool.[30,223,228] By means of studies of extracorporeal irradiation of the blood in patients with nonhematologic disorders, the total size of the extravascular pools has been estimated to be about thirty times that of the circulating pool,[1,84] and the total exchangeable lymphocyte pool in normal man has been estimated at between 100 and 200 × 10⁹ cells.[84] Surface counting has shown that lymphocytes which leave the blood to enter extravascular sites are found first in the liver, then in the spleen, and later in the marrow.[117,228]

The proliferative rate of lymphoid tissue in man has not been extensively documented. Thoracic duct drainage data have given estimates of a production rate of between 0.6 and 1.4 × 10⁹ lymphocytes per day,[14,204] which is a small fraction of the total exchangeable pool. The cell cycle parameters of dividing cells in human lymphoid tissue are similar to, or a little shorter than, those found in other human tissues,[209,210,242] but the number of cells synthesizing DNA is small[208-210,247] so that the per cell production rate is low. As Ford and Gowans point out, the principal drive for proliferation of cells which belong to the long-lived recirculating pool is exposure to antigen.[90] Considerable variation between sites and between individuals may therefore be expected.

Leukemic Lymphocyte Kinetics

The fundamental kinetic abnormality in chronic lymphocytic leukemia is the relentless accumulation of large numbers of small lymphocytes.[13,67,237] The per cell production rate is very low, but the total production by the expanded lymphoid mass may well be greatly increased.[208] Reinfused, isotopically labeled, autologous lymphocytes leave the blood in a manner similar to that seen in normals, with a rapid early equilibration and a complex disappearance pattern of the remaining cells.[30,117,153,208,211,221,223] As in normals, it is probable that these cells are equilibrating with several extravascular pools, present at least partly in the liver, spleen, and marrow[117,221] as well as in lymph nodes.[30] CLL lymphocytes accumulate more slowly than normal in the marrow.[117] The readily exchangeable pool, relative to the circulating pool, is either the same as[208,223] or smaller than [30,117] normal. Similar estimates of the size of the readily exchangeable lymphocyte pool have been derived by analyzing data from CLL patients being treated with extracorporeal irradiation of the blood (ECIB)[208,211]

The possibility that lymphocyte recirculation from blood to lymph might be abnormal in chronic lymphocytic leukemia has been suggested from studies of thoracic duct lymph.[14,18,31,192] In chronic lymphocytic leukemia, the number of lymphocytes in the thoracic duct is less than in the blood, whereas normally the concentrations in the two sites are roughly equal.[31] Isotopic studies of reinfused lymphocytes also suggest an impaired egress of cells from the CLL blood compared with normal blood.[117] Some workers have reported a delayed, as well as a reduced, recirculation of lymphocytes in chronic lymphocytic leukemia,[18] whereas others have found a normal recirculation time.[31] It has been suggested that possibly impaired recirculation may be a fundamental defect in chronic lymphocytic leukemia[208,237] and that this impairment might result from an abnormality of the lymphocyte surface.[237]

Virtually none of the small lymphocytes, and very few of the large lymphocytes, in CLL blood label initially with ³HTdR in vivo.[247] In patients without splenomegaly and with only moderate lymphocytosis, labeled cells enter the blood over the next 3–7 days after injection, indicating the presence of a small pool of proliferating cells.[247] By contrast, the blood activity of patients with splenomegaly and more marked lymphocytosis shows no evidence of cell proliferation; in these, the vast majority of lymphocytes are nonproliferating. That the spleen serves as a reservoir for these nonproliferating cells is suggested by the return of a proliferative pattern in a patient following splenectomy.[247] The great variability of cell proliferation in chronic lymphocytic leukemia is also shown by differences in the rates at which lymphocyte counts rise in untreated patients.[208]

REFERENCES

1. Andersen V, Bjerrum O, Ranek L: Studies on lymphocytes during extracorporeal irradiation of the blood in patients with active cirrhosis. Scand J Haematol 7:471, 1970.

2. Arbenz U: Zytokinetische Untersuchung einer aleukämischen akuten myeloischen Leukämie. Acta Haematol (Basel) 46:157, 1971.

3. Athens JW, Haab OP, Raab SO, Mauer AM, Ashenbrucker H, Cartwright GE, Wintrobe MM: Leukokinetic studies. IV. The total blood, circulating and marginal granulocyte pools and the granulocyte turnover rate in normal subjects. J Clin Invest 40:989, 1961.

4. _____, _____, _____, Boggs DR, Ashenbrucker H, Cartwright GE, Wintrobe MM: Leukokinetic studies. XI. Blood granulocyte kinetics in polycythemia vera, infection and myelofibrosis. J Clin Invest 44:778, 1965.

5. _____, Raab SO, Haab OP, Mauer AM, Ashenbrucker H, Cartwright GE, Wintrobe MM: Leukokinetic studies. III. The distribution of granulocytes in the blood of normal subjects. J Clin Invest 40:159, 1961.

6. _____, _____, _____, Boggs DR, Ashenbrucker H, Cartwright GE, Wintrobe MM: Leukokinetic studies. X. Blood granulocyte kinetics in chronic myelocytic leukemia. J Clin Invest 44:765, 1965.

7. Baccarini M, Killmann S-A: Cytokinetic studies in chronic myeloid leukaemia: Evidence for early presence of abnormal myeloblasts. Scand J Haematol 9:283, 1972.

8. Banerjee TK, Senn H, Holland JF: Comparative studies on localized leukocyte mobilization in patients with chronic myelocytic leukemia. Cancer 29:637, 1972.

9. Baserga R: Mitotic cycle of ascites tumor cells. Arch Pathol 75:156, 1963.

10. _____, Gold R: The uptake of tritiated thymidine by newly transplanted Ehrlich ascites tumor cells. Exp Cell Res 31:576, 1963.

11. Boll I, Kühn A: Granulocytopoiesis in human bone marrow cultures studied by means of kinematography. Blood 26:449, 1965.

12. Benckhuijsen C: Chemotherapy and the life cycle of leukaemic cells. Folia Med Neerl 12:74, 1969.

13. Bierman HR: Hypothesis: The leukemias—proliferative or accumulative? Blood 30:238, 1967.

14. _____, Byron RL Jr, Kelly KH, Gilfillan RS, White LP, Freeman NE, Petrakis NL: The characteristics of thoracic duct lymph in man. J Clin Invest 32:637, 1953.

15. _____, Kelly KH, Byron RL, Marshall GJ: Leucapheresis in man. I. Haematological observations following leucocyte withdrawal in patients with nonhaematological disorders. Br J Haematol 7:51, 1961.

16. _____, Marshall GJ, Kelly KH, Byron RL: Leucapheresis in man. II. Changes in circulating granulocytes, lymphocytes and platelets in the blood. Br J Haematol 8:77, 1962.

17. _____, _____, _____, _____: Leucapheresis in man. III. Hematologic observations in patients with leukemia and myeloid metaplasia. Blood 21:164, 1963.

18. Binet JL, Villeneuve B, Becart R, Logeais Y, Laudat JP, Mathey J: Temps de passage dans le canal thoracique des lymphocytes du sang de la leucémie lymphoïde chronique. Nouv Rev Fr Hématol 7:621, 1967.

19. Boggs DR: The cellular composition of inflammatory exudates in human leukemias. Blood 15:466, 1960.

20. _____: The kinetics of neutrophil leukocytes in health and disease. Sem Hematol 4:359, 1967.

21. _____, Athens JW, Cartwright GE, Wintrobe MM: The kinetics of neutrophils in exudates of patients with chronic myelocytic leukemia (CML). (Abstract). Clin Res 13:124, 1965.

22. Bohne F, Haas RJ, Fliedner TM, Fache I: The role of slowly proliferating cells in rat

bone marrow during regeneration following hydroxyurea. Br J Haematol 19:533, 1970.

23. Bond VP, Fliedner TM, Cronkite EP, Rubini JR, Brecher G, Schork PK: Proliferative potentials of bone marrow and blood cells studied by *in vitro* uptake of H^3-thymidine. Acta Haematol 21:1, 1959.

24. _____, _____, _____, _____, Robertson JS: Cell turnover in blood and blood-forming tissues studied with tritiated thymidine, in Stohlman F Jr (ed): The Kinetics of Cellular Proliferation. New York, Grune & Stratton, 1959.

25. Bradley TR, Metcalf D: The growth of mouse bone marrow cells *in vitro*. Aust J Exp Biol Med Sci 44:287, 1966.

26. Brandt L: Differences in the proliferative activity of myelocytes from bone marrow, spleen and peripheral blood in chronic myeloid leukaemia. Scand J Haematol 6:105, 1969.

27. _____, Schnell C-R: Granulopoiesis in bone marrow and spleen in chronic myeloid leukaemia. Scand J Haematol 6:65, 1969.

28. Brehaut LA: A delay in the G_2 period of cultured human leucocytes after treatment with rubidomycin (daunomycin). Cell Tissue Kinet 2:311, 1969.

29. Bremer K, Fliedner TM: RNA metabolism of circulating lymphocytes studied in man after autotransfusion and *in vitro* ^{3}H-cytidine labelling. Acta Haematol (Basel) 45:181, 1971.

30. _____, _____, Schick P: Kinetic differences of autotransfused, ^{3}H-cytidine labeled blood lymphocytes in leukemic and nonleukemic lymphoma patients. Eur J Cancer 9:113, 1973.

31. _____, Schick P, Wack O, Theml H, Brass B, Heimpel H: Rezirkulation von Lymphozyten bei Patienten mit malignen lymphatischen Systemerkrankungen. Blut 24:215, 1972.

32. Brown CH, Carbone PP: *In vitro* growth of normal and leukemic human bone marrow. J Natl Cancer Inst 46:989, 1971.

33. Brubaker LH, Spivak JL, Perry S: Nonequivalence of ^{3}H- and ^{32}P-labeled diisopropylfluorophosphate for the study of granulocyte kinetics. J Lab Clin Med 72:747, 1968.

34. Buckner D, Graw RG Jr, Eisel RJ, Henderson ES, Perry S: Leukapheresis by continuous flow centrifugation (CFC) in patients with chronic myelocytic leukemia (CML). Blood 33:353, 1969.

35. Buckton KE, Court Brown WM, Smith PG: Lymphocyte survival in men treated with x-rays for ankylosing spondylitis. Nature 214:470, 1967.

36. Burke PJ, Owens AH Jr: Attempted recruitment of leukemic myeloblasts to proliferative activity by sequential drug treatment. Cancer 28:830, 1971.

37. Carmel R, Coltman CA: Serum vitamin B_{12}-binding capacity and muramidase changes with cyclic neutropenia induced by cytosine arabinoside. Blood 37:31, 1971.

38. Cartwright GE, Athens JW, Haab OP, Raab SO, Boggs DR, Wintrobe MM: Blood granulocyte kinetics in conditions associated with granulocytosis. Ann NY Acad Sci 113:963, 1964.

39. _____, _____, Wintrobe MM: The kinetics of granulopoiesis in normal man. Blood 21:164, 1964.

40. Chan BWB, Hayhoe FGJ: Changes in proliferative activity of marrow leukemic cells during and after extracorporeal irradiation of blood. Blood 37:657, 1971.

41. Chan SH, Metcalf D, Gunz FW: Serum inhibitors of colony stimulating factor in leukaemia, in Vincent PC (ed): The Nature of Leukaemia. Sydney, Australian Cancer Society, 1972.

42. _____, _____, Stanley ER: Stimulation and inhibition by normal human serum of colony formation *in vitro* by bone marrow cells. Br J Haematol 20:329, 1971.

43. Chervenick PA, Boggs DR: Granulocyte kinetics in chronic myelocytic leukemia. Ser Haematol 1:24, 1968.

44. _____, _____: Bone marrow colonies: Stimulation *in vitro* by supernatant from incubated human blood cells. Science 169:691, 1970.

45. _____, _____: *In vitro* growth of granulocytic and mononuclear cell colonies from blood of normal individuals. Blood 37:131, 1971.

46. Cheung WH, Rai KR, Sawitsky A: Characteristics of cell proliferation in acute leukemia. Cancer Res 32:939, 1972.

47. Chikkappa G, Galbraith PR: Studies on the exchange of leukocytes between blood and bone marrow in chronic myelogenous leukemia. Can Med Assoc J 97:64, 1967.

48. Clarkson BD: Review of recent studies of cellular proliferation in acute leukemia. Natl Cancer Inst Monogr 30:81, 1969.

49. _____, Fried J, Strife A, Sakai Y, Ota K, Ohkita T: Studies of cellular proliferation in human leukemia. III. Behavior of leukemic cells in three adults with acute leukemia given continuous infusions of ^{3}H-thymidine for 8 or 10 days. Cancer 25:1237, 1970.

50. _____, Ohkita T, Ota K, Fried J: Studies of cellular proliferation in human leukemia. I. Estimation of growth rates of leukemic and normal hematopoietic cells in two adults with acute leukemia given single injections of tritiated thymidine. J Clin Invest 46:506, 1967.

51. _____, Ota K, O'Connor A, Karnofsky DA: Production of granulocytes by the spleen in chronic granulocytic leukemia (CGL). (Abstract). J Clin Invst 42:924, 1963.

52. _____, Strife A, Fried J, Sakai Y, Ota K, Ohkita T, Masuda R: Studies of cellular proliferation in human leukemia. IV. Behavior of normal hematopoietic cells in 3 adults with acute leukemia given continuous infusions of ^{3}H-thymidine for 8 or 10 days. Cancer 26:1, 1970.

53. Cowan DH, Clarysse A, Abu-Zahra H, Senn JS, McCulloch EA: The effect of remission induction in acute myeloblastic leukemia on efficiency of colony formation in culture. Ser Haematol 2:179, 1972.

54. Craddock CG: Kinetics of lymphoreticular tissue, with particular emphasis on the lymphatic system. Sem Hematol 4:387, 1967.

55. _____: Kinetics of monocytes and macrophages, in Williams WJ, Beutler E, Erslev AJ, Rundles RW (eds): Hematology. New York, McGraw-Hill, 1972, Chap 88.

56. _____, Nakai GS: Leukemic cell proliferation as determined by in vitro deoxyribonucleic acid synthesis. J Clin Invest 41:360, 1962.

57. Cronkite EP: Kinetics of leukemic cell proliferation. Sem Hematol 4:415, 1967.

58. _____: Kinetics of leukemic cell proliferation, in Dameshek W, Dutcher RM (eds): Perspectives in Leukemia. New York, Grune & Stratton, 1968.

59. _____: Acute leukemia: Is there a relationship between cell growth kinetics and response to chemotherapy? Proc Natl Cancer Conf 6:113, 1970.

60. _____: Granulopoietic models: Effect on chemotherapy. N Engl J Med 282:683, 1970.

61. _____, Bond VP, Fliedner TM, Killmann S-A: The use of tritiated thymidine in the study of haemopoietic cell proliferation, in Wolstenholme GEW, O'Connor M (eds): Ciba Foundation Symposium on Haemopoiesis. London, Churchill, 1960.

62. _____, Fliedner TM: Granulocytopoiesis. N Engl J Med 270:1347, 1964.

63. _____, Fliedner TM, Bond VP, Rubini JR, Brecher G, Quastler H: Dynamics of hemopoietic proliferation in man and mice studied by H^3-thymidine incorporation into DNA, in Progress in Nuclear Energy, series VI, vol 2, Biological Sciences. London, Pergamon Press, 1959.

64. _____, Moloney W, Bond VP: Radiation leukemogenesis. An analysis of the problem. Am J Med 28:673, 1960.

65. _____, Vincent PC: Granulocytopoiesis. Ser Haematol 4:3, 1969.

66. _____, _____: Granulocytopoiesis, in Stohlman F Jr (ed): Hemopoietic Cellular Proliferation. New York, Grune & Stratton, 1970.

67. Dameshek W: Chronic lymphocytic leukemia—An accumulative disease of immunologically incompetent lymphocytes. Blood 29:566, 1967.

68. _____: Riddle: What do aplastic anemia, paroxysmal nocturnal hemoglobinuria (PNH) and "hypoplastic" leukemia have in common? Blood 30:251, 1967.

69. Deinard AS, Page AR: An improved method for performing neutrophil survival studies. Blood 36:98, 1970.

70. DeVita VT: Cell kinetics and the chemotherapy of cancer. Cancer Chemomotherapy Rep 3:23, 1971.

71. Dicke KA, Platenburg MGC, van Bekkum DW: Colony formation in agar: In vitro assay for haemopoietic stem cells. Cell Tissue Kinet 4:463, 1971.

72. Dornfest BS, Lobue J, Handler ES, Gordon AS, Quastler H: Mechanisms of leukocyte production and release. I. Factors influencing release from isolated femora. Acta Haematol 28:42, 1962.

73. _____, _____, _____, _____, _____: Mechanisms of leukocyte production and release. II. Factors influencing leukocyte release from isolated perfused rat legs. J Lab Clin Med 60:777, 1962.

74. Dresch C, Najean Y, Beauchet J: In vitro ^{51}Cr and ^{32}P-DFP labeling of granulocytes in man. J Nucl Med 12:774, 1971.

75. Duvall CP, Carbone PP, Bell WR, Whang J, Tjio JH, Perry S: Chronic myelocytic leukemia with two Philadelphia chromosomes and prominent peripheral lymphadenopathy. Blood 29:652, 1967.

76. _____, Perry S: The use of 51-chromium in the study of leukocyte kinetics in chronic myelocytic leukemia. J Lab Clin Med 71:614, 1968.

77. Ernst P, Andersen V, Killmann S-A: Cell cycle effect of extracorporeal irradiation of the blood in acute myeloid leukaemia. Scand J Haematol 8:21, 1971.

78. _____, Killmann, S-A: Effect of anti-leukemic drugs on cell cycle of human leukemic blast cells *in vivo*. Preliminary report. Acta Med Scand 186:239, 1969.

79. _____, _____: Perturbation of generation cycle of human leukemic blast cells by cytostatic therapy *in vivo*: Effect of corticosteroids. Blood 36:689, 1970.

80. _____, _____: Perturbation of generation cycle of human leukemic myeloblasts *in vivo* by methotrexate. Blood 38:689, 1971.

81. Evert CF, Mauer AM: A discrete model of the kinetics of the mitotic cycle in acute leukemia, in Caldwell DK, Dawson B (eds): Fourth Annual Simulation Symposium. Record of Proceedings. New York, Gordon and Breach, 1971.

82. Feinendegen LE: Tritium-labeled molecules in Biology and Medicine. New York, Academic Press, 1967.

83. Fialkow PJ, Thomas ED, Bryant JI, Neiman PE: Leukaemic transformation of engrafted human marrow cells *in vivo*. Lancet 1:251, 1971.

84. Field EO, Sharpe HBA, Dawson KB, Andersen V, Killmann S-A, Weeke E: Turnover rate of normal blood lymphocytes and exchangeable pool size in man, calculated from analysis of chromosomal aberrations sustained during extracorporeal irradiation of the blood. Blood 39:39, 1972.

85. Fliedner TM, Bremer K, Pretorius F, Drücke B, Cronkite EP, Fache I: Utilisation de la thymidine et de la cytidine tritiees pour l'étude du turnover et du métabolisme des lymphocytes chez l'homme. Nouv Rev Fr Hématol 8:613, 1968.

86. _____, Calvo W, Haas R, Forteza J, Bohne F: Morphologic and cytokinetic aspects of bone marrow stroma, in Stohlman F Jr (ed): Hemopoietic Cellular Proliferation. New York, Grune & Stratton, 1970.

87. _____, Cronkite EP, Killmann S-A, Bond VP: Granulocytopoiesis. II. Emergence and pattern of labeling of neutrophilic granulocytes in humans. Blood 24:683, 1964.

88. _____, _____, Robertson JS: Granulocytopoiesis. I. Senescence and random loss of neutrophilic granulocytes in human beings. Blood 24:402, 1964.

89. _____, Hoelzer D, Seidel HJ, Harriss EB, Kuske B: Kinetics of erythropoiesis in acute leukaemia in man, rats and mice, in Vincent PC (ed): The Nature of Leukaemia. Sydney, Australian Cancer Society, 1972.

90. Ford WL, Gowans JL: The traffic of lymphocytes. Sem Hematol 6:67, 1969.

91. Gabutti V, Pileri A, Tarocco RP, Gavosto F, Cooper EH: Proliferative potential of out-of-cycle leukaemic cells. Nature 224:375, 1969.

92. Galbraith PR: Studies on the longevity, sequestration and release of the leukocytes in chronic myelogenous leukemia. Can Med Assoc J 95:511, 1966.

93. _____, Chikkappa G, Abu-Zahra HT: Patterns of granulocyte kinetics in acute myelogenous and myelomonocytic leukemia. Blood 36:371, 1970.

94. Gavosto F: The proliferative kinetics of the acute leukaemias in relation to their treatment. Eur J Clin Biol Res. 15:1042, 1970.

95. _____, Gabutti V, Masera P, Pileri A: The problem of anaemia in the acute leukaemias. Kinetic study. Eur J Cancer 6:33, 1970.

96. _____, Maraini G, Pileri A: Proliferative capacity of acute leukaemic cells. Nature 187:611, 1960.

97. _____, Masera P, Gabutti V: Cinetica proliferativa delle cellule di leucemia acuta. Haematol Lat 12:497, 1969.

98. _____, Pileri A, Bachi C, Pegoràro L: Proliferation and maturation defect in acute leukaemia cells. Nature 203:92, 1964.

99. _____, _____, Gabutti V, Masera, P: Cell population kinetics in human acute leukaemia. Eur J Cancer 3:301, 1967.

100. _____, _____, _____, _____: Non-self-maintaining kinetics of proliferating blasts in human acute leukaemia. Nature 216:188, 1967.

101. _____, _____, _____, Tarocco RP, Masera P, Ponzone A: Unusual blast proliferation and kinetics in acute lymphoblastic leukaemia. Eur J Cancer 5:343, 1969.

102. _____, _____, Pegoràro, L: Proliferation kinetics of acute leukaemia cells in relation to the chemotherapy. Acta Genet Med Gemellol 17:30, 1968.

103. _____, _____, Ponzone A, Masera P, Tarocco RP, Gabutti V: Different blast kinetics in acute myeloblastic and acute lymphoblastic leukaemia. A hypothesis of different stem cell origin. Acta Haematol (Basel) 41:215, 1969.

104. Godwin HA, Zimmerman TS, Perry S: Peripheral leukocyte kinetic studies of acute leukemia in relapse and remission and chronic myelocytic leukemia in blastic crisis. Blood 31:686, 1968.

105. Gowans JL, Knight EJ: The route of recirculation of lymphocytes in the rat. Proc Roy Soc (Biol) 159:257, 1964.

106. Gordon AS, Neri RO, Siegel CD, Dornfest BS, Handler ES, Lobue J, Eisler M: Evidence for a leukocytosis inducing factor. Acta Haematol (Basel) 23:323, 1960.

107. Greenberg ML, Chanana AD, Cronkite EP, Giacomelli G, Rai KR, Schiffer LM, Stryckmans PA, Vincent PC: The generation time of human leukemic myeloblasts. Lab Invest 26:245, 1972.

108. _____, _____, _____, Schiffer LM, Stryckmans PA: Tritiated thymidine as a cytocidal agent in human leukemia. Blood 28:851, 1966.

109. Greenberg PL, Nichols WC, Schrier SL: Granulopoiesis in acute myeloid leukemia and preleukemia. N Engl J Med 284:1225, 1971.

110. Gunz FW: Studies of leukaemic blood in vitro with special reference to the effect of some therapeutic agents. Ph.D. thesis, University of Cambridge, Cambridge, England, 1949.

111. Haas RJ, Bohne F, Fliedner TM: On the development of slowly-turning-over cell types in neonatal rat bone marrow. (Studies utilizing the complete tritiated thymidine labeling method complemented by C-14 thymidine administration). Blood 34:791, 1969.

112. _____, _____, _____: Cytokinetic analysis of slowly proliferating bone marrow cells during recovery from radiation injury. Cell Tissue Kinet 4:31, 1971.

113. Harriss EB, Hoelzer D: DNA synthesis time in leukaemic cells as measured by the double labelling and the percentage labelled mitoses methods. Cell Tissue Kinet 4:433, 1971.

114. Harris J, Freireich EJ: In vitro growth of myeloid colonies from bone marrow of patients with acute leukemia in remission. Blood 35:61, 1970.

115. Harris JW, Meyskens F, Patt HM: Biochemical studies of cytokinetic changes during tumor growth. Cancer Res 30:1937, 1970.

116. Haskill JS, McNeill TA, Moore MAS: Density distribution analysis of in vivo and in vitro colony forming cells in bone marrow. J Cell Physiol 75:167, 1970.

117. Hersey P: The separation and ^{51}chromium labeling of human lymphocytes with in vivo studies of survival and migration. Blood 38:360, 1971.

118. Hoelzer D, Harriss EB, Fliedner TM, Heimpel H: The turnover of blast cells in peripheral blood after in vitro ^{3}H-cytidine labelling and retransfusion in human acute leukaemia. Eur J Clin Invest 2:259, 1972.

119. Holden D, Lichtmann H: Paroxysmal nocturnal hemoglobinuria with acute leukemia. Blood 33:283, 1969.

120. Huber C, Huber H, Schmalzl F, Braunsteiner H: Decreased proliferative activity of erythroblasts in granulocytic stem cell leukaemia. Nature 229:113, 1971.

121. Hughes WL, Bond VP, Brecher G, Cronkite EP, Painter RB, Quastler H, Sherman FG: Cellular proliferation in the mouse as revealed by autoradiography with tritiated thymidine. Proc Natl Acad Sci (USA) 44:476, 1958.

122. Iscove NN, Senn JS, Till JE, McCulloch EA: Colony formation by normal and leukemic marrow cells in culture: Effect of conditioned medium from human leukocytes. Blood 37:1, 1971.

123. Jaffé RH: Morphology of the inflammatory defense reactions in leukemia. Arch Pathol 14:177, 1932.

124. Jenkins DE Jr, Hartmann RC: Paroxysmal nocturnal hemoglobinuria terminating in acute myeloblastic leukemia. Blood 33:274, 1969.

125. Kaufmann RW, Schechter GP, McFarland W: Paroxysmal nocturnal hemoglobinuria terminating in acute granulocytic leukemia. Blood 33:287, 1969.

126. Killmann S-A: Proliferative activity of blast cells in leukemia and myelofibrosis. Morphological differences between proliferating and non-proliferating blast cells. Acta Med Scand 178:263, 1965.

127. _____: Acute Leukemia: The kinetics of leukemic blast cells in man. Ser Haematol. 1: 38, 1968.

128. _____: Acute leukemia: Development, remission/relapse pattern, relationship between normal and leukemic hemopoiesis, and the "sleeper-to-feeder" stem cell hypothesis. Ser Haematol. 1: 103, 1968.

129. _____: A hypothesis concerning the relationship between normal and leukemic hemopoiesis in acute myeloid leukemia, in Stohlman F Jr (ed): Hemopoietic Cellular Proliferation. New York, Grune & Stratton, 1970.

130. _____: A biased view on the relapse and remission phase of acute myeloid leukaemia, in Vincent PC (ed): The Nature of Leukaemia. Sydney, Australian Cancer Society, 1972.

131. _____, Cronkite EP, Bond VP, Fliedner TM: Estimation of phases of the life cycle of

leukemic cells from *in vivo* labeling in human beings with tritiated thymidine. Proceedings of the Ninth Congress of the International Society of Hematology. New York, International Society of Hematology, 1962.

132. _____, _____, Robertson JS, Fliedner TM, Bond VP: Estimation of phases of the life cycle of leukemic cells from labeling in human beings *in vivo* with tritiated thymidine. Lab Invest 12:671, 1963.

133. _____, Karle H, Ernst P, Andersen V: Return of human leukemic myeloblasts from blood to bone marrow. Acta Med Scand 189:137, 1971.

134. Krogh Jensen M, Killmann S-A: Chromosome studies in acute leukaemia. Evidence for chromosomal abnormalities common to erythroblasts and leukaemic white cells. Acta Med Scand 181:47, 1967.

135. _____, _____: Additional evidence for chromosome abnormalities in the erythroid precursors in acute leukaemia. Acta Med Scand 189:97, 1971.

136. Kurnick JE, Robinson WA: Colony growth of human peripheral white blood cells *in vitro*. Blood 37:136, 1971.

137. Kurth D, Athens JW, Cronkite EP, Cartwright GE, Wintrobe MM: Leukokinetic studies. V. Uptake of tritiated diisopropylfluorophosphate by leukocytes. Proc Soc Exp Biol Med 107:422, 1961.

138. Lajtha LG, Gilbert CW, Guzman E: Kinetics of haemopoietic colony growth. Br J Haematol 20:343, 1971.

139. _____, Oliver R, Gurney CW: Kinetic model of a bone-marrow stem-cell population. Br J Haematol 8:442, 1962.

140. _____, Pozzi LV, Schofield R, Fox M: Kinetic properties of haemopoietic stem cells. Cell Tissue Kinet 2:39, 1969.

141. Lala PK, Patt HM: Cytokinetic analysis of tumor growth. Proc Natl Acad Sci (USA) 56:1735, 1966.

142. Lampkin BC, Nagao T, Mauer AM: Drug effect in acute leukemia. J Clin Invest 48:1124, 1969.

143. _____, _____, _____: Synchronization of the mitotic cycle in acute leukaemia. Nature 222:1274, 1969.

144. _____, _____, _____: Synchronization and recruitment in acute leukemia. J Clin Invest 50:2204, 1971.

145. Lewis SM, Dacie JV: the aplastic anaemia—paroxysmal nocturnal haemoglobinuria syndrome. Br J Haematol 13:236, 1967.

146. Lin MS, Bouroncle BA: The size and transit time of non-dividing subpool of precursor cells in acute leukemia. Blood 29:63, 1967.

147. Lind DE, Vincent PC, Gunz FW: The non-equivalence of mouse and human marrow culture in the assay of granulopoietic stimulatory factors. J Cell Physiol 83:35, 1974.

148. _____, _____, _____: Granulopoietic activity of human leukemic leukocytes for human and murine marrow colony growth *in vitro*. In preparation.

149. Lucas LS, Whang JJK, Tjio JH, Manaker RA, Zeve VH: Continuous cell culture from a patient with chronic myelogenous leukemia. I. Propagation and presence of Philadelphia chromosome. J Nat Cancer Inst 37:753, 1966.

150. McCredie KB, Hersh EM, Freireich EJ: Cells capable of colony formation in the peripheral blood of man. Science 171:293, 1971.

151. McCulloch EA, Till JE: Leukaemia considered as defective differentiation. Complementary *in vivo* and culture methods applied to the clinical problem, in Vincent PC (ed): The Nature of Leukaemia. Sydney, Australian Cancer Society, 1972.

152. McMillan R, Scott JL: Leukocyte labeling with ^{51}chromium. I. Technic and results in normal subjects. Blood 32:738, 1968.

153. _____, _____, Marino JV: The *in vivo* survival of leukocytes labeled *in vitro* with radioactive chromate. (Abstract). Blood 28:1009, 1966.

154. Marsh JC, Perry S: The granulocyte response to endotoxin in patients with hematologic disorders. Blood 23:581, 1964.

155. Mauer AM: Remission of disease in acute lymphoblastic leukaemia: Mechanisms and meaning, in Vincent PC (ed): The Nature of Leukaemia. Sydney: Australian Cancer Society, 1972.

156. _____, Athens JW, Ashenbrucker H, Cartwright GE, Wintrobe MM: Leukokinetic studies. II. A method for labeling granulocytes *in vitro* with radioactive diisopropylfluorophosphate. J. Clin Invest 39:1481, 1960.

157. _____, _____, Warner HR, Ashenbrucker H, Cartwright GE, Wintrobe MM: An analysis of leukocyte radioactivity curves obtained with radioactive diisopropylfluorophosphate (DFP^{32}), in Stohlman F Jr (ed): The Kinetics of Cellular Proliferation. New York, Grune & Stratton, 1959.

158. _____, Evert CF Jr, Lampkin BC, McWilliams NB: Cell kinetics in human acute lymphoblastic leukemia: Computer

simulation with discrete modeling techniques. Blood 41:141, 1973.

159. _____, Fisher V: Characteristics of cell proliferation in four patients with untreated acute leukemia. Blood 28:428, 1966.

160. _____, _____: Comparison of the proliferative capacity of acute leukaemia cells in bone marrow and blood. Nature 193:1085, 1962.

161. _____, _____: *In vivo* study of cell kinetics in acute leukaemia. Nature 197:574, 1963.

162. _____, Jarrold T: Granulocyte kinetic studies in patients with proliferative disorders of the bone marrow. Blood 22:125, 1963.

163. _____, Lampkin BC, Evert CF, McWilliams NB: Cell kinetic patterns in human acute leukemia: Evidence for control mechanisms. Bibl Haematol 39:1014, 1973.

164. _____, _____, Nagao T: Prospects for new directions in therapy of acute lymphoblastic leukemia, in Stohlman F Jr (ed): Hemopoietic Cellular Proliferation. New York, Grune & Stratton, 1970.

165. Mendellsohn ML: Autoradiographic analysis of cell proliferation in spontaneous breast cancer of C3H mouse. III. The growth fraction. J. Natl Cancer Inst 28:1015, 1962.

166. Metcalf D, Chan SH, Gunz FW, Vincent P, Ravich RBM: Colony-stimulating factor and inhibitor levels in acute granulocytic leukemia. Blood 38:143, 1971.

167. _____, _____, Stanley ER, Moore MAS, Gunz FW, Vincent PC: Regulation of normal and leukaemic granulocytic cells by colony stimulating factor (CSF), in Vincent PC (ed): The Nature of Leukaemia. Sydney, Australian Cancer Society, 1972.

168. _____, Moore MAS, Shortman K: Adherence column and buoyant density separation of bone marrow stem cells and more differentiated cells. J Cell Physiol 78:441, 1971.

169. Miller JFAP, Sprent J: The role of T and B lymphocytes in tumour immunity, in Vincent PC (ed): The Nature of Leukaemia. Sydney, Australian Cancer Society, 1972.

170. Mitani M, Okochi K: A H³-thymidine autoradiographic study of cell proliferation in patients with acute leukemia in childhood. Tumor Res 2:67, 1967.

171. Monti A, Maloney MA, Weber CL, Patt HM: Comparison of cell renewal in normal and leukemic states. (Abstract). Blood 18:793, 1961.

172. Moore MAS, Williams N, Metcalf D: Characterization of *in vitro* colony forming cells in acute and chronic myeloid leukaemia, in Vincent PC (ed): The Nature of Leukaemia. Sydney, Australian Cancer Society, 1972.

173. Morley AA: A neutrophil cycle in healthy individuals. Lancet 2:1220, 1966.

174. _____, Baikie AG, Galton DAG: Cyclical leucocytosis as evidence for retention of normal homeostatic control in chronic granulocytic leukaemia. Lancet 2:1320, 1967.

175. _____, Carew JP, Baikie AG: Familial cyclical neutropenia. Br J Haematol 13:719, 1967.

176. _____, King-Smith EA, Stohlman F Jr: The oscillatory nature of hemopoiesis, in Stohlman F Jr (ed): Hemopoietic Cellular Proliferation. New York, Grune & Stratton, 1970.

177. _____, Rickard KA, Howard D, Stohlman F Jr: Studies on the regulation of granulopoiesis. IV. Possible humoral regulation. Blood 37:14, 1971.

178. _____, Stohlman F Jr: Cyclophosphamide-induced cyclical neutropenia. An animal model of a human periodic disease. N Engl J Med 282:643, 1970.

179. Moxley JH, Perry S, Weiss GH, Zelen M: Return of leucocytes to the bone marrow in chronic myelocytic leukaemia. Nature 208:1281, 1965.

180. Ottesen J: On the age of human white cells in peripheral blood. Acta Physiol Scand 32:75, 1954.

181. Ogawa M, Fried J, Sakai Y, Strife A, Clarkson BD: Studies of cellular proliferation in human leukemia. VI. The proliferative activity, generation time, and emergence time of neutrophilic granulocytes in chronic granulocytic leukemia. Cancer 25:1031, 1970.

182. Paran M, Sachs L, Barak Y, Resnitzky P: *In vitro* induction of granulocyte differentiation in hematopoietic cells from leukemic and non-leukemic patients. Proc Natl Acad Sci (USA) 67:1542, 1970.

183. Perillie PE, Finch SC: The local exudative cellular response in leukemia. J Clin Invest 39:1353, 1960.

184. Perry S: Proliferation of myeloid cells. Ann Rev Med 22:171, 1971.

185. _____, Irvin GL, Whang J: Studies of lymphocyte kinetics in man. Blood 29:22, 1967.

186. _____, Moxley JH: Investigations of leu-

cocyte kinetics in normal and leukaemic individuals by means of scintillation counting. Nature 209:882, 1966.

187. _____, _____, Weiss GH, Zelen M: Studies of leukocyte kinetics by liquid scintillation counting in normal individuals and in patients with chronic myelocytic leukemia. J Clin Invest 45:1388, 1966.

188. Pegrum GD: Observations on the *in vitro* growth of peripheral leucocytes from patients with myeloproliferative disorders. Br J Haematol 12:689, 1966.

189. Pluznik DH, Sachs L: The cloning of normal "mast" cells in tissue culture. J Cell Comp Physiol 66:319, 1965.

190. Quagliana JM, Cartwright GE, Wintrobe MM: Paroxysmal nocturnal hemoglobinuria following drug-induced aplastic anemia. Ann Intern Med 61:1045, 1966.

191. Reisner EH Jr: Tissue culture of bone marrow. III. Myelostimulatory factors in serum of patients with myeloproliferative diseases. Cancer 20:1679, 1967.

192. Reizenstein P, Werner B: Normal and leukemic cell production in man. Acta Med Scand 185:27, 1969.

193. Rickard KA, Morley A, Howard D, Garrity M, Stohlman F Jr: Stem cell stimulatory properties *in vitro* of an agar colony-stimulating factor. Proc Soc Exp Biol Med 136:608, 1971.

194. _____, Rencricca NJ, Shadduck RK, Monette FC, Howard DE, Garrity M, Stohlman F Jr: Myeloid stem cell kinetics during erythropoietic stress. Br J Haematol 21:537, 1971.

195. _____, Shadduck RK, Howard DE, Stohlman F Jr: A differential effect of hydroxyurea on hemopoietic stem cell colonies *in vitro* and *in vivo*. Proc Soc Exp Biol Med 134:152, 1970.

196. _____, _____, Morley A, Stohlman F Jr: *In vitro* and *in vivo* colony technic in the study of granulopoiesis, in Stohlman F Jr (ed): Hemopoietic Cellular Proliferation. New York, Grune & Stratton, 1970.

197. Robinson WA, Entringer MA, Otsuka AL: *In vitro* studies in acute granulocytic leukaemia in humans, in Vincent PC (ed): The Nature of Leukaemia. Sydney, Australian Cancer Society, 1972.

198. _____, Kurnick JE, Pike BL: Colony growth of human leukemic peripheral blood cells *in vitro*. Blood 38:500, 1971.

199. _____, Pike BL: Leukopoietic activity in human urine. The granulocytic leukemias. N Engl J Med 282:1291, 1970.

200. _____, _____: Colony growth of human bone marrow cells *in vitro*, in Stohlman F Jr (ed): Hemopoietic Cellular Proliferation. New York, Grune & Stratton, 1970.

201. Rubini JR, Bond VP, Keller S, Fliedner TM, Cronkite EP: DNA synthesis in circulating blood leukocytes labeled *in vitro* with H^3-thymidine. J Lab Clin Med 58:751, 1961.

202. Rubinow SI, Lebowitz JL, Sapse AM: Parameterization of *in vivo* leukemic cell populations. Biophys J 11:175, 1971.

203. Safier S, Cottier H, Cronkite EP, Jansen CR, Rai KR, Wagner HP: Studies on lymphocytes. VI. Evidence showing different generation times for cytologically different lymphoid cell lines in the thoracic duct of the calf. Blood 30:301, 1967.

204. Sarles HE, Smith GH, Fish JC, Remmers AR: Observations concerning human lymphocyte homeostasis during prolonged thoracic duct lymph diversion. Tex Rep Biol Med 25:573, 1967.

205. Saunders EF, Lampkin BC, Mauer AM: Variation of proliferative activity in leukemic cell populations of patients with acute leukemia. J Clin Invest 46:1356, 1967.

206. _____, Mauer AM: Re-entry of non-dividing cells into a proliferative phase in acute childhood leukemia. J Clin Invest 48:1299, 1969.

207. Sandberg AA, Kikuchi Y, Crosswhite LH: Mitotic ability of leukemic leukocytes in chronic myelocytic leukemia. Cancer Res 24:1468, 1964.

208. Schiffer LM: Kinetics of chronic lymphocytic leukemia. Ser Haematol 1:3, 1968.

209. _____: Human lymphocyte proliferation: DNA synthesis time. Cell Tissue Kinet 4:585, 1971.

210. _____: Observations on the *in vitro* measurement of human lymphocyte DNA synthesis time. Cell Tissue Kinet 4:597, 1971.

211. _____, Chanana AD, Cronkite EP, Greenberg ML, Okuyama S, Rai KR, Robertson JS, Stryckmans PA, Vincent PC: A readily accessible compartment of lymphocytes in chronic lymphocytic leukemia: Examination by three techniques. Physiologist 10:299, 1967.

212. Schumacher HR, McFeely AE, Maugel TK: The acute leukemic cell. IV. DNA synthesis in peripheral blood and bone marrow. Am J Clin Pathol 56:508, 1971.

213. Scott JL, McMillan R, Davidson JG, Marino JV: Leukocyte labeling with ^{51}chro-

mium. II. Leukocyte kinetics in chronic myeloid leukemia. Blood 38:162, 1971.

214. Senn JS, McCulloch EA, Till JE: Comparison of colony-forming ability of normal and leukaemic human marrow in cell culture. Lancet 2:597, 1967.

215. Shadduck RK, Nunna NG, Krebs J: Granulocyte colony-stimulating factor. II. Relationship to in vivo granulopoiesis. J Lab Clin Med 78:53, 1971.

216. _____, Winkelstein A, Nunna NG: Cyclic leukemic cell production in CML. Cancer 29:399, 1972.

217. Shohet SB, Gardner FH: Tissue culture of primitive human myeloid cells for the study of cellular proliferation. Preliminary report on a growth inhibitor in the heated serum of two patients with chronic myelogenous leukaemia (CML) following splenic irradiation. Blood 31:180, 1968.

218. Skipper HE: Kinetic behavior versus response to chemotherapy. Natl Cancer Inst Monogr 34:2, 1971.

219. _____, Perry S: Kinetics of normal and leukemic leukocyte populations and relevance to chemotherapy. Cancer Res 30:1883, 1970.

220. Spivak JL, Brubaker LH, Perry S: Intravascular granulocyte kinetics in acute leukemia. Blood 34:582, 1969.

221. _____, Perry S: Lymphocyte kinetics in chronic lymphocytic leukaemia. Br J Haematol 18:511, 1970.

222. Stohlman F Jr: Cell cycle kinetics in leukemia. Blood 36:809, 1970.

223. Stryckmans PA, Chanana AD, Cronkite EP, Greenberg ML, Schiffer LM: Studies on lymphocytes. IX. The survival of autotransfused labeled lymphocytes in chronic lymphocytic leukemia. Eur J Cancer 4:241, 1968.

224. _____, Cronkite EP, Fache J, Fliedner TM, Ramos J: Deoxyribonucleic acid synthesis time of erythropoietic and granulopoietic cells in human beings. Nature 211:717, 1966.

225. _____, Delalieux G, Manaster J, Socquet M: The potentiality of out-of-cycle acute leukemic cells to synthesize DNA. Blood 36:697, 1970.

226. Thomas ED, Bryant JI, Buckner CD, Clift RA, Fefer A, Johnson FL, Neiman P, Ramberg RE, Storb R: Leukaemic transformation of engrafted human marrow cells in vivo. Lancet 1:1310, 1972.

227. Till JE, McCulloch EA: A direct measurement of the radiation sensitivity of normal mouse bone marrow cells. Radiat Res 14:213, 1961.

228. Torelli UL, Vaccari GL, Curci G, Mauri C: Studies on lymphocyte kinetics in hematologically normal subjects. Acta Haematol 46:129, 1971.

229. Todo A: Proliferation and differentiation of hematopoietic cells in hematologic disorders. Report III. In vitro radioautographic study of leukemia including erythroleukemia. Acta Haemat Jap. 31:947, 1968.

230. Tyler RW, Everett NB: Radioautographic study of cellular migration using parabiotic rats. Blood 39:249, 1972.

231. Uchida T: Leukokinetic studies in peripheral blood. II. Granulocyte kinetics in chronic myeloid leukemia. Acta Haemat Jap 34:186, 1971.

232. Vincent PC: Granulocytes and monocytes, in Hardisty RM and Weatherall D (eds): Blood and Its Disorders. Oxford, Blackwell, 1974.

233. _____, Borner G, Chanana AD, Cronkite EP, Greenberg ML, Joel DD, Schiffer LM, Stryckmans P: Studies on lymphocytes. XIV. Measurement of DNA synthesis time in bovine thoracic duct lymphocytes by analysis of labeled mitoses and by double labeling, before and after extracorporeal irradiation of the lymph. Cell Tissue Kinet 2:235, 1969.

234. _____, Cronkite EP, Greenberg ML, Kirsten C, Rai KR, Schiffer, LM: Leukocyte kinetics in chronic myeloid leukemia. (Abstract). Proceedings of the Twelfth International Congress of Hematology. New York, International Society of Hematology, 1968, p 41.

235. _____, _____, _____, _____, Schiffer LM, Stryckmans PA: Leukocyte kinetics in chronic myeloid leukemia. I. DNA synthesis time in blood and marrow myelocytes. Blood 33:843, 1969.

236. _____, Crossen P, Budendieck M, Mellor J, Gunz FW: Use of hydroxyurea in an attempt to induce synchronous cell division in acute myeloblastic leukaemia. (Abstract). Proceedings of the Thirteenth International Congress of Hematology, Munich, J. F. Lehmanns Verlag, 1970, p 226.

237. _____, Gunz FW: Control of lymphocyte level in the blood Lancet 2:342, 1970.

238. Wagner HP: Proliferative Eigenschaften blastärer Elemente im Knochenmark von Kindern mit akuter lymphoidzelliger Leukämie. Schweiz Med Wochenschr 98:1690, 1968.

239. _____, Cottier H: Blast cell proliferation in a child with acute leukemia: Results of a preliminary study using tritiated thymidine for pulse-labeling *in vivo*. Eur J Cancer 3:343, 1967.

240. _____, _____, Cronkite EP: Variability of proliferative patterns in acute lymphoid leukemia of children. Blood 39:176, 1972.

241. _____, _____, _____, Cunningham L, Jansen CR, Rai KR: Studies on lymphocytes. V. Short *in vivo* DNA synthesis and generation time of lymphoid cells in the calf thoracic duct after simulated or effective extracorporeal irradiation of circulating blood. Exp Cell Res 46:441, 1967.

242. _____, Eckman L: Proliferative characteristics of thoracic duct lymphoid cells in man. (Abstract). Proceedings of the Thirteenth International Congress of Hematology. Munich, J. F. Lehmanns Verlag, 1970, p 206.

243. Weiner HL, Robinson WA: Leucopoietic activity in human urine following operative procedures. Proc Soc Exp Biol Med 136:29, 1971.

244. Whang-Peng J, Perry S, Knutsen T: Maturation and phagocytosis by chronic myelogenous leukemia cells *in vitro*. A preliminary report. J Natl Cancer Inst 38:969, 1967.

245. _____, _____, _____, Gart JJ: Cell cycle characteristics, maturation and phagocytosis *in vitro* of blast cells from patients with chronic myelocytic leukemia. Blood 38:153, 1971.

246. Worton RG, McCulloch EA, Till JE: Physical separation of hemopoietic stem cells from cells forming colonies in culture. J Cell Physiol 74:171, 1969.

247. Zimmerman TS, Godwin HA, Perry S: Studies of leukocyte kinetics in chronic lymphocytic leukemia. Blood 31:277, 1968.

9

Pathology of the Leukemic Tissue

In Chapter 6, we have summarized some of the studies bearing on the problem of the fundamental nature of leukemic cells and the ways in which they differ from their normal counterparts. In this chapter, we will discuss the changes in the tissues which arise as a direct or indirect consequence of altered cellular activity. Because anatomic structure is intimately connected with physiologic function, we shall also describe some of the clinical disturbances arising from structural alterations in the organs.

Leukemia produces changes primarily by means of an excessive proliferation of neoplastic cells or by their infiltration into foreign sites. In either instance there is an accumulation in the tissues of abnormal cells and often damage to or destruction of normal cells. Whether leukemia spreads by metastasis or multicentric "autochthonous" new growth has been hotly debated in the older literature, but is of no material importance for our purpose here. Secondary changes often arise in leukemic tissues as the result of infection, hemorrhage, or ischemia. More and more frequently, too, the effects of therapy are seen in biopsy material or, more often, at autopsy. The increasingly intensive treatment given particularly to patients with acute leukemia produces its own complications, and both obstructs and obscures the changes wrought by the disease itself. It is now commonplace for pathologists to be faced with autopsy material which shows few or no signs of remaining leukemia, so that the final diagnosis rests on clinical and laboratory findings in life without the benefit of pathologic confirmation.

INVOLVEMENT OF THE HEMATOPOIETIC AND LYMPHATIC ORGANS

The Spleen

The changes in the most important of these organs, the bone marrow, are fully described in Chapter 10. The liver, spleen, and lymph nodes are enlarged in the majority of patients, especially in those with the chronic leukemias. In adults with acute leukemia they may be less prominent. Among ninety-seven cases of acute leukemia

223

in patients over 50, no less than 44 percent failed to demonstrate clinical enlargement of any of these organs at any stage of their course.[78] In the series of Boggs et al.[16] the spleen was not palpable at diagnosis in 14 percent of patients with acute lymphocytic leukemia and in 40 percent of those with acute granulocytic leukemia, the liver in 26 and 46 percent, and the lymph nodes in 24 and 53 percent, respectively. There is a strongly positive correlation between the degrees of splenomegaly and hepatomegaly.

At autopsy, the weight of the spleen in acute leukemia was given as 368–428 gm in adults by Krumbhaar and Stengel,[107] 335–670 gm by Kirshbaum and Preuss,[105] and 150–980 gm by Gunz and Hough[77] (normal 100–150 gm). In chronic granulocytic leukemia, the spleens are often much larger, with an average weight of 1696 gm, as given by Krumbhaar and Stengel,[107] and of 1500 gm as given by Amromin.[1] Very large spleens are not exceptional in this type of leukemia; we have seen several examples of spleen weights in excess of 4000–5000 gm. The size of the spleen in

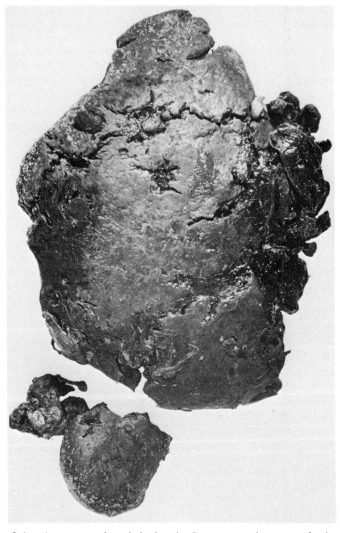

Fig. 9-1.   Acute granulocytic leukemia. Spontaneously ruptured spleen.

chronic lymphocytic leukemia is variable, but most commonly falls intermediately between that in acute and in chronic granulocytic leukemias (950 gm[105]). Very large spleens are sometimes found in the lymphosarcoma type of chronic lymphocytic leukemia.

The enlarged spleen generally preserves the shape of the normal organ. Its consistency varies. It is usually soft, sometimes almost diffluent in acute leukemia, but firm or even hard in the chronic granulocytic form. Ischemic infarction is common in the latter form (33 percent[107]), either because of extreme sequestration of leukocytes and thrombocytes, or because a greatly enlarged spleen outgrows its blood supply. An infarcted spleen may become adherent to the abdominal wall, as well as to other surrounding structures.

Occasional instances of spontaneous rupture of the spleen have been reported.[56,134,168] In 1966 a total of 32 acceptable cases had appeared in the world literature.[168] Nearly all were diagnosed postmortem, although successful removal of the ruptured organ has been accomplished during life, as in a personally observed case.

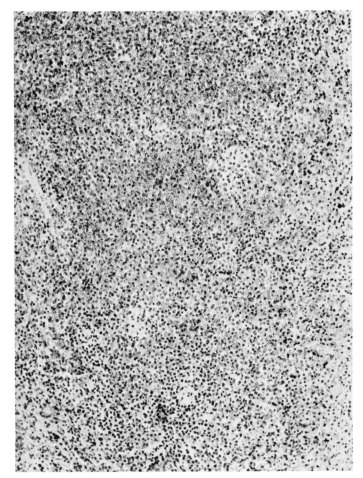

Fig. 9-2.   Acute granulocytic leukemia. Low-power view of spleen. Note massive infiltration of pulp.

Case report.   A 54-year-old man was being investigated for acute granulocytic leukemia before the beginning of therapy, when he was awakened from
sleep by an intense upper abdominal pain and developed signs of intraabdominal
hemorrhage. At operation, a 250-gm spleen, which was found to have been ruptured "as if by an explosion," was removed. (Fig. 9-1) Histologically, there was
extreme infiltration of the red pulp, with compression of the Malpighian follicles. Hemorrhage had occurred beneath the capsule which was itself infiltrated
and stripped off the pulp (Figs. 9-2 and 9-3).

Microscopically, the leukemic spleen shows more or less advanced infiltration
of the pulp with the type-specific cells. In acute leukemia the findings differ in the
various types. A characteristically uniform proliferation occurs in acute
lymphocytic leukemia, with involvement of the sinusoids and the red pulp and either
disappearance or enlargement of the Malpighian corpuscles (Fig. 9-4). In acute
granulocytic leukemia there is compression of the corpuscles, although some
remnants are found even in advanced cases (Figs. 9-5 and 9-6).[77,106] In chronic
granulocytic leukemia there is generally a uniform infiltration by myeloid cells of all

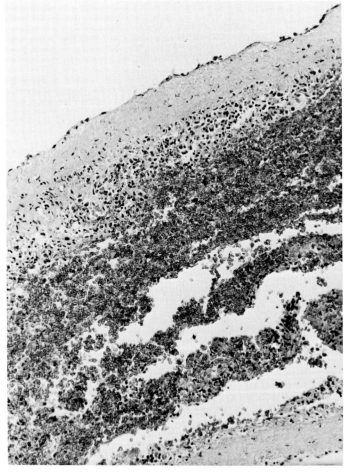

Fig. 9-3.   Acute granulocytic leukemia. Low-power view of spleen shows hemorrhage
beneath infiltrated capsule which led to stripping of the capsule and spontaneous rupture.

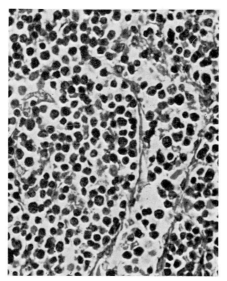

Fig. 9-4. Acute lymphocytic leukemia. Section of spleen showing uniform intra- and extrasinusoidal proliferation of blasts in pulp. × 570.

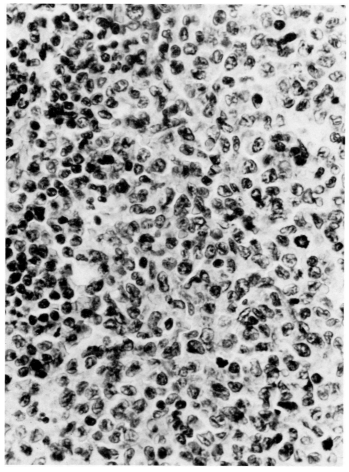

Fig. 9-5. Acute granulocytic leukemia. Spleen shows massive infiltration with early granulocytes.

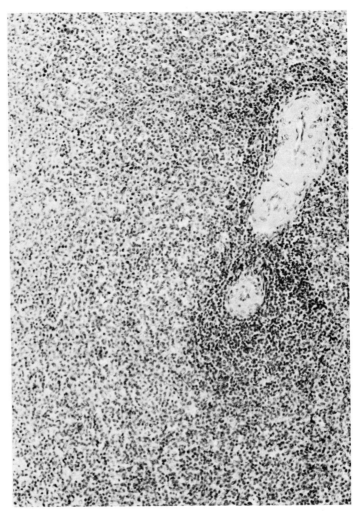

Fig. 9-6. Acute granulocytic leukemia. Medium-power view of spleen shows infiltration of pulp with compression of a Malpighian corpuscle.

ages, although sometimes early erythroid cells as well as megakaryocytes may be prominent (Fig. 9-7). Such cases merge into the category of pure myeloid metaplasia. Some fibrosis of the splenic pulp is usually present and may be quite advanced (Fig. 9-8). In chronic lymphocytic leukemia the spleen sections present the uniform picture of massed small lymphocytes, without any remaining Malpighian corpuscles. Iron pigment may be prominent where there has been much hemolysis.

The Liver

The changes in the *liver* are comparable to those in the spleen. Enlargement of the organ may be considerable in some of the chronic leukemias, but rarely as massive, relative to its normal size, as that of the spleen. Characteristically the outline of the organ is smooth (Fig. 9-9); if it is nodular, the diagnosis is unlikely to be leukemia. In acute leukemia hepatic enlargement is generally moderate, and when it

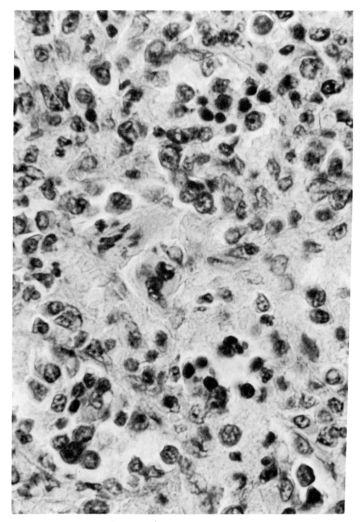

Fig. 9-7. Chronic granulocytic leukemia. Spleen shows infiltration with myeloid and early erythroid cells. (High power.)

occurs it may not be due to leukemic infiltration but to hyperplasia or hypertrophy of the normal parenchymal cells.[57]

Microscopically, a leukemic liver shows infiltration in and around the portal tracts in the chronic lymphocytic type, but diffusely throughout the sinusoidal system in the chronic granulocytic type (Fig. 9-10). In acute leukemia the picture varies, although prominent intrasinusoidal accumulations (Fig. 9-11), in addition to portal tract infiltrates, are found in the acute granulocytic type.[77] There is no confirmation[106] for the statement[69,70,71] that in all *lymphogenous* forms of leukemia the infiltration of both liver and spleen begins in, and spreads from, the local lymphatic vessels, and that this anatomic fact distinguishes these forms from the *myelogenous* varieties.

In acute leukemia, portal fibrosis of varying degree may be found. This was earlier believed to be a result of therapy with folic acid antagonists,[31] but it has more

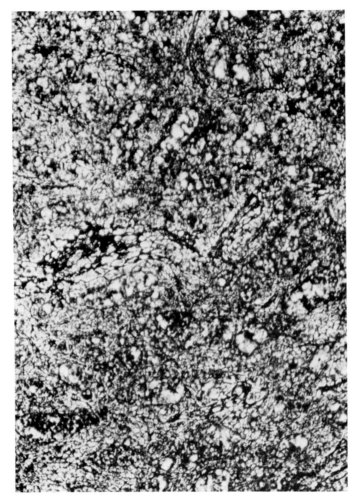

Fig. 9-8. Chronic granulocytic leukemia. Medium-power view of spleen shows massive fibrosis. Reticulin stain.

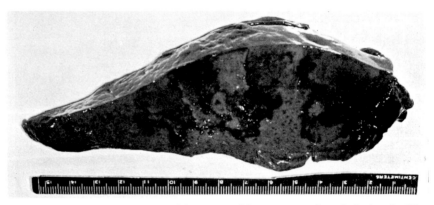

Fig. 9-9. Liver from a 36-year-old woman with acute granulocytic leukemia. There is no enlargement, but a marked disturbance of the normal pattern is present, resulting from massive leukemic infiltration.

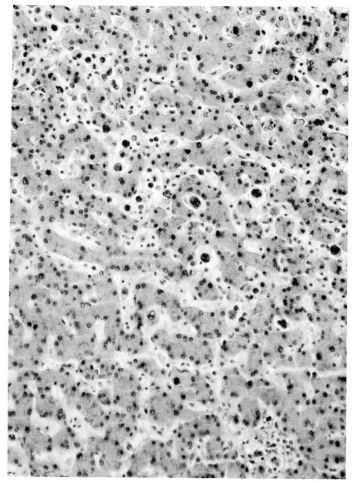

Fig. 9-10.   Chronic granulocytic leukemia. Liver shows gross infiltration throughout the sinusoids. (Medium power.)

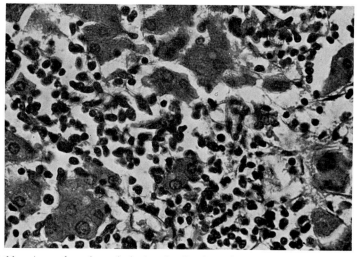

Fig. 9-11.   Acute lymphocytic leukemia. Section of liver shows infiltration of a portal tract and of sinuses. × 570.

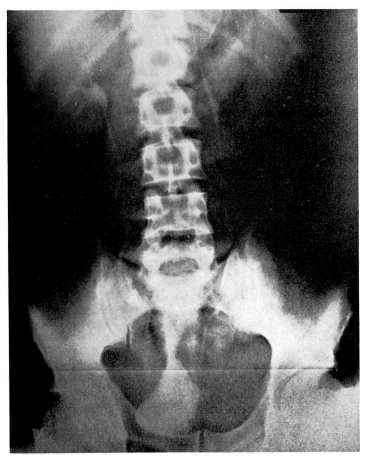

Fig. 9-12. An intravenous pyelogram from a 53-year-old male with chronic lymphocytic leukemia. Note displacement of both ureters and marked compression of bladder, owing to encroachment by large masses of lymph nodes.

recently been shown to be unassociated with any particular form of therapy.[181] It apparently arises as a sequel to portal tract infiltration with leukemic cells. Nonspecific changes such as fatty metamorphosis, cholestasis, and hemosiderosis are common in leukemic livers, either as the result of the disease process or of its treatment.

The Lymph Nodes

Enlargement of the lymph nodes is caused either by their infiltration with leukemic cells or by actual proliferation within the nodes, as in the chronic lymphocytic type. Not all enlarged nodes show leukemic changes: in some there may be signs of inflammation or even suppuration. The normal microscopic structure of lymph nodes is gradually lost in leukemia; this occurs early in some acute and in most cases of chronic lymphocytic leukemia, but only after metamorphosis or blastic change in the chronic granulocytic type. In both acute and chronic granulocytic leukemia, the Malpighian corpuscles remain visible, though diminished in

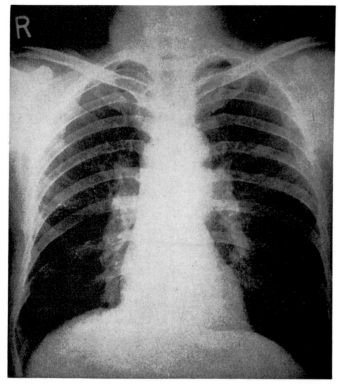

Fig. 9-13. Chronic lymphocytic leukemia. Chest x-ray shows hilar lymphadenopathy.

size by the growth of pathologic cells in the pulp and sinusoids. In chronic lymphocytic leukemia all vestiges of corpuscles are lost in late cases. Infiltration of the capsule often occurs in this type. Its presence or absence does not, as has often been stated, make possible a histologic distinction between *leukemia* and *lymphosarcoma*. When spread of leukemic lymphocytes into and through the capsule occurs, the enlarged nodes become adherent to each other and to surrounding tissues, a frequent finding in late cases of chronic lymphocytic leukemia (Figs. 9-12, 9-13, and 9-14). The early leukemic lymph node is freely mobile.

INVOLVEMENT OF THE BONES, JOINTS, AND MUSCLES

The frequency with which leukemia affects the bones, especially in children, is described in Chapter 10. The changes are most easily visualized radiographically in the long bones, especially in areas where the most rapid growth occurs (around the knees, wrists, ankles, and, less frequently, the elbows, shoulder, and hip).[185]

The commonest histologic change in bones involved by leukemia is an attenuation of the trabeculae which become slender, with irregular borders lined with giant osteoclasts. Actual erosion of the cortex is less frequent and follows penetration of the endosteal lining by leukemic tissue. It is not clear why this does not occur each time leukemic tissue begins to proliferate in a bony cavity. Widening of the cortical Haversian canals and their plugging with leukemic cells may sometimes lead to in-

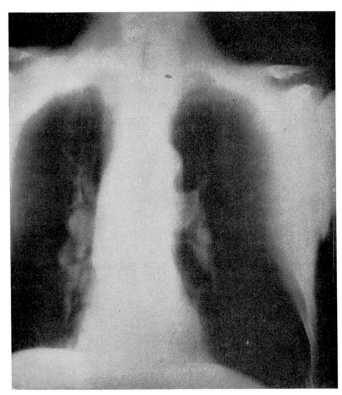

Fig. 9-14. Same patient seen in Fig. 9-13. Chest tomogram shows hilar lymphadenopathy.

terference with the blood supply,[95] bony necrosis, and even spontaneous fractures.
Infarction and necrosis of bone segments was found by Nies et al. in 15 percent of
autopsies in acute lymphocytic leukemia.[128] Great pain is common in bone infarction.[9,108] Infarction is much rarer in acute granulocytic leukemia.

Rarely, osteosclerosis occurs in leukemia, while periosteal involvement, though
less common than osteolysis, is rather characteristic and has attracted a good deal
of attention. Periosteal thickening, as seen in radiograms (see below) is usually
thought to result from mechanical "lifting" and irritation of the membrane by
leukemic infiltrates,[48,95,100,173] but this has been disputed.[186] Whatever the
mechanism, spicules of new bone are laid down beneath the heavily infiltrated periosteum; surrounding structures like muscles or ligaments may also become invaded
by leukemic cells. The newly laid down bone—when examined by such biophysical
methods as the polarizing microscope, microradiography, or roentgen diffraction—
does not differ structurally from normal bone in the same subject.[4]

Clinically, the bony changes are first detected by radiography, with or without
pain as a symptom, and like the several histologic pictures that have been described,
the x-ray findings, too, are variable.[122,174] Four main types may be seen.

Transverse bands of diminished density. These are seen at the end of the
metaphysis of the long bones (Fig. 9-15). This is a common finding in acute leukemia
of children. However, below the age of two, it may also occur in so many other con-

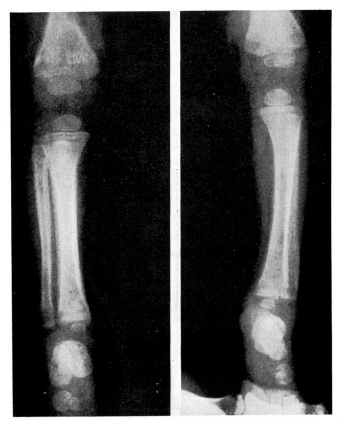

Fig. 9-15. Bone lesions seen in a 9-month-old female with acute lymphocytic leukemia. The x-ray of legs shows rarified transverse lines at lower end of femora and both ends of tibiae, as well as marked periosteal reaction of tibia and fibula. (Courtesy of Dr. Alice Ettinger, X-ray Department, New England Center Hospital, Boston.)

ditions that it is, in effect, a rather nonspecific sign which merely indicates ill-health. Above the age of two, it strongly suggests the diagnosis of leukemia.[185] Although the pathologic basis of the translucent lines is not entirely clear,[84] they probably represent a combination of local activity by leukemic cells and of general interference with bone metabolism.

Osteolytic lesions. Sometimes but not always, osteolytic lesions arise from the transverse bands, and involve both the medullary cavity and the cortex, give a moth-eaten appearance of the bones, and lead in advanced cases to spontaneous fractures. This is the commonest radiographic lesion, although actual fractures are rare (Figs. 9-16 and 9-17), except, of course, in myeloma. Lesions of this kind are sometimes found in chronic granulocytic leukemia, usually when the disease has undergone metamorphosis.[29]

Osteosclerotic lesions. With or without accompanying osteolytic ones, the osteosclerotic lesions are the least common of the bony lesions in leukemia. They are occasionally found in monocytic and lymphocytic leukemia, in both acute and

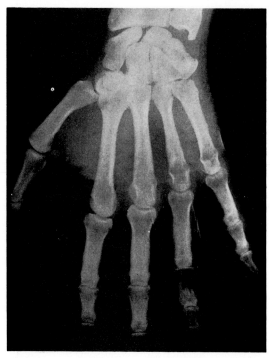

Fig. 9-16. Bone lesions seen in a 38-year-old male with chronic granulocytic leukemia. Terminal blast crisis after 2 years. X-ray shows lytic lesions of radius and second phalanx of fourth finger. (Courtesy of Dr. Alice Ettinger, X-ray Department, New England Center Hospital, Boston.)

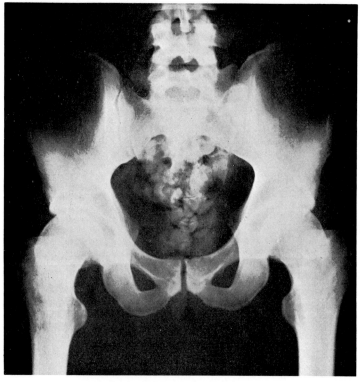

Fig. 9-17. Bone lesions seen in a 25-year-old male with acute granulocytic leukemia. X-ray of pelvis and upper femora shows multiple osteolytic lesions. (Courtesy of Dr. Alice Ettinger, X-ray Department, New England Center Hospital, Boston.)

236

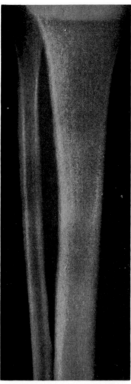

Fig. 9-18. Subacute granulocytic leukemia in a 67-year-old female. Onset with sudden pain and swelling of knees. X-ray of leg bones taken 4 months after onset of symptoms, shows periosteal infiltration in both tibia and fibula. (Courtesy of Dr. Alice Ettinger, X-ray Department, New England Center Hospital, Boston.)

chronic forms, but are rare in granulocytic leukemia, a rather surprising finding in view of the frequency of nonleukemic myelosclerosis with bony changes.[186]

Subperiosteal new bone formation. This is quite common, especially in the long bones, but may also be found in the ribs and the miniature long bones of the hands and feet (Figs. 9-18 and 9-19). In addition, a condition closely resembling, if not identical to the "idiopathic" Legg-Perthes' disease, is seen not infrequently in childhood cases of acute granulocytic leukemia. Aseptic necrosis of the femoral head has been reported.[18]

Generalized osteoporosis is a frequent finding in acute childhood leukemia and is usually, though not invariably, associated with steroid therapy. It occurred in 16 percent of the patients in one series,[166] but is reversible when remission occurs and steroids are discontinued.

None of the x-ray lesions are by themselves diagnostic, though they can be sufficiently characteristic to raise the suspicion of leukemia in the mind of an alert radiologist. Such diseases as infantile scurvy, rickets, syphilis, or septic osteomyelitis can produce very similar appearances, but today these are infrequently encountered. Several of the congenital anemias, notably thalassemia, can give rise to confusing appearances, and, in older patients, carcinomatous metastases and myeloma must be excluded.

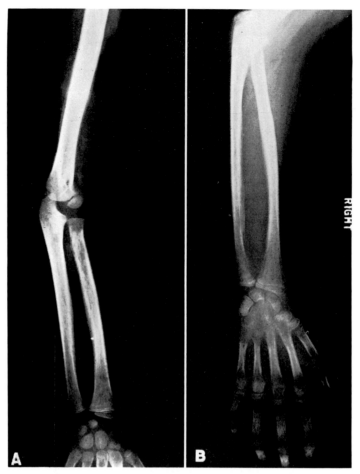

Fig. 9-19. A. Bone lesions in an 11-year-old female with subacute lymphocytic leukemia. She had a 9-month history of "rheumatism" with joint swellings. X-ray of left arm shows marked osteolytic changes and periosteal reaction. B. X-ray of right forearm of same patient shows periosteal reaction. (Courtesy of Dr. Alice Ettinger, X-ray Department, New England Center Hospital, Boston.)

Both the transverse metaphyseal lines and the osteolytic lesions can disappear with successful chemotherapy of the underlying disease (Figs. 9-20 and 9-21).[45, 164, 165] In the prechemotherapy era, treatment consisted of local irradiation by means of x-rays or radium,[35] or even of simple immobilization of the affected part[150]; interestingly enough, healing of lesions was stated to occur under this regimen. Even if healing is not complete under treatment, the lesions may cease to progress, and the more advanced erosions may not appear.[164, 165]

Chloromas

These tumorous manifestations of leukemia have already been mentioned in Chapter 3, but at this stage it will be convenient to give a more detailed account of them. Chloromas are green, tumorous masses consisting of primitive white blood

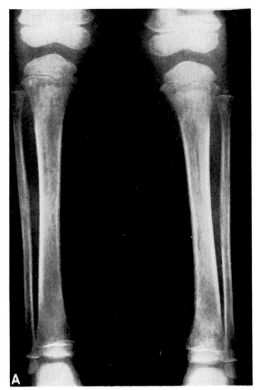

Fig. 9-20. Acute lymphocytic leukemia in a 3½-year-old male. X-ray of lower legs shows rarification of ends of bones and some periosteal reaction. (Courtesy of Dr. Alice Ettinger, X-ray Department, New England Center Hospital, Boston.)

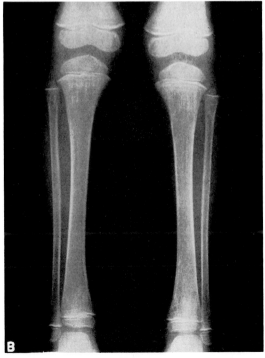

Fig. 9-21. Same patient as seen in Figure 9-20. X-ray of leg taken 8 months later, during which time folic acid antagonists had been given and a clinical remission produced. Picture shows almost complete recalcification of bone lesions. (Courtesy of Dr. Alice Ettinger, X-ray Department, New England Center Hospital, Boston.)

239

cells. They are almost invariably associated with acute granulocytic leukemia and occur much more frequently in children and young adults than in old people.[143]

Green tumors were first described by Burns before 1823.[24] King, in 1853, initiated the term *chloroma*.[104] Von Recklinghausen recognized histologic similarities between chloromas and leukemia,[144] but it was Dock who, in 1893, first linked chloroma with leukemia.[43] Lehndorff, in 1910, divided cases into myeloblastic and lymphoblastic chloromas,[109] but most later writers have accepted the view that chloromas are always myeloblastic, although occasional cases in monocytic leukemia have also been reported.[76] A unique case of chloroma with eosinophilia was described by Seemann and Sajzewa.[160]

The majority of chloromas are associated with an increased peripheral white cell count and a high percentage of myeloblasts, but there are many variations, and aleukemic forms occur. Obvious chloromatous lesions may precede the onset of leukemia by many months.[182] The characteristic green color of the chloroma has been one of the minor mysteries of pathology. The color fades rapidly when exposed to air and assumes a dirty yellow tinge, but the original color can be restored by hyposulfite or hydrogen peroxide. In ultraviolet light, there is an intense red fluorescence which has naturally been suspected of being caused by porphyrins. Protophorphyrin in large amounts has been isolated,[156,157] and shown to be responsible for at least part of the fluorescence; it appears to be synthesized by the tumor. The green color and the fluorescence do not, however, appear to be related since the green fraction can be separated from the fluorescent one. Besides protoporphyrin, chloromas contain a high concentration of verdoperoxidase,[157] and this, rather than the presence of the hemoglobin breakdown product choleglobin (as suggested by Humble),[89] may account for the green color. It is clear, at any rate, that the pigment is associated with the abnormal metabolism of the tumor cells rather than with their structural composition as such.

Chloroma usually occurs in bone, but almost any organ in the body may be affected. The bones of the face and cranium are characteristically involved. The green masses are adherent to the sutures, grow under, over, and into the dura, and fill the orbits, the paranasal sinuses, and the mastoids. Chloroma of the orbit has been found with surprising frequency in some non-European populations.[27] The sternum is next in frequency as a site of chloroma.[103,152] Here, large sheets of tumor grow from the under surface of the bone and may invade the muscles, pleurae, and, occasionally, the myocardium. Ribs, vertebrae, and pelvis are also frequently involved, but chloromas of long bones are less common.

The brain and spinal cord are never directly involved, but tumors arising from nearby structures, such as the dura mater, may press on these organs and cause symptoms. Of the other organs, the kidneys are most frequently the seat of chloroma.[103] Green nodules may be present, usually in the cortex, or the whole organ may be diffusely green. Other favorite sites are the lymph nodes (whose enlargement has been known to give rise to pressure signs), the testes, and the ovaries. Liver, spleen, bone marrow, pancreas, thyroid, breasts, and intestines are less commonly affected. We have seen a case of gross chloromatous invasion of the cecum and appendix, both of which were distinctly green and the former perforated. In one of our patients, an ovarian tumor was removed; 4 months later, the blood picture, which had previously been essentially normal, showed the presence of acute granulocytic leukemia. Review of the ovarian neoplasm revealed the characteristic features of chloroma. Chloromatous growths everywhere show a great tendency to expand, invade, and destroy, that is, they have truly malignant characteristics. Their symptoms are due both to the general leukemic process and to local spread.

Histologically, the tumors are composed of sheets of uniform cells of characteristic blastic appearance, with large primitive nucleolated nuclei and scanty, usually agranular cytoplasm. The peroxidase stain may be positive or negative. Mitotic figures are frequent. The fibrous stroma is very scanty, the reticulum is absent, but the vascular supply is usually good. Occasionally, tumors composed of myeloid or monocytic cells are encountered which do not show the green color.[12,25,109] These have been termed myelobastoma,[72,143] but except for the absence of pigment, they have all the characteristics of chloroma and the same significance. In some cases,[76] a number of the tumors are green while others are not, indicating a very close relationship, if not identity, between the two types.

Infiltration of *skeletal muscle* is often found if looked for at autopsy, but it produces no symptoms. When symptoms such as muscular weakness, wasting, or fibrillation occur in leukemia, these are usually the result of therapy, though disuse atrophy is common in advanced cases. Vincristine can cause muscle atrophy indirectly through its toxic action on motor nerves. The corticosteroids may be responsible for an actual myopathy whose degree is related to the total dosage of the drugs.[136,184] The histologic changes, such as vacuolization of muscle fibers and proliferation of sarcolemmic nuclei, are usually minimal and reversible, while clinical symptoms may be extremely severe, especially in the muscles of the pelvis and lower limbs.

INVOLVEMENT OF THE NERVOUS SYSTEM

Clinical signs and symptoms of central nervous system (CNS) involvement were rare before the introduction of successful chemotherapy of acute childhood leukemia, but postmortem studies had long before shown a high proportion of cases with leukemic lesions in the CNS. Since nearly all chemotherapeutic agents fail to penetrate the blood-brain barrier, leukemic foci can grow unhindered while systemic manifestations of leukemia are held in check. Hence, CNS manifestations have become one of the most frequent signs in acute leukemia; their incidence in children rose from 4–40 percent between 1948 and 1960, and of the children with CNS symptoms, 54 percent were in hematologic remission at onset.[51] That CNS involvement might be one of the penalties of increased survival in leukemia was realized as early as 1957.[170] In children with acute lymphocytic leukemia, up to 75 percent of those surviving for 4 years will develop clinical evidence of meningeal involvement.

The anatomic lesions of the CNS are well described in the older literature (Fig. 9-22).[37,88,110,158] In one series of 67 patients with brain lesions,[110] the cerebral hemispheres were involved in 61 percent, the region of the basal ganglia in 46 percent, the brain stem in 31 percent, and the cerebellum in 28 percent. Less frequently, there was involvement of the cerebral or spinal meninges or of the spinal cord. In a more recent series,[137] the incidence of significant anatomic CNS involvement was 27.1 percent. In addition to those already mentioned, cranial nerve lesions are common (Fig. 9-23) and peripheral nerve lesions less so (Fig. 9-24).

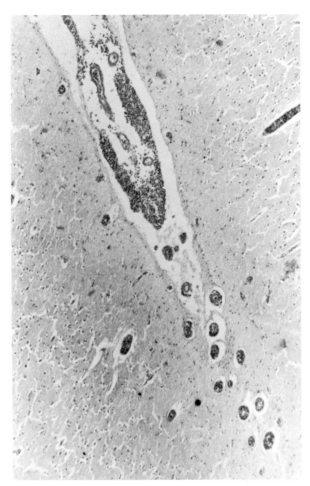

Fig. 9-22.   Acute granulocytic leukemia. Small perivascular foci of leukemic infiltration are seen in the cerebral medulla.

The type of lesion is variable. There may be multiple, small, infiltrative foci consisting of masses of leukemic cells (Fig. 9-25), with a tendency to grow, coalesce, and form obvious rounded patches of 2 cm or more in diameter. The meninges are frequently affected,[162] with focal or patchy thickening and plaque formation. This gives an almost invariable pleocytosis in the cerebrospinal fluid, usually with the presence of leukemic cells (94 percent[129,130]), although clinical symptoms may be absent for long periods. Once symptoms develop, however, 70 percent are due to meningeal involvement,[80] the great majority of them pointing to the cerebral but a few to the spinal meninges.[171] Meningeal leukemic deposits may lead to irritation and sometimes to actual infiltration of the cranial nerves (Fig. 9-23), or less often of the peripheral nerves (Fig. 9-24). In other cases, destruction of cranial nerve nuclei leads to lower motor neuron lesions.[88] Chloromas in the spinal canal may press on the cord and cause sudden paraplegia.

In 1960, intracranial hemorrhage was found to be responsible for 49 percent of deaths in an autopsy series, mostly of acute leukemia[75] and, even in 1968, it was stated to be the most important cause of death in leukemia.[127] Because of the changing methods of treatment, it is doubtful if this high proportion will be main-

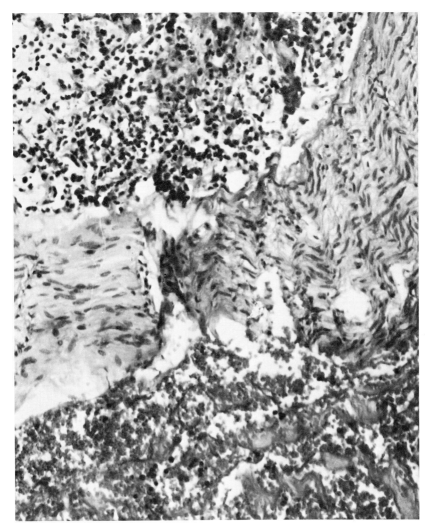

Fig. 9-23. Acute granulocytic leukemia. Longitudinal section of the facial nerve shows compression and infiltration by leukemic cells. Patient had facial palsy.

tained in the future. Hemorrhage may be produced by at least two mechanisms: most commonly, it is associated with a severe thrombocytopenia, and when this is the case, the primary source of bleeding is always either subdural or subarachnoid. It may be multifocal or originate in a single vessel. Its severity may range from widespread petechiae or small local effusions, probably unassociated with the patient's death, to massive fatal hemorrhages. Subarachnoid hemorrhages often penetrate to the ventricles and into the cerebral parenchyma. Another cause of hemorrhage is infiltration of the white matter of the brain with leukemic cells, beginning with plugging of the smaller cerebral arteries with leukocytes (leukostasis), and subsequent spread of the cells through the vessel walls which become weakened and eventually rupture (Figs. 9-25, and 9-26). This mechanism operates particularly in patients with acute leukemia who have very high leukocyte counts (300,000 per cubic millimeter of blood or more).[59,77] According to Freireich et al.,[58] the rate of fatal intracranial hemorrhage in patients with acute leukemia and very high leukocyte

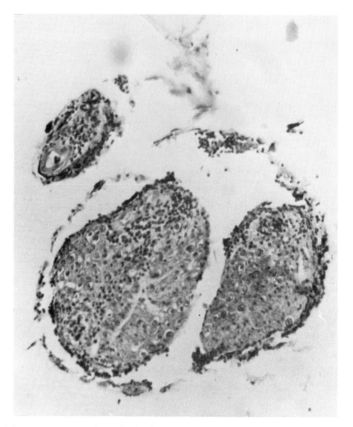

Fig. 9-24. Acute granulocytic leukemia. Cross section of peripheral nerve shows infiltration by leukemic cells.

counts reaches 69 percent. Significantly, bleeding in this group occurs even in the absence of thrombocytopenia.[137]

In a series of 1864 patients with leukemia, seen between 1926 and 1956, Diamond found 105 (5.6 percent) with signs of neurologic involvement,[41,183] a proportion of which were clinically silent. Thirteen of them had spinal compression, fifty-one cerebral involvement, seventeen infiltration of the pituitary (mostly asymptomatic), and eight cerebrospinal infections. There were also 140 patients with intracranial hemorrhage and thirty-one with herpes zoster. In Hunt's series,[90] the commonest neurologic complication of leukemia was "hydrops," a severe increase in intracranial pressure without focal signs, caused by blocking of the cerebral foramina by leukemic tissue or sometimes from proliferation of leukemic cells in the subarachnoid space. In a recent analysis of clinicopathologic features based on 170 of 417 children with acute leukemia, the following classification of syndromes was used:

1. Symptomatic meningeal with cerebrospinal fluid pleocytosis but without focal signs.
2. Cerebrospinal fluid pleocytosis without symptoms or signs.
3. Multiple focal abnormalities with pleocytosis.
4. Spinal radiculopathy or cauda equina involvement, usually with pleocytosis.
5. Isolated cranial nerve dysfunction with pleocytosis.

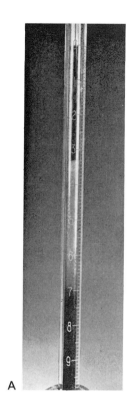
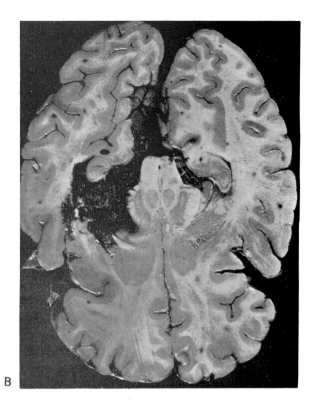

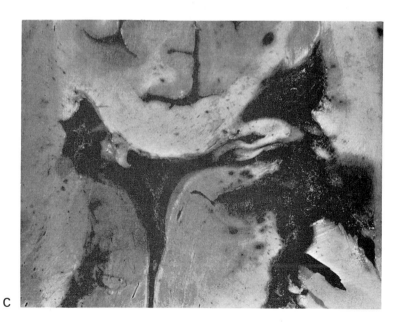

Fig. 9-25. Acute granulocytic leukemia. Cerebral hemorrhage in a patient with an extremely high leukocyte count. A. Hematocrit tube shows a buffy coat exceeding the packed red cells in thickness. B. Brain, horizontal section. C. Brain, coronal section through third ventricle.

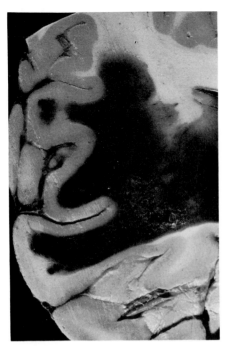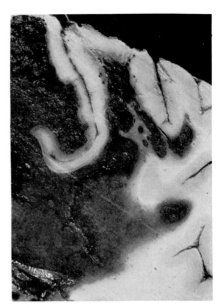

Fig. 9-26. Two views of brain from another patient with acute leukemia and an extremely high leukocyte count, shows leukemic infiltration surrounded by hemorrhage. The incidence of brain hemorrhage in acute leukemia with very high leukocyte counts seems far greater than in other cases.

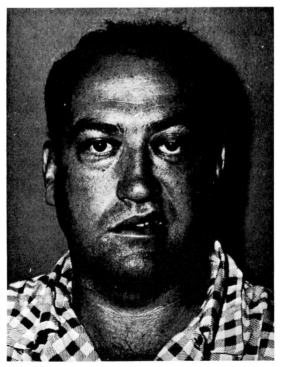

Fig. 9-27. Acute granulocytic leukemia in a 28-year-old male. Right facial palsy occurred at onset, and the patient died 3 weeks later.

6. Hypothalamic syndrome with pleocytosis.
7. Posterior fossa disease with pleocytosis.
8. Cerebral hemisphere disease without pleocytosis.[147]

Headache, vomiting and papilledema are much the most common clinical signs, with cranial lesions next in order of frequency.[80,91] Among the cranial nerves the most likely to be affected is the facial nerve.[41,42,147] Facial palsy (Fig. 9-27) is usually sudden and complete. Initially, it is usually unilateral but it may become bilateral; clinical improvement may occur under treatment.

Other signs of cranial nerve involvement are impairment of the eye movements,[60,158,175] the result of involvement of the third and sixth nerves; other disturbances of vision (optic nerve[110]), pain in the trigeminal distribution from invasion of the Gasserian ganglion,[175] and auditory and vestibular disturbances. Papilledema may result from direct involvement of the optic nerve,[85,139] or from a general rise in the intracranial pressure; as mentioned above, this is one of the most frequent signs of CNS leukemia. Pain and alterations in the limb reflexes have also been described, presumably as a consequence of invasion of the spinal meninges[62] or of the spinal nerve roots.[34,123,151,154,171] Peripheral neuritis is occasionally noted in leukemia, particularly in acute leukemia, and it may be the initial symptom. In the leukemias, peripheral neuropathy occurs most commonly when vincristine is used in the therapy of acute leukemia.[101] It begins with disturbances in nerve conductivity, causes changes in the reflexes, especially loss of ankle jerks, and, in advanced cases, lower motor neuron paralyses and sometimes sensory disturbances. The affected nerves show segmental myelin degeneration.[1]

The hypothalamic syndrome occurs occasionally in children undergoing long-term therapy. It is characterized by a voracious appetite, excessive weight gain, and secondary symptoms such as difficulty in walking. Meningitis as a complication of leukemia was formerly rare but is now more likely to be found as a result of energetic myelosuppressive therapy. It is usually part of a general septicemic condition. Any of the common gram-positive bacteria may be responsible, as well as gram-negative bacteria such as *Escherichia coli, Pseudomonas aeruginosa* or *Klebsiella;* or fungi such as *Cryptococcus neoformans,* etc. Among rare neurologic complications of leukemia is the Guillain-Barré syndrome.[1]

Herpes zoster appears to be much more common among patients with leukemia, especially the chronic lymphocytic form, than in the general population.[63] This is discussed in Chapter 10. Craver and Haagensen postulate the existence of a fairly widespread neurotropic virus ("pool" of virus) with which a large proportion of the normal population is infected, and which is capable of producing lesions in the afferent portions of the reflex arc when it is disturbed by leukemic invasion.[35] Though herpes zoster occurs usually in adults, particularly in those of advanced age, childhood cases have been described as well.[102] The appearance of herpes zoster, rapidly followed by leukemic infiltration of the skin in the same distribution, has been reported.[94]

Recently a disorder called *progressive multifocal leukoencephalopathy* has been found as a complication of some cases of chronic lymphocytic leukemia, lymphosarcoma, and Hodgkin's disease. Whether this is the result of a virus infection (particles resembling papova viruses having a regular crystalline arrangement have been found in several patients[142]), perhaps associated with a depressed immunologic mechanism, or possibly an autoimmune reaction against brain tissue is not clear at this time.[5,7,26,30,146]

INVOLVEMENT OF THE SKIN

The skin shows abnormalities in a large percentage of patients with leukemia. The commonest of these are hemorrhages, varying in size from petechiae to large ecchymoses. Nonhemorrhagic lesions are subdivided by some authors into true leukemic, nonproliferative, and tumorous varieties, according to the presence or absence of specific histologic findings. There is not, however, a strictly valid dividing line since transitions from rashes to tumors occur quite frequently. The purpuric lesions are often infiltrated with leukemic cells,[53] particularly in acute lymphocytic and myelomonocytic leukemias.

Skin lesions usually appear in the course of a well-established, previously diagnosed case of leukemia. Sometimes, however, they may present as the first sign of the disease, and some time may elapse before the systemic disease becomes obvious. Such cases may present great diagnostic difficulties, even when skin biopsies are available. It used to be said that monocytic leukemia probably shows a higher incidence of skin lesions than does any other type of leukemia. According to one dermatologist, although this form represents only 1.5 percent of all cases of leukemia, it is responsible for the great majority of the leukemic tumors and rashes.[38] Probably the picture of the incidence of leukemia observed in dermatologic practice is somewhat one-sided, but the relative frequency of skin involvement in the monocytoid forms cannot be doubted. Specific leukemic skin involvement was found in 5.5 percent of ninety cases of chronic granulocytic leukemia and in 8.3 percent of sixty cases of chronic lymphocytic leukemia, as well as in 13.9 percent of lymphosarcomas.[49] In the leukemias of adults, skin involvement is surprisingly common. It occurred in 13 percent of one series of ninety-seven cases.[78] It is much rarer in children, occurring in 2.6 percent of 122 patients in one series.[21] Although the relative incidence of dermatologic involvement may be highest in acute myelomonocytic leukemia, there is little question that in absolute numbers most cases of skin disturbances in leukemia occur in chronic lymphocytic leukemia.

The dermatologic lesions of acute leukemia are extremely varied in appearance and distribution, as is shown in a comprehensive study by Bluefarb.[14] The lesions may be either localized to one area, generalized from the beginning, or spread from a single site over much of the body. There may be a resemblance to a particular type of disease in the beginning but a change to an entirely different appearance at a later stage.[68,119] The lesions may remain constant in size, progress, or even regress, either spontaneously or as a result of treatment.[61] It has been stated that typical leukemic infiltration may be found in apparently normal skin.[6]

Pruritus is the commonest prodromal symptom in generalized leukemic rashes, and is often responsible for a scaling exfoliation of the skin found in many cases of mycosis fungoides and lymphocytic leukemia.[49] There may be a scaly lichenoid change, at times indistinguishable from psoriasis,[61] or the eruption may resemble that of pityriasis rosea. Advanced general lesions include exfoliative dermatitis and erythrodermatitis,[118] and, in extreme cases, the *homme rouge* of chronic lymphocytic leukemia (see Chapter 10). Histologically, such patients show a dense

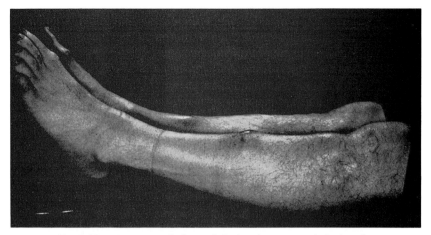

Fig. 9-28. Tumorous lesions of the legs in monocytic leukemia.

leukemic infiltration of the cutis, especially of the upper and middle layers, and there may be considerable edema separating the infiltrates from the epidermis.

Tumorous infiltrations are of frequent occurrence (Fig. 9-28). There may be only a single lesion or they may be multiple. These may take the form of papules, nodules, or plaques, and strikingly resemble in arrangement and pattern the cutaneous metastases of visceral neoplasms.[38] The tumors appear to lie in the skin or subcutaneously, and may vary in color from a light pink via red and brown to a dusky blue. Their size also varies and, in the older literature, is given in terms of glass pinheads, peas, raisins, damsons, lentils, cherries and peanuts, and in more subdued modern papers as "sometimes exceeding 3 cm in diameter."[61] Very much larger, solitary lesions of up to 15 cm in length have been described in cases of monocytic leukemia,[53] and these are liable to ulceration. Histologically, tumorous lesions tend at first to occur around blood vessels, hair follicles, or sebaceous glands, and, when fully developed, are usually sharply circumscribed and sometimes encapsulated. Such nodules are situated deep in the dermis and as a rule the dermal appendages remain undisturbed, although they may at times be invaded and destroyed. The epidermis rests intact (Fig. 9-29).

Bullae are sometimes noticed in the early stages of leukemic skin infiltration.[68, 159] A distribution of leukemic lesions in the vicinity of enlarged lymph nodes has been remarked upon by some authors,[49] although lymphadenopathy in cases of leukemic skin lesions may not be caused by leukemic infiltration but by nonspecific secondary changes (lymphadenitis dermatopathica). Others have commented on the frequency with which the face is spared, even when rashes are widespread over the rest of the body.[61, 149]

INVOLVEMENT OF THE GASTROINTESTINAL TRACT

Leukemic changes in the gastrointestinal tract have long been known to be common but clinically silent. Owing to the longer survival following the advent of modern chemotherapy, they have become more common and liable to give rise to symptoms, some of them of a catastrophic nature. In Kirshbaum and Preuss's 1943

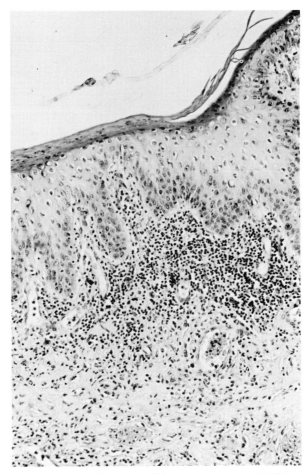

Fig. 9-29. Acute granulocytic leukemia. Skin shows a nodule of infiltration in dermis.

series, 13 percent of autopsied leukemias showed gastrointestinal changes,[105] and in another series, the stomach was involved in 5.7 percent.[33] Lesions were found from the cardia to the rectum, but the esophagus was nearly always clear. This, too, has changed. Chronic lymphocytic leukemia was the commonest form to cause gastric and intestinal lesions. Macroscopically, the gastric lesions were described as diffuse or localized, the former usually leading to enlargement of the stomach with great thickening of the mucosal rugae and the assumption of a strangely brainlike (encephaloid) appearance.[17,124,134] In the localized variety, there were one or more firm nodules of varying size under the mucosa; superficial ulceration or central umbilication, the result of necrotic changes, might occur. In the duodenum and intestine, leukemic lesions were plaquelike or polypoid masses, some of them of large size and ulcerating, or even leading to intussusception.[87] Microscopically, most gastrointestinal lesions show dense leukemic infiltrates in the mucosa and submucosa, with occasional lymphocytic infiltrates reaching and piercing the muscularis mucosae. At other times, there may be large aggregations of lymphocytes resembling lymph nodes in the mucosa and submucosa,[17] and Peyer's patches may become enlarged and infiltrated by leukemic cells, even in granulocytic leukemia (Fig. 9-30).

There was little, if any, relationship between the anatomic extent of the gast-

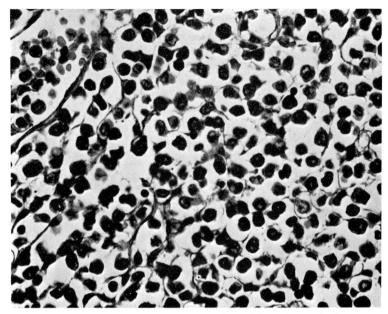

Fig. 9-30. Acute granulocytic leukemia. Section of Peyer's patch shows complete replacement of normal lymphocytes with primitive cells. × 480.

rointestinal lesions and the clinical symptoms. Mostly, in fact, no symptoms point to any gastric or intestinal abnormalities, and very large unsuspected growths were sometimes surprisingly discovered at autopsy.[177] In other patients, mild and nonspecific complaints such as indigestion or diarrhea might lead to a radiologic investigation and the disturbing discovery of extensive filling defects simulating carcinoma, especially in chronic lymphocytic leukemia,[7,17,19,98] although chronic granulocytic leukemia in the chronic phase could produce a similar picture.[28] How silent such lesions may be over very long periods was illustrated by a mass near the pylorus found at operation in a man with chronic lymphocytic leukemia. This was left *in situ,* the patient surviving free from symptoms for another 7 years.[93]

Like those in the stomach, uncomplicated leukemic lesions in the bowel were found to be mostly silent. They might affect any part of the intestines, their frequency increasing from the duodenum to the ileum;[140] diarrhea was an occasional symptom.[40,98]

The rather low-key picture of gastrointestinal leukemia painted by early authors has been changing considerably in recent years, as pointed out by Cornes et al.,[33] Prolla and Kirsner,[140] Amromin and Solomon,[2] and others. There can be little doubt that this is largely a result of the use of more radical forms of treatment, although greater awareness of the diagnostic possibilities must have also played a part. In addition, it has become obvious that gastrointestinal symptoms in leukemia can be caused by other coincidentally present diseases. Cornes discovered 32 peptic ulcers in 585 patients with leukemia (5.5 percent),[32] and there is a not infrequent association between chronic lymphocytic leukemia and carcinoma of the colon.[92]

The use of steroids and of cytotoxic drugs has brought with it an increasing tendency to peptic ulceration, with risk of hemorrhage and perforation, and to infections, especially by fungi. Many of the symptoms which may plague leukemia patients under treatment now arise from involvement of the gastrointestinal tract. Lesions of the mouth and throat will be discussed below. The esophagus has become

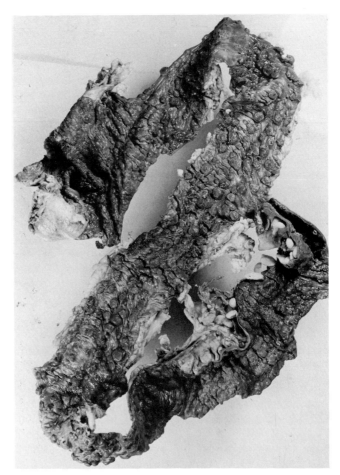

Fig. 9-31. Acute granulocytic leukemia. Colon shows necrotizing enteropathy with general ulceration.

a much more prominent site of pathologic changes than formerly. Petechiae and ecchymoses are frequently seen, leukemic infiltration may range from lesions of microscopic size to areas several centimeters in diameter, and, most distressingly, fungal esophagitis—nearly always caused by *Candida*—is found in up to 10 percent of patients with acute leukemia at autopsy.[140] Pseudomembranous esophagitis, resembling that in the intestine, occurs occasionally, and perforations have been seen. In the stomach, hemorrhages of varying degrees of severity may arise from steroid administration, leukemic infiltration, or associated diseases; they are often a part of a general hemorrhagic state. The most serious of the intestinal lesions is pseudomembranous enterocolitis which is also known as necrotizing enteropathy (Fig. 9-31).[2] This frequently fatal condition is seen in leukemia and lymphoma, as well as various other conditions characterized by shock, septicemia, or vascular stasis. In leukemia, in addition to these general predisposing factors, there is mucosal infiltration with or without necrosis due to therapeutic agents, and often an association with thrombocytopenia or with traumatic, stercoral, or decubitus mucosal erosions. Microscopically, there is necrosis of the leukemic infiltrates and normal tissues, with hemorrhage, stripping of the mucosa, and production of a

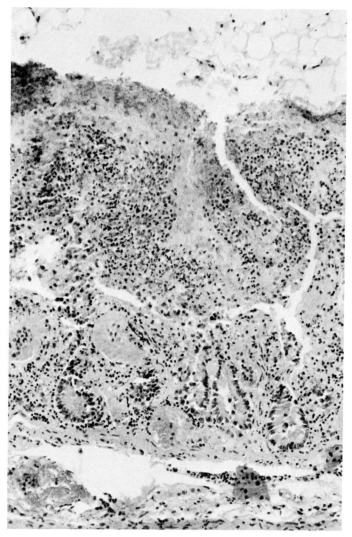

Fig. 9-32.   Acute granulocytic leukemia. Section of ileum affected by necrotizing enteritis. Pseudomembrane shows necrosis of infiltrated mucosa.

pseudomembrane (Fig. 9-32). Gangrene, perforation of the affected bowel, and peritonitis may follow, as well as intraperitoneal hemorrhage.[140] Moniliasis may occur anywhere in the gastrointestinal tract, though it is commonest in the esophagus. It may cause multiple local lesions in various sites and be part of a general disseminated moniliasis. Nearly always, gastrointestinal symptoms appear during relapse of the leukemia, but at times they may suddenly become evident during a seemingly complete remission.[52]

INVOLVEMENT OF THE HEART

Infiltration of the heart with leukemic cells is very frequently found at autopsy both in acute and chronic leukemia, occurring in 34 percent of the patients reported by Kirshbaum and Preuss[105]; 30 percent in the more recent series of Javier et al.,[96]

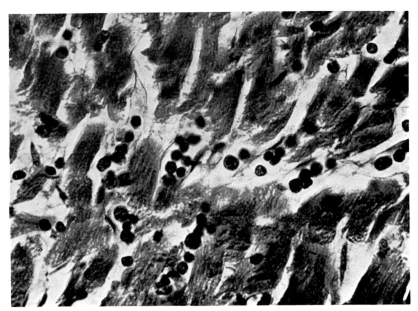

Fig. 9-33. Acute lymphocytic leukemia. Section of the heart muscle shows interstitial infiltration with blasts. × 570.

and 37 percent in that of Roberts et al.[148] However, reports of clinical disturbances of the heart action in leukemia patients stemming from the underlying pathologic condition are extremely rare. This fact may be partly explained by incomplete examination of the patients, but it is more probable that such cardiac lesions are truly silent. The lesions are usually myocardial and consist only of small interstitial foci, many of microscopic size (69%: Javier et al.[96]) (Figs. 9-33 and 9-34), and

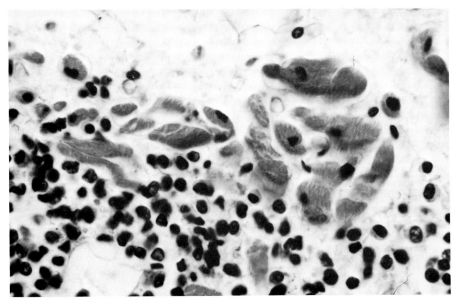

Fig. 9-34. Acute granulocytic leukemia. Infiltration of the myocardium is more advanced.

clinical symptoms would only be expected if they were so diffuse as to weaken the heart muscle in general, or so placed that they happened to involve a particularly sensitive portion of the myocardium. The most likely effect of leukemic infiltration would be interference with the conduction mechanism in cases where the bundle of His has been damaged. A few such reports have been published,[1, 13] though histologic proof has not always been available.

Other studies include a series of eight patients with leukemia reported by Aronson and Leroy.[3] Of these, five had signs of right- or left-sided heart failure and all showed abnormalities of the electrocardiogram, although, in two of the asymptomatic patients, such abnormalities were only borderline. These abnormalities did not constitute a diagnostic pattern and the autopsy findings were equivocal. Thus, advanced infiltrations of all layers of the heart with leukemic cells were found in four of the five patients with heart failure, the myocardium being especially involved in one. The other four patients showed merely congestion and engorgement of the small vessels of the myocardium with leukemic cells, small foci of interstitial hemorrhage in two and severe fatty changes in another. In another case,[44] a man showed undoubted evidence of acute granulocytic leukemia, together with complete heart block; autopsy revealed diffuse and focal infiltration of the interventricular septum. It thus appears likely that leukemic infiltration of the heart may lead to clinical symptoms; possibly more such cases might be discovered if specifically looked for. A paper by Bregani and Perrotta claims, in fact, that in 34 of 143 cases of leukemia there was evidence of either clinical, radiologic, or electrocardiographic abnormalities of the heart, and that in 15 of these the leukemia itself was responsible for these signs.[22] Heart failure is, of course, not uncommon in leukemias, resulting not from specific lesions but from myocardial degeneration from long-continued anemia, coupled, usually, with arterial disease. To these abnormalities must be added others caused by the effects of new drugs such as daunorubicin (see Chapter 17).

Petechiae or ecchymoses are very common in the endocardium, myocardium, and epicardium. Minute embolic mycotic abscesses are sometimes found in septicemic states, and these have become relatively common since the advent of the more recent chemotherapeutic agents. Infectious lesions of the myocardium were found by Roberts in 31 of 420 autopsies (7 percent), and were associated with recent infections in all but two of the cases.[148]

Massive involvement of the pericardium is occasionally found in leukemia (see Chapter 10).[10, 148, 180] In several cases of leukemia observed by us, there were clinical signs pointing to pericarditis, while at postmortem examination considerable thickening and roughening of both layers of the membrane were found. Microscopically, there was leukemic infiltration of the epicardium and pericardium, with deposition of fibrin and proliferation of fibroblasts.

INVOLVEMENT OF THE MOUTH AND THE RESPIRATORY SYSTEM

The Mouth and Throat

Lesions of the mouth and throat are among the commonest manifestations of acute leukemia and are not unknown among the chronic varieties. Most of these have already been referred to, but a summary, drawn from a painstaking paper by

Love,[112] may be given here. This author examined the abnormalities occurring in the ears, nose, throat, and larynx in a group of 153 patients with various leukemias and found the following:

Eighty-two patients had oral lesions: of these, thirty-three had bleeding gums; seven partial necroses; eight petechial hemorrhages in the mouth; fourteen ulcerative stomatitis; five very pale gums; two swollen, but not bleeding, gums; and four necroses of the cheek. Nine patients first presented with uncontrollable bleeding following a tooth extraction. There were thirty-four patients with inflamed and twenty-four with ulcerating tonsils. Three were first diagnosed as having leukemia as a result of a disastrous hemorrhage following tonsillectomy. Epistaxis was a very common occurrence in this series, but only two patients had actual leukemic infiltration of the nasal mucosa. In the ear, hemorrhages of varying kinds are the usual signs of leukemia; they may take place in the middle or internal ear or in both, thus giving rise to deafness and labyrinthine disturbances. Five of Love's patients had necroses and petechial hemorrhages in the larynx,[112] and another early case report concerns a patient with chronic granulocytic leukemia who died from laryngeal obstruction, the result of edema of the glottis with massive leukemic infiltration of the vocal cords.[179]

Love's report was published in 1936. Since then the oral manifestations of leukemia have become greatly modified, largely because of the newer forms of therapy, including not only the antibiotics and antimetabolites but the corticosteroids. These have had the twofold effect of producing lesions of their own, notably oral ulcerations, and of extending the survival of a number of patients and thus permitting the development of leukemic lesions. A paper written in 1958 makes an interesting contrast with the older publication.[46] Of thirty-eight patients with various leukemias, mostly acute, all but eight had some oral abnormalities. Five patients were edentulous; of these, only two were affected. Of the thirty affected patients, twenty had gingivitis, seventeen had gingival hypertrophy, one had Vincent's gingivitis, sixteen had bleeding from the mouth, fifteen had ulceration of the mouth and gums, and fourteen had petechiae in the oral mucosa. Gingival hypertrophy is especially characteristic of the monocytic varieties and may be quite gross. This is caused, not only by leukemic infiltration and proliferation, but also by secondary infections with the various mouth organisms whose spread is abetted by the lack of leukocytes, a common occurrence in patients in relapse and those having vigorous chemotherapy. Ulceration of the lips, gums, cheeks, palate, and oropharynx produces distressing symptoms. Many pathogenic and normally nonpathogenic bacteria, as well as fungi—especially monilia—are found in such patients. Extensive lesions may occur, and even noma—actual gangrene of the lips and surrounding structures—is once again a possibility, as it was in former days.

Although rare, leukemic infiltration of the larynx—especially the vocal cords— may be of clinical importance because it may cause respiratory obstruction.[99,163] This may also result from a hemorrhage into the walls of the larynx.

The Lungs

The lungs are not infrequently affected in leukemia as judged by postmortem findings: Kirshbaum and Preuss report a 13 percent incidence[105]; Green and Nichols report a 27 percent incidence[73]; and Bodey et al., a 62 percent incidence.[15] Clinical symptoms arising from such involvement are less common, with 7 percent being reported by Green and Nichols.[73] It is often difficult at postmortem to be certain that pulmonary changes are caused by leukemic infiltration rather than by associated conditions such as infection or infarction. In the classification of Green and Nichols,[73] the leukemic changes may be parenchymatous—either diffuse or nodular—or nonparenchymatous; the latter group includes bronchial, peribronchial, pleural, and subpleural lesions, as well as infarction. The commonest involvement is that of the pleurae, and pleural effusions, either serous or serosanguinous, occur. Far more often, however, these are infectious in nature or they follow heart failure. Pleural effusions occur especially in chronic lymphocytic leukemia, in 64 percent of patients in one series.[54]

Pulmonary lesions are seen macroscopically as isolated nodules, confluent and pneumonia-like, or as miliary lesions of the lung parenchyma; while microscopically, leukemic invasions, at first perivascular, may follow the capillaries, infiltrate the interalveolar septa, or encroach upon the alveoli themselves (Figs. 9-35 and 9-36).[82,97,125,138,187]

In an unusual case of chronic lymphocytic leukemia,[74] death was apparently due to extensive leukemic infiltration which produced an alveolar-capillary block and simulated the Hamman-Rich syndrome. Resnick et al. have reported a similar case.[145] In several of our patients with chronic granulocytic leukemia who were treated with busulfan,[132] pulmonary involvement suggesting the Hamman-Rich syndrome was seen. Whether this was caused by the leukemia or a reaction to the therapeutic agent was not completely clear,[178] although both patients showed other features of busulfan intoxication (see Chapter 17). More commonly, respiratory symptoms are produced by enlargement of intrathoracic lymph nodes which may be sufficiently large to produce obstruction of the bronchi or even the trachea.[111] We have seen several such cases. Respiratory symptoms, particularly in chronic lymphocytic leukemia, are usually a result largely of chronic infection of the nasal sinuses and the bronchopulmonary tract. Infections are caused in large measure by the striking antecedent infiltration of the pulmonary tissues by massive numbers of leukemic lymphocytes. The increasing importance of fungal pulmonary lesions and their association with new forms of therapy have been well documented.[167]

MIKULICZ'S SYNDROME

This syndrome, first described by Mikulicz in 1892,[116] consists of a bilateral, symmetrical, painless enlargement of the lacrimal and salivary glands, with symptoms caused by the mechanical enlargement of these organs—interference with vision, and possibly some difficulty in hearing, as well as of mastication because of dryness in the mouth. It occurs chiefly in chronic lymphocytic leukemia, lymphosarcoma, and Hodgkin's disease, though cases have also been described in children with acute leukemia.[155] There seems to be no question, besides, that an *idiopathic* variety exists which is sometimes familial. In this, no connection with leukemia has been shown, but a variety of other conditions, including tuberculosis, sarcoidosis, and syphilis have been incriminated as being primarily responsible: it should, perhaps, be called Mikulicz's *disease*. There are some indications that both the idiopathic cases and those associated with the lymphoproliferative disorders may be

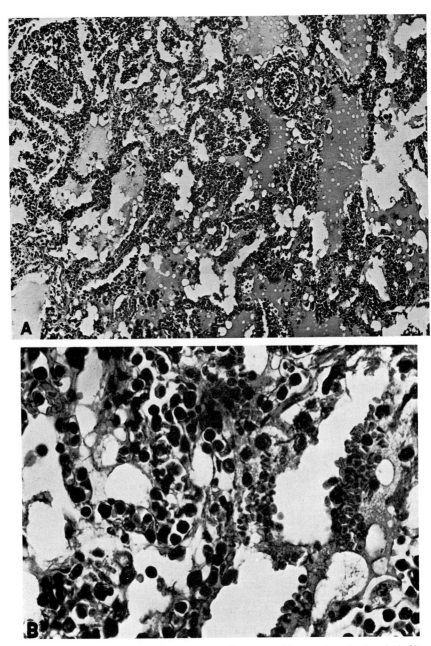

Fig. 9-35. Acute granulocytic leukemia. Sections of lungs show leukemic infiltration. A. × 118; B. × 480.

of immunologic origin. Morgan[120] and Morgan and Castleman[121] have suggested the possibility that the syndrome may be closely related to and, in fact, perhaps identical with the Sjögren syndrome—the Mikulicz-Sjögren syndrome. This may occasionally be the case, but it is certainly true that the sicca syndrome of Sjögren (dry mouth, dry eyes, rheumatoid arthritis, etc.), is only rarely associated with chronic lymphocytic leukemia or lymphosarcoma, whereas in the Mikulicz syndrome, this is more commonly the case (see also Chapter 12). In any event, it is becoming clear that a number of idiopathic or toxic disorders may precede systemic manifestations of leukemia by months or years,[153] during which period the blood may be practically normal and the marrow, if examined, nondiagnostic.[86] Parotid gland biopsy may show a striking lymphoid proliferation, which may indicate either an autoimmune type of reaction (as in the graft rejection phenomenon) or an actual lymphoproliferative disease such as chronic lymphocytic leukemia or lymphosarcoma. This again brings up the question of the resemblance, if not identity, of some autoimmune disorders with what is generally viewed as the neoplastic lymphoid proliferation of chronic lymphocytic leukemia.

The glandular swellings of salivary tissue readily respond to local x-irradiation, and the patient's condition may remain perfectly normal for years, thus producing the appearance of a successfully treated idiopathic case. However, after an indefinite lapse, lymph node enlargement may begin and lymphocytic invasion of the blood and marrow may then be demonstrated. The leukemia then takes its accustomed course with or without recurrent enlargement of the lacrimal and salivary glands.

OCULAR INVOLVEMENT

Conscientious examination of the fundus of the eye will reveal retinal changes in a large proportion of cases of leukemia of all kinds. In the majority of these, no ocular symptoms will, however, be present, although various kinds of visual impairment—most commonly complaints of "floating" specks or patches—may be noted by the patient, especially when changes have appeared suddenly or involve the macular region. The retinal appearances are most often nonspecific in type, although late cases may show characteristic findings.

Owing to the increasing frequency of neurologic manifestations of leukemia, papilledema is nowadays a common abnormality found in the fundus.[23] This is as a rule merely a sign of increased intracranial pressure but may signify leukemic infiltration of the optic nerve. In the older literature, papilledema is rarely mentioned as occurring in leukemia. Among a total of 138 patients with leukemia seen at the Mayo Clinic,[20] there were 89 (65 percent) whose retina was to some extent abnormal, and among 82 other leukemics, 35 (43 percent) had retinopathies.[114] The commonest change in the former series was engorgement of the retinal veins which occurred without other abnormalities in 27 and accompanied hemorrhages or exudates in 35 patients. Ten patients had definite leukemic appearances, attributed to infiltration of the choroid or retina with leukocytes and consisting of silvery streaks sheathing the peripheral portions of the veins, or of white nodules surrounded by hemorrhages. In these patients, the optic disk was nearly always blurred or slightly swollen. Hemorrhages unaccompanied by other changes occurred in only eight patients, and another eight showed the pale disk and retina of anemia only. In these, the pale color of the blood in the veins was quite striking.

The nature and extent of these lesions depends greatly on the degree of anemia present, and it is difficult to separate the effects of anemia from those of the leukemia itself. Dilatation of the veins is an early but quite nonspecific change and is followed by hemorrhages and exudates. Hemorrhages may be of various kinds, their appearance depending chiefly on their precise site in the retina; superficial hemorrhages tend to be flame-shaped as they spread among the bundles of optic nerve fibers, while deeper ones appear as dots and blots.[39] Some have white centers which

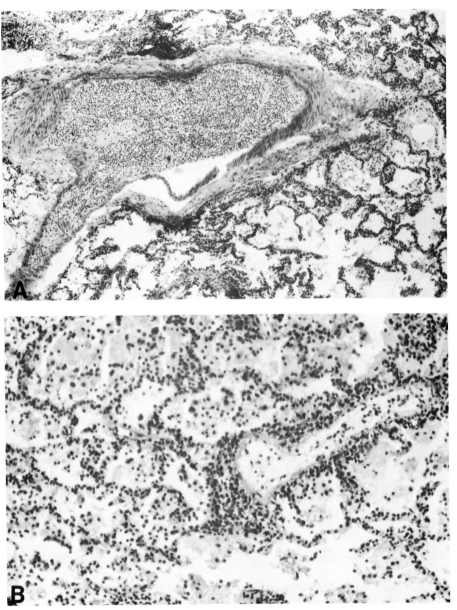

Fig. 9-36. Appearance of lung in acute granulocytic leukemia. A. Pulmonary vein is choked with vast numbers of leukemic cells. B. terminal bronchiole is surrounded by leukemic infiltration. C. Pulmonary venule and capillaries are distended with leukemic cells. D. Early pneumonic consolidation.

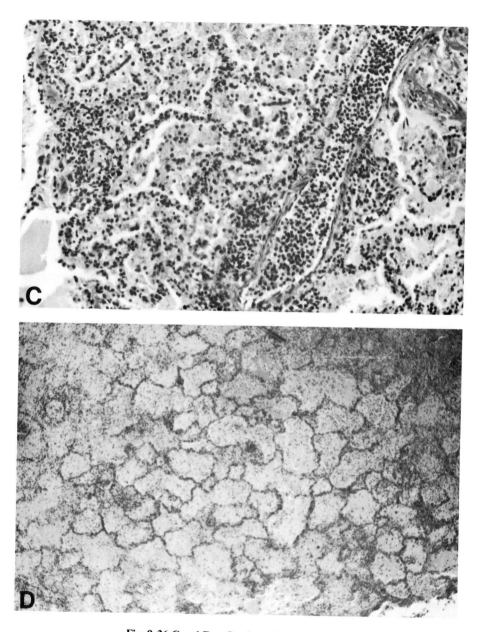

Fig. 9-36 C and D.   See legend, facing page.

have often been called pathognomonic of leukemia though they may occur in other conditions. So-called cotton-wool exudates are found occasionally but are certainly not limited to leukemia; perivenous sheathing and white, hard, nodular exudates are, however, thought to be characteristic of the disease, and when associated with extreme venous dilatation and multiple hemorrhages form a suggestive diagnostic picture.

Correlation between retinal changes and the clinical stage of the disease, including blood count, is difficult.[113] They are commonest in acute and in chronic granulocytic leukemia (70 and 87 percent of cases, respectively) but less so in chronic lymphocytic leukemia (20 percent, as reported by Borgeson and Wagener[20]). They may occur with high or low leukocyte counts or hemoglobin levels and have been seen as early as 3 weeks after the supposed onset of the disease while being absent in a patient with a 10-year history. Borgeson and Wagener believe that the presence of many immature cells may predispose to the development of lesions.[20] The same authors failed to find a definite correlation between retinal hemorrhages and the platelet level, although it is clear that they may occur as part of the findings in a generalized thrombocytopenic purpura. Provided the leukemia itself is susceptible to successful therapy, even advanced retinal lesions may disappear completely as the patient's condition improves. Involvement of the conjunctivae and the sclerae is sometimes seen (Fig 9-37). Massive subconjunctival infiltration responding to chemotherapy has been described in a child with acute lymphocytic leukemia.[133] Diffuse choroidal infiltration has been described by Amromin.[1] Retinal micro-aneurisms have been found postmortem in a high proportion of patients with chronic leukemia, but not in those with acute leukemia.[47]

Not uncommonly, unilateral or bilateral proptosis may occur in leukemia. This may be due to retro-ocular hemorrhages, to leukemic infiltration of the orbit or,

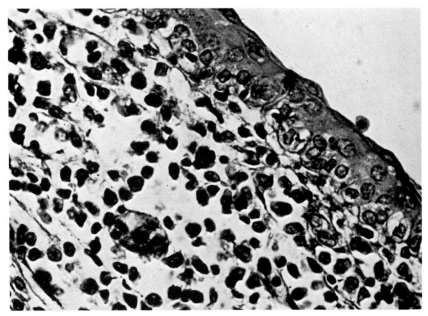

Fig. 9-37. Acute granulocytic leukemia. Section of sclera and conjunctiva shows infiltration. × 570.

sometimes, to a benign inflammatory "pseudotumor."[1] Glaucoma caused by infiltration of the limbus has been reported as the first sign in chronic lymphocytic leukemia.[66]

INVOLVEMENT OF THE UROGENITAL TRACT

The kidneys are found involved in the majority of cases of leukemia coming to autopsy, there being as a rule a diffuse infiltration (Figs. 9-38 to 9-40).[83,131] Uric acid crystals are often found in the pyramids and pelvis, especially in chronic granulocytic leukemia, as mentioned in Chapter 14, where we also quote reports of sudden renal failure occurring during therapy and resulting from tubular blockage by uric acid crystals. If such cases are excepted, there is no evidence that leukemic infiltration alone leads to impairment of renal function, and in the series of cases in which kidney function tests were systematically performed, no abnormalities were found which could not be explained by preexisting disease.[64,131] The special type of renal tubular involvement in myeloma is discussed in Chapter 13.

Occasional patients with leukemia in remission develop overt renal involvement. This is analogous to the involvement of the brain during remission (see page 00) and arises from foci of leukemic tissue surviving in the kidneys, even though the neoplastic cells have been suppressed in other sites. In one such case, a boy of 6, who was in complete remission from his acute leukemia for 4½ years, developed urinary symptoms and was found to have stony hard testicles, extremely thick, partially obstructed ureters, and very large kidneys. The blood and bone marrow examinations at this time were normal. Treatment with aminopterin resulted in partial improvement of the urogenital lesions, but, eventually, renal failure and recurrence of the generalized leukemic process resulted in death. Mathé has shown, by means

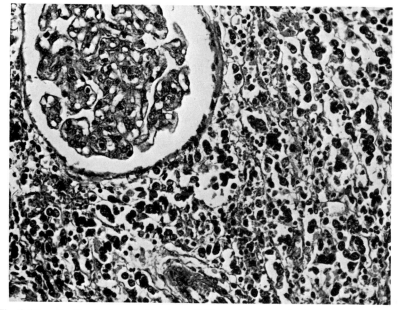

Fig. 9-38. Erythroleukemia. Section of kidney shows cortical infiltration. × 400.

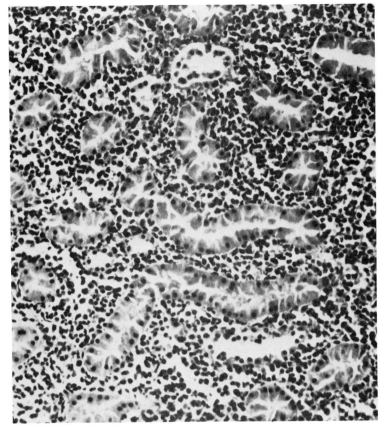

Fig. 9-39.   Acute granulocytic leukemia. Gross infiltration of renal medulla.

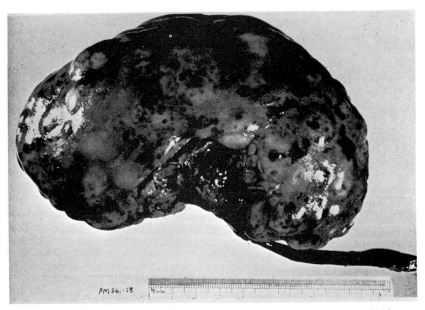

Fig. 9-40.   Acute lymphocytic leukemia. Diffuse leukemic infiltration of kidney.

of multiple routine organ punctures in patients in apparently complete remission, that foci of leukemia frequently survive in clinically obscure sites.[115] This fact undoubtedly accounts for the increasing frequency of testicular involvement in leukemia, particularly the acute forms in which clinical symptoms related to the testis not uncommonly appear during hematologic remissions.[65,79]

Impairment of renal function is frequently found in patients under treatment with antibiotics, many of which have a nephrotoxic activity (among them, amphotericin B,[8] kanamycin, gentamicin, polymyxin, and cephaloridin).

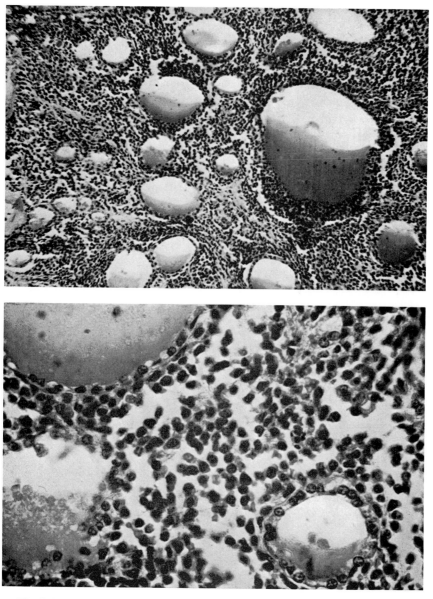

Fig. 9-41. Chronic lymphocytic leukemia. Note involvement of thyroid gland.

INVOLVEMENT OF OTHER ORGANS

Practically every organ has, at times, been found to be affected in the leukemic process. In most cases such changes were found at postmortem on routine examination of the tissues, having given rise to no clinical symptoms during life. One example is the thyroid gland (Fig. 9-41). Among 188 patients this showed small foci of leukemic cells in 34 (18.3 percent), none of whom had any symptoms referable to the thyroid.[126] Occasional patients may experience difficulty as a result of leukemic proliferation in unusual sites such as the prostate[55,117] or the bladder neck.[81] The leukemic proliferation being a generalized process, and the blood cells being found in every part of the body, indications of involvement, whether histologic or clinical, are to be expected in every tissue of the body. It can, therefore, truly be said that the lesions of leukemia are protean.

REFERENCES

1. Amromin GD: Pathology of Leukemia. New York, Hoeber, 1968.

2. _____ , Solomon RD: Necrotizing enteropathy. A complication of treated leukemia or lymphoma patients. JAMA 182:23, 1962.

3. Aronson SF, Leroy E: Electrocardiographic findings in leukemia. Blood 2:356, 1947.

4. Ascenzi A, Marinozzi V: Some biophysical aspects of changes in bone in blood diseases. Am J Clin Pathol 30:187, 1958.

5. Aström KE, Mancall EL, Robinson EP Jr: Progressive multifocal leuko-encephalopathy. Brain 81:93, 1958.

6. Barney RE: Leukemic myelosis associated with specific nodules in the skin; report of case and review of literature. Arch Dermat 27:725, 1933.

7. Behar A: Progressive multifocal leukoencephalopathy in a case of acute lymphatic leukemia. Israel J Med Sci 1:650, 1965.

8. Bell NH, Andriole VT, Sabesin SM, Utz JP: On the nephrotoxicity of Amphotericin B in man. Am J Med 33:64, 1962.

9. Bengtsson V, Hagmar B, Kutti J: Bone marrow infarction in a case of aleukemic lymphocytic leukemia. Acta Med Scand 188:1, 1970.

10. Bichel J: Lymphatic leukemia and lymphatic leukemoid states in cancer of the stomach. Blood 4:759, 1949.

11. Bierman HR, Perkins EK, Ortega P: Pericarditis in patients with leukemia. Am Heart J 22:417, 1952.

12. Birk L: Ein interessanter Fall von Leukämie. St Petersb Med Wochenschr 7:337, 1883.

13. Blotner H, Sosman MS: X-ray therapy of the heart in a patient with leukemia, heart block and hypertension; report of a case. N Engl J Med 230:793, 1944.

14. Bluefarb SM: The Cutaneous Manifestations of the Benign Inflammatory Reticuloses. Springfield, Thomas, 1961.

15. Bodey GP, Powell RD Jr, Hersh EM, Yeterian A, Freireich EJ: Pulmonary complications of acute leukemia. Cancer 19:781, 1966.

16. Boggs DR, Wintrobe MM, Cartwright GE: The acute leukemias. Medicine 41:163, 1962.

17. Boikan WS: Leukemic changes of the gastro-intestinal tract. Arch Intern Med 47:42, 1931.

18. Boksenbaum M, Mendelson CG: Aseptic necrosis of the femoral head associated with steroid therapy. JAMA 184:262, 1963.

19. Boquien Y, Kernéis JP, Guénel J: Leucémie lymphoïde avec tumeur gastrique terminale après quatre ans et demi d'évolution. Arch Mal App Digest 47:1217, 1958.

20. Borgeson EJ, Wagener HP: Changes in the eye in leukemia. Am J Med Sci 177:663, 1929.

21. Brandberg O: Studien über das klinische Bild der Leukose und der sog. leukämoiden Reaktionen im Kindesalter. Acta Paediatr 30 (suppl 1), 1943.

22. Bregani P, Perrotta P: The heart in leukemia. Clinical and electrocardiographic aspects. Folia Cardiol 19:193, 1960.

23. Brégeat P, Hammard H: Les manifestations oculaires des leucoses. Arch Ophthalmol 26:13, 1966.

24. Burns A: in Lucas F Jr, Cook EJ (eds): Ob-

servations on the Surgical Anatomy of the Head and Neck. Baltimore, Cushing & Jewitt, 1823, p 386.

25. Campbell ACP, Henderson JC, Croom JH: Monocytic leukaemia with myeloid hyperplasia and localized tumour formation. J. Pathol Bacteriol 42:617, 1936.

26. Cavanagh JB, Greenbaum D, Marshall AHE, Rubinstein LJ: Cerebral demyelination associated with disorders of the reticuloendothelial system. Lancet 2:524, 1959.

27. Cavdar AO, Gözdasoglu S, Arcasoy A, Demirag B: Chloroma-like ocular manifestations in Turkish children with acute myelomonocytic leukaemia. Lancet 1:680, 1971.

28. Cavins JA, Levin HS, Day HJ: Chronic myelogenous leukemia with gastric infiltration. Report of a case simulating carcinoma of the stomach. N Engl J Med 260:1111, 1959.

29. Chabner BA, Haskell CM, Canellos GP: Destructive bone lesions in chronic granulocytic leukemia. Medicine 48:401, 1969.

30. Chandor SB, Forno LS, Wivel NA: Progressive multifocal leucoencephalopathy. J Neurol Neurosurg Psychiatr 28:260, 1965.

31. Colsky J, Greenspan EM, Warren TN: Hepatic fibrosis in children with acute leukemia after therapy with folic acid antagonists. Arch Pathol 59:198, 1955.

32. Cornes JS: Multiple primary cancers: Primary malignant lymphomas and carcinomas of the intestinal tract in the same patient. J Clin Pathol 13:483, 1960.

33. ———, Jones TG, Fisher GB: Gastroduodenal ulcerations and massive hemorrhage in patients with leukemia, multiple myeloma, and malignant tumors of lymphoid tissue. Gastroenterology 41:337, 1961.

34. Cornil L, Olmer D, Olmer J: Paralysie ascendante de Landry avec Leukocytomyélie et syndrome de Froin au cours d'une leucémie myéloïde. Sang 6:114, 1932.

35. Craver LF, Copeland MM: Changes of the bones in the leukemias. Arch Surg 30:639, 1935.

36. ———, Haagensen CD: A note on the occurrence of herpes zoster in Hodgkin's disease, lymphosarcoma and the leukemias. Am J Cancer 16:502, 1932.

37. Critchley M, Greenfield JG: Spinal symptoms in chloroma and leukaemia. Brain 53:11, 1930.

38. Davies JHT: Dermatological aspects of blood diseases, in Wilkinson, JF (ed): Modern Trends in Blood Diseases. New York, Hoeber, 1955, p. 66.

39. Dawson DBH: Changes in the fundus in diseases of the blood, in: Wilkinson JF (ed): Modern Trends in Blood Diseases. New York, Hoeber, 1955, p 212.

40. Debray J, Sarakinos M: Les localisations digestives des hémopathies malignes. Sang 29:572, 1958.

41. Diamond HD, Williams HM, Craver LF: The pathogenesis and management of neurological complications of malignant lymphomas and leukemia. Acta Unio Int Contra Cancrum 16:831, 1960.

42. Diamond IB: Leukemic changes in the brain. A report of fourteen cases. Arch Neurol Psychiatr 32:118, 1934.

43. Dock G: Chloroma and its relation to leukemia. Am J Med Sci 106:152, 1893.

44. Dresdale DT, Spain D, Perez-Pina F: Heart block and leukemic cell infiltration of interventricular septum of heart. Am J Med 6:530, 1949.

45. Dresner E: The bone and joint lesions in acute leukaemia and their response to folic acid antagonists. Quart J Med 19:339, 1950.

46. Duffy JH, Driscoll EJ: Oral manifestations of leukemia. Oral Surg 11:484, 1958.

47. Duke JR, Wilkinson CP, Sigelman S: Retinal microaneurysms in leukaemia. Br J Ophthalmol 52:368, 1968.

48. Ehrlich JC, Forer S: Periosteal ossification in myelogenous leukemia; report of case associated with acute rheumatic fever. Arch Intern Med 53:938, 1934.

49. Epstein E, MacEachern K: Dermatologic manifestations of the lymphoblastomaleukemia group. Arch Intern Med 60:867, 1937.

50. Epstein EH Jr, Levin DL, Croft JD Jr, Lutzner MA: Mycosis fungoides—survival, prognostic features, response to therapy, and autopsy findings. Medicine 15:61, 1972.

51. Evans AE: Central nervous system involvement in children with acute leukemia. A study of 921 patients. Cancer 17:256, 1964.

52. Everett CR, Haggard ME, Levin WC: Extensive leukemic infiltration of the gastrointestinal tract during apparent remission in acute leukemia. Blood 22:92, 1963.

53. Fairburn EA, Burgen ASV: The skin lesions of monocytic leukaemia. Br J Cancer 1:352, 1947.

54. Falconer EH, Leonard ME: Pulmonary involvement in lymphosarcoma and lymphocytic leukemia. Am J Med Sci 195:294, 1938.

55. Flaherty SS, Cope HE, Shecket HA:

Prostatic obstruction as the presenting symptom of acute monocytic leukemia. J Urol 44:488, 1940.

56. Flood MJ, Carpenter RA: Spontaneous rupture of the spleen in acute myeloid leukaemia. Br Med J 1:35, 1961.

57. Frei E III, Fritz RD, Price E, Moore EW, Thomas LB: Renal and hepatic enlargement in acute leukemia. Cancer 16:1089, 1963.

58. Freireich EJ, Thomas LB, Frei E III, Fritz RD, Forkner CE Jr: A distinctive type of intracerebral hemorrhage associated with "blastic crisis" in patients with leukemia. Cancer 13: 146, 1960.

59. Fritz RD, Forkner CE Jr, Freireich EJ, Frei E III, Thomas LB: Association of fatal intracranial hemorrhage and "blastic crisis" in patients with acute leukemia. N Engl J Med 261:59, 1959.

60. Garvey PH, Lawrence JS: Facial diplegia in lymphatic leukemia. JAMA 101:1941, 1933.

61. Gates O: Cutaneous tumors in leukemia and lymphoma. Arch Dermatol 37:1015, 1938.

62. Gauld WR: Leukaemia presenting with neurological manifestations. Lancet 1:939, 1948.

63. Gelfand MI: Herpes zoster with a varicelliform eruption and parotitis in chronic leukemia. JAMA 145:560, 1951.

64. Gilbert EF, Rice EC, Lechaux PA: Renal function in children with leukemia. A clinical and pathological study. Am J Dis Child 93:150, 1957.

65. Givler RL: Testicular involvement in leukemia and lymphoma. Cancer 23:1290, 1969.

66. Glaser B, Smith JL: Leukaemic glaucoma. Br J Ophthalmol 50:92, 1966.

67. Glatt W, Weinstein A: Acropachy in lymphatic leukemia. Radiology 92:125, 1969.

68. Goeckerman WH, Montgomery H: Cutaneous lymphoblastoma. Report of two unusual cases. Arch Dermatol 24:383, 1931.

69. Goldberg GM, Rubenstone AI: A study of malignant lymphomas and leukemia. I. The significance of liver portal space "infiltration" in lymphogenous leukemia (with reference to the involvement of the lymphatics). Cancer 13:513, 1960.

70. _____, _____: A study of malignant lymphomas and leukemias. II. A diagnostic approach to lymphogenous leukemia and myelogenous leukemia with reference to the involvement of the lymphatics. Cancer 13:520, 1960.

71. _____, Ungar H: Lymphatics of spleen in leukemia; with reference to so-called infiltration of vessel walls. Lab Invest 7:146, 1958.

72. Gralnick HR, Dittmar K: Development of myeloblastoma with massive breast and ovarian involvement during remission in acute leukemia. Cancer 24:746, 1969.

73. Green RA, Nichols NJ: Pulmonary involvement in leukemia. Am Rev Resp Dis 80:833, 1959.

74. _____, _____, King EJ: Alveolar-capillary block due to leukemic infiltration of the lung. Am Rev Resp Dis 80:895, 1959.

75. Groch SN, Sayre GP, Heck FJ: Cerebral hemorrhage in leukemia. Arch Neurol Psychiatr 2:439, 1960.

76. Gump ME, Hester EG, Lohr OW: Monocytic chloroma. Arch Ophthalmol 16:931, 1936.

77. Gunz FW, Burry AF: Cellular types in acute leukaemia: Diagnosis and significance. J Clin Pathol 16:325, 1963.

78. _____, Hough RF: Acute leukemia over the age of fifty. A study of its incidence and natural history. Blood 11:882, 1956.

79. Haggar RA, MacMillan AB, Thompson DG: Leukemic infiltration of testis. Can J Surg 12:197, 1969.

80. Haghbin M, Zuelzer WW: A long-term study of cerebrospinal leukemia. J Pediatr 67:23, 1965.

81. Hermann HB, Goldberg MM, Salerno FM: Leukemic infiltration of the bladder neck in a female patient. J Urol 83:51, 1960.

82. Herold K, Michel W: Pulmonale Veränderungen bei chronischer Leukämie. Dtsch Arch Klin Med 197:596, 1950.

83. Heuchel G, Vom Dahl D: Leukaemie und Niere. Blut 5:390, 1959.

84. Hilbish TF, Besse BE Jr, Lusted LB, Daves ML, Thomas LB, Forkner CE: Acute leukemia. Skeletal manifestations in children and adults. Arch Intern Med 104:741, 1959.

85. Hill E: Papilledema and intracranial complications of leukemia. Am J Ophthalmol 15:1127, 1932.

86. Hird AJ: Mikulicz's syndrome. Br Med J 2:416, 1949.

87. Hoffmann M: Ueber Veränderungen des Magen-Darmkanales bei Leukämie. Inaug Diss Friedrichs Universität, 1905.

88. Howell A, Gough J: Acute lymphatic leukaemia with facial diplegia and double abducens palsy. Lancet 1:723, 1932.

89. Humble JG: The aetiology of chloroma and the nature of the green pigment. A report of three cases. Q J Med 15:299, 1946.

90. Hunt WE, Bouroncle BA, Meagher HN:

Neurologic complications of leukemias and lymphomas. J Neurosurg 16:135, 1959.

91. Hyman CB, Bogle JM, Brubaker CA, Williams K, Hammond D: Central nervous system involvement by leukemia in children. Blood 25:1, 13, 1965.

92. Hyman GA, Ultmann JE, Slanetz Ch A: The association of chronic lymphocytic leukemia or lymphoma and carcinoma of the colon. Correlation with blood type A, in: Proceedings of the Ninth Congress of the International Society of Hematology, Mexico City, 1962. New York, Grune & Stratton, 1963.

93. Ikeda K: Gastric manifestations of lymphatic aleukemia (pseudoleukemia gastrointestinalis). Am J Clin Pathol 50:167, 1931.

94. Jadassohn J: Leukämische Infiltrate in Zosternarben. Zentralbl. Haut-u Geschl-Krankh 20:741, 1926.

95. Jaffé HL: Skeletal manifestations of leukemia and malignant lymphoma. Bull Hosp Joint Dis 13:217, 1952.

96. Javier BV, Yount WJ, Crosby DJ, Hall TC: Cardiac metastases in lymphoma and leukemia. Dis Chest 52:481, 1967.

97. Joachim H, Loewe L: Atypical acute myeloid leukemia with unusual pulmonary manifestations. Am J Med Sci 174:215, 1927.

98. Jones EI: Intestinal ulceration in myelogenous leukaemia. Lancet 1:174, 1940.

99. Jones RV, Shalom AS: Laryngeal involvement in acute leukaemia. J Laryngol Otol 82:123, 1968.

100. Karelitz S: Unusual forms of periosteal elevation. Am J Dis Child 33:394, 1927.

101. Karon MR, Freireich EJ, Frei E III: A preliminary report on vincristine sulfate—a new active agent for the treatment of acute leukemia. Pediatrics 30:791, 1962.

102. Keidan SE, Mainwaring D: Association of herpes zoster with leukemia and lymphoma in children. Clin Pediatr 4:13, 1965.

103. Kendel EV: Chloroma. Arch Intern Med 59:691, 1937.

104. King A: A case of chloroma. Monthly J Med 17:97, 1853.

105. Kirshbaum JD, Preuss FS: Leukemia. A clinical and pathologic study of one hundred and twenty-three fatal cases in a series of 14,400 necropsies. Arch Intern Med 71:777, 1943.

106. Kostich ND, Rappaport H: Diagnostic significance of the histologic changes in the liver and spleen in leukemia and malignant lymphoma. Cancer 18:1214, 1965.

107. Krumbhaar EB, Stengel A: The spleen in the leukemias. Arch Pathol 34:117, 1942.

108. Kundel DW, Brecher G, Bodey GP, Brittin GM: Reticulin fibrosis and bone infarction in acute leukemia. Implications for prognosis. Blood 23:526, 1964.

109. Lehndorff H: Chlorom. Ergeb Inn Med Kinderheilkd 6:221, 1910.

110. Leidler F, Russell WO: The brain in leukemia. Arch Pathol 40:14, 1945.

111. Levison VB: Respiratory obstruction in acute leukaemia. Lancet 1:1151, 1955.

112. Love AA: Manifestations of leukemia encountered in otolaryngologic and stomatologic practice. Arch Otolaryngol 23:173, 1936.

113. Mahneke A, Videbaek A: On changes in the optic fundus in leukaemia. Aetiology, diagnostic and prognostic role. Acta Ophthalmol 42:201, 1964.

114. Marshall RA: A review of lesions in the optic fundus in various diseases of the blood. Blood 14:882, 1959.

115. Mathé G, Schwarzenberg L, Mery AM, Cattan A, Schneider M, Amiel JL, Schlumberger JR, Poisson J, Wajcner G: Extensive histological and cytological survey of patients with acute leukaemia in "complete remission." Br Med J 1:640, 1966.

116. Mikulicz-Radecki J von: Ueber eine eigenartige symmetrische Erkrankung der Thränen-und Mund-Speicheldrüsen, in: Beitr. zur Chirurgie. Festschrift gewidm. T. Billroth. Stuttgart, 1892, pp 610–630.

117. Mitch WE Jr, Serpick AA: Leukemic infiltration of the prostate: a reversible form of urinary obstruction. Cancer 26:1361, 1970.

118. Montgomery H: Exfoliative dermatosis and malignant erythroderma; value and limitations of histopathologic studies. Arch Dermatol 27:253, 1933.

119. _____, Watkins CH: Monocytic leukemia. Cutaneous manifestations of the Naegeli and Schilling types; hemocytologic differentiation. Arch Intern Med 60:51, 1937.

120. Morgan WS: Mikulicz-Sjögren syndrome. Cabot case record 86–1962. N Engl J Med 267:1367, 1962.

121. _____, Castleman B: Clinicopathologic study of "Mikulicz's disease." Am J Pathol 29:471, 1953.

122. Moseley JE: Patterns of bone change in the leukemias and myelosclerosis. Mt Sinai J Med NY 18:1, 1961.

123. Murphy JP, Brody BS: Nerve root infiltration in myelogenous leukemia. JAMA 115:1544, 1940.

124. Nagel W: Beitrag zur Frage der Magen-Darmveränderungen bei der lymphatischen Leukämie. Zentralbl Allg Pathol 88:259, 1952.

125. Nathan DJ, Sanders M: Manifestations of acute leukemia in the parenchyma of lungs. N Engl J Med 252:797, 1955.

126. Naylor B: Secondary lymphoblastomatous involvement of the thyroid gland. Arch Pathol 67:432, 1959.

127. Nieri RL, Burgert EO, Groover RV: Central-nervous-system complications of leukemia. A review. Mayo Clinic Proc 43:70, 1968.

128. Nies BA, Kundel DW, Thomas LB, Freireich EJ: Leukopenia, bone pain, and bone necrosis in patients with acute leukemia. A clinicopathologic complex. Ann Intern Med 62:698, 1965.

129. ———, Malmgren RA, Chu EW, Del Vecchio PR, Thomas LB, Freireich EJ: Cerebrospinal fluid cytology in patients with acute leukemia. Cancer 18:1385, 1965.

130. ———, Thomas LB, Freireich EJ: Meningeal leukemia. A follow-up study. Cancer 18:546, 1965.

131. Norris HJ, Wiener J: The renal lesions in leukemia. Am J Med Sci 241:512, 1961.

132. Oliner H, Schwartz R, Rubio F, Dameshek W: Interstitial pulmonary fibrosis following busulfan therapy. Am J Med 31:134, 1961.

133. O'Rourke JF, O'Connor GR: Unusual ocular involvement in acute lymphatic leukemia. Arch Ophthalmol 57:585, 1957.

134. Pearson B, Stasney J, Pizzolato P: Gastrointestinal involvement in lymphocytic leukemia. Arch Pathol 35:21, 1943.

135. Pease JC, Ward-McQuaid JN: Splenic rupture in leukaemia. Br Med J 1:293, 1961.

136. Perkoff GT, Silber R, Tyler FH, Cartwright GE, Wintrobe MM: Studies in disorders of muscle. XII. Myopathy due to the administration of therapeutic amounts of 17-hydroxysteroids. Am J Med 26:891, 1959.

137. Phair JP, Anderson RE, Namiki H: The central nervous system in leukemia. Ann Intern Med 61:863, 1964.

138. Polli E, Papagni L, Nicodemia E: Il polmone leucemico. Clin Med 38:1477, 1957.

139. Poncet F: Rétinite leucocythémique. Arch Physiol (2nd series) 1:496, 1874.

140. Prolla JC, Kirsner JB: The gastrointestinal lesions and complications of the leukemias. Ann Intern Med 61:1084, 1964.

141. Rappaport, H: Atlas of Tumor Pathology. Sec. III, Fasc. 8. Washington, D.C., Armed Forces Institute of Pathology, 1960.

142. Rausing A, Axelsson U: Progressive multi-focal leukoencephalopathy in chronic lymphatic leukemia—caused by polyoma virus? Scand J Haematol 7:184, 1970.

143. Reardon, G, Moloney WC: Chloroma and related myeloblastic neoplasms. Arch Intern Med 108:864, 1961.

144. Von Recklinghausen, FD: Chloroma. Versamml Dtsch Natur und Aerzte. 58:241, 1885.

145. Resnick ME, Berkowitz RD, Rodman T: Diffuse interstitial leukemic infiltration of the lungs producing the alveolar-capillary block syndrome. Am J Med 31:149, 1961.

146. Richardson EP Jr: Progressive multifocal leukoencephalopathy. N Engl J Med 265:815, 1961.

147. Rice MS, Murphy ML: Different neurologic syndromes in acute leukemia, lymphosarcoma and reticulum cell sarcoma in childhood. Proc Am Assoc Cancer Res 8:56, 1967.

148. Roberts WC, Bodey GP, Wertlake PT: The heart in acute leukemia. A study of 420 autopsy cases. Am J Cardiol 21:388, 1968.

149. Rolleston HD, Fox W: A case of atypical myeloid leukaemia with nodular infiltration of the skin. Br J Dermatol 21:377, 1909.

150. ———, Frankau CHS: Acute leukaemia simulating caries of the spine. Lancet 1:173, 1914.

151. Rosenblath W: Ueber Chlorom u. Leukämie. Dtsch Arch Klin Med 72:1, 1902.

152. Ross RR: Chloroma and chloroleukemia. Am J Med 18:671, 1955.

153. Rowe SN: Mikulicz's syndrome with chronic lymphatic leukemia. N Engl J Med 202:863, 1930.

154. Sauer C: Ein Beitrag zur Kenntniss der Chlorome. Virchows Arch pathol Anat 215:341, 1914.

155. Schaffer AJ, Jacobson AW: Mikulicz's syndrome. A report of ten cases. Am J Dis Child 34:327, 1927.

156. Schultz J, Schwartz S: The chemistry of experimental chloroma. II. Isolation of crystalline protoporphyrin, its origin and relation to other porphyrins. Cancer Res 16:565, 1956.

157. ———, Shay H, Gruenstein M: The chemistry of experimental chloroma. I. Porphyrins and peroxidases. Cancer Res 14:157, 1954.

158. Schwab RS, Weiss S: The neurologic aspect of leukemia. Am J Med Sci 189:766, 1935.

159. Scutt R: Bullous lesions in leukaemia. Br Med J 1:139, 1952.

160. Seemann G, Sajzewa A: Ein Fall von

Chloromyelose mit ungewöhnlicher Eosinophilie. Folia Haematol 37:258, 1928.

161. Shanbrom E, Finch SC: The auditory
manifestations of leukemia. Yale J Biol
Med 31:144, 1958.

162. Shaw RK, Moore EW, Freireich EJ,
Thomas LB: Meningeal leukemia. A syndrome resulting from increased intracranial
pressure in patients with acute leukemia.
Neurology 10:823, 1960.

163. Shilling BB, Abell MR, Work WP:
Leukemic involvement of the larynx. Arch
Otolaryngol 85:658, 1967.

164. Silverman FN: The skeletal lesions in
leukemia. Clinical and roentgenographic observations in 103 infants and children, with a
review of the literature. Am J Roentgenol
Radium Ther Nucl Med 59:819, 1948.

165. ――――: Treatment of leukemia and allied
disorders with folic acid antagonists: Effect
of aminopterin on skeletal lesions.
Radiology 54:665, 1950.

166. Simmons CR, Harle TS, Singleton EB: The
osseous manifestations of leukemia in
children. Rad Clin N Am 6:115, 1968.

167. Stefanini M, Allegra S: Pulmonary
mucormycosis in acute histiocytic leukemia. N Engl J Med 256:1026, 1957.

168. Stephens PTJ, Hudson P: Spontaneous
rupture of the spleen in plasma cell
leukemia. Can Med Assoc J 100:31, 1969.

169. Stites TB, Ultmann JE: Spontaneous
rupture of the spleen in chronic lymphocytic
leukemia. Cancer 19: 1587, 1966.

170. Sullivan MP: Intracranial complications in
leukemia. Pediatrics 20:757, 1957.

171. ――――: Leukemic infiltration of meninges
and spinal nerve roots. Pediatrics 32:63,
1963.

172. Summers JE, Johnson WW, Ainger LE:
Childhood leukemic heart disease. A study
of 116 hearts of children dying of leukemia.
Circulation 40:575, 1969.

173. Taylor HK: Periosteal changes in case of
lymphocytic leukemia. Radiology 6:523,
1926.

174. Thomas LG, Forkner CE Jr, Frei E III,

Besse BF, Stabenau JR: The skeletal lesions
of acute leukemia. Cancer 14:608, 1961.

175. Trömner E, Wohlwill F: Über Erkrankungen des Nervensystems, insbeson-
dere der Hirnnerven, bei Leukämie. Dtsch Z
Nervenheilkd 100:233, 1927.

176. Wagner ML, Rosenberg HS, Fernbach DJ,
Singleton EB: Typhlitis: A complication of
leukemia in childhood. Radiology 109:341,
1970.

177. Wahl HR, Hill JH: Gastric lesions in Hodg-
kins' disease and leukemia. Am J Pathol
32:235, 1956.

178. Ward HN, Konikov N, Reinhard EH:
Cytologic dysplasia occurring after
busulfan (Myleran) therapy. Ann Intern
Med 63:654, 1965.

179. Warthin AS: Death due to leukaemic
infiltration of the larynx; priapism persistent post mortem, myeloid thromboses in
the corpora cavernosa: Fatal hemorrhage
from spleen after prolonged radiotherapy.
Int Clin (19th series) 4:280, 1909.

180. Wendkos MH: Leukemic pericarditis. Am
Heart J 22:417, 1941.

181. Wetherley-Mein G, Cottom DG: Portal
fibrosis in acute leukaemia. Br J Haematol
2:345, 1956.

182. Wiernik PH, Serpick AA: Granulocytic sarcoma (chloroma). Blood 35:361, 1970.

183. Williams HM, Diamond HD, Craver LF:
The pathogenesis and management of neurological complications in patients with malignant lymphomas and leukemia. Cancer
11:76, 1958.

184. Williams RS: Triamcinolone myopathy.
Lancet 1:698, 1959.

185. Willson JKV: The bone lesions of childhood
leukemia. A survey of 140 cases. Radiology
72:672, 1959.

186. Windholz F, Foster SE: Bone sclerosis in
leukemia and in nonleukemic myelosis. Am
J Roentgenol Radium Ther Nucl Med
61:61, 1949.

187. Zampori O, Almici C: Les manifestations
pulmonaires leucémiques. Presse Med
66:1685, 1958.

III

Clinical and Laboratory Features

10

Clinical and Laboratory Features
of the Leukemias

This chapter deals with both the clinical and laboratory features of the leukemias. For ease of reading and reference, the clinical and laboratory aspects are discussed in two consecutive sections, first, for the leukemias in general, and then separately for each of the main kinds. In actual practice, whether for diagnostic or other purposes, it is rarely possible to accept even that degree of separation of the clinical and laboratory aspects. Nor does consideration necessarily proceed in that sequence. The diagnostic possibility of leukemia may first be raised by a chance finding in a laboratory test undertaken for some quite different reason. In such a case, and in others, there may be a complete absence of positive clinical findings, in history or on examination. Nevertheless, although laboratory findings are usually the more important in the leukemias, the clinical and laboratory features can never be considered separately, nor necessarily in the conventional order. In all cases, and especially in the presence of diagnostic uncertainty, the clinical findings may have to be considered in regard to their compatibility with the laboratory findings, and not just at one point in the natural history of the disease. For these reasons, a rigid separation of clinical and laboratory aspects is not desirable and is not intended in this chapter, even at the cost of some repetition. Similarly, since understanding of many clinical features depends on an appreciation of the underlying pathology, there must be some overlap with the content of Chapter 9, where the pathology of the leukemic tissue is discussed in detail.

It is less common than it once was to regard the leukemias as variants of a single disease in accordance with some kind of unitarian theory. This was an understandable attitude when greatest emphasis was placed on an elevated peripheral blood leukocyte count with immature leukocytes, and some common clinical features at diagnosis. A few specific or semispecific laboratory findings, a better appreciation of natural history, and, above all, major differences in response to very different forms of treatment, all make it desirable to regard the leukemias as several distinct diseases with some features in common. Before considering these common features it is as well to recognize some areas of special difficulty in the classification, differentiation, and diagnosis of the leukemias. Most of these difficulties arise from either a lack of specific laboratory findings or from the occurrence of a continuous spectrum of cases between two clearly distinct extremes, the extremes being currently accepted as representing two different disease entities. These nosological dilemmas are no more common in the leukemias than in other diseases of imperfectly understood etiology such as glomerulonephritis, chronic hepatitis, or the so-called collagen diseases. Some of the special problems arising in the leukemias are discussed in greater detail in Chapters 3, 6, and 11.

In a proportion of cases of acute leukemia in both children and adults it may be impossible to decide whether the leukemic cells arise from the granulocytic, lymphocytic, or other recognizable cell-line. The mere assignment of these cases to a stem cell or undifferentiated category is of doubtful advantage. In children, such cases may show the nuclear reactions of lymphocytic cells when examined for aryl sulphatase-positivity.[189] In children and adults, when differentiation is not possible, a better guide to prognosis and treatment may be the patient's age (Chapter 19), assuming the younger to be lymphocytic and the older nonlymphocytic. Epidemiologic studies suggesting that undifferentiated cases in childhood have a significantly worse prognosis than those of lymphocytic type[144] have not yet been confirmed as to their full significance for prognosis and treatment. In other cases it may, in the short run, be impossible to distinguish between aplastic anemia with some abnormal cells in the peripheral blood or marrow, and acute leukemia in the subleukemic or so-called aleukemic phase.[287] This difficulty is usually resolved by repeated studies at varying time-intervals, while reserving diagnosis and limiting treatment to supportive measures appropriate to both disorders. Obviously, in that particular dilemma the mere presence of some clinical features of acute leukemia may resolve the problem. Thus, lymphadenopathy, splenomegaly, or bone pain would suggest a diagnosis of acute leukemia, despite equivocal findings in blood and bone marrow.

LEUKEMOID REACTIONS

Apart from these special diagnostic problems in relation to the acute leukemias, there are many diseases in which the peripheral blood findings, and even the bone marrow, may suggest acute leukemia. In infectious mononucleosis at all ages; and in other viral infections, especially in children, leukemoid peripheral blood findings may occur. It is less common in these infections to find concomitant anemia or thrombocytopenia, still less common to have bone marrow findings of leukemia, and rare that the clinical features should be consonant with leukemia. In these and similar diagnostic problems involving acute leukemia, the suggestive evidence is usually found in the peripheral blood. All other features of the case, clinical and other, should then be considered, taking into account, if possible, any changes in the positive evidence which occur over a period of time. If this is done it will commonly be found that the sum of the evidence falls short of reasonable diagnostic certainty, especially if both positive and negative evidence is considered. Because of the nature of current therapy in acute leukemia a degree of diagnostic accuracy approaching certainty is desirable. Nevertheless, no system of discriminant analysis analogous to those used in suspected thyrotoxicosis and hypothyroidism[92,305] has been devised for the diagnosis of acute leukemia.

Similar problems arise less commonly than they once did from leukemoid reactions secondary to syphilis, tuberculosis, and pyogenic infections, but the earlier literature of leukemia includes many interesting examples.[143] The problems may be formidable or even insoluble at a particular time. Two useful principles should be followed where clinical and hematologic evidence falls short of reasonable diagnostic certainty. First, where another disorder is obvious such as infection,[285,293] bone marrow recovery from depression, or even megaloblastic anemia,[264,349,381] the evidence for coexisting leukemia should be viewed with special reserve. Second, in these and other conditions the progressive features usual in acute leukemia are commonly lacking. Accordingly, repeated clinical and hematologic examination over a period of time may resolve the diagnostic problem. This is especially true of the leukemoid blood picture in myelofibrosis: here, the clinical and hematological findings may remain unchanged over many years.

Not all the diagnostic problems arise in relation to acute leukemia but these are considered in greater detail below. Leukemoid peripheral blood pictures, simulating in some measure chronic granulocytic leukemia, may arise in myelofibrosis and polycythemia vera, especially after splenectomy, as well as in certain infections. Conventional bone marrow examination is only rarely of great discriminatory value in these problems. Marrow cytology does not differ significantly in the more difficult cases; and myelofibrosis, making marrow examination difficult or impossible, may occur in all three diseases. The alkaline phosphatase activity of peripheral blood neutrophils (NAP) is more useful and the discovery of the Philadelphia chromosome (Ph[1]) has added a new specific diagnostic criterion for chronic granulocytic leukemia. In one patient of our own, the peripheral blood picture simulated chronic granulocytic leukemia so closely as to be unexceptionable. The NAP was high and the Ph[1] was not present. Subsequent events revealed lymphosarcoma with a remarkable granulocyte response to bone marrow involvement, including the spectrum of granulocytes, from blast cell to mature polymorph, so suggestive of chronic granulocytic leukemia.

Relatively fewer diagnostic problems arise in relation to chronic lymphocytic leukaemia. When they do, they are generally of two kinds. A chance finding of minimal lymphocytosis in peripheral blood may raise the question of the diagnosis, yet the number and normal appearance of bone marrow lymphocytes may not be decisive. There is in chronic lymphocytic leukemia no specific criterion like the Ph[1] in chronic granulocytic leukemia, or semispecific finding like the blast cells of acute leukemia. More useful diagnostic criteria than any now available may be provided by the current studies on the different B and T components of the lymphocytic population in chronic lymphocytic leukemia. At present, this is not an urgent need since treatment of the disease is such that patients with equivocal findings are commonly not regarded as being in need of treatment. The same is true of the second diagnostic difficulty in relation to the chronic lymphocytic form. In some patients with minimal involvement of the blood and bone marrow it may be impossible to decide between chronic lymphocytic leukemia and lymphocytic lymphosarcoma (see Chapter 12). Lymph node histology is of no value in distinguishing between the two conditions, if, indeed, they are two separate conditions. Fortunately, these dilemmas rarely give rise to serious problems in management. Current treatment of the two conditions is not radically different (Chapter 18). The only difficulty arises from the fact that, while it is acceptable current practice to leave untreated an asymptomatic case of chronic lymphocytic leukemia, lymphosarcoma with or without symptoms is regarded as calling for treatment. More recently, this conservative management of early chronic lymphocytic leukemia has properly been questioned.[151]

CLINICAL FEATURES OF THE LEUKEMIAS

Most of the clinical features common to all the leukemias are dependent on the basic features of the diseases—interference with normal production of erythrocytes, leukocytes, and platelets; and the increased mass of tissue in the bone marrow and at other sites. Anemia, neutropenia, and thrombocytopenia are, respectively, the principal determinants of malaise, infection, and hemorrhage as presenting symptoms. The increased mass of hematopoietic tissue readily accounts for the splenomegaly, hepatomegaly, lymphadenopathy, tumors at other sites, and bone pain which may be the first detectable manifestations of the disease. The associated metabolic changes—including the common increase in basal metabolic rate (Chapter 14)—are less well understood. In the leukemias, as in other neoplastic diseases, metabolic changes may account for the common presenting symptoms of undue tiredness or nonspecific malaise, even in the absence of anemia or infection.

The problems of preleukemic states are different in each of the leukemias and so will be dealt with later. Nevertheless, it may be pointed out here that, as discussed in Chapter 5, the development of leukemia is a multistage process. It is likely that the progression through the different stages goes on at different rates in individual patients. If this is so, an immediately preleukemic stage of relatively longer duration might account, not only for the hematologic findings of the preleukemic syndrome, but also for otherwise unexplained prodromal symptoms in some patients.

The Onset of Leukemia

This may be abrupt or insidious, clearly dependent on the progress of the disease or apparently precipitated by intercurrent illness. Failure to recover from some infection is a common occurrence leading to diagnosis in all forms of leukemia, especially chronic lymphocytic and acute leukemia in children. In general, the rate of evolution of the clinical and hematologic picture is more rapid in acute leukemias of all kinds, and less so in the chronic disorders. There are some exceptions to this rule, notably those cases of chronic granulocytic leukemia presenting only at the stage of metamorphosis or acute transformation, the whole of the chronic phase having been silent.[150,307]

A history of recent malaise or tiredness may be obtained only in retrospect when the patient has presented on account of some more compelling symptom or dramatic occurrence. Such a history may be obtained in all forms of leukemia at diagnosis. It is generally of longer duration in the elderly with acute leukemia,[177] than in children. Manifestations referable to anemia, either by way of symptoms or unusual pallor, are the commonest features of the leukemias at diagnosis. Next most common is hemorrhage, which is usually, but not invariably, due to thrombocytopenia (see Chapter 14). In one series of 480 cases of acute leukemia of all ages, hemorrhage was a presenting feature in 15 percent of the patients.[351] Hemorrhage or bruising was the principal presenting symptom in 16 percent of a series of cases of acute leukemia in childhood.[421] In yet another series, mostly of adults, 73.3 percent of the acute and 31.2 percent of the chronic cases had hemorrhage at some stage, if not at diagnosis.[237]

Hemorrhages usually take the form of purpura or ecchymoses, and bleeding from mucous membranes. Of the latter, epistaxis is most common, followed by bleeding from gums, bronchial tree, gastrointestinal tract, or uterus. Subconjunctival hemorrhages are less common, and hematemesis and hematuria are relatively rare. In most cases where hemorrhage is obvious at other sites, retinal hemorrhages will be found on ophthalmoscopic examination. Rarely, presentation is due to sudden impairment of vision from massive retinal or vitreous hemorrhage. Hemorrhage into the middle or inner ear may determine the occurrence of deafness or tinnitus as initial manifestations.[387] In other cases, a diagnosis of leukemia may follow unexplained postoperative bleeding, occurring commonly after dental extraction[351] or tonsillectomy. Cerebral hemorrhage is less common as a presenting feature.

Reference has already been made to presentation with infection or because of failure of symptomatic recovery after infection. There seems little doubt that patients with leukemias are more prone to infections. This liability is probably related mainly, if not wholly, to neutropenia, and bacterial infections are most common at presentation. There seems to be a special liability in all forms of leukemia to typical and atypical infection with the virus of herpes simplex.[303] Typical herpes zoster is common in chronic lymphocytic leukemia but rare in the acute and chronic granulocytic forms.[373] Later in the course of the disease other viral infections including infectious mononucleosis, and mycoses may occur, but these are rare as presenting manifestations.

Other Clinical Features

Splenomegaly. Splenomegaly is the rule in chronic granulocytic leukemia, usual in chronic lymphocytic leukemia, and present in only a proportion of cases of acute leukemia. Of these last, splenomegaly is relatively more common in acute lymphocytic leukemia in childhood and is found much less frequently in acute granulocytic leukemia in adults. In all forms of leukemia, but especially in the chronic granulocytic form, an enlarged spleen is liable to infarction giving rise to pleuritic-type pain, often referred to the left shoulder. Rarely, a friction rub may be audible on auscultation. Some splenic infarctions may be clinically silent, as is suggested by the frequent finding of old infarcts at necropsy in patients without a clinical history suggesting such events. Relatively silent infarction may account for the spleen which is transiently tender to palpation but not spontaneously painful. In other cases, such tenderness may be due to rapid enlargement of the organ with tension in the capsule. That this is at least a possible mechanism of splenic pain is suggested by the occasional occurrence of spontaneous splenic rupture.[342] This calamity, giving rise to abdominal pain and shock, more commonly results from trauma to the spleen.

Minor degrees of splenomegaly may be defined by a plain x-ray of the abdomen, even when it cannot be felt or even percussed with confidence, or, better still, it can be outlined by scanning, using a technetium colloid. In chronic lymphocytic and acute leukemias, splenomegaly is commonly but not invariably associated with palpable lymphadenopathy.

Hepatomegaly. This occurs in all kinds of leukemia but is more common and more marked in chronic granulocytic and lymphocytic forms at presentation, than it is in the acute leukemias. It rarely gives rise to symptoms of pain or tenderness, or evidence of hepatic dysfunction. If jaundice does occur, it is usually late in the course of the disease or indicative of symptomatic hemolytic anemia, especially in chronic lymphocytic leukemia. Portal fibrosis, too, (see Chapter 9) may occur late in the course of acute leukemia but apparently not at first presentation.

Renal involvement. This is common in all kinds of leukemia,[404] but only rarely gives rise to symptoms or functional impairment. Grossly enlarged kidneys may sometimes be palpable, and pressure from leukemic lymph nodes or other masses may lead to hydronephrosis.[323] Renal involvement in leukemia most often takes the form of asymmetrical but diffuse infiltration found at necropsy, but undetected in life. In 50 percent of cases of leukemia of all kinds, leukemic involvement of kidneys has been found.[75,237] Mild proteinuria is the commonest effect in life but occasionally chronic, or even acute renal failure may result.[179] Hematuria may occur as well, but is generally a late, rather than an early, phenomenon. It may depend on the presence of both thrombocytopenia and leukemic infiltration of the kidneys or urinary tract.

The most common and life-threatening renal complications of the leukemias arise not from direct leukemic involvement but from secondary metabolic consequences. Of these, the most common is due to increased uric acid excretion leading to uric acid calculi and even to uric acid nephropathy, resulting in acute or chronic renal failure. Acute renal failure is especially liable to occur from this cause during rapid dissolution of lymphoid masses by treatment.[243,394] It is not so well appreciated that the same complication may arise in the patient already in remission,[50] or even at presentation. The frequency of this complication has been greatly reduced by the prophylactic use of allopurinol.

Rarely, renal impairment in the leukemias may result from secondary amyloidosis in chronic lymphocytic leukemia or from hypercalcemia complicating chronic lymphocytic, chronic granulocytic, or acute lymphocytic leukemias.[21,208,238,308]

Recent interest in muramidase (lysozyme) levels in blood and urine in monocytic and myelomonocytic leukemia (see Chapter 14) has been followed by the detection of a hitherto unsuspected renal effect. It may well be common in those forms of acute leukemia. The effects are mainly tubular and may result in marked hypokalemia.[302] Glomerular impairment may also occur, with uremia.[336]

Lymphadenopathy. Usually detected by the patient, lymphadenopathy is a common presenting feature (Fig. 10-1.). It occurs most frequently in acute lymphocytic leukemia in children and in chronic lymphocytic leukemia but may be a presenting feature in any of the leukemias, except chronic granulocytic leukemia in the chronic phase. In acute leukemia in adults there is considerable variation in the reported frequency of lymphadenopathy, as well as of splenomegaly and hepatomegaly, at diagnosis. These differences are likely to be due to differences in criteria of enlargement as much as to differences in the age composition of the series. Older subjects[177] tend to have less organ enlargement than younger adults.[350] Where lymphadenopathy is found at any stage in the natural history of chronic granulocytic leukemia, it is the mark of metamorphosis, and some other evidence of that change—including the peripheral blood picture of acute transformation—will commonly be present. In all the leukemias lymphadenopathy is painless. Its occurrence and degree often suggest the diagnosis of chronic lymphocytic leukemia in adults or of the acute lymphocytic form in children, but these are never by

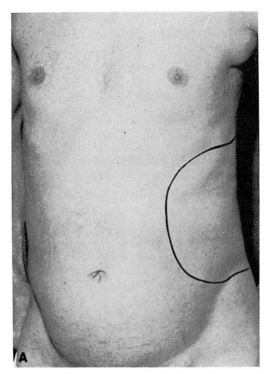

Fig. 10-1. A 53-year-old male with chronic lymphocytic leukemia. Note enlarged axillary lymph nodes and the outline of an enlarged spleen.

themselves diagnostic. In both conditions there is the expected correlation between the occurrence of lymph node enlargement and splenomegaly.

Bone pain.   Clinical features arising from expansion of the bone marrow mass are most common in acute leukemia in childhood. They may also occur in acute leukemia in adults, and in chronic granulocytic leukemia at metamorphosis,[14] with or without the peripheral blood findings of acute transformation. In childhood acute leukemia, involvement of bone or periosteum may account for a clinical picture at diagnosis which simulates rheumatic fever.[117,331] Less commonly, the bone and joint pains are localized to one or two joints.[117] Bone pain was a presenting symptom in 11 percent of cases of acute lymphocytic and undifferentiated acute leukemias, mainly in children.[351] In contrast, it was much less common in other varieties of acute leukemia, chiefly in older subjects. In another series of 50 cases of acute leukemia in children, bone pain was a principal presenting symptom in only two children.[421] We believe the frequency of this symptom at diagnosis of acute leukemia in children to have been overemphasized in the past. On the other hand, bone pain, sometimes severe, may occur in relapse without radiologic explanation.

Tenderness on fingertip pressure over the sternum has long been accepted as a valuable early sign in acute leukemia at all ages. The discerning physician knows to attach no significance to this when it can be elicited only over the lower sternum. Recently, after a systematic study, doubt has been cast on the value of this sign in leukemia.[273]

Extramyeloid tumors at presentation. As presenting symptoms, apart from lymphadenopathy, splenomegaly, hepatomegaly, and bone pain, clinical manifestations arising from extramyeloid proliferation of leukemic tissue are rare. The older literature[143] gives the impression that tumors at other sites were formerly much more common in the leukemias. This may well be fallacious, born of selective reporting and a greater interest in unusual clinical features when treatment was so unrewarding. Furthermore, it is obvious that all the leukemias were formerly diagnosed much later in their natural history; and only the chronic leukemias were greatly influenced by subsequent treatment. There are other difficulties in the assessment of the many older reports of unusual tumors or organ infiltrations in the leukemias. It is often impossible to establish the variety of the leukemia; and even more often the stage of the disease, early or terminal, is obscure. All these uncertainties are well exemplified by the difficulties in assessing the nature and frequency of neurologic involvement in the leukemias in the recent past. This is of particular interest in view of the increased frequency of these complications in acute lymphocytic leukemia in children, and to a lesser extent in other forms of acute leukemia at all ages.

Nervous system. Obvious involvement of the nervous system by leukemia is rare at time of diagnosis. Some cases of acute leukemia in children and adults may present with cerebral hemorrhage, which may be fatal. Meningeal involvement was once thought to be rare in acute leukemia, but in recent years an increasing number of cases has been found in children. Its frequency is obviously related to the duration of the disease, and so to otherwise successful treatment. The clinical and laboratory features of neurologic involvement in acute lymphocytic leukemia in childhood are discussed below. Nevertheless, it must be pointed out here that it is more than likely that meningeal involvement by acute lymphocytic leukemia in childhood is common at diagnosis, despite the lack of obvious clinical indications.[446] It is at present standard clinical practice to assume meningeal involvement in acute lymphocytic leukemia in children and give appropriate "prophylactic" treatment (see Chapter 18). In the future, it may be of importance to detect and assess subclinical meningeal leukemia, rather than to assume its presence. Meningeal involvement remains rare in acute granulocytic leukemia in childhood, in all forms of acute leukemia in adults,[20] and in the chronic leukemias.[245]

Involvement of the nervous system by leukemia may take many forms other than meningeal leukemia. The first known account was by that remarkable man, Allan Burns, and was published in 1811.[61] His case is usually regarded as one of chloroma (see below), arising in the bones and dura of the skull. In general, neurologic complications in leukemia, apart from meningeal leukemia, are caused either by leukemic proliferation or by bleeding, leading to hematoma formation and pressure effects.[200,455] There are a surprisingly large number of reports of leukemic involvement of the spinal cord. In one collected series of instances of spinal epidural leukemia, it was the presenting manifestation in 28 of 42 cases, most but not all of them contained in reports published before treatment for acute leukemia became effective.[450] Progressive paraplegia was the commonest feature, preceded in half the cases by nerve root pain in the back or legs. In a minority, paraplegia with disturbance of the anal and urinary sphincters preceded root pain. About half the patients in this study had cranial nerve involvement as well.

Leukemic involvement of the nervous system may account for the clinical findings of meningitis, encephalitis, monoplegia, hemiplegia, paraplegia, convulsions, or involvement of either cranial or peripheral nerves, motor or sensory. The relatively uncommon hypothalamic syndrome in acute lymphocytic leukemia in childhood is discussed elsewhere (see Chapter 9).[6,22] At presentation all are more common in the acute form than in any other kind of leukemia. Even so, and before the increased incidence of neurologic complications in treated cases of acute leukemia in childhood became evident, Hayhoe[188] wrote, "Neurological complications, apart from those due to cerebral haemorrhage, are sufficiently rare in acute leukaemia for them to be reported as curiosities. An awareness of them is important but they are not likely to be met frequently."

That statement is more or less true of extramyeloid leukemic proliferation at other sites. All are rare at time of diagnosis and the site may determine their detection, by giving rise to a palpable tumor or by obvious interference with some body function.

Chloroma. Reference has already been made to the first description of chloroma by Allan Burns in 1811, giving rise in that case to neurologic manifestations.[61] As with so much of the earlier literature of leukemias, chloromas were admirably reviewed by Forkner in 1938.[143] Recently, there has been a revival of interest in chloroma.[251] This has been prompted by appreciation of its association with forms of acute leukemia other than the granulocytic form[279]; its occasional appearance years before blood or bone marrow evidence of acute leukemia; its relatively greater frequency in Africa and its similarity in this and in other respects with Burkitt's lymphoma. Forkner attributed the first appreciation of the association between the greenish tumors which constitute chloroma and acute leukemia to Dock.[113] The characteristics described were the greenish color of the tumors, obvious on section and fading on exposure, and the blood and bone marrow findings of acute leukemia, which it now seems may be present later rather than earlier in its course. Chloroma is more closely associated with acute granulocytic leukemia than with other forms, although apparently typical examples have been reported with the blood and bone marrow findings of acute monocytic leukemia[357] and acute myelomonocytic leukemia.[357] It is not clear what essential difference exists between typical cases and those distinguished only by the fact that the extramyeloid tumors lack the green color. These have been called myeloblastomas.[168,344] Like chloromas, they are usually associated with acute granulocytic leukemia and may be present at diagnosis of acute leukemia or appear later. It is said[168] that chloroma and myeloblastoma may coexist in the same patient. An especially high incidence of chloromatous and nonchloromatous tumors, commonly located about the orbit, has been reported from Uganda, in association with acute granulocytic leukemia,[105,419] from Egypt in association with it and the acute myelocytic form,[301] and most recently from Turkey, as a presenting feature in acute myelomonocytic leukemia[69]—all in children.

Chloromas, whether typical or atypical, occur most often in children and young adults; and in males more often than in females. The tumors may or may not be solitary. They have been described at many sites but seem to occur most commonly in the periosteum, especially in the periosteum in relation to the orbit and paranasal sinuses. At these sites, and where they occur as epidural or meningeal tumors,[90] they readily give rise to clinical manifestations, and thus may be the presenting feature leading to the diagnosis of acute leukemia. Chloromas also occur at other sites in bones and soft tissues. In bones, apart from those of the skull and vertebral column, they have a predilection for the ribs, sternum, and pelvis, but may also be found in the long bones. Chloromas of soft tissues have been reported in the thyroid, thymus, breasts, pancreas, liver, kidneys, spleen, lymph nodes, uterus, ovaries, testes, urinary bladder, gastrointestinal tract, and the bone marrow itself.[143]

The symptoms of chloroma are those of the underlying acute leukemia, with additional manifestations depending on the site(s) of the tumor. When these occur in internal organs such as liver or ovaries, they are commonly discovered only at necropsy. Their radiologic appearances in bones do not differ from those of nonchloromatous leukemic masses, or, indeed, from those of nonleukemic lesions such as secondary neuroblastoma or even osteomyelitis.[232] Biopsy of accessible lesions may be helpful in diagnosis in that it reveals both the suggestive, if not diagnostic, histology and, macroscopically, the greenish color of the freshly cut tumor. Nevertheless, in the blood and bone marrow, the critical diagnostic findings are usually those of acute leukemia.

Apparently indistinguishable tumors, lacking only the green coloration, may occur in acute lymphocytic leukemia in children[301] and in adults, and in the chronic granulocytic form at metamorphosis[70] but not in the chronic phase. In acute lymphocytic leukemia of childhood these nonchlorotic tumors seem to occur especially around the orbit but this is not so in the chronic granulocytic form.

Other extramyeloid tumors. As has been noted, the distribution of chloromatous and nonchloromatous leukemic tumors is difficult to establish because some manifest their presence more readily than others. It is now obvious that extramyeloid leukemia, whether discrete tumors or diffuse infiltration, is common and widespread, at least in acute leukemia. Until recently the extent of leukemia was of little real interest unless it gave rise to complications or, more particularly, to unusual clinical features. This is no longer so, if only because of the improved treatment of acute leukemia in childhood. There is a new interest in extramyeloid leukemia as an obstacle to effective treatment, or even cure. It is seen as constituting additional sites for attack by aggressive therapy; as pockets of potentially resistant disease, even when marrow remission has been induced; and later, as sites of recrudescence and bases for leukemic recolonization despite seemingly satisfactory remission maintenance.[391] This new interest in extramyeloid leukemia in relation to apparently successful treatment is discussed later (see Chapter 18).

Eye. Reference has already been made above to nonchloromatous leukemic tumors around the eye, with evidence of an especially high incidence in children with acute leukemia in Egypt,[301] Turkey,[69] and Uganda.[105] Although an apparent rarity elsewhere in the world, this mode of presentation has been reported in an infant with acute promyelocytic leukemia.[91] An orbital tumor not involving bone gave rise to proptosis. Before the diagnosis of acute leukemia was established the differential diagnosis included neuroblastoma and rhabdomyosarcoma.

Apart from hemorrhages of retina, vitreous, and conjunctiva, the commonest ocular lesion in the leukemias is choroidal infiltration. It rarely gives rise to clinical signs, either at presentation or later.[278] Although this occurs most often in acute leukemia it seems likely that the commonest, nonhemorrhagic, clinical feature involving the eye in leukemia is as part of Mikulicz's syndrome (Chapter 9). This is a painless swelling, commonly bilateral and symmetrical, involving the lacrimal and salivary glands. It occurs most often in chronic lymphocytic leukemia and lymphosarcoma but has been reported in the acute form as well.[370] Mikulicz's syndrome associated with leukemia or lymphosarcoma is to be distinguished from the idiopathic form of the syndrome which is relatively rare. In one series of 38 cases,[339] 24 were associated with leukemia. In recent years there has been an understandable tendency to confuse the syndromes of Mikulicz and Sjögren or to regard them as identical. In part, this arises from the association of both with malignant lymphomas of one kind or another.[198,413]

Other ophthalmologic manifestations of the leukemias include visual loss due to involvement of the optic nerve and ophthalmoplegia resulting from lesions of the third, fourth and sixth cranial nerves.

Ear. Auditory manifestations in the leukemias are common, but rarely obtrusive. Impaired hearing often passes undetected, especially if it is unilateral or occurs in an elderly patient. One study of a hundred consecutive cases of leukemia revealed auditory signs or symptoms in 32, and 27 of these were attributable to leukemia.[387] In six patients the auditory manifestations preceded the diagnosis of leukemia. The auditory complications were, in general, attributable to hemorrhage, infiltration, or infection. Hemorrhage occurred especially in acute leukemia, and infiltration in chronic lymphocytic leukemia, while infection was associated with all types. Such an incidence of auditory manifestations may seem surprisingly high, but in another review of 148 patients, 25 had symptoms related to the ear.[120]

An appeal has recently been made[253] for the closer study and reporting of cases of leukemia with involvement of the inner ear: correlation of clinical findings and histology at necropsy may improve knowledge of the function of the inner ear.

Larynx and pharynx. Laryngeal manifestations in leukemia have not been reported other than as late features of the disease. Aphonia from pressure on the recurrent laryngeal nerve may occur in chronic lymphocytic leukemia with mediastinal lymphadenopathy. More often, aphonia is caused by laryngeal infiltration or ulceration in the later stages of acute leukemia.[217] When this occurs, laryngeal involvement is rarely isolated and other oropharyngeal and respiratory tract disease is usually obvious. It has been suggested that laryngeal infiltration may be more frequent and extensive in the acute granulocytic than in the acute lymphocytic form.[372] Tracheostomy may be needed. Aphonia in leukemia—especially acute leukemia and the later stages of chronic lymphocytic and granulocytic leukemias—should not be carelessly ascribed to candidiasis, even if it also is present.

Oropharyngeal lesions of one kind or another were presenting manifestations in 13 percent of a series of 580 AL patients.[351] They were relatively most common in acute "monocytic" leukemia (29 percent), least common in acute lymphocytic leukemia (5 percent). It is our experience that acute monocytic leukemia is often diagnosed by dentists on the finding of gingival swelling (Fig. 10-2). This remarkable feature is commonest in this form of AL but may also occur in other varieties. It may be confused with gingival hypertrophy caused by the use of hydantoins to control epilepsy, but bleeding and other features do not accompany the drug effect. Apart from bleeding and swollen gums, buccal and pharyngeal ulceration may also

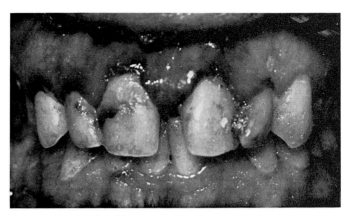

Fig. 10-2. Gingival swelling in acute leukemia.

occur in the acute form. Tonsillar enlargement may occur in chronic lymphocytic and acute leukemia, especially of the lymphocytic variety. With the exception of tonsillar enlargement in the former, usually without infection or ulceration, oropharyngeal involvement occurs in the chronic leukemias only at the stage of metamorphosis in chronic granulocytic leukemia, or as candidiasis.

Nasal infiltration and obstruction. This is a rare manifestation which does occur in acute leukemia. In one patient it was a presenting manifestation.[367]

Gastrointestinal tract. With the exception of lesions of mouth, esophagus, and the anorectal region, leukemic involvement of the alimentary system giving rise to symptoms has attracted relatively little attention. This is probably because such symptoms usually occur shortly before death, when the clinical picture may be dominated by anemia, bleeding, or infection. Gastrointestinal symptoms must be rare as presenting manifestations in all the leukemias, in contrast to their frequency in lymphosarcoma. The frequency of both leukemic and nonspecific lesions at necropsy has been described in Chapter 9. In one series of 264 patients seen at necropsy, 39 had gross leukemic lesions and 49 had nonleukemic lesions of the gastrointestinal tract.[84] In life, the clinical diagnoses for these patients included peptic ulcer, gastric carcinoma, typhoid, ulcerative colitis and carcinoma of the rectum. Thirty-six patients had massive bleeding from the gastrointestinal tract, which was the immediate cause of death in twenty. In two others, death was due to intestinal perforation. In this series, leukemic gastrointestinal lesions at necropsy were twice as frequent in acute leukemias of all kinds than they were in chronic granulocytic or lymphocytic leukemias.

Esophageal lesions. Such lesions are common in all forms of leukemia, occurring late in the disease but not at presentation. Most are due to candidiasis giving rise to dysphagia and retrosternal pain. In some patients, candidiasis may not be evident elsewhere and the diagnosis is thus not made in life. Esophageal ulceration without candidiasis may also occur. Microscopic infiltration of the esophagus is relatively common in acute leukemias, but only rarely gives rise to gross lesions and clinical manifestations.[160]

Perianal and anorectal lesions. These have recently attracted a great deal of attention, and it seems likely that a real increase in incidence has occurred.[374] In recognized cases of acute leukemia these usually occur as perianal abscesses, sometimes with fistula in ano or anal fissure.[384] Anorectal abscess may also occur as a presenting manifestation in acute leukemia.[350,437] As complications in diagnosed cases, they are much more common in acute than in either chronic granulocytic or lymphocytic forms. They are especially liable to occur in cases classified as acute "monocytic" leukemia and acute myelomonocytic leukemia. It remains uncertain whether the infection arises in an area of leukemic infiltration or is merely a special local manifestation of a general liability to infection, consequent upon neutropenia. A considerable proportion of the patients have preexisting anal or rectal lesions unrelated to leukemia. Some have symptoms such as constipation, diarrhea or gastrointestinal hemorrhage, suggesting infection or leukemic infiltration above the anorectal region.

Local treatment of these anorectal abscesses is a debatable subject. As with all infections in leukemia, the first consideration is to induce remission of the leukemia if the patient is in relapse. If possible, incision and drainage of any abscess should be postponed until remission has been induced.

The heart and pericardium. The occurrence of diffuse and focal infiltration of the myocardium is discussed in Chapter 9. The reported frequency at necropsy in adults and children with acute leukemia ranges from 30–44 percent.[213,237,352,411] Clinical manifestations in these cases were infrequent and inconspicuous. The most common was the occurrence of cardiac hypertrophy and decompensation, although observations differ inexplicably on this point.[352,411] Those who find cardiac hypertrophy relate its occurrence, at least in childhood acute leukemia, to anemia of long standing. Leukemic infiltration in children at necropsy is apparently more common in acute granulocytic leukemia, and is directly related to the peripheral blood leukocyte count. It is obviously difficult to separate these associations from the lesser efficacy of treatment in acute granulocytic leukemia than in acute lymphocytic leukemia. Electrocardiographic changes in life are frequent but minor and mostly nonspecific in nature. Changes indicative of focal myocardial damage are rare in relation to its occurrence at necropsy. Evidence of left ventricular hypertrophy is more frequent, as are nonspecific ST-segment and T-wave changes.

Understandably, leukemic infiltration of the myocardium in acute leukemia does not give rise to cardiac manifestations at diagnosis. In contrast, pericardial involvement may be responsible for the presenting symptoms of AL in children and in adults.[23,210,352] The clinical picture may be that of pericarditis with typical chest pain, or of pericardial tamponade.

Secondary infection as a cause of cardiac complications in the leukemias has recently been emphasized.[7] Septic myocarditis with frank abscesses may occur, as well as infective endocarditis from gram-positive and -negative organisms, or fungi. These findings are rarely diagnosed in life, presumably because the clinical picture at the time of their occurrence is dominated by more conspicuous terminal features.

Reference is made elsewhere (Chapters 9 and 17) to iatrogenic cardiac complications following the use of daunorubicin in the treatment of acute leukemia. Arrhythmias, congestive cardiac failure, and myocardial infarction may occur in patients who receive more of the drug than 35 mg per kg of body weight, however the dose may be fractionated. Cardiac complications are more likely to occur in the elderly treated with daunorubicin.[33] It is not known whether the occurrence of these complications is related to the presence of previously silent leukemic involvement of the myocardium.

Cardiac involvement of a quite different kind occurs as a feature of that debatable entity, eosinophilic leukemia.[459] The rarity of this disease and the variation among patients makes generalizations about it hazardous, and dogmatic statements unjustified. It is discussed more fully later (page 340), especially its relationship to chronic granulocytic leukemia. Whatever their relationship or its status as a leukemia, there can be no doubt about a very special association between marked blood and bone marrow eosinophilia and mural thrombi or endomyocardial fibrosis.[27,226,352] In some patients the cardiac manifestations predominate and they are regarded as instances of primary cardiac disease such as Loffler's fibroplastic parietal endocarditis,[270] or Davies's endomyocardial fibrosis with blood and bone marrow eosinophilia.[106] In others, a primary diagnosis of eosinophilic leukemia is made and evidence of cardiac involvement, even at necropsy, may be no more than is to be expected in acute leukemia.[26] Its clinical and laboratory features and course may suggest acute leukemia[26,459]: in other cases the course is longer and the disease may simulate a variant of the chronic granulocytic form—as some cases may indeed be. The clinical features at presentation are frequently those of congestive cardiac failure, as well as tachycardia, arrhythmias, cardiomegaly, murmurs, and a gallop rhythm.

Cardiac involvement in chronic lymphocytic leukemia and typical chronic granulocytic leukemia is obviously rare. In both diseases it must be much more common as a finding at necropsy than as a lesion giving rise to clinical manifestations.[38,213,412] The unresolved questions of eosinophilic leukemia and cardiac disease have been mentioned above. Consideration of the few published reports of chromosome studies in eosinophilic leukemia are inconclusive. Five such cases seem to have been described.[136,164,174,242] The Philadelphia chromosome (Ph¹) has been found in one patient in whom cardiac disease did not occur: of the four Ph¹-negative patients, two had cardiac disease[242] and two did not.[164]

The bronchi and lungs.   Leukemic infiltration of the respiratory tissues is certainly to be found at necropsy,[7] but clinical expression of this usually takes the form of resulting infection, infarction, or hemorrhage. Rarely, extensive infiltration in chronic lymphocytic leukemia may give rise to alveolar-capillary block as in the Hamman-Rich syndrome, and findings of pulmonary alveolar proteinosis have been noted at necropsy.[7]

It seems unlikely that significant lung changes occur in CGL in the chronic phase of granulocytic leukemia, except after treatment with busulfan. This is expressed as pulmonary fibrosis, again simulating the Hamman-Rich syndrome, as judged by clinical and radiologic criteria, as well as on tests of respiratory function. This syndrome seems to depend on busulfan-induced changes in bronchial mucosa and alveoli. Similar changes have been found at necropsy in the pancreatic acini of busulfan-treated subjects, but without any disorder of pancreatic function having been noted during the patient's lifetime.[236]

The thymus.   There have been many reports of acute leukemia coexisting with significant thymic enlargement in both children and adults. In some cases upper mediastinal obstruction or radiologic detection of a mediastinal mass has led to the diagnosis of leukemia.[8] In other cases, thymoma has manifested itself clinically, only after leukemia has been diagnosed and treated. In all the cases reported, the leukemia has been acute, and in most, but not all, clearly lymphocytic in type. It is not possible to distinguish those rare cases from the generality of acute leukemia, except as regards the thymic involvement. The relationship of the two is obscure but it seems likely, despite the role of the thymus in some animal leukemias, that thymic involvement in man is no more significant than the occasional leukemic enlargement of other extramyeloid tissues.

Breast. Leukemic infiltration of the female breast is another rare feature of acute leukemia. It has been the presenting manifestation in several reported cases,[41] in addition to one of our own patients. The associated leukemias have been described as lymphocytic[233] and granulocytic.[168] Most of the patients have been postpubertal, but one instance in an infant has been reported as well.[216] The breast tumors may simulate a breast abscess or carcinoma, but bilateral involvement may suggest the true diagnosis.

Gonadal involvement. Infiltration of testes and ovaries has been reported in acute leukemia,[7,168] but not as presenting manifestations. There seem to be no special liability to early involvement of the gonads such as exists in Burkitt's lymphoma in children.[60] Nevertheless, testicular infiltration occurring during blood and bone marrow remission in children with acute lymphocytic leukemia has recently attracted attention.[138,259,282] In some cases it has been detected clinically as a unilateral testicular tumor, but needle biopsy of the apparently unaffected testis has shown leukemic infiltration. Some of the patients with appreciable testicular tumors have been long-term survivors, so that testicular infiltration may be a very important example of residual disease.

Priapism. Usually attributed to thrombosis or stasis in the corpus cavernosum, priapism has long been recognized as a painful and distressing feature of chronic granulocytic leukemia. It is probably much less common than the number of case reports would suggest. Although apparently more common in this form of leukemia, it has also been reported in the chronic lymphocytic form,[87] and in acute leukemia.[209] It has been described in prepubertal CGL and AL patients[171,209,434]; and as a presenting manifestation in both diseases. If simpler measures fail, and leukemic remission cannot be induced quickly, local radiotherapy is the treatment of choice. Recently, there has been a favorable account of the use of the defibrinating agent ancrod, with success in 50 percent of patients.[328] Since the agent is not proteolytic it is believed that its favorable effect in leukemic priapism results from an alteration in blood viscosity.

Skin manifestations. Undoubtedly, the commonest skin manifestations in all the leukemias are hemorrhages. The most common single factor in their causation is thrombocytopenia (Chapter 14). They vary from petechial spots, through purpura and ecchymoses to subcutaneous hematomas. In addition, patients with leukemia are liable to the whole range of cutaneous drug eruptions since they usually receive antileukemic drugs during most of their life after diagnosis, as well as other agents for hyperuricemia, pain, anxiety, infection, and cardiac decompensation. They are at least as liable as others to skin disorders unrelated to either leukemia or drug therapy. It is our experience and that of others[221] that most skin rashes occurring in patients with leukemias are not related to the leukemia, are nonspecific, and usually transient. Nevertheless, the old terms *leukemic* and *leukemid* rashes persist, and are confusing and not especially useful. They should be abandoned. There is a special obstacle to our understanding of skin lesions in leukemia in that there is a reluctance to biopsy these lesions because of the risks of hemorrhage and infection. By analogy with what is now known about asymptomatic leukemic infiltration in other organs, it is likely that involvement of the skin—at least before treatment and in relapse—is much more common than the frequency of clinical manifestations would suggest.

Specific skin lesions of leukemia do occur and seem to depend in almost all cases on direct leukemic infiltration of the skin. They include pruritus, prurigo-like papules, erythrodermia, and tumors which range from minute, nonitchy papules (Fig. 10-3) to large, ulcerating masses. The lesions may arise at one site and spread, or be generalized from their first appearance. They may be presenting symptoms or appear only later, especially in relapse whether preterminal or not. In two very large series of AL patients of all ages,[50,351] skin rashes were present at diagnosis in 6 percent in both series. In one of these studies, an additional 2 percent of patients developed skin manifestations in their lifetime. Despite some differences between reported series,[50,351] cutaneous manifestations seem to be more common in acute "monocytic" leukemia, of all the varieties of acute leukemia. There may also be a relationship between incidence and age. In one series of children with acute leukemia skin infiltration was found at diagnosis in 2 of 50 patients: in comparison, it was present in 13 percent of a series of 97 patients, all over the age of 50.[177] This greater incidence in the elderly may be correlated with the type of acute leukemia which occurs in older people, rather than with age per se.

In the chronic leukemias, cutaneous manifestations of the leukemia occur in the granulocytic form only at the stage of metamorphosis, and even then they are

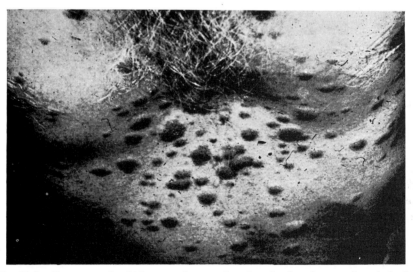

Fig. 10-3. Large papular lesions on the anterior chest in chronic granulocytic leukemia at metamorphosis (Courtesy of Dr. James F. Patterson, New England Center Hospital, Boston.)

rare in our experience. Skin lesions are much more common in the lymphocytic form. In that disease, pruritus may be the presenting complaint. Later in the course, multiple skin nodules—especially around the head and neck—and generalized erythrodermia (*l'homme rouge*) may occur. Mycosis fungoides (page 351) may rarely occur, although that puzzling condition is much more often associated with either Hodgkin's disease or reticulum cell sarcoma.

Patients with chronic lymphocytic leukemia are notoriously prone to herpes zoster (Fig. 10-4) which may be especially severe and associated with an unusual degree of general upset. In this connection it should be remembered that, except in

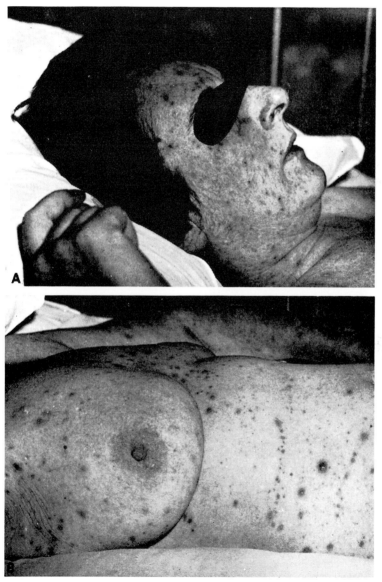

Fig. 10-4. Severe generalized herpes zoster with a varicelliform rash in a patient with chronic lymphocytic leukemia.

remission, all patients with acute leukemia and chronic lymphocytic leukemia have a special liability to infections, including those of the skin. In the treatment of cutaneous lesions in patients with leukemia, whether due to leukemic infiltration or not, the first object should be to induce hematologic remission.

The dermatologic manifestations of the leukemias have been reviewed in great detail by Bluefarb in his monograph, *Leukemia Cutis*.[45]

Course of the Leukemias

This remains extremely variable despite improvements in specific and nonspecific treatment. Some generalizations can be made for the individual diseases and these will be discussed later. It may, however, be said of all the leukemias that, in regard to course and median survival, the difference between the acute and chronic varieties is now much less than it once was. While treatment of the chronic disorders has made little progress recently, there have been major advances in the treatment of acute leukemia, especially the lymphocytic form in childhood. The median survivals of children with ALL and adults with CGL are now about equal, and their clinical courses less dissimilar.

Hemorrhage and anemia are now less important principal causes of death than they once were, mainly because of the availability of whole blood transfusion, and, more recently, of platelets. They remain important contributory causes, especially when death seems to result from a summation of adverse effects, usually including those of infection.[195] Anemia and hemorrhage being less important than they once were, infections are more important, despite greatly improved chemotherapy in infection. Patients may be longer at risk of infection; and iatrogenic neutropenia and immune suppression are now added to the naturally occurring neutropenia and immunological impairment of the leukemia.

The kinds of infection which beset the patient with leukemia have changed and seem likely to continue to do so.[263] Most occur in the untreated state, after treatment has begun but before remission is induced, or in relapse. Recently, there has been an increasing number of reports of fatal infections in acute leukemia in remission, especially in the childhood lymphocytic form. In one series, 5.2 percent of children died of infection while in hematologic remission.[393] Most of the infections were pneumonias, some viral, some fungal, and some bacterial. Immunosuppressive cytotoxic therapy, rather than granulocytopenia, seems to be the major determining factor. Infections with gram-positive organisms, particularly *Staphylococcus aureus,* are much less important than formerly. Gram-negative organisms are now more important, especially *Pseudomonas aeruginosa, Escherichia coli,* Proteus and Klebsiella. Of nonbacterial infections, candidiasis is the most common, with aspergillosis, mucormycosis, cryptococcosis, histoplasmosis, and infection with *Torulopsis glabrata* occurring less often.[49] Other infections reported with significant frequency in patients with leukemias include nocardiosis,[461] *Pneumocystis carinii,*[127,298] and *Listeria monocytogenes.*[48] Atypical mycobacterial infection,[276] *Aeromonas hydrophila* septicemia,[1] and generalized vaccinia[275,431] have also been described.

The most common forms of infection are pneumonia and septicemias, sometimes seen in conjunction with endocarditis, meningitis, and pyemic abscess formation. In one remarkable case of disseminated candidiasis, hypersplenism limiting remission in a patient with acute leukemia is said to have been cured by splenectomy, followed by treatment with amphotericin B.[47] The Budd-Chiari syndrome due to invasion of the hepatic veins by *Aspergillus* has been described.[462] Nevertheless, the lungs are probably the most important single site of infection in the leukemias, and the causal organism is commonly not identified in life.[49]

It has recently been suggested that leukemic patients with gram-negative septicemia are protected from the generalized Shwartzman reaction by their common neutropenia, granulocytes being essential for the reaction.[240] This deficiency is said to explain the absence of reports of disseminated intravascular coagulation in septicemia complicating acute leukemia.

Human cytomegalovirus has been isolated many times from children with acute leukemia,[10, 186, 206] but the infection seems to be asymptomatic and its significance is doubtful. In contrast, in adults with acute leukemia in remission, a syndrome has been described in which pyrexia and splenomegaly with atypical mononuclear cells in the peripheral blood appear.[231] Its occurrence has been associated with laboratory evidence of intercurrent infection with cytomegalovirus, toxoplasmosis, or infectious mononucleosis. This syndrome may obviously cause difficulties by suggesting recrudescence of the leukemia.

Reactivation of quiescent tuberculous infection may occur in the leukemias. This is especially liable to happen in older patients treated with corticosteroids in addition to other immunosuppressant agents.

Although catastrophic hemorrhage or overwhelming infection may still be immediate causes of death in the leukemias, they usually occur against a background of other hematologic, infective, or metabolic disorders. There is still room for further improvement in supportive therapy in the leukemias. Nevertheless, major improvements in survival and quality of life seem more likely to come from improved treatment of the leukemia itself, despite the disturbing reports of fatal infections in remission.

LABORATORY FEATURES OF THE LEUKEMIAS

The leukemias are differentiated by their laboratory features; accordingly, these findings are best discussed with regard to each kind of leukemia separately. Nevertheless, a few general principles may be stated. The relationship and relative places of clinical and laboratory findings have already been discussed (page 275). It cannot be said too often that examination of a well-made peripheral blood film stained by a Romanowsky stain is the most important single diagnostic tool in the leukemias. Nevertheless, the clinical features of the disease must also be considered, along with the other findings in the peripheral blood, and the bone marrow appearances. Bone marrow findings may be confirmative or even diagnostic in the acute leukemias and chronic lymphocytic leukemias: in the chronic granulocytic form the bone marrow appearances are seldom more than consistent with a diagnosis best made on the peripheral blood findings. Where doubts exist as to the significance or nature of abnormal cells in peripheral blood or bone marrow, repeated comparison of the two preparations with particular regard to any atypical cells is especially helpful. Where abnormal cells are few, or where diagnosis may depend on the occurrence of a spectrum of cells, the self-discipline of a differential leukocyte count is recommended. Account should be taken of the sampling error in making and spreading a blood film, and of the statistical aspect of differential leukocyte counts.[362] Where abnormal cells in the peripheral blood are few, their identification or characterization may be aided by examination of a buffy coat preparation.[96] Despite their usefulness in this regard, buffy coat preparations should not be allowed to give false impressions as to the relative numbers of any cells seen.

BONE MARROW BIOPSY

This procedure is essential in every case of leukemia or suspected leukemia. The marrow findings are always important, whether they are diagnostic as they often are in acute leukemia, or refutatory as in some leukemoid reactions. In the acute and chronic lymphocytic leukemias, the bone marrow appearances commonly have greater diagnostic value; in the chronic granulocytic form, commonly less. Even in the last disease, where diagnosis may seem certain on the clinical and peripheral blood findings, marrow examination should not be neglected. If diagnosis seems nearly certain on other grounds the bone marrow should nevertheless be studied critically, as to its consistency with the other findings. In addition, even if diagnosis is not in question, the results of marrow examination constitute part of the preliminary assessment of every case of leukemia. It is essential to know of other marrow changes which may coexist with leukemia, such as megaloblastic change, iron deficiency, marrow hypoplasia, or myelofibrosis. If a diagnosis of leukemia is in doubt, and a reversible marrow change such as iron deficiency or megaloblastic erythropoiesis is found, reassessment after treatment of the lesser disorder is often desirable. Although rarely of diagnostic primacy—except sometimes in chronic granulocytic leukemia—cytogenetic studies may be desirable (see Chapter 6) and are best carried out on bone marrow.

Apart from diagnosis, bone marrow findings are of increasing importance in acute and chronic lymphocytic leukemias for assessing the degree of leukemic involvement. This provides a useful baseline observation for comparison with findings during treatment (Chapter 18). Conversely, the proportion of normal marrow elements, megakaryocytes, erythrocyte and granulocyte precursors, may influence immediate treatment.

Marrow aspirate should be examined by all the basic methods in every case of leukemia—in trail preparations,[96] so-called squash preparations,[104] by embedding and sectioning of particles,[78] and staining for iron.[96] Failure to aspirate by a competent operator is itself significant. It may indicate myelofibrosis, increased cohesion of a marrow dominated by abnormal cells, or marrow changes consequent upon previous radiotherapy. If the marrow tap is not completely dry the best preparations possible be made of any marrow blood which may have to be forcibly expelled from the marrow needle. If a satisfactory marrow sample is not aspirated, trephine biopsy should be considered, especially if the diagnosis is in doubt or if chronic granulocytic leukemia is suspected. In our hands, the trephine described by Sacker and Nordin[365] has proved satisfactory.

Blast cells. In many ways the term *blast cell* is an unfortunate one, whether or not it is qualified by the adjective "leukemic." It implies an identity between leukemic cells and normal hematopoietic cells showing little or no differentiation. It also conveys to the inexperienced the idea that there are cells more or less specific for the acute leukemias and of primary diagnostic import in those diseases. In fact, as already pointed out, a diagnosis of acute leukemia must be made on all the clinical and hematological features, positive and negative. Clinical features may be nonspecific, or even totally absent in patients in whom a hematological abnormality is a chance finding. Even when abnormal cells, acceptable as leukemic, are present in both peripheral blood and bone marrow, a diagnosis of acute leukemia should be made only with care and reservation in the absence of anemia and thrombocytopenia, or of even one of these findings.

A leukemic blast cell is easily described as an undifferentiated cell which is usually of the same size or larger than normal peripheral blood lymphocytes or neutrophils (Fig. 10-5). The nuclear chromatin is commonly fine in pattern. Multiple, large nucleoli may be seen, even in the Romanowsky-stained preparation, although more readily with Chromotrope 2R and a Romanowsky stain.[158,366] The nuclear outline may be round or lobulated. Intermediate forms with shallow indentations or deep pseudoindentations—the Rieder cell—may occur in some cases. The nuclear-cytoplasmic ratio may be high as in acute lymphocytic leukemia or relatively low as in acute myelomonocytic leukemia, with acute granulocytic leukemia and erythroleukemia intermediate in this regard. The most important fact to emerge from such a description of the leukemic cell in acute leukemia is its nonspecificity and the range of possible appearances. This has already been mentioned in the discussion of leukemoid reactions. In some cases of acute leukemia of all varieties the leukemic cells may be indistinguishable from normal blood or bone marrow cells. When this is so they are *leukemic cells* only in the context in which they are seen and the term *blast cell* may be especially inappropriate. The whole subject of the morphology and cytochemistry of the acute leukemias was critically

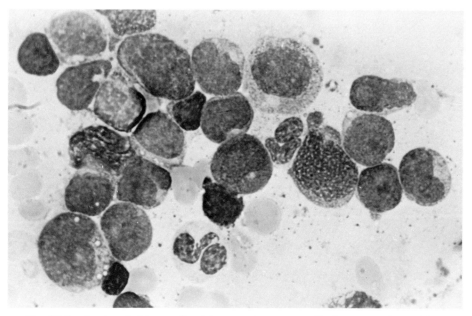

Fig. 10-5. Leukemic blast cells with normal marrow cells from a patient with acute myelomonocytic leukemia.

considered by Hayhoe, Quaglino, and Doll in 1964[191] (see Chapter 6). Since that date there have been advances in cytochemistry but these have had relatively little impact in practice. The morphology of blood and bone marrow cells, including leukemic cells, is considered in great detail by Miale.[288]

There are some other indications for a diagnosis of acute leukemia which may sometimes be seen on examination of Romanowsky-stained preparations of blood or bone marrow. Auer rods or bodies are apparently abnormal aggregations of peroxidase-positive granules occurring in leukemic cells which may or may not be otherwise recognizable as of the granulocyte series or, alternatively, of so-called myelomonocytes. In Romanowsky-stained preparations of blood and bone marrow they appear as red-stained rods. They seem to be specific for leukemic cells of acute granulocytic or acute myelomonocytic leukemia. Accordingly, especially in cases of diagnostic difficulty, they are worth searching for; and, since they may be infrequent, a prolonged and careful search for them is often required. They are sometimes very large inclusion bodies, round or oval in shape, but of the same staining reaction as the more typical rod forms. Of similar significance for a diagnosis of acute granu-locytic leukemia, is the rarer occurrence of the acquired Pelger anomaly (Fig. 10-6) of hyposegmentation of the granulocyte nucleus. When it does occur, it is usually much more readily detected than are Auer rods. It is rarely difficult to show by family studies or otherwise that this interesting abnormality is acquired and not inherited. When acquired it is commonly indicative of acute granulocytic leukemia, but not invariably so.[19,116] In acute granulocytic leukemia, the anomaly may be found, not only in obviously leukemic cells, but also in apparently normal mature granulocytes: the phenomenon may disappear in remission and reappear in re-lapse.[193] The acquired or pseduo-Pelger anomaly has also been described in

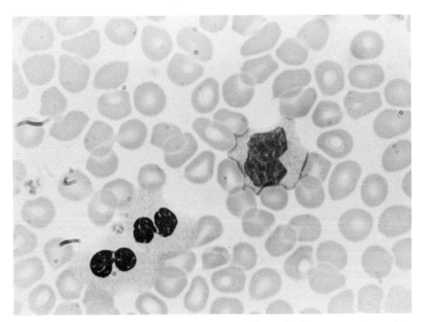

Fig. 10-6. Pseudo-Pelger cells with a leukemic cell from a patient with acute myelomonocytic leukemia.

chronic granulocytic leukemia, in nonleukemic myeloproliferative disorders, and in Fanconi's hypoplastic anemia.

Less specific indications of a possible diagnosis of acute leukemia include the occurrence of mitotic figures in the peripheral blood, and erythrophagocytosis by cells of the granulocytic or monocytic series in peripheral blood or bone marrow. When the presence of many smear cells, especially in the peripheral blood, is not explained by infection or technical shortcomings in making the preparations, acute or chronic lymphocytic leukemia may be suspected. Still less specific is the finding of many smear cells or damaged cells consisting of "naked nuclei" devoid of cytoplasm. These naked nuclei show a relatively structureless nuclear chromatin, often with the nucleoli especially obvious. They are more commonly derived from lymphocytes and monocytes, normal or leukemic, or from frankly leukemic blast cells than from apparently normal cells of the granulocyte series. Smear cells and naked nuclei are often seen in infections or can be accounted for by unsatisfactory methods of preparation of blood films. Where these explanations are not readily acceptable, the possibility of acute or chronic lymphocytic leukemia should be considered.

The name of Rieder cells has been given to both CLL lymphocytes and AGL leukemic cells of atypical nuclear form. In Rieder cells, a nucleus which is normally round or oval may show folding, indentation, cloverleaf form or pseudo-lobulation. An occasional cell of this kind is unlikely to be significant, but many such may suggest a leukemia.

In the chronic phase of chronic granulocytic leukemia the individual cells are indistinguishable from normal, whether in blood or bone marrow. The characteristic of the disease is the occurrence in the peripheral blood of a continuous spectrum of granulocytes from the most primitive to the mature polymorph. At this stage, too, many apparently normal basophils may occur. These cells are often poorly demonstrated in Romanowsky-stained preparations, the characteristic granules being dissolved out in fixation and staining.[300] After metamorphosis, the peripheral blood picture is especially variable and almost any of the described anomalies of leukocytes may occur.

The individual lymphocytes of chronic lymphocytic leukemia most commonly have the appearance of normal, small lymphocytes. Sometimes they are especially fragile and give rise to many smear cells or naked nuclei. Rarely, they are larger than normal lymphocytes, with relatively more cytoplasm, less condensed nuclear chromatin, and more obvious nucleoli. When of this appearance they may be mistaken for the leukemic cells of acute lymphocytic leukemia. This error is usually avoided by consideration of other features of the case, especially the age of the patient. Even typical chronic lymphocytic leukemia is excessively rare in childhood, and chronic lymphocytic leukemia with atypical cells in the peripheral blood does not occur. On the other hand, the development of acute lymphocytic leukemia in children previously diagnosed as having lymphosarcoma is well recognized.[284,410]

In a minority of adults with chronic lymphocytic leukemia, the leukemic cells in the peripheral blood have the appearance described above, in contrast to the small cell with little cytoplasm and pyknotic nuclear chromatin more commonly seen. Such cases have been described as chronic lymphosarcoma cell leukemia[204] because of the similarity of these cells to those seen in lymph node imprint preparations from typical cases of large cell lymphosarcoma. Whether called chronic lymphosarcoma cell leukemia or leukosarcoma the differentiation has long been regarded as one of morphological significance only. More recently, it has been shown to be associated with a more rapid course and shorter survival than typical chronic lymphocytic leukemia.[377,463]

Although the small CLL lymphocytes are not readily distinguished from normal small lymphocytes in Romanowsky-stained preparations, differentiation may be possible. Indeed, computer recognition of these cells in asymptomatic chronic lymphocytic leukemia has recently been described[212]: the same technique has been used to distinguish the cells of lymphosarcoma cell leukemia.[448] The CLL lymphocytes have been shown to differ from normal lymphocytes in their susceptibility to lethal effects of colchicine in vitro.[422,423] It remains to be seen whether attempts to distinguish so-called B and T lymphocytes may have similar discriminatory value in detecting abnormality of the small lymphocytes in chronic lymphocytic leukemia.[453]

Like cytochemistry, studies of muramidase or lysozyme production (Chapter 14) have been used mainly to distinguish cytological variations of acute leukemia in patients showing little recognizable cellular differentiation. Their use seems to be limited to this purpose rather than for the diagnosis of acute leukemia per se, if this is in doubt.

In doubtful cases of acute leukemia chromosomal studies may be of value in demonstrating abnormal aneuploidy, or even an abnormal clone, with or without a marker chromosome (Chapter 6). Absence of chromosomal abnormality does not, of course, exclude the diagnosis. On the other hand, a diagnosis of chronic granulocytic leukemia may be confirmed by the finding of the Ph[1] chromosome in bone marrow or unstimulated peripheral blood cultures. Typical chronic granulocytic leukemia is excluded by the absence of the Ph[1] from direct and uncultured chromosome preparations made from bone marrow. Atypical Ph[1]-negative cases of the disease certainly occur and are discussed elsewhere (page 334).

SPLENIC PUNCTURE

In the earlier editions of this book, the place of splenic puncture in the diagnosis of the leukemias was critically but favorably assessed. This assessment was based on the considerable experience of the method of Dr. William Dameshek, some of it reported elsewhere.[73] He concluded that splenic puncture is a diagnostic procedure of minor importance in the leukemias, and not to be undertaken in all patients as a matter of course. In addition, a palpable spleen and the absence of any hemorrhagic tendency are prerequisites for the use of this technique. The latter requirement may now be less difficult to satisfy since platelet concentrates are readily available. Previously, the difficulties in interpretation of aspirated material were recognized and reference was made to the troublesome lack of information about the aspirate obtained from normal spleens (Fig. 10-7).

Dameshek had found splenic puncture of value in two clinical situations: "Cases of splenomegaly and anemia, with or without the presence of immature cells in the blood, when a marrow aspiration has failed to yield adequate specimens and a diagnosis of myelosclerosis or myeloid metaplasia is to be differentiated from that of leukemia of the granulocytic variety."[102] Since that was written considerable advances have been made in the diagnosis of chronic granulocytic leukemia mainly consequent upon the discovery of the Ph[1] chromosome. It is rare for chronic granu-

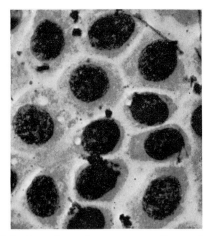

Fig. 10-7. Splenic aspirate shows a group of serosal cells. × 1800.

locytic leukemia to occur without diagnostic findings in the peripheral blood film (page 328). When it does happen, the Ph[1] can generally be demonstrated in direct chromosome preparations of bone marrow aspirate or unstimulated cultures of peripheral blood (page 146). In the exceedingly rare coincidence of chronic granulocytic leukemia with an atypical peripheral blood picture, with no cells capable of mitosis in unstimulated culture, and marrow aspiration made impossible by myelofibrosis,[169] splenic puncture might be of value (Fig. 10-8). Certainly the Ph[1] chromosome can be found in CGL spleen cells,[399] but its demonstration in aspirated material has not been reported. Furthermore, most hematologists now believe that myelosclerosis is best diagnosed by demonstration of increased connective tissue in sections of bone obtained by trephine biopsy. Splenic aspirate indicative of myeloid metaplasia of the spleen has less specific diagnostic value (Fig. 10-9).

Dameshek's second statement[102] is also liable to amendment. He recognized a second group of patients in whom splenic puncture is of value:

Cases of splenomegaly but without characteristic blood or marrow findings,

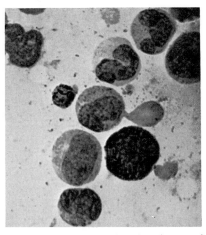

Fig. 10-8. Splenic aspirate from a patient with chronic granulocytic leukemia. × 1800.

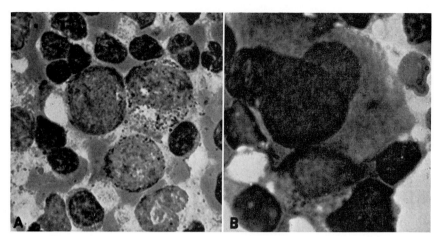

Fig. 10-9. Splenic aspirate from a patient with myeloid metaplasia showing (A) granulocyte precursors, and (B) a megakaryocyte. Both, × 1800.

and with absence of enlarged lymph nodes or other obvious physical abnormalities which might lead to the establishment of a diagnosis. In this group a sizeable proportion may, by means of splenic puncture, be shown to be suffering from one of the leukosarcomas, particularly lymphosarcoma or Hodgkin's disease.

Here, too, the situation has changed considerably since 1964. Abnormality on abdominal lymphangiography[219] may provide a relatively simple and reasonably reliable indication for laparotomy and diagnostic biopsy of intraabdominal lymph nodes in these very patients. Furthermore, there is now a greater willingness than formerly to embark upon splenectomy as a diagnostic measure in just the kind of clinical problem outlined.[2,396]

To summarize, it seems that the importance of splenic puncture in the differential diagnosis of the leukemias and related disorders has lessened because of the development of alternative diagnostic methods. It retains some place in unusual cases, but its utility is probably in need of fresh assessment. Unfortunately, the diagnostic problems in which it may be most useful arise infrequently, and considerable experience is required for the confident interpretation of the relatively small samples obtained by aspiration. There may be a place for technical innovations in splenic puncture, including the use of the cytocentrifuge.[443]

PREGNANCY AND LEUKEMIA

The coincidence of pregnancy and leukemia is rare. The literature on the subject consists of many individual case reports and a few valuable reviews.[11,187,297] Nevertheless, some authors have personally observed eight,[145] and others four cases[309,358] of acute leukemia in pregnancy. As might be expected from the known age-incidence of the main types of leukemia, cases of acute leukemia and pregnancy outnumber those of chronic granulocytic leukemia and pregnancy.[309] For the same reason, the coincidence of chronic lymphocytic leukemia and pregnancy is extremely rare. A series of 203 cases reported between 1955 and 1965 has been reviewed[309]: in 20 percent of patients with the acute form and 67 percent of those with chronic granulocytic leukemia the onset of leukemia, and in many cases its diagnosis, preceded pregnancy. Now that remissions are more easily obtained in adults with acute leukemia, the incidence of pregnancy may well increase. During the past few years four of our own patients became pregnant shortly after achieving their first remission in acute leukemia.

The diagnosis of pregnancy in patients with leukemia may be delayed because amenorrhea is accepted as a consequence of the disease or of its treatment by agents such as busulfan, 6-mercaptopurine, or methotrexate. Conversely, it is probable that in many patients a diagnosis of leukemia has been complicated or delayed by known pregnancy. Attention has been drawn to the simulation of acute leukemia by megaloblastic anemia of pregnancy.[264] This may have been a more common error in the past than it is now. In some cases of chronic granulocytic leukemia, the diagnosis has followed detection of symptomless splenomegaly at abdominal examination prompted by evidence of pregnancy.[124] In other instances, symptomless chronic granulocytic leukemia has been diagnosed when splenomegaly, masked in late pregnancy, has been detected only after delivery.

Generalizations on the effects of pregnancy on the course of leukemia are naturally difficult regarding acute leukemia. In chronic granulocytic leukemia it seems likely that the course of the disease is relatively little influenced, however it is treated.[122,274] Knowing the natural history of acute leukemia in women of childbearing age, it is difficult to believe that the effects are other than adverse. Certainly, there is no good evidence of a beneficial effect. On balance, pregnancy seems more likely to have an overall deleterious effect, if only because of the restraint on vigorous antileukemic treatment imposed by knowledge of pregnancy and concern for the fetus. In addition, the risk of complications of leukemia, especially hemorrhagic complications, must be heightened. When the question of termination of pregnancy is considered, the risk of bleeding complicating such termination may be as great as the risk of allowing pregnancy to go to term.[5,145] Despite the recent slight improvements in the treatment of acute leukemia in adults, there are few reports of long survival after pregnancy. This contrasts with chronic granulocytic leukemia where two women, at least, are known to have had two successful pregnancies each during the course of their disease.

The risks to the fetus of leukemia in pregnancy can only be increased. Stillbirths and neonatal deaths are certainly common,[11,274] although these may now be less frequent than they once were, if only because of the improved management of abnormal bleeding. Whether the risk to the child is increased by antileukemic treatment is less certain. There are now many reports of the birth of live, normal children after treatment of maternal chronic granulocytic leukemia by busulfan in the usual doses, even in the first trimester.[122] Low birth weight and transient anemia and neutropenia seem to be the only hazards. In contrast—but again without very firm evidence—it is accepted that in acute leukemia, chemotherapy should be avoided in the first trimester. Even later in pregnancy there must be a natural inclination to minimize treatment possibly harmful to the fetus, especially in regard to known teratogenic agents such as methotrexate. Nevertheless, we know of no recorded instance of congenital abnormality attributable to the treatment of maternal leukemia in pregnancy. It is inherently difficult to prove a causal relationship, even if abnormality occurs, especially in view of the high frequency of intrauterine and neonatal death in the children of leukemic mothers, whether or not the mothers have received specific antileukemic treatment.

When a woman with leukemia becomes pregnant or when leukemia is diagnosed in a woman known to be pregnant, there is a very special need for counseling the patient and her husband (Chapter 20). The risk of termination has been mentioned above: when this has been explained, the decision rests with the patient. Questions as to the effect on the mother should be answered as optimistically as truth allows. Questions as to possible hazards to the child are more difficult to answer, the truth being that fetal risks are much greater than in a normal pregnancy. In our four patients who became pregnant while in remission, we advised termination because of the possible teratogenic risk to the fetus of chemotherapy and our unwillingness, in the interests of the mothers, to modify the treatment they were receiving.

The special question of the possibility of the child having leukemia is more easily answered. We know of only three reported instances of leukemia in children born to mothers with leukemia. Allowing for selective recording of such cases, and accepting that over 300 cases of leukemia in pregnancy have been reported,[309] the risk is less than 1 in 100. Even in the reported cases, the development of leukemia in the child might have been a chance occurrence. This seems most likely where acute leukemia was diagnosed at the age of 16 in a child whose mother had chronic granulocytic leukemia in pregnancy.[211] In the other two reported cases, chance is rather less likely as a basis for acute leukemia in one mother and child when the diagnosis was made in the child at the age of nine months[86] and 5 months in another.[32] The need for follow-up of children born to mothers with leukemia has been stressed,[11] but this should be looked upon as research to be carried out discreetly and without alarming the subject.

Obviously, there is a particular need for sound and acceptable advice on contraception where leukemia of any kind is diagnosed in a woman who is not unquestionably infertile.

Preleukemia

This term was first used by Block, Jacobson, and Bethard in 1953.[43] As generally used, it refers most often to conditions known to be associated with a very high risk of leukemia. Obviously, only in retrospect can it be used with absolute truth or certainty. In this way, preleukemia describes a recognizable disorder with a known or suspected relationship to one of the leukemias which was observed in a patient who has since developed leukemia. More loosely, it is used to describe a detectable disorder believed to be a precursor of leukemia in a patient who has not yet developed leukemia. Used in this way, the term implies an assumption which cannot be admitted, since no so-called preleukemic condition is followed, even in all patients who survive long enough, by the development of frank leukemia.

The concept of preleukemia is justified theoretically by the fact that induction of leukemia, like the induction of other neoplasms, is almost certainly a multistage process.[114] This being so, it is very likely that some of the stages in induction, especially the later stages, may give rise to detectable effects in some patients. The concept also rests on the observed fact that some conditions (see Chapter 5), such as trisomy 21, Bloom's syndrome, Fanconi's hypoplastic anemia, and ataxia telangiectasia, as well as individuals who have been exposed to high doses of ionizing radiation, all have a greatly increased risk of developing acute leukemia, and the irradiated subjects, chronic granulocytic leukemia as well. In all these, the preleukemic state is recognizable and the risk of leukemia can be calculated. Their status as preleukemic conditions is unquestioned, except in the strict sense of the word: there can be no certainty that any particular patient will develop leukemia, and most never do so. The term *preleukemia* is applied more often to ill-defined conditions which resemble in some ways, or which are possibly indistinguishable from, states known sometimes to precede the development of leukemia.

It is now accepted that the myeloproliferative states (see Chapter 11)—especially myelofibrosis and polycythemia vera—sideroblastic anemia,[190] aplastic anemia,[115] some cytopenic or pancytopenic states, and paroxysmal nocturnal hemoglobinuria (PNH)[65,101,214] are preleukemic, at least in some patients. It is not known whether instances of sideroblastic anemia, aplastic anemia, and PNH which are preleukemic, differ at the beginning from the generality of these conditions. There have now been many studies, mainly cytochemical and cytogenetic, intended to detect preleukemic changes with certainty. More recently, a maturation defect has been demonstrated in bone marrow cultures,[165,386] and this may provide the basis of a diagnostic test.

The question of preleukemia arises most often in middle-aged or elderly patients with evident bone marrow dysfunction. The clinical features are commonly those of anemia, thrombocytopenia, or increased liability to infection, apparently attributable to neutropenia. Splenomegaly and lymphadenopathy are unusual. In addition to the cytopenias in the peripheral blood there may be evidence of qualitative dysfunction of the bone marrow. Of these, the most relevant to the concept of preleukemia is the presence of abnormal leukocytes. These may be atypical or frankly abnormal mononuclear cells, in some cases indistinguishable from leukemic blast cells. They rarely predominate as is common in the peripheral blood in overt leukemia. In addition to the leukocytes resembling blast cells, other abnormal leukocytes may be seen, such as pseudo-Pelger–Huët cells.[229] Qualitative changes are often not confined to the leukocytes.[267] Giant platelets and nucleated erythrocytes may be found, and the latter may be sideroblasts or show some degree of megaloblastic change.

In conditions recognized as preleukemic, the bone marrow findings are highly variable. They may be those of frank myelofibrosis with myeloid metaplasia (MMM) (see Chapter 11), but more commonly, bone marrow is aspirated with difficulty. It may be of normal cellularity or hypoplastic.[31,287] The bone marrow commonly shows frank dysfunction, whether or not it is reflected in the peripheral blood. The dysfunction may take the form of maturation arrest in the granulocyte precursors—abnormal megakaryocytes, and megaloblastic or sideroblastic erythropoiesis. The abnormal cells in the peripheral blood, suggesting a diagnosis of acute leukemia, are often present in the marrow too, but not usually in numbers sufficient to justify such a diagnosis.[203] Cytogenetic studies of bone marrow in preleukemia rarely yield conclusive results. Gross aneuploidy or the dominance of an abnormal cell line may weigh in favor of diagnosis of acute leukemia. More commonly, a normal chromosome constitution is found, or lesser abnormalities, which are difficult to interpret. A normal finding does not, of course, exclude the emergence of frank acute leukemia. The most difficult cytogenetic finding to interpret is the presence of a cell-line with numerical abnormality of the C-group chromosomes: these may persist for years without the other features of the disease warranting a diagnosis of acute leukemia.[359,418] Nevertheless, it has been shown that, in recognized preleukemic conditions, the presence of chromosomal abnormality increases the probability of the development of acute leukemia.[313] However, if acute leukemia does not develop within a period of a few months after the appearance of the preleukemic features, the ultimate risk declines. Apparently, some aneuploid cell lines are relatively stable. Preleukemic patients with such bone marrow cell abnormalities may live for years and die without ever developing acute leukemia.[269] Analogous lack of predictive value has been demonstrated in preleukemia, in regard to enzymatic abnormalities in erythrocytes and granulocytes.[119] On the other hand, strong PAS positivity in marrow erythroblasts may favor a diagnosis of erythroleukemia in a sideroblastic marrow.[190]

In preleukemia, the diagnostic question is usually one of acute leukemia. It rarely arises in the chronic lymphocytic or granulocytic forms and is rarely an urgent question in the former (page 343). In preleukemia, low neutrophil alkaline phosphatase values in the peripheral blood alone cannot be accepted as justifying a diagnosis of chronic granulocytic leukemia.[201] If the Ph[1] chromosome is simultaneously present in marrow cells the possibility is greatly increased.[415] Nevertheless, a chromosome morphologically indistinguishable from the Ph[1] has been found in the bone marrow cells of heavily irradiated individuals years after radiation exposure, without the emergence of chronic granulocytic leukemia.[162,296]

Acute Leukemia

Acute leukemia occurs at all ages (see Chapter 4). Acute lymphocytic leukemia predominates in childhood, and the various forms of acute granulocytic leukemia are more common in adults at all ages. Acute lymphocytic leukemia is not peculiar to children, nor is acute granulocytic leukemia found exclusively in adults, although the association between age and cytological type is a strong one. The relative frequency of both types in any population depends, therefore, on the age structure of the population and on its standards of medical care, especially that available to the elderly.[115]

Even before any attempt was made to distinguish between cytological types of acute leukemia, chronic and acute forms of the leukemias had to be distinguished. Such differentiation came relatively late in the history of the leukemias; and, until quite recently, the distinctions tended to be overlooked by all but physicians with a special interest in the field. In the early years of its history leukemia was most often diagnosed in association with gross splenomegaly, so that diagnosis of the chronic forms predominated. Only in 1847 did Virchow distinguish between splenic and lymphatic leukemias, emphasizing the occurrence of lymph node enlargement in the latter. Recognition of acute leukemia as a separate type of leukemia came still later.[188] Differentiation of cytological types of acute leukemia is among the most sophisticated of medical diagnostic procedures and remains imperfect, even today. The validity of some cytological differentiations within the disease are well-established in regard to reliability and significance for natural history and response to treatment. These subdivisions of acute leukemia are the subdivisions observed in Chapters 3 and 18 and in the account of the clinical and laboratory features of acute leukemia which follows. Other cytological differentiations are not well established, with respect to either practicability or significance[163,281]: these may be mentioned further but will not be allowed to influence the classification adopted or the sequence of description.

The term *acute* now applies with varying degrees of validity to the different forms of acute leukemia. As originally used, it referred to onset and clinical course in the average case, as well as to the undifferentiated or primitive form of the leukemic cells. These connotations remain in regard to the untreated patient but the validity of the adjective *acute* is now questionable when referring to the survival of the optimally treated case of acute lymphocytic leukemia, at least in childhood. Paradoxically, the duration and quality of life of the average ALL patient is now better than that of the average patient with chronic leukemia, whether granulocytic or lymphocytic. This being so, the physician should exercise discretion in use of the term *acute,* especially when speaking to patients and relatives who can be expected to understand it in one sense only.

ACUTE LYMPHOCYTIC LEUKEMIA

The natural history of acute lymphocytic leukemia has been profoundly influenced by successful treatment. Even its presenting manifestations have probably been changed, at least in the medically more advanced societies, by earlier diagnosis than formerly prevailed.[143] As a result, patients now more commonly than before have nonspecific symptoms and a diagnostic peripheral blood picture, confirmed by bone marrow findings (Fig. 10-10). Serious hemorrhagic and infective complica-

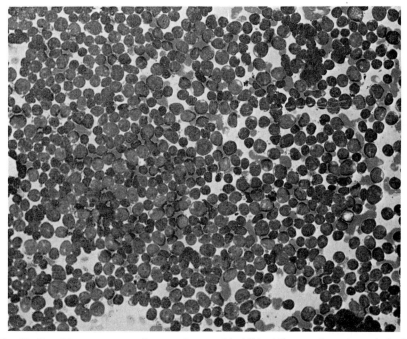

Fig. 10-10. Marrow smear from a 4-year-old child with acute lymphocytic leukemia. The marrow is almost solely composed of uniform blast cells. × 400.

tions, severe anemia, and obvious splenomegaly and lymphadenopathy are seen less often at diagnosis than in the past. Chloromas (page 283), gross organomegaly, cerebral hemorrhage, CNS leukemia,[132] arthralgia,[371,403] and metabolic complications such as hypercalcemia,[308] hypocalcemia,[3] and hyperuricemia[348] are more often seen later in the disease. These and other less common features of acute lymphocytic leukemia are seen, especially in patients who fail to achieve remission on treatment, or when more successfully treated patients subsequently relapse.

The typical child with acute lymphocytic leukemia has had nonspecific symptoms of tiredness, fever, or general malaise for a week or so. Pallor and easy bruising may have been noted by the parents. On examination, these observations may be confirmed and extended by the physician who may also discover lymphadenopathy, splenomegaly, hepatomegaly, and bone tenderness.[456] Abnormalities of gait may occur as a consequence of bone or joint pain. In one recent study of 191 children with acute lymphocytic leukemia, radiologic changes in bones were found at diagnosis in 21 percent.[13] This study used stricter criteria than had been used by others who found a higher incidence.[451] Such radiologic changes nevertheless correlate poorly with the occurrence of bone pain (see page 281) and seem to have little or no prognostic value. In contrast, other evidence of extramyeloid involvement seems to have a bad prognostic significance.[185] Other factors of proved prognostic significance include various findings on hematologic investigation (see below) and the age of the patient, especially if a child. Remission is induced twice as frequently in ALL children aged 1–10 years than in children aged over 10 years at diagnosis. Under the age of 1 year the prognosis is even worse than that for those over the age of 10, remission being induced in only 18 percent in one large series of cases.[457] This, in part, reflects the especially poor prognosis in cases accepted as instances of congenital leukemia (see page 325).

The diagnostic laboratory findings in acute leukemia in general have already been discussed (see page 293). Some relatively uncommon features may be of disproportionate interest or importance. With improved overall results in the treatment of acute lymphocytic leukemia, it is possible to discern some findings associated with a particularly poor prognosis. Thus, in the United States, or at least in Tennessee, Negro children with acute lymphocytic leukemia have a worse prognosis than do Caucasian children.[438] The reasons for these differences are probably socioeconomic rather than racial. Other bad prognostic features in this disease include very high leukocyte counts, severe thrombocytopenia at diagnosis, and the occurrence and degree of organ infiltration by leukemic cells.[185] In one series, 10 percent of children with acute lymphocytic leukemia had mediastinal involvement,[185] presumably arising in the thymus and/or hilar lymph nodes. Acute lymphocytic leukemia and thymoma seem to be common coincidences and are almost certainly two manifestations of the one disease.[8] Gross splenic involvement in acute lymphocytic leukemia is relatively uncommon and does not usually give rise to blood cell sequestration and the accepted findings of hypersplenism. Nevertheless, this has been described, and apparently successfully treated by splenectomy.[89]

In view of the accepted immunologic role of the normal lymphocyte, it is surprising that acute lymphocytic leukemia is not more often associated with monoclonal gammopathy (see Chapter 13). Its apparent infrequency may be due to failure to initiate the essential studies of serum proteins. It certainly occurs[268,407] in childhood acute lymphocytic leukemia and apparently in older patients with other forms of acute leukemia as well.[81]

CYTOLOGIC DIFFERENTIATION OF ACUTE LEUKEMIAS

In the past there has been more confusion than order resulting from attempts at cytologic differentiation of acute leukemia. Terminology was inconsistent and idiosyncratic. In addition, criteria for differentiation were inadequate and there was all too little agreement between authors. Much of this confusion resulted from overconfidence and lack of appreciation of observer error. Furthermore, while the treatment of acute leukemia was virtually ineffective there was relatively little incentive to greater accuracy. With the development of more effective treatment from 1948 onward, certain differences in therapeutic response have emerged, notably between the acute lymphocytic and granulocytic leukemias. There are now very good reasons of major clinical importance for differentiating one type of acute leukemia from another. With continued improvement in the treatment of all acute leukemias, new differences in response to particular forms of therapy seem to be emerging (see Chapter 18), and these seem likely to become more, rather than less, important.

The most significant single step in cytologic differentiation of acute leukemia was marked by the publication in 1964 of the study by Hayhoe, Quaglino, and Doll.[191] This study was a comprehensive exploration of possible characteristics of acute leukemia, both in Romanowsky-stained preparations, and using cytochemical techniques. Even more important was the fact that, in assessing the value of these characteristics, statistical methods were used. The main conclusions are summarized in Table 10-1. More recently, the whole field has been critically reviewed in the light of newer knowledge.[189a] The main conclusions of that review are summarized in Tables 10-1 through 10-5. Furthermore, as discussed below, other workers are now using the same techniques, and results are available which indicate the limits of confidence of the methods. Unfortunately, the reliability of the range of tests recommended by Hayhoe and Cawley,[189a] is likely to be higher in the hands of any group of workers sufficiently interested to explore their value, than in mere day-to-day use.

It seems likely that in the very near future techniques other than those reviewed by Hayhoe and Cawley[189a] will find a place in the cytologic differentiation of acute leukemia. Thus, the same authors have reviewed their own and others' experience of electron microscopy of blood and bone marrow cells in acute leukemia (see Chapter 6). Electron microscopic techniques are unlikely ever to be routinely used for this purpose, except in a few centers, but they may provide a basis for simpler techniques of differentiation for general use. On the other hand, it must be admitted that in an analogous situation electron microscopic methods have established themselves as being of direct diagnostic value and essential to therapeutic decisions in renal disease.

Other methods which may provide a basis for more accurate cytologic differentiation in acute leukemia are constantly being described. Unfortunately, it must be accepted that their evaluation, preferably at the hands of several groups of workers, will take several years. One promising method which may provide a means of differentiating acute lymphocytic from nonlymphocytic leukemia depends on differences in intracellular hydrogen transport between normal lymphocytes and

Table 10-1

Defining Characteristics of Value in the Classification of Acute Leukemia

Type	Group Discriminating Features	
	Romanowsky Stain Features	*Cytochemical Features*
Acute lymphocytic leukemia (ALL)	Nuclear-cytoplasmic ratio high Nuclei not indented or twisted Erythroblasts not present in peripheral blood Erythroblasts not predominant in bone marrow	5% or less of cells Sudan positive 5% or less of cells peroxidase positive Neutrophil alkaline phosphatase (NAP) score normal or high PAS score in erythroblasts polychromatophilic and oxyphilic, low
Acute granulocytic leukemia (AGL)		
Myeloblastic and promyelocytic (AGL)	Cell outlines not irregular Nuclear-cytoplasmic ratio not high Monocytes form less than 1% of nucleated cells of the peripheral blood Erythroblasts not predominant in the marrow	Neutrophil alkaline phosphatase (NAP) score is low. Invariably more than 5% and usually more than 85% of cells are Sudan black positive which is of a strong local or heavy overall type More than 5% of cells are peroxidase positive
Myelomonocytic (AMML)	Nuclei indented and twisted Monocytes form more than 1% of the nucleated cells of the peripheral blood Nuclear-cytoplasmic ratio not high Erythroblasts not present in the peripheral blood Erythroblasts not predominant in the marrow	More than 5% and less than 85% of cells show Sudan black positivity which is of a more finely granular type than in myeloblastic leukemia
Erythroleukemia (EL)	Cell outlines irregular Nuclear-cytoplasmic ratio not high Erythroblasts present in the peripheral blood Erythroblasts predominant in the marrow	PAS score high More than 5% of cells Sudan black positive More than 5% of cells peroxidase positive

From Hayhoe et al.,[191] and Hayhoe and Cawley.[189a] (With permission.[189a])

Table 10-2

Additional Features in Acute Lymphocytic Leukemia

Romanowsky Features	Cytochemical Features
Lymphocytes frequently exceed 1% of marrow cells.	The PAS reaction in primitive cells is not diffuse, but present as coarse granules or blocks against a negative cytoplasmic background in at least a few and often many cells.
Nucleolar number tends to be low (1–2).	
Auer rods are absent.	
Rieder cells are frequent.	
Agranular or hypogranular polymorphs not found.	May show nuclear staining for aryl sulphatase.
Acquired pseudo-Pelger-Huet not found.	Acid phosphatase in general lower than in myeloblastic or myelomonocytic leukemia
Promyelocytes uncommon although a few may be present.	
Monocytes and promonocytes are uncommon.	Naphthol AS-D chloroacetate esterase negative
	Naphthol AS-D acetate and alpha naphthyl acetate esterases negative or weakly positive
	Extramitochondrial dehydrogenases active (e.g., lactate, malate)
	Intramitochondrial dehydrogenases depressed (e.g., succinate, glutamate)

From Hayhoe and Cawley.[189a] (With permission.)

Table 10-3

Additional Features in Acute Granulocytic Leukemia (Myeloblastic and Promyelocytic)

Romanowsky Features	Cytochemical Features
Cells more regular in size	PAS reaction negative in many cells, but some show a diffuse tinge with or without superimposed fine granules.
Nucleolar number tends to be higher (3–5).	
Auer rods present	
Rieder cells uncommon	Naphthol AS-D chloroacetate esterase positive (increasing positivity with increasing maturity) but alpha naphthol acetate esterase negative. Naphthol AS-D acetate esterase reaction positive (particularly in promyelocytes and myelocytes) but less so than in monocytoid cells. Naphthol AS-D acetate esterase activity not inhibited by sodium fluoride (see monocytic cells)
Agranular or hypogranular polymorphs may be seen.	
Acquired pseudo-Pelger-Huet anomaly may be seen.	
Abnormal eosinophils may be seen	
Promyelocytes nearly always present and often predominant.	
	Other cytochemical methods as yet of little value

From Hayhoe and Cawley.[189a] (With permission.)

Table 10-4
Additional Features in AMML

Romanowsky Features	Cytochemical Features
Nucleolar number tends to be higher (3–5)	Peroxidase reaction of monocyte precursors usually negative
Auer rods present	
Agranular or hypogranular polymorphs may be seen.	PAS reaction variable; some cells negative, but some may show diffuse tinging with fine granules superimposed.
Acquired pseudo-Pelger-Huet anomaly may be seen.	Alpha naphthol acetate esterase positive.
Abnormal eosinophils may be present.	Naphthol AS-D acetate esterase is more positive than in granulocytic cells and is inhibited by sodium fluoride, unlike the positivity in the granulocytic series.
Promyelocytes often present, but not predominating	
Thrombocytopenia less frequent than in other acute leukemias	Naphthol AS-D chloroacetate esterase negative

From Hayhoe and Cawley.[189a] (With permission.)

leukemic lymphoblasts.[409] At present, that differentiation is the one of major importance in acute leukemia (see Chapter 18). Fortunately, other recent innovations hold promise for its greater accuracy. Thus, it seems likely that estimation of fetal hemoglobin (HbF) may provide a means of differentiating lymphocytic from nonlymphocytic acute leukemias. HbF commonly accounts for 2 percent or more of hemoglobin in acute granulocytic leukemia and less than 2 percent in acute lymphocytic leukemia. It is of interest that a single case of acute "monoblastic" leukemia studied in this way yielded a result in the acute lymphocytic range. The rationale of this differentiation technique may lie in the involvement of all marrow stem lines, including erythropoietic cells, in the leukemic change in acute granulocytic but not in acute lymphocytic leukemia.

Despite their value in the study of other aspects of the leukemias, chromosome

Table 10-5
Additional Features in Erythroleukemia

Romanowsky Features	Cytochemical Features
Cell outlines irregular	Heavy PAS positivity, granular or diffuse, is present in red cell series at all stages of maturity.
Nuclear-cytoplasmic ratio not high	
Erythroblasts present in peripheral blood	
Erythroblasts predominant in the marrow	Abnormal granulocytic precursors present show PAS positivity resembling that in myeloblastic leukemia
Promyelocytes usually present	
Auer rods may be found in granulocytic precursors	More than 5 percent of cells Sudan black positive
Abnormal eosinophils may be seen	More than 5 percent of cells peroxidase positive
	Alpha naphthol acetate esterase strongly positive
	Strong paranuclear unipolar acid phosphatase activity

From Hayhoe and Cawley.[189a] (With permission.)

studies (see Chapter 6) have not provided a reliable basis for cell-type differentiation in acute leukemia. In contrast, there is some evidence that the adenosine deaminase phenotype, as studied in leukemic blast cells, may have distinguishing value.[44] By this means it seems possible that acute myelomonocytic leukemia, on the one hand, may be differentiated from the acute lymphocytic and granulocytic leukemias on the other. Similarly, myeloperoxidase-deficient neutrophils may be characteristic of the latter, and of chronic granulocytic leukemia after metamorphosis.[68]

In cytologic differentiation of AL it took years for the unreliability of cytogenetic studies to be established. The whole question may now have to be reexamined using the recently introduced chromosome-banding techniques. Similarly, the newer methods mentioned above will take some time to evaluate. As an example of the time, care, and scepticism appropriate to this field of hematology, attention may be drawn to published experience of observations on nuclear arylsulfatase activity. Early reports suggested that by this method the acute lymphocytic and granulocytic forms might always be distinguished,[128,255] but more recent experience makes this hope seem remote.[325]

The obvious practical value of cell-type differentiation in acute leukemia lies mainly in the differences in prognosis of the various types, and in differences in optimal treatment which are discussed in Chapter 18. Stated briefly, the prognosis, including response to treatment, is better in acute lymphocytic than in acute granulocytic leukemia at all ages. The latter, acute myelomonocytic leukemia, and erythroleukemia may at present be considered as members of one group, in regard to both survival without treatment and survival with optimal treatment. Their rarity and the lack of correspondence of diagnostic criteria make it presently unjustifiable to be more specific about acute myelomonocytic and erythroleukemia, other than simply accepting them as variants of acute granulocytic leukemia. The same reservations should be employed in statements about even rarer entities such as promyelocytic leukemia (see page 315) and acute histiocytic leukemia or "true" acute monocytic leukemia (see page 23). Some workers question the existence of a separate class of undifferentiated acute leukemias.[55] Their feeling is that in any series this class is made up of cases of both lymphocytic and granulocytic leukemias (or one of their subtypes), which, because of predictable biologic variation and the imperfections of diagnostic criteria, cannot confidently be assigned to either of the main types. Others[144] find the undifferentiated category to behave, in a variety of ways, more like acute granulocytic than acute lymphocytic leukemia. This is an important point since, until recently, at least in children, the practice has been to equate acute lymphocytic and undifferentiated acute leukemia, whether the latter is called stem cell leukemia or by some other name.

Presently, the broadest valid classification of practical value is probably that of the two classes, acute lymphocytic and acute nonlymphocytic leukemia. Nevertheless, it is unlikely that differences within the latter broad group are without significance. Accordingly, every effort should be made to explore these differences and assess their significance for etiology, natural history, and response to treatment.

Inseparable from the problems of cytologic differentiation in acute leukemia are questions as to the significance of age. In the first year of life, in both sexes, the incidence of acute granulocytic leukemia is almost equal to that of acute lymphocytic leukemia; at the ages of 4–6 years it is one-fifth as great. The incidence of the latter is less than that of the former after the age of 14 and remains so at older ages. In old age, when the incidence of AGL is highest in Western countries, acute lymphocytic leukemia is relatively uncommon.[115] These relative age incidences should be considered with what we know of the efficacy of treatment in acute leukemia, that of acute lymphocytic leukemia being obviously more successful than the treatment of acute granulocytic leukemia. It can then be seen why the median survival in optimally treated children in the age group 3–10 may be better than 5 years (see Chapter 18): it is notably less in children under the age of 1 year (page 306) and in those over the age of 10 at diagnosis. In adults, in whom acute granulocytic leukemia predominates and the lymphocytic form is uncommon, half achieve remission on optimal therapy and median survival is of the order of 6 months. Can these differences be explained by the cell types of acute leukemia or does age per se play a part? At present, this question cannot be answered. There can be little doubt that at all ages the acute granulocytic form responds less often and less well to treatment than do the acute lymphocytic leukemias. On the other hand, it seems that children with the former may respond more favorably than adults; and adults with acute lymphocytic leukemia probably, but not certainly (see Chapter 18), have a poorer therapeutic response than do children with ALL.

Two points of great practical importance emerge on the question of the relationship of age to cytologic type in acute leukemia. When doubt exists as to cell type, the patient's age, which is never in question, should be given greater weight. Between the age of 1 and 15, doubtful cases of acute leukemia can be regarded as the lymphocytic type and over the age of 20, as the granulocytic type. Secondly, regardless of cell type the response to the current therapy of acute leukemia is worse in older adults and the optimal therapy for younger adults may be quite inappropriate for those over the age of 60, or even younger.

Critical evaluation of cytologic diagnosis in AL.   In the past, there have been too many dogmatic statements on the subject of criteria for cell-type differentiation in acute leukemia, often depending on the whim of individual observers or authors. Unfortunately, such statements are still being made and papers published in which the cytologic criteria used are barely described. In a recent study by Brincker and Jensen,[55] the degree of agreement between two independent observers was explored in 87 cases of acute leukemia. They used blood and bone marrow preparations— stained only by the May–Grunwald–Giemsa method, and classified by the morphological criteria of Hayhoe, Quaglino, and Doll.[191] In this investigation 21.8 percent of cases were unclassified without any reservation, and 13.8 percent were unclassified with some reservations. The corresponding figures for the earlier work of Hayhoe and his colleagues,[191] using both morphological and cytochemical criteria, were 11.0 percent and nil. In the light of these studies it should not be assumed, as it often is, that all cases of acute leukemia can be confidently assigned to a cell class without error. Indeed, it is certain that the error in day-to-day practice is probably much greater than 20 percent, and not very much less when cytochemical methods are used in addition to morphological criteria.

ACUTE GRANULOCYTIC (MYELOCYTIC; MYELOBLASTIC) LEUKEMIA

This term and its near-synonyms were, until recently, used to denote one of the two main divisions of acute leukemia—the other being acute lymphocytic leukemia. Following the partial recognition as variants, or even as separate entities of acute myelomonocytic leukemia, acute promyelocytic leukemia, and erythroleukemia, acute granulocytic leukemia has become a narrower concept and is less frequently diagnosed. The current confusion is compounded by its continued use as a generic term for the whole group. In this section, as elsewhere in this book, it is used as a generic term for acute granulocytic leukemia as a whole, and, more specifically, for what other authors call *acute myeloblastic leukemia.* This latter term is coming to denote the residuum of acute granulocytic leukemia, not otherwise distinguished by the special prominence of promyelocytes and disseminated intravascular coagulation, monocytosis, or of conspicuous disorder of erythropoiesis. Since the narrower use of this term and of the term *acute myeloblastic leukemia,* is relatively recent, care must be taken in the interpretation of older, as distinct from more recent, writings.

Used in the narrower sense, acute granulocytic leukemia occurs at all ages with peaks in its age incidence occurring around the age of 5 years, in late adolescence, and then increasing steadily with advancing years.[115] As noted above, it is the common form of acute leukemia in adults, and both its untreated natural history and survival in the optimally treated patient tend to be shorter than for acute lymphocytic leukemia at all ages. Onset may be sudden or insidious. More rapid onset tends to be associated with the presence of its more serious complications, by way of infection, hemorrhage, or anemia. In the absence of such complications, the evolution of the clinical picture may be slow, especially in the elderly. There are no characteristic clinical findings. Enlargement of spleen, lymph nodes, and liver are much less common, and slighter in degree than they are in acute lymphocytic leukemia. Skin involvement and other extramyeloid proliferation may be seen. When these occur in or around bones, especially the bones of the base of the skull, they are sometimes called chloromas (see page 283). Bone tenderness is common, but its value as a diagnostic sign has been questioned.[273] Diagnosis most often follows hematologic investigation prompted by nonspecific symptoms of tiredness, pallor, and malaise, or by the common complications of infection or hemorrhage. Pyrexia may occur in the absence of demonstrable infection but it is prudent to regard it as usually indicative of infection and to investigate accordingly.

Diagnosis of acute granulocytic leukemia is usually made on examination of a blood film. Confirmation is by bone marrow examination and review of the clinical and laboratory findings for consistency. The differential diagnosis of acute leukemia in general is reviewed elsewhere (see page 323). In acute granulocytic leukemia, the diagnosis may be rendered more difficult by normal or low leukocyte counts with relatively few leukemic cells in the peripheral blood. Anemia and thrombocytopenia are almost invariable. In their absence, the case may be regarded as *preleukemic,* especially if leukemic cells in the peripheral blood are few. Such cases may also sometimes be called *smouldering leukemia,* especially in the elderly. The use of both terms should be restrained and their true meaning always questioned. The diagnostic features of the blood and marrow leukemic cells are set out in Tables 10-1 and 10-3. As will be seen, the features may be summarized as those of grossly disordered but quantitatively conspicuous granulopoiesis, without the additional features denoting the myelomonocytic, promyelocytic, or erythroleukemic varieties. The leukemic cells are regular in size with round nuclei and numerous visible nucleoli. Auer rods are characteristically present and both agranular polymorphs and pseudo-Pelger cells occur. Rieder cells are uncommon but their presence, or the

presence of indistinguishable cells, does not exclude a diagnosis of acute granulocytic leukemia (Fig. 10-11). The neutrophil alkaline phosphatase activity is usually
low, but most of the leukemic cells are commonly Sudan black positive. Other
cytochemical features are of lesser value in establishing a cell-type diagnosis of
acute granulocytic leukemia.

Chromosomal abnormalities occur in about half of those with acute granulocytic leukemia, but seem to have neither distinguishing nor prognostic value. Their
demonstration may have some diagnostic value where the whole question of acute
leukemia is in doubt (page 149). The occurrence of chromosomal aberrations, and
their failure to change in therapeutically induced remission has some bearing on the
question of two or more marrow cell populations in acute granulocytic

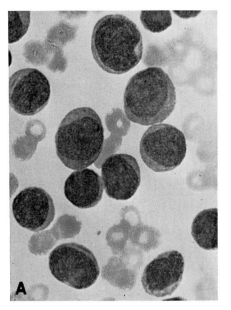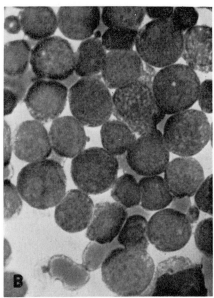
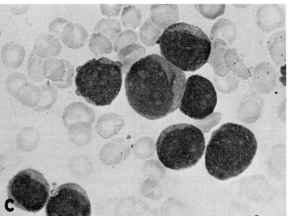

Fig. 10-11. Acute granulocytic leukemia. A. Blast cells in the peripheral blood. B. Blast
cells in the bone marrow. C. Auer body in the cytoplasm of the largest blast cell. A, B, C, ×
1100.

leukemia.[17,234] It is also relevant to the potential and strategy of treatment in the disease.[77] In the untreated patient, or even in patients initially responsive to treatment, death usually results from infection, hemorrhage, or a combination of these. Anemia per se is a less common cause of death than it formerly was because of the availability and ready use of blood transfusion. Blood components other than erythrocytes are less easily replaced (see Chapter 18). CNS involvement, once rare in acute granulocytic leukemia, is increasingly seen as a later complication. Pulmonary infarction and hemorrhage are now being recognized as terminal events with much greater frequency.[449]

ACUTE PROMYELOCYTIC LEUKEMIA

This form cannot be distinguished clearly from the commonest form of acute granulocytic leukemia, sometimes called acute myeloblastic leukemia. In all cases of acute granulocytic leukemia abnormal promyelocytes are found in varying number in the peripheral blood (Table 10-3): in the promyelocytic form they predominate. Acute promyelocytic leukemia is rare, and we are not aware of the disease having been reported in childhood. Because of the uncertain diagnostic criteria and the difficulty of distinguishing it from the granulocytic form in general, it is impossible to estimate its true frequency. Certainly, its recognition as a variety of acute granulocytic leukemia and its diagnosis in many individual cases is caused not by its ill-defined cytological features but to the occurrence of its most notorious complication—hemorrhage.

Acute promyelocytic leukemia was rarely described as a separate entity before the early 1960s. When it was, it was usually classified as a variety of acute granulocytic leukemia occurring in adults, presenting with epistaxis, bleeding gums, or even more serious hemorrhages. The hemorrhagic tendency was quickly found not to be mainly or solely attributable to thrombocytopenia. Low fibrinogen levels were found to be its most striking laboratory feature (see Chapter 14). In due course, with the improved definition and recognition of disseminated intravascular coagulation,[327] this has been found to be especially common in acute promyelocytic leukemia. As Pitney has pointed out,[327] disseminated intravascular coagulation is not peculiar to acute promyelocytic leukemia among the acute granulocytic leukemias: recognition of the association has possibly led to a double bias in ascertainment. As a consequence, the possibility of disseminated intravascular coagulation is especially considered and investigated in cases of acute granulocytic leukemia with the clinical and hematological features of the acute promyelocytic form; and its demonstration has come to be accepted as a feature favoring a diagnosis of the latter disease in otherwise undistinguished cases of acute granulocytic leukemia. In fact, disseminated intravascular coagulation in acute leukemia is not peculiar to acute promyelocytic leukemia, or even to the acute granulocytic form.

Apart from its striking hemorrhagic tendency, the promyelocytic form has other characteristics. The cytologic features are not clearly separate from those of acute granulocytic leukemia in general (Table 10-3), although myeloblasts are often said to be lacking in the bone marrow. Clinically, splenomegaly, lymphadenopathy, and hepatomegaly are perhaps uncommon. This variety seems to run an especially rapid course but this may be due to its complication by hemorrhage.[340] The syndrome of disseminated intravascular coagulation with secondary fibrinolysis seems to respond to heparin therapy,[170] but the overall effect on survival is slight. Other hematologic features in acute promyelocytic leukemia are leukopenia, giving rise to a relatively "aleukemic" peripheral blood picture; and very high serum vitamin B_{12} levels in the absence of liver damage.[338] This last finding is commonly found together with increased serum vitamin B_{12}-binding capacity but is not peculiar to acute promyelocytic leukemia among the acute granulocytic leukemias.

ACUTE MYELOMONOCYTIC LEUKEMIA

There is no doubt that the introduction of this term, *acute myelomonocytic leukemia,* if not the recognition of the variant of acute leukemia has come about relatively recently (see Chapter 3).[143] In the earlier literature most cases of this variant of acute granulocytic leukemia were described as acute monocytic leukemia, and some continue to be so described, at least until recently. Acute myelomonocytic leukemia is to be identified with the so-called Naegeli type of acute leukemia[306] since that author emphasized the occurrence of monocytes and leukemic granulocytes together. Wider recognition of this form of acute granulocytic leukemia is probably a consequence of the more general use of bone marrow biopsy in the investigation of acute leukemia. In acute myelomonocytic leukemia the peripheral blood leukocytes may be dominated by abnormal monocytes and the bone marrow by abnormal granulocytes. Naegeli was a strong exponent of the doctrine of a common origin for monocytes and granulocytes as well as drawing attention to this association in acute myelomonocytic leukemia. His feeling on this point seems to have been vindicated by more recent studies,[257] although other interpretations are not lacking.[435] Despite its relatively long history, even under the misleading name of acute monocytic leukemia, acute myelomonocytic leukemia is a relatively new concept and most of the literature is recent. Many cases now so named were obviously in the past regarded as instances of acute granulocytic leukemia without qualification, and not as examples of acute monocytic leukemia. Consequently, they are now being recognized at all ages, including childhood.[266]

Clinically, the acute myelomonocytic form cannot be distinguished from the generality of acute granulocytic leukemia. Since the occurrence of gingival involvement, oral sepsis, and skin lesions have long been recognized as features of so-called monocytic leukemia, it is to be expected that these complications are now seen to have a special association with acute myelomonocytic leukemia. Otherwise it has no particular clinical features so that its diagnosis depends on hematologic features (Table 10-4). Among these the low nuclear-cytoplasmic ratio and the indented and convoluted nuclei of the leukemic cells are especially useful. In addition, the leukemic cells show an especially fine Sudan black positivity, helping to distinguish it from the generality of acute granulocytic leukemia. In keeping with the concept of its close relationship to acute granulocytic leukemia in general are the many features of disordered granulopoiesis. Among these, the presence of Auer rods, pseudo-Pelger cells, and relatively agranular polymorphs are easily recognizable (Fig. 10-12). Serum muramidase levels[302] and serum vitamin B_{12} values are said to be especially high.[67,464] Nevertheless, these statements, as well as the finding of relatively low neutrophil alkaline phosphatase levels in acute myelomonocytic leukemia should be treated with reserve in view of its uncertain differentiation from acute granulocytic leukemia in general. The current tendency is to classify as acute myelomonocytic leukemia not merely cases of acute granulocytic leukemia with conspicuous monocytosis but most cases in which leukemic change is not largely

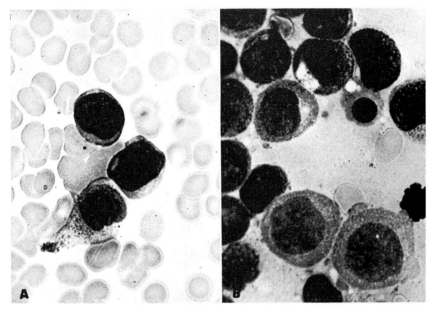

Fig. 10-12. Acute myelomonocytic leukemia. A. Blasts in peripheral blood with monocyte features conspicuous. B. Abnormal granulopoiesis in bone marrow. Both × 1100.

confined to the granulocyte series. As a result, disordered erythropoiesis as well as monocytosis tend to be special features of acute myelomonocytic leukemia. Recently, a special liability to immunological disorder has been reported in children with acute myelomonocytic leukemia.[64]

ERYTHROLEUKEMIA

This condition is discussed in Chapter 11. The term is regarded as synonymous with acute erythremic myelosis or the acute form of Di Guglielmo's syndrome. As such it has features in common with both the myeloproliferative disorders as defined in Chapter 11, and with acute leukemia, being acceptable as a variant of acute granulocytic leukemia. It is thus a difficult disease entity to define and to separate clearly from its congeners. In the past, it seems likely to have been under-diagnosed.[143] Wider attention was drawn to it in 1958 by Di Guglielmo. The largest reported series is one of 20 cases studied by Scott and his colleagues.[383] With greatly increased awareness of the condition, it now seems likely that it is overdiagnosed. In our experience many cases of acute granulocytic and myelomonocytic leukemia with megaloblastoid erythropoiesis are so classified. In fact, relatively few cases would be acceptable examples of erythroleukemia if the criteria summarized in Table 10-5 were adhered to.

The most important of the criteria, and those now most commonly ignored,[325] are that erythroblasts should be present in the peripheral blood and should predominate in the bone marrow (Fig. 10-13). Observance of these criteria ensures that other forms of acute leukemia with disordered erythropoiesis are not accepted as instances of erythroleukemia. Nevertheless, it is recognized as a mixed form of acute leukemia as is exemplified by inclusion of abnormalities of the granulocyte series in the criteria. The most useful of the cytochemical features is the heavy PAS

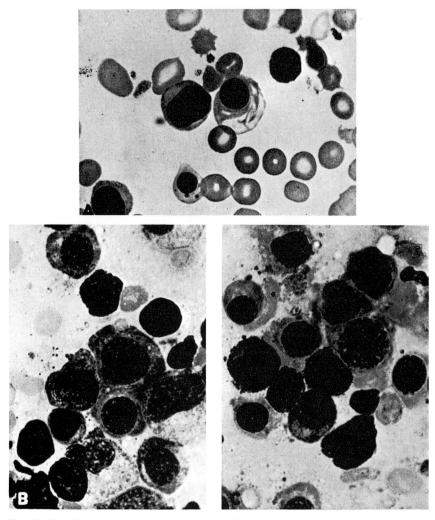

Fig. 10-13. Erythroleukemia. A. Peripheral blood showing erythroblasts. B. Bone marrow erythroblasts. × 1100. C. Bone marrow showing erythroblasts with megaloblast features. A, B, C, × 1100.

positivity of the erythroblasts. This feature is also seen in the abnormal granulocytes commonly present.

Erythroleukemia has no special cytogenetic abnormality to distinguish it from the other forms of acute granulocytic leukemia (Fig. 10-14). It is similarly undistinguished regarding its age incidence and its response to treatment. Indeed, it has an especially sinister reputation among the various forms of acute granulocytic leukemia in respect to its resistance to therapy. In our experience, this reputation is unwarranted since a few cases respond unusually well and enjoy an unusually long survival. It may be that these very cases approximate more closely to the chronic rather than to the acute form of erythremic myelosis (Chapter 11), or even to the refractory sideroblastic anemias.[97,190] In differential diagnosis, deficiency of vitamin B_{12} or folate should be excluded, as should hemolytic anemia with folate deficiency.

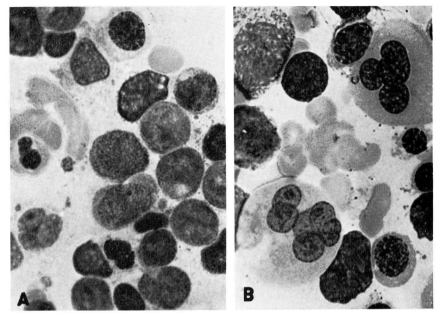

Fig. 10-14. Erythroleukemia. A. Bone marrow showing erythroblasts and myeloblasts. B. Bone marrow showing grossly aberrant erythroblasts. Both, × 1100.

SPECIAL CLINICAL FEATURES IN CYTOLOGIC TYPES OF ACUTE LEUKEMIA

Some symptoms and signs in acute leukemia may be related to the age incidences of the main cytologic types. Others seem to be related to the cytologic type regardless of the age of the patient. However, none of these features is specific enough or frequent enough in its occurrence to have great discriminating value by comparison with the hematologic features.[176] These clinical features and some less common modes of presentation in acute leukemia have recently been reviewed by Israels in the light of his great experience.[205]

The frequency of lymph node enlargement and splenomegaly in childhood acute lymphocytic leukemia may be related more to the plasticity of lymphoid tissue in children than to cell type. In the same way, pain in bones and joints, and radiologic changes in bones in childhood may be attributed to the readier expansion of bone marrow at that age. Analogous changes occur in younger patients with hemolytic anemia, presumably for the same reason. The same ready expansion of hematopoiesis may account for the gross hepatomegaly more often seen in children with acute leukemia than in adults.

On the other hand, cell type rather than age appears to be related to the occurrence of skin lesions in acute leukemia. These are more frequent in acute granulocytic leukemia and its variants than in acute lymphocytic leukemia. Skin lesions are thus more common in younger children with acute granulocytic leukemia than in older children with acute lymphocytic leukemia. Similarly, gingival infiltration is uncommon in children with the latter and relatively common in the granulocytic form at all ages. It is not a feature peculiar to so-called monocytic leukemia but may have a special association with acute myelomonocytic leukemia. It certainly seems likely that patients with that variety of acute leukemia have a special liability to oral and rectal sepsis. This liability may depend on the deficiency of myeloperoxidase in even apparently normal neutrophils in some cases of acute granulocytic leukemia.[68]

As discussed elsewhere (see Chapter 14), bleeding in acute leukemia is mainly dependent on platelet levels, and to a lesser extent on the occurrence of disseminated intravascular coagulation. The latter mechanism may operate, especially in the promyelocytic variety of acute granulocytic leukemia, and so be the basis of that disorder's unquestioned association with serious hemorrhagic complications.[82, 167, 340] Since it is by no means confined to acute promyelocytic leukemia, disseminated intravascular coagulation cannot be used as a distinguishing characteristic.[170, 197]

Central nervous system (CNS) leukemia. Central nervous system leukemia was once rare, at least clinically, if not at careful postmortem examination. Now it is commonplace in acute lymphocytic leukemia and of slight but growing frequency in acute granulocytic leukemia, and even in chronic granulocytic leukemia after metamorphosis. Its clinical occurrence seems to depend not directly on the cell type of acute leukemia but in part at least on the duration of survival. In short, its greatly increased incidence and emergence as a major clinical problem depends paradoxically on the improved efficacy of treatment in acute lymphocytic leukemia. In 1938, Forkner described neurologic disorders in leukemia "as by no means rare."[143] Even then, attention was drawn to the discrepancy between gross and microscopic evidence of frequent involvement of the nervous system and the rarity of associated clinical manifestations. The increase in the frequency of frank clinical manifestations of CNS leukemia seems to date from the advent of effective chemotherapy in 1948.[57] Between 1947 and 1960, its incidence increased tenfold.[132] In one recent study of acute leukemia in childhood 50 percent of the patients developed CNS leukemia.[446] This important problem is now the subject of a vast number of publications, and the literature has recently been critically reviewed.[57, 108] Because of its special relevance to the efficacy of systemic treatment of acute lymphocytic leukemia, as well as the problems in therapy it itself presents, CNS leukemia is considered in some detail in Chapter 18.

It seems likely that in many, if not most cases of acute leukemia, and certainly in the acute lymphocytic form, leukemic seeding of the CNS has already occurred at the time of diagnosis. In the past, in most patients, these seeds remained clinically silent although they could readily be found at autopsy. Even with modern therapy of acute lymphocytic leukemia these seeds must persist, probably unaffected by most antileukemic therapy, behind the blood-brain barrier. Furthermore, since modern therapy has resulted in greatly improved survival in acute leukemia, the CNS leukemic deposits are given time to proliferate and possibly seed more widely in the nervous system, so as to give rise to clinical manifestations. Clinical manifestations result most commonly from meningeal leukemia, although at autopsy involvement of the brain substance is even more common.[57, 260] Time for proliferation seems to be a critical factor in the development of meningeal leukemia. Since this is more often available in acute lymphocytic leukemia than in the acute granulocytic type, because of the striking difference in the efficacy of treatment in the two forms, meningeal leukemia is much more common in the former than in the latter. Since acute lymphocytic leukemia is the predominant form of acute leukemia in childhood, meningeal leukemia is at present mainly a problem of acute lymphocytic leukemia in childhood. Although this seems to depend on cytology and resulting duration of survival, it remains possible that the age of the patient itself may have some effect on the risk of development of meningeal leukemia. An age-effect is difficult to demonstrate, separate from the cytological type of acute leukemia and the duration of survival. Other factors which have been related to the occurrence of CNS leukemia are a direct correlation with the total leukocyte count and the presence of lymph node enlargement; and an inverse correlation with the initial platelet count.[446] It is believed that the total leukocyte count and extramyeloid proliferation reflect the leukemic cell mass and that this, in turn, determines the number and size of leukemic seeds. The platelet count may determine the occurrence of minute intracranial hemorrhages whereby leukemic cells find their way to the CNS both before diagnosis and between diagnosis and the induction of remission. An additional factor other than longer survival may play a part in the recent increase in frequency of CNS leukemia. This increase is not readily explained by improved survival and greater awareness of the complication: it is possible that more recently introduced treatment may, by immunosuppression or some other effect, in addition to its effect on survival, contribute to the occurrence of CNS leukemia.

Seeding by minute intracranial hemorrhage and resulting passage of the blood-brain barrier is not the only pathogenic mechanism proposed for extension of leukemia to the CNS. Since deposits are at autopsy found much more commonly in the dura than in the arachnoid, direct extension from the bone marrow has been suggested.[299] However, there are many good reasons why autopsy findings may not provide a reliable indication of the mechanism of extension to the CNS. Most obviously, they are late rather than early findings and they reveal a state which usually follows a long period of treatment, some of which may have been initially successful. The same objection applies to some more recent autopsy findings which have led to the suggestion that leukemic invasion of the CNS occurs from the superficial arachnoid veins into the arachnoid trabeculae.[333]

It is understandable that the details of the pathogenesis of CNS leukemia should be difficult to elucidate. The site of the disease is relatively inaccessible and the initial lesions are minute, if not microscopic. In addition, the remarkable capacity of the lesions to remain clinically silent has been demonstrated in many studies.[260,310] Cytogenetic studies have shown that the leukemic cells recovered from cerebrospinal fluid (CSF) have basically the same characteristic chromosomal aberrations as are demonstrable in bone marrow.[280] Even more important is the fact that these same findings demonstrate continuing clonal evolution of leukemic cell-lines in CSF.[17] In some patients, this evolution is indistinguishable from that going on in the bone marrow; in others, the findings are consistent with continuing evolution in the CNS and possible recolonization of the bone marrow by new and resistant cell-lines.

As has already been pointed out, most clinical episodes of CNS leukemia are of meningeal leukemia. In acute lymphocytic leukemia they occur with about equal frequency in children in hematologic relapse and in children judged to be in hematologic remission. The median time from diagnosis to the first episode of meningeal leukemia is apparently about 9 months.[183] There is an increasing number of episodes with longer survival as might be expected since very few cases occur early in the course of acute leukemia and meningeal leukemia has been shown to be strongly survival-dependent. It seems likely that there is a point of equilibrium in the relationship of survival in acute leukemia to the probability of development of CNS leukemia. Up to this point there is an increasing liability to develop CNS leukemia whether in hematologic relapse or remission. On the other hand, very long-term survivors have rarely manifested meningeal leukemia.[424] This is in keeping with the fact that the survival of those with CNS leukemia after their first episode is shorter than in matched cases of equivalent survival differing only in not having meningeal leukemia. As might be expected, those who develop meningeal leukemia early in their course are usually among the short-term survivors. There are obvious reasons for these observations: first, meningeal leukemia has, like any other intracranial neoplasm, its own considerable effect on mortality. Death commonly results from increased intracranial pressure, sometimes from sudden respiratory arrest. Second, as indicated by the cytogenetic studies cited above, leukemic cells may persist behind the blood-brain barrier, protected from the effects of otherwise effective systemic antileukemic therapy (see Chapter 18). With or without fresh cytogenetic evolution having occurred in the CNS deposits, cells from these deposits may recolonize the bone marrow and lead to hematological relapse. It is possible that the CNS is not the only site of such "sanctuary" for leukemic cells at times of otherwise successful antileukemic therapy. Liver, kidneys, gonads, and other tissue may harbor leukemic cells while the patient with acute lymphocytic leukemia is in apparently complete remission.[282,310] At present, however, the CNS is the best-known site and meningeal leukemia its recognized and recognizable manifestation. Consequently, there are justifiable hopes that more effective antileukemic therapy aimed at leukemic cells in their CNS sanctuary will have a beneficial effect on survival and possible cure rate in acute lymphocytic leukemia in general (see Chapter 18).[398,424]

In the diagnosis of meningeal leukemia a high index of suspicion is the first prerequisite, since the most common symptoms are nonspecific (Table 10-6). Nausea, vomiting, headache, and lethargy are not uncommon in sick people, children or adults, and are readily attributable to side effects of treatment. Patients and the parents of patients adopt the explanation with apparent alacrity. Nevertheless, proper awareness of the possible significance of these symptoms may lead to diagnosis. The most common physical sign is papilledema present in about half the

Table 10-6

Frequency of the Commoner Manifestations of Meningeal Leukemia

Symptoms	%	Signs	%	CSF findings	%
Nausea and vomiting	63	Papilledema	49	Pressure (>200 mm water)	84
Headache	61	Separation of sutures	34	Cells (>10 per cu mm)	89
Lethargy	35	Hydrocephalus	7	Glucose (<50 mg per 100 ml)	52
Visual disturbance	20	Facial nerve palsy	22	Protein (>45 mg per 100 ml)	40
Auditory disturbance	9	Peripheral nerve palsy	5		
Psychiatric symptoms	20	Pupillary changes	20		
Irritability	20	Reflex changes	40		
Vertigo	15	Hemiparesis	5		
Coma	17	Rigidity	22		
Convulsions	15	Ataxia	6		
		Abnormal EEG	56		

Based on Broder and Carter.[52]

patients. Even in its absence, diagnosis may follow examination of the CSF prompted by these apparently nonspecific symptoms. Once papilledema has occurred the appearance of the optic discs may not return to normal, and it may be an unreliable sign in second or later episodes or suspected episodes of meningeal leukemia. In meningeal leukemia the presence of papilledema is not a contraindication to cautious lumbar punctures with removal of a small volume of CSF. Nevertheless, although lumbar tap has a therapeutic value, it should be carried out with restraint in the presence of papilledema.

Some relatively rare manifestations of CNS leukemia include a presentation which suggests multifocal leukoencephalopathy with transient hemiparesis, tremor, and ataxia.[224] Presumably, too, reflex, auditory, and pupillary changes result from direct cerebral involvement rather than from the meningeal leukemia. Despite the value of CSF changes in confirming a diagnosis of meningeal leukemia, and despite the fact that it is the preponderant form of CNS leukemia, the possibility of cerebral leukemia without CSF changes should be considered.[343] Treatment with intrathecal antileukemic agents and/or radiotherapy must not be withheld because of apparently normal CSF pressure and other findings. The frequency of such misleading findings has been greatly reduced by the introduction of the cytocentrifuge.[118, 239] This elegant piece of equipment yields technically superior preparations for Romanowsky and other staining methods. It makes it possible to identify leukemic cells in CSF even when they are present in very small numbers.

Confusion may sometimes arise as to the role of side effects of antileukemic treatment and CNS leukemia in the genesis of certain signs and symptoms. Obesity, increased appetite, and behavioral changes caused by leukemic infiltration of the hypothalamus may be mistaken for the side effects of corticosteroids. Similarly, encephalopathy from the intrathecal administration of methotrexate for meningeal leukemia (Chapter 18) may be mistaken for the effects of cerebral leukemia, as well as of hemorrhage or infection.[230]

In summary, the most useful clinical indications of meningeal leukemia are headache and an increase of cells in the CSF. Abnormal cells may be found in the asymptomatic patient with a normal CSF cell count; and this finding is an indication for treatment. Less commonly, both the CSF cell count and morphology may be normal in a patient with severe cerebral leukemia. The CSF glucose and protein values are less useful indications of meningeal leukemia than are the CSF pressure and the number and morphology of its cells.

Less than 10 percent of cases of meningeal leukemia occur in acute granulocytic leukemia or in chronic granulocytic leukemia after metamorphosis.[245] With longer survival, resulting from improved treatment, these leukemias may be expected to contribute a larger proportion of cases of meningeal leukemia in the future. Evidence of the efficacy of intrathecal methotrexate in meningeal leukemia complicating acute granulocytic leukemia is contradictory. It may be effective as an antileukemic agent for meningeal leukemia when given intrathecally, when it would not be expected to be effective if given systemically for acute granulocytic leukemia (see Chapter 18).[385]

DIFFERENTIAL DIAGNOSIS OF ACUTE LEUKEMIA

Some general principles, especially the need to consider clinical and laboratory findings together, have already been stated (see page 275). Regardless of the cytologic type of acute leukemia, some problems of differential diagnosis occur with particular frequency. Aplastic anemia or hypoplastic anemia may often be confused with acute leukemia, especially when, in addition to pancytopenia, the peripheral blood contains some atypical leukocytes which may be accepted as blast cells. In hypoplastic states these cells are rarely so numerous in the bone marrow as to justify a diagnosis of acute leukemia. As for clinical features, hemorrhage and infection may be common to both acute leukemias and hypoplastic anemias. On the other hand, enlargement of spleen, lymph nodes, and liver, and the occurrence of bone pain suggests acute leukemia. In a small proportion of patients, both adults and children, in whom this diagnostic problem arises, it may be accepted as insoluble at any particular time. The two conditions may for the moment be indistinguishable. This is especially understandable in view of the possible relationship of aplastic anemia to acute leukemia, and the occurrence of aplastic or hypoplastic states as preleukemic manifestations (see page 302). The answer generally lies in serial observations. In acute leukemia, the features suggesting that diagnosis, whether in blood, bone marrow, or both, are likely to become rapidly more conspicuous, while in aplastic anemia, they may disappear or persist unchanged.

Leukemoid reactions to infection or those occurring in the recovery phase following transient bone marrow depression may closely simulate acute leukemia at all ages. Only when there has been antecedent marrow hypofunction are leukemoid reactions likely to be associated with anemia and thrombocytopenia, certainly of the degree usual in acute leukemia. Nevertheless, especially difficult problems may arise in children with lymphocytic leukemoid reactions to viral infection, which may closely simulate acute lymphocytic leukemia. As with hypoplastic states, leukemoid reactions are rarely accompanied by organ enlargement. Similarly, the features in the peripheral blood which suggest AL are hardly ever matched by equally suggestive evidence in bone marrow. If they are, the answer usually lies with the very different time courses of the two conditions. Acute leukemia is usually more or less rapidly progressive, whereas leukemoid reactions are commonly transient. Consequently, serial clinical and hematologic assessments over a fairly short time will usually resolve the difficulty.

Refractory anemias, including the sideroblastic anemias in adults, may simulate acute leukemias. Indeed, differentiation may be temporarily impossible since refractory anemia and sideroblastic erythropoiesis may be features of true acute leukemias. Again, the difference in time course is most likely to provide the answer where careful assessment of all the features, clinical and laboratory, fails to do so. In a proportion of elderly patients—and it is in this age group that the difficulty most often arises—differentiation may be impossible, even over a protracted period of observation. Although immediate and accurate diagnosis is always desirable for prognosis and for explanation to the patient, in these very cases there is little or no urgency for therapeutic decisions. Aggressive treatment of so-called smouldering leukemia in those over 60 is probably contraindicated (see Chapter 18). Regarding the prognosis in these situations, the prudent course is either to give the patients and relatives the more optimistic diagnosis or to discuss the problem frankly. The latter course is preferred if the diagnostic problem is of other than short duration.

In children with acute lymphocytic leukemia the clinical picture may simulate either rheumatic fever or acute rheumatoid arthritis. The confusing features are commonly bone and joint pain and even true arthritis. The blood and bone marrow findings in the nonleukemic disorders are rarely truly leukemoid. Again, the time course of the diseases usually resolves the problem quickly. Use of antiinflammatory drugs may be a critical diagnostic test. Osteolytic lesions in bone point to acute leukemia.

In children, too, neuroblastoma may simulate acute leukemia. The simulation is especially close in bone marrow where neuroblastoma cells may be indistinguishable from leukemic blasts and present in such numbers as to justify a diagnosis of acute leukemia if the peripheral blood findings are not given due weight. Such cells rarely occur in peripheral blood although there is often a leukoerythroblastic picture. Radiologic studies of bone are commonly not helpful since the findings in neuroblastoma may simulate those of acute leukemia.[182] The problem is readily resolved by the findings in the bone marrow of the pseudorosettes characteristic of neuroblastoma.[375] An abdominal mass displacing a kidney may be found, and the occurrence in it of calcification alone is sufficient to differentiate it from spleen.

The peripheral blood picture in infectious mononucleosis may simulate acute lymphocytic leukemia. The diagnostic confusion rarely has any other basis than in the peripheral blood lymphocytosis with splenomegaly, lymphadenopathy, and fever. The lymph nodes in the latter disease are rarely tender. Anemia and thrombocytopenia may certainly occur in mononucleosis but bone marrow findings suggestive of leukemia of any kind hardly ever do. Similarly, the serologic findings of mononucleosis are not found in acute leukemia. Transient diagnostic confusion may occur between infectious mononucleosis and chronic lymphocytic leukemia. The age incidence of the two diseases is, however, radically different and the confusion is rare and unlikely to persist.

In summary, leukemia in all its forms rarely presents great difficulty in differential diagnosis. When it does, the difficulty often arises from faulty hematologic techniques especially in making, staining, and examining blood films and bone marrow preparations. If these preparations are less than completely satisfactory, and the opportunity exists to make better ones, the first step in resolving diagnostic difficulty is to replace suboptimal blood and bone marrow preparations with the best that can be made. Particular caution is advised in making a diagnosis of any kind of leukemia, if the evidence of leukemia is minimal or if other disease is obviously present. Where both causes for scepticism exist a diagnosis of leukemia is rarely tenable. The demonstration of cytogenetic abnormality as a confirmatory test, especially for acute leukemia has proved disappointing. Chromosomal aberrations may be present in preleukemic conditions (page 303) where a diagnosis of acute leukemia is not justified; and in the very cases where help is most needed, a marrow sample adequate for chromosomal studies may not be obtained.

CONGENITAL LEUKEMIA

This is a rare and poorly defined group of cases, of special interest in relation to the etiology of acute leukemia. The difficulty of definition arises from the variation in criteria for recognition as congenital. Strictly speaking, leukemia should be present at birth and, if diagnosed later, it should be reasonably certain that it was present at birth and would have been demonstrable if the appropriate diagnostic steps had been taken. In fact, while some authors employ the more strict criterion, others recognize *congenital leukemia* as being synonymous with "leukemia in the newborn period."[397] There is a special and understandable tendency for authors to be more liberal in their recognition of congenital leukemia, diagnosed later where there is a family history of leukemia or associated congenital abnormalities. The best recognized of the latter is of course trisomy 21 (see Chapter 5).[34,115,406] Acute leukemia in the neonatal period has also been described in association with trisomy 13–15,[369] absence of radii,[408] the Ellis-van Creveld syndrome,[289] patent ductus arteriosus,[408] the Klippel-Feil syndrome,[408] atrial and ventricular septal defects,[144,408] and the Bonnevie-Ullrich syndrome.[334] These coincidences should for some purposes, be distinguished from the other associations of a congenital abnormality with acute leukemia in which the congenital abnormality seems to lead to an unduly high risk of leukemia developing later than the neonatal period.

The associations of certain familial and congenital abnormalities with acute leukemia, regardless of the age of development, are discussed in Chapter 5 and have been reviewed in their various aspects.[15,115,144,249,290,291] They include conditions depending on known abnormalities of chromosome number such as trisomy 21 and trisomy 13–15. In some similar associations the chromosomal abnormality is a special liability to chromosomal breakage as in ataxia telangiectasia, Fanconi's hypoplastic anemia, and Bloom's syndrome. In others, there are no recognizable chromosomal aberrations, such as neurofibromatosis,[144] Marfan's syndrome,[144] familial ectodermal dysplasia,[144] osteogenesis imperfecta,[156] and Poland's syndrome (congenital absence of pectoralis major with other abnormalities of hand, arm, or thorax).[439] In addition to these and other less well established associations of familial and congenital abnormalities with acute leukemia, we ourselves have noted similar associations with the rare juvenile forms of chronic granulocytic leukemia, both Ph^1-positive and -negative (see page 334).

Congenital leukemia which is strictly congenital is said to be almost exclusively of the acute granulocytic type.[397] In earlier reviews of the condition, only 4 of 32 cases were described as lymphocytic in one series,[345] and 2 of 21 in another.[326] In contrast to these observations is a recently described series of 32 cases of acute leukemia diagnosed in the first year of life. All were seen at a single hospital over a 20-year period.[139] Of this series, 23 had acute lymphocytic and 9 acute granulocytic leukemias of one variety or another. The difference between the distribution of cytologic types of acute leukemia in this series and the earlier reviews may depend on age at diagnosis, most of the more recent series being not strictly cases of congenital leukemia. If congenital leukemia is accepted as embracing all cases diagnosed in the first year of life, then a few cases of the rare juvenile variety of chronic granulocytic leukemia would be so regarded.[346,414] Apart from this possible association as to cytological type, the only other recognized peculiarities of congenital leukemia are the frequency of skin infiltration[76,345] and the poor prognosis. The latter feature may be largely caused by the unfavorable cytologic type of acute leukemia. Cases of congenital acute lymphocytic leukemia are too rare to allow reliable assessment to be made of the efficacy of modern treatment.[139]

The differential diagnosis of acute leukemia in the newborn has few special difficulties once the disease is suspected. The usual criteria apply as to bone marrow findings and appropriate doubt in the absence of anemia and thrombocytopenia. As with young children in general, the newborn may have leukemoid reactions to infection which may simulate acute leukemia closely. For example, a similar leukemoid reaction has been described in folate deficiency.[250] Nevertheless, leukemoid reactions can usually be differentiated from acute leukemia by the absence of organ infiltration and thrombocytopenia, and the bone marrow findings. Misdiagnosed leukemoid reactions probably account for most of the reported instances of spontaneous remission of acute leukemia, many of which have been among neonates.[110]

A particular diagnostic difficulty arises regarding the occurrence of acute leukemia in newborn children with trisomy 21. There have now been several reports of spontaneous recovery from congenital acute leukemia in trisomy 21.[25,129,354,356] It seems most likely that these are especially convincing leukemoid reactions. There is other evidence of abnormal control of bone marrow activity in trisomy 21.[235,295,445] It has been erroneously thought that acute leukemia in trisomy 21 is mainly, or even exclusively, acute granulocytic leukemia. In fact, acute granulocytic leukemia predominates in mongols developing acute leukemia in the first year of life, as it does in other children of that age. Taking the association of trisomy 21 and acute leukemia as a whole, in a review of published cases, acute lymphocytic leukemia was found to predominate.[354]

Chronic Granulocytic Leukemia

Chronic granulocytic leukemia generally follows a more predictable natural history than either acute leukemia or chronic lymphocytic leukemia. Since the discovery of the Philadelphia chromosome (Ph[1]) in 1960, it has been the subject of many studies. These have used the unique chromosomal aberration as a label for the leukemic cell and, more recently, as a diagnostic criterion for the clearer delineation of chronic granulocytic leukemia from related diseases which may simulate it. Use of the Ph[1] has led to a better understanding of the natural history of the disease, but not of its usual etiology (see Chapter 5). Unfortunately, after 13 years, this exciting and challenging discovery has not made any real difference to the treatment of the disease, which remains unsatisfactory.

Chronic granulocytic leukemia occurs at all ages although most but not all of the rare childhood cases are variants of the disease distinguished by absence of the Ph[1] chromosome, and by other features as well. The greatest incidence is in the age group 40–60, and it is slightly more common in men than in women (see Chapter 4).[115]

Case history. A typical case of CGL may occur in a male aged 45. The most likely presenting symptoms are undue tiredness and some weight loss.[382] Other patients may be aware of painless splenomegaly and, in some, splenomegaly is first discovered after splenic infarction. This usually gives rise to a sharp pain of sudden onset in the left hypochondrium, left lower chest, or left shoulder, which is aggravated by respiration so as to suggest pleurisy. After a day or so the pain passes off or loses its commanding quality and is succeeded by a dull ache over the enlarged spleen. In some instances of splenic infarction, the abdominal pain is more diffuse and lacks the pleuritic features, although it is usually of sudden onset.

Other less common presenting symptoms are those of anemia if the hemoglobin level is below 10 gm, which is unusual; or hemorrhagic phenomena. The latter may take the form of easy bruising or undue bleeding on slight injury or minor surgery, and are often difficult to explain. Even less common, but still not rare, presenting features are those of hernia or ankle edema, presumably caused by splenomegaly and resultant increased intra-abdominal pressure.

About 20 percent of otherwise typical CGL patients are symptom-free when the diagnosis is made.

On examination of a typical patient there is usually surprisingly little to find. Splenomegaly is the commonest feature and its absence should suggest a special need for critical scrutiny of the evidence for chronic granulocytic leukemia. The spleen may be so large as to extend across the midline and have its lower pole in the pelvis; in otherwise typical patients it may be detectable only on radiological examination. If recent infarction has occurred, the spleen may be tender and, if the infarction is very recent, a friction rub may be heard. The liver may or may not be enlarged. Lymphadenopathy is not a typical finding, and its presence suggests that the disease is no longer in the chronic phase. Bone pain or tenderness on pressure is of similar significance. Hemorrhagic phenomena are common, even in the chronic phase, and usually take the form of cutaneous ecchymoses or purpura; other skin lesions are rare.

The blood findings in a typical patient usually include a leukocytosis of 100,000 per cubic millimeter or more. The differential leukocyte count is typical, showing a continuous spectrum of granulocytes—from blasts to segmented neutrophils—with no marked preponderance of either form (Table 10-7). Blood basophils are commonly increased and account for up to 10 percent of leukocytes. Typically, neutrophil alkaline phosphatase activity is absent or greatly reduced. Anemia is normochromic and normocytic, and moderate in degree, rarely being less than 9 gm. Platelet levels are usually raised or normal (Fig. 10-15).

Bone marrow is aspirated with ease, the marrow is hypercellular with an increased number of megakaryocytes and fat spaces are usually absent (Fig. 10-16). Erythropoiesis is normoblastic. Granulocytes predominate as in the pe-

Table 10-7

Chronic Granulocytic Leukemia

Typical Findings in Peripheral Blood and Bone Marrow

Blood		Bone Marrow	
Hemoglobin	11.0 gm	Cellularity	increased
PCV	31%	Fat spaces	absent
Reticulocytes	2%	Megakaryocytes	increased
Platelets	600,000/cu mm		
		G:E ratio	20:1
WBC	150,000/cu mm	Erythropoiesis	normoblastic
Mature neutrophils	60%	Iron stores	present
Metamyelocytes	20	Lymphocytes and	
Myelocytes	20	plasma cells	few
Promyelocytes	8		
Blasts	3	Cytogenetics:	
Basophils	5	46 Ph[1]-positive	
Eosinophils	2	in 90%-100% of cells	
Lymphocytes	4		
Monocytes	6		
Neutrophil alkaline			
phosphatase activity			
low or absent			

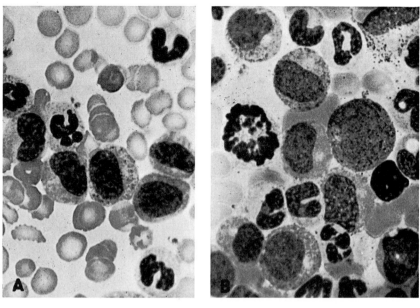

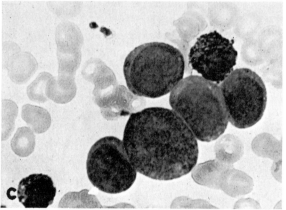

Fig. 10-15. Chronic granulocytic leukemia. A. Peripheral blood in the chronic phase. B. Bone marrow in the chronic phase. C. Bone marrow at metamorphosis. A, B, C, × 1100.

ripheral blood, but again without preponderance of any one part of the spectrum from blast cell to mature polymorph. Cytogenetic studies on bone marrow will show 90–100 percent of mitoses, depending on criteria of scoring, to be Ph^1-positive.

There are few other common findings of diagnostic significance in typical cases of chronic granulocytic leukemia in the chronic phase. Blood uric acid levels may be raised and serum vitamin B_{12} levels are almost invariably raised.[24,355] The latter abnormality is secondary to a greatly increased level of transcobalamin I, the major B_{12}-binding protein.[194]

In proportion as the clinical and other features at presentation in a suspected case of chronic granulocytic leukemia deviate from the described mode, the veracity of the diagnosis should be questioned. Of particular importance as rare or inconsis-

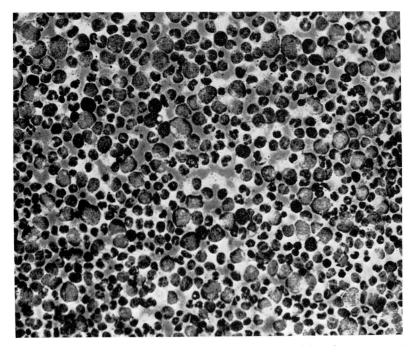

Fig. 10-16.   Chronic granulocytic leukemia. Bone marrow with no fat spaces. × 400.

tent clinical findings are the absence of splenomegaly, conspicuous hemorrhagic phenomena, lymphadenopathy, or extramyeloid tumors other than splenomegaly or hepatomegaly. Of analogous significance are severe anemia or thrombocytopenia; a leukocyte count of less than 100,000 per cubic millimeter not explained by treatment; an excess of blast cells or other deviation from the continuous spectrum of granulocytes in blood or bone marrow; inability to aspirate marrow; a normal or raised neutrophil alkaline phosphatase score; or absence of the Ph[1] chromosome. Some of these findings—clinical and laboratory—are of greater significance than others. Thus, the absence of the Ph[1] chromosome is more important than the presence of conspicuous hemorrhagic phenomena; and deviation from the continuous spectrum of granulocytes is more important than the absence of splenomegaly. Some combinations of inconsistent findings are especially significant: absence of splenomegaly alone is not conclusive, but absence of splenomegaly with lymph node enlargement weighs heavily against a diagnosis of chronic granulocytic leukemia in the chronic phase. The most frequent problems in differential diagnosis are in distinguishing chronic granulocytic leukemia in the chronic phase from chronic granulocytic leukemia in metamorphosis[14,151] or from unusual instances of myelofibrosis with myeloid metaplasia (see Chapter 11).

METAMORPHOSIS

It has long been recognized in the majority of cases of chronic granulocytic leukemia that death is preceded by a change—often a dramatic one—in the character of the disease. In some cases, possibly in the majority, there is reason for describing this change as a *blast cell crisis,* and seeming to equate it with acute granulocytic leukemia arising *de novo.* Indeed, in rare cases of chronic granulocytic leukemia, differentiation may be very difficult, especially if the chronic phase has been silent and had gone undiagnosed.[52,307] Such cases have been mistakenly reported as instances of acute leukemia with the Ph[1] chromosome.[280,355] In the earlier literature,[143] while the more striking changes in the peripheral blood in some patients were recognized, emphasis was placed on the refractory state in terminal chronic granulocytic leukemia. This state was characterized by the failure of previously effective treatment. In fact, this is the most constant single feature of the terminal stages of chronic granulocytic leukemia in which many other features— clinical, hematologic, and cytogenetic—may occur. Because of their number and variety, and to avoid undue attention being given to one nonessential aspect, we prefer the term *metamorphosis*, instead of *blast cell crisis* or its synonyms.[14]

The clinical and hematologic features of metamorphosis were admirably described by Bernard and his colleagues before the discovery of the Ph[1] chromosome.[35] Common clinical features, apart from resistance to previously effective treatment, are increasing malaise and weight loss, pyrexia without infection, rapidly increasing splenomegaly and hepatomegaly, lymphadenopathy, and the appearance of extramyeloid tumors. The range of possible hematologic changes is even greater. Indeed, metamorphosis should be suspected whenever there occurs any departure from the pattern of hematologic findings usual in the chronic phase of chronic granulocytic leukemia, which cannot be accounted for by treatment or a second disease.[16] The total leukocyte count may rise, or fall inexplicably, with a preponderance of less mature cells, whether blasts or promyelocytes. Such a preponderance may obviously disturb the spectrum of granulocytes previously present in the blood. The spectrum may also be broken by the relative disappearance of one type in the sequence of granulocyte development. The neutrophil alkaline phosphatase activity may rise to normal or abnormally high levels.[235] Other leukocyte changes such as monocytosis, and the appearance of giant myelocytes may occur.[121] At metamorphosis, the usual change in peripheral blood platelet levels is a new and unexplained thrombocytopenia, but more rarely thrombocytosis occurs. Rapidly worsening anemia is the rule.[152,225] If the bone marrow is examined at this time it is likely to show predominance of blast cells or promyelocytes, disturbance of erythropoiesis, and perhaps an apparent monocytosis (Fig. 10-15C). Frequently, aspiration in patients in whom marrow has previously been aspirated with ease, becomes difficult or impossible at metamorphosis.

The occurrence at metamorphosis of all these clinical and hematologic changes in chronic granulocytic leukemia may be correlated with cytogenetic changes.[318,402] In general, this is the appearance in bone marrow of a chromosomal aberration additional to the Ph[1] chromosome (see Chapter 6). The reported range of additional chromosomal aberrations is a wide one. Perhaps the most common new abnormality is the appearance of a cell-line with not one but two Ph[1] chromosomes. In some cases, a remarkable range of related cell lines has been demonstrated, usually in bone marrow, [94,173,401] but sometimes in peripheral blood[85] and spleen.[401] In a few cases, these many and varied cell-lines can be seen to be derived from one another by known mechanisms of chromosomal change.[172] The one common feature of all these cell-lines is their derivation from a parent line with no detectable abnormality other than the Ph[1] chromosome. The clinical relevance of these demonstrations of cytogenetic evolution and clonal proliferation is that they provide a rationale for the events at metamorphosis in chronic granulocytic leukemia. This cytogenetic diversity is presumably the basis of the many and varied clinical and hematologic features of metamorphosis, including the well-recognized hematologic findings of blastic transformation. Above all, the cytogenetic diversity provides a rationale for the poor results of treatment of chronic granulocytic leukemia at this stage (see Chapter 18).

Unusual clinical features in the chronic phase.   Most but not all of the unusual clinical and other features described in chronic granulocytic leukemia may be accounted for by diagnostic error or iatrogenic effects. By far, the most common error in this regard is failure to appreciate the onset of metamorphosis, usually because of the absence of the accepted feature of blast cell transformation. Thus, many of the unusual clinical and hematologic features described in the earlier literature, without qualification as to the stage of the disorder, occurred in patients after metamorphosis. This is especially true of lymphadenopathy, cutaneous involvement, and extramyeloid proliferation generally, apart from hepatosplenomegaly. These must be excessively rare in the chronic phase of the disease, if they occur at all. In our experience, their appearance is commonly accompanied by or followed soon after by features of frank metamorphosis. Even in some more recently described cases with unusual findings, suspicion must often exist that more obvious features of metamorphosis would have been noted had the patients been observed more closely for longer periods. It is also our experience that atypical clinical and hematologic features in the chronic phase occur much more often in the unusual and debatable Ph[1]-negative cases (see Chapter 6) than in the more usual Ph[1]-positive cases. This is true of Ph[1]-negative cases in both children[184] and adults.[136,447]

These reservations notwithstanding, certain unusual clinical features may occur, although rarely, in the chronic phase of chronic granulocytic leukemia. Absence of demonstrable splenomegaly is especially common in early cases of chronic granulocytic leukemia diagnosed by accident. In cases of longer standing, splenomegaly may regress so as to become imperceptible after treatment: in such patients, persistent regression is commonly associated with longer and more complete remission. Absence of frank splenomegaly is not incompatible with the occurrence of splenic infarction. In this way, some patients present with what may at first seem to be inexplicable upper abdominal pain.

Additional clinical features at metamorphosis.   Bone pain is commonly due to osteolytic bone lesions. When these occur, they are usually an indication of metamorphosis, or even of frank blastic change.[70] Less commonly, radiologically demonstrable osteolytic lesions and bone pain may occur in cases in the chronic phase which seem to remain so for many months.[70] The obvious question arises whether the bony lesions herald metamorphosis and death, being the site of the first evolution of the new autonomous cell-line with the Ph[1] and additional chromosomal aberration. It seems to be an acceptable general rule to regard any extramyeloid proliferation in chronic granulocytic leukemia, other than in spleen or liver, as evidence of metamorphosis. In some cases, the interval may be long between the detection of the first feature of metamorphosis and the appearance of additional evidence.

Lymphadenopathy,[123,153,420] cutaneous infiltration,[420] cardiac involvement,[412] meningeal involvement,[245] and leukemic arthropathy[403] all illustrate the rule that extramyeloid infiltration commonly spells metamorphosis. As such, each indicates evolution of the disease and worsening of the prognosis. Splenomegaly and hepatomegaly have already been mentioned as exceptions to the rule, both being usual in cases unquestionably in the chronic phase. Presumably, both liver and spleen may be regarded as alternative sites of hematopoiesis, rather than frankly abnormal sites such as the skin or myocardium. Obviously sternal tenderness, as an indication of expansion of bone marrow volume at a normal site, is not an indication of metamorphosis, occurring commonly in the chronic phase. In contrast, the rare occurrence of priapism in the chronic phase of chronic granulocytic leukemia might seem to be an exception. As an exception, it is more apparent than real, since here the leukemic involvement is not extravascular, but is caused by thrombosis or sludging in the penile cavernous tissue.[87] It occurs in 1 percent or so of patients, in the chronic phase as well as after metamorphosis.

When the whole course of chronic granulocytic leukemia is considered, abnormal bleeding is most common after metamorphosis. At that time, thrombocytopenia is usually the most conspicuous cause although, as in all the leukemias, other hemostatic deficiencies may have a contributory role.[197] Nevertheless, severe hemorrhage may occur in the chronic phase with normal or increased platelet levels, and not uncommonly leads to diagnosis of chronic granulocytic leukemia. It may be spontaneous, follow injury or surgical operation, or take the form of menorrhagia (Chapter 14).

Lymphadenopathy, splenomegaly, and histological findings at metamorphosis may lead to a mistaken diagnosis of coexisting chronic granulocytic leukemia and malignant lymphoma or reticulum cell sarcoma (see page 338).

After exposure to ionizing radiation. Within the category of apparently typical chronic granulocytic leukemia, some subgroups may be discerned, even in the chronic phase. Patients in whom ionizing radiation has played a part in the genesis of the leukemia may be distinguished only because of their history of significant radiation exposure. Since not all so exposed develop leukemia, in no single patient is it possible to say with certainty that chronic granulocytic leukemia—or acute leukemia which follows more commonly—is caused by radiation exposure. Obviously, the probability is high in the case of closely exposed survivors of the atomic bomb at Hiroshima or Nagasaki; or in someone developing chronic granulocytic leukemia 3–7 years after radiotherapy involving irradiation of a considerable volume of bone marrow in high doses. Conversely, the probability is low, even in an atomic bomb survivor who develops the disease 25 years later, or in someone whose special radiation exposure has been confined to diagnostic radiology. Apart from their history, probable radiation-induced chronic granulocytic leukemias differ in no clear-cut way from the non-radiation-caused chronic granulocytic leukemias. It has been suggested[222] that they run a relatively slower, more benign course than comparable cases of chronic granulocytic leukemia without radiation exposure, but the number of cases on which this belief is based is small. Certainly, most well-studied cases with a high probability of being radiation induced have had the Ph[1] in bone marrow.[222,415,426,452] In a proportion of these patients, nonspecific chromosomal changes have been demonstrated in peripheral blood lymphocytes[222] and in bone marrow.[223] In some individuals who have survived heavy irradiation exposure without as yet manifesting leukemia, the observed chromosomal changes in bone marrow include an unduly small G-group chromosome indistinguishable from the Ph[1] (see Chapter 6).

45, XO, Ph[1]-positive cases.   The first instance of this variant of chronic granulocytic leukemia was described in 1962.[12] It is, of course, distinguished by cytogenetic criteria but seems to have the clinical characteristic of running an unusually long and relatively benign course. At least 12 such cases have now been described.[154,427] Since all occurred in males, it has been assumed that the missing chromosome in the Ph[1]-positive cells in these cases is the Y chromosome. This has recently been proved by use of a fluorescent staining technique.[154]

Ph[1]-negative chronic granulocytic leukemia in adults.   Generalizations about either the clinical or hematologic features of Ph[1]-negative chronic granulocytic leukemia are on especially uncertain ground. In the early days of human cytogenetic studies, typical cases were so described because of absence of the Ph[1] from cultures of peripheral blood. Presumably, many of these patients carried the Ph[1] in bone marrow cells, but some erroneously described as Ph[1]-negative are still cited as such long after the source of error has come to be appreciated. The converse error is to adopt unduly lax criteria for a diagnosis of chronic granulocytic leukemia, and to accept questionable instances of the disease as being Ph[1]-negative cases. These have most commonly been instances of myelofibrosis with myeloid metaplasia with unusually high leukocytosis (Chapter 11). Nevertheless, apparently typical cases of chronic granulocytic leukemia without the Ph[1] do occur. In our experience these are very rare, but instances multiply as diagnostic criteria are relaxed, especially as regards the occurrence of the full spectrum of granulocytes in the peripheral blood. Nevertheless, some centers have reported 12–29 percent of their cases of chronic granulocytic leukemia as Ph[1]-negative.[136,447] These patients are on average older, respond poorly to busulfan, and have a shorter median survival than Ph[1]-positive cases.[150,151] For these reasons they may be referred to special centers such as those reporting surprisingly high frequencies. Their hematologic peculiarities include lower leukocyte counts, fewer basophils, and more severe anemia and thrombocytopenia. Other differences between Ph[1]-negative and Ph[1]-positive patients seem to be emerging from studies of lysozyme levels in tissues and body fluids. In the untreated state, Ph[1]-negative patients have been shown to have muramidasuria and elevated leukocyte muramidase levels, unlike Ph[1]-positive cases.[321] This difference is not to be confused with the regular finding of elevated serum muramidase levels in Ph[1]-positive cases.[262] Marked muramidasuria may occur after treatment in both Ph[1]-positive and Ph[1]-negative chronic granulocytic leukemia.[425] Galton and Spiers[150] have suggested that Ph[1]-negative cases in adults should be described as subacute. While we deplore further multiplication of names for leukemias, this suggestion has some merit. No modification of standard treatment used for typical chronic granulocytic leukemia has been reported or even suggested for these Ph[1]-negative cases.

Chronic granulocytic leukemia in childhood.   Chronic granulocytic leukemia is rare in childhood. In most large series it accounts for only 1.3–5 percent of patients under the age of 10, with an overall average of 3.4 percent. The age incidence shows a peak at about the age of 3 years. About half are Ph[1]-positive patients who seem to respond to busulfan and run a course more or less indistinguishable from that in adults. The rest are Ph¹-negative and may be distinguished from the typical cases by several points of difference (Table 10-8). The clinical and hematologic differences have now been described by several authors.[184,346]

The Ph¹-negative variety may be regarded not as true chronic granulocytic leukemia but as a variant of acute myelomonocytic leukemia with an associated nonleukemic neutrophil response, or a leukemic granulocytic component as is postulated in typical acute myelomonocytic leukemia. The name *subacute juvenile myelomonocytic leukemia* has been suggested for it, but it has not gained general acceptance and rightly so. It would be unfortunate if it did. Now that the justification for differentiating between acute and chronic forms of leukemia is becoming more questionable, it would be regrettable to reintroduce an intermediate step in the acute-chronic scale. At present we prefer to call it juvenile chronic granulocytic leukemia or, better still, if the facts allow, Ph¹-negative chronic granulocytic leukemia in childhood.

Congenital abnormalities of all kinds are excessively common in both Ph¹-positive and Ph¹-negative cases in childhood. In the Ph¹-negative form, persistent high levels of fetal hemoglobin have been described.[283] Apart from this association with congenital abnormalities, Ph¹-positive patients have more or less typical clinical and hematologic features at diagnosis. Because of their relative rarity, generalizations are hazardous, but it does seem that at this age, even otherwise typical patients have a relatively rapid course to metamorphosis and death.

Myelofibrosis before and after metamorphosis. Myelofibrosis may occur early or late in the disease. When it is found at diagnosis, early in the chronic phase of chronic granulocytic leukemia, myelofibrosis is not associated with any particular clinical finding other than difficulty in or failure to aspirate bone marrow. Such patients may as a group be slightly more anemic than is common. On the other hand, the neutrophil alkaline phosphatase activity is usually absent or low as in typical CGL; and they do not have the teardrop poikilocytes so commonly seen in primary myelofibrosis.[169] The Ph¹ is present, although it may be demonstrable only in unstimulated cultures of peripheral blood, because of failure to obtain a marrow

Table 10-8

Comparison of Ph¹-Positive and Ph¹-Negative Chronic Granulocytic Leukemia in Childhood

	Ph¹-positive	Ph¹-negative
Age	Older	Younger
Splenomegaly	+	+
Lymphadenopathy	−	+
Infections	−	++
Hemorrhage	+	++
Congential abnormalities	++	++
Leukocyte count	Higher	Lower
Thrombocytopenia	+	++
Monocytosis	−	+
Response to busulfan	+	±
Survival	Short	Shorter

From Baikie, unpublished observations.

sample by aspiration. Ph^1-negative myelofibrosis with myeloid metaplasia is discussed in Chapter 11. Ph^1-positive cases, with myelofibrosis present in the early stages of the chronic phase, do not differ from more typical cases with cellular marrow in regard to natural history and response to treatment.

The implications of myelofibrosis developing late in chronic granulocytic leukemia are quite different. Again the cases are Ph^1-positive and the features and natural history of the disease have not, until then, differed from those of typical chronic granulocytic leukemia. Myelofibrosis developing late is apparently a mark of metamorphosis. In some patients, it is accompanied by frank blastic transformation.[169,420] In all patients there is failure of previously effective treatment and other less constant clinical features of metamorphosis. Additional chromosomal abnormalities appear, especially cells which are doubly Ph^1-positive. Anemia and thrombocytopenia are usual; the previously low or normal neutrophil alkaline phosphatase activity commonly becomes elevated.

Iatrogenic induction of metamorphosis. It is understandable that, since almost all cases of chronic granulocytic leukemia recognized in the chronic phase are treated and later undergo metamorphosis, the role of treatment in inducing this change has been questioned. The suggestion is, at first glance, a reasonable one. Busulfan and x-irradiation are known to cause both point mutations and grosser chromosomal damage of the kind likely to hasten the evolution of aneuploid and Ph^1-positive cells from a previously Ph^1-positive yet diploid population. Positive evidence of such a harmful effect is not available and must be difficult or impossible to obtain. The hypothesis certainly does not justify withholding treatment in the chronic phase of the disease, whether by busulfan or x-irradiation. On the other hand it should prompt a search for new methods of treatment in the chronic phase of the disease (see Chapter 18). There is some evidence that, of the two standard modes of treatment of the chronic phase of chronic granulocytic leukemia, x-irradiation may be more potent than busulfan in the induction of metamorphosis.[241,286] There is some similarly inconclusive evidence that once an aneuploid Ph^1-positive cell-line has evolved, treatment with either busulfan or x-irradiation may select in favor of such a line, and against the diploid Ph^1-positive cell, characteristic of the chronic phase of the disease.[317] The evidence is certainly inconclusive in regard to a positive harmful effect by busulfan or radiotherapy at this stage of the disease. Nevertheless, both are without beneficial effect once metamorphosis has occurred, so that a case may be made for their earlier abandonment as soon as metamorphosis is detected.[18]

The suggestion that metamorphosis is actually caused by treatment given in the chronic phase is not a reasonable one. It is well known that the disease in some patients (see page 331) is first diagnosed after metamorphosis so that the patients have never before received treatment. The possibilities of treatment hastening metamorphosis, or influencing the patient's course unfavorably once metamorphosis has occurred, is much more difficult to disprove. This topic is given new importance by the increasing number of reports of the development of acute leukemia and other second neoplasms in patients with Hodgkin's disease, other malignant lymphomas, and myeloma treated by both radiotherapy and chemotherapy.[71,304] In some of these patients the apparently radiation-induced second disease has been, as might be expected, Ph^1-positive chronic granulocytic leukemia; in others the radiation-induced chronic granulocytic leukemia was apparently Ph^1-negative.[452]

Other iatrogenic effects. The most common unwanted effects of treatment in chronic granulocytic leukemia, whether by busulfan or radiotherapy, is bone marrow depression and hypoplasia. Where this effect is severe, death is usual. If the patient should survive, long-term remission is common, often without further treatment.[149] This beneficial effect has been related to the reappearance in the bone marrow of Ph[1]-negative cells.[140]

Other undesirable but less obvious effects have been attributed to busulfan therapy (see Chapters 17 and 18). The most commonly reported of these is so-called *busulfan lung*,[458] first described as a form of diffuse interstitial pulmonary fibrosis in 1961.[314] *The clinical syndrome* with its characteristic histological findings at biopsy or autopsy has not been described in untreated chronic granulocytic leukemia. Indeed, it seems to occur only after 1 year or more of continuous busulfan treatment.[98] Not every patient given continuous busulfan develops this complication. The clinical features are most commonly increasing dyspnea and unproductive cough. Radiologic changes in lung, suggesting generalized or patchy infiltration or fibrosis, may be detected before symptoms. In some patients, the clinical onset is acute with pyrexia and adventitious breath sounds. The earliest histologic changes are apparently in the lining cells of the lung alveoli which become greatly enlarged. This is followed by deposition of fibrin and later by fibrosis. Changes similar to those in the alveolar cells may be demonstrable in biopsy specimens of bronchial mucosa. Recently, indistinguishable changes in bronchial mucosa have been found in chronic granulocytic leukemia not treated with busulfan, but occurring three times as frequently in patients treated with busulfan. Similar cytological aberrations in the pancreas were found in busulfan-treated patients only.[236] In one patient, 12 years of continuous busulfan therapy was followed by pulmonary fibrosis with widespread heterotopic ossification.[244] Some of the earlier changes seem to be partly reversible on cessation of busulfan.

Although the side effects of long-term busulfan therapy most obviously involve the lung, it seems likely that the underlying cellular changes are much more generally distributed in epithelial cells. Cytomegaly, multinucleated cells, nuclear vacuolization and inclusion bodies have been demonstrated in the liver, pancreas, uterine cervix, skin, urinary tract, intestinal mucosa and in several endocrine glands, including the adrenals. Thus, it is of particular interest that an Addisonian-like syndrome has been described in chronic granulocytic leukemia. The clinical features include cutaneous pigmentation, weakness, weight loss, nausea and anorexia, but biochemical evidence of adrenal insufficiency is usually lacking. In contrast, some authors have found low plasma and urinary steroid levels indicative of adrenocorticotrophic hormone deficiency in clinically indistinguishable cases.[429] The same authors have argued against this syndrome being busulfan-induced although their patients have received busulfan, admittedly some time before. We know of no reports of this Addisonian-like syndrome occurring in chronic granulocytic leukemia without a history of busulfan therapy at some time. In some patients, the dose and duration of busulfan therapy have been such as to suggest that the syndrome may be an inherent, if rare, complication of CGL.[324]

Other features of chronic granulocytic leukemia, best explained as uncommon side effects of busulfan therapy, include gynecomastia, infertility, and cataracts. Myasthenia gravis with an anterior mediastinal tumor has been reported, attributed to an autoimmune response to busulfan; but the case was not typical of chronic granulocytic leukemia.[112]

Gaucher cells. The occurrence in the bone marrow of large storage cells was first described by Albrecht in 1966.[4] Systematic review of bone marrow aspirates, after their initial demonstration in a single patient, revealed these large cells in about 15 percent of CGL patients. By both light and electron microscopy studies they seemed to be identical with the cerebroside storage cells of Gaucher's disease.[155,227] In no case of chronic granulocytic leukemia have these cells been numerous enough in bone marrow aspirate to suggest a diagnosis of primary storage disease, even omitting consideration of the usual features of chronic granulocytic leukemia. It seems likely that the storage material in these cells in chronic granulocytic leukemia is derived from cells of the granulocyte series, and its occurrence is a reflection of the high rate of granulocyte turnover. In Gaucher's disease, in contrast, the accumulation of glucocerebroside may reflect enzyme deficiency rather than increased metabolism.

More recent studies using high-power electron microscopy have demonstrated differences between the storage cells in chronic granulocytic leukemia and those diagnostic of Gaucher's disease.[258] The relationship of the storage cells in both these diseases to storage cells found in the bone marrow in thalassemia[166] and the syndrome of the sea-blue histiocyte,[392] is uncertain. Gaucher-like storage cells have also been described in the bone marrow of acute leukemia in childhood.[454]

COEXISTING CHRONIC GRANULOCYTIC LEUKEMIA AND MALIGNANT LYMPHOMA

There have been many reports of the coincidence of chronic granulocytic leukemia and one or other of the malignant lymphomas. Especially among the earlier reports the leukemia is sometimes described as "granulocytic leukemia" and was, in fact, acute leukemia and not chronic granulocytic leukemia.[143,252] It is now obvious that in most of these cases, and in some in which the leukemia was indeed chronic granulocytic leukemia, it was likely to have been induced by radiotherapy given for the antecedent lymphoma (see page 336). In some instances it has been Ph^1-positive,[136] and in others apparently Ph^1-negative.[452] Even more often, confusion has obviously arisen from a mistaken diagnosis of lymphoma of one kind or another occurring late in the course of the disease, when lymphadenopathy, splenomegaly, extramyeloid tumors, and histologic appearances of undifferentiated sarcoma have been properly attributable to the metamorphosis of chronic granulocytic leukemia.[147,218,417]

A further source of confusion may be cases such as the one already cited in which extensive bone marrow involvement by lymphosarcoma resulted in a peripheral blood picture closely simulating chronic granulocytic leukemia (see page 277). These explanations of reported and known cases notwithstanding, true chronic granulocytic leukemia and malignant lymphoma may well coexist without the coincidence being indicative of any special etiologic relationship.

BASOPHILIC LEUKEMIA

This rare and debatable entity was first described by Lazarus in 1905.[256] In 1938, Forkner was able to review 11 reported cases of basophilic leukemia in man.[143] He referred to mast cell leukemia, only as a disease of cats, and regarded basophilic leukemia as a variant of chronic granulocytic leukemia. Forkner's view of basophilic leukemia seems to be confirmed by more recent case reports. On the other hand, a few cases of so-called mast cell leukemia have since been reported in man, having features suggesting a variant of acute leukemia rather than chronic granulocytic leukemia.[126,146,442] This differentiation of basophilic leukemia from tissue mastocytosis and mast cell leukemia is in accord with what is now known of the fundamental differences between the blood basophil and the tissue mast cell,[341] despite their apparent similarities.

The only remaining doubts as to the status of basophilic leukemia as a variant of chronic granulocytic leukemia arise from its rarity, the usual occurrence of extreme basophilia only at metamorphosis, and the frequency of milder degrees of basophilia in otherwise unexceptionable cases. Basophilia of up to 10 percent is not uncommon in untreated chronic granulocytic leukemia and even higher percentages may be found following response to treatment in patients still in the chronic phase of their disease. The level of blood basophilia is often underestimated in Romanowsky-stained preparations (Fig. 10-17) but may be more certainly assessed in preparations stained with toluidine blue.[379] This difficulty in the assessment of blood basophilia makes it impossible to know if cases with higher basophil levels in the chronic phase, whether untreated or after treatment, are the cases which tend to show more extreme basophilia at metamorphosis. These possible associations are well illustrated in two more recently reported cases of "basophilic leukemia," both acceptable as instances of chronic granulocytic leukemia.[246] Some doubts as to this classification have arisen from the failure to demonstrate the Ph[1] chromosome and a normal neutrophil alkaline phosphatase level in the same patient. Since the chromosome preparation is said to have been unsatisfactory and the normal neutrophil alkaline phosphatase level was found at apparent metamorphosis, this objection is invalid. More recently, a typical case of basophilic leukemia with the Ph[1] has been described.[294]

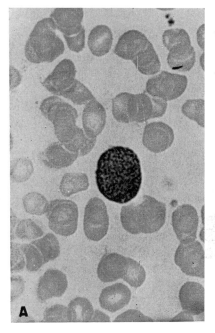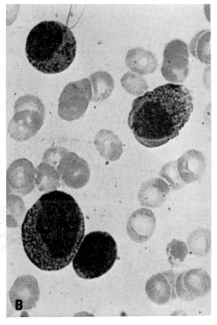

Fig. 10-17.   Basophilic leukemia showing abnormal basophils. × 1100.

Basophilic leukemia as a variant of chronic granulocytic leukemia seems to be distinguished mainly by the levels of basophils in blood and bone marrow. No definite clinical difference can be distinguished from findings in chronic granulocytic leukemia patients but two patients have had either late-onset asthma with high blood histamine levels,[390] or probable asthma,[246] while a third patient had a multiplicity of symptoms attributable to histamine excess.[460] A worse prognosis than average for chronic granulocytic leukemia is sometimes associated with the basophilic variant but may be caused by its common detection at the stage of metamorphosis. Urticaria pigmentosa and a special liability to hemorrhage seem to be concomitants of mast cell leukemia as a variant of acute leukemia, rather than of basophilic leukemia as a variant of chronic granulocytic leukemia.[126,341]

EOSINOPHILIC LEUKEMIA

This rare condition has been discussed briefly (see page 288) with reference to the occurrence of both endomyocardial fibrosis and mural thrombus in cases diagnosed as eosinophilic leukemia. Scott's series of 160 cases of chronic granulocytic leukemia included 2 cases regarded as eosinophilic leukemia.[382] The literature has been reviewed many times[54,134]; and most recently by Benvenisti and Ultmann, who also reported five cases of their own and took account of the diagnostic value of both the Ph[1] chromosome and neutrophil alkaline phosphatase values.[29]

There can be little doubt that many of the previously reported cases of eosinophilic leukemia did not have leukemia but rather an unusually marked eosinophilic response to another primary disease process. The most common of these were probably parasitic infestations, Löffler's endocarditis,[270] Davies's endomyocardial fibrosis,[106] polyarteritis nodosa,[40] or so-called disseminated eosinophilic col-

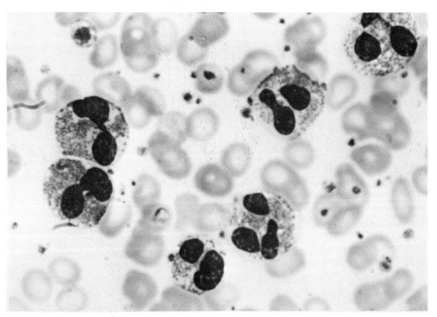

Fig. 10-18. Eosinophilic leukemia (Ph[1]-negative) showing mature neutrophils in the peripheral blood. × 1200.

lagen disease.[130] Indeed, even today, these and other possibilities including transient eosinophilic reactions to drugs should be excluded, so far as is possible, before a diagnosis of eosinophilic leukemia is made, even tentatively. This is often no easy matter because, even in cases acceptable as instances of eosinophilic leukemia there may be evidence of cardiac involvement, neurological features, respiratory symptoms, and arteriolar thrombosis. The differential diagnosis is further complicated by the fact that in many cases otherwise acceptable as examples of eosinophilic leukemia, the eosinophils in blood, bone marrow, and other tissues are mostly mature and may include few forms earlier than myelocytes (Figs. 10-18 and 10-19).

There can be little diagnostic certainty about the majority of reported cases of eosinophilic leukemia. Nevertheless, acceptable instances have been described, some with features suggesting acute leukemia, and others more readily regarded as variants of chronic granulocytic leukemia. We ourselves have seen examples of both, as well as patients for whom confident diagnosis was not practicable, even at autopsy. Benvenisti and Ultmann[29] go further and accept acute, immature or subacute, and chronic forms, distinguished by the maturity or immaturity of the eosinophils in blood, bone marrow, and tissues. The cases classified as acute may also have chloromatous tumors and a very rapid course; the chronic cases include some classified as variants of chronic granulocytic leukemia and others with myelofibrosis which Benvenisti and Ultmann regard as unusual examples of a nonleukemic, myeloproliferative disorder. Some cases have features suggestive of polychthemia vera.

The Ph[1] chromosome has been demonstrated in at least two patients,[174,228] but was absent in others.[29,136,164] As already pointed out, there is no clear-cut correlation between Ph[1] status and the occurrence of cardiac involvement (Fig. 10-20). The Ph[1]-negative patients had an abnormal acrocentric chromosome in a small proportion of

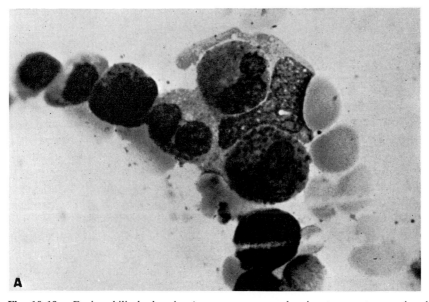

Fig. 10-19. Eosinophilic leukemia. A marrow smear showing two mature eosinophils, an eosinophilic metamyelocyte and a myelocyte having both basophilic and eosinophilic granules. × 1400.

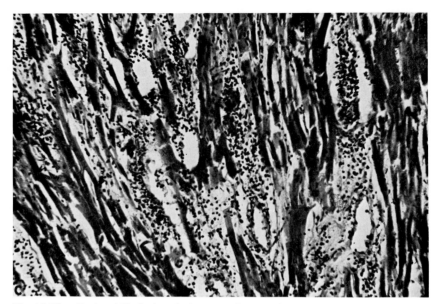

Fig. 10-20. Eosinophilic leukemia (same patient as Fig. 10-19). Heart muscle shows disruption by infiltrating eosinophils. × 140.

metaphases, but no evidence of cardiac complications.[164] In another patient with cardiac involvement and haematologic features suggesting a variant of CGL, the Ph[1] was not found; instead, an unduly short Y chromosome of doubtful significance was found.[142] Reported neutrophil alkaline phosphatase values are few but have been normal, even in the presence of the Ph[1] chromosome.[174] Consequently, we must conclude that, even using the most recent criteria, eosinophilic leukemia is difficult to diagnose as a leukemia and, once accepted as such, even more difficult to relate to the accepted diagnostic criteria for acute leukemia, chronic granulocytic leukemia, or the nonleukemic myeloproliferative disorders.

CHRONIC NEUTROPHILIC LEUKEMIA

This disease is rarely diagnosed. In one series of patients with leukemias of all kinds,[382] which might be expected to include an undue proportion of atypical cases, there were 3 cases of chronic neutrophilic leukemia and 160 of chronic granulocytic leukemia. It seems to occur in older patients and its course is said to be more prolonged than that of typical chronic granulocytic leukemia. Marked splenomegaly with a lesser degree of hepatomegaly are usual, but lymph node enlargement does not occur. The total leucocyte count is generally lower than 100,000 per cubic millimeter, and 90 percent or more are mature neutrophils. This latter feature distinguished the patients in the earlier case reports[143] from patients with typical chronic granulocytic leukemia. In reviewing the literature, Forkner pointed out the occurrence of leukemic changes in bone marrow, spleen, liver, and other organs,[143] indistinguishable from those in chronic granulocytic leukemia, despite the very different peripheral blood picture. Other distinguishing features in cases studied more recently include absence of the Ph[1] chromosome,[361,416] and elevated neutrophil alkaline phosphatase levels.[207,361,416] A very high serum vitamin B_{12} level was found in one case, as in chronic granulocytic leukemia. Bone marrow is aspirated with ease and myelofibrosis is not a feature. The absence of immature granulocytes in the peripheral blood, serves to distinguish the condition from chronic granulocytic leukemia without the Ph[1] chromosome. The persistence of the leucocytosis in the peripheral blood, splenomegaly, and the absence of a primary cause distinguish chronic neutrophilic leukemia from unusually marked leukemoid reactions. It is probably best regarded as a form of myeloproliferative disorder (Chapter 11), despite its name.

Chronic Lymphocytic Leukemia

Chronic lymphocytic leukemia (CLL) has a median age of onset of 55 (see Chapter 4) and there is a male preponderance of 2:1.[115] In Western countries it is intermediate in incidence between the more common acute leukemia and less common chronic granulocytic leukemia. In Japan and other Eastern countries it is relatively less common. It is of rare occurrence before the age of 40 and excessively rare in childhood.[66,368] It is more variable in clinical features and natural history than either acute leukemia or chronic granulocytic leukemia and, unlike them, it is apparently not induced by even high doses of radiation.[39] Another point of difference is the absence of visible chromosomal abnormalities in chronic lymphocytic leukemia (see Chapter 6). These and other differences have led to the questioning of its neoplastic nature. Because of our increasing appreciation of the immunological function of lymphocytes, it was called an immunoproliferative disorder by Dameshek in 1966,[99] but later he characterized it as "an accumulative disease of immunologically incompetent lymphocytes."[100] Certainly, aberrations of immunological function are more common in it than in the other leukemias.[36]

Its onset is insidious as judged by continued observations of accidentally diagnosed cases. Such cases are said to account for from 10–25 percent of diagnoses in Western countries.[148,382] Serial studies of untreated cases, accidentally discovered and otherwise, suggested two main patterns of progression in chronic lymphocytic leukemia. In Galton's type-I trend,[148] the peripheral blood lymphocyte count increased throughout the observation period, which was generally ended by a need for treatment dictated by the appearance of symptoms in a previously asymptomatic patient. A continuous increase in lymphocyte levels was found in the other patients designated as showing type-IIa and -IIb trends. In type IIa, the rise occurred early in the period of observation and then ceased; in type-IIb trend the lymphocyte levels fluctuated above and below a mean value. In both type-I and -II trends, increasing lymphocytosis was associated with increasing lymphadenopathy, splenomegaly, and the appearance of symptoms; and splenomegaly was associated with impairment of bone marrow function. Galton does not claim that these patterns indicate two forms of chronic lymphocytic leukemia. It seems more likely that he detected two or three stages which may occur in the natural history of the same disease process. Apart from the basic significance of these patterns for the pathogenesis of chronic lymphocytic leukemia, their recognition in individuals has obvious relevance for prognosis and treatment. A much more elaborate classification into fourteen types has been proposed, on the basis of a study of involvement of bone marrow, lymph nodes, spleen, and liver in 365 cases.[80] The study itself is a valuable one, but the classification is too complex to be of practical use.

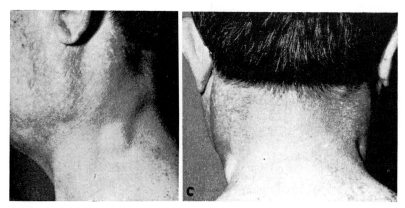

Fig. 10-21.   Chronic lymphocytic leukemia. Cervical lymphadenopathy.

A typical CLL patient is likely to be a man aged 55 who has recently noted enlarged, nontender, cervical lymph nodes (Fig. 10-21). Examination by his physician has revealed lymphadenopathy in other lymph node groups, splenomegaly, and tonsillar enlargement. Hematologic investigation shows a leukocyte count of 50,000 per cubic millimeter, 98 percent of these being small lymphocytes or smear cells. There is neither anemia nor thrombocytopenia. The bone marrow is diffusely infiltrated with small lymphocytes and the fragile smear cells derived from these. Sometimes in bone marrow the lymphocytes may spread more readily than in peripheral blood so that they appear larger (Fig. 10-22), with more cytoplasm and open nuclear chromatin with obvious nucleoli. A mistaken diagnosis of acute lymphocytic leukemia may be made if blood and bone marrow are not compared and contrasted and if due consideration is not given to the other clinical and hematologic facts.

If constitutional symptoms are present at diagnosis they are most likely to be those of undue tiredness, weight loss, and, if anemia is present, dyspnea on exertion

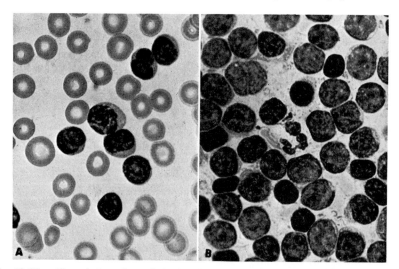

Fig. 10-22.   Chronic lymphocytic leukemia. A. Peripheral blood. B. Bone marrow in the same patient. Note difference in appearance in the two preparations. Both, × 1100.

or angina. The elderly patient with chronic lymphocytic leukemia is especially likely to have myocardial ischemia unmasked by moderate anemia. It is unusual for the patient to be aware of his splenomegaly—probably a reflection of the moderate and slow enlargement of that organ in chronic lymphocytic leukemia. Abdominal pain from splenic enlargement or infarction is rare. Where constitutional symptoms are most marked they are likely to be associated with more severe anemia.

There are many other modes of presentation leading to a diagnosis of chronic lymphocytic leukemia, the range of presenting features being greater here than in any other kind of leukemia. In some, the clinical picture may be dominated by a single manifestation or complication of the disease so that chronic lymphocytic leukemia may not at first glance be obvious. Such may be the case when the presenting clinical picture is dominated by hemolytic anemia, thrombocytopenic purpura, skin involvement, respiratory or other infection, herpes zoster, or reaction to insect bites or smallpox vaccination. However, the association of some of these features with chronic lymphocytic leukemia is so frequent and so well known as to suggest the underlying disease. An even more obvious picture is the presentation of the advanced case of chronic lymphocytic leukemia. Here lymphadenopathy is marked and may be visible as well as palpable in all peripheral lymph node groups. The patient may be aware of splenomegaly, although the organ rarely reaches the extremes of enlargement commonly found in chronic granulocytic leukemia and in myelofibrosis with myeloid metaplasia. Such a patient will often be in a hypermetabolic state, even in the absence of infection, and may show marked weight loss. Advanced cases, whether at diagnosis or late in the course of already diagnosed and treated disease, may have a variety of other features depending on lymphoid proliferation at particular sites. Bone pain may arise from localized proliferations or from progressive skeletal infiltration.[382] Involvement of abdominal lymph nodes is common and may give rise to intestinal obstruction or urinary obstruction, as well as being commonly accompanied by pain and fever. In contrast, mediastinal lymph nodes are less frequently enlarged in chronic lymphocytic leukemia than in lymphosarcoma and the other lymphomas: when they are enlarged they may cause bronchial obstruction or be accompanied by pulmonary infiltration. Thymic enlargement is rare, as is upper airway obstruction[141] and esophageal infiltration.[160] Hepatomegaly is the rule in advanced cases and jaundice may occur terminally, either because of hepatic infiltration or biliary obstruction. Other features include cutaneous tumors and other skin lesions (Fig. 10-23),[45] Mikulicz's syndrome (see pages 285 and 446), orbital involvement, tinnitus and deafness.[387] A rare complication peculiar to chronic lymphocytic leukemia is acropachy—finger-clubbing, symmetrical destruction of the terminal phalanges, and edema of the overlying skin.[62, 161]

Although uric acid levels are raised in chronic lymphocytic leukemia, both gout and uric acid nephropathy are less common than in acute leukemia or chronic granulocytic leukemia.

AUTOIMMUNE HEMOLYTIC ANEMIA

The anemia of chronic lymphocytic leukemia is not of simple causation. Bone marrow involvement by lymphocytes probably limits the erythropoietic response to anemia in many cases. The most severe anemias are usually Coombs' positive autoimmune hemolytic anemias[95] with the usual evidence of increased erythrocyte

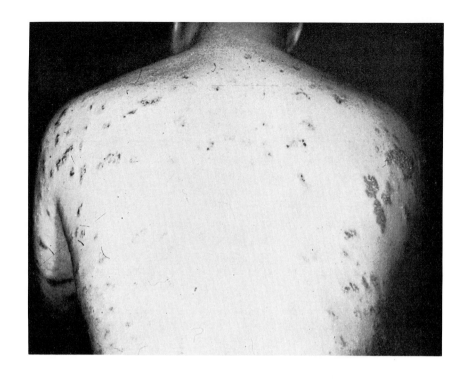

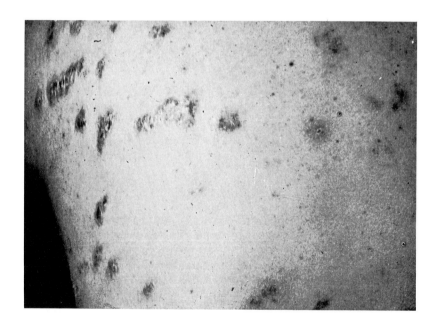

Fig. 10-23. *See legend, facing page.*

346

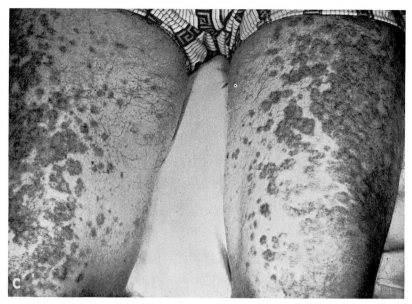

Fig. 10-23. Chronic lymphocytic leukemia. Skin lesions. (Courtesy of Dr. James F. Patterson, New England Center Hospital, Boston.)

destruction and increased erythropoiesis in the bone marrow (Fig. 10-24).[353] Not all the hemolytic anemias in chronic lymphocytic leukemias are direct Coombs' positive. In some cases, antibody may not be demonstrable on the surface of erythrocytes but may be free in serum and found only by the indirect Coombs' test or by testing enzyme-treated erythrocytes against the patient's serum. Rarely, the autoimmune nature of the anemia may be assumed only from the occurrence of acquired spherocytosis demonstrable as increased osmotic fragility. In other more problematical cases, the evidence is even more tenuous, depending on the patient's response to a trial of corticosteroid. This is, indeed, uncertain evidence since the primary disease may itself respond to corticosteroid therapy alone. Nevertheless, in all cases of chronic lymphocytic leukemia with significant anemia not due to a discernible and remediable cause such as bleeding, iron deficiency, or megaloblastic change, corticosteroid should be tried (see Chapter 18), whether abnormal antibodies are or are not found. This belief, arising from personal experience, has recently been given a rational basis by the demonstration of significant amounts of IgG antibody on the surface of erythrocytes, but well below the threshold of the conventional antiglobulin test.[157]

It has been suggested that autoimmune reactions in chronic lymphocytic leukemia, giving rise to hemolytic anemia, thrombocytopenic purpura, and vasculitis, may be triggered by treatment with alkylating agents or x-irradiation.[199,265] The evidence for this is largely circumstantial and it ought not to be allowed to influence decisions on treatment or the choice of treatment. This is all the more true since it is well known that autoimmune hemolytic anemia may not only be a presenting feature in chronic lymphocytic leukemia, but may precede evidence of it or of lymphosarcoma by many years, even when such evidence is carefully sought. This is strikingly exemplified by a personally observed patient.[107]

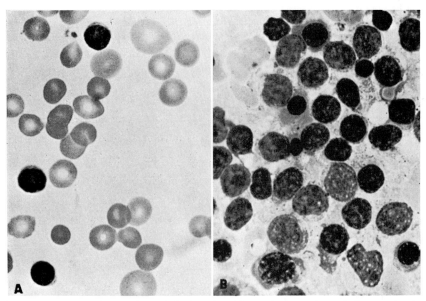

Fig. 10-24. Chronic lymphocytic leukemia with autoimmune hemolytic anemia. A. Peripheral blood showing spherocytes. B. Bone marrow with increased erythropoiesis. Both, × 1100.

Case report. A 46-year–old male presented with a history of symptoms of anemia for 5 months. He had a severe hemolytic anemia with a positive direct Coombs' test, the adsorbed antibody being especially active at 4°C. There was a remarkable hemolytic crisis, during which no reticulocytes were found in the peripheral blood, and the bone marrow contained few red cell precursors and a preponderance of cells of the granulocyte series—a transient, pure, red cell aplasia. At this stage the patient was treated by blood transfusion and corticotrophin. After 6 days, active erythropoiesis was resumed, and the patient made a good recovery. There was no evidence of lymphoproliferative disease in blood or bone marrow, and no lymphadenopathy. There was, however, marked splenomegaly so that splenectomy was carried out shortly after the hemolytic crisis. The histologic appearances in the spleen were those of hemolytic anemia only. Thereafter, evidence of hemolysis disappeared; the patient remained well without treatment and the antiglobulin test became negative several years later. During all this time the clinical and hematologic features were constantly scrutinized for evidence of other disease, since it was felt that this was an instance of symptomatic hemolytic anemia. Fourteen years after splenectomy the patient developed hepatomegaly and lymphadenopathy with symptoms of anemia. He had a leukocytosis of 13,000 per cubic millimeter, almost all the leukocytes being mature lymphocytes. Attempts at aspirating bone marrow were repeatedly unsuccessful. A diagnosis of lymphoproliferative disease, probably chronic lymphocytic leukemia was made and the patient died 15 years after his first presentation with hemolytic anemia.

In this patient the interval between presentation with hemolytic anemia and the development of evidence of lymphoproliferative disease was remarkably long.

Nevertheless, this sequence is fairly common, so that chronic lymphocytic leukemia or lymphosarcoma should be suspected in any elderly patient with apparently idiopathic hemolytic anemia and a positive antiglobulin test, especially if lymph node enlargement is present or splenomegaly is unusual in degree.

When anemia does develop in chronic lymphocytic leukemia, no assumptions should be made as to its causation until blood loss, iron deficiency, vitamin B_{12} deficiency, and deficiency of folic acid have been excluded. The last should never be overlooked. Malabsorption of folic acid is often present in chronic lymphocytic leukemia without megaloblastic anemia or clinically obvious gastrointestinal involvement.[329] Presumably, deficiency is especially likely to occur in patients with increased requirements arising from symptomatic hemolytic anemia.

THROMBOCYTOPENIC PURPURA

Patients with chronic lymphocytic leukemia may present with severe thrombocytopenic purpura,[125] in an analogous way to the more common presentation with autoimmune hemolytic anemia. Demonstration of platelet antibodies being what it is, the autoimmune basis for the secondary disorder may be less certain than in cases of severe anemia with a positive antiglobulin test. Where anemia and thrombocytopenia coexist and the antiglobulin test on red cells is positive, it may be reasonable to assume an autoimmune basis for both secondary disorders, as in the idiopathic Evans' syndrome,[133] not associated with chronic lymphocytic leukemia. In such a situation, treatment with corticosteroid or by splenectomy is indicated, as well as more specific treatment of the chronic lymphocytic leukemia (see Chapter 18), if that diagnosis has been confirmed.

SKIN LESIONS

These are discussed in their pathologic aspect in Chapter 9. They are seemingly more common in chronic lymphocytic leukemia than in any other form of leukemia. Certainly, skin manifestations are more common in CLL than in chronic granulocytic leukemia. The apparently greater frequency of skin lesions in chronic lymphocytic than in acute leukemia may be due to the longer average survival of patients with the former: the incidence of skin lesions in the monocytic varieties of acute leukemia must be close to that in chronic lymphocytic leukemia. The true frequencies of skin lesions in leukemias are difficult to determine, depending as they do on the hazards of ascertainment, selective reporting, and duration of survival. Of Scott's series of 212 patients with chronic lymphocytic leukemia, 7 percent had skin lesions as presenting features, but many of these were infective, and specific leukemic lesions were much less common.[382] In contrast, it seems likely that as many as 50 percent of CLL patients may have skin symptoms or visible lesions in the course of their disease.

Dermatologic manifestations may occur early or late in the course of the disease. In either case, but especially when occurring early, they may lead to presentation and diagnosis. Leukemia cutis in chronic lymphocytic leukemia, as in other forms of leukemia, depends basically on the infiltration of the dermis by leukemic cells (see Chapter 9). This gives rise to the specific leukemic lesions of the skin which may be localized or generalized. If localized, they usually appear first on the face and scalp, upper trunk or extremities, and tend to become generalized. Their progression or regression parallels the progression or therapeutic control of the basic disease process. This infiltration may lead to erythroderma with exfoliation in some cases, to papules, nodules, plaques, (Fig. 10-25), or even to frank tumors which may ulcerate.[45] Symmetrical nodules on the face may give rise to a remarkable leonine appearance. Rarely, several types of lesion may coexist in the same patient; and the clinical picture may be further confused by hemorrhagic lesions, visible lymphadenopathy, or herpes zoster. The infiltrative lesions—whether papules, tumors, or lesions of intermediate size—are usually red or reddish blue in

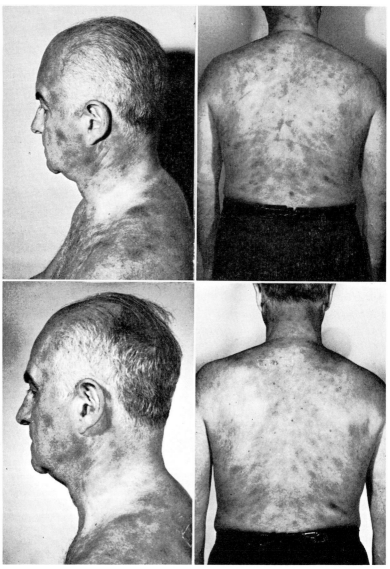

Fig. 10-25. Chronic lymphocytic leukemia. Top, a 63-year-old man with macules, papules, and small nodules, most of them with purpuric discoloration. Bottom, improvement after corticosteroid therapy.

color, and neither itchy nor painful. In contrast, leukemic enythroderma or so-called leukemia cutis universalis is intensely itchy, especially where erythroderma is accompanied by exfoliation. Generalized erythroderma gives rise to the charac-teristic appearance of *l'homme rouge* in which erythroderma is invariable, and skin thickening and exfoliation with pruritus are common.

Leukemic erythroderma, like the more obviously infiltrative lesions, may be lo-calized or generalized. If generalized, it is more likely to be associated with frank clinical and hematologic evidence of chronic lymphocytic leukemia. As in all specific leukemic lesions of the skin, diagnosis is established on the basis of the leukemia, preferably with the results of skin biopsy.

Mycosis fungoides is a term usually reserved for a characteristic spectrum of skin lesions with typical histologic appearances readily differentiated from those of skin involvement in chronic lymphocytic leukemia.[131] Nevertheless, in chronic lymphocytic leukemia when erythroderma, nodules, and ulcerating tumors coexist, the clinical picture may be indistinguishable from that of mycosis fungoides (Fig. 10-26), so that differentiation is only possible on skin biopsy and identification of the diagnostic features of chronic lymphocytic leukemia. True mycosis fungoides may have a relationship to Hodgkin's disease, lymphosarcoma, and reticulum cell sar-coma which is still debatable.[131] Also to be differentiated from chronic lymphocytic leukemia with skin manifestations is the rare Sézary syndrome (see page 444), in which pruritus, erythroderma, skin thickening, and lymphadenopathy may coexist with a typical blood picture.[93,248]

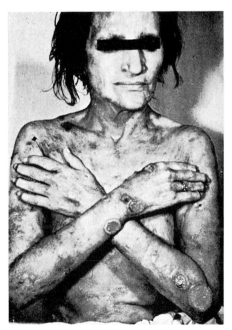

Fig. 10-26. Typical lesions of mycosis fungoides. (Courtesy of Dr. James F. Patterson, New England Center Hospital, Boston.)

Nonspecific skin lesions in chronic lymphocytic leukemia are either hemorrhagic in character, indirectly related to the disease as are iatrogenic rashes, or not
obviously infiltrative with their relationship to chronic lymphocytic leukemia only
rarely proved by biopsy. In the last class are pruritus, prurigolike papules, urticaria,
and bullae. A special association exists between chronic lymphocytic leukemia and
herpes zoster.[388] The association is not understood, although the current trend is to
regard it as a special reflection of the impaired immunologic status in chronic
lymphocytic leukemia, whether treated or not.[373] Other explanations have depended
on the occasional demonstration of leukemic infiltration of posterior nerve roots or
on the triggering effect of local radiotherapy. Herpes zoster may be a presenting
feature in the undiagnosed and untreated patient.[382] When it does occur, it may be
severe with unusually marked constitutional upset, and, in some patients, with a
generalized varicelliform rash.[9] Cutaneous leukemic infiltration may occur in the
scars of treated herpes zoster, as it may in other scars.[79]

Herpes simplex infections are especially common in chronic lymphocytic
leukemia and may lead to diagnosis of the leukemia.[303] Oral as well as cutaneous lesions may be present, and persistent necrotic ulcers of the skin may occur, especially just before death.

The special liability to infection in chronic lymphocytic leukemia may also be
reflected in recurrent pyogenic lesions of skin such as impetigo, furunculosis, or
cellulitis. These, too, may be presenting features, but occur more commonly late in
the course of the disease when the immunologic impairment is usually worst.

Patients with chronic lymphocytic leukemia are especially liable to unusual
reactions to smallpox vaccination and the bites of mosquitoes and other insects,[444]
as well as to herpes zoster. Because smallpox vaccination or revaccination may result in generalized vaccinia, as well as in a severe necrotic local reaction, it should be
avoided. If it is unavoidable, attenuated vaccine should be used and the patient
should be warned of the need to report any unusual reaction. Alternatively, he
should be protected by the administration of hyperimmune gamma globulin at time
of vaccination.

Special precautions should be taken against insect bites by susceptible patients
with chronic lymphocytic leukemia, and the possibility of superimposed pyogenic infection not forgotten.

Attention has recently been drawn to a high incidence of skin rashes in patients
with chronic lymphocytic leukemia treated with ampicillin.[63] This is analogous to
the occurrence of similar side effects in infective mononucleosis, and is presumably
caused by an aberration of lymphocyte immune function.

INFECTIONS

The special liability of CLL patients to infection has been long recognized. It
may well have been heightened by the therapeutic use of corticosteroids and of
forms of treatment leading to worsening of neutropenia. In addition, most forms of
treatment used in chronic lymphocytic leukemia have immuno-suppressive effects of
some kind. The most common infective complications involve the skin and the
respiratory system; but septicemia, endocarditis, urinary tract infections, cellulitis,
and a variety of viral and fungal infections may also occur. Though most common
late in the course of the disease, when natural progression may be followed by iatro-

genic effects in worsening neutropenia and further reducing the immune response, infections may occur as presenting manifestations. In one large series, repeated infections, mainly bacterial infections of skin and respiratory tract, were the presenting features in 13.2 percent of patients.[382] A common occurrence is an episode of pneumonia in an elderly person—perhaps only one of several over a few months—with the resulting clinical examination leading to finding of splenomegaly and lymphadenopathy; or hematologic investigation revealing lymphocytosis. Urinary tract infections are commoner in women than in men. Skin infections may take the form of impetigo or furunculosis (see page 349),[45] or even pyoderma gangrenosum.[322] Pyogenic infections of existing herpetic lesions or of the untoward reactions to smallpox vaccination or insect bites may also occur.

There can be little doubt that, before the advent of antibacterials and, even today in underdeveloped societies, elderly people with chronic lymphocytic leukemia commonly died of their complicating infections without the primary disease being diagnosed.

Pain is an uncommon symptom except when due to complicating infection or hemorrhage. Abdominal pain as a presenting symptom was found in 6.6 percent of patients in one series.[382] Bone pain is rare, but may occur in the presence of skeletal infiltration which is usually diffuse,[88] leading to generalized osteoporosis rather than to discrete bone tumors. Vertebral collapse may occur, and this painful complication may be impossible to differentiate from an iatrogenic effect where corticosteroids have been used in high doses, or over a long period.[56]

IMMUNOLOGIC ABNORMALITIES

As with most immunologic abnormalities in human disease, those occurring in chronic lymphocytic leukemia are as yet only imperfectly understood. This is true of the impairment of immunologic response, which is generally related to the stage and severity of the disease. It is equally true of the aberrant responses believed to underlie autoimmune disease in chronic lymphocytic leukemia, which are even more capricious in occurrence. Of these latter, autoimmune hemolytic anemia and thrombocytopenia are the most common (pages 345 and 349), but vasculitis, thyroiditis, rheumatoid disease, the Mikulicz-Sjögren syndrome, and systemic lupus erythematosus have all been observed.[100]

The crudest evidence of immunologic impairment is the clinical evidence of greatly increased liability to infection. While not discounting the role of neutropenia in some patients, this was early associated with hypogammaglobulinemia,[363,432] demonstrable in about 50 percent of patients at all stages of the disease. In one recent study,[137] some abnormality of immunoglobulins was found in all 54 patients studied by quantitative methods. Most have marked reduction in IgG and IgM levels, the reductions being related to both the duration of the disease and the duration of treatment. Low levels of IgA also occur. Liability to infection may be particularly related to low IgG levels, but these rarely occur alone. In the circumstances, it is difficult to withhold gamma globulin in the treatment of chronic lymphocytic leukemia complicated by serious infection (see Chapter 18), but objective evidence of its therapeutic value is lacking.[56]

As well as showing progressive reduction in immunoglobulin levels affecting

IgG, IgM, and IgA, a very few patients will have a paraprotein.[178] In one study this was found in 6 of 54 cases,[137] including paraproteins of IgG, IgM, and IgA classes: one patient had both an IgM and an IgA paraprotein. Many cases of chronic lymphocytic leukemia have been described with the monoclonal IgM paraprotein (see Chapter 13) which suggests Waldenström's macroglobulinemia.[208,465] Differential diagnosis in such cases may be difficult or even impossible. Relatively marked peripheral blood lymphocytosis favors a diagnosis of chronic lymphocytic leukemia: Bence Jones proteinuria and prominent manifestations of hyperviscosity syndrome may point to Waldenström's macroglobulinemia. In the present state of knowledge, it is probably best to accept that cases falling between the two readily recognized disorders do occur.

The relationship between, and relative importance of, impairment of humoral and cellular immune mechanisms in chronic lymphocytic leukemia are difficult to assess. The effects on cellular immunity are much more difficult to measure than are the immunoglobulin changes as a reflection of humoral impairment. The two may indeed be more closely interdependent than is currently believed. Nevertheless, the reduced response of CLL lymphocytes in vitro, by way of transformation by phytohemagglutinin (PHA) and other mitogens, is generally accepted as reflecting impaired cellular immunity.[312,378,389] This impaired response is favorably affected by successful treatment,[220] but further impaired by progressive disease or during active treatment, especially with prednisolone and chlorambucil in combination.[180]

NATURAL HISTORY

The course of chronic lymphocytic leukemia is more variable and less predictable than that of any other form of leukemia. Some cases progress rapidly despite early treatment, while at the other extreme, some remain quiescent for years, or may even go into apparently complete remission after limited treatment.[74,181] Twenty-year survival is not uncommon, and one instance of survival for 17 years after diagnosis and 28 years from probable onset has been reported.[405] Prognosis and survival are discussed in detail in Chapter 19. Both duration and quality of life after diagnosis bear only a general relationship to the stage of the disease at the time of diagnosis, or the time of first treatment. Some apparently advanced cases—as judged by splenomegaly, lymphadenopathy, and evidence of impaired bone marrow function—may respond rapidly and apparently completely to even conservative treatment[181], while other apparently early cases may advance unrelentingly, despite energetic treatment. The trends in natural history discerned by Galton (see page 343) are only some of the patterns of progression which may occur.[148] Cases in which the disease remains benign over many years despite no treatment are certainly common. Their occurrence is no excuse for failure to observe and reassess such patients regularly, and not less often than one in 3–6 months, as well as warning them of the special risks of infection. Death may result from overwhelming infection, commonly respiratory or septicemic, after only a brief illness. Fatal hemorrhage, usually from the gastrointestinal tract, may occur in the severely thrombocytopenic. Neutropenia and thrombocytopenia may result from the natural progression of the disease with increasing splenomegaly and bone marrow involvement: both are often worsened by side effects of chemotherapy or radiotherapy. In addition, corticosteroids especially in high dosage, may further impair resistance to infection.

In the absence of the commonly fatal complications of infection and hemorrhage, the patient's deterioration may follow another pathway. A hypermetabolic state with progressive wasting apparently may result from rapidly increasing masses of lymphoid tissue with deteriorating bone marrow function. The hypermetabolic state (see Chapter 14) and weight loss may suggest a diagnosis of hyperthyroidism, but specific evidence, both clinical and laboratory, is lacking. The possibility of a superimposed opportunistic infection—whether bacterial, fungal, or viral—may be less readily excluded. Dameshek likened the stage of chronic lymphocytic leukemia to runt disease, the graft-versus-host reaction in animals.[100] The analogy is apt, but remains incomplete without more immunologic evidence. The frequency and severity of intestinal malabsorption in terminal chronic lymphocytic leukemia, which might well explain many of the features of this syndrome, do not appear to have been adequately studied.[329]

ACUTE LEUKEMIC TERMINATION

As with chronic granulocytic leukemia, the terminal stages of chronic lymphocytic leukemia are commonly marked by the failure of previously effective treatment. Unlike the former, any hematologic change which might be described as acute transformation of a formerly chronic leukemia is not a regular feature of chronic lymphocytic leukemia. Such changes do occur, but rarely. In one study,[277] it occurred in two of 340 cases of chronic lymphocytic leukemia, although it has been found more commonly by others.[109,254,315] In some of these patients it is likely that the terminal acute leukemia was separate and radiation-induced by treatment given for chronic lymphocytic leukemia; in other cases acute leukemia may have arisen by chance as a second and unrelated neoplasm[337]; in some, it may represent a rare evolution of the primary chronic lymphocytic leukemia.[320] As is now also becoming obvious in myeloma (see Chapter 13), and Hodgkin's disease (see Chapter 12), the possibility of the induction of acute leukemia by the treatment of chronic lymphocytic leukemia with chemotherapeutic agents such as cyclophosphamide, chlorambucil, and even prednisolone must arise.

OTHER NEOPLASMS

There is evidence that in chronic lymphocytic leukemia a second primary neoplasm other than acute leukemia may occur more often than can be accounted for by chance.[30,175,202] The second neoplasm is most commonly of skin, but carcinomas at other sites also occur. It remains uncertain whether this is an indication of increased liability to neoplastic change per se, possibly genetically determined. Another possibility is a higher rate of ascertainment of a second neoplasm in elderly patients already under closer medical supervision because of known chronic lymphocytic leukemia. It seems likely that typical chronic lymphocytic leukemia may coexist with both Hodgkin's disease[51,141] and reticulum cell sarcoma[159,347] more often than is explained by chance. The name of Richter's syndrome has been given to the latter association. Both associations have been the subject of speculation on the coincidental occurrence of two separate diseases, common etiological mechanisms, or transformation of one disorder into a second. Recently, interest has centered on the possibility that impaired immunosurveillance in the primary disease may predispose to the development of a second neoplasm. This is discussed further in relation to the lymphoproliferative disorders in Chapter 12. Similar considerations apply to the development of a second neoplasm, acute leukemia, or reticulum cell sarcoma, in myeloma (see page 477).

DIFFERENTIAL DIAGNOSIS

Given adequate examination of peripheral blood and bone marrow, the diagnosis of chronic lymphocytic leukemia is rarely difficult. Without these results, the differential diagnosis after clinical examination alone may include all those conditions in which lymph node enlargement, localized or generalized, and splenomegaly, may occur. For this reason alone, examination of blood and bone marrow is essential in all but a few instances of lymphadenopathy and splenomegaly, certainly before lymph node biopsy. The blood and bone marrow findings may provide conclusive evidence of chronic lymphocytic leukemia in a patient with lymphadenopathy or splenomegaly: lymph node biopsy is rarely helpful or necessary in such a patient.

A sustained, peripheral blood lymphocyte count of 5,000 per cubic millimeter, with increased bone marrow lymphocytes probably justifies a diagnosis of chronic lymphocytic leukemia in an adult over the age of 40. In children and younger adults, in whom these findings may accompany or follow viral infection, autoimmune disease, and drug sensitivity reactions, the possibility of chronic lymphocytic leukemia hardly arises. In the older patient, in whom diagnostic difficulty does arise, the need for a firm diagnosis leading to a decision on treatment is unlikely to be urgent. Such a patient may be observed over a period and examination of blood and bone marrow repeated several times if necessary.

Real difficulty may arise in differentiating small cell or lymphocytic lymphosarcoma (see page 438) with involvement of blood and bone marrow, from chronic lymphocytic leukemia, the blood and marrow involvement in such patients being less than those typically found in CLL. In these patients, the lymphocytes in blood and bone marrow are small and indistinguishable from those in typical chronic lymphocytic leukemia. It is doubtful if differentiation is possible and, if so, if it has any significance for treatment or prognosis. On the other hand, it is generally accepted that large cell lymphosarcoma with a leukemic blood picture can be differentiated from chronic lymphocytic leukemia. Furthermore, such patients have now been shown to have a worse prognosis than CLL patients so that a different approach to treatment may be indicated.[377,463]

In studies on lymph node lymphocytes, it is possible to differentiate between chronic lymphocytic leukemia and lymphosarcoma by the occurrence of chromosomal abnormalities in the latter and their absence in the former.[400] The value of this difference in distinguishing the two diseases in equivocal cases has not been explored. In general, however, cytogenetics has a limited place in the differential diagnosis of chronic lymphocytic leukemia because of the absence of chromosomal changes in the disease as such (see Chapter 6).

Rarely, diagnostic difficulty may arise in distinguishing atypical cases of myeloma and Waldenstrom's macroglobulinemia from chronic lymphocytic leukemia. The occurrence of paraproteins in blood and urine weighs against a diagnosis of the last named, but does not exclude it. Conversely, leukemic peripheral blood findings, and lymph node and splenic enlargement favor a diagnosis of chronic lymphocytic leukemia. In a minority of patients, differentiation may be impossible and meaningless since truly transitional disease may occur. In atypical cases of myeloma, the common occurrence of chromosomal aberrations in peripheral blood and bone marrow may have diagnostic value.[103]

LABORATORY FINDINGS

A diagnosis of chronic lymphocytic leukemia depends mainly on the persistence of an increased number of lymphocytes in peripheral blood and bone marrow. More than 5000 lymphocytes per cubic millimeter, with a corresponding lymphocytosis in bone marrow establishes the diagnosis. Because it may be counted, the lymphocytosis in the blood is more readily assessed than lymphocytosis of marrow. The individual lymphocytes are not usually abnormal in appearance and they lack the pleomorphy commonly seen in reactive, as distinct from leukemic, lymphocytosis. They are usually indistinguishable from mature, small lymphocytes, with dense nuclear chromatin, nucleoli well masked by perinucleolar chromatin, and a very thin rim of cytoplasm. The cytoplasm is readily lost in spreading the blood film. Even more marked fragility may result in a variable number of smear cells, damaged in different degrees. Apart from cytoplasmic loss, the nucleus may be altered so as to lose its normal chromatin pattern, stain more lightly with Romanowsky stains, and reveal its nucleoli. More extreme change gives rise to disordered smears of altered chromatin, sometimes called *basket cells,* and barely recognizable as of cellular structure: these are more common in the acute leukemias than in chronic lymphocytic leukemia. In some cases, the lymphocytes in blood and bone marrow are not obviously fragile, but the nuclear chromatin appears even more pyknotic than usual and the nucleoli even more effectively concealed than in the normal lymphocyte. These have been called grumelée cells, presumably from the French *se grumelér,* meaning to clot or condense.

In other cases of chronic lymphocytic leukemia the lymphocytes are frankly abnormal and more obviously fragile. They are larger than normal lymphocytes with more abundant basophilic cytoplasm, relatively open nuclear chromatin, and obvious nucleoli. Such cells are often called lymphosarcoma cells (see page 438) because of their resemblance to those seen in lymph node imprints of lymphosarcoma; and because they sometimes appear in the blood in the later stages of lymphosarcoma (see Chapter 12). The association of these cells with a more aggressive form of chronic lymphocytic leukemia, known as lymphosarcoma cell leukemia, has been discussed (see page 356). In extreme instances they may be mistaken for blast cells of acute lymphocytic leukemia. In children with lymphosarcoma, leukemic transformation is common[410] and the cytology and natural history are those of a variant of acute lymphocytic leukemia especially resistant to treatment.

Although other changes in the peripheral blood film may be found in chronic lymphocytic leukemia, none is diagnostic. A variable but small proportion of atypical mononuclears, or large lymphocytes, may be present. The granulocytes are usually normal in appearance if reduced in absolute and relative numbers. In more advanced cases, granulocytes may be found with difficulty in a white cell picture of depressing uniformity. The acquired Pelger-Huët anomaly has been described in a single case of chronic lymphocytic leukemia.[192] Platelets may be obviously reduced in number, and variable in size. Erythrocytes are usually normochromic and normocytic, but anisocytosis is common, depending on the degree of marrow involvement by lymphocytes. Other red cell changes depend on the presence of hemolysis and are related in degree to the level of hemolytic activity. In extreme instances, autoagglutination, spherocytosis, polychromasia, and reticulocytosis may be obvious. Premature delivery from the bone marrow may give rise to nucleated red cells and immature granulocytes in the peripheral blood, as well as polychromatic red cells and reticulocytosis. When folate deficiency complicates chronic lymphocytic leukemia, with or without symptomatic hemolytic anemia, erythrocyte precursors in the peripheral blood may be megaloblastic.[72,329] The possibility of coincidental iron or vitamin B_{12} deficiency should be remembered, as well as the special risk of folic acid deficiency.

Bone marrow. Examination of the bone marrow in chronic lymphocytic leukemia is essential for the proper assessment of the case, if not for diagnosis. All the usual methods of examination should be employed (see page 294). Not infrequently, no discrete particles are aspirated or a dry tap yielding no aspirate at all is the result. In some patients this is explained by the occurrence of myelofibrosis which is nevertheless much less common in chronic lymphocytic leukemia than in chronic granulocytic leukemia or in Waldenström's macroglobulinemia. In other patients, myelofibrosis is absent but difficulty in aspiration is probably explained by the increased cohesion of a marrow packed with leukemic lymphocytes.

In chronic lymphocytic leukemia an obvious excess of marrow lymphocytes is seldom lacking. Difficulty rarely arises in deciding if the number of lymphocytes is excessive or not. When it does, the marrow examination should be repeated after a lapse of weeks or months, unless the patient's situation is urgent, when it may be repeated at once at a second site. In a few patients marrow lymphocytosis may be found, even before the lymphocytosis in peripheral blood alone warrants the diagnosis. The bone marrow lymphocytes may be diffusely or patchily distributed. Normal marrow elements are reduced in proportion as the marrow is replaced by leukemic lymphocytes. This replacement aside, erythropoiesis and granulopoiesis generally remain qualitatively normal. Disordered erythropoiesis is more likely to occur if anemia is severe. If folic acid deficiency is present, erythropoiesis may be frankly megaloblastic: in other patients folic acid deficiency is associated with normoblastic or so-called macronormoblastic erythropoiesis. When symptomatic hemolytic anemia is present, erythrocyte precursors may outnumber lymphocytes. Megakaryocytes may be found with difficulty, or not at all, in advanced cases. They may be fallaciously underrepresented in marrow aspirate obtained with difficulty which contains no discrete particles.

In chronic lymphocytic leukemia, as in other lymphoproliferative diseases, increased numbers of mast cells may be found in the bone marrow but their significance is unknown.[311]

Lymph nodes. Surgical biopsy of enlarged lymph nodes in chronic lymphocytic leukemia is not necessary for diagnosis. Furthermore, it adds nothing to the assessment of the patient's disease unless a second disease is suspected. Undoubtedly, aspiration biopsy of lymph nodes is generally a poor substitute for surgical biopsy. Accordingly, it is hard to see any place for it in the diagnosis or treatment of chronic lymphocytic leukemia. As with splenic puncture, more favorable assessments have been made, but the crucial test is that the procedure has not found favor, although first described many years ago.[440] The interpretation of findings in samples obtained by aspiration is obviously extremely difficult (Fig. 10-27), with a formidable error.[42,261,271,433]

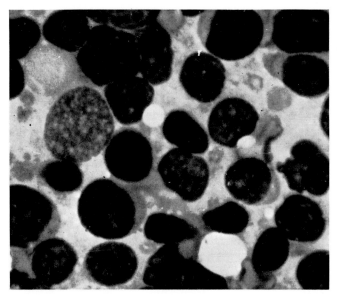

Fig. 10-27.   Lymph node aspirate from an enlarged cervical node shows small and medium lymphocytes. The aspirate did not aid diagnosis. × 1400.

Splenic puncture.   The value of splenic puncture in the diagnosis of the leukemias and related disorders with splenomegaly has been discussed (see page 298). In experienced hands it may have some place in the diagnosis of chronic lymphocytic leukemia but this must be very limited indeed. Where lymphocytosis in blood and marrow is demonstrated, and a diagnosis thus established, splenomegaly is to be expected. Where the diagnostic criteria are not satisfied by the blood and bone marrow findings, a predominance of abnormal lymphocytes in splenic aspirate suggests a diagnosis of lymphosarcoma. Obviously, considerable experience is needed to distinguish with confidence between normal lymphocytes, and small lymphocytes which are likely to be present in the spleen in both lymphocytic lymphosarcoma and chronic lymphocytic leukemia.

Other hematologic findings.   The most common and troublesome complication of chronic lymphocytic leukemia is the occurrence of anemia. In 10–25 percent of patients it is apparently autoimmune in pathogenesis, although anemia of some kind occurs before death in all in whom the disease runs its natural course. In autoimmune hemolytic anemia the direct antiglobulin test is generally positive due to IgG and complement.[135] The antibody may also be present in serum and is of warm type. The serological findings thus correspond to those commonly found in idiopathic acquired hemolytic anemia.[95] It seems likely that an autoimmune mechanism may underlie those instances of anemia, or reduced erythrocyte survival in chronic lymphocytic leukemia without anemia, in which present serological methods may fail to demonstrate immunological abnormality.[157] Increased osmotic fragility of erythrocytes and obvious spherocytosis may be indications of occult serological abnormality. Certainly they are more common features in patients with positive antiglobulin tests or other serological abnormalities. Mechanical fragility, too, may be increased but the correlation between increased fragility, osmotic or mechanical, and visible morphologic change is not close.[95]

The frequency with which reduced erythrocyte survival has been demonstrated in chronic lymphocytic leukemia has varied from one study to another.[59,319,430] These differences may be due in part to the use of different methods—the Ashby technique, radiochromium labeling, and radiochromium labeling with surface counting. Other reasons for such differences may be the few patients studied and the different composition of each series in regard to the stage of the disease and other evidence of hemolysis. Despite these differences, it is obvious that in chronic lymphocytic leukemia significant reduction of erythrocyte life span may be present, with or without more blatant evidence of hemolysis.

Reference has been made (see page 349) to the occurrence of folic acid deficiency, with or without megaloblastic erythropoiesis. Analogous deficiency of vitamin B_{12} seems to be excessively rare.

Blood chemistry. There are no consistent or diagnostic changes in blood chemistry in chronic lymphocytic leukemia in the absence of complicating disease. The occurrence of increased uric acid levels and their renal complications have been mentioned. The frequency of this metabolic aberration makes blood uric acid estimation an essential in the initial assessment of the disease. In addition, it should be carefully monitored during active treatment leading to the reduction of lymphoid tissue. In such situations, especially, the occurrence of acute renal failure and of calculi should be remembered, even in the presence of an apparently satisfactory urinary volume.

Elevation of serum bilirubin, sometimes sufficient to give rise to obvious jaundice, occurs in three situations in chronic lymphocytic leukemia. In the presence of very active erythrocyte destruction, hemolytic jaundice without bilirubinuria may be found. The serum level of conjugated bilirubin may be raised, with bilirubinuria, in the presence of massive hepatic infiltration, or by biliary obstruction, commonly by enlarged lymph nodes at the porta hepatis. Changes in serum immunoglobulin levels have been outlined earlier (page 353) in relation to their consequences by way of increased liability to infection.

(Chronic) Histiocytic Leukemia

Because of their rarity and lack of specific diagnostic features it must be doubtful if all the cases described under these terms—chronic histiocytic leukemia; chronic monocytic leukemia; chronic myelomonocytic leukemia; chronic erythromonocytic leukemia; leukemic reticuloendotheliosis; chronic reticulolymphocytic leukemia; "hairy" cell leukemia—represent distinct disease entities, or are to be accepted as synonyms for a single disorder. There has been an understandable tendency on the part of authors to emphasize the similar features of the groups of cases they describe, and to make light of the points of difference. When the main series are reviewed, certain points in common and many differences emerge. While it is unlikely that each of the names cited above represents a separate disease, it is equally unlikely that one entity can embrace all. Two or more separate diseases seem likely, without dismissing the possibility of a continuous spectrum with graded variation in some features (see Chapter 21).

Most of the published reports concern elderly males. The presenting features are commonly those of anemia, thrombocytopenia, or liability to infection. Splenomegaly is usually present, while hepatomegaly and lymphadenopathy are much less frequent features. There may be leukopenia with a relative excess of large mononuclear cells which, by various authors and for a variety of unconvincing reasons, have been regarded as abnormal monocytes, lymphocytes, or reticulum cells. The picturesque term, *hairy cell,*[330,376] refers, unfortunately, to the appearance of living cells by phase-contrast microscopy: in stained preparations they are usually accepted as atypical large lymphocytes.[360] The same cells have been described in bone marrow, spleen, and sometimes in lymph nodes, when these tissues have been studied. In some series granulopoietic proliferation in marrow has been especially conspicuous, suggesting the name of (chronic) myelomonocytic leukemia.[201,364] The course of the disease, or these diseases, seems to be a lengthy one, with a median survival of 3 years from diagnosis. In view of the evidence of a long initial course with nonspecific manifestations, the average duration of the disease is probably very much longer. No treatment other than blood transfusion, the management of complications and, in a few patients, the administration of adrenal corticosteroids, has been shown to have any effect. It seems likely that even today, and more commonly in the past, many patients die with their disease undiagnosed. Especially in the past, this may commonly have resulted from hemorrhage or infection in the long preleukemic period.

As mentioned above, particular features emerge from the descriptions of particular authors. These special features are clinical, hematologic, histologic, cytologic, and cytogenetic. In some they depend on how the series has been collected and when it was reported. If the patients were all followed to death, the long course and gradual deterioration may be emphasized; if they are diagnosed early in the disease, the lack of features justifying a diagnosis of leukemia may be conspicuous. Some cases have been described in children.[316] The frequency of infections, rectal and oral lesions, including ulceration and gingival hypertrophy, has been emphasized.[395] Skin lesions other than infections seem to occur late in the disease.[395] Most reports show that marrow has been aspirated with ease,[201] but in some aspiration has been successful only with difficulty.[53] Megaloblastic and sideroblastic features in erythropoiesis have been described.[58] Some authors report that the bone marrow is dominated by abnormal mononuclear cells as seen in the peripheral blood, while others describe a few such cells among marked granulopoietic proliferation.[201,267] In one series of 15 cases, low neutrophil alkaline phosphatase values were noted[201,292]; and three of nine male patients had 45 XO cell-lines in bone marrow only. Characterization of the leukemia by the cytologic features of the abnormal cells has been proposed.[330,360] Because of the superficial similarity of the leukemic cells to reticulum cells they were sought unsuccessfully in 100 cases of reticulum cell sarcoma.[330] This result suggests that chronic histiocytic leukemia, as defined by the presence of hairy cells, is not closely related to the malignant lymphomas. Nevertheless, a continuous spectrum including histiocytosis X and histiocytic medullary reticulosis (see Chapter 12) cannot be discounted.

It must be admitted that some cases described as chronic histiocytic leukemia, or by a synonym, could at some stage of the disease be quite differently diagnosed. Thus, the term *preleukemia* (see page 302) can readily be applied to its long chronic stage. Conversely, if seen only terminally, some indistinguishable cases may be regarded as examples of acute leukemia of one kind or another. In some instances it has been described as acute monocytic leukemia[332] or histiocytic leukemia.[215] In one study, the obvious analogy with metamorphosis of chronic granulocytic leukemia has been suggested.[292]

REFERENCES

1. Abrams E, Zierdt CH, Brown JA: Observations on *Aeromonas hydrophila* septicaemia in a patient with leukaemia. J Clin Pathol **24,** 491, 1971.

2. Aisenberg AC, Goldman JM, Raker JW, Wang CC: Spleen involvement at the onset of Hodgkin's disease. Ann Intern Med 74:544, 1971.

3. Alberts DS, Serpick AA, Thomson WL: Hypocalcemia complicating acute leukemia. Cancer Res 17:399, 1969.

4. Albrecht M: "Gaucher-Zellen" bei chronisch-myeloischer Leukämie. Blut 13:169, 1966.

5. Allan J: Leukaemia and pregnancy. Br Med J 2:1080, 1954.

6. Al-Rashid RA: Hypothalamic syndrome in acute childhood leukemia. Clin Pediatr 10:53, 1971.

7. Amromin GD: Pathology of Leukemia. New York, Hoeber, 1968, pp 241–246.

8. Andersen V, Pedersen H: Thymoma and acute leukaemia. Acta Med Scand 182:581, 1967.

9. Anderson D: Severe zoster associated with leuchaemia. Med J Austr 2:126, 1948.

10. Armstrong D, Haghbin M, Balakrishnan SL, Murphy ML: Asymptomatic cytomegalovirus infection in children with leukemia. Am J Dis Child 122:404, 1971.

11. Ask-Upmark E: Leukaemia and pregnancy. Acta Med Scand 170:635, 1961.

12. Atkin NB, Taylor MC: A case of chronic myeloid leukaemia with a 45-chromosome cell-line in the blood. Cytogenetics 1:97, 1962.

13. Aur, RJA, Westbrook HW, Riggs W: Childhood acute lymphocytic leukemia: Initial radiological bone involvement and prognosis. Am J Dis Child 124:653, 1972.

14. Baikie AG: Chromosomes and leukaemia. Acta Haematol 36:157, 1966.

15. ———: Chromosomal aspects of leukaemia, in: Proceedings of the Eleventh Congress of the International Society of Haematology. Sydney, Government Printer, 1966, p 198.

16. ———: Chronic granulocytic leukaemia: The metamorphosis of a conditioned neoplasm to an autonomous one in: Proceedings of the Fourth Congress of the Asian and Pacific Society of Hematology. Nagoya, Japan, International Society of Hematology, Asian-Pacific Division, 1969, p 197.

17. ———: What is a leukaemic remission? The evidence from cytogenetic studies, in Vincent PC (ed): The Nature of Leukaemia. Sydney, Government Printer, 1972, p 231.

18. ———: Chronic granulocytic leukaemia. Med J Austr. 2:12, 1974.

19. ———, Gillis EM, King MJ: Polymorph alkaline phosphatase activity in the PelgerHuët anomaly. Lancet 1:670, 1963.

20. ———, Spiers ASD: Methotrexate in meningeal leukaemia. Lancet 2:259, 1967.

21. Ballard HS, Marcus AJ: Hypercalcemia in chronic myelogenous leukemia. N Engl J Med 282:663, 1970.

22. Barak Y, Liban E: Hypothalamic hyperphagia, obesity and disturbed behaviour in acute leukaemia. Acta paediatr 57:153, 1968.

23. Battle CU, Bonfiglio TA, Miller DR: Pericarditis as the initial manifestation of acute leukemia: Report of a case. J Pediatr 75:692, 1969.

24. Beard MF, Pitney WR, Sanneman EH: Serum concentrations of vitamin B_{12} in patients suffering from leukemia. Blood 9:789, 1954.

25. Behrman RE, Sigler AT, Patchefsky AS: Abnormal hematopoiesis in two of three siblings with mongolism. J Pediatr 68:569, 1966.

26. Bengtsson E: Eosinophilic leukemia—an immunopathological reaction? Acta Paediatr 57:245, 1968.

27. Bentley HP, Reardon AE, Knoedler JP, Krivit W: Eosinophilic leukemia. Am J Med 30:310, 1961.

28. Benvenisti DS, Sherwood LM, Heinemann HO: Hypercalcemic crisis in acute leukemia. Am J Med 46:976, 1969.

29. ———, Ultmann JE: Eosinophilic leukemia: Report of five cases and review of the literature. Ann Intern Med 71:731, 1969.

30. Beresford O: Chronic lymphatic leukaemia associated with malignant disease. Br J Cancer 6:339, 1952.

31. Bernard J: Les aplasies pré-léucemiques. Nouv Rev Fr Hématol 9:41, 1969.

32. ———, Jacquillat C., Chavelet F, Boiron M, Stoitchkov J, Tanzer J: Leucémie auguë d'une enfant de 5 mois née d'une mère atteinte de leucémie aiguë au moment de l'accouchement. Nouv Rev Fr Hématol 4:140, 1964.

33. ———, Jacquillat C, Weil M, Boiron M, Tanzer J: Present results on daunorubicine, *in* Mathé G (ed): Advances in the Treatment

of Acute (Blastic) Leukemias. London, Heinemann, 1970, p 3.

34. _____, Mathe G, Delorme JC, Barnoud O: Les leucoses des très jeunes enfants (leucos de nouveau-né, leucos du premier semestre de la vie, leucos associées à des malformations congenitales. Arch Fr Pediatr 12:470, 1955.

35. _____, Séligmann M, Kvicala R; La transformation aiguë de la leucémie myéloide chronique. Rev Fr Etud Clin Biol 4:1024, 1959.

36. Bergsagel DE: The chronic leukemias: A review of disease manifestations and the aims of therapy. Can Med Assoc J 96:1615, 1967.

37. Bichel J: Lymphatic leukemia and lymphatic leukemoid states in cancer of the stomach. Blood 4:759, 1949.

38. Bisel HF, Wroblewski F, LaDue JS: Incidence and clinical manifestations of cardiac metastases. J Am Med Assoc 153:712, 1953.

39. Bizzozzero OJ, Johnson KG, Ciocco A: Radiation-related leukemia in Hiroshima and Nagasaki, 1946–1964. N Engl J Med 274:1095, 1966.

40. Blackburn CR: Periarteritis nodosa simulating eosinophilic leukemia. Am J Med Sci 220:313, 1950.

41. Blackwell B: Acute leukaemia presenting as a lump in the breast. Br J Surg 50:769, 1963.

42. Block M: Comparative study of lymph node cytology by puncture and histopathology. Acta cytol 11:139, 1967.

43. _____, Jacobson LO, Bethard WF: Preleukemic acute human leukemia. J Am Med Assoc 152:1018, 1953.

44. Bloom GE: Leukocyte adenosine deaminase phenotypes in acute leukemia. Cancer 29:1357, 1972.

45. Bluefarb SM: Leukemia Cutis. Springfield, Ill., Thomas, 1960, pp 41–78.

46. Bodey GP: Fungal infections complicating acute leukemia. J Chron Dis 19:667, 1966.

47. _____, de Jongh D, Isassi A, Freireich EJ: Hypersplenism due to disseminated candidiasis in a patient with acute leukemia. Cancer 24:417, 1969.

48. _____, Hersh EM, Freireich EJ: Recurrent listeria monocytogenes meningitis in a patient with acute leukemia. Cancer 21:619, 1968.

49. _____, Powell RD, Hersh EM, Yeterian A, Freireich EJ: Pulmonary complications of acute leukemia. Cancer 19:781, 1966.

50. Boggs DR, Wintrobe MM, Cartwright GE:

The acute leukemias: Analysis of 322 cases and review of the literature. Medicine 41:163, 1962.

51. Bonadonni G, Monfardini S, Pizzetti F: Simultaneous diagnosis of Hodgkin's disease and chronic lymphocytic leukemia. Lymphology 1:88, 1968.

52. Bornstein RS, Nesbit M, Kennedy BJ: Chronic myelogenous leukemia presenting in blastic crisis. Cancer 30:939, 1972.

53. Bouroncle BA, Wiseman BK, Doan CA: Leukemic reticuloendotheliosis. Blood 13:609, 1958.

54. Bousser J: Eosinophilie et leucémie. Sangre 28:553, 1957.

55. Brincker H, Jensen KB: Cytomorphological classification of acute leukaemias. Dan Med Bull 19:215, 1972.

56. Clinicopathological conference: A case of chronic lymphocytic leukaemia. Br Med J 1:546, 1970.

57. Broder LE, Carter SK: Meningeal Leukemia. New York, Plenum Press, 1972.

58. Broun GO: Chronic erythromonocytic leukemia. Am J Med 47:785, 1969.

59. Brown GM, Elliott SM, Young WA: The haemolytic factor in anaemia of lymphatic leukemia. J Clin Invest 30:130, 1951.

60. Burkitt DP, Wright DH: Burkitt's Lymphoma. Edinburgh, Livingstone, 1970, pp 20–21.

61. Burns A: Observations on the Surgical Anatomy of the Head and Neck. Edinburgh, Bryce, 1811, p 369.

62. Calvert RJ, Smith E: Metastatic acropachy in lymphatic leukemia. Blood 10:545, 1955.

63. Cameron SJ, Richmond J: Ampicillin hypersensitivity in lymphatic leukaemia. Scott Med J 16:425, 1971.

64. Cannat A, Seligmann M: Immunological abnormalities in juvenile myelomonocytic leukaemia. Br Med J 1:71, 1973.

65. Carmel R, Coltman CA, Yatteau RR, Costanzi JJ: Paroxysmal nocturnal hemoglobinuria with erythroleukemia. N Engl J Med 283:1329, 1970.

66. Casey TP: Chronic lymphocytic leukaemia in a child presenting at the age of two years and eight months. Australas Ann Med 17:70, 1968.

67. Catovsky D, Galton DAG, Griffin C: The significance of lysozyme estimations in acute myeloid and chronic monocytic leukaemia. Br J Haematol 21:565, 1971.

68. _____, _____, Robinson J: Myeloperoxidase-deficient neutrophils in acute myeloid leukaemia. Scand J Haematol 9:142, 1972.

69. Cavdar AO, Arcasoy A, Gözdasoğlu S, Demirağ B: Chloroma-like ocular manifestations in Turkish children with acute myelomonocytic leukaemia. Lancet 1:680, 1971.

70. Chabner JB, Haskell CM, Canellos GP: Destructive bone lesions in chronic granulocytic leukemia. Medicine 48:401, 1969.

71. Chan, BWM, McBride JA: Hodgkin's disease and leukemia. Can Med Assoc J 106:558, 1972.

72. Chanarin I, Dacie JV, Mollin DL: Folic-acid deficiency in haemolytic anaemia. Br J Haematol 5:245, 1959.

73. Chatterjea JB, Meza Arrau C, Dameshek W: Splenic puncture. Br Med J 1:987, 1952.

74. Chervenick PA, Boggs DR, Wintrobe MM: Spontaneous remission in chronic lymphocytic leukemia. Ann Intern Med 67:1239, 1967.

75. Chomé J, Saglier P: Particularités histologiques de la participation rénale dans les hémopathies malignes. J Urol Med Chir 66:846, 1960.

76. Christie RW, Bergwall WL: Congenital leukemia. J Indiana State Med Assoc 57:749, 1964.

77. Clarkson BD: Acute myelocytic leukemia in adults. Cancer 30:1572, 1972.

78. Clayden EC: Practical Section Cutting and Staining, 4th ed. London, Churchill, 1962.

79. Cleland JB; Leukaemic infiltrations. Br Med J 2:1191, 1935.

80. Coeur P, Revol L, Viala J–J, Croizat P: Considérations statistiques sur l'atteinte on l'intégrité des organes hématopoïétiques au cours de la leucémie lymphoide chronique. Sem Hôp Paris 47:2171, 1971.

81. Constantoulakis M, Phocas E, Theodoropoulos G: Atypical leukaemia of long duration with monoclonal hypergammaglobulinaemia. J Clin Pathol 23:156, 1970.

82. Cooperberg AA: Acute promyelocytic leukemia. Can Med Assoc J 97:57, 1967.

83. _____, Neiman, GMA:Fibrinogenopenia and fibrinolysis in acute myelogenous leukemia. Ann Intern Med 42:706, 1955.

84. Cornes, JS, Jones TG: Some important clinical and pathological features of leukaemic lesions in the gastro-intestinal tract. Proc R Soc Med 55:702, 1962.

85. Court Brown WM, Tough IM: Cytogenetic studies in chronic myeloid leukemia. Adv Cancer Res 7:351, 1963.

86. Cramblett HG, Friedman JG, Najjar S: Leukemia in an infant born of a mother with leukemia. N Engl J Med 259:727, 1958.

87. Craver LF: Priapism in leukemia. Surg Clin North Am 13:472, 1933.

88. _____, Copeland MM: Changes of the bones in the leukemias. Arch Surg 30:639, 1935.

89. Crist WM, Ragab AH, Vietti TJ: Hypersplenism in a child with acute lymphatic leukemia. Cancer 31:1328, 1973.

90. Critchley M, Greenfield JG: Spinal symptoms in chloroma and leukaemia. Brain 53:11, 1930.

91. Crombie AL: Proptosis in leukaemia. Br J Ophthalmol 51:101, 1967.

92. Crooks J, Murray IPC, Wayne EJ: Statistical methods applied to the clinical diagnosis of thyrotoxicosis. Q J Med 28:211, 1959.

93. Crossen PE, Mellor JEL, Finley AG, Ravich RBM, Vincent PC, Gunz FW: The Sézary syndrome. Cytogenetic studies and identification of the Sézary cell as an abnormal lymphocyte. Am J Med 50:24, 1971.

94. _____, _____, Vincent PC, Gunz FW: Clonal evolution in human leukaemia. Cytobios 4:29, 1971.

95. Dacie JV; The Haemolytic Anaemias: Congenital and Acquired, 2nd ed, Part III, Secondary or Symptomatic Haemolytic Anaemias. London, Churchill, 1967, p 729.

96. _____, Lewis SM: Practical Haematology, 4th ed. London, Churchill, 1968, p 88.

97. _____, Smith MD, White JC, Mollin DL: Refractory normoblastic anaemia: A clinical and haematological study of seven cases. Br J Haematol 5:56, 1959.

98. Dahlgren S, Holm G, Svanborg N, Watz R: Clinical and morphological side-effects of busulfan (Myleran) treatment. Acta Med Scand 192:129, 1972.

99. Dameshek W: Immunocytes and immunoproliferative disorders, in The Thymus: Experimental and Clinical Studies. London, Churchill, 1966.

100. _____: Chronic lymphocytic leukemia—an accumulative disease of immunologically incompetent lymphocytes. Blood 29:566, 1967.

101. _____: What do aplastic anemia, paroxysmal nocturnal hemoglobinuria (PNH) and "hypoplastic" leukemia have in common? Blood 30:251, 1967.

102. _____, Gunz F: Leukemia, 2nd ed. New York, Grune & Stratton, 1964, p 301.

103. Dartnall J, Mundy GR, Baikie AG: Cytogenetic studies in myeloma. Blood 42:229, 1973.

104. Davidson LSP, Davis LJ, Innes J: Studies in

104. refractory anaemia. I. The technique and interpretation of sternal puncture biopsies. Edinburgh Med J 50:226, 1943.

105. Davies JNP: In Roulet FC (ed): Symposium on Lymphoreticular Tumours in Africa. Basel, Karger, 1964, p 67.

106. _____, Ball JD: The pathology of endomyocardial fibrosis in Uganda. Br Heart J 17:337, 1955.

107. Davis LJ, Kennedy AC, Baikie AG, Brown A: Haemolytic anaemia of various types treated with ACTH and cortisone: Report of ten cases, including one of acquired type in which erythropoietic arrest occurred in crisis. Glasgow Med J 33:263, 1952.

108. d'Eramo N, Levi M: Neurological Symptoms in Blood Diseases. Translated by John Iliffe. London, Harvey Miller and Medcalf, 1973.

109. Diamond HD, Craver LF, Woodard HQ, Parks GH: Radioactive phosphorus. I. In the treatment of lymphatic leukemia. Cancer 3:778, 1950.

110. Diamond LK, Luhby LA: the pattern of spontaneous remissions in leukemia in childhood: A review of 26 remissions in 300 cases. Am J Med 10:236, 1951.

111. Di Guglielmo G: Acute erythremic disease, in, Proceedings of Sixth International Congress of Hematology. New York, Grune & Stratton, 1958, p 33.

112. Djaldetti M, Pinkhas J, DeVries A, Kott E, Joshua H, Dollberg L: Myasthenia gravis in a patient with chronic myeloid leukemia treated by busulphan. Blood 32:336, 1968.

113. Dock G: Chloroma and its relation to leukemia. Am J Med Sci 106:152, 1893.

114. Doll R: The age distribution of cancer: implications for models of carcinogenesis. J R Statist Soc (Series A) 134:133, 1971.

115. _____: The Epidemiology of Leukaemia. London, Leukaemia Research Fund, 1972.

116. Dorr AD, Moloney WC: Acquired pseudo-Pelger anomaly of granulocytic leukocytes. N Engl J Med 261:742, 1959.

117. Dresner E: The bone and joint lesions in acute leukaemia, and their response to folic acid antagonists. Q J Med 43:339, 1950.

118. Drewinko B, Sullivan MP, Martin T: Use of the cytocentrifuge in the diagnosis of meningeal leukemia. Cancer, 31, 1331, 1973.

119. Dreyfus B, Rochant H, Sultan C: Anémies réfractaires: enzymopathies acquises des cellules souches hématopoiétiques. Nouv Rev Fr Hématol 9:65, 1969.

120. Druss JG: Aural manifestations of leukemia. Arch Otolaryngol 42:267, 1945.

121. Dubois-Ferrière H: Etude cytologique de la transformation aiguë d'une leucémie myélocytaire chronique. Acta Haematol 39:249, 1968.

122. Dugdale M, Fort AT: Busulfan treatment of leukemia during pregnancy. J Am Med Assoc 199:131, 1967.

123. Duvall CP, Carbone PP, Bell WR, Whang J, Tjio JH, Perry S: Chronic myelocytic leukemia with two Philadelphia chromosomes and prominent peripheral lymphadenopathy. Blood 29:652, 1967.

124. Earll JM, May RL: Busulfan therapy of myelocytic leukemia in pregnancy. Am J Obstet Gynecol 92:580, 1965.

125. Ebbe S, Wittels B, Dameshek W: Autoimmune thrombocytopenic purpura ("ITP" type) with chronic lymphocytic leukemia. Blood 19:23, 1962.

126. Efrati P, Klajman A, Spitz H: Mast cell leukemia? Malignant mastocytosis with leukemia-like manifestations. Blood 12:869, 1957.

127. Einzig S, Hong R, Sharp HL: Successful treatment of pneumocystis carinii in an immunologically deficient acute lymphatic leukemic patient. Cancer 23:658, 1969.

128. Ekert H, Denett X: An evaluation of nuclear sulphatase activity as an aid to the cytological diagnosis of acute leukaemia. Australas Ann Med 15:152, 1966.

129. Engle RR, Hammond GD, Eitzman DV, Pearson H, Krivit W: Transient congenital leukemia in 7 infants with mongolism. J Pediatr 65:303, 1964.

130. Engfeldt B, Zetterström R: Disseminated eosinophilic collagen disease. Acta Med Scand 153:337, 1956.

131. Epstein EH, Levin DL, Croft JD, Lutzner MA: Mycosis fungoides: survival, prognostic features, response to therapy and autopsy findings. Medicine 15:61, 1972.

132. Evans AE: Central nervous system involvement in children with acute leukemia. Cancer 17:256, 1963.

133. Evans RS, Takahashi K, Duane RT, Payne T, Liu CK: Primary thrombocytopenic purpura and acquired hemolytic anemia. Arch Intern Med 87:48, 1951.

134. Evans TS, Nesbit RR: Eosinophilic leukemia; Report of a case with autopsy confirmation; review of literature. Blood 4:603, 1949.

135. Eyster ME, Jenkins DE: Erythrocyte coating substances in patients with positive

direct antiglobulin reactions. Correlation of γ G globulin and complement coating with underlying diseases, overt hemolysis and response to therapy. Am J Med 46:360, 1969.

136. Ezdinli EZ, Sokal JE, Crosswhite L, Sandberg AA: Philadelphia chromosome-positive and -negative chronic myelocytic leukemia. Ann Intern Med 72:175, 1970.

137. Fiddes P, Penny, R, Wells JV, Rozenberg MC: Clinical correlations with immunoglobulin levels in chronic lymphatic leukaemia. Aust. N. Z. J. Med., 4, 346, 1972.

138. Finkelstein JZ, Dyment PG, Hammond GD: Leukemic infiltration of the testes during bone marrow remission. Pediatrics 43:1042, 1969.

139. _____, Higgins GR, Rissman E, Nixon GW: Acute leukemia during the first year of life: Presentation, chemotherapy and clinical course. Clin Pediatr 11:236, 1972.

140. Finney R, McDonald GA, Baikie AG, Douglas AS: Chronic granulocytic leukaemia with Ph[1] negative cells in bone marrow and a ten year remission after busulphan hyperplasia. Br J Haematol 23:283, 1972.

141. Firestone FN, Robinson MF: Upper airway obstruction: a rare presentation of chronic lymphocytic leukemia. Chest 61, 505.

142. Flannery EP, Dillon DE, Freeman MCV, Levy JD, D'Ambrosio U, Bedynek JL: Eosinophilic leukemia with fibrosing endocarditis and short Y chromosome. Ann Intern Med 77:223, 1972.

143. Forkner CE: Leukemia and Allied Disorders. New York, Macmillan, 1938.

144. Fraumeni JF, Manning MD, Mitus WJ: Acute childhood leukemia: Epidemiologic study by cell type of 1263 cases at the Children's Cancer Research Foundation in Boston, 1947–65. J Natl Cancer Inst 46:461, 1971.

145. Frenkel EP, Meyers MC: Acute leukemia and pregnancy. Ann Intern Med 53:656, 1960.

146. Friedman BI, Will JJ, Frieman DG, Braunstein H: Tissue mast cell leukemia. Blood 13:70, 1958.

147. Fukuda T: Neoplastic reticulosis associated with chronic myelogenous leukemia. Virchows Arch Zell Pathol 345:310, 1968.

148. Galton DAG: The pathogenesis of chronic lymphocytic leukemia. Can Med Assoc J 94:1005, 1966.

149. _____: Chemotherapy of chronic granulocytic leukemia. Sem Hematol 6:323, 1969.

150. _____, Spiers ASD: Progress in the Leukemias, in Brown EB, Moore CV (eds): Progress in Hematology, vol. VII. New York, Grune & Stratton, 1971, p 371.

151. _____, _____: Progress in the leukemias, in Brown EB, Moore CV (eds): Progress in Hematology, vol. VII. New York, Grune & Stratton, 1971, p 379.

152. Gardikas C, Thomopoulos D, Hatzioannou J, Kanaghinis HT, Jordanoglou J, Lyberatos K: Some data concerning the onset of the acute myeloblastic crisis in chronic myeloid leukaemia. Acta Haematol 46:201, 1971.

153. Garfinkel LS, Bennett DE: Extramedullary myeloblastic transformation in chronic myelocytic leukemia simulating a coexistent malignant lymphoma. Am J Clin Pathol 51:638, 1969.

154. Garson OM, Milligan WJ: The 45, XO, Ph[1] subgroup of chronic granulocytic leukaemia. Scand J Haematol 9:186, 1972.

155. Gerdes J, Marathe RL, Bloodworth JMB, MacKinney AA: Gaucher cells in chronic granulocytic leukemia. Arch Pathol 88:194, 1969.

156. Gilchrist GS, Shore NA: Familial leukemia and osteogenesis imperfecta. J Pediatr 71:115, 1967.

157. Gilliland BC, Leddy JP, Vaughan JH: The detection of cell-bound antibody on complement-coated human red cells J Clin Invest 49:898, 1970.

158. Gillis EM, Baikie AG: Method for demonstration of nucleoli in lymphocytes and other blood and bone marrow cells. J Clin Pathol 17:573, 1964.

159. Givler RL: Lymphocytic leukemia with coexistent localized reticulum cell sarcoma. Cancer 21:1184, 1968.

160. _____: Esophageal lesions in leukemia and lymphoma. Am J Dig Dis 15.31, 1970.

161. Glatt W, Weinstein A: Acropachy in lymphatic leukemia. Radiology 92:125, 1969.

162. Goh K-O: Smaller G chromosome in irradiated men. Lancet 1:659, 1966.

163. _____: Classifying acute leukemias. Ann Intern Med 76:325, 1972.

164. _____, Swisher SN, Rosenberg CA: Cytogenetic studies in eosinophilic leukemia. Ann Intern Med 62:80, 1965.

165. Golde DW, Cline MJ: Human preleukemia: Identification of a maturation defect in vitro. N Engl J Med 288:1083, 1973.

166. Gordon GB, Hyun BH, Kuhn ML: Pathogenesis of the foam cell in thalassemia. Lab Med 10:398, 1969.

167. Gralnick HR, Bagley J, Abrell E: Heparin treatment for the hemorrhagic diathesis of acute promyelocytic leukemia. Am J Med 52:167, 1972.

168. _____, Dittmar K: Development of myeloblastoma with massive breast and ovarian involvement during remission in acute leukemia. Cancer 24:746, 1969.

169. _____, Harbor J, Vogel C: Myelofibrosis in chronic granulocytic leukemia. Blood 37, 152, 1971.

170. _____, Marchesi S, Givelber H: Intravascular coagulation in acute leukemia: Clinical and subclinical abnormalities. Blood 40: 709, 1972.

171. Graw RG, Skeel RT, Carbone PP: Priapism in a child with chronic granulocytic leukemia. J Pediatr 74:788, 1969.

172. Grouchy J de, Nava C de: A chromosomal theory of carcinogenesis. Ann Intern Med 68:381, 1968.

173. _____, _____, Feingold J, Bilski-Pasquier G, Bousser J: Onze observations d'un modèle précis d'évolution caryotypique au cours de la leucémie myéloide chronique. Eur J Cancer 4:481, 1968.

174. Gruenwald H, Kiossoglou KA, Mitus WJ, Dameshek W: Philadelphia chromosome in eosinophilic leukemia. Am J Med 39:1003, 1965.

175. Gunz FW, Angus HB: Leukemia and cancer in the same patient. Cancer 18:145, 1965.

176. _____, and Burry AF: Cellular types in acute leukaemia: Diagnosis and significance. J Clin Pathol 16:325, 1963.

177. _____, Hough RF: Acute leukemia over the age of fifty: A study of its incidence and natural history. Blood 11:882, 1956.

178. Hallen J: Discrete gammaglobulin (M-) components in serum. Clinical study of 150 subjects without myelomatosis. Acta Med Scand (suppl. 462), 1966.

179. Hamburger J, Richet G, Crosnier J, Funck-Brentano JL, Antoine B, Ducrot H, Mery JP, de Montera H: Nephrology, p. 933. Philadelphia: Saunders 1968.

180. Han T: Studies of correlation of lymphocyte response to phytohemagglutinin with the clinical and immunologic status in chronic lymphocytic leukemia. Cancer, 31:280, 1973.

181. _____, Ezdinli EZ, Sokal JE: Complete remission in chronic lymphocytic leukemia and leukolymphosarcoma. Cancer 20:243, 1967.

182. Hansman CF, Girdany BR: The roentgenographic findings associated with neuroblastoma. J Pediatr. 51:621, 1957.

183. Hardisty RM, Norman PM: Meningeal leukaemia. Arch Dis Child 42:411, 1967.

184. _____, Speed DE, Till M: Granulocytic leukaemia in childhood. Br J Haematol 10:551, 1964.

185. _____, Till MM: Acute leukaemia 1959–64: Factors affecting prognosis. Arch Dis Child 43:107, 1968.

186. Harnden DG, Elsdale TR, Young DE, Ross A: The isolation of cytomegalovirus from peripheral blood. Blood 30:120, 1967.

187. Harris LJ: Leukaemia and pregnancy. Can Med Assoc J 68:234, 1953.

188. Hayhoe FGJ: Leukaemia: Research and Clinical Practice. London, Churchill, 1960, p 218.

189. _____: Cytochemical aspects of leukemia and lymphoma. Sem Hematol 6:261, 1969.

189a. _____, Cawley JC: Acute leukaemia: cellular morphology, cytochemistry and fine structure. Clinics Hematol 1:49, 1972.

190. _____, Quaglino D: Refractory sideroblastic anaemia and erythraemic myelosis: possible relationship and cytochemical observations. Br J Haematol 6:381, 1960.

191. _____, _____, Doll R: The Cytology and Cytochemistry of Acute Leukaemias. London, Her Majesty's Stationery Office, 1964.

192. Heinivarra O, Kaipainen WJ: Pelger-Hüet anomaly in lymphocytic leukaemia. Acta Haematol 25:375, 1961.

193. Hennekeuser HH, Fischer R, Talke H, Mainzer K: Pseudo-Pelger-Zellen vom homozygoten Typ bei unreifzelliger myeloischer Leukämie. Dtsch Med Wochenshr 94:2284, 1969.

194. Herbert V: Diagnostic and prognostic values of serum vitamin B_{12} binding proteins. Blood 32:305, 1968.

195. Hersh EM, Bodey GP, Nies B, Freireich EJ: Causes of death in acute leukemia. JAMA 193:99, 1965.

196. Hillestad LK: Acute promyelocytic leukaemia. Acta Med Scand 159:189, 1957.

197. Hirsh J, Buchanan J, de Gruchy GC, Baikie AG: Hypofibrinogenaemia without increased fibrinolysis in leukaemia. Lancet 1:418, 1967.

198. Hornbaker JH, Foster EA, Williams GS, Davis JS: Sjögren's syndrome and nodular

reticulum cell sarcoma. Arch Intern Med 118:449, 1966.

199. Hotchkiss DJ; Hemolytic anemia and thrombocytopenia (ITP type) in chronic lymphocytic leukemia following nitrogen mustard therapy. Cancer 19:803, 1966.

200. Hunt WE, Bouroncle BA, Meagher JN: Neurologic complications of leukemias and lymphomas. J Neurosurg 26:135, 1959.

201. Hurdle ADF, Garson OM, Buist DGP: Clinical and cytogenetic studies in chronic myelomonocytic leukaemia. Br J Haematol 22:773, 1972.

202. Hyman GA: Increased incidence of neoplasia in association with chronic lymphocytic leukaemia. Scand J Haematol 6:99, 1969.

203. Ibbott JW, Whitelaw DM, Thomas JW: The significant percentage of blast cells in the bone marrow in the diagnosis of acute leukaemia. Can Med Assoc J 82:358.

204. Isaacs, R: Lymphosarcoma cell leukemia. Ann Intern Med 11:657, 1937.

205. Israëls MCG: Diagnosis and clinical picture of acute leukaemia. Clin Haematol 1:115, 1972.

206. Jack I, Todd H, Turner EK: Isolation of human cytomegalovirus from the circulating leucocytes of a leukaemic patient. Med J Austr 1:210, 1968.

207. Jackson IM, Clark RM: A case of neutrophilic leukemia. Am J Med Sci 249:72, 1965.

208. Jaeger M, Lapp R: Complex Waldenström's syndrome associated with chronic lymphoid leukemia. Helv Med Acta 35:266, 1970.

209. Jaffe N, Kim BS: Priapism in acute granulocytic leukemia. Am J Dis Child 118:619, 1969.

210. _____, Traggis DG, Tefft M: Acute leukemia presenting with pericardial tamponade. Pediatrics 43:461, 1970.

211. Jannini P: Familial leukemias (chronic and acute) in two successive generations (In Spanish). Sangre 12:331, 1967. (Cited in Leuk Abstr 16:64, 1968.

212. Jarkowski TL, Layton JM, Bahr GF, Wied GL, Bellamy, JC, Bartels PH: Computer recognition of cells from asymptomatic lymphocytic leukemia. I. Methodologic study. Acta Cytol 15:147, 1971.

213. Javier BV, Yount WJ, Crosby DJ, Hall TC: Cardiac metastases in lymphoma and leukemia. Dis Chest 52:481, 1967.

214. Jenkins DS, Hartmann RC: Paroxysmal nocturnal hemoglobinuria terminating in acute myeloblastic leukemia. Blood 33:274, 1969.

215. Johnson DE, Griep JA, Baehner RL: Histiocytic leukemia following lifelong infection and thrombocytopenia: Histologic, metabolic and bactericidal studies. J Pediatr 82:664, 1973.

216. Jones FS, Numainville LJ, Hause WA: Leukemia in a three-month-old infant with chloromatose features. Blood 5:773, 1950.

217. Jones RV, Shalom AS: Laryngeal involvement in acute leukaemia. J Laryngol Otol 82:123, 1968.

218. Joseph RR, Zarafonetis CJD, Durant JR: "Lymphoma" in chronic granulocytic leukemia. Am J Med Sci 251:417, 1966.

219. Juttner H-U, Miller WE, Kiely JM, Scanlon PW, Harrison EG: Influence of lymphography in determining extent of disease in patients with lymphoma. Mayo Clin Proc 48:249, 1973.

220. Kagan AR, Johnson RE: Evaluation of therapy in chronic lymphocytic leukemia using in vitro lymphocyte transformation. Radiology 88:352, 1967.

221. Kahanowicz-Feierberg J, Ziprkowsky L: Dermatological manifestations of leukemia (in Hebrew). Harefuah 77:408, 1969. (Cited in Leuk. Abstr 18:88, 1970).

222. Kamada N: The effects of radiation on chromosomes of bone marrow cells: III. Cytogenetic studies on leukemia in atomic bomb survivors. Acta Haematol Jap 32:87, 1969.

223. _____, Tsuchimoto T, Uchino H: Smaller G chromosomes in the bone-marrow cells of heavily irradiated atomic-bomb survivors. Lancet 2:880, 1970.

224. Kanner SP, Wiernik PH, Serpick AA, Walker MD: CNS leukemia mimicking multifocal leukoencephalopathy. Am J Dis Child 119:264, 1970.

225. Karanas A, Silver RT: Characteristics of the terminal phase of chronic granulocytic leukemia. Blood 32:445, 1968.

226. Karle H, Videbaek A: Eosinophilic leukaemia or a collagen disease with eosinophilia. Dan Med Bull 13:41, 1966.

227. Kattlove HE, Williams JC, Gaynor E, Spivack M, Bradley RM, Brady RO: Gaucher cells in chronic myelocytic leukemia: An acquired abnormality. Blood 33:379, 1969.

228. Kauer GL Jr, Engle RL Jr: Eosinophilic leukaemia with Ph¹-positive cells. Lancet 2:1340, 1964.

229. Kaur J, Catovsky D, Valdimarsson H,

Jensson O, Spiers ASD: Familial acute myeloid leukaemia with acquired Pelger-Huët anomaly and aneuploidy of C group. Br Med J 4:327, 1972.

230. Kay HEM, Knapton PJ, O'Sullivan JP, Wells, DG, Harris RF, Innes EM, Stuart J, Schwartz FCM, Thompson EN: Encephalopathy in acute leukaemia associated with methotrexate therapy. Arch Dis Child 47:344, 1972.

231. Keating MJ, Penington DG: Infections resembling infectious mononucleosis in adult acute leukaemia. Aust NZ J Med 3:101, 1973.

232. Kemp TA, Williams ER: Chloroma. Br J Radiol 14:157, 1941. (Quoted by Hayhoe, 1960).

233. Kennedy J, Bornstein R, Brunning RD, Oines D: Breast involvement in acute lymphatic leukemia. Cancer 25: 693, 1970.

234. Killman S-A: A biased view on the relapse and remission phase of acute myeloid leukaemia, in Vincent PC (ed): The Nature of Leukaemia, Sydney: NSW Government Printer, 1972, p 205.

235. King MJ, Gillis EM, Baikie AG: Alkaline phosphatase activity of polymorphs in mongolism. Lancet 2:1019, 1962.

236. Kirschner RH, Esterley JR: Pulmonary lesions associated with busulfan therapy of chronic myelogenous leukemia. Cancer 27:1074, 1971.

237. Kirshbaum JD, Preuss FS: Leukemia: A clinical and pathologic study of 123 fatal cases in a series of 14,400 necropsies. Arch Intern Med 71:777, 1943.

238. Knisley RE: Hypercalcemia associated with leukemia. Arch Intern Med 118:14, 1966.

239. Komp DM: Cytocentrifugation in the management of central nervous system leukemia. J Pediatr 81:992, 1972.

240. _____, Donaldson MH: Sepsis in leukemia and the Shwartzman reaction. Am J Dis Child 119:114, 1970.

241. Korbitz BC, Reiquam CW: Radiation therapy in chronic granulocytic leukaemia. Lancet 1:794, 1967.

242. Krauss S, Sokal JE, Sandberg AA: Comparison of Philadelphia chromosome-positive and -negative patients with chronic myelocytic leukemia. Ann Intern Med, 61, 625, 1964.

243. Kritzler RA: Anuria complicating the treatment of leukemia. Am J Med 25:532, 1958.

244. Kuplic JB, Higley CS, Niewoehner DE: Pulmonary ossification associated with long-term busulfan therapy in chronic myeloid leukemia. Am Rev Resp Dis 106:759, 1972.

245. Kwaan HC, Pierre RV, Long DL: Meningeal involvement as first manifestation of acute myeloblastic transformation in chronic granulocytic leukemia. Blood 33:348, 1969.

246. Kyle RA, Pease GL: Basophilic leukemia. Arch Intern Med 118:205, 1966.

247. _____, Schwartz RS, Oliner HL, Dameshek W: A syndrome resembling adrenal cortical insufficiency associated with long-term busulfan (Myleran) therapy. Blood 28:497, 1961.

248. Labaze JJ, Moscovic EA, Pham TD, Azar HA: Histological and ultrastructural findings in a case of the Sézary syndrome. J Clin Pathol 25:312, 1972.

249. Lachmann D, Zweymuller E: Konnatale und neonatale Leukämien. Auswertung der Weltliteratur. Wien Klin Wochenscher 82:28, 1970.

250. Lahey ME, Beier FR, Wilson JF: Leukemia in Down's syndrome. J Pediatr 63:189, 1963.

251. Leading Article. Chloroma Confusion. Lancet 1:1099, 1973.

252. Laszlo J, Grode HE: Granulocytic leukemia and reticulum cell sarcoma. Cancer 20:545, 1967.

253. La Venuta F, Moore JA: Involvement of the inner ear in acute stem cell leukemia. Ann Otol. Rhinol. Laryngol 81:132, 1972.

254. Lawrence JH, Low-Beer BVA, Carpender JWJ: Chronic lymphatic leukemia: a study of 100 cases treated with radioactive phosphorus. J Am Med Assoc 140:585, 1949.

255. Lawrinson W, Gross S: Nuclear arylsulfatase activity in primitive hemic cells. Lab Invest 13:1612, 1964.

256. Lazarus A: In Nothnagel's Encyclopedia of Practical Medicine, vol. IX. Philadelphia, Saunders, 1905. (Quoted by Forkner.)

257. Leder LD: Der Blutmonocyt. Berlin, Springer, 1967.

258. Lee RE, Ellis LD: The storage cells of chronic myelogenous leukemia. Lab Invest 24:261, 1971.

259. Leef F, Kende G, Ramot B: Testicular leukemia. Pediatrics 45:338, 1970.

260. Leidler F, Russell WO: The brain in leukemia. A clinico-pathologic study of twenty cases with a review of the literature. Arch Pathol 40:14, 1945.

261. Lennert K: Lymphknoten: Cytologie und Lymphadenitis. Berlin, Springer, 1961.

262. Levi JA, Speden JB, Vincent PC, Gunz FW: Studies of muramidase in haematological disorders: serum and marrow muramidase in leukaemia. Pathology 5:59, 1973.

263. Levine AS, Graw RG, Young RC: Management of infections in patients with leukemia and lymphoma: Current concepts and experimental approaches. Sem Hematol 9:141, 1972.

264. Levine PH, Hamstra RD: Megaloblastic anemia of pregnancy simulating acute leukemia. Ann Intern Med 71:1141, 1969.

265. Lewis FB, Schwartz RS, Dameshek W: X-radiation and alkylating agents as possible "trigger" mechanisms in the autoimmune complications of lymphoproliferative disease. Clin Exp Immunol 1:3, 1966.

266. Li FP, Jaffe N, Mitus WJ, Moloney WC, Fraumeni JF: Epidemiology of acute myelomonocytic leukemia in children. Cancer 31:516, 1973.

267. Linman JW: Myelomonocytic leukemia and its preleukemic phase. J Chron Dis 22:713, 1970.

268. Linqvist KJ, Ragab AH, Osterland CK: Paraproteinemia in a child with leukemia. Blood 35:213, 1970.

269. Lisker R, De Gutiérrez AC, Velázquez-Ferrari M: Longitudinal bone marrow chromosome studies in potential leukemic myeloid disorders. Cancer 31:509, 1973.

270. Löffler W: Endocarditis parietalis fibroplastica mit Bluteosinophilie. Schweiz Med Wochenschr 66:817, 1936.

271. Lucas PF: Lymph node smears in the diagnosis of lymphadenopathy: A review. Blood 10:1030, 1955.

272. Lusher JM: Chloroma as a presenting feature of acute leukemia. Am J Dis Child 108:62, 1964.

273. McAndrew GM, Ogston D, Dawson AA: An evaluation of sternal tenderness as a sign of leukaemia. Acta Haematol 43:309, 1970.

274. McGoldrick JL, Lapp WA: Leucemia and pregnancy; cash report and review of literature. Am J Obstet Gynecol 46:711, 1943.

275. MacKenzie NG, Chapman OW, Middleton PJ: Progressive vaccinia with chronic lymphatic leukaemia: A case report. NZ Med J 70:324, 1969.

276. McNutt DR, Fudenberg HH: Disseminated scotochromogen infection and unusual myeloproliferative disorder. Ann Intern Med 75:737, 1972.

277. McPhedran P, Heath CW: Acute leukemia occurring during chronic lymphocytic leukemia. Blood 35:7, 1970.

278. Martin B: Infiltration of the iris in chronic lymphatic leukaemia. Br J Ophthalmol 52:781, 1968.

279. Mason TE, Demaree RS, Margolis CI: Granulocytic sarcoma (chloroma), two years preceding myelogenous leukemia. Cancer 31:423, 1973.

280. Mastrangelo R, Zuelzer WW, Ecklund PS, Thompson RI: Chromosomes in the spinal fluid: evidence for metastatic origin of meningeal leukemia. Blood 35:227, 1970.

281. Mathé G, Pouillart P, Sterescu M, Amiel JL, Schwarzenberg L, Schneider M, Hayat M, de Vassal F, Jasmin C, Lafleur M: Subdivision of classical varieties of acute leukaemia: Correlation with prognosis and cure expectancy. Rev Eur Etud Clin Biol 16:554, 1971.

282. _____, Schwarzenberg L, Mery AM, Cattan A, Schneider M, Amiel JL, Schlumberger JR, Poisson J, Wajcner G: Extensive histological and cytological survey of patients with acute leukaemia in "complete remission." Br Med J 1:640, 1966.

283. Maurer HS, Vida LN, Honig GR: Similarities of the erythrocytes in juvenile chronic myelogenous leukemia in fetal erythrocytes. Blood 39:778, 1972.

284. Maxwell GM: Twelve cases of lymphoblastomata in children. Arch Dis Child 29:155, 1954.

285. Medd WE, Hayhoe FGJ: Tuberculous miliary necrosis with pancytopenia. Q J Med 24:351, 1955.

286. Medical Research Council's Working Party for Therapeutic Trials in Leukaemia. Chronic granulocytic leukaemia: Comparison of radiotherapy and busulphan therapy. Br Med J 1:201, 1968.

287. Melhorn DK, Gross S, Newman AJ: Acute childhood leukemia presenting as aplastic anemia: The response to corticosteroids. J Pediatr 77:647, 1970.

288. Miale JB: Laboratory Medicine: Hematology, Saint Louis, Mosby, 1972, Chapter 3.

289. Miller DR, Newstead GJ, Young LW: Perinatal leukemia with a possible variant of the Ellis-van Creveld syndrome. J Pediatr 74:300, 1969.

290. Miller RW: Relation between cancer and congenital defects in man. N Engl J Med 275:85, 1966.

291. _____: Childhood cancer and congenital defects: a study of U.S. death certificates during the period 1960–1966. Pediatr Res 3:389, 1969.

292. Milligan WJ: Personal communication, 1973.

293. Mills SD: Conditions mistaken for leukemia in children. Minn Med 37:44, 1954.

294. Mitrakul C, Othaganond B-O, Manothai P, Bhanichayabhongsa S: Basophilic leukemia. Report of a case. Clin Pediatr 8:178, 1969.

295. Mittwoch U: The leukocyte count in children with mongolism J Ment Sci 104:457, 1958.

296. Modan B, Padeh B, Jallner H, Akstein E, Meytes D, Czerniak P, Ramot B, Pinkhas J, Modan M: Chromosomal aberrations in polycythemia vera. Blood 35:28, 1970.

297. Moloney WC: Management of leukemia in pregnancy. Ann NY Acad Sci 114:857, 1964.

298. Moore DL, Carnahan CE, Mills SD, Burgert EO: Pneumocystis carinii pneumonitis complicating leukemia. Mayo Clin Proc. 44:162, 1969.

299. Moore EW, Thomas LB, Shaw RK Freireich EJ: The central nervous system in acute leukemia. Arch Intern Med 105:141, 1960.

300. Moore JE, James GW: A simple direct method for absolute basophil leucocyte count. Proc Soc Exp Biol Med 82:601, 1953.

301. Mortada A: Bilateral exophthalmos and lymphoblastic aleukaemic leukaemia. Br J Ophthal 52:68, 1968.

302. Muggia FM, Heinemann HO, Farhangi M, Osserman EF: Lysozymuria and renal tubular dysfunction in monocytic and myelomonocytic leukemia. Am J Med 47:351, 1969.

303. Muller SA, Herrmann EC, Winkelmann RK: Herpes simplex infections in hematologic malignancies. Am J Med 52:102, 1972.

304. Mundy GR, Baikie AG: Myeloma treated with cyclophosphamide and terminating in reticulum cell sarcoma. Med J Austr 1:1240, 1973.

305. Murray IPC: The clinical diagnosis of thyroid disease. Med J Austr 1:827, 1964.

306. Naegeli E: Blutkrankheiten und Blutdiagnostik. Berlin, Springer, 1923.

307. Neerhout RC: Chronic granulocytic leukemia: Early blast crisis simulating acute leukemia. Am J Dis Child 115:66, 1968.

308. Neiman RS, Li HC: Hypercalcemia in undifferentiated leukemia: possible production of a parathormone-like substance by leukemic cells. Cancer 30:942, 1972.

309. Nicholson HO: Leukaemia and pregnancy. A report of five cases and discussion of management. J Obstet Gynaec Br Commonw 75:517, 1968.

310. Nies BA, Malmgren RA, Chu EW, Del Vecchio PR, Thomas LB, Freireich EJ: Cerebrospinal fluid cytology in patients with acute leukemia. Cancer 18:1385, 1965.

311. Nixon RK: The relation of mastocytosis and lymphomatous disease. Ann Intern Med 64:856, 1966.

312. Nowell PC: Differentiation of human leukemic leukocytes in tissue culture. Exp Cell Res 19:267, 1960.

313. _____: Marrow chromosome studies in "preleukemia": further correlation with clinical course. Cancer 28:513, 1971.

314. Oliner H, Schwartz R, Rubio F, Dameshek W: Interstitial pulmonary fibrosis following busulfan (Myleran) therapy. Am J Med 31:134, 1961.

315. Osgood EE, Seaman AJ: Treatment of chronic leukemias: Results of therapy by titrated, regularly spaced total body radioactive phosphorus or roëntgen irradiation. JAMA 150:1372, 1952.

316. Pearson HA, Diamond LK: Chronic monocytic leukemia in childhood. J Pediatr 53:259, 1958.

317. Pedersen B: Karyotype profiles in chronic myelogenous leukaemia: Influence of therapy on progression of disease. Acta Pathol Microbiol Scand 67, 463, 1966.

318. _____: Relation between karyotype and cytology in chronic myelogenous leukaemia. Scand J Haematol 8:494, 1971.

319. Pengelly CDR, Wilkinson JF: The frequency and mechanism of haemolysis in the leukaemias, reticuloses and myeloproliferative diseases. Br J Haematol 8:343, 1962.

320. Péquignot H, Levy J-P, Girerd R, Cocheton J-J, Reut J-C: Transformation aigue terminale d'une leucémic lymphoide chronique. Sem Hôp Paris 46:2678, 1970.

321. Perillie PE, Finch SC: Muramidase studies in Philadelphia-chromosome-positive and chromosome-negative chronic granulocytic leukemia. N Engl J Med 283:456, 1970.

322. Perry HO, Winkelmann RK: Bullous pyoderma gangrenosum and leukemia. Arch Dermatol 106:901, 1972.

323. Persky L, Newman AJ, Tucker AS: Urologic manifestations of childhood leukemia. J Urol 107:1073, 1972.

324. Persson S, Söderström N: Adrenocortical insufficiency in chronic leukaemia. Acta Haematol 27:345, 1962.

325. Petersen HS: Anerythraemic Di

Guglielmo's syndrome. Acta Med Scand 193:363, 1973.

326. Pierce M: Leukemia in the newborn infant. J Pediatr 54:691, 1959.

327. Pitney WR: Disseminated intravascular coagulation. Sem Hematol 8:65, 1971.

328. ———: Thrombosis: Anticoagulant and thrombolytic therapy, in Hoffbrand AV and Lewis SM (eds): Haematology: Tutorials in Postgraduate Medicine, vol. II. London, Heinemann, 1972, p. 628.

329. ———, Joske RA, Mackinnon NL: Folic acid and other absorption tests in lymphosarcoma, chronic lymphocytic leukaemia and some related conditions. J Clin Pathol 13:440, 1960.

330. Plenderleith IH: Hairy cell leukemia. Can Med Assoc J 102:1056, 1970.

331. Poynton FJ, Lightwood R: Lymphatic leukaemia with infiltration of the periosteum, simulating acute rheumatism. Lancet 1:1192, 1932.

332. Pretlow TG: Chronic monocytic dyscrasia culminating in acute leukemia. Am J Med 46:130, 1969.

333. Price RA, Johnson WW: The central nervous system in childhood leukemia. Cancer 31:520, 1973.

334. Pridie G, Dimitrescu-Pirvu D: Laucemie acutasi sindrom Bonnevie-Ulrich la un nounascut. Pediatria (Bucur) 10:345, 1961.

335. Propp S, Lizzi FA: Philadelphia chromosome in acute lymphocytic leukemia. Blood 36:353, 1970.

336. Pruzanski W, Platts ME: Serum and urinary proteins, lysozyme (muramidase), and renal dysfunction in mono- and myelomonocytic leukemia. J Clin Invest 49:1694, 1970.

337. Puech A, Izarn P, Olivier G, Emberger J-M: Leucémie myéloblastique, mode de terminaison d'une leucémie lymphoïde chronique. J Med Montpellier 2:508, 1967.

338. Rachmilewitz D, Rachmilewitz EA, Polliack A, Hershko C: Acute promyelocytic leukaemia: A report of five cases with a comment on the diagnostic significance of serum vitamin B_{12} determination. Br J Haematol 22:87, 1972.

339. Radding J: Northwest Med 49:772, 1950. (Cited by Durham RH: Encyclopedia of Medical Syndromes. New York; Hoeber, 1960, p 32.)

340. Rand JJ, Moloney WC, Sise HS: Coagulation defects in acute promyelocytic leukemia. Arch Intern Med 123:39, 1969.

341. Rappaport H: Tumors of the Hemopoietic System. Washington, D.C., Armed Forces Institute of Pathology, 1966.

342. Ravich RBM, Reed CS, Stephens FO, Vincent PC, Gunz FW: Spontaneous rupture of the spleen in acute myeloid leukaemia. Med J Austr 1:90, 1971.

343. Rawbone RG, Shaw MT, Bagshawe KD: Intracranial leukaemia and the cerebrospinal fluid. Br Med J 2:444, 1972.

344. Reardon G, Moloney WC: Chloroma and related myeloblastic neoplasms. Arch Intern Med 108:864, 1961.

345. Reimann DL, Clemmens RL, Pillsbury WA: Congenital acute leukemia. J Pediatr 46:415, 1955.

346. Reisman LE, Trujillo JM: Chronic granulocytic leukemia of childhood. J Pediatr 62:710, 1963.

347. Richter MN: Generalized reticular cell sarcoma of lymph nodes associated with lymphatic leukemia. Am J Pathol 4:285, 1928.

348. Rieselbach RE, Dentzel CJ, Cotlove E, Frei E, Freireich EJ: Uric acid excretion and renal function in the acute hyperuricemia of leukemia. Am J Med 37:872, 1964.

349. Ritchie GM: Extensive myeloid response during folic acid therapy in megaloblastic anaemia of pregnancy. J Clin Pathol 5:329, 1952.

350. Rivers SL, Whittington RM, Gendel R, Patno ME: Acute leukemia in the adult male: natural history. Cancer 16:249, 1963.

351. Roath S, Israëls MCG, Wilkinson JF: The acute leukaemias: A study of 580 patients. Q J Med 33:257, 1964.

352. Roberts WC, Buja LM, Ferrans VJ: Löffler's fibroplastic parietal endocarditis, eosinophilic leukemia, and Davies' endomyocardial fibrosis: The same disease at different stages? Pathol Microbiol 35:90, 1970.

353. Rosenthal MC, Pisciotta AV, Komninos ZD, Goldenberg H, Dameshek W: The autoimmune hemolytic anemia of malignant lymphocytic disease. Blood 10:197, 1955.

354. Rosner F, Lee SL: Down's syndrome and acute leukemia: myeloblastic or lymphoblastic? Am J Med 53:203, 1972.

355. ———, Schreiber ZA: Serum vitamin B_{12} and vitamin B_{12} binding capacity in chronic myelogenous leukemia and other disorders. Am J Med Sci 263:473, 1972.

356. Ross JD, Moloney WC, Desforges JF: Ineffective regulation of granulopoiesis masquerading as congenital leukemia in a mongoloid child. J Pediatr 63:1, 1963.

357. Ross RR: Chloroma and chloroleukemia. Am J Med 18:671, 1955.

358. Rothberg H, Conrad ME, Cowley RG: Acute granulocytic leukemia in pregnancy: report of four cases with apparent acceleration by prednisone in one. Am J Med Sci 237:194, 1959.

359. Rowley JD, Blaisdell RK, Jacobson LO: Chromosome studies in preleukemia: I. Aneuploidy of group C chromosomes in three patients. Blood 27:782, 1966.

360. Rubin AD, Douglas SD, Chessin LN, Glade PR, Dameshek W: Chronic reticulo-lymphocytic leukemia. Am J Med 47:149, 1969.

361. Rubin H: Chronic neutrophilic leukemia. Ann Intern Med 65:93, 1966.

362. Rumke CL: Variability of results in differential cell counts on blood smears. Triangle 4:154, 1960.

363. Rundles RW, Coonrad EV, Arends T: Serum proteins in leukemia. Am J Med 16:842, 1954.

364. Saarni MI, Linman JW: Myelomonocytic leukemia: disorderly proliferation in all marrow cells. Cancer 27:1221, 1971.

365. Sacker LS, Nordin BEC: A simple bone biopsy needle. Lancet 1:347, 1954.

366. Salsbury AJ: Nucleolar staining in the differentiation of acute leukaemias. Br J Haematol 13:768, 1967.

367. Sandford DM, Becker GD: Acute leukemia presenting as nasal obstruction. Arch Otolaryngol 85:124, 1967.

368. Sardemann H: Chronic lymphocytic leukaemia in an infant. Acta Paediatr 61:213, 1972.

369. Schade H, Schoeller L, Schultze KW: D-trisomie (Patau-syndrome) mit kongenitaler myeloischer Leukaemie. Med Welt 50:2690, 1962.

370. Schaffer AJ, Jacobsen AW: Mikulicz's syndrome, a report of ten cases. Am J Dis Child 34:327, 1927.

371. Schaller J: Arthritis as a presenting manifestation of malignancy in children. J Pediatr 81:793, 1972.

372. Schilling BB, Abell MR, Work WP: Leukemic involvement of larynx. Arch Otolaryugol 85:658, 1967.

373. Schimpff S, Serpick A, Stoler B, Rumack B, Mellin H, Joseph JM, Block J: Varicella-zoster infection in patients with cancer. Ann Intern Med 76:241, 1972.

374. Schimpff SC, Wiernik PH, Block JB: Rectal abscesses in cancer patients. Lancet 2:844, 1972.

375. Schneider KM, Becker JM and Krasna IH: Neonatal neuroblastoma. Pediatrics 36:359, 1965.

376. Schrek R, Donnelly WK: "Hairy" cells in blood in lymphoreticular neoplastic disease and "flagellated" cells of normal lymph nodes. Blood 27:199, 1966.

377. Schrek R, Donnelly WJ: Cytology in lymphosarcoma cell leukemia. Am J Clin Pathol 55:646, 1971.

378. Schrek R, Rabinowitz Y: Effects of Phytohemagglutinin on rat and normal human blood cells. Proc Soc Exp Biol Med 113:191, 1963.

379. Schubert JCF, Martin H: Beobachtungen an sieben Kranken mit Blutmastzell-Leukämie. Klin Wochenschr 46:929, 1968.

380. Schwartz DL, Pierre RV, Scheerer PP, Reed EC, Linman JW: Lymphosarcoma cell leukemia. Am J Med 38:778, 1965.

381. Sclare G, Cragg J: A leukaemoid blood picture in megaloblastic anaemia of the puerperum. J Clin Pathol 11:45, 1958.

382. Scott RB: Leukaemia: Chronic lymphatic leukaemia. Lancet 1:1162, 1957.

383. Scott RB, Ellison RR, Ley AB: A clinical study of twenty cases of erythroleukemia (Di Guglielmo's syndrome). Am J Med 37:162, 1964.

384. Sehdev MK, Dowling MD, Seal SH, Stearns MW: Perianal and anorectal complications in leukemia. Cancer 31:149, 1973.

385. Seligman BR, Rosner F, Lee SL, Ritz ND: Clinical meningeal leukemia in acute myelocytic leukemia. NY State J Med 72:1855, 1972.

386. Senn JS, Pinkerton PH: Defective in vitro colony formation in human bone marrow preceding overt leukaemia. Br J Haematol 23:277, 1972.

387. Shanbrom E, Finch SC: The auditory manifestations of leukemia. Yale J Biol Med 31:144, 1958.

388. ———, Miller SH, Harr H: Herpes zoster in hematologic neoplasias: some unusual manifestations. Ann Intern Med 53:523, 1960.

389. Sharman C, Crossen PE, Fitzgerald PH: Lymphocyte number and response to phytohaemagglutinin in chronic lymphocytic leukaemia. Scand J Haematol 3:375, 1966.

390. Shohet SB, Blum SF: Coincident basophilic chronic myelogenous leukemia and pulmonary tuberculosis associated with extreme elevation of blood histamine levels

and maturity onset asthma. Cancer 22:173, 1968.

391. Silverstein MN, Bayrd ED: Nonmeningeal extramedullary relapse in leukemia. Arch Intern Med 123:401, 1969.

392. _____, Ellefson DR, Ahearn EJ: The syndrome of the sea-blue histiocyte. N Engl J Med 282:1, 1970.

393. Simone JV, Holland E, Johnson W: Fatalities during remission of childhood leukemia. Blood 39:759, 1972.

394. Sinks LF, Newton WA, Nagi NA, Stevenson TD: A syndrome associated with extreme hyperuricemia in leukemia. J Pediatr 68:578, 1966.

395. Sinn CM, Dick FW: Monocytic leukemia. Am J Med 20:588, 1956.

396. Skarin AT, Davey FR, Moloney WC: Lymphosarcoma of the spleen. Arch Intern Med 127:259, 1971.

397. Smith CH: Blood Diseases of Infancy and Childhood, 3rd ed. St. Louis; Mosby, 1972.

398. Spiers ASD: Cure as the aim in therapy for the acute leukaemias. Lancet 2:473, 1972.

399. _____, Baikie AG: Chronic granulocytic leukaemia: Demonstration of the Philadelphia chromosome in cultures of spleen cells. Nature 208:497, 1965.

400. _____, _____: Cytogenetic evolution and clonal proliferation in acute transformation of chronic granulocytic leukaemia. Br J Cancer 22:192, 1968.

401. _____, _____: Cytogenetic studies in the malignant lymphomas and related neoplasms. Cancer 22:193, 1968.

402. _____, _____: Anomalies of the small acrocentric chromosomes in human tumour cells. Austr NZ J Med 2:188, 1972.

403. Spilberg I, Meyer GJ: The arthritis of leukemia. Arthritis Rheum 15:630, 1972.

404. Sternby NH: Studies in enlargement of leukaemic kidneys. Acta Haematol 14:354, 1955.

405. Stevens AR: Lymphatic leukemia for perhaps 28 years. N Engl J Med 281:448, 1969.

406. Stewart A: Aetiology of childhood malignancies. Br Med J 1:452, 1961.

407. Stoop JW, Zegers BJM, Van der Heiden C, Ballieux RE: Monoclonal gammopathy in a child with leukemia. Blood 32:774, 1968.

408. Stransky E: Perinatal leukemia. Acta Paediatr Acad Sci Hung 8:121, 1967. (Cited by Smith CH, 1972.)

409. Stuart J, Simpson JS, Mann JR: Intracellular hydrogen transport systems in acute leukaemia. Br J Haematol 19:739, 1970.

410. Sullivan MP: Leukemic transformation in lymphosarcoma of childhood. Pediatrics 29:589, 1962.

411. Sumners JE, Johnson WW, Ainger LE: Childhood leukemic heart disease: A study of 116 hearts of children dying of leukemia. Circulation 40:575, 1969.

412. Suryaprasad AG, Van Slyck EJ, James TN: The sinus node in chronic granulocytic leukemia. Chest 61:494, 1972.

413. Talal N, Bunim JJ: The development of malignant lymphoma in the course of Sjögren's syndrome. Am J Med 36:529, 1964.

414. Tan KH, Tan TS: Chronic myeloid leukaemia in children. Singapore Med J 9:39, 1968.

415. Tanaka N, Ito K, Kamada N, Okada K: A case of atomic bomb survivor with chronic granulocytic leukemia in the early stage. J Kyushu Hematol Soc 13:124, 1963.

416. Tanzer J, Harel P, Boiron M, Bernard J: Cytochemical and cytogenetic findings in a case of chronic neutrophilic leukaemia of mature cell type. Lancet 1:387, 1964.

417. Taylor JJ, Evans DW: Lymphosarcoma during the course of myeloid leukaemia. Postgrad Med J 44:558, 1968.

418. Teasdale JM, Worth AJ, Corey MJ: A missing group C chromosome in the bone marrow cells of three children with myeloproliferative disease. Cancer 25:1468, 1970.

419. Templeton AC: Tumors of the eye and adnexa in Africans of Uganda. Cancer 20:1689, 1967.

420. Theologides A: Unfavorable signs in patients with chronic myelocytic leukemia. Ann Intern Med 76:95, 1972.

421. Thompson RB, Walker W: Study of 50 cases of acute leukaemia in childhood. Br Med J 1:1165, 1962.

422. Thomson AER, O'Connor TWE, Wetherley-Mein G: Killing and characterizing action of colchicine in vitro on lymphocytes in chronic lymphocytic leukaemia. Scand J Haematol 9:231, 1972.

423. _____, Robinson MA: Cytocidal action of colchicine in vitro on lymphocytes in chronic lymphocytic leukaemia. Lancet 2:868, 1967.

424. Till MM, Hardisty RM and Pike MC: Long survivals in acute leukaemia. Lancet 1:534, 1973.

425. Tischendorf RW, Ledderose G, Müller D, Wilmanns W: Heavy lysozymuria after X-irradiation of the spleen in human chronic myelocytic leukaemia. Nature 235:274, 1972.

426. Tough IM: Cytogenetic studies in cases of chronic myeloid leukaemia with a previous history of radiation, *in* Hayhoe FJG (ed): Current Research in Leukaemia. Cambridge, Cambridge University Press, 1965, p47.

427. _____, Jacobs PA, Court Brown WM, Baikie AG, Williamson ERD: Cytogenetic studies on bone-marrow in chronic myeloid leukaemia. Lancet 1:844, 1963.

428. Tjio JH, Whang J: Chromosome preparations of bone marrow cells without prior in vitro or in vivo colchicine administration. Stain Technol 37:17, 1962.

429. Tobin MS, Kyung S-K, Kossowski WA: Adrenocorticotrophic hormone deficiency in chronic myelogenous leukemia after treatment. N Engl J Med 282:187, 1970.

430. Ultmann JE: The role of the spleen in the hemolytic anemia of cancer patients. Cancer Res 18:959, 1958.

431. _____: Generalized vaccinia in a patient with chronic lymphocytic leukemia and hypogammaglobulinemia. Ann Intern Med 61:728, 1964.

432. _____, Fish W, Osserman E, Gellhorn A: The clinical implications of hypogammaglobulinemia in patients with chronic lymphocytic leukemia and lymphocytic lymphosarcoma. Ann Intern Med 51:501, 1959.

433. _____, Koprowska I, Engle RL: A cytological study of lymph node imprints. Cancer 11:507, 1958.

434. Vadakan VV, Ortega J: Priapism in acute lymphoblastic leukemia. Cancer 50:373, 1972.

435. Van Furth R: Mononuclear phagocytes. Oxford, Blackwell, 1970.

436. Walker IR, Ali MAM: Hemoglobin abnormalities in neoplastic hematological disorders. Can Med Assoc J 108:843, 1973.

437. Walsh G, Stickley CS: Acute leukemia with primary symptoms in the rectum. Southern Med J 96:684, 1934.

438. Walters TR, Bushore M, Simone J: Poor prognosis in Negro children with acute lymphocytic leukemia. Cancer 39:210, 1972.

439. _____, Reddy BN, Bailon A, Vitale LF: Poland's syndrome associated with leukemia. J Pediatr 82:889, 1973.

440. Ward GR: Bedside Hematology: An Introduction to the Clinical Study of So-called Blood Diseases and of Allied Disorders. Philadelphia, Saunders, 1914.

441. Warthin AS: A case of lymphatic leukemia with histological picture resembling that of Hodgkin's disease. Trans Assoc Am Physicians 21:465, 1906.

442. Waters WJ, Lacson PS: Mast cell leukemia presenting as urticaria pigmentosa; report of a case Pediatrics 19:1033, 1957.

443. Watson PA: A slide centrifuge: An apparatus for concentrating cells in suspension onto a microscope slide. J Lab Clin Med 68:494, 1966.

444. Weed RI: Exaggerated delayed hypersensitivity to mosquito bites in chronic lymphocytic leukemia. Blood 26:257, 1965.

445. Weinberger MM, Oleinick A: Congenital marrow dysfunction in Down's syndrome. J Pediatr 77:273, 1970.

446. West RJ, Graham-Pole J, Hardisty RM, Pike MC: Factors in the pathogenesis of central-nervous-system leukemia. Br Med J 3:311, 1972.

447. Whang-Peng J, Canellos GP, Carbone PP, Tjio JH: Clinical implications of cytogenetic variants of chronic myelocytic leukemia (CML). Blood 32:755, 1968.

448. Wied GL, Bahr GF, Griep J, Rappaport H, Bartels PH: Computer discrimination of blood cells from two cases of "leukemic" lymphosarcoma. Acta Cytol 13:688, 1969.

449. Wiernik PH, and Serpick AA: Pulmonary embolus in acute myelocytic leukemia. Cancer 24:581, 1969.

450. Wilhyde DE, Jane JA, Mullan S: Spinal epidural leukemia. Am J Med 34:281, 1963.

451. Willson JKV: The bone lesions of childhood leukemia: a survey of 140 cases. Radiology 72:672, 1959.

452. Wilson BD, Van Slyck EJ: Coexistent lymphosarcoma and chronic granulocytic leukemia. Cancer 19:809, 1966.

453. Wilson JD, Nossal GJV: Identification of human T and B lymphocytes in normal peripheral blood and in chronic lymphocytic leukaemia. Lancet 2:788, 1971.

454. Witzleben CL, Drake WL, Sammon J, Mohabbat OM: Gaucher's cells in acute leukemia of children. J Pediatr 76:129, 1970.

455. Wolcott GJ, Grunnet ML, Lahey ME: Spinal epidural hematoma in a leukemic child. J Pediatr 77:1060, 1970.

456. Wolff JA: Acute leukaemia in children. Clin Haematol 1:189, 1972.

457. _____, Brubaker CA, Murphy ML, Pierce MI, Severo N: Prednisone therapy of acute childhood leukemia: Prognosis and duration of response in 330 treated patients. J Pediatr 70:626, 1967.

458. Woodliff HJ, Finlay-Jones LR: Busulphan lung. Med J Austr 2:719, 1972.

459. Yam LT, Li CY, Necheles TF, Katayama I:

Pseudoeosinophilia, eosinophilic endocarditis and eosinophilic leukemia. Am J Med 53:193, 1972.

460. Youman JD, Taddeini L, Cooper T: Histamine excess symptoms in basophilic chronic granulocytic leukemia. Arch Intern Med 131:560, 1973.

461. Young LS, Armstrong D, Blevins A, Lieberman P: Nocardia asteroides infection complicating neoplastic disease. Am J Med 50:356, 1971.

462. Young RC: The Budd-Chiari syndrome caused by aspergillus. Arch Intern Med 124:754, 1969.

463. Zacharski LR, Linman JW: Chronic lymphocytic leukemia versus chronic lymphosarcoma cell leukemia. Am J Med 47:75, 1969.

464. Zittoun R, Bernadou A, Zittoun J, Cadiou M, Degos L: Leucémie myélo-monocytaire subaiguë. Sem Hôp Paris 48:1965, 1972.

465. Zlotnick A, Robinson E: Chronic lymphatic leukemia associated with macroglobulinemia. Israel J Med Sci 6:365, 1970.

11

Clinical and Laboratory Features
of the Myeloproliferative Disorders

In this chapter we shall discuss a group of conditions characterized by the self-perpetuating (i.e., neoplastic) proliferation of one or more lines of bone marrow elements: The erythroblast-erythrocyte, myeloblast-granulocyte, megakaryocyte-platelet, and reticulum cell-fibroblast series. Recent work (reviewed in Chapter 8) has clearly shown that the first three of these lines are derived from a common stem cell. Whether the last has the same origin is doubtful, for cytogenetic studies have suggested that fibroblastic proliferation may be a secondary phenomenon.[268] The term *myeloproliferative disorders* (*disorders* being the key word), first used by us in 1951 and 1956,[56,58] signifies that the proliferation is abnormal and the essence of the pathologic process, and that it is without a recognizable cause. It occurs in varying degrees in the marrow, and in such sites as the spleen or liver. Sometimes one cell-line predominates, at other times there appears to be a combination of several lines. We include in the group chronic as well as acute granulocytic leukemia; polycythemia vera; myelosclerosis with myeloid metaplasia; thrombocythemia; the Di-Guglielmo syndrome; as well as many intermediate conditions. The collective term does not, of course, imply that all these conditions need have the same causation or that, in fact, we are often in a position to determine their origin; it does, however, imply that clinically, hematologically, and perhaps etiologically they have much in common and that "mixed up" conditions and transitions between them are quite frequent. Perhaps the most useful subdivision within this large group is between the obviously leukemic conditions and those of less clearly neoplastic nature.

Proliferations of the marrow cells may be divided into (*1*) benign, nonneoplastic, and (*2*) self-perpetuating, and probably, neoplastic types. The first are due to known causes, ordinarily acute and ordinarily self-limited. They may involve the red cells, white cells, or platelets—either singly or *in toto*. A benign, granulocytic proliferation is most commonly seen in the pyogenic infections, in which, in response to a known bacterial agent, a striking increase in granulocyte production by the marrow takes place; when the infection is terminated, the marrow reverts to its original status. Total, benign proliferation occurs in response to acute blood loss, whether by hemorrhage or hemolysis. Here, the entire marrow may be said to respond *en*

377

Table 11-1
Myeloproliferative Disorders—Types

Chronic	Polycythemia Vera
	Myelosclerosis with Myeloid Metaplasia
	Chronic Granulocytic Leukemia
	Thrombocythemia
Acute	Di Guglielmo Syndrome
	Erythremic Myelosis
	Erythroleukemia
	Acute Granylocytic Leukemia
	Acute Myelosclerosis with Myeloid Metaplasia

masse, and there is not only erythroblastic proliferation but an increase in granulocytes, megakaryocytes, and platelets as well. With the cessation of blood loss, the
marrow reverts to its original status. These are myeloproliferative *reactions* and are
not included under the myeloproliferative disorders as we have described them. The
latter are proliferations of one, two, or several of the marrow cell series—either
within the marrow or in potential marrow (yellow marrow, spleen, liver)—without
discernible cause, and having a self-perpetuating character. Once the proliferation
has begun, there is no tendency to revert to the original status; in many instances,
the process appears to become accelerated as it continues. As with the benign
processes, the self-perpetuating forms may be confined to a single cell type, but
more commonly several cell-lines may proliferate either simultaneously or at different times. We have used the all-inclusive term *the myeloproliferative syndromes*
for the various "idiopathic" or "agnogenic" proliferations—single or multiple—
arising from bone marrow cells. They may be classified (as we have done in Tables
11-1 and 11-2), with the reservation constantly in mind that transitional forms and
transformations may occur, thus making the exact pigeonholing of a given state at
times a rather difficult matter. Parenthetically, it may be observed that nature has
but little regard for our often highly artificial classifications. Thus, a given condition
may partake simultaneously of some of the features of one, two, or three "different"
disorders. This is particularly true of the myeloproliferative disorders. Figure 11-1
illustrates diagrammatically our conception of the interrelationships in this group.

Table 11-2
Myeloproliferative Disorders—Classified as to Degree of Cellular Proliferation

	RBC	WBC	Megakaryocyte-Platelet	Reticulum Cell	Potential (Metaplastic) Bone Marrow
Polycythemia vera	+++	++	++(+)	+	+
Myelosclerosis—Myeloid metaplasia	–	+(+)	++(+)	+++	+++
Chronic granulocytic leukemia	+	+++	++	+	+
Thrombocythemia	±	±	+++	+	+
Di Guglielmo syndrome	++(+)	++(+)	+(–)	–	–
Acute granulocytic leukemia	–	+++	–	–	–

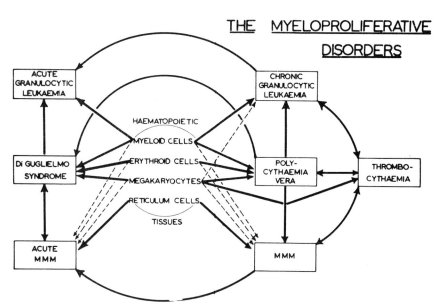

Fig. 11-1.   Schema of possible relationships in the myeloproliferative disorders. In the center are shown the hematopoietic tissues, on the right, the chronic, and on the left, the acute myeloproliferative disorders. *Arrows* from center show cell systems principally involved. Arrows connecting disorders denote transitions which have been observed. (Reproduced from Gunz,[106] courtesy of the publisher.)

The history of the conditions which we now term *myeloproliferative* is of some interest. It is a story of long-continued efforts to delineate newly discovered syndromes, to determine the identity or disparity of clinical or pathologic appearances, and to discern the essential nature of hematologic abnormalities. Even today, no absolute diagnostic criteria are known, and the acquisition of such new parameters as the neutrophil alkaline phosphatase and the presence of the Philadelphia (Ph[1]) chromosome, though adding some objective characters, has still failed to resolve entirely the prevailing uncertainties. Examples of such checkered nosologic careers are myelosclerosis with myeloid metaplasia and the Di Guglielmo syndrome.

Some years after the first descriptions of leukemia, cases became known which displayed most of the usual features of chronic granulocytic leukemia, but at the same time also some striking peculiarities, such as relatively low leukocyte counts and reduced marrow cellularity. These, as well as rather similar cases occurring in the course of polycythemia vera, were at first regarded as variants of leukemia. Further experience produced increasing numbers of patients with fibrotic or sclerotic marrow changes, a remarkable degree of splenomegaly, and immature leukocytes and erythroblasts in the blood. Evidently, a new syndrome or group of syndromes had been born and was christened with a galaxy of names such as "leukanemia," "leukoerythroblastic anemia," "erythremia," "thrombocythemia," "myelofibrosis," "myelosclerosis," "megakaryocytic splenomegaly," and dozens more, according to the features which first caught the authors' attention. Whether they were all identical among themselves, the tendency became to separate and distinguish them from granulocytic leukemia on the assumption that they had a different pathologic nature. Our own preference has settled on the term *myelofibrosis with myeloid metaplasia (MMM)*. It was found at an early stage that this could be associated with other disorders, especially polycythemia vera, but sometimes also with tuberculosis or carcinomatosis. Its relation to leukemia is discussed below.

From about 1920 onward, reports began to appear (at first from Italy) which described another group of conditions characterized by an abundance of erythroblasts in the blood and a course varying from extreme acuteness to one of many years' duration. At first thought to be hemolytic anemias, these cases showed many of the features of leukemia, mostly acute, but at the other extreme of their spectrum they seemed to impinge on myelosclerosis and even aplastic anemia. The relation of these "erythremias" or "erythroleukemias" to leukemia, polycythemia, and MMM became of increasing interest, but as more and more papers appeared, the outlines became blurred rather than clarified. Only in relatively recent years was it realized that though there are recognizable syndromes, they may, and often do, interchange among each other in a kaleidoscopic fashion, and that clinical dogma has a rather unimportant part to play in their description and analysis. The concept of the myeloproliferative disorders is, in fact, a dynamic one, and accounts of definite disease entities must to some extent be artificial. Nevertheless, the overall picture can only be built up from that of its components, and this we shall attempt to do in the following pages.

CHRONIC MYELOPROLIFERATIVE DISORDERS

Myelofibrosis with Myeloid Metaplasia

In 1870, Heuck reported the case of a 24-year-old butcher who died after an illness of more than 1 year.[126] He had a greatly enlarged spleen and liver and a severe anemia. Examination of his blood showed that his "colorless corpuscles" were far more numerous in relation to the colored ones than was usual in normal people. It was arranged to have them counted, and the result was 1.2 million colored and 400,-000 colorless corpuscles in 1 cu mm of blood. Figures of about the same order were repeatedly found later in the disease. This, then, seemed clearly to be a case of "splenic" leukemia as it was then understood.

An autopsy produced the findings customary in such cases. There were, however, two unusual features. First, the bones examined, particularly the femur and humerus, had an abnormally thick and very firm corticalis. The marrow cavity was very narrow and completely permeated by small, bony spicules, forming a very fine meshwork from which only tiny fragments of pale, red, coarse, fibrous marrow could be extracted. The fibrosis was confirmed microscopically, and Heuck commented that there was "an osteosclerosis of the whole skeleton which led to a considerable diminution of the marrow." The second unusual feature was the composition of the juice which could be scraped from the cut surfaces of the spleen and liver; this contained very numerous nucleated red blood cells.

Heuck's paper appeared at a time when the leukemias were still generally regarded as being either of splenic or lymphatic origin, but when isolated authors such as Neumann had begun to emphasize the importance of the marrow in such cases. Heuck thought that his finding of osteosclerosis spoke against the "myelogenous" origin of leukemia. Neumann countered with the ingenious theory that the marrow might have been hyperplastic before becoming sclerotic and might, therefore, have originated the leukemic process after all.[203] Neumann thus became the first protagonist of the hypothesis of the "burnt-out" marrow.

Another case resembling that of Heuck was published by Schmorl in 1904.[235] Both cases were regarded by their authors as leukemia ending in osteosclerosis, and there seems little doubt about the correctness of this interpretation, at least in Heuck's patient. However, a different view was taken by Donhauser in 1908.[76] His patient had splenomegaly; the blood showed little anemia; there was a leukocyte count of only 11,550, a differential count which was "suggestive of nothing" and no nucleated red cells. There was here no question of leukemia; and the autopsy demonstrated myelofibrosis and myeloid metaplasia. Donhauser concluded that some toxin had probably produced a chronic inflammatory change in the bone marrow which was thus the primary focus of disease and owing to its "enormous sclerosis . . . lost its hematopoietic powers . . . and the spleen . . . reverted to its fetal power to form blood." In other words, the spleen compensated for the failure of the bone marrow.

Even at this early stage, there were already two opposing points of view which have yet to be reconciled: either MMM is a disease, akin to leukemia and affecting marrow, spleen, and probably other reticuloendothelial organs simultaneously or in sequence,[12,38,43,89,113,125,127,136,137,170,186,204,221,229] or it has a distinctive nature of its own and is different from leukemia[27,144,164,231,251]; a view recently restated in considerable detail by Ward and Block[274] and by Gilbert.[101] A second controversy was long current over the question whether the splenic myeloid metaplasia was primary or compensatory. This seems at last to have been settled.

THE TYPICAL HISTORY

Case report. In March 1948, a 62-year-old man noticed a slight pain below the left breast, which was diagnosed as a virus infection of the lung and which cleared spontaneously. He remained well until September 1948, when there was again pain, with a sense of fullness and pressure in the left upper abdomen. This was subsequently found to be the result of an enlarged spleen. A blood count taken in November 1948 showed a hemoglobin level of 84 percent and a leukocyte count of 19,000 per cubic millimeter, with 60 percent neutrophil polymorphs, 8 percent myelocytes, and 6 percent myeloblasts. A needle biopsy of the sternal marrow produced a rather dilute marrow with a small percentage of immature myeloid and erythroid cells and a few megakaryocytes. A diagnosis of chronic granulocytic leukemia was made and a series of x-ray treatments given to the spleen. These diminished the splenic size, and by March 1949, following a series of blood transfusions, the blood count showed a hemoglobin level of 65 percent and a white cell count of 3,600 per cubic millimeter. At this stage the patient was admitted to our hospital for further study.

Examination revealed a well-developed man without any abnormal physical signs except for a spleen which was just palpable on deep inspiration, and a liver edge protruding two fingerbreadths below the costal margin. The blood showed a hemoglobin level of 11.7 gm per 100 ml; red blood cell count, 3.2 million per cubic millimeter; reticulocytes 2 percent, platelets 419,000 per cubic millimeter; leukocyte count 3,000 per cubic millimeter, with 62 percent

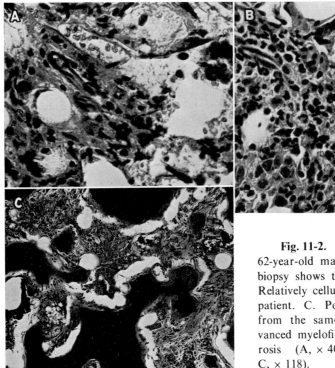

Fig. 11-2. A. Myelofibrosis in a 62-year-old male. Marrow trephine biopsy shows the sclerotic area. B. Relatively cellular area in the same patient. C. Postmortem specimen from the same patient shows advanced myelofibrosis and osteosclerosis (A, × 400; B, × 400; and C, × 118).

neutrophils and 1 percent metamyelocytes. There was one erythroblast per 100 leukocytes. Attempts at bone marrow aspiration were unsuccessful. A surgical biopsy produced a varied picture in different parts of the sections: areas of myelosclerosis alternated with hyperplastic areas, in which many early cells were found, especially erythroblasts and megakaryocytes, but few myeloid cells (Fig. 11-2). Among the results of additional investigations were a serum bilirubin level of 1.3 mg per 100 ml, and a fecal urobilinogen output of 251 mg per day, both of which were thought to indicate some degree of increased hemolysis. The diagnosis appeared to lie between myelosclerosis with myeloid metaplasia of the spleen and chronic granulocytic leukemia. A definite, though slight, hemolytic component was apparently present.

The patient was seen again in April 1950, having had no treatment in the interval. He had been feeling fairly well but tired rather easily. His main complaint was a dragging sensation in the abdomen. The spleen was now found to be greatly enlarged. The hemoglobin level was 10 gm per 100 ml, a red blood cell count of 3.8 million per cubic millimeter, reticulocytes 5.1 percent, platelets 900,000 per cubic millimeter. The leukocytes were 28,000 per cubic millimeter with 41 percent neutrophils, 10 percent metamyelocytes, 1 percent myelocytes, 7 percent myeloblasts, and an occasional erythroblast. The serum cholesterol was 160 mg per 100 ml, and the serum uric acid 7.4 mg per 100 ml. X-rays showed for the first time early osteosclerosis of the lumbar and cervical spines and the pelvis. The diagnosis now seemed definitely one of osteosclerosis and myelofibrosis with myeloid metaplasia of the spleen.

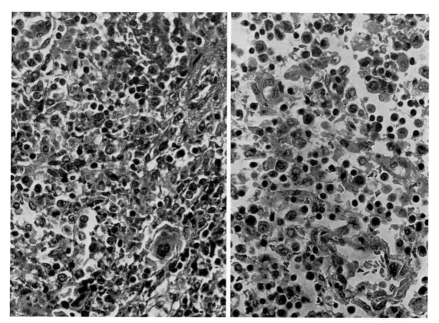

Fig. 11-3. Myeloid metaplasia. Section of spleen shows foci of myeloid and erythroid cells and megakaryocytes (× 480).

Fig. 11-4. Myeloid metaplasia. Lymph node shows almost complete replacement by myeloid tissue; no obvious lymphoid tissue left (× 480).

By August 1950, the patient was complaining bitterly of pain in the splenic area and the spleen was found to extend to the iliac crest and to be tender. He was weak and tired, with a hemoglobin level of 8 gm per 100 ml, a red blood cell count of 3.3 million per cubic millimeter, a hematocrit level of 28 percent, platelets 597,000 per cubic millimeter, leukocytes 23,000 per cubic millimeter, with 3 percent metamyelocytes, 3 percent myelocytes, 6 percent myeloblasts, and 17 erythroblasts per 100 leukocytes. There was no definite indication of increased hemolysis. A marrow aspiration produced only a few "primordial cells." A splenic puncture was carried out and showed, in addition to many lymphocytes, some erythroblasts and numerous early granulocyte precursors.

For the rest of his life the patient remained in a rather pitiful condition. Some temporary relief from the discomfort produced by the huge spleen was afforded by several local applications of x-rays, and transfusions were given to combat the increasing anemia. He died on April 1, 1951, 3 years and 2 months after he noted his first abnormal symptoms. An autopsy showed massive myeloid metaplasia of the spleen, liver, and lymph nodes, and myelofibrosis with osteosclerosis. Findings are illustrated in Figures 11-2 through 11-4. There was also pulmonary edema, cholelithiasis, and benign prostatic hypertrophy.

This case report illustrates the classical triad of findings in MMM: First, fibrosis of the marrow, initially patchy and later generalized; second, great enlargement of the spleen, as a result of myeloid metaplasia, with lesser involvement of the liver; and third, leukoerythroblastic anemia.[270,271] There was, at first, a moderate anemia with immature granulocytes and erythroblasts present from an early stage of the disease (Fig. 11-5). At times there was also a mild thrombocytosis. Symptoms

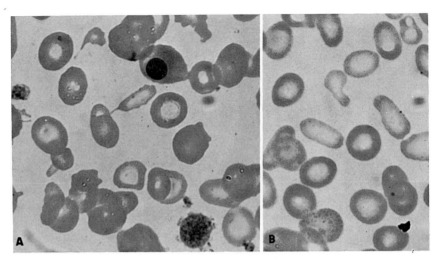

Fig. 11-5. A. Myelofibrosis and myeloid metaplasia. Blood film shows characteristic picture. Note erythroblast, giant platelet, and marked poikilocytosis with teardrop forms. B. Same as A. Note poikilocytosis and stippled red cell (A and B, × 1800).

were mild for a long time, and terminally were caused mainly by the massive enlargement of the spleen. Treatment was, on the whole, ineffective.

MMM typically occurs in middle-aged and elderly people (mean age 58.4 years[244] or 60.2 years[219]) although a few cases have been found in children.[230] We have observed two apparently congenital cases, and a youngster aged 10 with the characteristic features of the disorder—splenomegaly and anemia—first noted at the age of 2 years. An insidious onset is the rule, with asthenia, loss of weight, and symptoms of anemia usually at the forefront. Not infrequently, the large spleen first gives rise to complaints, including a "weight" in the abdomen, a sense of unusual fullness after eating, and, sometimes, sudden sharp pain lasting for several days and due to infarction with perisplenitis. Occasionally (in 14 percent of patients),[49] hemorrhagic manifestations may be the presenting feature, while in about 20 percent there is bone pain, especially in the legs. In contrast to this rather striking clinical picture, it is not uncommon to see patients in whom splenomegaly is an accidental discovery, who have no clinical symptoms, and in whom the condition may persist unchanged for years before manifestations of the disease appear.[219]

Patients with MMM are often pale and sometimes slightly jaundiced, although not infrequently—particularly in those with previous polycythemia—a plethoric appearance may be present. Splenomegaly is nearly always found and is usually gross. Some of the largest spleens are seen in this condition. Hepatomegaly of moderate to marked degree is usually present. There are few other physical abnormalities. Radiologic signs occur in about two-thirds of the cases and consist of either patchy or diffuse osteosclerosis, or, less specifically, of generalized osteoporosis. There may be irregular, lytic defects in close association with areas of increased density—often resembling the lesions of Paget's disease. The bony cortex often shows generalized thickening and appears unusually dense; extreme forms are reminiscent of the "marble-bone" disease of infancy and osteopetrosis of adults.

The blood shows a normocytic, normochromic anemia of varying severity. It may be hypochromic if there has been much bleeding. Whether or not hypochromia exists, the red cells are characteristically misshapen, with much anisocytosis and poikilocytosis, and the almost invariable presence of "teardrop" cells; these have some diagnostic significance (Fig. 11-5). The anemia often has a complex origin, with elements due to inadequate marrow, ineffective erythropoiesis, increased hemolysis, iron deficiency, and sometimes an added folic acid deficiency.[94, 132, 256] The erythrocyte reduced glutathione, glucose-6-phosphate dehydrogenase and 6-phosphogluconic dehydrogenase are often increased,[102] probably because the red cell population is younger than normal in these patients.[16] The leukocyte count is nearly always increased as the result of an increase in mature neutrophils, usually also with a few to moderate numbers of myelocytes and often some myeloblasts. The latter cells may be present year after year in concentrations of 2-5 percent of the total leukocyte count, and atypical mononuclear cells—often difficult to distinguish from leukemic blasts—may contribute up to 15 percent of the leukocytes. Nucleated red cells are very often present and may be more numerous than the immature granulocytes. The total leukocyte count ordinarily does not exceed 20,000–50,000 per cubic millimeter,[49, 130, 285] but may be as high as 75,000–100,000 per cubic millimeter. The total blood granulocyte pool is enlarged in MMM, and its marginated part disproportionately so.[10]

Elevated numbers of platelets are often present, particularly in the earlier stages; the platelet level, as measured in the thrombocytocrit, may measure from 1–5 percent. High platelet levels may persist until close to the end of the disease, when thrombocytopenia may occur, but some early cases may also show reduced platelet counts. Platelet function is often abnormal, for example, their adhesiveness.[67] Abnormal as well as giant platelets are usually present, and fragments of megakaryocytes are seen at times.[38] In the later stages, leukopenia may also occur.

The marrow is characteristically difficult to obtain by puncture aspiration. Penetration of the bone is difficult, and aspiration produces a dry tap or a hypocellular preparation with fibrous strands and perhaps masses of platelets. Trephine biopsy reveals paucity or absence of most parenchymatous elements, although megakaryocytes may be abnormally plentiful; there is a great increase in reticulum tissue, and at times a laying down of new atypical bone.

DISTINCTIONS BETWEEN MMM AND CHRONIC GRANULOCYTIC LEUKEMIA

In classic cases these two conditions are readily distinguished. The most immediately obvious difference is in the blood picture, chronic granulocytic leukemia having a higher total leukocyte count and a spectrum of more immature granulocytes. Nevertheless, when all these features are compared, the two conditions are found to be strikingly alike in many instances. The insidious onset, splenomegaly, anemia, and occasional hemorrhagic complications[28, 175, 187, 258] are just as characteristic of MMM as of chronic granulocytic leukemia. Hematologically, too, there may be little to distinguish them. Relatively low leukocyte counts in MMM are by no means universal; levels of 100,000 per cubic millimeter or even higher may be found, and although the more mature members of the granulocyte series predominate, enough myelocytes and even blasts are often present to raise serious suspicions of leukemia. The anemia, too, is very similar and often has a hemolytic element, more commonly in MMM[201] than in chronic granulocytic leu-

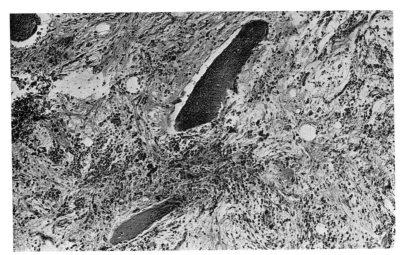

Fig. 11-6. Marrow section shows almost complete myelosclerosis (× 118).

kemia.[127,150,236] The serum B_{12} may be elevated in MMM but rarely to the degree found in chronic granulocytic leukemia (see Chapter 14).[19]

Naturally, the diagnosis is most often made by a study of the marrow, and nothing could be more dissimilar than the appearances in classic cases of the two disorders: On the one hand, the complete replacement of the hematopoietic elements by connective tissue, either fibrous or osseous or both (Fig. 11-6); on the other, vast collections of leukopoietic cells, both mature and immature, obliterating

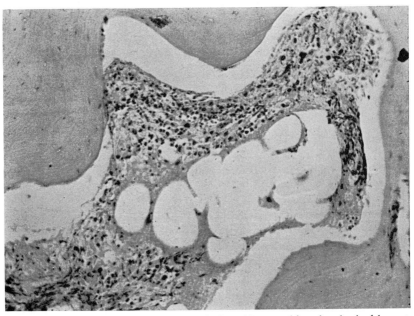

Fig. 11-7. Chronic granulocytic leukemia in a 33-year-old male who had been treated with busulfan for 2 years with good remissions. Relapse occurred with great splenomegaly and the marrow was difficult to aspirate. Marrow trephine biopsy, shows osteosclerosis and myelofibrosis, with many megakaryocytes (× 140).

the normal fat spaces, and often accompanied by increased numbers of megakaryocytes. Difficulties arise, however, in those not infrequent cases which are either
atypical or not fully developed when first seen. As is now clearly recognized, the
marrow in MMM may show changes ranging from near normality, via increasing
degrees of hyperplasia of one or more cell-lines, to partial or complete fibrosis and
sclerosis,[129,215] and numerous cases have been reported in which a very cellular
marrow accompanied splenomegaly, undoubtedly caused by myeloid metaplasia.[23,38,125,139,186] The usually active centers of hematopoiesis, the flat bones,
etc., may become sclerotic first, while the normally inactive yellow marrow may simultaneously be hyperplastic.[206] Sclerosis or myeloid hyperplasia may therefore be
discovered according to the site from which marrow is taken, and conclusions cannot necessarily be based on the results of a single aspiration. To these difficulties
must be added another, namely, the fact that some degree of fibrosis frequently
forms part of the marrow changes in chronic granulocytic leukemia, even early in its
course[21,34,44,137,151,228,234] and more frequently, in its terminal phase (Fig. 11-7).[104]

The changes in the spleen which occur in MMM are said by some authors [28,139]
to be characteristic, and splenic puncture should probably be carried out more often
than it is, although this procedure seems to have an unjustified reputation of being
dangerous. In typical cases of MMM, the splenic punctate resembles normal
marrow, with numerous immature red cells and granulocytes, as well as
megakaryocytes, being present, in contrast to the monotonously granulocytic aspirate of typical chronic granulocytic leukemia. However, here also many exceptions occur,[144,175,187] and the diagnosis may remain in doubt. Biopsy of lymph nodes
occasionally helps,[4] and in several of our patients the discovery of myeloid cells and
megakaryocytes in liver biopsy sections led to the diagnosis of general myeloid
metaplasia.

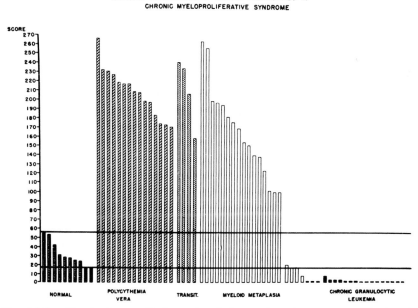

Fig. 11-8. Chart shows alkaline phosphatase of mature neutrophils in chronic
myeloproliferative syndrome. (Reproduced from Mitus et al.,[189] courtesy of the publisher.)

In recent years, two new tests have been used extensively in the diagnosis of the myeloproliferative disorders. The earlier one is the semiquantitative estimation of neutrophil alkaline phosphatase which has already been discussed in Chapter 6. An all but uniformly low concentration of this enzyme has been found in chronic granulocytic leukemia by cytochemical methods,[149,166,183,190,191] but in MMM, though many cases have NAP values in the high range, the concentration is quite variable, high to abnormally low values having been reported (see Fig. 11-8). If, therefore, the neutrophil alkaline phosphatase is high, the presence of leukemia can be excluded with some confidence, but a low score is of little diagnostic value by itself: certainly, the diagnosis should not be made in obscure cases simply on the basis of this single, nonspecific laboratory test.

The discovery of the Ph[1] chromosome (see Chapter 6) has added another and more decisive differential test. While all undoubted cases of chronic granulocytic leukemia in adults are Ph[1]-positive, the classic case of MMM is clearly negative, although a variety of inconstant chromosomal abnormalities have been described in MMM.[148,185,192,214,282] The difficulty lies in the few intermediate cases which some authors have designated as Ph[1]-negative chronic granulocytic leukemia, but which may closely resemble the more active forms of MMM. While individual diagnostic problems can thus be resolved by the discovery of the Ph[1] chromosome, its absence does not suffice to classify the case as nonleukemic. This is further discussed below.

It has been reported that, like neutrophil alkaline phosphatase, the periodic acid-Schiff (PAS)-positive material in mature neutrophils is diminished in chronic granulocytic leukemia, whereas it is usually elevated in MMM, as well as in polycythemia vera.[96]

As noted above, although hyperuricemia and gout may occur in all of the chronic myeloproliferative disorders, the highest incidence by far is in MMM. Hickling has convincingly correlated the serum uric acid level with the number of megakaryocytes, which are nearly always high in MMM[128]: Certainly the highest serum uric acid levels (commonly in excess of 10 mg per 100 ml) are found in this disorder, and the passage of uric acid stones in untreated patients has, in our experience, been limited to MMM. Treatment of chronic granulocytic leukemia with x-rays or chemotherapy may also give rise to the same symptoms.

In summary, typical and fully developed cases of MMM can be clearly distinguished from those of classic chronic granulocytic leukemia, but atypical forms exist which cannot readily be classified. These often appear intermediate between what might be termed the *two polar conditions*, and thus suggest the possibility of transitions between them. Before this possibility is further discussed, the two closely related conditions of polycythemia vera and thrombocythemia will be considered.

POLYCYTHEMIA VERA

Originally described by Vaquez in 1892 as a "special form of cyanosis" accompanied by excessive and persistent hyperglobulia,[269] polycythemia vera shows as its most characteristic clinical features easy fatigue, weakness, dyspnea, vertigo, headache, and pruritus. Severe itching, often unbearable, occurs after bathing in about 50 percent of all patients. Erythromelalgia and thrombotic phenomena, particularly of the lower extremities, are common. An appearance of plethora with striking redness of the face, distension of the retinal veins, congestion of the conjunctivae, nasal, and oral mucosae, peripheral vasodilation and cyanosis, splenomegaly, and hepatomegaly are the commonest physical abnormalities.[36,55] The spleen is palpable in over 80 percent of patients in true polycythemia.[218] In some, the organ is barely palpable while in others it seems to occupy the greater part of the abdomen. Unusually large spleens, if seen in polycythemia, are almost invariably signposts to the future development (or recognition) of hematologic complications such as MMM or acute leukemia.[264] Examination of the blood shows a gross erythrocytosis, a great elevation of the red cell mass, a moderate leukocytosis with counts ranging from 10,000 to 20,000 per cubic millimeter in 60 percent of patients, and a moderate to marked thrombocytosis. The platelet count is usually two to five times normal, but may be as high as 5 million per cubic millimeter or more. At these very high levels, platelet counts are more than usually inaccurate; the best estimates are then made by means of the "thrombocytocrit," that is, the percentage of platelets in the upper, cream-colored layer in the centrifuged hematocrit tube. The marrow is very hyperplastic, and in 50 percent of patients it shows an increased thickness of the reticulin network. As long ago as 1908, Osler noted an "extraordinary increase" in the total volume of blood and thought that this overproduction of erythrocytes by the marrow was entirely analogous to leukemia, both affections being associated with "states of morbid activity in the bone marrow."[211] In the same year, Parkes Weber drew attention to the granulocytic hyperplasia, which is a constant feature of polycythemia, and stressed that this might actually exceed the erythroid hyperplasia in extent.[279] That the megakaryocytic system is also hyperplastic, and, like the myeloid and erythroid precursors, produces excessive numbers of descendant cells, was stressed by Minot and Buckman[189] and numerous observers since then (Fig. 11-9). Polycythemia vera is, in fact, a panmyelopathy with the blood showing a "pancytosis."[55] It gives the impression as if all "stops" in blood production in the bone marrow had been pulled.

The natural course of polycythemia vera is not easy to determine as there are

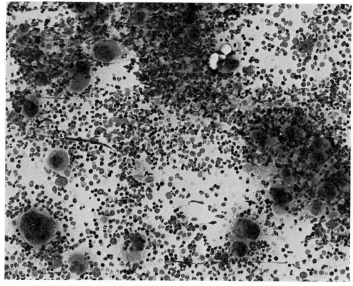

Fig. 11-9. Polycythemia vera. Marrow smear shows numerous megakaryocytes (× 200).

very few untreated patients. Initially, the evolution is slow, and the date of onset can rarely be pinpointed. By the time the diagnosis is made, the disease process has probably been going on for a number of years; the fact that the patient has become aware of symptoms generally indicates a fairly advanced stage, and by then the disease is no longer the benign one as which it is so often regarded. It has been said that in the absence of treatment fewer than 50 percent survive more than 2 years after diagnosis, but this seems an unduly drastic statement. Modan shows a median survival of 9 years for patients untreated by radio- or chemotherapy.[192]

Treatment prolongs life considerably, although opinions vary by how much. The uncertainty is, in part, accounted for by the varied ways in which survival times are expressed, some as averages, others as medians. Some authors include living and deceased patients, others only those deceased, while some quote predicted survival times for their whole series. Furthermore, times are sometimes calculated from onset, sometimes from diagnosis, or first treatment. *Onset* is variably defined, but hardly likely to coincide with the actual beginning of the pathologic process: If used as a precise date, it "often coincides with the date of first treatment or referral,"[209] and, as mentioned above, this is probably years later than the true onset. Some published median survival times of treated patients are as follows: 11 years,[36,278] 11.4 years,[62] 12 years,[161] 13 years,[276] 13.3 years,[156] 13.6 years,[218] 170 months,[209] and 14.5 years.[264] It seems certain that treatment prolongs life. However, life-table methods of charting results have clearly established that, even with treatment, the prognosis of survival of patients with polycythemia vera is considerably worse than that of "normal" people of the same ages.[110,161,218]

In this chapter we are particularly concerned with the relationship of polycythemia vera to other members of the myeloproliferative group. A tendency has lately arisen to speak of the "hematologic complications" of polycythemia vera, and to include among them MMM and the various leukemias. There is controversy in the literature regarding both the frequency of such "complications" and their relationship to the therapy of polycythemia vera.

In every series of patients with polycythemia vera there are some who, treated or untreated, sooner or later develop anemia and pass into a clinical state entirely different from that obtaining until then. According to Wasserman and Bassen,[277] this change occurs in all patients who survive the polycythemic phase sufficiently long, but such has not been the general experience.

This novel character of the disease begins to assert itself after periods of a few, to as many as 15 or 20, years from its known onset. The spleen develops progressive enlargement and may reach a huge size. The hemoglobin level, which had been grossly increased, begins to fall until eventually an actual anemia supervenes. Concurrently, the leukocyte count, which had been normal or moderately elevated, tends to rise further, and immature granulocytes—metamyelocytes, myelocytes, and myeloblasts—appear in the blood. These are often accompanied by a variable number of nucleated red cells. The platelets, which had been unusually numerous, may still further increase in number or they may diminish to thrombocytopenic levels. These changes, which are illustrated in Figure 11-10, were usually interpreted by early authors as signaling the onset of leukemia.[103,111,112,121,189,260] Jacobson and Smith summed up this interpretation by stating that "it is well known that chronic leukemia and especially myelogenous leukemia occur in about 10 plus percent of all cases of polycythemia even though no x-ray therapy or ^{32}P is given."[140]

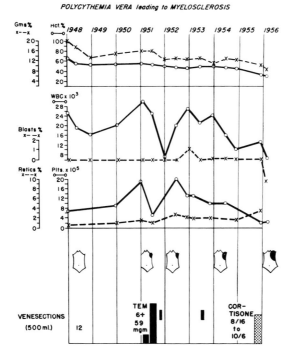

Fig. 11-10. Originally, a mild polycythemia vera treated only with venesections in a 50-year-old male. Gradual onset of myelofibrosis occurred, characterized by increasing splenomegaly, with anemia, leukocytosis, and thrombocytosis.

By contrast, as early as 1922, some workers had doubts about the precise classification of such cases and thought that they might be dealing with a "midgroup between erythremia and myelogenous leukemia."[216] As new tests, particularly marrow and splenic puncture biopsies, became available, it was discovered that the marrow was often fibrotic, and that myeloid tissue appeared in the spleen; the syndrome of myelosclerosis was, in fact, present, and statements now appeared to the effect that most, if not all of the reported cases of leukemia in the wake of polycythemia vera were actually examples of MMM. As a result of its long-continued, frantic overactivity the marrow had become "spent" or "burnt-out," and the spleen and, perhaps, other organs such as the liver had apparently taken over the manufacture of blood cells.[27,231,237]

There are now few proponents of this compensatory theory. Myeloid metaplasia is present in the spleen well before the marrow becomes fibrotic.[27,125,189] Marrow reticulum is increased at an early, and even at an untreated stage.[81,226] Splenic fibrosis occurs simultaneously with myeloid metaplasia,[43,139] and MMM has been known to develop "backwards" into polycythemia vera,[171] all of which facts suggest that MMM develops *coincidentally* with polycythemia vera and not as a compensatory process.

The incidence of MMM in patients with polycythemia vera is not easy to determine. Earlier authors[36,181,253] did not distinguish it clearly from chronic granulocytic leukemia; some more recent ones[110,161] include it with leukemia in a group termed *marrow failure*. In those papers in which MMM is listed separately as a cause of

Table 11-3

Incidence of MMM and Acute Leukemia in Polycythemia Vera

Authors and References	MMM		Acute Leukemia	
	Percentage of Patients	Radiation (+) or other treatment (−)	Percentage of Patients	Radiation (+) or other treatment (−)
Arthur (9)	3.5	+	7.8	+
Dameshek (58)			12.9	+
Dameshek (58)			2.6	−
Halnan and Russell (107)	3.7	+	−	+
Lawrence et al. (158)	25.0	+	14.4	+
Modan and Lilienfeld (193, 194)	4.5	−	0.8	−
Modan and Lilienfeld (193, 194)	3.5–10	+	11.6	+
Osgood (209)			14.0	+
Perkins et al. (218)	2.5	−	−	−
Reed (223)	17.2	+	5.8	+
Szur and Lewis (255)	7.0	+	1.8	+
Tubiana et al. (264)	6.0	+	10.8	+
Wasserman (276)			11.0	+
Watkins et al. (278)			2.5	+

death in polycythemia vera, the incidence ranges from 2.5–25 percent (Table 11-3), but in these series many patients were still alive, and the actual incidence is probably higher. Clearly, the transition occurs whether or not the patient has had treatment.

Although *chronic* granulocytic leukemia was formerly said to follow polycythemia vera fairly frequently, confusion with MMM must have been frequent, and by present diagnostic standards few of these cases would be acceptable. In our own experience, MMM is a far more common sequel than chronic granulocytic leukemia which is, in fact, a rare occurrence. There are a few reports on Ph[1]-positive leukemia following polycythemia vera,[8,119,138] and the occasional occurrence of this complication is, therefore, not to be doubted following extensive radiotherapy. A further source of confusion is the occasional occurrence of mild erythrocytosis in early chronic granulocytic leukemia.

Acute granulocytic leukemia is now recognized (next to MMM) as possibly the commonest hematologic sequel of polycythemia vera. This recognition has been slow in dawning, mainly because acute and chronic leukemia and MMM were long confused with each other, or not separated. Papers published since 1964 (Table 11-3) show an incidence of acute leukemia varying from zero to 14 percent. These figures should be interpreted with some reservations since the patient material, selection, length of follow-up, and, particularly, therapy have varied greatly. Whatever the numerical relationships, it is important to realize that acute leukemia can and does follow polycythemia vera. Such a change is sometimes accompanied by the acquisition of new, abnormal chromosome clones, but the precise significance of such events is uncertain since some patients have abnormal clones without showing any signs of changing to leukemia.[146,188,273] From the practical, as well as the theoretical, point of view, the salient question is whether acute leukemia is a "natural" sequel of polycythemia vera or whether it has always been induced by therapy.

Since there are practically no untreated patients with polycythemia vera, it is at best possible to obtain an indirect answer to this question. For many years, the treatment of choice in most clinics has been by means of ionizing radiations, at first in the form of x-rays to the spleen, the long bones, or the whole body, but for the past 20 years or more, it has almost exclusively been ^{32}P. It has been abundantly demonstrated (see Chapter 5) that ionizing radiations are themselves leukemogenic, and as early as 1928, Harrop[111] and others began voicing suspicions that the onset of leukemia in polycythemia vera might be radiation-induced. Statistical studies have been carried out ever since then, especially in the past 10 years, but although the case for an iatrogenic origin of the leukemias has become much stronger, the statistics of incidence are still in considerable confusion and the risks uncertain. Table 11-3 shows the incidence of acute leukemia in several series of patients with polycythemia vera, all of them recorded since 1964. Earlier work[11, 140, 160, 181, 225, 237, 253, 254] is difficult to interpret and will not be considered here. The largest recent series is that analyzed by Modan and Lilienfeld[193, 194]; this is drawn from seven American and Canadian clinics, some of which treated polycythemia vera by means of radiation while others used either phlebotomy alone or combined with various chemotherapeutic agents. These authors found that the incidence of leukemia in the radiation-treated series was over 10 percent and in the controls less than 1 percent; it increased with the higher doses of radiation given but did not depend on the length of survival alone. These results appeared to provide strong evidence to show that many, if not all, acute leukemias in patients with polycythemia vera were radiation-induced.

Supporting the data of Modan and Lilienfeld, were those of Perkins et al.,[218] who reported the largest single series of polycythemia vera patients treated without radiation, but by other means—phlebotomy, thio-TEPA, pyrimethamine, nitrogen mustard, busulfan, triethylenemelamine (TEM), etc. Not a single case of acute leukemia occurred. The conclusion seems inescapable that radiation increases the chances of leukemia, and Modan and Lilienfeld showed that there was no difference in that respect between ^{32}P and x-rays. It seems certain that the liability of patients with polycythemia vera to suffer radiation-induced leukemia is substantially greater than that of normal individuals.

Although these general conclusions must be accepted, the detailed results from different quarters are puzzling. Thus, at least four groups,[107, 223, 255, 278] with a total of 434 patients treated by radiation, report very low leukemia figures, probably not significantly raised over those in Modan and Lilienfeld's "no radiation" series. Others report much higher incidences. Osgood has pointed out the importance of using patient groups with a comparable age and sex distribution, and similar length of observation.[209] Dose, nature, and mode of administration of the radiation are of obvious significance, and length of observation and selection of material introduce other variables. These difficulties can be overcome only by means of carefully controlled prospective studies; and until results from such studies become available, the exact risk of radiation leukemogenesis in polycythemia vera must remain uncertain, although it cannot be denied that a well-defined risk is present.

The same is true for the treatment of polycythemia vera by means of chemotherapy. This modality has been in use for far shorter periods than radiation, and although few cases of acute leukemia have been reported in patients treated with chemotherapeutic agents, the eventual risk cannot as yet be assessed with any degree of certainty.[24, 178, 196]

Whether the risk of developing acute leukemia should be incurred by treating polycythemia vera with ^{32}P may be a philosophical question: Osgood has shown that treatment with ^{32}P prolongs life on the average by a number of years compared with treatment by means of other modalities.[209,210] It would appear from his findings that though more patients will die from leukemia when ^{32}P is used, they will do so at a relatively advanced stage, whereas the risk of a relatively early death from causes other than leukemia may be increased when ^{32}P is withheld. Osgood's figures do not, of course, show the possible shortening of life span of those patients dying of acute leukemia 2–5 years after radiation therapy is given, and it is of little value to the man dying of acute leukemia to know that the *average* life span for the group is increased. At this time, each physician must weigh these risks for himself, always with the understanding that their precise magnitude is still subject to considerable doubt. Certainly, it is our feeling that in younger patients ^{32}P should be used only in special circumstances. Prospective studies now in progress are likely to provide more definite guidance on the prognosis of polycythemia vera when treated by various means, and on the associated risks.

THROMBOCYTHEMIA

The term *thrombocythemia* is used in varying senses by many different authors, and the literature is extremely confusing. In particular, thrombocythemia is frequently equated with *thrombocytosis,* a general designation for a rise in the platelet count. In order to have any meaning whatever, the term should be confined to instances where the platelet count is persistently elevated to at least three times the normal value.[163] Such values may be found in the course of polycythemia vera, in chronic granulocytic leukemia, and in MMM, and it is evident that the thrombocythemia here is part and parcel of the general picture of increased myeloid activity obtaining in these conditions. Diagnostic difficulties may arise when the thrombocythemia is unduly prominent.

In addition to these cases, others occur more rarely, in which an extremely high platelet count appears to be the central feature of the condition. Very occasionally, these present clinically as purely thrombotic conditions ("essential thrombophilia"[205]). More commonly, patients with such platelet levels (up to 5 million per cubic millimeter or higher) have symptoms of hemorrhagic disease, with bleeding from the mucosae and into the tissues and body cavities recurring over long periods, and with only occasional thromboses. This syndrome was termed *thrombocythemia hemorrhagica* by Epstein and Goedel in 1934[90] and has since been described in at least 100 patients.[23,91,224,248,250,283] and repeatedly reviewed.[106,212,243] Case histories are characterized by persistent bleeding from mucous membranes, notably those of the gastrointestinal tract, and nearly always by slight to moderate splenomegaly. Occasionally, there is splenic atrophy.[177] Hematologically, there are thrombocytosis, a high neutrophilia, and anemia of varying degree. The anemia is characteristically hypochromic because of prolonged bleeding resulting in iron deficiency. In the intervals between bleeding there may be a mildly polycythemic state. The marrow shows a general hyperplasia, and the large groups of megakaryocytes producing huge masses of platelets are an extraordinary sight. Blood smears seem to be overrun by masses of platelets; bits of megakaryocytes are often seen (Fig. 11-11).

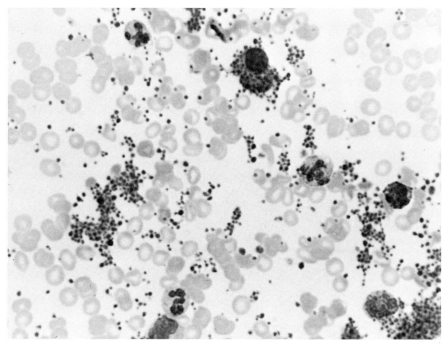

Fig. 11-11. Blood film from patient with hemorrhagic thrombocythemia shows numerous platelets.

The cause of the bleeding is not understood. Its severity is closely correlated with the height of the platelet count,[106] but although various abnormalities of platelet function can be demonstrated[173] and the platelet chemistry may also be disturbed,[200] the changes are inconstant and variable, and the bleeding phenomenon still presents one of the enigmas in this challenging field.

There is no conclusive pathologic evidence to show that thrombocythemia hemorrhagica is a distinctive primary condition, and such terms as *primary*, *idiopathic*, or *essential* thrombocythemia are probably inaccurate. The close connection between thrombocythemia, polycythemia vera, and MMM seems quite obvious. Transitions and overlaps among them are common, so that it is often uncertain where one begins and the other ends. *Thrombocythemia hemorrhagica* is, however, a useful term as it defines fairly well a *clinical* syndrome in which the prognosis is more or less predictable and the treatment fairly well defined. Hematologically and pathologically, it appears to be one of the chronic myeloproliferative disorders, characterized as it is by a pronounced proliferation of all the myeloid elements—megakaryocytes, erythroid and granulocytic cells—and sometimes by myeloid metaplasia in the spleen and liver as well.

Whether there is any justification for calling this condition "megakaryocytic leukemia," as has been suggested by some authors, is a matter of taste or interpretation. There can be no question that the magnitude of the megakaryocytic proliferation, with the appearance in the blood of not only masses of platelets but of bits of megakaryocytes, is indicative of a neoplastic proliferation of the megakaryocyte-platelet line. On the other hand, at least in the chronic cases, there is little, if any, infiltration of organs other than those that are normally hematopoietic. True megakaryocytic or megakaryoblastic leukemia is rare and is either associated with, or closely resembles, the acute granulocytic form.[30,65 ,100] The various chronic forms of the myeloproliferative syndrome may all be classed as neoplastic, but are probably best thought of as relatively benign "first cousins." It is however, not unusual for MMM to terminate as acute granulocytic leukemia[87] and Silverstein and Linman report as many as 25 percent of deaths in agnogenic myeloid metaplasia to be due to this complication.[245]

INTERRELATIONSHIPS

The three more or less well-defined conditions, MMM, polycythemia vera, and thrombocythemia have been briefly surveyed. In all of them there is general hyperplasia of the myeloid elements, either in the marrow or in the other hematopoietic tissues, or both. The clinical pictures are varied, to be sure, but numerous transitions between them, as well as between the hematologic appearances, have been noted. In some instances, there is a close relationship to granulocytic leukemia. Are these then entities, or should they be regarded as divergent manifestations of a single underlying process?

Niles et al., in 1959, made a critical study of a group of 69 patients diagnosed as having "myeloproliferative diseases," their purpose being to decide if the commonly accepted clinical, hematologic, and pathologic criteria of diagnoses were sufficiently precise to enable clear distinctions to be made.[204] Twelve patients had acute granulocytic leukemia, 41 chronic granulocytic leukemia, 3 MMM, and 13 PV; the authors concluded that at least at postmortem examination the conditions were not distinct entities, that their limits were poorly defined, and that transitional cases, rather than typical ones, were the rule. They suggested, however, that possibly clearer distinctions could be made with the aid of more refined diagnostic methods.

Our own experience with such patients is similar. Anyone who has seen a large number of patients with these disorders must have been struck by the diversity of syndromes encountered, a diversity which has led to the introduction of such a profusion of names and epithets that their unraveling becomes nearly impossible. However, there is obviously a common bond: polycythemia and the various syndromes characterized chiefly by an excess of megakaryocytes and platelets all show a *total* proliferation of all hematopoietic elements of the marrow, at least at some stage of their course.

Polycythemia vera may be taken as the central member of the group, because a panmyelosis is always found in this condition. Its progression to MMM is a frequent (some say inevitable) and well-recognized stage of its natural history. Very significantly, the opposite course—a change from MMM or leukemia to polycythemia—may also be found occasionally.[32,171] The inclusion of MMM in the myeloproliferative disorders remains a problem only if we confine ourselves to the terminal stages. There is no evidence to support the theory that it represents a kind of marrow failure in which the spleen plays a compensatory role. In the human, the reticuloendothelial organs do not seem to resume their total activity of hematopoiesis in those clear cases of marrow destruction in which a compensatory activity would be most desirable, as, for instance, in aplastic anemia.[2] Furthermore, contrary to the opinion of many authors (Hickling[127] and others), removal of the "compensating" spleen in MMM is by no means always a fatal mistake, but instead

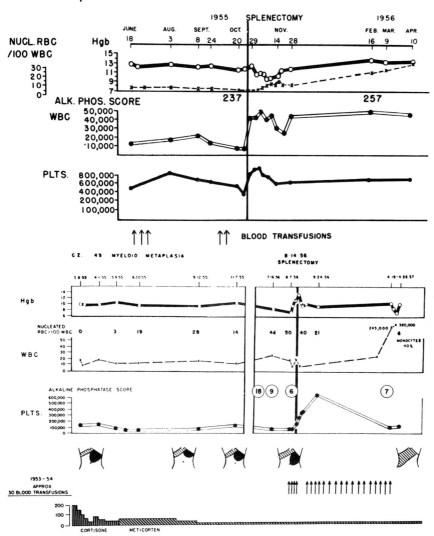

Fig. 11-12. Charts showing blood counts of two patients with myelofibrosis and myeloid metaplasia of the spleen who had splenectomies. Both showed substantial temporary improvement following the operation.

it can lead to clinical and hematologic improvement in properly chosen cases (Fig. 11-12).[57,66,197,238,280]

Case report. A 50-year-old male was in his normal state of health when he was by chance found to have a tumor in the left upper abdomen. At operation, this proved to be an enlarged spleen which was removed. Section showed that it was the seat of advanced myeloid metaplasia. Blood counts were then done and showed a mild leukoerythroblastic anemia. Marrow puncture gave a dry tap. The patient lived another 18 years, during the last few of which he required occasional blood transfusions. His death was caused by pneumonia.

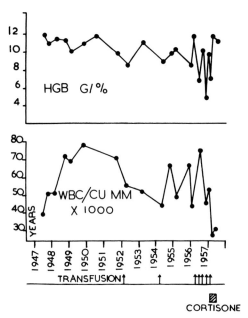

Fig. 11-13. MMM in a 50-year-old male who had had splenectomy in 1939. The patient survived until 1957.

At autopsy, there was advanced but patchy myelofibrosis and osteosclerosis with myeloid hyperplasia of the liver (Fig. 11-13).

Splenic myeloid metaplasia may coexist with hyperplasia of the marrow. This provides the strongest argument in favor of the view that MMM, like polycythemia, is a panmyelopathy in which hematopoietic tissue proliferates *en masse* in many sites including the marrow and spleen. Eventually, the chief emphasis in MMM falls on the proliferation, possibly as a secondary event, of the connective tissue element with ensuing marrow fibrosis and osteosclerosis; this is accompanied by reduced cellularity of the hematopoietic organs—whether they have been crowded out or burnt out is not clear. We have alluded elsewhere to the physician's desire, whether conscious or not, to make a definite diagnosis and thus to put the case into the proper pigeonhole. Sometimes the problem of the indefinite diagnosis is solved if the patient is watched long enough. In others, a supposedly accurate diagnosis can be more inaccurate than the rather vague classification, chronic or acute myeloproliferative disorder. The controversy between the "lumpers" and "splitters" will probably always continue as there are merits on both sides.

Although the close relationship between polycythemia vera, MMM and thrombocythemia is clear, their relation to chronic granulocytic leukemia still deserves examination. It has been stated by many that there is a fundamental dichotomy, chronic granulocytic leukemia being somehow quite distinctive when compared with the others. The most important evidence for this has been seen in the behavior of the neutrophil alkaline phosphatase and the presence of the Philadelphia chromosome. Thus, the question must be examined if, by virtue of these two parameters or any others, it is possible to separate chronic granulocytic leukemia from MMM and its cousins and to recognize it as a distinctive and homogeneous entity.

Case report. A 35-year-old married female was examined in February 1967 and a diagnosis of chronic granulocytic leukemia was made because of splenomegaly and the following blood count: Hemoglobin 10.0 gm per 100 ml; leukocytes, 280,000 per cubic millimeter, with a predominance of neutrophils and myelocytes; platelets 380,000 per cubic millileter. From March 1967 onward, the patient was treated with a daily dose of 4 mg of busulfan, and showed a prompt response. The leukocyte count had fallen to 2000 per cubic millimeter and the platelets to 75,000 per cubic millimeter in July, when treatment was discontinued. She then felt well, although her hemoglobin level remained at 9–10 gm per 100 ml. In December 1967, the leukocyte count was 8,500 per cubic millimeter with a normal differential count; and the platelets had increased to 220,000 per cubic millimeter.

In mid-February 1968, her symptoms returned, with increasing tiredness, dyspnea, pallor, night sweats, and abdominal pain. On March 15, she was admitted to our hospital. She was pale and feverish with a 15-cm splenomegaly

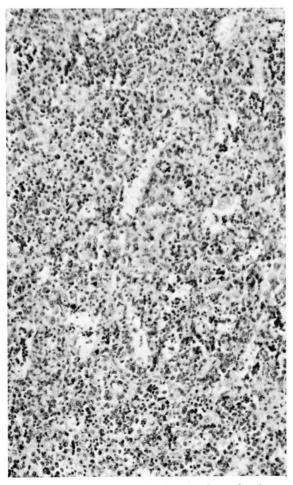

Fig. 11-14. Chronic granulocytic leukemia. Section of spleen after splenectomy showing myeloid metaplasia.

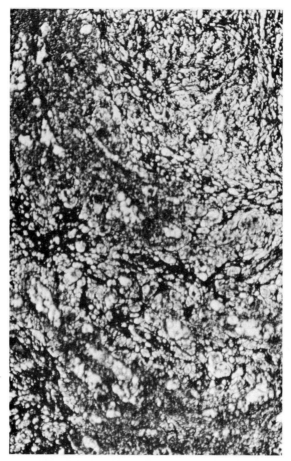

Fig. 11-15. Chronic granulocytic leukemia in same patient. Section of spleen after splenectomy. Reticulin stains showing fibrosis.

and 5-cm hepatomegaly. The hemoglobin level was 7.5 gm per 100 ml, and the leukocyte count was 256,000 per cubic millimeter (neutrophils 46 percent; basophils 10 percent, myelocytes 36 percent, blasts 5 percent), the platelet count was 380,000 per cubic millimeter. The neutrophil alkaline phosphatase score was 0. Treatment with busulfan, in a daily dose of 8 mg, was begun on March 27, and on April 16 the leukocyte level was 8,000 per cubic millimeter, the platelets 220,000 per cubic millimeter, the spleen measured 9 cm, and the hemoglobin level was 10 gm per 100 ml.

The patient was clinically much improved and afebrile. Marrow aspiration was attempted from two sites but only two minute, hypercellular fragments were obtained. These showed plentiful erythroid and myeloid precursors and, probably, increased megakaryocytes and basophils. Splenic aspiration yielded clear evidence of myeloid metaplasia, with many erythroblasts and megakaryocytes, as well as myeloid precursors.

The leukocyte count now began to rise again, reaching 100,000 per cubic millimeters on May 12. At this stage, a 1-day blood culture without phytohemagglutinin (PHA) showed the presence of the Ph[1] chromosome in all

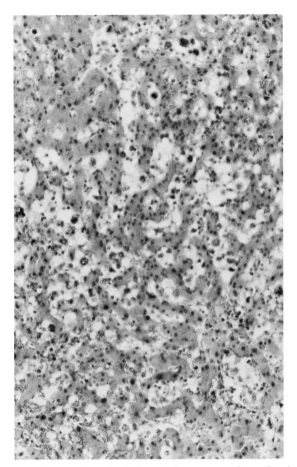

Fig. 11-16. Chronic granulocytic leukemia in same patient. Section of liver shows myeloid metaplasia.

identifiable mitoses. The count fell gradually with the recommencement of busulfan therapy, but the spleen continued to increase in size, reaching 24 cm below the costal margin by mid-June and causing considerable distress. Splenectomy was carried out on July 2, resulting in relief of the patient's symptoms, but postoperative complications caused her death on July 15, 1968. Sections of the spleen showed advanced myeloid metaplasia and fibrosis (Figs. 11-14 and 11-15), as did the liver (Fig. 11-16) and lymph nodes at autopsy. The marrow was partly very hyperplastic (Fig. 11-17), partly fibrotic. Very large numbers of megakaryocytes, often immature, were present throughout many of the organs.

Comment. This patient showed the signs and symptoms of chronic granulocytic leukemia, with splenomegaly, a characteristic blood count, low neutrophil alkaline phosphatase score, the Ph[1] chromosome, and a rapid response to busulfan therapy. The remissions, however, were only partial (with no rise in hemoglobin level, and residual splenomegaly) and short lived. In the later stages, the patient was found to have myelofibrosis and pronounced myeloid metaplasia, and biopsy and

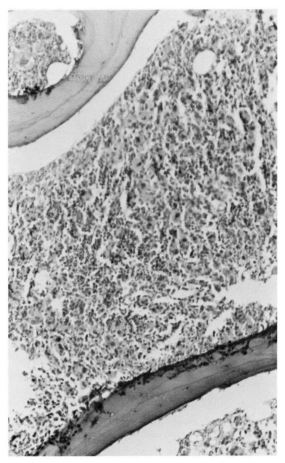

Fig. 11-17. Chronic granulocytic leukemia in same patient. The postmortem marrow section shows hyperplasia with numerous megakaryocytes.

autopsy findings showed chronic granulocytic leukemia and MMM. Here, then, was a patient in whom features of both diseases coexisted.

A total of seven similar cases has been reported by Krauss[151] and by Pennelli et al.[217] Other authors had patients showing a transition from Ph[1]-positive leukemia to MMM.[44,247] In Hiroshima, following the detonation of an atomic bomb, there was an increase in the number of cases of MMM as well as of leukemia.[5] Benzene may cause myelosclerosis as well as leukemia.[222] The suggestion of a close clinical, as well as an etiologic, connection is thus strong.

The neutrophil alkaline phosphatase score is quite variable in MMM (see page 387). In chronic granulocytic leukemia, it certainly tends to be very low, but this is by no means constant, for a rise to normal or even high levels may occur in remission, during intercurrent infections, and in the terminal blastic phase. Thus, the neutrophil alkaline phosphatase level does not distinguish between the two disorders. Neither is it possible to rely on the Ph[1] chromosome as a final arbiter. Quite apart from what may be termed *hybrid* cases such as those just discussed, every large series of chronic granulocytic leukemias has a proportion of patients (about 10 percent or less of the total) in whom the hematologic findings are typical but the Ph[1] is absent.[261,281] Similarly, in childhood, there is a form of chronic granulocytic leukemia with Ph¹-positive cells and another, often called the juvenile form, with similar hematologic features but an absence of the Ph¹.[109,226] Both the adult and juvenile forms of Ph¹-negative chronic granulocytic leukemia are stated to have a worse prognosis than the positive variants.[281] Are the two variants, in fact, the same disease? If they are, then the Ph¹ chromosome is not the absolute criterion for the presence of leukemia; if not, then there must be myeloproliferative disorders intermediate between genuine chronic granulocytic leukemia and MMM. This is not simply a matter of semantics, for if there are transitions from one disease to the other, as well as patients exhibiting the characteristics belonging to both or lying intermediate between them, then it seems difficult, indeed, to draw hard and fast lines between monolithic "entities." In this connection, it is highly significant that the Ph¹ chromosome occurs, not only in myeloid, but also in erythroid precursors,[220] and probably in megakaryocytes, as is further discussed in Chapter 6.

To us, the conclusion seems inescapable that MMM, polycythemia vera, and thrombocythemia belong to a close-knit group of diseases which are related in a most intimate way, so much so that their segregation is often difficult and the transformation of one into another commonplace. Even chronic granulocytic leukemia, although in most cases distinguishable by means of its possession of the Ph¹ and a very low neutrophil alkaline phosphatase score, may on occasion have features which suggest one or several of the other myeloproliferative disorders. Diversity among the various myeloproliferative disorders may be due, not so much to fundamental differences between them as to the effects of differing growth rates among the cell-lines which together constitute the rather complex bone marrow structure, and to secondary reactions in response to neoplastic transformation. The group of myeloproliferative disorders is probably neoplastic in nature, with growth rates varying in degree from extreme chronicity or benignity to excessive acuteness. So far we have considered the more chronic disorders. In the next section we shall deal with the acute ones, and with transitions between chronic and acute disorders.

ACUTE MYELOPROLIFERATIVE SYNDROMES

Whereas the course in most cases of chronic granulocytic leukemia, polycythemia vera, MMM, and thrombocythemia is measured in periods of years, some other myeloproliferative disorders proceed much more rapidly and their course may be only a matter of months or at most a year. These may be classed as acute cases; in these, many of the proliferating cells of the blood and marrow are primitive. As with the chronic cases, the proliferation may involve a single cell-line, though increasing experience suggests that combined proliferations of several cell-lines— either simultaneous or in sequence—are much more common.

The Di Guglielmo Syndrome and Its Relation to MMM and Polycythemia Vera

This group of morbid conditions of the blood, to which the name of Giovanni Di Guglielmo has been attached, forms the subject of one of the most confused chapters in modern hematology. The volume of descriptive and analytical literature is quite out of proportion to the rarity of the condition, a fact which stems largely from the pertinacity with which a comparatively small number of cases has been assessed, reassessed, classified, and reclassified by a multiplicity of authors, led by Di Guglielmo, who himself produced a whole series of classifications embracing at different times very different groups of diseases.

In March 1962, a few months after Di Guglielmo's death, there appeared what may be regarded as his scientific testament, the large volume entitled *Le Malattie Eritremiche ed Eritroleucemiche.*[75] In it, he distinguishes between "acute erythremia" which he first described in 1926[71] and regarded as a "pure" disease of the erythron, and "erythroleukemia," which made its debut as early as 1917[69] in a paper, which already contained the germ of the idea of a "panmyelopathy," and which in 1920 was considerably expanded.[70] Much later still (1958), Di Guglielmo acknowledged that acute erythremia, too, was a "polyphasic myeloproliferative disease,"[74] a disease which passed from an almost pure red cell neoplasia through a mixed leukoerythroblastosis (erythroleukemia) to the picture of pure granulocytic (myeloblastic) leukemia. The reverse progression, from pure leukemia to pure erythremia, might also occur, although rarely.

Di Guglielmo described the bone marrow of acute erythremia as showing the following five features[74]: (*1*) hypercellularity; (*2*) proliferation of the erythroblasts which might comprise more than 90 percent of the marrow cells; (*3*) inversion of the leukoerythroblastic ratio, in most cases to lower than 1:1; (*4*) maturation arrest of the erythroblasts; and (*5*) abnormalities of the erythroblasts such as gigantism, polyploidy, or "neoplastiform monstrosities." Such findings, without some concomitant changes in the myeloid cells, are very unusual, and cases of pure erythremia are indeed of great rarity, even in the older literature. Moeschlin, who calls them "genuine erythroblastosis," rejects most of those described, including even the first one of Di Guglielmo himself. Writing in 1940, Moeschlin accepts only five.[17,72,73,159,213] Of these, one was termed *chronic* by the author and had a history of 4 years duration, a fact which exemplifies the almost insurmountable difficulties of classifying these diseases.[17] There are many more cases which fall into the "polyphasic" group, beginning with an erythroblastic proliferation and ending as typical acute granulocytic leukemia. Verloop et al.,[272] who described the history of a man with such an illness, made the suggestion that the longer the patient's survival, the greater the chance of an acute granulocytic transformation taking place; this would perhaps explain the increasing numbers of "mixed" cases appearing in the literature, as individuals with anemia are kept alive for lengthy periods by transfusions and other therapeutic means.

In our own experience with cases of the Di Guglielmo syndrome, as we prefer to call it, the pure examples of erythremic myelosis are rare, but on the other hand the *syndrome*, in which erythroblastic and myeloblastic proliferations are mixed is fairly common, almost certainly because the condition arises in the multipotential stem cells, and not in those unilaterally committed to erythropoiesis. We have developed the concept that, except in very acute or fulminating cases, the disease usually passes through three stages. At first there is a *pure* (more correctly *preponderant*) erythroblastic proliferation with all the various abnormalities occurring as Di Guglielmo described them. Even at this stage, a few myeloblasts may be found in the blood, together with foci of myeloblastic proliferation in the marrow. In a few months or in a few years—depending upon the intrinsic character of the disease— the myeloblasts increase in number, both in the marrow and in the blood; this is now the mixed phase of erythroleukemia; many cases are of this type when first observed. The last stage is characterized by a preponderant or almost complete myelo-blastosis, almost identical with that seen in the metamorphosis of chronic granu-locytic leukemia or in acute myeloblastic leukemia. Thus, there are (*1*) acute erythremia; (*2*) erythroleukemia; and (*3*) acute myeloblastic leukemia in successive stages. We use the inclusive term *Di Guglielmo syndrome* for all of them, realizing that mixed transitional forms are probably much more common than the pure forms of erythremic myelosis, which have been so widely emphasized. Examples of such mixed cases, showing varying proportions of erythroblasts and immature granulocytes at different stages, as well as occasionally considerable numbers of megakaryocytes in the marrow[199] and platelets in the blood, have been recorded by Verloop et al.[272]; Shively and Dorrance[241]; Mackenzie and Stephenson[174]; Martin and Bayrd[179]; Blackburn and Lajtha[26]; Emery[88]; Magalini and Ahstrom[176]; Crowley et al.[51]; Sheets et al.[240]; Scott et al.[239]; and Haranghy et al.[108] and Harwerth,[113] who discuss the conditions in monographs. These cases have usually been classified as erythroleukemia by the authors.

The more acute cases may be very difficult to distinguish from acute hemolytic anemia, since both conditions may display extreme proliferation of the erythroblasts and be rapidly fatal. Although a distinction can often be drawn by means of the direct Coombs' test, which is positive in many of the acute hemolytic anemias and negative in erythremic myelosis, this is not absolutely diagnostic. More recent studies indicate that a mild degree of increased hemolysis may be demonstrated by appropriate tests, such as the estimation of the serum haptoglobin, the ^{51}Cr red cell survival time, and the fecal urobilinogen output. As is shown below (see page 408), the paradox of an enormous erythroid hyperplasia, associated with an apparently slight need for it in the form of only mildly increased hemolysis, may be explained by a neoplastic type of red cell proliferation with ineffective erythropoiesis on the basis of arrested maturation and perhaps other intracellular disturbances.[202] Thus, the abnormal erythroblastic hyperplasia is essentially futile, since simultaneously the red cells of the blood continue to decline. Several patients have been described in whom splenectomy was carried out either under the mistaken impression that a nonleukemic hemolytic anemia was present, or in the attempt to stop excessive hemolysis and thus prolong the life of a patient with definite leukemia.[88,272] The re-sults of operative intervention have been uniformly unsuccessful.

The following Case report illustrates some of the points which have been men-tioned.

Case report. A 53-year-old carpenter, complaining of a rather sudden onset of weakness and tiredness in December 1954, was found to be anemic. Be-tween January and April 1955, he was given eleven transfusions as well as liver extract and other hematinics. When seen by us in June 1955, he showed marked pallor and moderate splenomegaly. His blood sample indicated the presence of a severe hemolytic anemia, with a hemoglobin of 7.2 gm per 100 ml, with 27 percent reticulocytes. The leukocyte count was 12,000 per cubic millimeter, with 7 percent myeloblasts. There were 56 erythroblasts per 100 leukocytes. The marrow was the site of marked normoblastic erythroid hyperplasia with a few megaloblastoid forms. Foci of cells interpreted as myeloblasts were seen. There was a hyperbilirubinemia; the direct Coombs' test was negative (Fig. 11-18).

Although the findings which suggested a diagnosis of "acquired" or

A.R., ♂ 53YRS. - DI GUGLIELMO'S SYNDROME

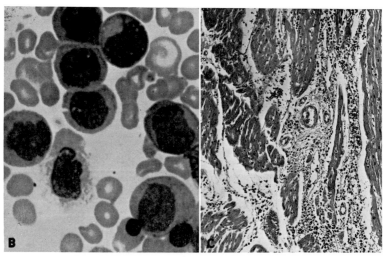

	6/22/55	7/5/55	8/25/55	1/5/56	3/19/56	6/9/56	8/9/56
RBC	2.11 M	3.90 M	2.68 M	2.55 M	2.22 M	3.02 M	2.59 M
Hgb	7.6 (49%)	11.6 (74%)	9.3 (60%)	8.8 (57%)	6.2 (40%)	9.6 (61%)	7.0
RETICS	27.1 %	14.5 %	15.5 %	9.2 %	8.8%	2.0 %	0.1%
PLATELETS	147,000	507,000	696,800	336,600	666,000	712,000	235,000
CORRECTED WBC	13,000	7,500	11,000	113,000	13,000	130,000	306,000
TOTAL # BLASTS	910 (7%)	225 (3%)	0	53,000(47%)	260 (2%)	44,200(14%)	257,000(84%)
TOTAL # NUCL. RBC	7,200 $\frac{56}{100 \text{ WBC}}$	8,250 $\frac{110}{100 \text{ WBC}}$	14,000 $\frac{127}{100 \text{ WBC}}$	60,000 $\frac{53}{100 \text{ WBC}}$	52,000 $\frac{400}{100 \text{ WBC}}$	94,900 $\frac{73}{100 \text{ WBC}}$	12,000 4%
MARROW CELLULARITY	2+ - 3+	3 +		4 +		4 +	
% BLASTS	0.4 %			30 %		40%	
% NUCL. RBC	60 %			21 %		37%	
WBC / RBC	2/3			4/1		2/1	
	▓▓▓▓▓▓	‖‖	TRANSFUSIONS	‖	‖	‖‖‖	
R_x				200mgm 6 MP 150mgm			

SPLENECTOMY
↑
7/2/55   ↑ 12/31/55   ↑ 1/13/56   ↑ 5/25/56

Fig. 11-18. A. Chart shows course of 53-year-old male with the Di Guglielmo syndrome.

Fig. 11-18 *(Continued).* B. Same patient as A. Blood shows myelomonocytic cells in the late stage of disease (× 1800). C. Same patient. Section of heart muscle shows infiltration between muscle bundles (× 118).

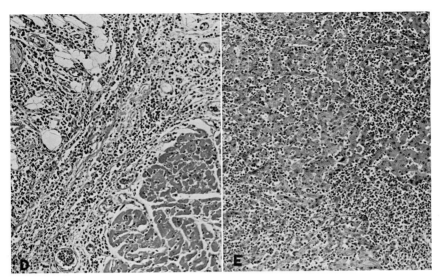

Fig. 11-18 *(Continued).* D. Same patient. Section of heart shows gross leukemic peri-carditis (× 118). E. Same patient. Section of liver shows widespread leukemic infiltration (× 118).

"autoimmune" hemolytic anaemia were somewhat atypical, particularly the marked erythroblastemia and the negative Coombs' test, splenectomy was car-ried out July 2, 1955. The spleen was enlarged and imprints and sections gave a picture compatible with myeloid metaplasia, that is, a focal growth of im-mature red cells and granulocytes, with preservation of the general archi-tecture of the organ.

Splenectomy was followed by an improvement in the anemia (Fig. 11-18), and a rise in the platelet count which had previously been subnormal. Concur-rently, the immature granulocytes disappeared from the blood, but there was no reduction either in the reticulocytosis or the erythroblastosis. Further mar-row examinations during the subsequent 3 months showed varying pictures, but all were characterized by a gross hyperplasia of both the erythroid and granu-locyte series, with sometimes one and sometimes the other predominating. There appeared no doubt that this was a rather acute leukemic process, either granulocytic or erythremic in nature.

For 6 months after splenectomy, the patient felt reasonably well without transfusions or medication, and continued to work as usual. In December 1955, he showed definite evidence of relapse. On January 5, 1956, the hemoglobin was 8.5 gm per 100 ml and the leukocyte count 113,000 per cubic millimeter, with 47 percent blast forms. There were 60,000 erythroblasts per cubic millimeter. Reticulocytes were 9.2 percent and platelets 336,000 per cubic millimeter. The patient was treated by transfusions and the administration of 6-mercaptopurine, and there was a rapid fall in the leukocyte count and in the percentage of blasts, but not in the erythroblasts in the blood or the reticulocy-tosis. The platelet count continued to rise to abnormally high levels. Clinically, there was little improvement; anemia persisted, and there was increasing hepatomegaly. The course remained downhill, and was interspersed with various acute episodes, one of which, in June 1956, suggested pericarditis. The blood count varied, but the percentage of very young and often abnormal granulocytes rose gradually, and the number of erythroblasts in the blood remained high. The patient expired on August 12, 1956. During the last month, the blood picture became that of a frank granulocytic leukemia of the myelomonocytic variety, and the percentage of erythroblasts diminished sharply (Fig. 11-18). Autopsy confirmed the diagnosis of acute granulocytic leukemia. There was widespread leukemic infiltration of many organs, particularly of the heart muscle and pericardium (Fig. 11-18). The total known duration of the illness was 21 months.

The patient showed at differing times the pictures of acquired hemolytic anemia, mixed erythroleukemia, and a pure granulocytic leukemia. Moreover, his spleen which had been removed 1 year before his death, presented the appearance usually found in myeloid metaplasia. Despite the great overgrowth of erythroblasts and granulocytes in the marrow, the number of megakaryocytes was persistently high, and the platelets in the blood were abnormally numerous until very shortly before death. This extreme hyperplasia of all three cell systems signified the existence of a panmyelosis rather than an overgrowth of any one cell-line. In many respects the picture resembled that found in fully developed cases of polycythemia vera. To be sure, there was an anemia instead of an erythrocytosis; this was partly the result of ineffective erythropoiesis and partly of hemolysis. Most of the immature cells were more primitive than those seen in polycythemia vera and appeared in greater numbers in the peripheral blood. Even with these findings, however, it seems likely that this condition was an acute manifestation of the same process which, when chronic, would present itself as polycythemia vera. An additional point of similarity is the occurrence of myeloid metaplasia in the course of both diseases.

The possible connection between polycythemia vera and erythroleukemia may be more clearly seen in the following case history, in which polycythemia was actually followed by an extremely acute erythroleukemia.

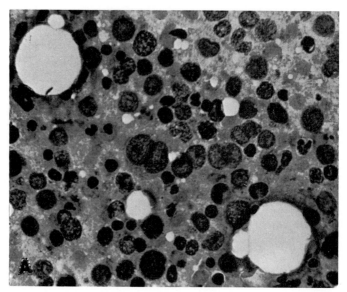

Fig. 11-19. A. Erythroleukemia following polycythemia vera. Marrow aspiration biopsy (× 700).

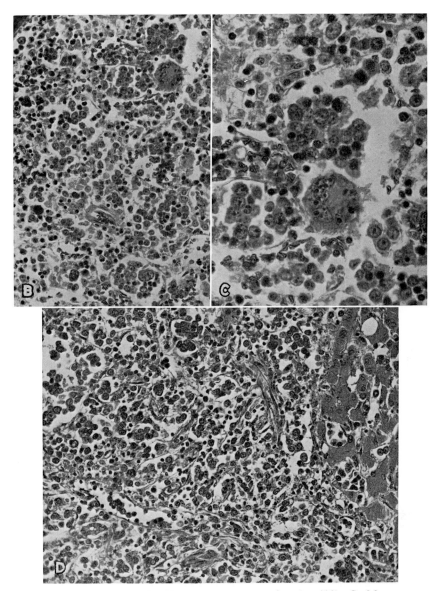

Fig. 11-19 *(Continued).*   B. Marrow autopsy section (× 400). C. Marrow autopsy section (× 700). D. Liver autopsy section (× 400).

Case report.   The patient, a psychiatrist aged 51, suffered a myocardial infarction in December 1950, and while convalescing from it in February 1951, was discovered to have an extremely high red cell count. The diagnosis of polycythemia vera was made and accepted by experienced hematologists. The patient was treated by venesections of 500 ml, at first daily, and then at gradually increasing intervals until blood was withdrawn at biweekly intervals. This man had never received treatment with x-rays, radiophosphorus, or chemotherapy and had never been professionally exposed to the action of ionizing radiations.

In January 1952, the patient became suddenly ill, with fever, increasing

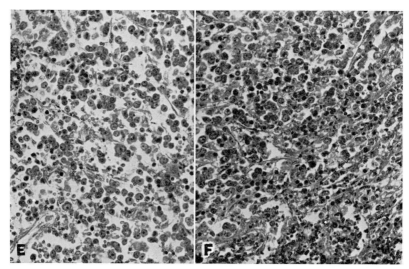

Fig. 11-19 *(Continued).* E. Lymph node autopsy section (× 400). F. Spleen autopsy section (× 400). All show massive infiltration with primitive leukemic cells and erythroblasts.

weakness, malaise, nausea, vomiting, and bone pains in the left leg. He himself felt his liver enlarging. On February 1, he developed bleeding from the gums and tongue and into the skin of the arms, chest, and abdomen. He was admitted under our care the following day. On examination, he was found to be feverish, extremely weak and pale, with icterus of the sclerae. The liver and spleen both extended to the iliac crest and were very tender on palpation. There were hemorrhages of the gums and ecchymoses of the extremities. The blood showed a hemoglobin level of 8.5 gm per 100 ml, with 1.2 percent reticulocytes, 65,000 platelets per cubic millimeter, and a leukocyte count of 32,000 per cubic millimeter with 68 percent neutrophils, 4 percent lymphocytes, 3 percent metamyelocytes, 7 percent promyelocytes, and 9 percent myeloblasts. There were 31 erythroblasts per 100 leukocytes in all stages of maturation, gross anisocytosis, macro- and microcytosis, and many unusual polychromatophilic erythrocytes. The marrow was hypercellular, with a predominance of blast forms (Fig. 11-19). Some of these appeared to be abnormal myeloblasts and others very early erythroblasts, often with multiple nuclei and bizarre nucleoli. There was an increase of mature erythroblasts, many of them abnormal. Megakaryocytes were present in normal numbers. On the basis of the blood and marrow findings a diagnosis of erythroleukemia was made. The patient died 2 days later. Autopsy showed an extreme infiltration of many organs (Fig. 11-19)—marrow, spleen, liver, kidneys, and lymph nodes—with primitive erythroblastic and leukemic cells, as well as multiple hemorrhages into the organs and from the mucous membranes.

This man showed typical features of polycythemia in 1951. A year later, he developed a fulminating acute leukemia which fulfilled Di Guglielmo's criteria of an acute erythroleukemia of the mixed type. Here, then, is an example of an acute myeloproliferative disorder succeeding a chronic one. The case is no longer unique for, since we described it in the first edition of this work, at least five more instances have been reported in which polycythemia vera was converted to the Di Guglielmo syndrome.[14,64,84,239,267] The analogy with the acute and chronic forms of granulocytic leukemia is obvious. Is not the conclusion likely that polycythemia vera and erythroleukemia may be different manifestations of the same underlying pathologic process?

NONACUTE FORMS OF THE DI GUGLIELMO SYNDROME

While most cases of the Di Guglielmo syndrome show features corresponding to those of acute granulocytic leukemia—short course, presence of many primitive cells in the blood and marrow, a relative resistance to therapy—others appear to be more chronic. They may or may not be characterized by a pronounced erythroblastosis in the blood; the marrow is generally dominated by proliferating erythroblasts, although an excess of other blasts is almost always found on careful examination. The clinical course may extend over a period of 2–5 years, and in some cases over a much longer period. This is a rather heterogeneous group whose demarcation from some other blood dyscrasias is often difficult to establish. Thus, the description of these cases varies greatly from clinic to clinic. We suspect that what we call the Di Guglielmo syndrome in our laboratories may be dubbed "primary refractory anemia," "refractory normoblastic anemia," "sideroblastic anemia," or "sideroachrestic anemia" in others. Clearly, in many instances of this disorder the leukemic process is relatively slowly progressive.

The patients described by Schwartz and Critchlow as having "chronic erythremic myelosis" probably fell into this category.[236] In some the disease was of exceedingly long duration, one patient surviving 10 years. They were characterized by a chronic "refractory" anemia, enlargement of the spleen and liver, and proliferation in the marrow of young erythroid cells that failed to mature. The blood showed anemia without marked reticulocytosis, thrombocytopenia without hemorrhagic phenomena, a normal or low leukocyte count with preponderance of immature granulocytes, and few or no erythroblasts. The marrow was composed of many erythroid forms, usually very immature and often abnormal, with active or slightly reduced granulopoiesis, sometimes resembling that seen in pernicious anemia; megakaryocytes were usually normal. An early case of this nature was described by Copelli in 1912.[45] Schwartz's cases resembled closely those of "refractory anemia" described by Bomford and Rhoads in 1941 and not regarded by them as leukemia.[29]

Some of the cases studied by us and others[13,59,259] were, like those of Schwartz and Critchlow,[236] of great chronicity with courses up to 10 years or more. A few patients were at first diagnosed as having MMM (Fig. 11-20). Others had been referred to us as having "refractory anemia" and at first sight they closely resembled some of Bomford's and Rhoads's patients.[29] Nucleated red cells in the blood were by no means a characteristic feature, although the marrow was crowded with red cell precursors. This seemed to us analogous to "aleukemic" leukemia, that is, "anerythroblastic" anemia. However, these patients all eventually developed frank leukemic signs. Here, obviously, is another area where several hematologic syndromes appear to meet, and conceivably longer observation might have revealed leukemia in Bomford's and Rhoads's patients as well.[29] Dacie and his colleagues have studied carefully seven patients with "refractory normoblastic anemia" whose clinical and hematologic features were very similar to those of our more chronic

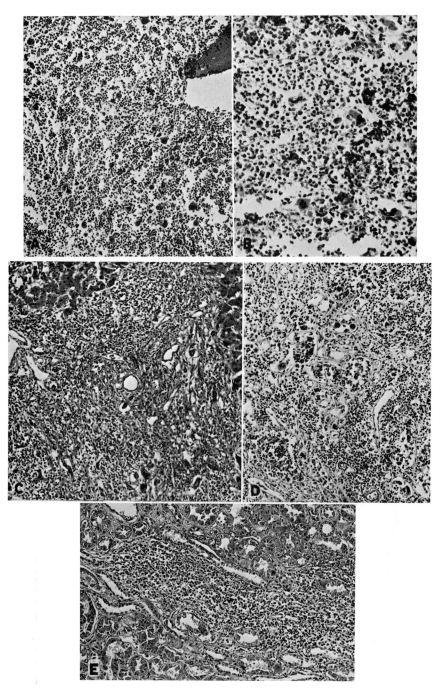

Fig. 11-20. Autopsy sections from patient diagnosed during life as having MMM. All sections show intense cellularity and extreme myeloid metaplasia. Total course of disease was 18 months. A. Marrow (× 118). B. Spleen (× 260). C. Liver (× 118). D. Lymph node (× 118). E. Kidney (× 118).

cases of the Di Guglielmo syndrome,[54] with the important difference that no signs of leukemia were seen, in spite of observation of up to 11 years, and no pathologic features pointing to leukemia could be discovered postmortem in the two patients who died. Similar findings have been published by Heilmeyer.[122] In such patients, a cytochemical study of the marrow may be helpful, particularly the periodic acid-Schiff (PAS) reaction which has been found by Hayhoe to show characteristic coarse stippling of part, or all, of the erythroblasts in many cases of the Di Guglielmo syndrome.[114,115] In refractory sideroblastic anemia, the PAS reaction is much less distinctive, but sometimes it nevertheless suggests a relationship between the two conditions.

Probably the most realistic way of classifying the erythroleukemias, on the one hand, and the refractory or achrestic anemias, on the other, is to regard them as the extremes of a spectrum of proliferative diseases involving the three principal hematopoietic cell-lines. All of these diseases are characterized by a general marrow hyperplasia and a failure to produce adequate numbers of normal red cells, granulocytes, and platelets. All of them may show changes in the erythroblastic series, including abnormal morphology, excessive sideroblastosis, changes in the red cell enzymes,[78,92] antigens,[233] and cytochemistry (see Chapters 6 & 14),[115] and failure of normal iron incorporation into the mature erythrocytes or "ineffective erythropoiesis."[249] All of them, too, may show hyperplasia of the granulocytic series, especially of its early members, and of the megakaryocytes. Abnormal chromosome clones have been described in erythroleukemia, as well as in sideroblastic anemias, and some of these have been remarkably similar (see Chapter 6).[65,118] Unquestionable transitions have occurred from a refractory anemic state to frank erythroleukemia,[15,25,60,242] and both the refractory anemias and erythroleukemias are almost invariably fatal. Until it becomes possible to characterize more precisely what constitutes leukemia—an object which has so far remained unattainable—it may be wise to regard all so-called refractory anemias as potentially neoplastic in nature, and to refrain from drawing any clear lines of demarcation.

It may also be advantageous, at least from a speculative point of view, to incorporate *paroxysmal nocturnal hemoglobinuria* (PNH) into the same group of myeloproliferative disorders.[61] Although this disease has for long been regarded as an unusual form of acquired red cell abnormality, it has been found in recent years to be closely related to other blood dyscrasias. Its first sign is not uncommonly pancytopenia resulting from marrow aplasia, while, conversely, established cases may proceed to severe or fatal marrow failure.[53,165,167] Lewis and Dacie suggested that an abnormal clone might arise in some marrows regenerating from an aplastic state,[167] and Dameshek believed that such clones might at times become self-replicating and eventually leukemic.[61] That PNH erythrocytes have a clonal origin has been positively established in at least one patient.[208] Patients in whom paroxysmal nocturnal hemoglobinuria was followed by acute granulocytic leukemia or erythroleukemia have been published,[37,133,142,145,275] but it is as yet unknown how often this transition occurs. However, it can certainly be argued that paroxysmal nocturnal hemoglobinuria is a panmyelopathy, and as such is closely related to other myeloproliferative disorders such as the Di Guglielmo syndrome.

The Di Guglielmo Syndrome and Pernicious Anemia

Probably the most significant morphologic difference between the refractory anemias and Di Guglielmo's syndrome is the relative scarcity of atypical and, especially, megaloblastoid erythroblasts in the former, and their abundance in the latter.[63] The resemblance to the megaloblastosis of pernicious anemia is often striking; moreover, both the Di Guglielmo syndrome and pernicious anemia, as well as many refractory anemias, show the same functional defect, namely, ineffective erythropoiesis, with a rapid plasma clearance time of injected ^{59}Fe, but with little iron incorporation into the red cells, together with hyperbilirubinemia in the presence of an almost normal red cell survival time; a phenomenon probably explained by a premature breakdown of the abnormal red cell precursors. It has also recently been shown that both pernicious anemia and the Di Guglielmo syndrome have very similar chromosomal abnormalities (multiple breaks) resulting from a disturbed DNA metabolism (premature arrest of DNA synthesis.)[50,117,184] In the Di Guglielmo syndrome, in a proportion of cases examined, as in other cases of acute leukemia, these changes are accompanied by other chromosomal abnormalities more directly associated with malignancy, such as aneuploidy, exchanges, and, in at least three instances, ring chromosomes (Fig. 11-21).[39,50,68,83,118,120,143,147]

The major hematologic difference between pernicious anemia and the Di Guglielmo syndrome is, of course, the response of the former to the administration

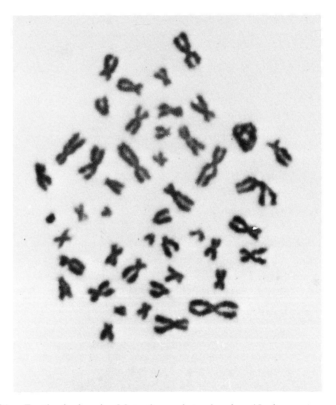

Fig. 11-21.   Erythroleukemia. Metaphase plate showing 45 chromosomes including a ring chromosome.

of vitamin B_{12}, and the complete resistance of Di Guglielmo patients whose serum B_{12} is normal or high. It would seem likely that in the latter the deficiency lies within the cell itself; conveivably, it may consist in the deletion of a specific enzyme concerned with vitamin B_{12} uptake or utilization. This is a distinct possibility, which would be in line with defects in some other types of neoplastic cells. In pernicious anemia, B_{12} administration causes the disturbed DNA metabolism to return to normal within 4 days at the most (Menzies, personal communication). If it were possible to pinpoint the presumed missing enzyme in the Di Guglielmo syndrome, then the same restoration of function might conceivably follow. At this point, successful substitution therapy for this highly intractable form of the acute myeloproliferative syndrome does not seem entirely beyond the bounds of possibility, especially since there is some evidence that the ostensibly neoplastic erythropoiesis in the Di Guglielmo syndrome is responsive to changes in erythropoietin concentration and, hence, not entirely autonomous in character (see Chapter 5).[3,95]

Acute Myelosclerosis with Myeloid Metaplasia

Although this disturbance is far more unusual than the typical chronic case of the disease, it nevertheless appears to be a definite entity.[18,168] Here, we are dealing with a condition in which anemia develops rapidly and is associated with the presence in the blood of 10–20 percent myeloblasts. In some patients, an extraordinary thrombocytosis may be present, at least initially, and associated with bits of megakaryocytes. The bone marrow shows a varying degree of fibrosis, foci of myeloblasts, and, in some patients, enormous numbers of megakaryocytes. Splenic puncture demonstrates myeloid metaplasia, although the leukocytes and, perhaps, the nucleated red cells are more primitive. Differential diagnosis between acute granulocytic leukemia, megakaryocytic leukemia, and the Di Guglielmo syndrome may be difficult, if not quite impossible, in some of these cases, and it might well be doubted if it is rational to attempt a rigid compartmentalization of these rare cases. Nature certainly does not.

Case report. A 64-year-old pearl merchant was found to have a mild anemia (with a hemoglobin level of 11.6 gm per 100 ml) in November 1956. In April 1957, his complaints of abdominal discomfort, night sweats, and fatigue led to a careful examination. The patient was found to be pale but not icteric. The liver edge was felt 7 cm and the spleen 2 cm below their respective costal margins. The blood findings included a hemoglobin level of 8.4 gm per 100 ml, with a hematocrit of 24 percent, and a leukocyte count of 8850 per cubic millimeter, with 66 percent mature neutrophils, 8 percent band forms, 20 percent lymphocytes, 3 percent monocytes, 2 percent basophils, and 1 percent eosinophils. Four nucleated red cells were seen per 100 leukocytes. Bone marrow punctures were dry. A surgical trephine biopsy revealed myelofibrosis. In November 1957, the spleen was at the umbilicus. The blood platelets numbered 240,000 per cubic millimeter (about half-normal by the indirect method); the differential count of the white cells showed: 71 percent mature neutrophils, 4 percent metamyelocytes, 8 percent myelocytes, 2 percent promyelocytes, 8 percent myeloblasts, 6 percent lymphocytes, and 1 percent eosinophils; occasional nucleated red cells were seen. The platelets varied greatly in size and shape, with many bizarre forms. Spleen puncture showed the characteristic features of myeloid metaplasia, with many early nucleated red cells and early granulocytes including myeloblasts. Alkaline phosphatase of the mature neutrophils was scored at 200, a very high level. Another bone marrow biopsy revealed myelofibrosis. The patient died on December 14, 1957, after an illness of approximately one year or less.

Case report.   A 74-year-old clothing merchant, previously in good health, developed fatigue and pallor in September 1957. He was found to have a hemoglobin level of 6.3 gm per 100 ml and a leukocyte count of 8500 per cubic millimeter. The diagnosis of aplastic anemia was made because it was found impossible to obtain marrow by puncture aspiration. Further history revealed that he often used a solution of carbon tetrachloride and benzene in spraying garments in his clothing store. In October 1957, the leukocyte count was 15,000 per cubic millimeter, with 52 percent mature neutrophils, 8 percent band forms, 4 percent metamyelocytes, 6 percent myelocytes, 4 percent myeloblasts, 17 percent lymphocytes, 4 percent monocytes, and 5 percent eosinophils. Two nucleated red cells were counted in 100 leukocytes. Several bone marrow punctures yielded unsatisfactory results. A Vim-Silverman needle biopsy of the posterior ilium disclosed marked myelofibrosis. The neutrophil alkaline phosphatase was scored at 110. Treatment with transfusions and prednisone was given. Despite this, there was rapidly increasing anemia and thrombocytopenia. On January 7, 1958, blood counts were as follows: a hemoglobin level of 5.5 gm per 100 ml, with 1.93 million red blood cells per cubic millimeter, 23,700 leukocytes per cubic millimeter, and 0.2 percent reticulocytes, and a platelet count of 24,800 per cubic millimeter. Differential count: 64 percent mature neutrophils, 9 percent band forms, 9 percent metamyelocytes, 4 percent myelocytes, 8 percent myeloblasts, 5 percent lymphocytes, and 1 percent eosinophils. The sedimentation rate was 149 mm per hour (Westergren). The patient's course was that of rapidly increasing anemia, fever, and mucous membrane and skin bleeding. He underwent numerous transfusions but eventually died in August 1958.

Case report.   A 62-year-old woman developed the characteristic features of polycythemia vera 4 years before being seen. She was treated with ^{32}P in a dosage of 6 mCi, resulting in an excellent remission for more than 3 years. However, she then developed increasing anemia and thrombocytopenic purpura. The blood showed pancytopenia and the marrow, a striking myelofibrosis. The entire acute terminal illness lasted for no longer than 3 months.

Case report.   A case illustrative of nature's mixup of diseases occurred in a male (Fig. 11-22) beginning with typical chronic granulocytic leukemia. Following busulfan therapy, the characteristic features of polycythemia vera were present. After a year, anemia, leukocytosis, nucleated red cells, and striking thrombocytopenia were present; the bone marrow now showed marked myelofibrosis. The anemia increased and the patient developed the acute features of the Di Guglielmo syndrome. He died eventually in myeloblastic crisis.

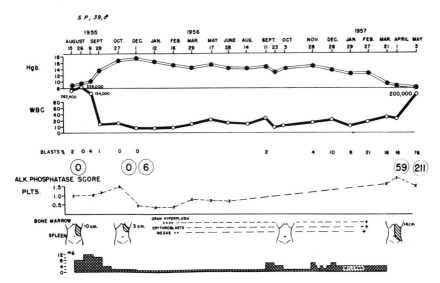

Fig. 11-22. Changing events in a case of chronic myeloproliferative disorder, beginning as chronic granulocytic leukemia in a 39-year-old male. Development of polycythemia vera (December 1955), myelosclerosis with myeloid metaplasia (December 1956), and myeloblast crisis (May 1957) followed by death. (Reproduced from Mitus et al.,[189] courtesy of the publisher.)

To summarize the section on the acute myeloproliferative syndromes, it has been shown that the Di Guglielmo syndrome has many features which make it difficult to distinguish from acute granulocytic leukemia; that it may follow upon a chronic myeloproliferative disorder, polycythemia vera and that its less acute forms may be almost indistinguishable from MMM and from the refractory anemias. Acute forms of MMM have been shown to exist, and to resemble acute leukemia and the Di Guglielmo syndrome. Clearly, the acute myeloproliferative disorders are also a closely knit group, overlapping among themselves, and with the chronic forms; and equally clearly, progress in research on one or the other of them must further knowledge of the group as a whole. Such progress is however impeded by their relative rarity and the marked variation of clinical and hematologic features among patients.

Leukemia, Tuberculosis, and Carcinomatosis

The relationship between leukemia and tuberculosis has been the subject of a great deal of research (see especially the review by Andre[7]). We consider the topic here because of the occasional occurrence of cases of myelofibrosis with myeloid metaplasia in which there is a strong indication that a coexistent tuberculous infection may have been of etiologic importance. Similarly, polycythemia vera sometimes occurs in the course of tuberculosis.[93, 105] In fact, the first patients in whom polycythemia was described had tuberculosis.[269] Finally, leukemoid reactions have been reported in tuberculous patients, and these are said to mimic leukemia—especially the acute variety—so closely that even very experienced hematologists have had trouble in making the correct diagnosis.[152]

The finding of two diseases in the same patient may represent nothing but coincidence. It may, on the other hand, mean that one condition has predisposed the organism to an attack by the other, if, indeed, the two were not basically caused by the same underlying mechanism, that is, the tubercle bacillus. Moreover, the presence of one disease may modify the usual manifestations of the other. These various possibilities all exist when MMM or leukemia are found together with tuberculosis.

The incidence of tuberculosis does not appear to be increased in patients with untreated leukemia when compared with the general population.[1,172] This makes it seem unlikely that leukemia itself predisposes the organism to attack by tuberculosis. Their occasional coexistence is most likely coincidental. If this is true, the next question is whether and how they influence each other.

TUBERCULOSIS AND MYELOFIBROSIS

Tuberculous foci are not infrequently discovered in the course of MMM. The first report came in 1908 from Donhauser, whose patient with MMM had tuberculosis of the mesenteric nodes.[76] By 1948, 91 patients with myelofibrosis had been reported in the literature, among whom 7 had active tuberculosis.[48] The tuberculosis and "idiopathic" cases resembled each other closely, both clinically and hematologically. The course of several of the former was very rapid, with pronounced signs of toxicity such as fever, night sweats, and loss of weight. Miliary tubercles were sometimes found, and when this occurred, there was a characteristic absence of the normal cellular reaction around them, and a paucity of giant cells. Many of the tubercles were teeming with bacilli.

The question arises whether tuberculosis may be an etiologic factor in MMM. This has been discussed at length.[7] It is unlikely to be so where there are only localized tuberculous lesions, as in the lungs or the lymph nodes, but the possibility deserves serious consideration in patients in whom the enlarged spleen itself contains tuberculous lesions, or where there are general miliary changes. Tuberculosis is capable, in certain instances, of causing a great deal of fibrosis in areas surrounding its lesions (reticulotrophic tuberculosis of Cazal,[40]), and occasionally myeloid metaplasia occurs around tuberculous foci in the spleen.[99] It is possible that some cases of MMM may represent similarly atypical reactions to the organism, as may certain cases of pancytopenia, which have been described in association with tuberculous infection.[182] The following case report illustrates these relationships and some of the questions raised by them.

> *Case report.* A 65-year-old man entered hospital because of a weight loss of 30 pounds during the past 8 months, and weakness for 2 months. Eight weeks before admission he had first noted pain in the left upper abdominal quadrant, and his spleen had then been found to be enlarged. He had become weaker and feverish, with night sweats. On examination, he appeared chronically ill and wasted, with a temperature of 101.8. There were some small, palpable, axillary lymph nodes, the liver edge was 10 cm below the right costal margin, and the spleen was palpable to the iliac crest. He had a mild normochromic anemia, a mild thrombocytopenia, and a leukocyte count of 17,000 per cubic millimeter, with 91 percent neutrophils and a few metamyelocytes and myelocytes. His sedimentation rate was raised, the bone marrow was hypocellular, and his chest x-ray normal.

He was thought to be suffering from either Hodgkin's disease or a collagen disorder, and a scalene node biopsy was carried out. In view of his rapidly deteriorating clinical state, treatment with prednisone, 100 mg daily, was begun immediately after the biopsy. After 2 days of therapy, the result of the lymph node biopsy became available, and this showed a granuloma with tissue necrosis, presumably tuberculous. The prednisone was immediately discontinued and full antituberculous therapy instituted. Soon afterward a second chest x-ray showed the presence of miliary tuberculosis.

The patient's clinical condition improved immediately after antituberculous therapy was commenced. Two months later, his temperature was normal and his symptoms had subsided. His chest x-ray was again clear. After 4 months he was clinically well and had gained 30 pounds. After 8 months he remained entirely symptom-free. However, his spleen was still extremely large, his red blood count was 6.0 million per cubic millimeter, and his leukocyte count 100,000 per cubic millimeter, mostly mature neutrophils. His neutrophil alkaline phosphatase score was in excess of 200.

This patient undoubtedly had widespread tuberculosis when first seen. He also had gross hepatosplenomegaly and a very fibrotic bone marrow. In view of his serious clinical state and hemorrhagic tendency, it was felt unwise to carry out either bone marrow or spleen biopsies. We do not, therefore, know for certain that he had myeloid metaplasia or myelofibrosis at that stage. Subsequently, all tuberculous manifestations cleared with specific therapy, but splenomegaly persisted and the blood strongly suggested a condition of MMM. Does the course of the disease in this patient mean that a tuberculous infection was initially responsible for the production of MMM, and that the latter remained irreversible, even when the original infection had cleared up? Or must we assume that both conditions originated independently, that one was cured but the other remained? There is no answer to this question at the moment. Somewhat similar cases have been described by Medd and Hayhoe,[182] and by Corr et al.[46] In none of these patients did the hematologic abnormalities regress following successful treatment of the coexisting tuberculosis. Possibly, therefore, tuberculosis might be capable of initiating myelofibrosis, and the MMM might become self-perpetuating at a later stage.

It remains to add that *carcinomatosis* of the bones is capable of inducing a syndrome simulating that of idiopathic MMM. This subject was reviewed by Lang.[154] As in other cases of myelosclerosis, there may be either patchy or diffuse fibrosis of the marrow and sclerosis of the bone,[198] and the spleen may be enormous, with gross myeloid metaplasia. The carcinoma may be so diffuse and anaplastic that there may be difficulty in diagnosing its primary site, or sometimes even in recognizing the small groups of cells as being epithelial in origin. The most likely primary sites are the prostate, breast, and stomach.[21,31] The association between myelosclerosis and systemic lupus erythematosus has been described by Lau and White, who suggested that the latter disease may occasionally cause marrow necrosis which is later followed by sclerosis.[155]

TUBERCULOSIS AND LEUKEMIA

The relationship between leukemia and tuberculosis is complex and several clinical groups may be distinguished.

Coexistence of leukemia and tuberculosis. Either disease may antedate the other. Perhaps the commonest event is the lighting up of an old tuberculous focus with a generalized spread after a patient has acquired leukemia or after the latter has been treated, particularly by means of steroids. Among 30 patients studied by Jaffe,[141] 3 had active tuberculosis. This author, as well as several others,[52,124,134,266] noted that there was an improvement in the leukemic blood picture when the tuberculosis supervened, and that at autopsy, only a few leukemic lesions might be seen. These findings are weakened by the fact that, in each reported instance, the patient had recently been treated by means of radiation or cytotoxic drugs, and it was therefore doubtful if the improvement was caused by the general tuberculosis or by the antileukemic therapy. We have seen a man with chronic lymphocytic leukemia who developed tuberculous meningitis. This was treated by means of streptomycin, *p*-aminosalicylic acid, and isonicotinic acid hydrazide. During this time, and without specific antileukemic therapy, the lymphocyte count fell from 450,000 to 45,000 per cubic millimeter. The marrow, however, showed no improvement. Experiences such as this make caution advisable before changes in the blood of leukemic patients are interpreted as suggesting improvement resulting from the advent of tuberculosis.

Miliary tuberculosis and leukemia. The literature contains a number of reports on patients with miliary tuberculosis and blood counts suggesting leukemia: for example, the presence of anemia, moderate to marked leukocytosis, and many immature granulocytes including blasts.[20,85,153,162] These were very virulent infections which rapidly led to death. At autopsy there were widespread miliary lesions, usually without much cellular reaction, and teeming with acid-fast bacilli. These cases were reported when there was no adequate therapy for miliary tuberculosis, and the question always arose whether leukemia was present as well as tuberculosis, or whether these were leukemoid reactions. No clear decisions could usually be made. Today, it is clear that these are double afflictions, with both tuberculosis and leukemia occurring in the same patient. If antituberculous treatment is given, the miliary lesions disappear, but the leukemia remains.[46,265] Miliary tuberculosis alone is very rarely accompanied by marked leukocytosis except in meningitic cases immediately before death.[22] There now seems little doubt that acute leukemoid reactions in tuberculosis, if they occur at all, must be of excessive rarity.

Relationship of Leukemia and PV to Other Hematologic Conditions

Since leukemia and polycythemia are moderately common diseases, it is to be expected that through the operation of the laws of chance, instances will occur in which they coexist with certain other blood diseases. Although the authors who have reported such cases have usually speculated about possible fundamental connections between the two conditions, it is difficult to accept any factor but coincidence as being operative. Instances of such combinations are the following: polycythemia vera and myelomatosis[33,123,157]; lymphocytic leukemia and pernicious anemia[180,227,262]; thalassemia and erythremic myelosis.[207]

The coexistence of lympho- and myeloproliferative disorders in the same patient may, conceivably, have more than chance significance.[82,123] Many otherwise typical cases of the Di Guglielmo syndrome, for instance, show abnormalities of the immunoglobulins,[92] and the same may occur in MMM. These could conceivably be the early stages of lymphoproliferative disease which, in most instances, would have little chance of developing fully. It should be remembered that not infrequently myelofibrosis occurs as part of a generalized lymphoproliferative syndrome.[79] Such patients do not, however, have splenic myeloid metaplasia, and these are therefore not lympho- and myeloproliferative disorders co-existing in the same patient.

There are a good many reports of chronic granulocytic leukemia or polycythemia vera in patients in whom pernicious anemia was also present. In earlier days, as has been previously mentioned, the distinction between leukemia and pernicious anemia was not always clearly appreciated, and it was only after the etiology and pathology of the latter condition had been clearly established in the late 1920s that it became possible to apply strict criteria to, at least, the diagnosis of pernicious anemia. Sinek and Kohn in 1930 reviewed the cases of so-called pernicious anemia occurring together with chronic granulocytic leukemia and accepted only one, to which they added another of their own.[246] A few more instances have since come to light in which either acute or chronic granulocytic leukemia followed in the wake of pernicious anemia.[252,257,263,284] These were well documented and there is thus no doubt that a number of patients with pernicious anemia have developed chronic granulocytic leukemia, and a prospective study has suggested that patients with pernicious anemia may have a slightly increased risk of developing chronic granulocytic leukemia.[26a] It does not seem possible, however, to suggest any causal connection between the two conditions; the only superficial resemblance is in the hyperplasia of the marrow which occurs in both, and which may have misled early observers, especially in Di Guglielmo's syndrome. In any case of doubt, a decision can be made by the determination of the serum vitamin B_{12} and the performance of the ^{60}Co B_{12} test (Schilling test). The B_{12} blood level in chronic granulocytic leukemia is, of course, greatly elevated.

Cases have occasionally been recorded of patients with untreated pernicious anemia who developed the features of polycythemia vera after treatment with liver extracts or vitamin B_{12}.[77,86,97,131] We have observed several such cases. Although a very high red cell count not infrequently follows successful treatment of pernicious anemia, the most searching investigations are required before these can be interpreted as polycythemia vera, and only very occasional cases will be found to fulfill the criteria of polycythemia.[41,169] It is likely that Galt et al.[97] have correctly assessed the course of events by suggesting that the stimulus for the medullary overproduction prevailing in all cases of PV is present in the combined cases from the beginning of the illness, but that it can only become operative when the nutritive factor (B_{12}) which is lacking in pernicious anemia, has been supplied, thus enabling the marrow to respond to both normal and abnormal stimuli toward cellular proliferation. Pernicious anemia following in the wake of polycythemia vera is of exceptional rarity and its presence is probably coincidental.[232] Yet another association of megaloblastosis with myeloproliferative disorders is seen occasionally in MMM. As in other conditions with continued overactivity of the hematopoietic cells, a relative folic acid deficiency may develop, and this can in itself lead to an intensification of the anemia.[135]

Of special interest is the association of leukemia with congenital familial marrow hypoplasia such as the Fanconi syndrome.[47,98] This is discussed in Chapter 5 which deals with leukemia etiology. In the same chapter, we mention also the recently discovered occurrence of acute leukemia in patients with myelomatosis treated by means of chemotherapy (see page 477). It seems highly probable that these associations did not occur on the basis of mere chance.

REFERENCES

1. Abbatt JD, Lea AJ: Leukaemia and pulmonary tuberculosis. Lancet 2:917, 1957.

2. Adams EB: Aplastic anaemia. Review of twenty-seven cases. Lancet 1:657, 1951.

3. Adamson JW, Finch CA: Erythropoietin and the regulation of erythropoiesis in Di Guglielmo's syndrome. Blood 36:590, 1970.

4. Amos JA, Goodbody RA: Lymph node and liver biopsy in the myeloproliferative disorders. Br J Cancer 13:173, 1959.

5. Anderson RE, Hoshino T, Yamamoto T: Myelofibrosis with myeloid metaplasia in survivors of the atomic bomb. Ann Intern Med 60:1, 1964.

6. André J: Hémopathies et Tuberculose. Toulouse, Imprim. Toulousaine, 1959.

7. Schwartz R, Dameshek W: Tuberculosis and myelosclerosis with myeloid metaplasia. Report of three cases. JAMA 178:1169, 1961.

8. Anstey L, Kemp NH, Stafford JL, Tanner RK: Leucocyte alkaline phosphatase activity in polycythaemia rubra vera. Br J Haematol 9:91, 1963.

9. Arthur K: Radioactive phosphorus in the treatment of polycythaemia. A review of ten years experience. Clin Radiol 18:287, 1967.

10. Athens JW, Haab OP, Boggs DR, Ashenbrucker H, Cartwright GE, Wintrobe MM: Leukokinetic studies. XI. Blood granulocyte kinetics in polycythemia vera, infection, and myelofibrosis. J Clin Invest 44:778, 1965.

11. DeBacker J, Lawrence JH: L'association de la leucémie à la polycythémie vraie. Presse Méd 59:461, 1951.

12. Baikie AG, Cunningham TA, McAlpine SG: Thrombocythaemia and thrombocytosis in the myeloproliferative syndromes. Scott Med J 3:26, 1958.

13. Baldini M, Fudenberg HH, Fukutake K, Dameshek W: The anemia of the Di Guglielmo syndrome. Blood 14:334, 1959.

14. Bank A, Larsen PR, Anderson HM: Di Guglielmo syndrome after polycythemia. N Eng J Med 275:489, 1966.

15. Barry WE, Day JJ: Refractory sideroblastic anemia. Clinical and hematologic study of ten cases. Ann Intern Med 61:1029, 1964.

16. Bartos H, Desforges JF, Moloney WC: Red cell enzymes in the anemia of myelofibrosis. Ann Intern Med 68:533, 1968.

17. Benedetti G: L'eritremia cronica (considerazioni su di un caso tipico di mielosi aneritremica cronica). Haematologica 19:229, 1938.

18. Bergsman KL, Van Slyck EJ: Acute myelofibrosis. An accelerated variant of agnogenic myeloid metaplasia. Ann Intern Med 74:232, 1971.

19. Better O, Brandstaetter S, Padeh B, Biann G: Myeloid metaplasia: Clinical, laboratory and cytogenetic observations. Israel Med J 23:162, 1964.

20. Betz H, Liégeois A: Pseudo-leucémie et tuberculose aiguë. Acta Clin Belg 8:219, 1953.

21. Bianchi C: Etiopatogenesi delle cosidette "mielosi croniche nonleucemiche" o "pseudoleucemiche." Medicina 4:253, 1954.

22. Biehl JP: Miliary tuberculosis. A review of sixty-eight adult patients admitted to a municipal general hospital. Am Rev Tuberc 77:605, 1958.

23. Bigelow FS: Serotonin activity in blood. Measurements in normal subjects, and in patients with thrombocythemia hemorrhagica, and other hemorrhagic states. J Lab Clin Med 43:759, 1954.

24. Bilski-Pasquier G, Blanc CM, Bousser J: Traitement de la polycythémie de Vaquez par le 1-4-bis (3 Bromopropionyl-Pipérazine). Etude de 36 cas. Presse Méd 76:1953, 1968.

25. Bjorkman SE: Chronic refractory anemia with sideroblastic bone marrow. Study of four cases. Blood 11:250, 1956.

26. Blackburn EK, Lajtha LG: Erythroleukemia. Blood 6:261, 1951.

26a. Blackburn EK, Callender ST, Dacie JV, Doll R, Girdwood RH, Mollin DL, Saracci R, Stafford JL, Thompson RB, Varadi S, Wetherley-Mein G: Possible association between pernicious anaemia and leukaemia: A prospective study of 1625 patients with a note on the very high incidence of stomach cancer. Int J Cancer 3:163, 1968.

27. Block M: Phylogenetic, embryologic and clinical aspects of myeloid metaplasia, in Proceedings of the sixth Congress of the

International Society of Hematology. New York, Grune & Stratton, 1958.

28. ———, Jacobson LO: Myeloid metaplasia. JAMA 143:1390, 1950.

29. Bomford RR, Rhoads CP: Refractory anaemia: Clinical and pathological aspects. Q J Med 10:175, 1941.

30. Von Boros J, Karenyi A: Über einen Fall von akuter Megakaryoblastenleukaemie, zugleich einige Bemerkungen zum Problem der akuten Leukaemie. Z Klin Med 118:697, 1931.

31. Bousser J, Piguet H, Dryll A: Les splénomégalies myéloïdes. Sem Hôp Paris 40:2711, 1964.

32. Braunsteiner H, Sailer S: Erythrocythaemia during the course of a chronic myeloid leukaemia. Wien Z Inn Med 42:10, 1961.

33. Brody JI, Beizer LH, Schwartz S: Multiple myeloma and the myeloproliferative syndromes. Am J Med 36:315, 1964.

34. Burston J, Pinniger JL: The reticulin content of bone marrow in haematological disorders. Br J Haematol 9:172, 1963.

35. Calabresi P: Myeloproliferative syndrome with leukemia preceding polycythemia vera: A case report. Blood 13:642, 1958.

36. ———, Meyer OO: Polycythemia vera, I and II. Ann Intern Med 50:1182, 1959.

37. Carmel R, Coltman CA, Jr, Yatteau RF, Costanzi JJ: Association of paroxysmal nocturnal hemoglobinuria with erythroleukemia. N Engl J Med 283:1329, 1970.

38. Carpenter G, Flory CM: Chronic non-leukemic myelosis. Report of a case with megakaryocytic myeloid splenomegaly, leukoerythroblastic anemia, generalized osteosclerosis and myelofibrosis. Arch Intern Med 67:489, 1941.

39. Castoldi E, Yam LT, Mitus WJ, Crosby WH: Chromosomal studies in erythroleukemia and chronic erythremic myelosis. Blood 31:202, 1968.

40. Cazal P: La tuberculose réticulotrope, forme maligne de la tuberculose ganglionnaire. Presse Méd 55:99, 1947.

41. Chalmers JNM, Richards W: Megaloblastic anaemia alternating with polycythaemia vera. Br Med J 1:540, 1961.

42. Chievitz E, Thiede T: Complications and causes of death in polycythaemia vera. Acta Med Scand 172:513, 1962.

43. Churg J, Wachstein M: Osteosclerosis, myelofibrosis and leukemia. Am J Med Sci 207:141, 1944.

44. Cohen SM: Chronic myelogenous leukemia with myelofibrosis. Arch Intern Med 119:620, 1967.

45. Copelli M: Di una emopatia sistemizzata rapresentata da una iperplasia eritroblastica (eritromatosi). Pathol Riv Quin Dicin 4:460, 1912.

46. Corr WP, Kyle RA, Bowie EJW: Hematologic changes in tuberculosis. Am J Med Sci 248:709, 1964.

47. Cowdell RH, Phizackerley PJR, Pyke DA: Constitutional anemia (Fanconi's syndrome) and leukemia in two brothers. Blood 10:788, 1955.

48. Crail HW, Alt HL, Nadler WH: Myelofibrosis associated with tuberculosis. A report of four cases. Blood 3:1426, 1948.

49. Croizat P, Revol L, Morel P, Mouriquand C1, Drapier Mme: A propos de 42 cas cliniques de réticulomyélose aleucémique essentielle. Sang 29:346, 1958.

50. Crossen PE, Fitzgerald PH, Menzies RC, Brehaut LA: Chromosomal abnormality, megaloblastosis, and arrested DNA synthesis in erythroleukaemia. J Med Genet 6:95, 1969.

51. Crowley LV, Munkittrick RC, Saunders RH Jr: Acute leukemia with erythroid hyperplasia of the bone marrow. Am J Clin Pathol 29:135, 1958.

52. Custer RP, Crocker WJ: The myeloleukaemoid blood picture associated with tuberculosis. Folia Haematol 46:359, 1932.

53. Dacie JV, Lewis SM: Paroxysmal nocturnal haemoglobinuria: variation in clinical severity and association with bone marrow hypoplasia. Br J Haematol 7:442, 1961.

54. ———, Smith MD, White JC, Mollin DL: Refractory normoblastic anaemia: A clinical and haematological study of seven cases. Br J Haematol 5, 56, 1959.

55. Dameshek W: Physiopathology and course of polycythemia vera as related to therapy. JAMA 142:790, 1950.

56. ———: Some speculations on the myeloproliferative syndromes. Blood 6:372, 1951.

57. ———: Splenectomy in myeloid metaplasia with myelosclerosis. Panels in therapy. Blood 10:550, 1955.

58. ———: The myeloproliferative disorders. Proc. Natl Cancer Cong, p. 383, 1957.

59. ———: The Di Guglielmo syndrome. Bull Tufts–N Engl Med Center 5:103, 1959.

60. ———: Sideroblastic anaemia. Is this a malignancy? Br J Haematol 11:52, 1965.

61. ———: Riddle: What do aplastic anemia, paroxysmal nocturnal hemoglobinuria (PNH) + "hypoplastic" leukemia have in common? Blood 30:251, 1967.

62. ———, Wasserman LR, Osgood EE, Gil-

bert HS, Laszlo J: The treatment of polycythemia vera. Blood 32:483, 1968.

63. _____, Baldini M: The Di Guglielmo syndrome (editorial). Blood 13:192, 1958.

64. Dammert K, Kaipanen WJ: Acute erythremic myelosis as a terminal stage of polycythemia vera. Acta Pathol Microbiol Scand 50:156, 1960.

65. De Grouchy J, De Nava C, Zittoun R, Bousser J: Analyses chromosomiques dans l'anémie sidéroblastique idiopathique acquise. Une étude de six cas. Nouv Rev Hématol 6:367, 1966.

65a. Demmler K, Burkhardt R, Prechtel K: Megakaryoblastische Myelose. Klin Wochenschr 48:1168, 1970.

66. Denef W, Desaive P, Leroux G, Betz H, Monnoyer E: De la splénectomie dans les myéloscléroses. Acta Chir Belg 58:141, 1959.

67. Didisheim P, Bunting D: Abnormal platelet function in myelofibrosis. Am J Clin Pathol 45:566, 1966.

68. DiGrado F, Teixeira Mendes F, Schroeder K: Ring chromosome in a case of Di Guglielmo syndrome. Lancet 2:1243, 1964.

69. Di Guglielmo G: Un caso di eritroleucemia. Folia Med 13:386, 1917.

70. _____: Eritroleucemia e piastrinemia. Folia Med 6:1, 36, 55, 81, 101, 1920.

71. _____: Eritremie acute. Boll Soc Med Chir Pavia 40:665, 1926.

72. _____: Le eritremie. Haematologica 9:301, 1928.

73. _____: Boll Soc Med Chir Catania 5:588, 1937. (Quoted by Moeschlin.)

74. _____: Acute erythremic disease, in Proceedings of the sixth Congress of the International Society of Hematology. New York, Grune & Stratton, 1958.

75. _____: Le Malattie Eritremiche ed Eritroleucemiche. Rome, Il Pensiero Scientifico, 1962.

76. Donhauser JL: The human spleen as an haematoplastic organ, as exemplified in a case of splenomegaly with sclerosis of the bone marrow. J Exp Med 10:559, 1908.

77. Douglas AS, Rifkind BM: Megaloblastic anaemia in association with polycythaemia vera. Scott Med J 9:469, 1964.

78. Dreyfus B, Rochant H, Sultan C: Anémies refractaires: Enzymopathies acquises Dés Cellules Souches Hématopoiétiques. Nouv Rev Hématol 9:65, 1969.

79. Duhamel G, Guerra L: Un syndrome hématologique difficile a définir: La myelofibrose lymphoïde. Étude nosologique de six observations. Presse Méd 74:585, 1966.

80. _____, Levy VG, Ouahnich M: Un cas de myélofibrose lymphoïde. Sem Hôp Paris 43:3450, 1967.

81. _____, Najman A, André R: L'Histologie de la moelle osseuse dans la maladie de Vaquez et le problème de la myelosclérose. Nouv Rev Hématol 10:209, 1970.

82. Durant JR, Tassoni EM: Coexistent Di Guglielmo's leukemia and Hodgkin's disease. A case report with cytogenetic studies. Am J Med Sci 254:824, 1967.

83. Dyment PG, Melnyk J, Brubaker CA: A cytogenetic study of acute erythroleukemia in children. Blood 32:997, 1968.

84. Eastman P, Wallerstein RO, Schrier SI: Polycythemia converted to Di Guglielmo's syndrome. JAMA 204:1141, 1968.

85. Eckel P: Ein Fall von Typhobacillose-Landouzy unter dem Bilde der aleukämischen Mikromyeloblastenleukämie. Med Klin 25:223, 1929.

86. Ellman P, Bowdler AJ: Pernicious anaemia and polycythaemia vera; a case report. Postgrad Med J 34:638, 1958.

87. Emberger JM, Wagner A, Izarn P: La terminaison en leucémie aiguë de l'ostéomyélofibrose avec métaplasie myéloïde hépato-splénique. Nouv Rev Hématol 9:375, 1969.

88. Emery JL: Erythraemic myelosis in a girl aged 13 years. J Pathol Bacteriol 63:395, 1951.

89. Emile Weil P, Clerc A: La splénomégalie chronique avec anémie et réaction myéloïde du sang. Sem méd 22:373, 1902.

90. Epstein E, Goedel A: Hämorrhagische Thrombocythämie bei vasculärer Schrumpfmilz. Virchows Arch Pathol Anat 293:233, 1934.

91. Fanger H, Cella LJ Jr Litchman H: Thrombocythemia: Report of three cases and review of the literature. N Engl J Med 250:456, 1954.

92. Finkel HE, Brauer MJ, Taub RN, Dameshek W: Immunologic aberrations in the Di Guglielmo syndrome. Blood 28:634, 1966.

93. Fitzpatrick WJ, Schwartz SO: Polycythemia secondary to tuberculosis of the spleen; report of case and review of the literature. Am Rev Tuber 60:660, 1949.

94. Forshaw J, Harwood L, Weatherall DJ: Folic-acid deficiency and megaloblastic erythropoiesis in myelofibrosis. Br Med J 1:671, 1964.

95. Gabuzda TG, Shute HE, Erslev AJ: Regulation of erythropoiesis in erythroleukemia. Arch Intern Med 123:60, 1969.

96. Gahrton G: The periodic acid-Schiff

reaction in neutrophil leukocytes in chronic myeloproliferative diseases. Scand J Haematol 3:106, 1966.

97. Galt J, Hunter RB, Hill JM: Pernicious anemia superseded by polycythemia vera. Report of a case. Am J Med Sci 223:61, 1952.

98. Garriga S, Crosby WH: The incidence of leukemia in families of patients with hypoplasia of the marrow. Blood 14:1008, 1959.

99. Gelin G: La Rate et ses Maladies. Paris, Masson, 1954.

100. _____, Wasserman LR: Remarques sur les mégakaryocytoses malignes. Sang 30:829, 1959.

101. Gilbert HS: A reappraisal of the "myeloproliferative disease" concept. Mt Sinai J Med NY 37:426, 1970.

102. Goswitz F, Lee GR, Cartwright GE, Wintrobe MM: Erythrocyte reduced glutathione, glucose-6-phosphate dehydrogenase, and 6-phosphogluconic dehydrogenase in patients with myelofibrosis. J Lab Clin Med 67:615, 1966.

103. Graham D: Erythraemia-polycythaemia rubra vera. Can Med Assoc J 42:281, 1940.

104. Gralnick HR, Harbor J, Vogel C: Myelofibrosis in chronic granulocytic leukemia. Blood 37:152, 1971.

105. Guild AA, Robson HN: Polycythaemia vera with tuberculosis and splenomegaly; report of a case. Edinburgh M. J., 57, 145, 1950.

106. Gunz FW: The myeloproliferative disorders. N Z Med J 57:428, 1958.

106a. _____: Hemorrhagic thrombocythemia: A critical review. Blood 15:706, 1960.

107. Halnan KE, Russell MH: Polycythaemia vera. Comparison of survival and causes of death in patients managed with and without radiotherapy. Lancet 2:760, 1965.

108. Haranghy L, Doczi P, Szekely K, Spielmann J: Klinik and pathologische Anatomie der Erythromyelosis Leukaemica. Budapest, Akademiai Kiado, 1959.

109. Hardisty RM, Speed EE, Till M: Granulocytic leukaemia in childhood. Br J Haematol 10:551, 1964.

110. Harman JB, Ledlie EM: Survival of polycythaemia vera patients treated with radioactive phosphorus. Br Med J 2:146, 1967.

111. Harrop GA Jr: Polycythemia. Medicine 7:291, 1928.

112. _____, Wintrobe MM: Polycythemia, in: Downey's Handbook of Hematology, vol. 4. Boston, Little, Brown, 1938, p 2365.

113. Harwerth HG: Akute und chronische Erythrämie (Erythromyelose) in Mohr und Staehelin R: Handbuch der Inneren Medizin, 5th ed., vol. 2, part 2. Berlin, Springer, p 735.

114. Hayhoe FGJ: Leukaemia. Research and Clinical Practice. London, Churchill, 1960.

115. _____, Quaglino D: Refractory sideroblastic anaemia and erythraemic myelosis: Possible relationship and cytochemical observations. Br J Haematol 6:381, 1960.

116. _____, _____, Doll R: The cytology and cytochemistry of acute leukaemias. London, H. M. Stationery Office, 1964.

117. Heath CW Jr: Cytogenetic observations in vitamin B_{12} and folate deficiency. Blood 27:800, 1966.

118. _____, Bennett JM, Whang-Peng J, Berry EW, Wiernik PH: Cytogenetic findings in erythroleukemia. Blood 33:453, 1969.

119. _____, Moloney WC: The Philadelphia chromosome in an unusual case of myeloproliferative disease. Blood 26:471, 1965.

120. _____, _____ Cytogenetic observations in a case of erythremic myelosis. Cancer 18:1495, 1965.

121. Hedinius: Erythrocytosis and leukocytosis. Svenska Lak Sällsk Forhandl 40:259, 1914. (Quoted by Pendergrass and Pancoast.)

122. Heilmeyer L: The sidero-achrestic anemias. Ger Med Mont 4:403, 1959.

123. Heinle EW Jr, Sarasti HO, Garcia D, Kenny JJ, Westerman MP: Polycythemia vera associated with lymphomatous diseases and myeloma. Arch Intern Med 118:351, 1966.

124. _____, Weir DR: Morphologic obliteration of chronic myeloid leukemia by active tuberculosis. Report of a case. N Engl J Med 207:450, 1944.

125. Heller EL, Lewisohn MG, Palin WE: Aleukemic myelosis. Chronic nonleukemic myelosis, agnogenic myeloid metaplasia, osteosclerosis, leuko-erythroblastic anemia and synonymous designations. Am J Pathol 23:327, 1947.

126. Heuck G: Zwei Fälle von Leukämie mit eigenthümlichem Blut-resp. Knochenmarksbefund. Virchows Arch Pathol Anat 78:475, 1879.

127. Hickling RA: Chronic non-leukemic myelosis. Q J Med 6:253, 1937.

128. _____: Leukaemia and related conditions and the blood-uric-acid. Lancet 1:175, 1958.

129. _____: The natural history of chronic non-leukaemic myelosis. Q J Med 37:267, 1968.

130. Hill JM, Duncan CN: Leukemoid reactions. Am J Med Sci 201:847, 1941.

131. Hinz CF Jr: Fatal polycythemia following

pernicious anemia treated with vitamin B_{12}. Ann Intern Med 47:544, 1957.

132. Hoffbrand AV, Chanarin I, Kremenchuzky S, Szur L, Waters AH, Mollin DL: Megaloblastic anaemia in myelosclerosis. Q J Med 37:493, 1968.

133. Holden D, Lichtman H: Paroxysmal nocturnal hemoglobinuria with acute leukemia. Blood 33:283, 1969.

134. Holler G: Beobachtung über die Wechselwirkung zwischen Leukämie und Tuberkulose im menschlichen Organismus. Klin Wochenschr 10:1663, 1931.

135. Hooey MA, Crookston JH, Squires AH: Myeloproliferative disease complicated by megaloblastic anemia and hyperuricemia. Can Med Assoc J 93:935, 1965.

136. Hutt MSR, Pinniger JL, Wetherley-Mein G: The myeloproliferative disorders with special reference to myelofibrosis. Blood 8:295, 1953.

137. _____, _____, _____: Myelofibrotic syndrome—its pathogenesis and treatment, in: Proceedings of the sixth Congress of the International Society of Hematology. New York, Grune & Stratton, 1958.

138. Israëls MCG: Treatment and prognosis of polycythaemia managed by non-radioactive methods. Proc R Soc Med 59:1100, 1966.

139. Jackson H Jr, Parker F Jr, Lemon HM: Agnogenic myeloid metaplasia of the spleen. A syndrome simulating other more definite hematologic disorders. N Engl J Med 222:985, 1940.

140. Jacobson LO, Smith TR: The evaluation of the present forms of treatment of polycythemia rubra vera. Am Pract., *3,* 267, 1949.

141. Jaffé RH: Tuberculosis and leukemia. Am Rev Tuberc 27:32, 1933.

142. Jenkins DE, Hartmann RC: Paroxysmal nocturnal hemoglobinuria terminating in acute myeloblastic leukemia. Blood 33:274, 1969.

143. Jensen KM: Chromosomal findings in two cases of erythro-leukaemia. Acta Med Scand 180:245, 1966.

144. Jordan HE, Scott JK: A case of osteosclerosis with extensive extramedullary hemopoiesis and a leukemic blood reaction. Arch Pathol 32:895, 1941.

145. Kaufmann RW, Schechter GP, McFarland W: Paroxysmal nocturnal hemoglobinuria terminating in acute granulocytic leukemia. Blood 33:287, 1969.

146. Kay HEM, Lawler SD, Millard RE: The chromosomes in polycythaemia vera. Br J Haematol 12:507, 1966.

147. Kiossoglou A, Mitus WJ, Dameshek W: Chromosomal aberrations in acute leukemia. Blood 26:610, 1965.

148. _____, _____, _____: Cytogenetic studies in the chronic myeloproliferative syndrome. Blood 28:24, 1966.

149. Koler RD, Seaman AJ, Osgood EE, Vanbellinghen P: Myeloproliferative diseases. Diagnostic value of the leukocyte alkaline phosphatase test. Am J Clin Pathol 30:295, 1958.

150. Korst DR, Clatanoff DV, Schilling RF: On myelofibrosis. Arch Intern Med 97:169, 1956.

151. Krauss A: Chronic myelocytic leukemia with features simulating myelofibrosis with myeloid metaplasia. Cancer 19:1321, 1966.

152. Kuzma JF: Moderator, Clinicopathological conference. Ann Intern Med 42:945, 1955.

153. Landon JF: Conditions simulating acute lymphatic leukemia (infections, mononucleosis, tuberculosis). Am J Med Sci 170:37, 1925.

154. Lang FJ: Myeloid metaplasia, in Downey H (ed): Handbook of Hematology, vol 3. New York, Hoeber, 1938, p 2105.

155. Lau KS, White JC: Myelosclerosis associated with systemic lupus erythematosus in patients in West Malaysia. J Clin Pathol 22:433, 1969.

156. Lawrence JH: Polycythemia. New York, Grune & Stratton, 1955.

157. _____, Rosenthal RL: Multiple myeloma associated with polycythemia. Report of four cases. Am J Med Sci 218:149, 1949.

158. _____, Winchell HS., Donald WG: Leukemia in polycythemia vera. Ann Intern Med 70:763, 1969.

159. Lazzaro G: Mielosi eritremica acuta. Haematologica 14:483, 1933.

160. Ledlie EM: The incidence of leukaemia in patients with polycythaemia vera treated by radioactive phosphorus. Clin Radiol 11:130, 1960.

161. _____: Treatment of polycythaemia by ^{32}P. Proc R Soc Med 59:1095, 1966.

162. Leibowitz S: Tuberculous sepsis with a myeloblastic blood picture. Arch Pathol 25:365, 1938.

163. Leitner St J: Über Thrombozythämien mit Megakaryozytenvermehrung im Knochenmark. Acta Med Scand 119:331, 1944.

164. Leonard BJ, Israëls MC, Wilkinson JF: Myelosclerosis. A clinico-pathological study. Q J Med 26:131, 1957.

165. Letman H: Possible paroxysmal nocturnal hemoglobinuria with pronounced pancyto-

penia, reticulocytopenia and without hemoglobinuria simulating aplastic anemia. Blood 7:842, 1952.

166. Leonard BJ, Israëls MC, Wilkinson JF: Alkaline phosphatase in the white cells in leukaemia and leukaemoid reactions. Lancet 1:289, 1958.

167. Lewis SM, Dacie JV: The aplastic anaemia-paroxysmal haemoglobinuria syndrome. Br J Haematol 13:236, 1967.

168. ———, Szur L: Malignant myelosclerosis. Br Med J 1:472, 1963.

169. Lind I: Pernicious anemia and polycythemia vera. Acta Med Scand 169:213, 1961.

170. Linman JW, Bethell FH: Agnogenic myeloid metaplasia. Am J Med 22:107, 1957.

171. Lopas H, Josephson AM: Myeloproliferative syndrome. Arch Intern Med 114:754, 1964.

172. Lowther P: Leukemia and tuberculosis. Ann Intern Med 51:52, 1959.

173. McClure PD, Ingram GIC, Stacey RS, Glass U H, Matchett MO: Platelet function tests in thrombocythaemia and thrombocytosis. Br J Haematol 12:478, 1966.

174. Mackenzie I, Stephenson AG: A case of erythremic myelosis (Di Guglielmo's anemia). Blood 7:927, 1952.

175. McMichael J, McNee JW: Leuco-erythroblastosis. Edinburgh Med J 43:303, 1936.

176. Magalini SI, Ahström L: Clinical and hematological aspects of acute erythromyelosis. J Pediatr 52:501, 1958.

177. Marsh GW, Lewis SM, Szur L: The use of ^{51}Cr-labelled heat-damaged red cells to study splenic function. II. Splenic atrophy in thrombocythaemia. Br J Haematol 12:167, 1966.

178. Martin H, Schubert JCF: Cytostatic treatment of polycythaemia vera with a methylbenzylhydrazine derivative. Ger Med Mon 11:315, 1966.

179. Martin WJ, Bayrd ED: Erythroleukemia, with special emphasis on the acute or incomplete variety. Report of five cases. Blood 9:321, 1954.

180. Mason J, Schwartz SO: The coexistence of pernicious anemia and chronic lymphatic leukemia. Ill Med J 96:197, 1949.

181. Masouredis SP, Lawrence JH: The problem of leukemia in polycythemia vera. Am J Med Sci 233:268, 1957.

182. Medd WE, Hayhoe FGJ: Tuberculous miliary necrosis with pancytopenia. Q J Med 24:351, 1955.

183. Meislin AG, Lee SL, Wasserman LR: Leukocyte alkaline phosphatase activity in hematopoietic disorders. Cancer 12:760, 1959.

184. Menzies RC, Crossen PE, Fitzgerald PH, Gunz FW: Cytogenetic and cytochemical studies on marrow cells in B_{12} and folate deficiency. Blood 28:581, 1966.

185. Merker H, Schneider G, Burmeister P, Wolf U: Chromosomentranslokation bei chronisch-myeloproliferativem Syndrom. Klin Wochenschr 46:593, 1968.

186. Merskey C: Chronic nonleukemic myelosis. Report of six cases. Arch Intern Med 84:277, 1949.

187. Mettier SR, Rusk GI: Fibrosis of the bone marrow (myelofibrosis) associated with leukemoid blood picture. Am J Pathol 13:377, 1937.

188. Millard RE, Lawler SD, Kay HEM, Cameron CB: Further observations on patients with a chromosomal abnormality associated with polycythaemia vera. Br J Haematol 14:363, 1968.

189. Minot GR, Buckman TE: Erythremia (polycythemia rubra vera). The development of anemia; the relation to leukemia; consideration of the basal metabolism, blood formation and destruction and fragility of the red cells. Am J Med Sci 166:469, 1923.

189a. Mitus WJ, Bergna LJ, Mednicoff IB: Atypical myeloblasts in acute leukemia. Clin Res Proc 5:149, 1957.

190. ———, Gherardi GJ, Mednicoff IB, Dameshek W: Cytochemistry of myelofibrosis with myeloid metaplasia in relation to spleen changes. Arch Pathol 67:188, 1959.

191. ———, Mednicoff IB, Dameshek W: Alkaline phosphatase of mature neutrophils in various "polycythemias". N Engl J Med 260:1131, 1959.

192. ———, Coleman N, Kiossoglou KA: Abnormal (marker) chromosomes in two patients with acute myelofibrosis. Arch Intern Med 123:192, 1969.

192a. Modan B: The polycythemic disorders. Springfield, Ill., Thomas, 1971.

193. ———, Lilienfeld AM: Leukaemogenic effect of ionising irradiation treatment in polycythaemia. Lancet 2:439, 1964.

194. ———, ———: Polycythemia vera and leukemia—the role of radiation treatment. Medicine 44:305, 1965.

195. Moeschlin S: Erythroblastosen, Erythroleukämien und Erythroblastämien. Folia Haematol 64:262, 1940.

196. Monto RW, TenPas A, Battle JD, Rohn

RJ, Louis J, Louis NB: A-8103 in polycythemia. JAMA 19:833, 1964.

197. Morrison M, Samwick AA, Rubinstein J, Swiller AI, Loewe L: Spleen aspiration in osteosclerosis and splenic hematopoiesis. Rationale of splenectomy. Acta Haematol 6:309, 1951.

198. Müller A, Werthemann H: Unter dem Bilde der sog. Leukanaemie verlaufende Karzinose des Knochenmarkes bei kleinem, versteicktem Mammakarzinom. Folia Haematol 46:429, 1932.

199. Muratore R, Follana R: Erythromyélose, leucose aiguë et panmyélose. Sem Hôp Paris 47:609, 1971.

200. Nachman RL, Horowitz HI, Silver RT: Platelet amino acid levels in essential thrombocytosis. Blood 27:715, 1971.

201. Nathan DG, Berlin NI: Studies of the production and life span of erythrocytes in myeloid metaplasia. Blood 14:668, 1959.

202. Necheles TF, Dameshek W: The Di Guglielmo syndrome: Studies in hemoglobin synthesis. Blood 29:550, 1967.

203. Neumann E: Ueber leukaemische Knochenaffektionen. Klin Wochenschr 17:281, 1880.

204. Niles NR, Koler RD, Johnson RL, Smith DD, Dunlap WJ: Myeloproliferative diseases. Clinical and pathologic study of 69 cases. Am J Clin Pathol 31:222, 1959.

205. Nygaard KK, Brown GE: Essential thrombophilia. Arch Intern Med 59:82, 1937.

206. Oechslin RJ: Osteomyelosklerose und Skelett. Acta Haematol 16:214, 1956.

207. Olshin I, Sawitsky A: Familial thalassemia and erythremic myelosis. Pediatrics 22:250, 1958.

208. Oni SB, Osunkoya BO, Luzzatto L: Paroxysmal nocturnal hemoglobinuria: Evidence for monoclonal origin of abnormal red cells. Blood 36:145, 1970.

209. Osgood EE: Polycythemia vera: Age relationships and survival. Blood 26:243, 1965.

210. _____: The case for ^{32}P in treatment of polycythemia vera, in Wasserman, LR, Dameshek W, Osgood EE, Gilbert HS, Laszlo J: The treatment of polycythemia vera: a panel discussion. Blood 32:483, 1968.

211. Osler W: A clinical lecture on erythraemia (polycythaemia with cyanosis, maladie de Vaquez). Lancet 1:143, 1908.

212. Ozer FL, Truax WE, Miesch DC, Levin WC: Primary hemorrhagic thrombocythemia. Am J Med 28:807, 1960.

213. Paradiso F, Reitano R: Studio clinico e anatomopatologico sulla malattia di Di Guglielmo. Haematologica 20:947, 1939.

214. Pawelski S, Maj St, Topolska P: Chromosomal abnormalities of spleen cells in osteomyelosclerosis. Acta Haematol 38:397, 1967.

215. Pegrum GD, Risdon RA: The haematological and histological findings in 18 patients with clinical findings resembling those of myelofibrosis. Br J Haematol 18:475, 1970.

216. Pendergrass EP, Pancoast HK: The close relationship of the erythrogenetic and leukogenetic functions of the bone marrow in disease. Report of a case of erythremia. The roentgen-ray treatment of erythremia. Am J Med Sci 163:797, 1922.

217. Pennelli N, Collarvo D, Cappuzzo GM: Contributo istopatologico alla conoscenze della megacariocitosi maligna. Tumori 54:291, 1968.

218. Perkins J, Israëls MCG, Wilkinson JF: Polycythaemia vera: Clinical studies on a series of 127 patients managed without radiation therapy. Q J Med 33:499, 1964.

219. Pitcock JA, Reinhard EH, Justus BW, Mendelsohn RS: A clinical and pathological study of seventy cases of myelofibrosis. Ann Intern Med 51:73, 1962.

220. Rastrick JM, Fitzgerald PH, Gunz FW: Direct evidence for presence of Ph¹ chromosome in erythroid cells. Br Med J 1:96, 1968.

221. Rathéry F: Splénomégalie du type myéloïde sans myélocythémie. Sem Méd 22:44, 1902.

222. Rawson R, Parker F Jr, Jackson H Jr: Industrial solvents as possible etiologic agents in myeloid metaplasia. Science 93:541, 1941.

223. Reed C: Polycythaemia rubra vera. Med J Austr 2:654, 1965.

224. Reid J: Haemorrhagic thrombocythaemia. Lancet 2:584, 1940.

225. Reinhard E: Critical evaluation of the harmful effects and dangers of radioactive isotope therapy, in Proceedings of the Sixth Congress of the International Society of Hematology. New York, Grune & Stratton, 1956.

226. Reisman LE, Trujillo JM: Chronic granulocytic leukemia of childhood. J Pediatr 62:710, 1963.

227. Rich ML, Schiff L: A case of pernicious anemia and chronic lymphatic leukemia. Ann Intern Med 10:252, 1936.

228. Roberts BE, Miles DW, Woods CG: Polycythaemia vera and myesclerosis. A

bone marrow study. Br J Haematol 16:75, 1969.

229. Robson HN: Myelosclerosis. A study of a condition also known as myelofibrosis, aleukemic myelosis, agnogenic myeloid metaplasia and other titles. Australas Ann Med 2:170, 1953.

230. Rosenberg HS, Taylor FM: The myeloproliferative syndrome in children. J Pediatr 52:407, 1958.

231. Rosenthal N, Erf LA: Clinical observations on osteopetrosis and myelofibrosis. Arch Intern Med 71:793, 1943.

232. Sage RE: Polycythemia rubra vera with pernicious anemia. Some observations on vitamin B_{12} metabolism. Blood 34:14, 1969.

233. Salmon C: Étude quantitative et thermo-dynamique de l'isohémagglutination. Methodes et résultats récents. Nouv Rev Hématol 5:191, 1965.

234. Sanerkin NG: Stromal changes in leukaemia and related bone marrow proliferation. J Clin Pathol 17:541, 1964.

235. Schmorl G: Leukämie mit Ausgang in Osteosklerose. Münch Med Wochenschr 51:537, 1904.

236. Schwartz SO, Critchlow J: Erythremic myelosis (Di Guglielmo's disease). Critical review with report of four cases and comments on erythroleukemia. Blood 7:765, 1952.

237. _____, Ehrlich L: The relationship of polycythemia vera to leukemia. A critical review. Acta Haematol 4:129, 1950.

238. Scott RB: Abstract. Q J Med 21:464, 1952.

239. Scott, RB, Ellison RR, Ley AB: A clinical study of twenty cases of erythroleukemia (Di Guglielmo's syndrome). Am J Med 37:162, 1964.

240. Sheets RF, Drevets CC, Hamilton HE: Erythroleukemia (Di Guglielmo's syndrome). Arch Intern Med 111:295, 1963.

241. Shively JA, Dorrance TO: Erythro-leukemia—a myeloproliferative disease. Report of a case. Am J Clin Pathol 25:282, 1955.

242. Silberman S, Krmpotic E: Refractory anaemia with leukaemic transformation and chromosome change—a case report. Acta Haematol 41:186, 1969.

243. Silverstein MN: Primary or hemorrhagic thrombocythemia. Arch Intern Med 122:18, 1968.

244. _____, Gomes MR, ReMine WH, Elveback LR: Agnogenic myeloid metaplasia. Arch Intern Med 120:546, 1967.

245. _____, Linman JW: Causes of death in agnogenic myeloid metaplasia. Mayo Clin Proc 44:36, 1969.

246. Sinek F, Kohn E: Gleichzeitiges Bestehen perniziöser Anämie und chronischer myeloischer Leukämie. Folia Haematol 42:180, 1930.

247. Smalley RV, Tassoni E, Durant JR: Chronic myeloid leukaemia and myelofibrosis. Lancet 2:393, 1966.

248. Spangberg J, Zettergren L: A case of thrombocythaemia essentialis. Acta Med Scand 135:176, 1949.

249. Steiner M, Baldini M, Dameshek W: Heme synthesis defect in "refractory" anemias with ineffective erythropoiesis. Blood 22:810, 1963.

250. Stenström NM: Three cases of mega-karyocytic leukaemia. Acta Med Scand (suppl) 246:234, 1950.

251. Stephens DJ, Bredeck JF: Aleukemic myelosis with osteosclerosis. Ann Intern Med 6:1087, 1933.

252. Sterne EH, Schiro H, Molle WE: Pernicious anemia complicated by myelogenous leukemia. Am J Med Sci 202:377, 1941.

253. Stroebel CF: Polycythemia vera. Am Pract Digest Treat 4:853, 1953.

254. _____, Treatment of polycythemia vera with radiophosphorus, in: Proceedings of the Sixth Congress of International Society of Hematology. New York, Grune & Stratton, 1957, p 359.

255. Szur L, Lewis SM: The haemorrhagical complications of polycythaemia vera and treatment with radioactive phosphorus. Br J Radiol 39:122, 1966.

256. _____, Smith MD: Red-cell production and destruction in myelosclerosis. Br J Haematol 7:147, 1961.

257. Tawast M, Siurala M: Transition of pernicious anaemia into chronic myeloid leukaemia. Acta Med Scand 154:211, 1956.

258. Thompson WP, Illyne CA: The clinical and hematologic picture resulting from bone marrow replacement. Med Clin North Am 24:841, 1940.

259. Thurm RH, Casey MJ, Emerson CP: Chronic Di Guglielmo syndrome. Am J Med Sci 253:399, 1967.

260. Tinney WS, Hall BE, Giffin HZ: Hematologic complications of polycythemia vera. Proc Staff Meet Mayo Clin 18:227, 1943.

261. Tjio JH, Carbone PP, Whang J, Frei E III: The Philadelphia chromosome and chronic myelogenous leukemia. J Natl Canc Inst 36:567, 1966.

262. Touw JF, Graafland CA: A case of aleukemic lymphatic leukemia with specific localizations and symptomatic pernicious anaemia. Acta Med Scand 102:124, 1939.

263. Townsend SR: Pernicious anaemia complicated by myelogenous leukaemia. Can Med Assoc J 61:417, 1949.

264. Tubiana M, Flamant R, Attie E, Hayat M: A study of hematological complications occurring in patients with polycythemia vera treated with ^{32}P (based on a series of 296 patients). Blood 32:536, 1968.

265. Twomey JJ, Leavell BS: Leukemoid reactions to tuberculosis. Arch Intern Med 116:21, 1965.

266. Ulrich H, Parks H: The relation between leukemia and tuberculosis. N Engl J Med 222:711, 1940.

267. Van den Bogaert P, Van Hove W: Polycythèmia vera suivie d'une erythroleucémie aiguë. Presse Méd 79:1685, 1971.

268. Van Slyck EJ, Weiss L, Dully M: Chromosomal evidence for the secondary role of fibroblastic proliferation in acute myeloproliferation. Blood 36:729, 1970.

269. Vaquez MH: Sur une forme spéciale de cyanose s'accompagnant d'hyperglobulie excessive et persistante. C R Soc Biol 44:384, 1892.

270. Vaughan JM: Leuco-erythroblastic anaemia. J Pathol Bacteriol 42:541, 1936.

271. _____, Harrison CV: Leuco-erythroblastic anaemia and myelosclerosis. J Pathol Bacteriol 48:339, 1939.

272. Verloop MC, Deenstra H, van der Hoeven LH: Erythroblastosis and leukemia. A case report illustrating variations in the clinical picture. Blood 7:454, 1952.

273. Visfeldt J: Primary polycythaemia. 2. Types of chromosome aberrations in 21 clones found in bone marrow samples from 50 patients. Acta Pathol Microbiol Scand (sect. A) 79:513, 1971.

274. Ward HP, Block MH: The natural history of agnogenic myeloid metaplasia (AMM) and a critical evaluation of its relationship with the myeloproliferative syndrome. Medicine 50:357, 1971.

275. Wasi P, Kruetrachue M, Na-Nakorn S: Aplastic anemia—paroxysmal nocturnal hemoglobinuria syndrome. Acute leukemia in the same patient. The first record of such occurrence. J Med Assoc Thai 53:656, 1970.

276. Wasserman LR: The treatment of polycythemia vera. Blood 32:483, 1968.

277. _____, Bassen F. Polycythemia. J Mt Sinai Hos 26:1, 1959.

278. Watkins PJ, Fairley GH, Scott RB: Treatment of polycythaemia vera. Br Med J 2:664, 1967.

279. Weber FP: Polycythaemia, erythrocytosis and erythraemia. Q J Med 2:85, 1908–1909.

280. Wetherley-Mein G, Jones NF, Pullan JM: Effects of splenectomy on red-cell production in myelofibrosis. Br Med J 1:84, 1961.

281. Whang-Peng J, Canellos GP, Carbone PP, Tjio JH: Clinical implications of cytogenetic variants in chronic myelocytic leukemia (CML). Blood 32:755, 1968.

282. Winkelstein A, Sparkes RS, Craddock CG: Trisomy of Group C in a myeloproliferative disorder. Report of case. Blood 27:722, 1966.

283. Woodrow JC, Cope S: Haemorrhagic thrombocythaemia treated with radioactive phosphorus. Br Med J 2:1069, 1955.

284. Woolley PB: Myelogenous leukaemia complicating pernicious anaemia. Lancet 1:85, 1944.

285. Wyatt JP, Sommers SC: Chronic marrow failure, myelosclerosis, and extramedullary hematopoiesis. Blood 5:329, 1950.

12

Clinical and Laboratory Features
of the Lymphoproliferative Disorders

The lymphoproliferative disorders, like the myeloproliferative ones considered in Chapter 11, form a group of diseases closely related to each other with frequent difficulties of demarcation between its members. Some of these may be acceptable as examples of true transitions from one form to another, but most are probably accounted for by the substantial diagnostic error arising from lack of specific diagnostic criteria. In such a situation both "lumping" and "splitting" are justifiable since, as Dameshek, in the second edition of this work, said in defense of lumping, "a narrow name becomes no longer an accurate one."

These disorders may be regarded as a complex where neoplasia, infection, and immunologic function and dysfunction meet, and appear to influence one another. Some, such as Hodgkin's disease, are initially localized in particular lymph nodes or organs, while others, such as acute and chronic lymphocytic leukemia are widey disseminated in blood and bone marrow: regarding dissemination, lymphosarcoma and Burkitt's lymphoma are usually intermediate between these extremes. Acute lymphocytic and chronic lymphocytic leukemias in their various aspects are discussed in other chapters, and a detailed consideration of the solid tumors is beyond the scope of this work. The purpose of this chapter is to discuss the lymphoproliferative disorders as a whole, with particular regard to their interrelationships, those manifestations of the more localized varieties which are seen in blood and bone marrow, and their relationship to other diseases not thought to be neoplastic in character.

At least two other aspects of normal lymphocyte activity should be remembered in any consideration of the lymphoproliferative diseases. These are the existence in normal animals, and probably in man, of several lymphocyte migration streams; and the heterogeneity of the lymphocyte population. The migration streams are probably both numerous and complex, the best evidence being for migration from bone marrow to lymphoid tissue, from lymphoid tissue to bone marrow, and from thymus to lymphoid tissue.[130] It is not known if all classes of lymphocytes participate equally in these and other migrations. If they do, it is surprising that any lymphoproliferative disease remains localized. Since some certainly remain localized for years, whether treated or not, it seems unlikely that all lymphocytes take part in these cellular migrations.

Differentiation of lymphocytes by morphologic criteria have long been known to be an oversimplification. Nevertheless, reliable criteria for differentiation have until recently been lacking. Even now it is obvious that lymphocytes cannot simply be divided into B and T categories believed to originate in bone marrow (or the bursa of Fabricius or its analog in man) and thymus, respectively. Despite the development of immunologic and other criteria for differentiating so-called B and T lymphocytes, it seems likely that neither is a functionally homogeneous group.

Reactive Lymphoid Proliferations

The lymphoid system, even more than the marrow, is scattered widely throughout the body. Very few tissues are devoid of small foci of lymphoid cells, and the bone marrow itself contains tiny lymphoid follicles. Large collections of lymphoid cells are found in the lymph nodes, spleen, thymus, Waldeyer's ring, and the Peyer's patches of the gastrointestinal tract. The functions of the lymphoid system and their underlying mechanisms have become much clearer in the past decade. As is more fully explained in Chapter 13, the basic function is protection, by both cell-mediated and humoral means, against a variety of microorganisms and other foreign materials, including those arising within the body but recognized as "nonself" in nature, a concept introduced by Burnet in 1958.[19] To such stimuli, the organism responds by means of a lymphocytosis, both local at the tissue level, and general, and the result is commonly rejection, whether of a virus infection, a heterologous transplant, or, possibly, a clone of autologous mutant cells. These are reactive and self-limiting phenomena like the neutrophil response to pyogenic infec-

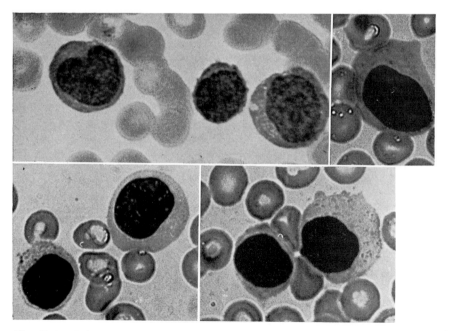

Fig. 12-1. Infectious mononucleosis. Various types of abnormal lymphocytes in peripheral blood.

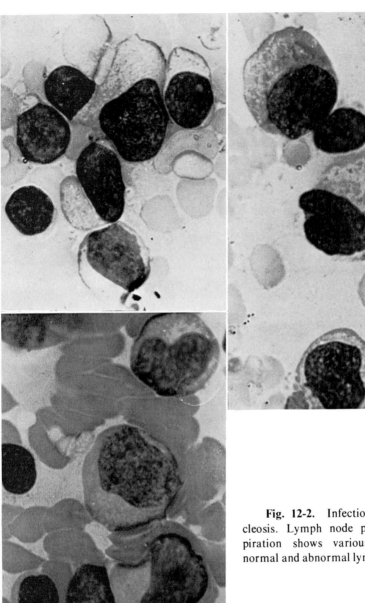

Fig. 12-2. Infectious mononucleosis. Lymph node puncture aspiration shows various types of normal and abnormal lymphocytes.

tions. The immunologic activities of the lymphocytes as displayed in such reactions include both the production of antibodies and a more direct cytotoxic activity.

INFECTIOUS MONONUCLEOSIS

This condition is of particular interest because it shows many of the hallmarks of a neoplastic lymphoproliferative reaction, including a blood picture strongly reminiscent of leukemia, and infiltration of many of the solid organs: yet the condition is self-limited and, as discussed in Chapter 5, almost certainly due to an identifiable cause, infection with the Epstein-Barr virus (EBV).[12,88] Figures 12-1, 12-2, and 12-3 show many of the features seen in the blood and lymph nodes of patients with infectious mononucleosis. Although in typical patients the blood picture is quite characteristic, there are notorious instances in which its differentiation from that of acute leukemia or lymphosarcoma cell leukemia (Chapter 10) is extremely difficult. Moreover, the findings in lymph node aspirates (Fig. 12-3) resemble those induced by the homograft rejection phenomenon (Fig. 12-4). In the tissues, invasion by normal lymphocytes often mimics that found in malignant neoplasms, particularly in the lymph nodes and spleen, where involvement of the capsule may lead to rupture of the organ.[63] Infectious mononucleosis has, on account of this proliferation of immature cells in blood and tissues, been likened to "a benign, self-limiting, virus-induced leukemia." It seems more likely that the cellular proliferation is part of an immune response to the EBV. Nevertheless, the possibility of more subtle relationships between infectious mononucleosis and neoplasms such as Burkitt's lymphoma and Hodgkin's disease may have some substance.

Infectious mononucleosis is invariably associated with nonspecific immunologic

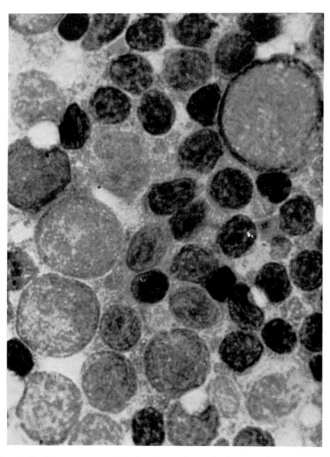

Fig. 12-3. Infectious mononucleosis. Lymph node impression smear made directly from freshly cut surface of biopsied node.

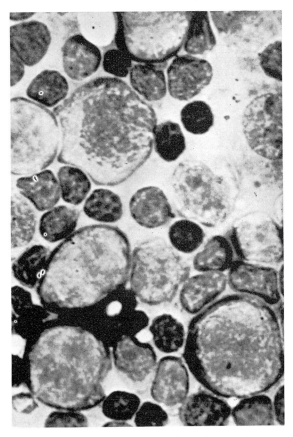

Fig. 12-4. Lymph node of a normal rabbit. A homologous skin transplant has been applied to one ear, resulting in enlargement of an adjacent lymph node. Impression smear shows a striking reaction with the presence of large numbers of very large primitive-appearing cells (immunoblasts). Although the picture resembles leukemia or lymphosarcoma closely, this is actually a reaction of immunization. There are many resemblances between immunologic and neoplastic proliferations of the complex of immunocytes.

reactions, including the heterophil sheep-cell antibody and, less frequently, positive serologic tests for syphilis, *Brucella melitensis,* and other organisms. Autoimmune reactions such as acquired hemolytic anemia or idiopathic thrombocytopenic purpura occur in a small proportion of patients, as they do in chronic lymphocytic leukemia and the lymphomas. Increases in serum IgM and IgG concentrations are almost invariable. Whether these are produced by the activity of proliferating abnormal lymphoid cells is not clear.

Infectious mononucleosis thus resembles both leukemia and lymphomas in some of its hematologic, histologic, and immunologic features. It differs from them in two fundamental respects: first, it has at least one known causative agent, the DNA virus of Epstein and Barr. Second, its course is always reversible. It may be surmised that progress in the leukemia-lymphoma field would be materially accelerated if the mechanism which causes reversal of the disease process in infectious mononucleosis could be more closely defined. Although there is little evidence that the EBV is implicated in human leukemogenesis,[97] its relationship to the disease process in infectious mononucleosis, as well as to the proliferation of lymphoid cell-lines in vitro (see Chapter 5), is of fundamental importance, for it may well be a model for the role of other oncogens in the production of neoplasia, including leukemia. The evidence for EBV having some causal role in Burkitt's lymphoma is almost as strong as the evidence that it is the primary if not the only cause of infectious mononucleosis.[5,41]

Other disorders caused by viruses or mycoplasmas, such as rubella or primary atypical pneumonia and even the protozoal infestation, toxoplasmosis, also result in various degrees of lymphoid proliferation and in the development of abnormal immunoglobulins. Thus, cold hemagglutinins, sometimes in high concentration, may arise in their course, and autoimmune hemolytic anemia follows occasionally.[30] These further examples of the association between self-limited lymphoid proliferations, with or without blood lymphocytosis, and the development of new and often abnormal immunoglobulins, are once again reactive phenomena, perhaps initially with a protective function. Similar reactions occur in the neoplastic lymphoproliferative conditions, but in response to no known stimulatory agent and without any obvious purpose. These will be considered in subsequent sections.

Neoplastic Proliferations: The Malignant Lymphomas

The neoplastic proliferations of the lymphoid cells may be classified as either localized tumors or generalized disorders, at least in regard to their early features, since all eventually become generalized. At present, they are not known to be caused by any specific identifiable agents; they have no known useful function, and their course is not self-limited or reversible, save by successful therapy. Table 12-1 shows a classification of this group of disorders based on the schema of Rappaport.[99]

Table 12-1
Classification of the Malignant Lymphoproliferative Disorders

Group	Predominant Component Cells	Initially Localized Tumors	Systemic Proliferative Disorders
1	Primitive reticular cell	Malignant lymphoma, undifferentiated. Burkitt's lymphoma	– – –
2	Histiocyte	Malignant lymphoma, histiocytic (reticulum cell sarcoma)	Malignant histiocytosis. Disseminated reticulum cell sarcoma
		Hodgkin's disease	– – –
3	Histiocyte and lymphocyte	Malignant lymphoma, mixed cell*	– – –
4	Poorly differentiated lymphocyte	Malignant lymphoma, poorly differentiated, lymphocytic*	Lymphosarcoma-cell leukemia
5	Differentiated lymphocyte	Malignant lymphoma, well-differentiated, lymphocytic*	Chronic lymphocytic leukemia; Waldenström's macroglobulinemia

*The localized tumors in Groups 3, 4, and 5 are also known as lymphosarcomas.

Most of what follows will relate to Groups 3–5 in Table 12-1. We omit consideration of Waldenström's macroglobulinemia which is discussed in Chapter 13. Burkitt's lymphoma is discussed here in its clinical and diagnostic aspects, and its etiologic significance is further considered in Chapter 5. Hodgkin's disease receives limited discussion in view of the rarity of its leukemic phase.

Like most classifications, that proposed in Table 12-1 is to some extent arbitrary. It is also incomplete. Thus, most of the solid lymphomas shown in the third column can be further subdivided into follicular (nodular) and diffuse varieties, with apparent differences in prognosis and response to therapy, as discussed below. The principal virtue of the classification is that it shows the possible relationships between the localized tumors and the corresponding generalized leukemic proliferations. It should be noted that the leukemias do not always *begin* as generalized disturbances—indeed, as mentioned in Chapter 5, it is not certain that they ever do. In the lymphoproliferative group, a transition from a localized to a generalized disease is commonly observed: the assessment of this transition is the reason for the accepted clinical practice of staging individual cases of lymphoproliferative disorders.[68] Early or late progression from the localized to the generalized stage is commonly associated with particular histologic features. Thus, it occurs early in poorly differentiated lymphocytic malignant lymphoma (ML) and relatively late in Hodgkin's disease (HD), especially cases of HD with particular histologic features.[70] Less commonly, the initially localized lymphoproliferative disorders may have a frankly leukemic phase. This is, of course, common in well-differentiated lymphocytic ML, as chronic lymphocytic leukemia; rare in HD,[12,68,112] and of inter-

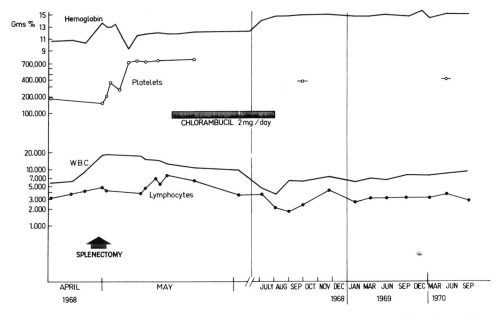

Fig. 12-5. A 64-year-old female presented with gross splenomegaly, lymphocytosis, mild anemia, and marrow showing lymphocytic infiltration. At splenectomy, the spleen showed well-differentiated lymphocytic lymphoma of the follicular variety. A short course of chlorambucil was given after operation. Patient remained in full unmaintained remission since then (64 months).

mediate frequency in poorly differentiated lymphocytic ML taking the form of lymphosarcoma cell leukemia.

The apparent initial site of any lymphoproliferative disease may be in a lymph node or, more rarely, in one of the solid organs. Localized lesions cannot be distinguished by histologic means from those associated with generalized or leukemic changes. One often finds cases of apparent chronic lymphocytic leukemia in which either certain groups of lymph nodes or the spleen are very prominently enlarged, giving the impression that the disease may have begun in these organs and thence spread to the marrow and blood. These are cases of originally unicentric lymphoma which have become disseminated. If the spleen is removed in such a patient, a regression of marrow invasion and of lymphocytosis in the blood may follow, especially when the lesions in the spleen show a follicular pattern: such patients have a particularly favorable prognosis.[1,33,62,113] Figure 12-5 shows the course of events in one such patient. The distinction is thus well worth making between patients having splenomegaly and a normal blood and marrow picture as primary manifestations, with leukemia appearing later on, and those showing generalized lymphadenopathy and a leukemic blood picture from diagnosis.

Observation of the features of primary lymphosarcoma of the spleen over a long period may present a "moving picture" of the development of the disease process (Fig. 12-6), rather than the more usual "snapshot" of a patient seen during a relatively short period. At first splenomegaly alone is observed, coupled frequently with various pancytopenias, the result of excessive margination of granulocytes or thrombocytes[124] and attributable to "hypersplenism." In carefully studied patients, neutropenia may be shown to be cyclical.[87] Later, the marrow becomes involved and shows abnormal cells similar to those of the spleen, to be followed eventually by a leukemic blood picture, often again with the same abnormal cells as are found in the spleen.

The leukemia that develops in lymphosarcoma in adults is usually chronic. Morphologically, it may be indistinguishable from chronic lymphocytic leukemia

MRS. A.H. – 8 YEAR COURSE OF PRIMARY LYMPHOSARCOMA OF SPLEEN
A "MOVING PICTURE"

JAN. 1947	APRIL 1947	MAY 1949	NOV. 1949	JULY 1950	JAN. 1954	MAY 1955	JULY 1955
		X-RAY R,		SPLENECTOMY			EXPIRED
CC: FATIGUE AND INDIGESTION. P.E: SLIGHT SPLENOMEGALY BLOOD: MODERATE PANCYTOPENIA		CC: FATIGUE AND INDIGESTION. P.E: INCREASING SPLENOMEGALY BLOOD: MARKED PANCYTOPENIA BONE MARROW: NORMAL HYPERPLASIA		CC: EXTREME FATIGUE, DRENCHING NIGHT SWEATS, PAIN IN LEFT FLANK. P.E: HUGE SPLEEN. BLOOD: MARKED PANCYTOPENIA SPLENIC PUNCTURE: LYMPHOSARCOMA. BONE MARROW: HYPERPLASIA OF ALL ELEMENTS SPLENECTOMY: 3½ YEAR REMISSION PATHOLOGY: LYMPHOSARCOMA (LYMPHOCYTIC LYMPHADENOSIS)		CC: FATIGUE, MODERATE NIGHT SWEATS. P.E: PALLOR. BLOOD: MARKED PANCYTOPENIA SEVERE HEMOLYTIC ANEMIA, MANY TRANSFUSIONS, TRANSFUSION REACTIONS BONE MARROW: CONSIDERABLE INFILTRATION	

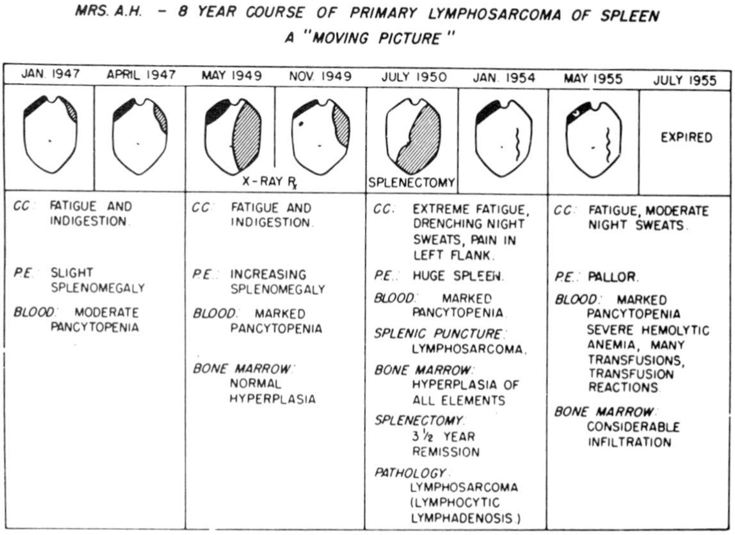

Fig. 12-6.   Late stage of lymphosarcoma.

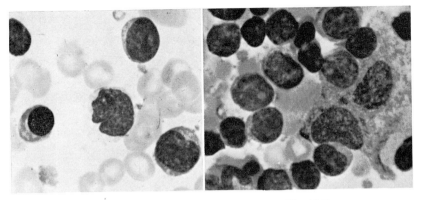

Fig. 12-7   Fig. 12-8

Fig. 12-7. Disseminated lymphosarcoma in a 71-year-old male. Original primary lesion occurred in the cervical lymph node; generalized lymphadenopathy occurred after 2 years without splenomegaly. The white blood cell count was 50,000 per cubic millimeter with 90 percent lymphocytes. In the blood film, the lymphocytes were mostly atypical lymphosarcoma cells with large, folded nuclei and with irregular outlines and prominent nucleoli (× 1400).

Fig. 12-8. Same patient as Fig. 12-7. Marrow film shows many lymphosarcoma cells, including a giant trinucleated reticular form (× 1400).

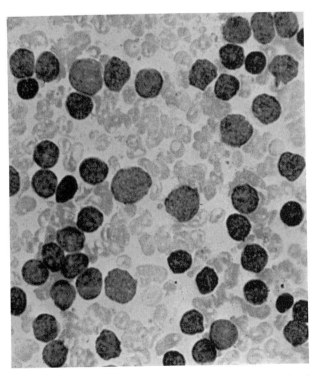

Fig. 12-9. Primary lymphosarcoma of spleen in a 40-year-old male with an essentially normal blood picture. Splenic aspiration showing many abnormal lymphocytes with relatively large, light-staining nuclei and prominent nucleoli (× 700).

439

(Chapter 10), but in a substantial number of patients the cells are less mature, with a less dense, nuclear chromatin pattern, frequent lobulation of the nucleus, and conspicuous nucleoli (Figs. 12-7 through 12-9). This form of lymphosarcoma cell leukemia[11,66] has been shown to have a considerably worse prognosis than chronic lymphocytic leukemia.[106,131] Correlation between hematologic and histologic findings shows that lymphosarcoma cell leukemias arise from poorly differentiated lymphocytic lymphomas, and that the outlook is worse when the involved lymph nodes show a diffuse rather than a nodular pattern.[105] When very poorly differentiated lymphosarcomas spread to the blood, the cells closely resemble lymphoblasts, but it is important to distinguish such cases from acute lymphocytic leukemia since they have a different response to therapy and often a better prognosis. In children, however, general lymphosarcomatosis not only looks hematologically like acute lymphocytic leukemia, but also has a similar clinical course[100] and responds poorly to the same treatment. Leukemic transformation of histiocytic lymphomas (reticulum cell sarcomas) is relatively rare and very resistant to therapy.[76]

BURKITT'S LYMPHOMA

Etiological factors in this disease, especially the role of the EBV, are discussed fully in Chapter 5. Apart from its remarkable features as a possible model of viral oncogenesis in man, it arouses particular interest because of its peculiarities of geographic distribution.[18] It is endemic in parts of tropical Africa and New Guinea and of low incidence in many other parts of the world. Where it is endemic, its incidence shows a remarkable proponderance in childhood and early adult life. In addition, its endemic occurrence is closely related to climatic factors of temperature and rainfall, suggesting a causal role for an insect vector, as well as the EBV.

The separate status of Burkitt's lymphoma as a malignant lymphoma is well established.[129] It is not to be regarded as a mere variant of one of the more widely distributed malignant lymphomas with some special features determined by geographic factors. Furthermore, despite the obvious parallel between Burkitt's lymphoma and acute lymphocytic leukemia in childhood, it is not merely a form of acute lymphocytic leukemia occurring under special conditions. Typical acute lymphocytic leukemia occurs in Uganda, where Burkitt's lymphoma has its highest incidence, at the same rate as in Western countries.[123]

The clinical peculiarities of Burkitt's lymphoma include the sites of its initial features in addition to its age incidence and geography. Involvement of face, jaws, abdominal organs, and other extralymphoid sites are common presenting manifestations, and generalized peripheral lymphadenopathy is rare. Untreated, the course is a rapid one with death commonly occurring within a few months. Central nervous system (CNS) involvement occurs in at least 60 percent of patients, and is even more common as a terminal feature. It usually takes the form of meningeal infiltration but direct infiltration of the brain through the base of the skull also occurs.[15]

A diagnosis of Burkitt's lymphoma depends on characteristic appearances in histologic sections and in imprints from tumor tissue,[18] with consonant clinical features. The hematologic findings are not diagnostic and, indeed, blood and bone marrow involvement may be lacking. In one series of 100 patients,[128] massive bone marrow infiltration by tumor cells was found in 8 patients and a lesser degree of marrow involvement in 8 more. Even in the patients with severe bone marrow involvement, spillover of tumor cells into the blood was slight, although most with marrow infiltration also had a leukoerythroblastic peripheral blood picture. In patients without obvious marrow involvement by tumor cells, bone marrow lymphocytes may be reduced in number. Anemia and thrombocytopenia are not features of Burkitt's lymphoma so that the disease is unlikely to be confused with acute lymphocytic leukemia. Especially in sporadic cases, occurring in arid or temperate climates, the diagnostic problem is commonly one of differentiating Burkitt's lymphoma from lymphocytic or histiocytic lymphoma.

One of the most remarkable aspects of this remarkable tumor is its degree of response to what would, for comparable neoplasms, be regarded as inadequate chemotherapy.[27]

HISTIOCYTIC MEDULLARY RETICULOSIS

This is a rare disease, first described by Scott and Robb-Smith in 1939.[109] Since then, fewer than a hundred cases have been described. It is of uncertain nosology, but has been likened to histiocytic malignant lymphoma on the one hand, and to histiocytic leukemia on the other. Patients commonly have generalized lymphadenopathy and hepatosplenomegaly. Bone marrow involvement is usual, but its focal occurrence may add to the diagnostic difficulty. A leukemic blood picture is uncommon but, when it does occur, it may be due to the occurrence of cells resembling either lymphoblasts[26] or histiocytes of demonstrable phagocytic capacity. More commonly, the diagnosis depends on demonstration of abnormal histiocytes in liver, the red pulp of spleen, and in the sinuses of lymph nodes.[110] Erythrophagocytosis and phagocytosis of cell debris, hemosiderin, and lipid also occur. As well as having enlargement of lymph nodes, liver, and spleen, patients are usually pyrexial, cachectic, anemic, and thrombocytopenic. Treatment is commonly unrewarding but corticosteroid therapy may result in transient symptomatic and even some objective improvement.

LYMPHOID MYELOFIBROSIS

An unusual syndrome, lymphoid myelofibrosis, has been described by Duhamel,[38,39] and is probably related to lymphosarcoma cell leukemia. In this condition, circulating atypical lymphocytes are associated with a pancytopenia, splenomegaly, and a marrow picture characterized by both lymphoid-histiocytic infiltration and striking myelofibrosis. Possibly this is a special form of malignant histiocytosis (see Table 12-1, Group 2). Related to it may be the condition termed *reticulolymphocytic leukemia* by Rubin and his colleagues.[101]

It will be seen that neither from the histologic nor the hematologic points of view is it possible to draw an absolutely clear distinction between the lymphocytic leukemias and the solid lymphomas as disease entities. In rare cases, there may be difficulty in distinguishing leukemia from lymphoma, especially if observed only at particular times in their natural history. Histologically, a biopsied lymph node, which is apparently the site of a primary proliferation of lymphocytes and thus diagnosed as well-differentiated malignant lymphoma, will be identical with another lymph node from a case of chronic lymphocytic leukemia in which there is generalized proliferation with an abnormal blood picture. Nor can the cells found in

Table 12-2
Age-Specific Incidence Rates Per 100,000 for Lymphoma (ICD 200) Standardized to European Populations (Males Only), for Registries with Populations-at-Risk over 1,000,000

CANADA, Alberta	4.7	NORWAY	4.5
CANADA, Quebec	4.1	POLAND, Cracow	2.5
DENMARK	4.0	POLAND, Katowice	1.6
ENGLAND, Birmingham	4.5	POLAND, Warsaw	1.8
ENGLAND, Liverpool	3.5	PUERTO RICO	4.8
ENGLAND, Oxford	4.7	ROMANIA	4.4
ENGLAND, Sheffield	4.0	SCOTLAND	3.8
ENGLAND, Southwest Region	5.0	SLOVENIA	2.7
FINLAND	2.6	SWEDEN	5.7
GERMANY (DDR)	4.0		
GERMANY (Hamburg)	3.7		
INDIA, Bombay	3.5		
ISRAEL	9.4	JAPAN, Miyagi	4.0
NEW ZEALAND (European)	6.9	JAPAN, Okayama	3.6

Based on data from Doll et al.[36]

the blood be distinguished in many instances. The same holds true for the less well-differentiated lymphomas, and the corresponding leukemias.

One curious discrepancy must, however, be mentioned in this context. Whereas, as stated in Chapter 4, chronic lymphocytic leukemia is much more rarely found in Japanese and other Oriental populations than in Western countries, this is not so in the case of the solid lymphomas. Table 12-2 shows the incidence of lympho- and reticulum cell sarcoma (International List of Causes of Death No. 200) in various localities, and it can be seen that in the two Japanese prefectures reporting incidence, these lymphomas were, unlike chronic lymphocytic leukemia, not less common than in North America or Europe. The reason for this discrepancy is not known at present. Nevertheless, it provides additional grounds for accepting as real the differences between leukemic and more localized forms of lymphoproliferative disease. Analogies, points of similarity, and even the occurrence of features of both forms in some patients should not at present be allowed to blind us to basic differences in occurrence, natural history, and response to treatment.

CYTOGENETIC FINDINGS

Several authors have used direct preparations or short-term cultures of lymph nodes to study the chromosomes in cases of lymphoma.[9,73,85,115] Lymph node preparations were employed because the simpler technique of culturing blood cells with phytohemagglutinin (PHA) was unsuccessful, the abnormal lymphoid cells in the lymphomas being unresponsive to PHA, like those in chronic lymphocytic leukemia (see Chapter 6). On the other hand, lymphocytes derived from nodes of many patients with lymphomas were found to divide spontaneously, thus yielding metaphases for analysis. Abnormalities have been discovered in a high proportion of lymphomas, their precise character being highly variable, as in acute leukemia (Chapter 6). In contrast, using the same methods, no chromosomal aberrations were found in chronic lymphocytic leukemia. The commonest abnormalities in the lymphomas were pseudo- and hyperdiploidy, with abnormal or extra chromosomes in all groups. Spiers and Baikie[116] found aberrations to be particularly common in the 17–18 group of chromosomes and raised the possibility that this group might play a special role in the genesis of some lymphomas.

When lymphocytes from the nodes of patients with Hodgkin's disease are examined in direct preparations or after 24-hour culture without PHA, two classes of cells are often found together: those with normal and abnormal chromosome complements.[85,115] It is probable that the former belong to normal lymphocytes while the abnormal figures characterize the tumor cells. Thus, lymph nodes in at least one of the lymphomas appear to contain a mixture of normal and neoplastic cells, and it seems likely that as the tumor grows, the abnormal cell populations increase at the expense of the normal one. It should be recalled (Chapter 10) that even in some cases of chronic lymphocytic leukemia there appears to be a similar double population, the normal cells increasing in proportion when remissions occur. As chronic lymphocytic leukemia has no visible chromosomal abnormalities, the demonstration of population shifts must be made by indirect means. By contrast, the interplay of normal and pathologic clones can be directly observed, at least in Hodgkin's disease.

As stated above, blood cultures in the presence of PHA do not usually show the abnormal clones which can be demonstrated in the lymph node cells of patients with lymphoma. The explanation for this difference is probably the fact that abnormal

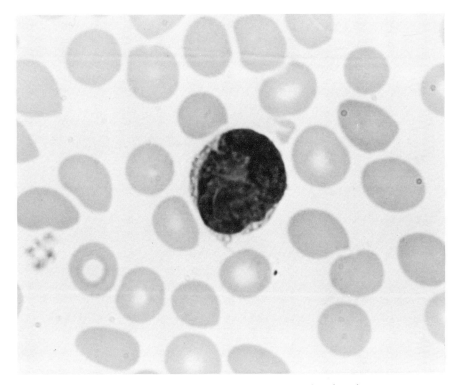

Fig. 12-10.   Sézary cell; note the large convoluted nucleus.

cells are only poorly stimulated, or not at all, by agents such as PHA.[25,92] This has been well demonstrated in chronic lymphocytic leukemia, but it appears also to hold true for the rare leukemic forms of the malignant lymphomas. Whether this is so because the abnormal lymphocytes are B cells which, unlike the thymus-derived T cells, are normally unresponsive to PHA, is not yet certain. Some evidence suggests that there may be T as well as B cell lymphomas (see Chapter 13).[95] Recently, demonstration of B cell characteristics in reticulum cell sarcoma has led to the suggestion that the tumor should be accepted as of lymphoid rather than reticulum cell origin.[118]

There is a rare exception to the rule that PHA has no stimulatory effect on aneuploid lymphoid cells. In the condition known as Sézary's syndrome,[47,111,121] a chronic skin disorder (erythroderma), in which large numbers of abnormal lymphoid cells are constantly circulating in the blood (Fig. 12-10), clones of grossly aneuploid cells have been found in PHA-stimulated blood cultures[29] (Fig. 12-11) and identified as belonging to the T cell class.[16,77] The cytogenetic characteristics of these abnormal cells suggest that they are neoplastic, and the fact that they are responsive to PHA is a clear indication that they belong to the lymphoid series. The Sézary syndrome is therefore definitely a lymphoid neoplasm or malignant lymphoma. Since its clinical manifestations are extremely chronic and the level of the abnormal lymphocytes in the blood tends to be almost unchanged over a period of years, it is likely that the neoplastic cells are responsive to normal control mechanisms. Sézary's syndrome may therefore be an example of that seemingly

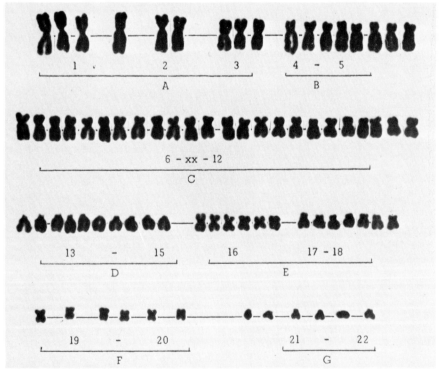

Fig. 12-11. Karyotype of Sézary cell from PHA-stimulated blood culture. There are 76 chromosomes including a marker chromosome.

unique phenomenon, a "conditioned" neoplasm of the lymphoid system. Whether a rather similar neoplasm, mycosis fungoides—which also has prominent skin manifestations—has similar cellular properties has not yet been determined.

Autoimmunity and the Lymphoproliferative Disorders

The basic facts of cell-mediated and humoral immunity are considered in Chapter 13. The relationship of autoimmune phenomena to the malignant lymphoproliferative disorders is of twofold interest. First, as is well recognized, autoimmune complications are common in this group of diseases. Second, the question has been raised whether the coincidence of autoimmune and lymphoproliferative conditions is indicative of a common causal mechanism in the emergence of a mutant lymphocyte clone, with both neoplastic characteristics and autoimmune activity.

AUTOIMMUNE COMPLICATIONS OF LYMPHOPROLIFERATIVE DISORDERS

By far the commonest of these is autoimmune hemolytic anemia. This complication (see Chapter 10) is frequent in chronic lymphocytic leukemia (affecting 10–15 percent of patients), but much less common in the solid lymphomas (affecting 1.7 percent).[30,67,96] Its precise causative mechanism is still unclear. It was originally believed that autoimmunization represented, at the cellular level, "an abnormal, self-replicating proliferation of cells producing an abnormal protein," that is, *abnormal* antibodies being made by *abnormal* cells in response to *normal* cells or tissue antigens.[32] As the concept of cell-mediated immunity became clearer, leukemic or lymphomatous cells were believed to react with autologous normal tissues in the fashion of a graft-versus-host reaction.[69] An obvious objection to this theory is that subsequent evidence has shown the neoplastic lymphocytes to be immunologically incompetent—as pointed out by Gorman,[53] and by Dameshek,[31]— and that, therefore, these cells are unlikely to have the capacity for reacting directly against red cell or other "self" antigens. It seems more probable that the autoimmune phenomena are due to lack of immune surveillance by the incompetent cells, and that this permits the growth of "forbidden" clones which are capable of reacting against the antigens. Whether impairment of immunosurveillance is an antecedent or a consequence of neoplastic change is still uncertain. Whatever the sequence may be, autoimmune hemolytic anemia occurs in consequence of the growth of a pathologic cell clone, and it is, moreover, a matter of rather common experience that the onset of sudden and violent hemolysis can be triggered by the application of chemo- or radiotherapy to previously untreated lymphoma patients: disastrous consequences have followed in several of our patients (Fig. 12-12). This complication may be an example of the breaking of immunologic tolerance, an event which has been demonstrated to occur in experimental animals as a result of various procedures including irradiation.[107]

Though much the commonest autoimmune complication, autoimmune hemolytic anemia is by no means the only one which can occur in the course of the lymphoproliferative conditions. Autoimmune ("idiopathic") thrombocytopenic purpura is not rare (Fig. 12-13),[40] although lacking a good diagnostic test like the antiglobulin test as applied to red cells. It is less well defined or readily diagnosed than

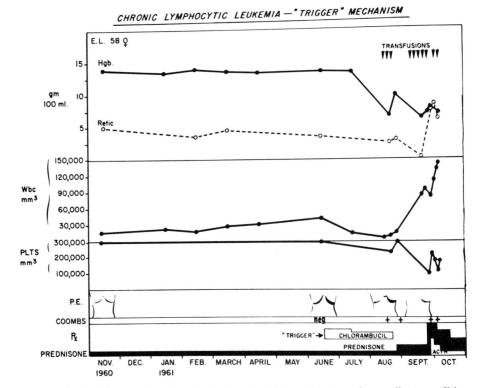

Fig. 12-12. Chronic lymphocytic leukemia. This patient was in excellent condition, taking 5-mg of prednisone daily as maintenance therapy. When the leukocyte count rose to 30,000 and the spleen became palpable, chlorambucil in an 8-mg dose was given daily. Severe autoimmune hemolytic anemia followed and, despite all therapeutic efforts, death occurred. We have seen similar occurrences following total-body x-ray therapy, the administration of nitrogen mustard, etc. These may represent trigger mechanisms touching off a graft-versus-host reaction, in which the immunologically competent graft may react against the host, as in runt disease (homologous disease).

autoimmune hemolytic anemia. It should be carefully distinguished from the thrombocytopenias of marrow depression, either due to the disease or its treatment. In the autoimmune cases, numerous megakaryocytes are present in the marrow, yet the platelets are greatly reduced. The platelet survival time is much shortened, indicating that the extrinsic factor attacking the platelets is of immunologic origin. It is also possible that the Mikulicz syndrome, which is occasionally seen in chronic lymphocytic leukemia, the polyarthritis of some patients, and the rapid wasting of others may have similar causal mechanisms. Objective evidence for the presence of autoimmune disease is the finding of lupus erythematosus cells, of antinuclear and antithyroid antibodies, all of which have been reported in some lymphomas.[64] These associations are discussed below.

AUTOIMMUNE DISEASE LEADING TO LYMPHOMA

The development of lymphomas in the wake of autoimmune disorders has been studied in at least two experimental systems. The New Zealand Black mouse (NZB) has a very high spontaneous rate of autoimmune hemolytic anemia, and its female F_1 hybrids, NZB/NZW, develop fatal renal disease, which has been likened to lupus

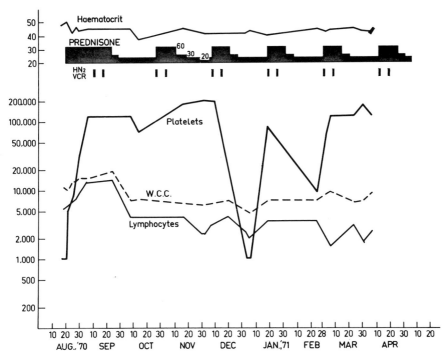

Fig. 12-13. A 65-year-old male presented with severe purpura and a platelet count of 1000 per cubic millimeter. He responded to steroid therapy and then was found to have disseminated lymphosarcoma, of the well-differentiated type. This was kept under control with combination chemotherapy.

nephritis, in a high proportion of cases. Treatment of both parental and hybrid animals with azathioprine leads to the development of lymphomas in as many as 75 percent of animals.[23] In the NZB/B1 strain Mellors found a 25 percent rate of spontaneous lymphoma, especially splenic tumors of reticulum cell origin, following on the occurrence of autoimmune hemolytic anemia,[81] and cell-free extracts from the tumors induced both autoimmune diseases and malignant lymphomas when injected into newborn Swiss mice.[83] When F_1 hybrids of the two strains C57B1 and DBA were injected with parenteral (C57B1) spleen cells, those animals escaping fatal runt disease developed autoimmune hemolytic anemia, which was followed by lymphomas in a high proportion of animals.[107] More extensive experiments in a similar system, employing BALB/c × AJ F_1 hybrids and injection with parental BALB/c spleen cells confirmed these findings; the incidence of lymphomas rising in step with the number of spleen cells injected.[3] It should be noted that the lymphomas in the hybrid mice proved to be of host origin.

The mechanism of lymphoma induction in experimental mice has not been clearly established. Mellors[82] thought it was due to an RNA virus which could be transmitted along with injected cells, but no virus was found in Schwartz's experiments.[3] Activation of a latent virus, when grafted parental cells injure host cells, appears a possibility; such an activated virus might continue to proliferate and provide the antigen responsible for the massive hyperplasia of lymphoid cells,[3] but at present this explanation is speculative.

In man, numerous instances have been recorded in which autoimmune conditions preceded, followed, or coexisted with lymphoproliferative disorders. The term *autoimmune disorder* has been variously and loosely employed. Miller, who reviewed the subject, included conditions ranging from diffuse connective tissue disease such as rheumatoid arthritis and disseminated lupus erythematosus to the nephrotic syndrome and ataxia telangiectasia.[86] He described 17 cases of associations between such conditions and lymphomas, and, in addition, he found a statistically increased incidence (1.86 versus 0.58 percent) of diffuse connective tissue disease in 264 patients with malignant lymphoma compared to 1863 with other solid tumors. On the other hand, statistics gathered from the literature lent no support to the hypothesis that patients with autoimmune diseases had an increased risk of developing leukemia or lymphoma.[89] A great deal obviously depends on the precise interpretation of what constitutes autoimmune disease. Certainly, many factors found in commonly accepted autoimmune conditions also occur in patients with lymphomas; among them are disturbances in immunoglobulin concentration[122] and the presence of antinuclear and complement-fixing factors.[120] Lupus erythematosus cells are not infrequently found. Sjögren's syndrome is associated with lymphomas in nearly 10 percent of patients.[74, 120] However, the exact classification of such cases is often difficult, and the dividing line between self-perpetuating autoimmune disorders and lymphoproliferative disorders may, at times, be very thin or even nonexistent. Thus, is "cold hemagglutinin" hemolytic anemia with a high concentration of macroglobulin, generalized lymphadenopathy, and lymphoid hyperplasia of lymph nodes, spleen, and liver a neoplastic process or is it a benign immunologic one? The same difficulty arises in a case described by Sage and Forbes,[103] in which a woman with a 12-year history of Sjögren's syndrome developed autoimmune hemolytic anemia, multiple antibodies, and an abnormal serum gamma globulin. The marrow was densely infiltrated with lymphocytes, which were also present in the blood, and these features persisted after treatment with azathioprine which controlled the hemolytic process.

Enough has now been published to make it highly probable that the association of autoimmune and lymphoproliferative disorders is not an accidental one. A consideration of the case material in this group is not, however, sufficient by itself to clarify the precise nature of the relationship, especially whether impaired immunosurveillance precedes or follows the appearance of the forbidden clone, whether of neoplastic or autoimmune activity. To obtain a clearer picture, it is necessary to consider the subject of tumor immunity and its significance for the lymphoproliferative disorders.

Tumor Antigens, Immunity, and Lymphoproliferation

The lymphoproliferative disorders form a key group where immunologic disturbances and neoplastic proliferations meet, a field in which much recent work has been done and knowledge is expanding rapidly. Working hypotheses have been put forward on the relationship between the lymphoid system, immunity, and malignancy.[21, 52] These hypotheses are based on a multiplicity of experimental and clinical findings, among them the existence of tumor antigens, well recognized in animals and becoming so in man; the increased incidence of neoplasms, especially lymphomas, in individuals with congenital defects of the immune system, and in those whose natural immunity has been deliberately suppressed; the frequent coexistence in the same patient of solid tumors and lymphomas or chronic lymphocytic leukemia; and the immunologic disturbances which occur so frequently in the course of the lymphomas. As a consequence of this work, the relatively old theory of tumor immunity[61] has recently been revived and the first attempts have been made to exploit immunologic mechanisms in a search for better therapy of solid tumors, lymphomas, and leukemia[7] (see also Chapter 18).

TUMOR ANTIGENS

The term *antigen* means, in this context, a component which distinguishes tumor cells from normal autologous cells and which can be demonstrated by means of immunologic techniques.[14] Tumor antigens (TAs) have been clearly shown in experimental animals to be of two kinds: first, those specified by oncogenic viruses, either RNA or DNA, which have already been alluded to in Chapter 5. The second class of tumor antigens in specified by the genome of the neoplastic cell itself, although in some tumor cells there is good evidence that virus DNA is actually incorporated into the genome of the neoplastic cell.[41] It is the second class of TAs with which this section is concerned. These new antigens arise either as a result of a cellular mutation, of viral or other origin, or because genes are expressed in the tumor which, though present in normal cells, are ordinarily repressed, at least in the adult. Most of the evidence on tumor antigens has been obtained in inbred animal strains by means of serologic methods; that is, antisera have been developed which react with tumor cells but not with normal cells from the same animal.

In man, the existence of tumor antigens has long been suspected, if only because of the occasional occurrence of "spontaneous" regressions in the growth of certain tumors[43]—especially melanomas and neuroblastomas—and of long-term remissions, after minimal treatment, in many patients with Burkitt's tumor[17] and a few with leukemia.[44] More positive, though not yet conclusive, evidence has come from laboratory studies by means of three basic techniques. The first and most powerful of these depends on the demonstration that cells from some tumors, when cultivated in vitro, can be inhibited or actually destroyed by the addition of autologous lymphocytes. This technique was first used with animal tumors but has been successfully adapted to human work and used to show tumor-cell-lymphocyte interactions in many solid tumors, including neuroblastoma, melanoma, and several carcinomas and sarcomas.[58-60] The existence of a cell-mediated immunologic reaction against autologous tumors has been accepted as evidence showing the presence of antigenic differences between these tumors and the lymphocytes from the same patients.

A second means of demonstrating the existence of tumor antigens has been by the mixed lymphocyte reaction.[6] This has been used especially in acute leukemia in which several authors have shown that, in a proportion of cases, lymphocytes are stimulated to DNA synthesis and transformation when cultured together with autologous leukemic blasts[4,48,56,71,75,98,125]; a reaction which could be reinforced if patients were "immunized" with their own leukemic cells after having attained remission.[57] It must, however, be admitted that the occurrence of lymphocyte transformation is not proof of an immunologic reaction since it can also be caused by nonspecific stimuli such as PHA, and, in at least one study, it was shown that no transformation occurred when lymphocytes from a number of normal children were cultured with the blasts of their leukemic identical twins.[102]

Serologic rather than cytologic techniques have been used as a third method of searching for tumor antigens in man; again, chiefly in leukemias and lymphomas, but also in melanomas. Antibodies against their own leukemic cells have been reported in the serum of some patients with acute leukemia[37] and melanoma.[45] Antisera produced in rabbits,[10,78,90] mice,[8] and primates[84] have been found to react specifically with leukemic cells or sections of tissue from patients with Hodgkin's disease, but not with normal cells. However, lymphocytes from normal newborns were able to react with antileukemia sera,[10] a finding which raises doubts as to the specificity of some of the reported antibodies.

Like many other problems, the demonstration and investigation of tumor antigens has been a relatively simple matter in animals because inbred strains were available whose immunologic and other characteristics were well recognized. In man, the situation is more complicated, and although much of the evidence is plausible, the very existence of tumor antigens, let alone their significance, cannot yet be taken to be firmly established. Many otherwise unexplained remissions in malignancies could be accounted for by the action of immunologic defenses against neoplastic cells, and some laboratory work is consistent with this interpretation. Positive proof has yet to be adduced, but critical trials of immunotherapy need not be delayed until proof is available (see also Chapter 18).

INCIDENCE OF NEOPLASIA IN IMMUNE DEFICIENCY

It has been clearly recognized in recent years, largely as the result of the work of Good and his colleagues,[51,91,94] that neoplasms—many of them lymphomas or leukemias—occur with unusual frequency in the rare, inherited, primary immunodeficiency diseases of man, including the Bruton type of x-linked agammaglobulinemia, ataxia telangiectasia, the Wiskott-Aldrich and Chediak-Higashi syndromes. In all, except the first of these conditions, both cellular and humoral immune mechanisms are impaired, and it is this combined deficiency which seems of particular relevance to the induction of neoplasia.[35] Similarly, patients with acquired rather than inherited immune deficiencies, and autoimmune disturbances, have a special propensity to develop neoplasms, particularly lymphomas and leukemias.[49,79,120] An increased susceptibility to the development of lymphomas and other neoplasms has become evident in patients exposed to prolonged immunosuppressive treatment especially after renal transplantations,[34,93,104,117,126,127] either because neoplastic or potentially neoplastic cells were transplanted along with the grafted kidney and given the opportunity of free dissemination, or because the patient's own mutant clones found no effective immunologic defenses. Acute leukemia develops with undue frequency in patients with myelomatosis, Hodgkin's disease, and chronic lymphocytic leukemia who have long survival after immunosuppressive treatment,[2,24,55,72,119] and carcinomas of skin, and perhaps those in other sites, are unduly common in patients with chronic lymphocytic leukemia (see Chapter 10) or lymphosarcoma; conditions which, as indicated in Chapter 13, are nearly always associated with immune deficiency.[13,28,54,65]

IMMUNOLOGIC DISTURBANCES IN LYMPHOMAS

These have already been discussed in detail (see page 445).

SUMMARY: LYMPHOMAS AND IMMUNITY

All the work quoted in the preceding paragraphs is consistent with the concept of immunosurveillance first suggested by Burnet,[19,20] and espoused by others—especially by Good and his group.[52] According to this concept, an essential function of the normal lymphoid system is the defense against foreign (nonself) cells; that is, all those carrying surface antigens which differ from the antigens of the host. Malignant cells carrying specific tumor antigens would be in accord with this concept, so that mutant clones capable of becoming malignant would normally be detected and eliminated by the lymphocytes, especially, but not exclusively, the thymus-dependent T cells.

Lack of immunologic competence could lead to malfunctioning of this surveillance mechanism, permitting the growth of neoplastic clones which would normally be destroyed: hence, the increased incidence of neoplasms in the many immunodeficient states mentioned above. The particular prevalence of lymphoproliferative neoplasms in immunodeficient states is of great interest in this connection since these tumors, above all, are accompanied by depression or perversion of components of the immune mechanisms. Indeed, as stated by Dameshek,[31] the frequent occurrence of autoimmune phenomena in the lymphomas might well be another result of a deficient immunosurveillance, with clones of mutant cells having "antiself" characteristics being allowed to proliferate, instead of being eliminated as in normal individuals. Whether, as postulated by Fudenberg,[50] the deficiency is specifically the result of a lack of T cell function or of a more wide-ranging disturbance, is not yet clear. What has become apparent, however, is the very close connection between immunologic disturbances and the lymphoproliferative disorders. It may well be that a more precise analysis of this connection will clarify the pathogenesis of other forms of malignant neoplasms.

REFERENCES

1. Ahmann DL, Kiely JM, Harrison EG Jr, Payne WS: Malignant lymphoma of the spleen. A review of 49 cases in which the diagnosis was made at splenectomy. Cancer 19:461, 1966.

2. Andersen E, Videbaek A: Stem cell leukaemia in myelomatosis. Scand J Haematol 7:201, 1970.

3. Armstrong MYK, Gleichmann E, Gleichmann H, Beldotti L, Andre-Schwartz J, Schwartz RS: Chronic allogeneic disease. II. Development of lymphomas. J Exp Med 132:417, 1970.

4. Bach ML, Bach FH, Joo P: Leukemia-associated antigens in the mixed leukocyte culture test. Science 166:1520, 1969.

5. Baikie AG, Kinlen LJ, Pike MC: Detection and assessment of case clustering in Bur-

kitt's lymphoma and Hodgkin's disease. Recent Results Cancer Res 39:201, 1972.

6. Bain B, Loewenstein L: Genetic studies on the mixed leukocyte reaction. Science 145:1315, 1964.

7. Baker MA, Taub RN: Immunotherapy of human leukemia. Mt Sinai J Med NY 39:548, 1972.

8. ———, ———: Production of antiserum in mice to human leukaemia-associated antigens. Nature 241:93, 1973.

9. Baker MC, Atkin NB: Chromosomes in short-term cultures of lymphoid tissue from patients with reticulosis. Br Med J 1:770, 1965.

10. Bentwich Z, Weiss DW, Sulitzeanu D, Kedar E, Izak G, Cohen I, Eyal O: Antigenic changes on the surface of lymphocytes

from patients with chronic lymphocytic leukemia. Cancer Res 32:1375, 1972.

11. Bethell FH: Lymphogenous (lymphatic) leukemia; diagnostic, prognostic and therapeutic considerations based on analysis of its morphologic and clinical variations. JAMA 118:95, 1942.

12. Bouroncle BA: Sternberg-Reed cells in the peripheral blood of patients with Hodgkin's disease. Blood 27:544, 1966.

13. Bousser J, Zittoun R, Simony D, Schaison G: L'association d'une leucose lymphöide à un cancer épithélial. Sem Hôp Paris 40:2721, 1964.

14. Boyse EA, Old LJ, Stockert E, Shigeno N: Genetic origin of tumor antigens. Cancer Res 28:1280, 1968.

15. Broder LE, Carter SK: Meningeal Leukemia. New York, Plenum, 1972.

16. Brouet JC, Flandrin G, Seligmann M: Thymus-derived nature of the proliferating cells in Sézary's syndrome. N Engl J Med 289:341, 1973.

17. Burkitt DP, Kyalwazi SK: Spontaneous remission of African lymphoma. Br J Cancer 21:14, 1967.

18. _____, Wright DH: Burkitt's Lymphoma. Edinburgh, Livingstone, 1970.

19. Burnet FM: The Clonal Selection Theory of Acquired Immunity. Nashville, Vanderbilt University Press, 1959.

20. _____: Immunological factors in the process of carcinogenesis. Br Med Bull 20:154, 1964.

21. _____: Auto-Immunity and Auto-Immune Disease. Lancaster, Medical and Technical, 1972.

22. _____: Implications of cancer immunity. Austr NZ J Med 3:71, 1973.

23. Casey TP: The development of lymphomas in mice with autoimmune disorders treated with azathioprine. Blood 31:396, 1968.

24. Catovsky D, Galton DAG: Myelomonocytic leukaemia supervening on chronic lymphocytic leukaemia. Lancet 1:478, 1971.

25. _____, Holt PJL, Galton DAG: Lymphocyte transformation in immunoproliferative disorders. Br J Cancer 26:154, 1972.

26. Clark BS, Dawson PJ: Histiocytic medullary reticulosis presenting with a leukemic blood picture. Am J Med 47:314, 1969.

27. Clifford P, Singh S, Stjernswärd J, Klein G: Long-term survival of patients with Burkitt's lymphoma: An assessment of treatment and other factors which may relate to survival. Cancer Res 27:2578, 1967.

28. Coeur P, Morel P, Gentilhomme O: L'association "cancer-leucémie lymphoïde chronique." Sem Hôp Paris 46:791, 1970.

29. Crossen PE, Mellor JEL, Finley AG, Ravich RBM, Vincent PC, Gunz FW: The Sézary syndrome. Am J Med 50:24, 1971.

30. Dacie JV: The Haemolytic Anaemias, Part II. Auto-Immune Haemolytic Anaemias, 2nd ed. London, Churchill, 1962, pp 534–541.

31. Dameshek W: Chronic lymphocytic leukemia—an accumulative disease of immunologically incompetent lymphocytes. Blood 29:566, 1967.

32. _____, Schwartz RS: Leukemia and autoimmunization—some possible relationships. Blood 14:1151, 1959.

33. Davey FR, Skarin AT, Moloney WC: Pathology of splenic lymphoma. Am J Clin Pathol 59:95, 1973.

34. Doak PB, Montgomerie JZ, North JDK, Smith F: Reticulum cell sarcoma after renal homotransplantation and azathioprine and prednisone therapy. Br Med J 4:746, 1968.

35. Doll R, Kinlen L: Immunosurveillance and cancer: epidemiological evidence. Br Med J 4:420, 1970.

36. _____, Muir, C, Waterhouse J (eds.): Cancer Incidence in Five Continents, vol. II, U.I.C.C. Berlin, Springer, 1970.

37. Doré JF, Motta R, Marholev L, Hrsak I, Colas de la Noue H, Seman G, Vassal F de, Mathé G: New antigens in human leukaemic cells, and antibody in the serum of leukaemic patients. Lancet 2:1396, 1967.

38. Duhamel G: Lymphoid myelofibrosis. About 10 further observations. Acta Haematol 45:89, 1971.

39. _____, Guerra L: Un syndrome hématologique difficile à définir: la myélofibrose lymphoïde. Etude nosologique de six observations. Presse Méd 74:585, 1966.

40. Ebbe S, Wittels B, Dameshek W: Autoimmune thrombocytopenic purpura ("ITP" type) with chronic lymphocytic leukemia. Blood 19:23, 1962.

41. Epstein MA, Achong BG: Various forms of Epstein-Barr virus infection in man: established facts and a general concept. Lancet 2:836, 1973.

42. Evans AS, Niederman JC, McCollum RW: Sero-epidemiologic studies of infectious mononucleosis with EB virus. N Engl J Med 279:1121, 1968.

43. Everson TC, Cole WH: Spontaneous Regression of Cancer. Philadelphia, Saunders, 1966.

44. Fairley GH: Immunity to malignant disease in man. Br Med J 2:467, 1969.

45. _____: Evidence for antigenicity in human tumours with reference to both melanoma and acute leukaemia. Br Med J 4:483, 1970.

46. Fitzgerald PH, Adams A: Chromosome studies in chronic leukemia and lymphosarcoma. J Natl Cancer Inst 34:827, 1965.

47. Fleischmajer R, Eisenberg S: Sézary's reticulosis. Its relationship with neoplasias of the lymphoreticular system. Arch Dermatol 89:9, 1964.

48. Fridman WH, Kourilsky FM: Stimulation of lymphocytes by autologous leukaemic cells in acute leukaemia. Nature 224:277, 1969.

49. Fudenberg HH: Immunologic deficiency, autoimmune disease and lymphoma: Observations, implications and speculations. Arthritis Rheum 9:464, 1966.

50. _____: Genetically determined immune deficiency as the predisposing cause of "autoimmunity" and lymphoid neoplasia. Am J Med 51:295, 1971.

51. Gatti RA, Good RA: Occurrence of malignancy in immuno-deficiency diseases. Cancer 28:89, 1971.

52. Good RA, Finstad J: Essential relationship between the lymphoid system, immunity, and malignancy. Nat Cancer Inst Monogr 31:41, 1969.

53. Gorman JG, Chandler JG: Is there an immunologically incompetent lymphocyte? Blood 23:117, 1964.

54. Gunz FW, Angus HB: Leukemia and cancer in the same patient. Cancer 18:145, 1965.

55. _____, Levi JA, Lind DE, Vincent PC: Development of acute leukaemia in a patient with lymphosarcoma. NZ Med J 78:71, 1973.

56. Gutterman JU, Mavligit G, McCredie KB, Bodey GP Sr, Freireich EJ, Hersh EM: Antigen solubilized from human leukemia: lymphocyte stimulation. Science 177:1114, 1972.

57. _____, _____, _____, Freireich, EJ, Hersh EM: Auto-immunization with acute leukemia cells: Demonstration of increased lymphocyte responsiveness. Int J Cancer 11:521, 1973.

58. Hellström I, Hellström KE, Sjögren HO, Warner GA: Demonstration of cell-mediated immunity to human neoplasms of various histological types. Int J Cancer 7:1, 1971.

59. _____, _____: Some aspects of the immune defense against cancer. I. In vitro studies on animal tumors. Cancer 28:1266, 1971.

60. _____, _____: Some aspects of the immune defense against cancer. II. In vitro studies on human tumors. Cancer 28:1269, 1971.

61. Héricourt J, Richet C: De la sérothérapie dans le traitement du cancer. CR Hebd Séanc Acad Sci Paris 121:567, 1895.

62. Hickling RA: "Giant follicle lymphoma of the spleen." A condition closely related to lymphatic leukaemia but apparently curable by splenectomy. Br Med J 2:787, 1964.

63. Hoagland RJ: Infectious Mononucleosis. New York, Grune & Stratton, 1967, pp 14–15.

64. Howqua J, Mackay IR: L. E. cells in lymphoma. Blood 22:191, 1963.

65. Hyman GA: Increased incidence of neoplasia in association with chronic lymphocytic leukaemia. Scand J Haematol 6:99, 1969.

66. Isaacs R: Lymphosarcoma cell leukemia. Ann Intern Med 11:657, 1937.

67. Jones SE: Autoimmune disorders and malignant lymphoma. Cancer 31:1092, 1973.

68. Kaplan HS: Hodgkin's Disease. Cambridge, Mass., Harvard University Press, 1972.

69. _____, Smithers DW: Auto-immunity in man and homologous disease in mice in relation to the malignant lymphomas. Lancet 2:1, 1959.

70. Keller AR, Kaplan HS, Lukes RJ, Rappaport H: Correlation of histopathology with other prognostic indicators in Hodgkin's disease. Cancer 22:487, 1968.

71. Knight SC, Moore GE, Clarkson BD: Stimulation of autochthonous lymphocytes by cells from normal and leukaemic cell lines. Nature 229:185, 1971.

72. Kyle RA, Pierre RV, Bayrd ED: Multiple myeloma and acute myelomonocytic leukemia. Report of four cases possibly related to melphalan. N Engl J Med 283:1121, 1970.

73. Lawler SD, Pentycross CR, Reeves BR: Chromosomes and transformation of lymphocytes in lymphoproliferative disorders. Br Med J 4:213, 1968.

74. Lehner-Netsch G, Barry A, Delage J-M: Leucémies et maladies auto-immunes: Syndrome de Sjögren et anémie hémolytique associés à la leucémie lymphoïde chronique. Can Med Assoc J 100:1151, 1969.

75. Leventhal BG, Halterman RH, Rosenberg EB, Herberman RB: Immune reactivity of

leukemia patients to autologous blast cells. Cancer Res 32:1820, 1972.

76. Lowenbraun S, Sutherland JC, Feldman MJ, Serpick AA: Transformation of reticulum cell sarcoma to acute leukemia. Cancer 27:579, 1971.

77. Lutzner MA, Emerit I, Durepaire R, Flandrin G, Grupper Ch, Pruniéras M: Cytogenetic, cytophotometric and ultrastructural study of large cerebriform cells of the Sézary syndrome and description of a small-cell variant. J Natl Cancer Inst 50:1145, 1973.

78. Mann DL, Rogentine GN, Halterman R, Leventhal B: Detection of an antigen associated with acute leukemia. Science 174:1136, 1971.

79. Medical Research Council, Working Party: Hypogammaglobulinaemia in the United Kingdom. Lancet 1:163, 1969.

80. Medical Research Council: Infectious mononucleosis and its relationship to EB virus antibody. Br Med J 4:643, 1971.

81. Mellors RC: Autoimmune disease in NZB/B1 mice. II. Autoimmunity and malignant lymphoma. Blood 27:435, 1966.

82. ———, Huang CY: Immunopathology of NZB/B1 mice. V. Virus like (filterable) agent separable from lymphoma cells and identifiable by electron microscopy. J Exp Med 124:1031, 1966.

83. ———, ———: Immunopathology of NZB/B1 mice. VI. Virus separable from spleen and pathogenic for Swiss mice. J Exp Med 126:53, 1967.

84. Metzgar RS, Mohanakumar T, Miller DS: Antigens specific for human lymphocytic and myeloid leukemia cells: Detection by nonhuman primate antiserums. Science 178:986, 1972.

85. Millard RE: Chromosome abnormalities in the malignant lymphomas. Eur J Cancer 4:97, 1968.

86. Miller DG: The association of immune disease and malignant lymphoma. Ann Intern Med 66:507, 1967.

87. Morley AA, Carew JP, Baikie AG: Familial cyclical neutropenia. Br J Haematol 13:719, 1967.

88. Niederman JC, McCollum RW, Henle G, Henle W: Infectious mononucleosis: Clinical manifestations in relation to the E.B. virus. JAMA 203:205, 1968.

89. Oleinick A: Analytical review: Leukemia or lymphoma occurring subsequent to autoimmune disease. Blood 29:144, 1967.

90. Order SE, Porter M, Hellman S: Hodgkin's disease: Evidence for a tumor-associated antigen. N Engl J Med 285:471, 1971.

91. Page AR, Hansen AE, Good RA: Occurrence of leukemia and lymphoma in patients with agammaglobulinemia. Blood 21:197, 1963.

92. Papac RJ: Lymphocyte transformation in malignant lymphomas. Cancer 26:279, 1970.

93. Penn I, Starzl TE: Malignant lymphomas in transplantation patients: A review of the world experience. Z Klin Pharmakol Theor Toxikol 3:149, 1970.

94. Peterson RDA, Kelly WD, Good RA: Ataxia-telangiectasia: Its association with a defective thymus, immunological deficiency disease and malignancy. Lancet 1:1189, 1964.

95. Piessens WF, Schur PH, Moloney WC, Churchill WH: Lymphocyte surface immunoglobulins. Distribution and frequency in lymphoproliferative diseases. N Engl J Med 288:176, 1973.

96. Pirofsky B: Autoimmunization and the Autoimmune Hemolytic Anemias. Baltimore, Md., Williams & Wilkins, 1969.

97. Pope JH, Walters MK, Scott W, Gunz FW: Antibody to Epstein-Barr virus in man in Australia and New Guinea. Internat J Cancer 12:689, 1973.

98. Powles RL, Balchin LA, Fairley GH, Alexander P: Recognition of leukaemia cells as foreign before and after autoimmunization. Br Med J 1:486, 1971.

99. Rappaport H: Tumors of the hematopoietic system. In: Atlas of Tumor Pathology, Sect. III, Fasc. 8. Washington, D.C.: Armed Forces Institute of Pathology, 1966.

100. Rosenberg SA, Diamond HD, Dargeon HW, Craver LF: Lymphosarcoma in childhood. N Engl J Med 259:505, 1958.

101. Rubin AD, Douglas SD, Chessin LN, Glade PR, Dameshek W: Chronic reticulolymphocytic leukemia. Am J Med 47:149, 1969.

102. Rudolph RH, Mickelson E, Thomas ED: Mixed leukocyte reactivity and leukemia: Study of identical siblings. J Clin Invest 49:2217, 1970.

103. Sage RE, Forbes IJ: A case of multiple autoimmune disease, lymphoid proliferation and hypogammaglobulinemia. Blood 31:536, 1968.

104. Schneck SA, Penn I: De novo brain tumours in renal-transplant recipients. Lancet 1:983, 1971.

105. Schnitzer B, Loesel LS, Reed RE: Lympho-

sarcoma cell leukemia. A clinicopathologic study. Cancer 26:1082, 1970.

106. Schrek R, Donnelly WJ: Cytology in lymphosarcoma cell leukemia. Am J Clin Pathol 55:646, 1971.

107. Schwartz RS, Beldotti L: Reactivation of homologous disease by x-irradiation. Science 140:171, 1963.

108. _____, _____: Malignant lymphomas following allogeneic disease: Transition from an immunological to a neoplastic disorder. Science 149:1511, 1965.

109. Scott RB, Robb-Smith AHT: Histiocytic medullary reticulosis. Lancet 2:194, 1939.

110. Serck-Hanssen A, Purchit GP: Histiocytic medullary reticulosis. Report of 14 cases from Uganda. Br J Cancer 22:506, 1968.

111. Sézary A, Bouvrain Y: Erythrodermie avec présence de cellules monstrueuses dans le derme et le sang circulant. Bull Soc Fr Dermatol Syphiligr 45: 254, 1938.

112. Sinks LF, Clein GP: The cytogenetics and cell metabolism of circulating Reed-Sternberg cells. Br J Haematol 12:447, 1966.

113. Skarin AT, Davey FR, Moloney WC: Lymphosarcoma of the spleen. Results of diagnostic splenectomy in 11 patients. Arch Intern Med 127:259, 1971.

114. Smith RT: Tumor-specific immune mechanisms. N Engl J Med 278:1207, 1268, 1326, 1968.

115. Spiers ASD, Baikie AG: Cytogenetic studies in the malignant lymphomas and related neoplasms. Results in twenty-seven cases. Cancer 22:193, 1968.

116. _____, _____: A special role of the group 17,18 chromosomes in reticuloendothelial neoplasia. Br J Cancer 24:77, 1970.

117. Starzl TE, Penn I, Putnam CW, Groth CG, Halgrimson CG: Iatrogenic alterations of immunologic surveillance in man and their influence on malignancy. Transplant Rev 7:112, 1971.

118. Stein H, Lennert K, Parwaresch MR: Malignant lymphomas of B-cell type. Lancet 2:855, 1972.

119. Steinberg MH, Geary CG, Crosby WH: Acute granulocytic leukemia complicating Hodgkin's disease. Arch Intern Med 125:496, 1970.

120. Talal N, Bunim JJ: The development of malignant lymphoma in the course of Sjögren's syndrome. Am J Med 36:529, 1964.

121. Taswell HF, Winkelmann RK: Sézary-syndrome—a malignant reticulemic erythroderma. JAMA 177:465, 1961.

122. Ultmann JE, Fish W, Osserman E, Gellhorn A: The clinical implications of hypogammaglobulinemia in patients with chronic lymphocytic leukemia and lymphocytic lymphosarcoma. Ann Intern Med 51:501, 1959.

123. Vanier TM, Pike MC: Leukaemia incidence in tropical Africa. Lancet 1:512, 1967.

124. Vincent PC: Haematological complications of lymphoma. Pathology 6:87, 1974.

125. Viza D, Davies DAL, Todd R, Bernard-Degani O, Bernard CL, Harris R: Mise en évidence, isolement et purification partielle d'antigènes leucémiques chez l'homme. Press Méd 78:2259, 1970.

126. Walder BK, Robertson MR, Jeremy D: Skin cancer and immunosuppression. Lancet 2:1282, 1971.

127. Wilson RE, Hager EB, Hampers CL, Carson JM, Merrill JP, Murray JE: Immunologic rejection of human cancer transplanted with a renal allograft. N Engl J Med 278:479, 1968.

128. Wright DH, Pike PA: Bone marrow involvement in Burkitt's tumour. Br J Haematol 15:409, 1968.

129. _____, Roberts M: The geographical distribution of Burkitt's tumour compared with the geographical distribution of other types of malignant lymphoma in Uganda. Br J Cancer 20:469, 1966.

130. Yoffey JM, Courtice FC: Lymphatics, Lymph and the Lymphomyeloid Complex. London, Academic Press, 1970, pp 41–46.

131. Zacharski LR, Linman JW: Chronic lymphocytic leukemia versus chronic lymphosarcoma cell leukemia. Analysis of 496 cases. Am J Med 47:75, 1969.

Ronald Penny, Michael A. McGrath,
and John B. Ziegler

13

Clinical and Laboratory Features
of the Paraproteinemias

Immune function is expressed either as humoral (antibody) or cell-mediated responses. There is now a large body of evidence[45] indicating that these two functions are performed by two separate cell classes which have distinct physiology and function. Thymus-derived cells are responsible for cell-mediated responses and are conveniently referred to as T cells.[224] Bone marrow-derived cells or B cells[224] are the precursors of the plasma cell-line and are responsible for antibody production.

A population of cells which arises in the embryonic yolk sac migrates to the fetal liver and later to the bone marrow, where it provides a source of immunological stem cells. These cells, which have the morphology of small lymphocytes, gain immunological competence by passing through the primary lymphoid organs, namely, the thymus[161] and bursa of Fabricius,[39] or its functional equivalent. Cells so programmed by the thymic microenvironment, T cells, are responsible for cell-mediated immunity (delayed hypersensitivity; immunity to intracellular organisms such as mycobacteria, fungi, protozoa, viruses; homograft rejection; tumor immunity; graft-versus-host reactivity). In contrast, bone marrow-derived lymphoid cells which enter the bursa of Fabricius or its yet-unidentified mammalian equivalent are programmed therein to respond to antigen with production of antibody.

T cells constitute about 60–70 percent of the small lymphocytes in peripheral blood, and constantly recirculate through lymphoid organs returning to venous blood via the thoracic duct lymph; these long-lived cells constitute the lymphoid population of the paracortical regions of lymph nodes and periarteriolar areas of spleen. B cells can be readily identified by immunoglobulin determinants which they carry at their surface; these cells constitute some 30–40 percent of circulating lymphocytes, are relatively short lived, and are mostly nonrecirculating. They are found in the lymphoid follicles and medullary cords of lymph nodes, in the red pulp and peripheral white pulp of spleen, and in lymphoid follicles adjacent to mucosae of respiratory and gastrointestinal tracts. Although circulating antibody is produced by lymphocytes and plasma cells, which are the progeny of B cells, it appears that in the humoral response to most antigens, T cells may be involved indirectly by facilitating or augmenting the response of the B cell to antigen.[45] Work on the relevance of T and B cells in man is however in progress.

IMMUNOGLOBULINS

Immunoglobulins are a heterogeneous population of proteins synthesized by lymphoid cells to function either as membrane receptors or as circulating antibodies. Antigen is generally, but not invariably, responsible for initiation of synthesis of circulating antibody. The immunogenicity of antigen in this respect and the genetic capacity of the host to respond to antigen have been reviewed.[14] The receptor antibody in the plasma membrane of lymphocytes probably plays a role in the recognition of antigen and the triggering of immune responses.[93]

Structure and Classes of Immunoglobulins

The basic unit or monomer of all immunoglobulins comprises four polypeptide chains, two identical heavy (H) and two identical light (L) chains (Fig. 13-1). A considerable amount of detailed information about the structure of immunoglobulins is available,[1,82,212] and is discussed briefly below. The amino acid sequence of each polypeptide chain (H or L) is divided into two regions[204]; one of these varies little from molecule to molecule and is referred to as the constant region (C_H or C_L). The other region exhibits the variability which is responsible for diversity of immunoglobulin antibody activity and is known as the variable region (V_H or V_L). Antigen-specificity is present in the variable regions. Treatment of the immunoglobulin molecule with proteolytic enzymes (for example, papain) separates it into two Fab fragments and one Fc fragment. The Fab fragments contain the variable regions and, therefore, bind antigen. The Fc fragment, which contains part of the C_H regions determines general biological functions, some of which are independent of antigen binding, such as in vivo survival time of whole molecule, membrane binding, and tissue distribution. Another property of the Fc region, which is strictly dependent on changes induced in the immunoglobulin molecule following exposure to antigen, involves complement fixation. Functions such as chemotaxis, phagocytosis, cytolysis, and inflammation are sequelae of complement fixation.

Immunoglobulins are classified according to specific antigenic characteristics of their H chains. These chains are named γ, α, μ, δ, ϵ, to correspond with the five main immunoglobulin classes, IgG, IgA, IgM, IgD, and IgE, respectively. Each class contains two types of L chains termed *kappa* (K) and *lambda* (λ). Features of each main class are shown in Table 13-1 and are briefly outlined below.

IgG comprises about 70 percent of the total serum immunoglobulins. Just under one-half of the total body IgG is distributed intravascularly. With antigenic stimulation, especially by protein antigens, IgM is formed first, and IgG antibody formation follows. IgG (except subclass IgG_4)[234] activates complement. IgG is the only class of immunoglobulins that crosses the placenta. Catabolism of IgG differs from that of the other immunoglobulin classes in that it is dependent on the serum concentration, so that high serum levels result in high catabolic rate and vice versa. The normal half-life of IgG in the circulation is about 21 days. Factors concerned in

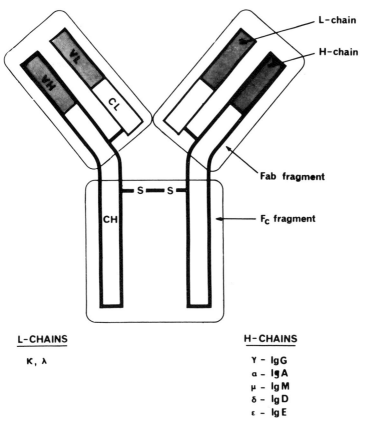

L-CHAINS

K, λ

H-CHAINS

Y - Ig G
α - Ig A
μ - Ig M
δ - Ig D
ε - Ig E

Fig. 13-1. Diagrammatic representation of the basic structure of the immunoglobulin molecule, showing two heavy (H) chains and two light (L) chains, each with a variable (V) and constant (C) region. The five heavy-chain classes and two light-chain classes are listed. Papain digestion results in one Fc and two Fab fragments.

Table 13-1
Characteristics of Serum Immunoglobulins

	IgG	IgA	IgM	IgD	IgE
H chain	γ	α	μ	δ	ϵ
L chain	K,λ	K,λ	K,λ	K,λ	K,λ
Subclasses	IgG_{1-4}	IgA_1, IgA_2	IgM_1, IgM_2	—	—
$(Ig)_n$	n = 1	n = 1, 2, ...	n = 5	n = 1	n = 1
Molecular weight	160,000	160,000– 300,000...	900,000	180,000	190,000
Sedimentation coefficient S_{20}	7	7,9,11,...	19	6.5	8
Carbohydrate content %	2.9	7.5	11.8	12	10.7
Serum concentration (mg/ml) (adult range)	6–16	1.2–4	0.6–1.6	20–50	0.1–0.4*
Intravascular distribution %	44	41	80	73	50
Intravascular half-life, (days)	21	5–6	5–6	3	2
Complement fixation	+	–	+	–	–
Synthetic rate (mg/kg/day)	31	27	5.7	0.4	–
Electrophoretic mobility	$\gamma_2-\alpha_2$	$\gamma_1-\beta_2$	$\gamma_1-\beta_2$	$\beta_2-\alpha_2$	$\gamma_1-\beta$

*μg/ml.

459

IgG metabolism are numerous, and include age, hormone levels, and normal microbial environment.[264,270]

IgA, although representing only 20 percent of all serum immunoglobulins, is by contrast the major serum immunoglobulin in external secretions, such as those of the gastrointestinal and respiratory tracts and colostrum. Unlike IgG, a proportion of serum and all of secretory IgA is in the form of polymers (usually dimers). The two IgA molecules in secretory IgA are linked by a transport piece (T piece) which is synthesized by glandular epithelium. All dimeric IgA molecules (serum and secretory) as well as IgM also have linked to their Fc portion a recently described constituent called a J chain.[103] Secretory IgA appears to provide antibody-mediated protection of the mucosal surfaces, but the precise mechanism remains unclear, especially as IgA molecules do not fix complement.

IgM is present as a polymer made up of five basic units, except in the sera of newborn infants and adults with some diseases, where monomeric 7S IgM has been found.[24] It constitutes about 5–10 percent of the serum immunoglobulins, and occurs mainly in the intravascular compartments. Antigenic challenge, especially with carbohydrate antigens, results in an early IgM response which, together with the greater ability of IgM than IgG to fix complement, endows the host with a potent defence mechanism. The half-life of serum IgM of 5–6 days is similar to that of IgA. The rate of synthesis is only one-sixth that of IgA and IgG, but the higher molecular weight determines that most remains in the circulation and thus serum levels are maintained.

IgD is a minor constituent of serum immunoglobulins and little is known of its specific antibody function.[251] IgE is the class to which reaginic or anaphylactic antibodies belong.[9,122] Being fixed to basophils and tissue mast cells, the molecule induces their degranulation following binding to antigen. Although recognizable clinically as an allergic reaction, this mechanism is probably a normal one in protective inflammatory responses of rapid onset.

Cellular Basis of Immunoglobulin Synthesis

Extracellular immunoglobulin is synthesized at a rate of about 2000 molecules per second per cell, mainly by cells having the morphological appearance of plasma cells. H and L chains are synthesized on separate membrane-bound polyribosomes and then pass into the cisternae of the endoplasmic reticulum. During transport of the chains along the cisternae, carbohydrate units are sequentially added and, just prior to secretion, the H and L chains are linked together by covalent disulfide bonds, probably in the Golgi apparatus (see Fig. 13-8).[277]

The mechanism involved in the genetic control of variability of the H and L chains has not been elucidated, although it is now held that two genes control the synthesis of each chain.[117,202] The individual is endowed with a potential for the production of antibody with varying specificities to meet a wide range of environmental antigens. Two mechanisms have been postulated to explain this potential: the germ-line theory, which assumes the total complement of genes coding for all possible V regions in the antibody to be present in the individual from conception; and the somatic mutation theory, in which mutation and selection generate the necessary V region diversity.[127,202]

PARAPROTEINS

A single plasma cell secretes only one species of immunoglobulin at a time, that is, one L- and H-chain class in balanced synthesis, although some recent work suggests that a cell may synthesize both IgM and IgG simultaneously at certain times.[173] The normal heterogeneous population of immunoglobulins is produced by a number of clones of plasma cells, each coding for a particular V and C region of L and H chains. A normal response of the immune system to antigenic challenge results in a population of immunoglobulins (antibodies) specific for the appropriate antigenic determinants, but belonging to more than one immunoglobulin class.

A paraprotein is a population of immunoglobulin molecules which is completely homogeneous with respect to L and H chain class and subclass, genetic markers, and, ultimately, primary amino acid sequence but which nevertheless may exhibit some heterogeneity because of varying degrees of polymerization. A paraprotein results from the expansion of a single clone of immunoglobulin-secreting cells, each cell synthesizing an identical whole immunoglobulin molecule, or its component L or H chain. Such a paraprotein can usually be recognized as a homogeneous band in the serum and/or urinary protein electrophoretogram (EPG) (see below). All evidence to date supports the view that paraproteins produced by the proliferation of a clone of cells are in every way identical to normal immunoglobulins. Paraproteins can even be induced in normal animals by repeated antigenic challenge.[134,198]

A variety of names has been used to describe a paraprotein: plasma cell dyscrasia; M-component; M-band; paraimmunoglobulin; monoclonal gamma- or immunoglobulin; spike; and band. None is terminologically ideal. Paraproteins have been recognized in many species besides man, including the mouse, Aleutian mink, dog, horse, cow, rabbit, pig, and cat.[64,69] Paraproteins may be composed of the whole immunoglobulin, or its H or L chain. Recently, "heavy chain diseases" have been reported with incomplete synthesis only of the γ, α, or μ chains, apparently due to extensive deletion of V and C amino acid residues at the V-C junction of the H chain[277] which, as a consequence, disrupts the immunoglobulin molecule. L chains may also occur in a free form (Bence Jones protein) either accompanying synthesis of the whole immunoglobulin molecule (due to imbalance of the H- and L-chain production) or representing the only product of the proliferating plasma cells.

Some paraproteins may represent only a half-molecule, that is, one H and one L chain per molecule.[112] Two or even three different paraproteins may occur in individual sera. Their presence may be coincidental but in some cases a true interrelation between the paraproteins has been revealed by biochemical analysis.[119,126,173]

Benign and Malignant Paraproteinemia

Paraproteinemia may be present only transiently, disappearing within a few weeks or months.[214,281] Transient paraproteins most commonly accompany infectious or hypersensitivity diseases, hyperimmunization, malignancy, and the insertion of heart valve prostheses. Those paraproteins that persist may be either benign or malignant.[35,96,109,179,180,193,221,283] The concept of benign paraproteinemia has been

Table 13-2
Diseases Associated with Paraproteinemia

Malignant	Benign
Myeloma	Primary amyloidosis
Macroglobulinemia	Autoimmune disease
Heavy-chain disease	Hepatobiliary disease
(γ-, α-, or μ-chain)	Lichen myxedematosus
Lymphoma	Primary cold-agglutinin disease
Leukemia	Chronic infection
Carcinoma	Miscellaneous

accepted in view of the persistence of paraprotein for many years without evidence of any underlying neoplastic disease. However, the term *benign paraprotein* has been applied by some authors to paraproteins occurring in the absence of any disease, and by others to paraproteins in the absence of malignant disease. The latter definition will be used in the present review. A list of diseases associated with paraproteins appears in Table 13-2. Features of the paraproteins favoring an association with malignancy are the presence of immunoglobulin fragments, reduction of normal serum immunoglobulins, a paraprotein concentration in excess of 1 gm per 100 ml[109] or 2 gm per 100 ml,[96] and a progressive rise of paraprotein concentration.[96,109] There is also ample evidence of benign paraproteins transforming over the years into malignant forms. The benign or malignant behavior of a plasma cell clone should be considered comparable to neoplasia of other somatic cell-lines. The benign form is nonprogressive, highly differentiated (only a whole immunoglobulin molecule, not fragments, is synthesized), and associated with a small tumor mass (low concentration of paraprotein). Formation and function of normal immunoglobulins are unaffected. The malignant form differs in each of these criteria.

The association of paraproteins with neoplasia of immunocompetent cells seems straightforward enough, but whether a similar association with carcinomas is real or coincidental is far from clear.[179,193] This association has been emphasized in carcinomas of the gastrointestinal tract, breast, prostate, and lung.[179] The difficulty is even greater with benign paraproteins where the list of associated disorders is a long one. Furthermore, the incidence of paraproteins in a random population over 70 years of age has been reported to be as high as 3 percent.[96] This tends to favor coincidental association of paraproteinemia in many of the benign disorders in the literature.

The distribution of immunoglobulin H-chain classes in the different disease groups is shown in Table 13-3. The incidence of the immunoglobulin classes in each

Table 13-3
Association and Incidence of Paraproteinemia and Disease

Disease Group	Paraprotein (Decreasing Order of Frequency)
Myeloma	IgG, IgA, L chain alone, IgD, no paraprotein, IgM, IgE
Macroglobulinemia	IgM
Lymphoma, Leukemia	IgM, IgG, IgA, Heavy chain α, γ, μ
Carcinoma	IgG, IgM, IgA
Benign	IgG, IgA, IgM

category is presented in order of frequency, as the actual percentages vary widely in different series.[109,110,179,193,283] The L-chain typing of paraproteins usually reveals a preponderance of Type K (1.5–2.0:1) except for IgD paraproteins where Type λ are more often present.[57,111]

Kinetics of Tumor Growth

In myeloma, in both mouse and man,[109] considerable effort has been made to measure mass and growth patterns of the tumor cells by a study of the rates of synthesis and catabolism of paraproteins in relation to the serum concentration. Hobbs[109] determined doubling times of serum paraprotein levels in humans, and growth patterns of ascitic plasma cell tumors in animals. He concluded that plasma cell tumors grow exponentially, and that there is a direct relationship between their mass and the serum paraprotein concentration. He calculated that the natural history of myelomas must be exceedingly long, the period from the onset of abnormal cell proliferation to the point of clinical diagnosis being up to 33 years for IgG myeloma. Salmon,[227] however, found a growth pattern in which the growth rate slows increasingly as the tumor mass enlarges (Gompertzian). If this model is a valid one, the natural history of myeloma could be much shorter and probably less than 5 years in most instances.

Pathogenesis of Plasma Cell Tumors

The pathogenesis of paraprotein production and of plasma cell tumors in animals and man is still only partly known, but appears to be determined by multiple factors, including the response to repeated antigenic stimulation of the immune system and certain genetically predetermined characteristics.[48,58,179,198] Experimental evidence derives from plasma cell tumors arising spontaneously in certain inbred strains of mice, or in chronic viral infection occurring in Aleutian mink and NZB mice. In addition, the remarkable inbred BALB/c mouse, utilized especially by Potter,[207,208] develops plasmacytomas after intraperitoneal injection of mineral oils or plastics. The induction of this tumor depends on the adjuvant effect of the injectant, on genetic factors, and the presence of commensal organisms particularly in the gastrointestinal tract. The paraproteins induced in BALB/c mice belong mainly to the IgA class and frequently show antibody activity to bacterial antigens. Furthermore, horses and rabbits repeatedly immunized with the same antigen produce paraproteins with specific antibody activity.[134]

Evidence on the pathogenesis of paraproteins in man is only indirect,[179,198] but includes the following:

1. The familial occurrence of myeloma or of abnormal immunoglobulin patterns.[222]
2. Repeated antigenic challenge from chronic infection, autoimmunity, or allergenic injections being reported in some patients with paraproteinemia.[198]
3. The incidence of paraproteins with autoantibody activity in humans (Table 13-4).[37,134,159]
4. The increased occurrence with aging of immunologic aberrations of all varieties.[83]

Table 13-4
Paraproteins with Antibody Activity

Paraprotein Class	Antigen or Hapten	Associated Clinical Features	References
IgG IgA	Streptolysin O	Recurrent streptococcal infection in some patients	261, 284
IgG	Staphylococcal protein	? Recurrent staphylococcal infection	159
IgM	Dinitrophenol	?	62
IgG	Dinitrophenol	?	257
IgM	Factor VIII	Bleeding diathesis	25
IgM	Nuclear protein	Rheumatoid arthritis	38
IgM IgA IgG	IgG	Rheumatoid arthritis, mixed cryoglobulinemia, immune complex vasculitis	13, 95, 129, 275
IgM	I red cell antigen	Hemolysis, Raynaud's phenomenon	123, 233
IgG	Transferrin	Iron storage disease	134
IgM IgA	Lipoprotein	Hyperlipidemia, Xanthomatosis	7, 8, 38, 60, 72, 80, 146
IgG	Lipoprotein	Normolipidemic Xanthomatosis	38, 146
IgG	Thyroglobulin	Myxedema Nodular goitre	38 261
IgM	Heparin	?	159
IgG	Cardiolipin	Positive Wassermann reaction	159
IgA IgM	Smooth muscle	?	261

It would appear in man, as in animals, that an interaction exists between constitutional and environmental factors leading to neoplastic change in the immune system (see Chapter 5).

Laboratory Identification of Paraproteins

The heterogeneous nature of normal serum immunoglobulins produces the well-recognized diffuse zone in the gamma (γ) region of the serum protein EPG whether performed on paper, cellulose acetate, starch, or polyacrylamide.[244] The most widely used supporting material is cellulose acetate, and since its introduction the EPG has become a routine investigative procedure, with the consequent revolution in the recognition and apparent incidence of paraproteinemias and in our appreciation of disease profiles.

Paraproteins are homogeneous with respect to L- and H-chain classes and are recognized because they present as a narrow, well-defined band in the EPG, most commonly located in the γ regions (Fig. 13-2). Occasionally, they migrate in the β or α regions; this applies in particular to IgA, IgD, and heavy chain paraproteins. Difficulty in their recognition may arise in the following circumstances:

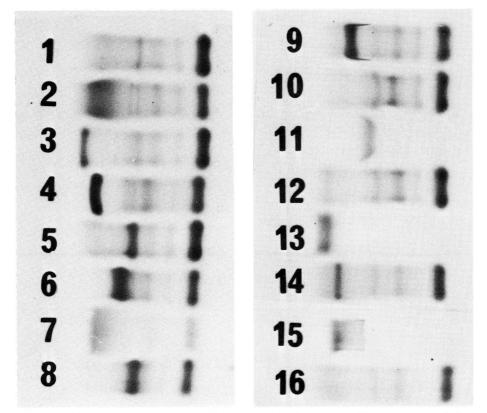

Fig. 13-2. Variety of patterns of immunoglobulin abnormalities seen on cellulose acetate protein electrophoresis. In each pattern, albumin is to the right and the γ region to the left. 1. Normal serum. 2. Diffuse polyclonal hypergammaglobulinemia. 3. γ-migrating IgG paraprotein. 4. γ-migrating IgG paraprotein showing slight heterogeneity of migration. 5. β-migrating IgG paraprotein and severe reduction of γ globulin. 6. β-migrating IgA paraprotein. 7. Urine of patient whose serum is shown in 6. γ-migrating Bence Jones paraprotein of different mobility to serum IgA paraprotein and present in greater concentration than urinary albumin. 8. α2-migrating IgA paraprotein with hypogammaglobulinemia. 9. γ-migrating IgM paraprotein showing uneven migration in cellulose acetate due to relative insolubility (euglobulin). 10. Serum hypogammaglobulinemia in a patient with myeloma whose urine (11) shows Bence Jones protein in the β-γ region. 12. γ-migrating Bence Jones protein in the serum of a patient with severe renal failure. 13. Urine EPG of patient whose serum is shown in (12) shows mobility of urinary Bence Jones protein identical to serum. 14. γ-migrating IgM cryoparaprotein. 15. Isolated purified IgM cryoparaprotein. 16. Serum supernatant from 14 after cryoparaprotein has been removed, to show how easily such a paraprotein settling to the bottom of the tube could be missed if care is not taken.

1. Paraproteins may be of low concentration as in IgD myeloma[57] or travel in the β or α regions.
2. Clear banding may be obscured, in part because of physicochemical aberrations which may cause cryoprecipitation, affect the degree of aggregation, or may reduce the solubility of the protein in the particular medium.
3. Sera may show diffuse hypergammaglobulinemia with restricted or "oligoclonal" heterogeneity.

4. Serum of myeloma patients may contain no paraprotein or show hypogammaglobulinemia.
5. Serum in heavy chain disease may be completely normal on EPG.

   Some of the more common patterns are shown in Figure 13-2. Qualitative
examination of the paraprotein band can give some indication of the immunoglobulin class, if attention is directed toward the location, height-width ratio,
absolute height (on densitometer analysis), and the density of normal "background"
immunoglobulin. Absolute confirmation must always depend on immunoelectrophoretic examination of the serum. The distribution of immunoglobulin classes in
different diseases is presented in Table 13-3. The identification of such classes by immunoelectrophoresis is also shown in Figure 13-3. It usually requires utilization of
both polyvalent antihuman serum antiserum and monospecific antisera directed

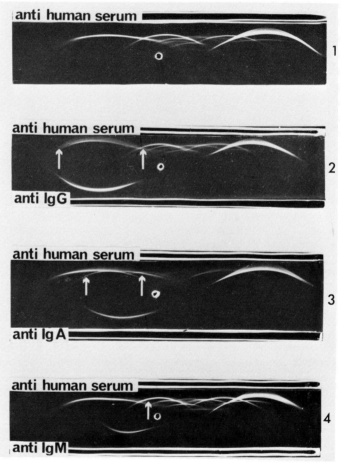

Fig. 13-3. Representative patterns of immunoelectrophoretic analysis of serum.
Albumin is to the right. 1. Normal serum. 2. IgG paraprotein showing characteristic precipitin arc (↑ ↑) and identification with monospecific anti-IgG antiserum. 3. IgA paraprotein
(↑ ↑) showing crossing of the normal IgG arc and identification with monospecific anti-IgA
antiserum. 4. IgM paraprotein, showing distortion of the anodal end of the normal IgG arc
(↑) by the abnormal precipitin band and identification by monospecific anti IgM antiserum.

against the H- and L-chain classes. Even more than with EPG, immunoelectrophoretic analysis requires considerable experience in interpretation.[92,184,221] Obvious paraproteins produce a dense precipitin arc of restricted mobility and sharp,
even contour (Figure 13-3), quite different in appearance from the more elongated
arc of typical normal immunoglobulins. A paraprotein arc will be comprised of only
one type of H and one type of L chain, indicating its monoclonal nature. In the heavy
chain diseases, heavy chains of α, γ, and μ class can be recognized by precipitation
with H chain-specific antiserum and nonprecipitation with L chain-specific antiserum.[78]

The need for the ultracentrifuge (Fig. 13-4) for characterization of paraproteins
has been greatly curtailed in recent years for two main reasons: first, the ability of
immunoelectrophoresis to identify paraproteins, and second, the use of gel filtration
procedures both by column and thin layer which readily give data about molecular
weights of paraproteins. Molecular weight determinations, however, are still useful
for research purposes.

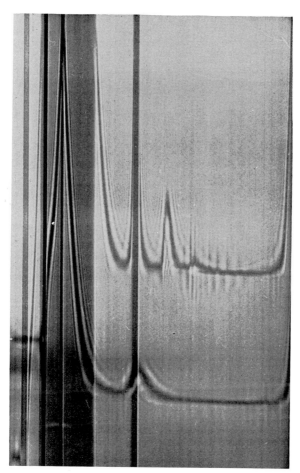

Fig. 13-4.   Macroglobulinemia. Ultracentrifuge tracing after 24 minutes at 52,640 rpm.
Upper line, Patient with macroglobulin peak to right of thin vertical line. *Lower line,* Normal
control serum.

BENCE JONES PROTEIN

Since 1848, a heat test of one form or another has been utilized for the detection of Bence Jones protein in the urine.[254] However, even such a simple procedure has intrinsic difficulties, particularly when the urine contains other proteins not exhibiting reversible thermoprecipitation. Consequently, the most informative approach is by electrophoretic analysis of concentrated urine. A dense homogeneous band is characteristic (see Fig. 13-2) and always occupies a position different from the whole paraprotein molecule in the serum. Immunoelectrophoretic precipitation of such a Bence Jones band with antiserum to the Fab fragment of K or λ chain will confirm that it comprises only L chains—that is, Bence Jones protein. Furthermore, urinary EPG identifies the presence of other proteins, such as albumin or the whole paraprotein, and establishes their relative proportions. Bence Jones protein may result in a distinct band in the serum EPG and be identified in the serum immunoelectrophoretogram if renal failure is severe enough to interfere with its excretion in the urine, or if Bence Jones protein polymerises such as to a tetramer.[94]

IMMUNE ASPECTS OF PARAPROTEINEMIAS

Paraproteins with Antibody Activity

There are many examples in the literature of human paraproteinemic sera with very high titers of a particular antibody activity; isolation of the paraprotein in these cases showed that the antibody activity was exclusively a property of that paraprotein and not of other serum proteins (Table 13-4).[159]

The etiology of this antibody is unclear. The paraprotein could arise from proliferation of a clone of plasma cells normally responsible for such antibody synthesis. The cellular proliferation could be induced by chronic antigenic stimulation,[102,134,159,198,206,238] or develop spontaneously. However, the antibody activity of a paraprotein could be coincidental and be explained by cross reactivity as in the case of dinitrophenol binding.[62] Whatever the uncertainty about etiology, the clinical expression of antibody function of paraproteins seems clear enough in a few situations, as revealed in Table 13-4.

Immunoglobulin Abnormalities

In myeloma, serum levels of normal polyclonal IgG, IgA, and IgM are reduced, irrespective of the class of the monoclonal paraprotein.[41,47,160,179] In myeloma characterized by elaboration of Bence Jones protein only, hypogammaglobulinemia is clearly evident (see Fig. 13-2, No. 10) as it is also when a β-migrating paraprotein is present (see Fig. 13-2, No. 5). In macroglobulinemia, reduction of normal immunoglobulin does occur, but is usually not as marked as in myeloma and involves IgA to a greater extent than IgG (see Fig. 13-2, No. 14).[108] The reduction of normal immunoglobulins both in myeloma and macroglobulinemia is secondary to the disease process and with successful therapy, immunoglobulin levels return toward normal.[179]

In these disorders, the synthetic rates of normal immunoglobulin are reduced, but while the catabolic rate of 7S immunoglobulin (IgG and IgA) is reduced in macroglobulinemia, it is accelerated in myeloma.[247] Specific antibody production has been clearly shown to be defective in multiple myeloma.[41,68,286] The primary antibody response to keyhole limpet hemocyanin has been studied in myeloma patients and found to be impaired.[99] Induction of antibody response is delayed, the switch from IgM to IgG antibody is accelerated, and antibody levels are poorly sustained. Secondary antibody responses are relatively unaffected.[100] In macroglobulinemia, IgM antibody synthesis is reduced,[203] and, therefore, both primary and secondary antibody responses are impaired.[68,100] However, the antibody production defect in macroglobulinemia tends to be less severe than in myeloma and is of lesser clinical significance.

CELL-MEDIATED IMMUNITY

Patients with myeloma show unimpaired delayed hypersensitivity to bacterial antigens,[41,100,285] and are readily sensitized to new antigens. In vitro lymphocyte response to PHA, an accepted criterion of T cell function, has been found to be intact in myeloma,[100,285] except in one study performed under highly artificial culture conditions.[228]

By contrast, patients with macroglobulinemia frequently show impaired T cell function, as indicated by lack of delayed hypersensitivity responses to bacterial antigens and impaired in vitro lymphocyte response to PHA.[228,285] Unlike myeloma serum, which does not affect DNA synthesis by normal lymphocytes,[228] some macroglobulinemic sera can impair the PHA response of normal lymphocytes.[285]

INFLAMMATION

Neutrophil function in vitro, as measured by phagocytosis of yeast particles and adhesiveness to glass bead columns, is impaired by paraproteins.[197] In vivo studies using the skin window technique[219] have shown impairment of neutrophil function in myeloma,[195,196] but not in macroglobulinemia.[285]

Clinical Effects of the Immune Deficiency

Bacterial infection is a common form of presentation of myeloma, and represents a major clinical problem in more than 50 percent of patients.[56,160] Defective defenses against infection which have been detailed above include reduced immunoglobulin levels, impaired antibody synthesis and enhanced antibody catabolism, impaired phagocytosis, and lack of participation of polymorphs in inflammatory responses.

While *Diplococcus pneumoniae* has, in the past, been found to be the most frequent cause of infection in myeloma, a recent study of 55 patients with myeloma[160] showed that pneumococcal infection did not occur and that most isolates were of gram-negative organisms with only 11 of 39 being streptococci or staphylococci. The most frequent infections reported were urinary tract infections, septicemia, and pneumonia. The focus of infection in septicemic patients was usually the urinary tract or lung. In contrast, infections usually associated with T cell defects occur infrequently in myeloma and then usually as a complication of corticosteroid or other immunosuppressive therapy. Intracellular parasitic infections are uncommon, although one case of toxoplasmosis and two of pneumocystis carinii infestation have been described[160]; there is no particular susceptibility to fungal and viral infection in myeloma.[179]

In macroglobulinemia, bacterial infection is infrequent and usually occurs only as a very late manifestation. The incidence of infection as a presenting feature was found to be only 7 percent.[149] Herpes zoster is a common feature, and Osserman points out the very frequent association of macroglobulinemia and tuberculosis.[179] These features are consistent with the observed frequency of T cell defects.

CLINICAL FEATURES OF MYELOMA

Myeloma is a disease of middle and old age, the mean age at diagnosis being 62 years for IgG myeloma or 65 for IgA. Where the paraprotein is IgD, or where Bence Jones protein only is produced, patients appear to be slightly younger. Males and females are equally affected, except in the case of IgD myeloma, where males predominate.[111] Diagnosis is generally preceded by a relatively asymptomatic period, which is variable in length but may be as long as 20 years.[174] Repeated bacterial infections, especially pulmonary, may occur for months or even years before clinical diagnosis.[180]

Skeletal pain is the most common presenting symptom, but infection, anemia, renal failure, hypercalcemia, hyperviscosity syndrome, neurological complications, or features attributable to amyloidosis may lead to diagnosis. Weakness and weight loss are very frequent complaints at presentation. The appearance, at first, of vague and, later, of increasing bone pain in an individual of the older age group with the appearance of pallor, and the lack of other abnormalities on physical examination would make one suspect the diagnosis of myeloma. The disease may continue at a more or less static level for 1 year, 2 years, or even longer, but sooner or later the various events listed below manifest themselves, due either to plasma cell infiltration or to the effects of paraprotein. Thus, spontaneous fractures, progressive renal failure, hemorrhagic disturbances, and numerous infections (especially pulmonary) supervene, making the course an ever-increasingly complex and difficult one. The patient eventually becomes bedridden as the result of numerous fractures, usually of the vertebrae, and of anemia and uremia. Hypercalcemia and hyperviscosity result in neurologic symptoms. The terminal event may be uncontrollable infection, hemorrhage, or renal failure, or less commonly, a leukemialike condition may occur, dominated by the appearance of large numbers of abnormal plasma cells in the blood.

The outcome of the treated disease depends on the immunoglobulin class involved, the mean survival being 35 months for IgG–K and only 11 months when L chains only are produced.[214] Paradoxically, it has been reported that when the serum concentration of paraprotein is relatively unaffected by therapy, prognosis is good compared to those patients in whom the immunoglobulin level falls rapidly[128] when treatment is given.

Skeletal Involvement

Skeletal pain. This is the most common presenting symptom and, at some time during the disease, it occurs in 90 percent of patients.[178] It usually takes the form of backache or chest pain of sudden onset due to pathologic fracture of the vertebra or rib. Fractures of long bones after minimal trauma are also common. With extensive skeletal involvement, bone deformity such as kyphoscoliosis may develop.

Osteoporosis. The most common radiological abnormality in myeloma is osteoporosis, occurring in 90 percent of patients.[267] It may be diffuse but particularly involves the spine (Fig. 13-5).[190] In one-quarter of patients, it is the only radiological abnormality of the skeleton.[178] Histological studies indicate that the osteoporotic appearance is due to diffuse infiltration of marrow spaces by myeloma tissue. In untreated myeloma, osteoporosis generally goes on to discrete osteolytic lesions.[180]

Osteolytic lesions. These lesions occur in almost two-thirds of patients, and are most frequent when Bence Jones protein only is produced by the tumor.[111,214] The most common sites of osteolytic lesions are the skull, mandible, spine, ribs, pelvis, clavicles, sternum, and proximal long bones. The appearance is of multiple "punched-out" lesions without osteoblastic reaction (see Fig. 13-5) or erosion of bone cortex by expansion of the medullary cavity.

Solitary skeletal lesions. In a small percentage of patients, these are the presenting symptoms.[179] Nearly two-thirds of these isolated lesions are found in a vertebra, pelvis, or femur.[278] Truly solitary lesions are, however, excessively rare. More often, isolated skeletal lesions which appear to be solitary myeloma tumors, are, in fact, found after detailed investigation to be associated with serum or urinary protein abnormalities, and marrow distant from the site of the lesion is frequently found to be involved. Patients who present with a solitary bone lesion may, after several years, develop disseminated disease, which is then clinically indistinguishable from typical myeloma.[273]

Hypercalcemia. This is found at presentation in one-third of patients with IgG myeloma and nearly twice as often in patients with IgA paraproteins or Bence Jones proteinuria only.[111,214] Bone destruction causes negative calcium balance and hypercalcuria. Hypercalcemia is associated with dehydration and oliguria and is potentiated by immobilization. Drowsiness, muscular hypotonia, nausea, and vomiting may be presenting symptoms attributable to hypercalcemia, accompanying either diffuse osteoporosis or discrete destructive bone lesions.

Osteosclerotic lesions. Such lesions are rare in multiple myeloma and only about 60 cases have been described.[154,170] The incidence of this type of lesion has been estimated to be 3 percent.[65,170] Osteosclerotic lesions are solitary in one-quarter of reported patients, and occur in the absence of lytic lesions in a similar proportion of patients.[170] Radiologic appearances have been described as discrete areas, either solitary or multiple; diffuse sclerosis (usually of a whole vertebra); or lytic lesions surrounded by a ring of sclerosis.[154] The serum alkaline phosphatase remains normal in almost all instances of osteoblastic lesions, and serum calcium is less often elevated in osteosclerotic myeloma than in classic myeloma with osteolytic lesions. Peripheral neuropathy may be associated with osteoblastic bone lesions.

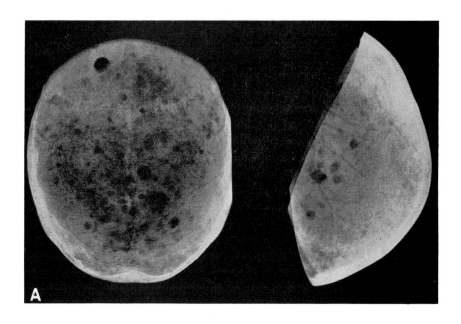

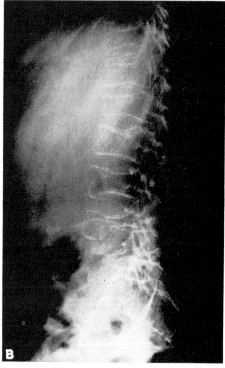

Fig. 13-5. Multiple myeloma. A. X-rays of skull taken postmortem show characteristic lesions. B. Lateral x-ray of lower spine shows marked general osteoporosis, with multiple compression fractures of the vertebral bodies. C. X-ray of pelvis shows multiple lytic lesions of all bodies. D. X-ray of humerus shows many osteolytic lesions. (Courtesy of Dr. G. L. Rolleston, Christchurch Hospital, Christchurch, New Zealand.)

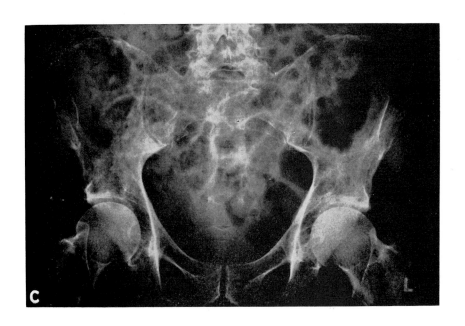

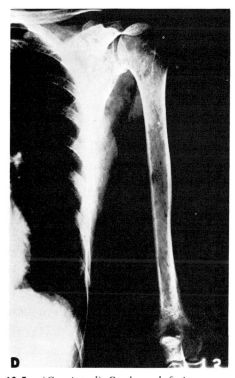

Fig. 13-5. *(Continued). See legend, facing page.*

Neurologic Manifestations

Neurologic complications occur in nearly 50 percent of patients with myeloma. Symptoms result from interference with the blood supply to nervous tissue by anemia and hyperviscosity, amyloid infiltration, pressure from expanding bony deposits or pathologic fractures, or direct invasion of the central nervous system (CNS) by tumor tissue. Metabolic factors affecting the CNS include hypercalcemia and uremia. In addition, a peripheral neuropathy unrelated to malignant invasion or amyloid infiltration is recognized.[265]

Spinal cord compression. Usually in the thoracic region, spinal cord compression occurs in 10 percent of patients with myeloma as the result of fractured vertebrae or pressure from extradural deposits of myeloma tissue.[243]

Nerve root compression. Nerve root compression causing radicular pain is a common presentation and is experienced by one-quarter of all patients at some stage of their illness. The pain most commonly involves a limb, but may occur in the thoracic region. Objective neurologic changes are found in about half these patients. The lesions are usually due to nerve compression by tumor mass, but symmetrical spinal nerve root symptoms may be the result of amyloid infiltration.

Intracranial and cranial nerve involvement. Such involvement by myeloma tissue is rare, even though the skull bones are a favorite site for myeloma deposits. Myeloma of the orbit[57,230] or retroorbital tissue[243] and isolated or multiple cranial nerve lesions have been described. The brain is a very infrequent site for myeloma tumors, but reports of solitary intracranial plasmacytomas have appeared.[163,266] Diffuse degenerative involvement of the nervous system with tumor deposits produces a rapidly progressive syndrome.[11]

PERIPHERAL NEUROPATHY

A symmetrical *peripheral neuropathy* is a rare but well-recognized manifestation of myeloma, there being at least 43 cases in the literature.[50,154,170,243,265] The incidence in one large series was almost 3 percent.[243] Invasion of nerve roots by myeloma tissue or deposition of amyloid in vasa nervorum, or, very rarely, in peripheral nerve tissue itself,[50] can produce isolated peripheral nerve lesions. Osteosclerotic bone lesions, a rare feature of myeloma (see above), have been found in association with half the cases of peripheral neuropathy that have been described, but no satisfactory explanation for this association can be offered.

EXTRAMEDULLARY PLASMACYTOMA

Myeloma is predominantly a tumor of bone marrow and, although small extramedullary foci of disease are found to be widespread at postmortem examination, it is rare for such metastases to be clinically detectable. The incidence of extraosseous tumors in IgG or IgA myeloma, was reported to be a little more than 1 percent,[111] although in another series,[61] six examples were found among 78 patients with myelomatosis. The incidence is higher in Bence Jones myeloma and, even more so (63 percent), in IgD myeloma.[111] A feature of IgD myeloma is the growth of large tumor masses from bones, particularly of the rib cage; tumor may occur in lymph nodes, liver, spleen, kidneys, subcutaneous tissues and orbit.[57]

In a review of 266 cases of extramedullary plasmacytoma, seventy-five percent presented in the upper airways.[278] These tumors have also been found arising in the gastrointestinal tract,[242] brain,[163] conjunctiva, and lung. Wiltshaw[278] considered that extramedullary plasmacytoma represented an entity distinct from myeloma, and one with a better prognosis, but Edwards and Zawadski denied this.[61] It is to be emphasized that full investigation and the passage of time show that many of these patients ultimately develop classic myeloma.

Hematologic Manifestations

Anemia of variable severity is found in nearly all patients. Factors contributing to anemia are marrow replacement by tumor, shortened red cell survival, blood loss, bone marrow suppression due to infection, renal failure, and drugs used for therapy. The hemoglobin may be reduced even further by plasma volume expansion caused by the paraprotein. Occasionally, folic acid deficiency is induced by the increased requirements of the malignant cells, together with a poor dietary intake.[113] *Leukopenia* or *thrombocytopenia* are seen in one-third of patients before therapy,[178] probably on the basis of marrow replacement. The *erythrocyte sedimentation rate* (ESR) is almost invariably very rapid when a serum protein abnormality is present, unless there is a large amount of cryoprecipitable protein; the ESR is normal in 10 percent of myeloma patients.[120] Examination of a *peripheral blood film* characteristically shows marked rouleaux formation, (Fig. 13-6) and background staining due to increased plasma protein concentration. Red blood cells are usually normocytic and normochromic, although macrocytosis caused by folic acid deficiency or hypochromia from chronic blood loss are occasionally found. *The differential leukocyte* count may show a relative lymphocytosis with a variable number of immature cells. A careful search will reveal circulating plasma cells in 50 percent of myeloma patients (Fig. 13-6).[84,215] Recently, the frequent presence of abnormal cells in peripheral blood in myeloma has been confirmed by DNA measurements[168] and by the results of unstimulated cultures.[49] Eosinophilia is occasionally found.[178] Fre-

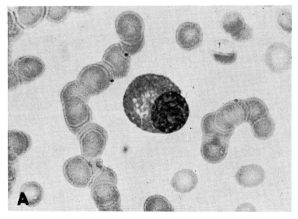

Fig. 13-6. Multiple myeloma. Peripheral blood, plasma cell, and rouleaux formation of red blood cells (X 1100).

quently, there are immature cells of both the red and white cell series giving a leukoerythroblastic picture.

  Bone marrow is usually easily aspirated through a thin soft cortex. In typical cases, fragments are hypercellular and more than 15 percent of nucleated cells are myeloma cells, which may occur in sheets or nests, but because of the multifocal nature of the disease relatively normal marrow may be sampled. Myeloma cells vary from typical, well-differentiated plasma cells to large, bizarre multinucleate cells and cell syncytia. Mitotic figures may be seen and cells with multiple nucleoli occur. The typical cell has an eccentric nucleus with chromatin in clumps which may even show a cartwheel arrangement. The abundant cytoplasm stains blue and a perinuclear halo is apparent (Fig. 13-7). Russell bodies are discrete cytoplasmic vacuoles (see below). A plasma cell whose cytoplasm is filled with such bodies is

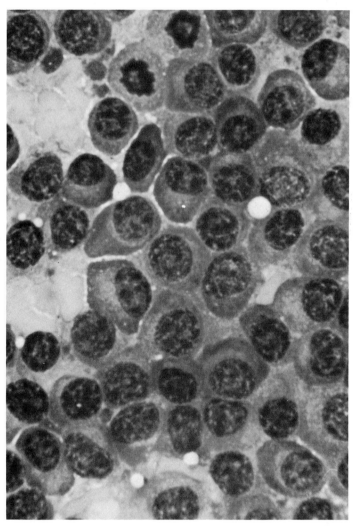

Fig. 13-7. Myeloma. Bone marrow shows plasma cells which are pleomorphic with variable nuclear chromatin, nucleoli, cytoplasmic staining, and volume.

called a *morula* or *Mott cell*. In some cases of IgA and, less often, of IgG myeloma, flame cells with abundant protein accumulations and thesaurocytes with degenerate nuclei are evident. Occasionally, cells in the marrow may be indistinguishable from lymphocytes and abnormal monocytes.

Electron microscopy of the myeloma cell (Fig. 13-8)[179] shows that the characteristic basophilia of cytoplasm is due to large amounts of endoplasmic reticulum to which is bound RNA (Fig. 13-8*A*). Gammaglobulin has been demonstrated within the endoplasmic reticulum. The flame cell appearance is due to distension of the endoplasmic reticulum with amorphous material which is presumably IgA incapable of being secreted. Degeneration of these cells, giving rise to the thesaurocyte appearance, may be necessary for release of this material.[153] Intracytoplasmic crystals have been shown to lie in the endoplasmic reticulum and to have a lamellar structure with periodicity of 100 Å; they are comprised of crystalline gamma globulin. The perinuclear halo is due to accumulations of Golgi vesicles. Russell bodies (Fig. 18-8*B*) are seen to be homogeneous electron-dense deposits within the endoplasmic reticulum. Thus, the characteristic distension of endoplasmic reticulum, as well as flame cell appearance, are attributable to the high rate of synthesis of protein which may be secreted from cells with difficulty.

PLASMA CELL LEUKEMIA

Although circulating plasma cells may be seen occasionally at any time in the disease, their presence in large numbers usually occurs in the terminal stages of myeloma. However, a very rare form of myeloma presents with a plasma cell leukemia, having clinical features and a course which distinguishes it from classic myeloma. Age, sex, incidence of skeletal lesions, and protein abnormalities indicate similarities with classic myeloma, but, in addition, hepatosplenomegaly, lymphadenopathy, thrombocytopenia, and bleeding occur. Response to therapy is poor. Two of the three reported patients with IgE myeloma[74,176] have had plasma cell leukemia without extensive spread of tumor at presentation and have had a good initial response to chemotherapy.

MULTIPLE MYELOMA AND ACUTE LEUKEMIA

Myeloma has a recognized association with a large number of neoplasms, particularly of the gastrointestinal tract, breast, and prostate, and the incidence of a second malignancy has been reported to be as high as 19 percent.[10,269] It would appear that either the myeloma is secondary to the other malignancy or both evolve from the same etiologic stimulus since similar tumor types are found in patients with asymptomatic plasma cell dyscrasias.[179] However, the relationship of acute leukemia and myeloma is apparently different. Acute leukemia is now a well-recognized complication of myeloma and appears to develop during the course of the latter. There are a large number of reports of acute granulocytic leukemia (either myeloblastic or myelomonocytic) appearing in patients with myeloma of $2\frac{1}{2}$–3 years' duration.[2,137,231] In other cases, sarcoma indistinguishable from reticulum cell sarcoma has followed treatment with cyclophosphamide or melphalan.[115,169]

It has been emphasized that most of these patients have received melphalan therapy for most of this time. In a personally observed case, however, cytotoxic therapy had not been given for 2 years prior to development of leukemia, and mel-

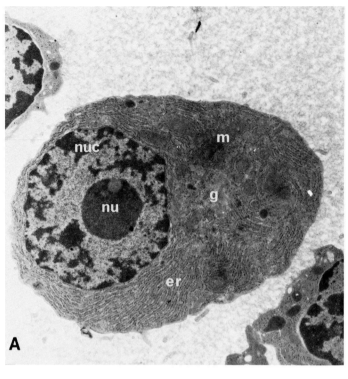

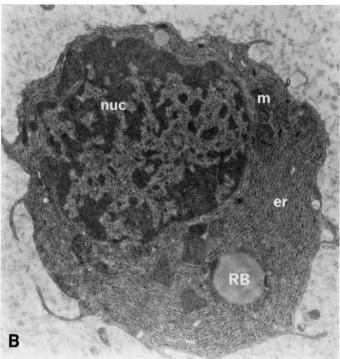

Fig. 13-8. Myeloma. Electron micrographs of plasma cells. A. The nucleus (nuc) contains coarse, clumped chromatin, with a prominent nucleolus (nu); increased Golgi apparatus (g) is also seen. B. Extensive rough endoplasmic reticulum (er) is well developed and has proceeded to Russell body formation (RB). Mitochondria (m) are scattered throughout the cytoplasm (X 10,000).

phalan had been given in small increments for 18 months prior to this. Myeloma may precede the leukemia by many years, and disease duration may be a major etiologic factor. However, the currently favored principal cause is prolonged cytotoxic therapy with melphalan or cyclophosphamide.

Although in the absence of satisfactory controls one cannot be certain of a direct relationship between melphalan therapy and the development of leukemia, the history of myeloma followed by acute leukemia was unrecorded prior to the use of melphalan.[231] The possible role of melphalan in leukemogenesis is unclear. It could depend on the immunosuppressive action of this agent, but this appears unlikely since leukemia has not been observed in renal allograft recipients in association with immunosuppressive therapy, even though there is a high incidence of other malignancies.[191] An alternative explanation may be the radiomimetic property of melphalan, and certainly the time relationships between the use of this drug in myeloma and the subsequent onset of leukemia are similar to those obtaining in radiation leukemogenesis (see Chapter 5).

CLINICAL FEATURES OF MACROGLOBULINEMIA

This disease is more common in males than females[148,149,180,263] and most patients are over 50 years of age. The most frequent presenting symptoms are weakness, weight loss, fever and associated symptoms which are caused by the pathologic effects of the paraprotein. These include dilutional anemia, hyperviscosity with impaired cerebral circulation and bleeding (see below). Infections are rarely the reason for presentation or diagnosis.[149] Enlargement of liver, spleen, or lymph nodes of mild degree are the most frequently found physical abnormalities and occur in a third to half the patients.[148,149] Mikulicz's syndrome (enlargement of salivary and lacrimal glands) may develop. Neurologic and retinal changes, purpura, and cardiovascular changes are described below.

In macroglobulinemia, in contrast to myeloma, skeletal lesions are not a prominent feature. Several patients with destructive bone lesions have been recorded,[273] but these must be considered to represent IgM myeloma (Table 13-3). Generalized osteoporosis is commonly seen but is not a dominant feature. Three of 40 patients in one series[148] had lytic bone lesions which were shown to consist of infiltrates of malignant lymphoid cells.

A normocytic normochromic anemia is usually present, partly as a result of marrow involvement in the pathologic process, partly because the plasma volume is increased because of paraproteinemia. The erythrocyte sedimentation rate is usually high and rouleaux formation prominent. There may be leukopenia and thrombocytopenia. A relative lymphocytosis may be seen and chronic lymphocytic leukemia has been recognized in association with macroglobulinemia on at least thirty occasions.[287] Eosinophilia is occasionally seen. Recent immunofluorescent studies on the blood lymphocytes in macroglobulinemia, chronic lymphocytic leukemia, and related lymphoproliferative diseases have utilized the lymphocyte surface immunoglobulin as markers of B cells. The overall problem is still far from resolution but it does appear that circulating lymphocytes in macroglobulinemia have monoclonal IgM on their surface with the same immunochemical characteristics as the serum paraprotein. In addition, some lymphocytes show intracytoplastic IgM.[212] The bone marrow contains large numbers of "plasmacytoid" lymphocytes,

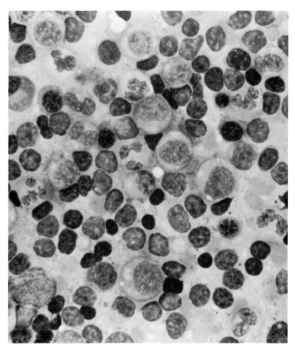

Fig. 13-9. Macroglobulinemia. Bone marrow cells showing morphologic variations from typical lymphocytes via intermediate forms (plasmacytoid lymphocytes) to typical plasma cells.

with an increase in small lymphocytes and, to a lesser extent, in plasma cells (Fig. 13-9). Although a spectrum varying from plasma cells to small lymphocytes may be found, the marrow in macroglobulinemia is usually clearly distinguishable from that in myelomatosis, with lymphocytic cells predominating in the former while normal and abnormal plasma cells predominate in the latter. Eosinophils and mast cells may be a prominent feature in the marrow of macroglobulinemia. Intranuclear PAS-positive globules are found in a large number of the plasmacytoid lymphocytes. Electron micrograph studies show that bone marrow lymphoid cells contain abundant endoplasmic reticulum, indicative of their role as immunoglobulin-producing cells.

The lymph nodes show diffuse replacement with lymphocytic lymphoma. The cells may resemble small lymphocytes or the typical plasmacytoid lymphocytes. The appearance of lymph nodes, liver, and spleen are usually indistinguishable from those in lymphosarcoma or chronic lymphocytic leukemia.

HEAVY-CHAIN DISEASES

These recently recognized paraproteinemic states are brought about by a malignant proliferation of immunoglobulin-producing cells which fail to synthesize intact Ig molecules. The serum contains an abnormal protein which resembles the Fc fragment of the Ig molecule. Heavy chain diseases of the IgG, IgA, and IgM type are now recognized and distinguishable clinically (Tables 13-3 and 13-5).

Table 13-5
Features of Heavy-chain Diseases

Heavy-chain Class	Gamma (γ)	Alpha (α)	Mu (μ)
Number of cases reported	20	10	4
Bacterial infection	+++	+	++
Palatal edema	Yes	No	No
Bone lesions	No	No	1 patient
Bowel lesions	No	Yes	No
Finding of amyloid	1 patient	No	2 patients
Peripheral blood	Lymphocytoid cells		Chronic lymphocytic leukemia, (3 patients)
Bone marrow	Eosinophilia Lymphocytoid cells Atypical plasma cells		Lymphocytosis
Normal serum immunoglobulins	Reduced	Reduced	Reduced
Abnormal urinary protein	Gamma chain	Alpha chain	Kappa chain

GAMMA-CHAIN DISEASE

About twenty cases have been described,[52,63,78,79,182,262,282] mostly occurring in middle-aged or elderly patients. Presentation is usually as a disseminated malignant lymphoma. Splenomegaly and generalized lymphadenopathy are usual and hepatomegaly is common. Involvement of lymphoid tissue of Waldeyer's ring produces characteristic palatal and uvular edema which is usually transient but may cause respiratory obstruction.[183] There may be fever, and recurrent bacterial infections, including septicemia, are usual. Infection is frequently the cause of death. Bone lesions have been reported in only one patient.

Examination of the peripheral blood shows anemia and leukopenia with atypical lymphocytoid or plasmacytoid cells in about half the patients. Thrombocytopenia is evident at presentation also in half the patients. The bone marrow aspirate may be indistinguishable from that of multiple myeloma, but usually it contains a large number of lymphocytoid cells resembling those seen in macroglobulinemia. Lymph node histology reveals a malignant lymphoma of mixed cellularity comprising plasma cells, lymphocytes, plasmacytoid cells, reticulum cells, and eosinophils so that the disease appears to be a variant of reticulum cell sarcoma.

Serum protein electrophoresis usually shows a broad peak in the β region accompanied by a reduction in gammaglobulin levels, reflecting the low levels of IgG, IgA, and IgM. The urine contains an abnormal protein identical with that found in serum.

ALPHA-CHAIN DISEASE

This is a malignant lymphoma involving usually the small intestine[240] and the respiratory tract in a single patient.[256] The clinical syndrome is quite distinctive. The patient is usually of Mediterranean origin and in the second to fourth decade of life. Earlier reports were mainly of Africans and Sephardic Jews, but recent reports describe patients of European or South American origin.[12,78,256]

Presentation is with a rapidly progressive disease, the predominant features of which are cachexia and diarrhea with severe steatorrhea unresponsive to gluten withdrawal. Barium studies of small bowel show thickened mucosal folds, dilated loops of bowel, and segmentation of barium. The histology is that of a diffuse lymphoplasmocytic infiltrate of small bowel and mesentery. Urine and serum contain an abnormal protein devoid of light chains, but reactive with anti α chain-specific antiserum.[239] Osteoporosis occurs but no destructive lesions of bone are seen. Although the course is usually one of rapid deterioration, spontaneous remissions have been described, and response to broad spectrum antibiotics such as tetracycline has been claimed.[223]

MU-CHAIN DISEASE

Seven years after it was predicted in 1963,[182] the first case of μ-chain disease was reported,[4,76] and three further cases have now been recognized.[77,129] Three of these patients had long-standing, chronic lymphocytic leukemia, and μ-chain disease represents a rare accompaniment of that disorder. The fourth patient had a lymphoproliferative disorder accompanied by μ-chain and monoclonal IgA in serum. In contrast to γ- and α-chain diseases, lymphoma is not usually a feature but bone lesions are observed. The report of Ballard describes a patient with a destructive bone lesion causing pathologic fracture of the neck of femur.[4] Hepatosplenomegaly is described. Amyloidosis was found in one patient and kappa Bence Jones protein in the serum or urine in two. The μ-chain is not found in urine. Bone marrow examination shows an infiltrate of plasma cells, mainly atypical forms and lymphocytes. The plasma cells contain vacuoles which are characteristic.

EFFECTS OF PARAPROTEINS

Many of the clinical and pathologic manifestations of paraproteinemia can be correlated with certain specific physicochemical properties of the individual paraproteins, in particular, their solubility, molecular structure, thermodynamic properties, viscosity, kinetics of polymerization, and degree of intermolecular association.[106,192] The resultant clinical expression of these properties, though complex, is specific for the individual paraprotein. The components and behavioral characteristics of blood which may be affected by the presence of paraproteins are listed below.[40,192]

1. Effects on:
   Erythrocytes
   Leukocytes
   Platelets
   Coagulation factors

        Other plasma constituents
        Blood viscosity
        Blood volume
  2. Cryoproperties
  3. Pyroproperties

Erythrocytes

Paraproteins result in an enhancement of erythrocyte aggregation and rouleaux formation. In vitro, this is responsible for the characteristically high erythrocyte sedimentation rate. Intravascular erythrocyte aggregation ("sludging") as seen in the conjunctival and skin microvasculature is considered the in vivo equivalent of a rapid sedimentation rate.[105,143,177] Increased erythrocyte aggregation may be either a result of direct cell-to-cell bridging by paraproteins, neutralization of the negative erythrocyte surface charge, or the formation of an adhesive layer over the erythrocyte membrane.[274] The phenomenon of aggregation is uninfluenced by anticoagulants.[155] Increased erythrocyte aggregation in the presence of a paraprotein is responsible for the granularity seen in blood and marrow films and on the walls of test tubes, and often leads to difficulty in crossmatching of blood, especially if the paraprotein is cryoprecipitable or behaves as a cold agglutinin.[132,255]

The formation of rouleaux occurs when the force of attraction between the cells is small and their surfaces are smooth so that they can readjust their relative positions after coming into contact. The minimum free surface of the cells is then in contact with the plasma.[225,274] Erythrocyte aggregation, including rouleaux formation, produces corpuscular aggregates of large volumes but relatively small surface area, with resultant acceleration in sedimentation rate. The presence of a low packed-cell volume will contribute to this high erythrocyte sedimentation rate.[279]

In the presence of marked plasma hyperviscosity, especially if the paraprotein is a cryoglobulin or cryogelglobulin, the sedimentation rate at room temperature may be relatively low due to the resistance offered to sedimentation by the plasma.[175] In these situations, the erythrocyte sedimentation rate will increase if measured at 37° C and will also paradoxically increase with the initial reductions in the amount of paraprotein following treatment. If the paraprotein behaves as a cold agglutinin, then the sedimentation rate will increase with a reduction in temperature.[143,232] Intravascular erythrocyte aggregation correlates with in vitro rouleaux formation, a high erythrocyte sedimentation rate, and elevated plasma viscosity.[155] This phenomenon can be directly observed in the microvasculature of the skin and in the bulbar conjunctivae.[51,143,177] It is especially marked following exposure to cold in cryoglobulinemia and in patients with cold agglutinins,[5,118] and may result in peripheral vascular insufficiency, ranging in severity from uncomplicated Raynaud's phenomenon to digital gangrene.[151]

Shortened erythrocyte survival with a negative direct Coombs' test is well documented and frequently associated with paraproteinemia.[29,179] This may result from an alteration in the rheologic properties of erythrocytes due to the nonspecific coating of these cells by the paraprotein.[29] Occasionally, paraproteins have antierythrocyte specificity, usually directed against the I surface antigen. These paraproteins behave as cold agglutinins and are almost invariably 19S IgM globulins of kappa-type light chains.[36,37,91,97,98,233] The symptoms are related to the in vivo activity of the autoantibody and consist of chronic hemolytic anemia, peripheral vascular insufficiency, and occasional attacks of cold-induced hemoglobinuria.

Leukocytes

Infections are a common and serious complication of paraproteinemia, especially septicemia, bronchopneumonia, or urinary tract infections.[160] The predisposition to recurrent infections arises from leukopenia,[56,118] leukocyte dysfunction,[197] abnormalities of humoral antibody levels and responses, and immunosuppressive therapy.

Leukocyte abnormalities demonstrated in paraproteinemias include a reduction of polymorph adhesiveness as measured with glass bead columns,[197] a reduction of phagocytosis of particles such as saccharated iron or yeast cells,[195-197] and impaired leukocyte emigration as observed by the skin window technique.[195,196] Leukopenia may be caused by marrow involvement, immunosuppressive therapy, or the presence of leukoagglutinins.[115,178] The adsorption of paraproteins to polymorphs may initiate the action of specific agglutinins,[115] thus adding a further factor to the impressive list of mechanisms responsible for impaired bacteriocidal activity in these patients.

Platelets

The association of paraproteinemia and serious hemostatic defects is well recognized.[73,186,199] However, in most patients the hemostatic defect is apparent only as a prolongation of the bleeding time.[196]

Abnormalities of platelet function which have been recorded in the presence of a paraprotein (Table 13-6) include interference with platelet adhesiveness to surfaces, interference with platelet aggregation by adenosine diphosphate or collagen, impaired release or activity of platelet factor 3, and defective clot retraction.[73,185,196] Sluggish pseudopodial formation and defective viscous metamorphosis of platelets have also been demonstrated.[16,185,186,226] Plasmapheresis is the most effective therapy when these in vitro defects are associated with obvious bleeding problems.[196] A rapid reduction in the concentration of paraprotein is paralleled by a reversal of abnormalities of platelet function and immediate clinical improvement. Abnormal platelet function may thus be due to the direct coating of platelets by paraproteins,[55,124,226] as shown by a number of studies including electron microscopy and fluorescent antibody techniques.[46,185,186] The paraprotein coat over the platelet probably results in changes in surface tension and interference with platelet surface macromolecules. When present, thrombocytopenia results either from dysfunction of a marrow infiltrated with malignant cells or depressed by cytotoxic therapy, or from the activity of platelet agglutinins and antiplatelet antibodies.[125,178]

Coagulation Factors

Some paraproteins cause hemostatic defects (Table 13-6) through their anticoagulant properties.[73,133,196,199,200,217,241,259] Inhibition of the thrombin-fibrinogen reaction is the most frequently observed abnormality.[44,81,133,140,196,217,241] The basis of

Table 13-6
Disordered Hemostasis in Paraproteinemia

Site of Disorder	Effect
Platelets	
	Thrombocytopenia
	Impaired platelet function
Coagulation factors	
	Abnormal thrombin-fibrinogen reaction, e.g., inhibition of fibrin monomer polymerization
	Antithrombin, heparinlike activity
	Antibodies and inhibitors of coagulation factors
	Reduced levels of coagulation factors
	Intravascular coagulation and consumption of coagulation factors
Fibrinolysis	
	Increased
	Impaired
Hyperviscosity	
	Reduced local availability of platelets and coagulation factors
	Endothelial shearing stresses
	Hypoxemic damage to vessel wall
	Endothelial coating by paraproteins, resulting in impaired diffusion of nutrients
	Capillary thromboses
Vessel Wall	
	Infiltration with amyloid
	Immune complex vasculitis (see Table 13-4)

this inhibition is probably interference with fibrin monomer polymerization.[31,34,133,139,213] In some cases this anticoagulant activity has been shown to be associated with the isolated paraprotein.[241,260] Characteristically, clots are gelatinous, bulky, and friable, clot retraction is poor, and thrombin times are prolonged. Paraproteins with antithrombin or heparinlike activity have also been reported.[70,81,133,139,167,172] These give rise to a prolongation of the thrombin time which is reversed by the addition of protamine sulphate. The mechanism of these effects is not clear, but may consist in the formation of complexes of thrombin-paraprotein or fibrinogen-paraprotein, thus altering the thrombin-binding capacity of fibrinogen. Paraproteins which inhibited specific coagulation factors and possibly acted as antibodies have also been reported.[25,89,171,172,268] Specific anti-factor VIII activity is the best documented example of this.[25,89]

Hemostatic defects in patients with paraproteinemias may also be secondary to the rare complication of disseminated intravascular coagulation, with consumption of coagulation factors and the appearance of circulating fibrin degradation products (FDP).[211] Complex clinical problems result from such disturbances of the clotting mechanism. Fibrinolytic activity is frequently increased in patients with paraproteinemia,[162,172,241,245] as demonstrated by raised FDP levels, lowered levels of normal inhibitors to streptokinase and urokinase, lowered antiplasmin levels, and abnormal euglobulin clot lysis or dilute blood clot lysis. In contrast, some patients have impairment of their fibrinolytic mechanism,[210,241] and this may contribute to thromboembolic complications.[27,81] As in other disease processes, whether the clinical expression is thromboembolism or hemorrhage depends upon the dynamic balance between increased fibrin deposition and increased fibrinolysis.

Patients with paraproteinemia are frequently subject to additional complications which may contribute to defective hemostasis.[199] These include renal failure, hepatic failure, and the effects of multiple blood transfusions or the administration of cytotoxic agents or salicylates. Plasmapheresis is an effective means of improving hemostasis when bleeding caused by coagulation factor abnormalities is a problem.[90,141,209,246] However, regular monitoring of coagulation function is essential during plasmapheresis because a reduction of normal coagulation factors may occur and necessitate replacement of the patient's plasma with fresh normal plasma.

Other Plasma Constituents

LIPOPROTEINS

The plasma lipids in myeloma are usually low or normal,[144,237] and the degree of atherosclerosis in myeloma is less severe than average.[249] Hyperlipidemia is a rare but well documented manifestation of paraproteinemia.[80] In some patients, the paraprotein has been shown to have autoantibody activity against the serum lipoprotein.[7,8,60,72]

Xanthomatosis has been seen in patients having hyperlipidemic[32,38,72,130,142,145,252] and normolipidemic paraproteinemia.[38,72,146] The xanthomas are typically of the soft eruptive variety and contain complexes of the paraprotein and lipoprotein.[110]

SODIUM

A low plasma sodium concentration has been found in about 8 percent of patients reported in one series of IgG myeloma.[107] It has been suggested that the sodium concentration is low either because the normal plasma water space is occupied by large amounts of paraprotein or because a high isoelectric point of the paraprotein allows it to act as a base at normal blood pH.[106]

COMPLEMENT

In some patients with an IgM paraprotein, depressions of the total serum hemolytic complement and of the first, second, and third complement components have been observed.[88] In a single patient with cold urticaria and an IgG-K cryoparaprotein[42,43] the induction of cold urticaria was accompanied by a drop in total serum complement and in the fourth (C_4) and third (C_3) complement components. In vitro studies demonstrated that the isolated cryoparaprotein inactivated both C_3 and C_4. One patient has been reported with a circulating 7S IgM which acted as an inhibitor of the first (C_1) complement component.[20]

Blood Viscosity

Many of the clinical features of paraproteinemia result from impairment of blood flow through the narrower vascular channels because of hyperviscosity of the blood.[151] A number of reviews of the factors affecting blood viscosity have recently

Table 13-7

Features of the Paraprotein Hyperviscosity Syndrome

Vascular Effects	Hypervolemia	Subjective Features	Disordered Hemostasis
Retina: Venous dilation and "trucking," retinal vein hemorrhages, and thromboses	Dilutional anemia Congestive cardiac failure	Lassitude, anorexia, muscle weakness	See Table 13-6
Central nervous system: headache, tinnitus, ataxia, dizziness, memory disturbance, thrombosis, coma.			
Peripheral Vasculature: Raynaud's phenomenon, claudication, gangrene			
Cardiac: cardiac failure			
Renal: renal failure			
Pulmonary: dyspnea, thromboembolism, pulmonary hypertension			
Skin and mucosa: subcutaneous and mucosal hemorrhages			
Venous system: edema, dependent plethora, varicose veins, deep vein thromboses			

been published.[19,53,158,216,248,271,272,276] These all stress the important role of immunoglobulins in the rheology of the blood. Paraproteinemia, by promoting cell-cell aggregation and protein-protein interaction, is a particularly potent cause of hyperviscosity, particularly when shear rates are low. Because of their physicochemical characteristics—especially size, shape, and intrinsic viscosity—19S IgM paraproteins and aggregated IgG_3 are more commonly associated with clinical hyperviscosity syndromes than are other immunoglobulins.[22,59,66,67,110,148,151] The clinical spectrum of the paraprotein hyperviscosity syndrome is illustrated in Table 13-7.

Because the retinal circulation is characterized by unique hemodynamic properties[116] any increase in blood viscosity tends to be apparent in it before other vascular beds. Distension, tortuosity and "trucking" of the retinal veins, multiple hemorrhages, venous occlusion, and papilledema are common accompaniments of hyperviscosity.[23,67,236,250,263] These changes may herald the onset of serious neurologic complications and indicate an urgent need for plasmapheresis to reduce the blood viscosity.[209,235]

The neurologic effects of blood hyperviscosity range in severity from headaches, tinnitus, vertigo, and ataxia, to coma.[59,67,148,263] Blood hyperviscosity may be the cause of otherwise unexplained neurologic symptoms or signs in any patient with paraproteinemia and must be considered, especially when the neurologic status is deteriorating. The problem is often urgent but the effects are rapidly reversible by plasmapheresis.[3,67,280]

Peripheral vascular insufficiency in paraproteinemia is also a direct result of blood hyperviscosity.[27,150,151] The temperature gradient at the periphery is an important factor in modifying the severity of vascular symptoms which may range from uncomplicated Raynaud's phenomenon to actual digital gangrene. Hyperviscosity due to paraproteinemia is a possible diagnosis whenever peripheral vascular insufficiency occurs suddenly in the presence of normal pulses.

Cardiac or renal failure may result from hyperviscosity and hypervolemia. Both conditions can be improved if the paraprotein concentration is reduced. The slow flow rates in the venous system, especially of the lower limbs, contribute to the clinical manifestations of the hyperviscosity syndrome, including edema, vague pains in the legs, varicose veins, and deep venous thromboses. Thromboembolism may be responsible for the respiratory symptoms and signs occasionally seen in these patients. Pulmonary capillary hyperviscosity and hypervolemia may contribute to a reduced pulmonary compliance and to ventilation-perfusion inequality as evidenced by impaired respiratory function tests.

Hypervolemia

A number of recent reports have stressed the association of paraproteinemia and blood hypervolemia.[104,147,151,258] A correlation has been found between the degree of blood viscosity in these patients and the increase in plasma volume. In plasma hypervolemia, the total red cell mass is greater than that predicted from the hematocrit and body weight. Attempts to increase the hematocrit by transfusion may, in these patients, result in a marked increase of viscosity, especially in vascular regions with low shear rates. This may be dangerous to the patient; therefore *whole blood* viscosity should be monitored during such procedures as plasmaphereses and blood transfusions.[138]

Cryoproteins

A number of paraproteins, especially of the IgM class, show a reversible precipitation on cooling.[17,150,220,263] The critical temperature for precipitation of such cryoproteins varies in different patients from $0°C$ to just below body temperature. The associated symptoms and signs are classically cold-dependent and resemble those due to hyperviscosity, with peripheral vascular insufficiency being the most prominent.

The molecular basis of the temperature-dependent solubility of cryoglobulins has not been explained. The mechanisms suggested include:

1. Polymerization through peptide and side-chain hydrogen bonds, hydrophobic bonds, and electrostatic forces.
2. Abnormalities in the chemical structure or spatial relationship of the molecules, resulting in insolubility at low temperatures through enhanced molecular polymerization.
3. Variations in the amount of carbohydrate associated with the polypeptide chains of the paraprotein molecules.
4. A deficiency of sulfhydryl groups in the globulins.

The presence of cryoglobulins often results in technical difficulties, for example, in blood crossmatching (see above). The interpretation of blood and bone marrow films and of tissue biopsies may be hindered by precipitation of the protein during preparation of the material. With marked cryoprecipitation the erythrocyte sedimentation rate if measured at room temperature, is relatively low, but paradoxically, it may rise if the amount of cryoprotein is reduced. Analyses of sera must be carried out at 37°C, for failure to observe this precaution may result in a marked reduction in the amount of paraprotein available for characterization, (see Fig. 13-2, Nos. 14-16).

Pyroglobulins

Paraproteins which precipitate on heating serum are termed *pyroglobulins*.[156,157,187-189,253] These proteins are very uncommon and are usually discovered after heating serum for serologic studies or by testing serum-containing paraproteins for heat lability in a search for such reactants. This property of heat precipitation has no known clinical significance.

AMYLOID

Amyloidosis[30,183] occurs more frequently in multiple myeloma than in most other neoplastic diseases, the reported incidence varying from 6-20 percent.[6,21,131,152] Amyloid in myeloma may be deposited in any organ or tissue. Its distribution in relation to blood vessels is more characteristically pericollagen than perireticulin in nature, in contrast to the amyloid associated with chronic infections. Amyloid in myeloma has also been noted in unusual sites such as the bone marrow,[136] pituitary,[66] intestine, skin, and skeletal muscle, including the tongue. Amyloid infiltration in cutaneous vessels may result in purpura (Table 13-6). Amyloid in association with macroglobulinemia is less common but has been reported.[15,33,75,148,218]

Recently, the immunoglobulin proteins have been shown to be the source of amyloid fibrils in many cases of human amyloidosis.[26,85-87] The amyloid proteins from different patients have been shown to share antigens with each other and with some coexisting Bence Jones proteins.[85,121] These immunochemical findings suggest that specific variable region sequences of the light chains are required for amyloid fibril formation. In myeloma patients with concurrent amyloidosis, the circulating paraproteins have been shown in one series to have a kappa- to lambda-chain ratio of about 2:3 and, in another series, of 1:2.[85,201] This is almost the reverse of the kappa- to lambda-light chain ratio of paraproteins in patients who have myeloma without amyloidosis. Lambda light chain may thus be more prone to form amyloid fibrils than kappa chains. Clinically, amyloid infiltration of the skin is to be differentiated from lichen myxedematosus (scleromyxedema). This condition is characterised by the presence of whitish, lichenoid macules in the skin which gradually coalesce and form plaques resulting in marked skin thickening together with a serum IgG paraprotein of very slow gamma mobility.[214]

RENAL DISEASE IN PARAPROTEINEMIA

Progressive renal insufficiency in paraproteinemia[64, 110] is a serious and common complication, but one which is largely preventable if the mechanisms are recognized. Clinically, it may present as acute renal insufficiency,[18, 205, 211] chronic renal failure, adult Fanconi syndrome with aminoaciduria, glycosuria, and hypophosphatemia,[101] renal tubular acidosis with reduced serum bicarbonate, hyperchloremia and hypokalemia,[164, 165] salt-losing nephritis, or nephrotic syndrome. Inexplicably, hypertension is a very uncommon component of the clinical spectrum associated with paraproteinemia.

When present in large amounts, Bence Jones protein may precipitate, forming casts of the renal tubules which result in tubular obstruction and interference with normal tubular cell function. Dehydration, as in fluid restriction in preparation for pyelography, and other causes of reduced renal blood flow, may lead to this complication in patients with Bence Jones proteinemia.

Urinary tract infections are common in paraproteinemias associated with lesions because of the impaired immunologic responses which have been described. The need for treatment is urgent because of the possibilities of both septicemia and progressive renal damage. Other factors which may contribute to renal insufficiency include amyloid deposition in the glomeruli and blood vessel walls, malignant cell infiltration of the kidney and the effects of hypercalcemia, rarely, with nephrocalcinosis. Hyperuricemia may be especially marked during effective cytotoxic therapy or radiotherapy. This may contribute to renal disease by causing nephrolithiasis, a predisposition to pyelonephritis, and the appearance of renal vascular complications. Renal tubular dysfunction presenting as the Fanconi syndrome or as renal tubular acidosis may be caused by direct interference with normal tubular cell function by the deposition of Bence Jones protein. Hyperviscosity in the renal microvasculature has also been considered as a possible factor in promoting tubular dysfunction. In a patient with myeloma who has received radiotherapy and who develops progressive renal insufficiency with proteinuria and hypertension, radiation nephritis must be considered.

In macroglobulinemia, clinical manifestations of renal damage are rare. The reported pathologic features of the kidney in this disease have included amyloidosis, intraglomerular deposits of IgM ("thrombi"),[166] interstitial lymphocytic and plasmacytic infiltration, and Bence Jones proteinuria.[263]

APPROACH TO PATIENTS WITH PARAPROTEIN

It will be apparent to the reader that a number of underlying diseases (see Table 13-2) may be associated with the finding of a paraprotein in the serum or urine, and the clinician's efforts must be directed toward distinguishing between these possibilities. From an analysis of many series,[109, 179, 193, 214, 283] some form of malignancy is likely to be responsible in 60–80 percent of patients.

The characteristics of the paraprotein itself—immunoglobulin class, concentration, the presence of immunoglobulin fragments (H or L chains)—and the degree of suppression of normal immunoglobulins are incomplete indicators of benignity or malignancy. The patient's history and physical examination may, of course, produce a self-evident diagnosis. Clinical features attributable to effects of paraproteins (see page 482) should be carefully assessed.

Laboratory investigations should include routine blood counts and chemical pathology tests. Diagnosis depends essentially on obtaining appropriate tissue for microscopy. Bone marrow may have to be aspirated from several sites, and histologic sections, as well as smears, may be useful because of the patchy distribution of myeloma in the medullary cavity. In the absence of peripheral lymph node enlargement, lymphangiography, venography or selective angiography may be of help in defining abnormal lymph nodes, especially in the abdomen. Skeletal surveys may localize certain myeloma deposits. Contrast studies of the gastrointestinal tract may reveal a carcinoma. Intravenous urography is risky in the patient with paraproteinemia, especially when Bence Jones protein is present, but such studies may be undertaken if strongly indicated, provided that the patient is not subjected to dehydration and the contrast dye is administered by slow intravenous infusion. In general, however, intravenous contrast dyes for any radiologic study carry grave risk of aggravating red cell aggregation in vivo, increasing whole blood hyperviscosity, and producing vascular occlusive episodes, especially in the brain or limbs.[151]

Lymph node biopsy, liver biopsy, or even laparotomy with splenectomy may be essential to achieve a diagnosis. By these means, one of the more common diseases will probably be diagnosed—myeloma, macroglobulinemia of Waldenström, lymphoma, or carcinoma. If no diagnosis has been reached, very careful follow-up of the patient is mandatory, even in that group of diseases which is provisionally considered benign, since transitions from benign to malignant forms are recognized. This involves close clinical supervision and regular examination of the serum for paraprotein concentration, and of the urine for the Bence Jones protein. In some patients, however, treatment directed toward reduction of concentration of the paraprotein will be necessary because of significant symptomatology attributable to the paraprotein such as hyperviscosity or cold-hemagglutinin disease.

The prognosis in the individual patient depends mainly on the prognosis of the underlying disease and less on the presence of the paraprotein. In myeloma, treatment (see Chapter 18) improves the survival unless irreversible renal or bone marrow failure is present. In macroglobulinemia, the prognosis is, in general, better than that in myeloma and is influenced predominantly by the degree and rate of infiltration of lymphoid tissues. In addition, the disease is more sensitive to chemotherapy and radiotherapy (see Chapter 18) than myeloma.

REFERENCES

1. Amos B (ed): Progress in Immunology, vol 1. New York, Academic Press, 1971.

2. Andersen E, Videbaek A: Stem cell leukaemia in myelomatosis. Scand J Haematol 7:201, 1970.

3. Bain B, Penny R: Multiple myeloma treated by plasmapheresis. Asian J. Med 7:435, 1971.

4. Ballard HS, Hamilton LM, Marcus AJ, Illes CH: A new variant of heavy chain disease (μ-chain disease). N Engl J Med 282:1060, 1970.

5. Barr DP, Reader GG, Wheeler CH: Cryoglobulinemia (report of two cases with discussion of clinical manifestations). Incidence and significance. Ann Intern Med 32:6, 1950.

6. Bayrd ED, Bennett WA: Amyloidosis complicating myeloma. Med Clin North Am 34:1151, 1950.

7. Beaumont J-L: Gamma-globulines et hyperlipidémies. L'hyperlipidémie par auto-anticorps. Ann Biol Clin (Paris) 27:611, 1969.

8. _____: Auto-immune hyperlipidemia. An atherogenic metabolic disease of immune origin. Rev Eur Etud Clin Biol 15:1037, 1970.

9. Bennich H, Johansson SGO: Structure and function of human immunoglobulin E. Adv Immunol 13:1, 1971.

10. Berg JW: Incidence of multiple primary cancers. 1. Development of further cancers in patients with lymphomas, leukemias and myeloma. J Natl Cancer Inst 38:741, 1967.

11. Bing J, Neal AV: Two cases of hyperglobulinaemia with affection of central nervous system on toxic-infectious basis. Acta Med Scand 88:492, 1936.

12. Bonomo L, Dammacco F, Marano R, Bonomo GM: Abdominal lymphoma and alpha chain disease: Report of three cases. Am J Med 52:73, 1972.

13. _____, _____, Tursi A, Trizio D: Waldenström's macroglobulinaemia with anti-IgG activity: A series of five cases. Clin Exp Immunol 6:531, 1970.

14. Borek F: Immunogenicity, in North-Holland Research Monographs: Frontiers of Biology, vol. 25. Amsterdam, North-Holland, 1972.

15. Brandt K, Cathcart ES, Cohen AS: Clinical study of 42 patients with amyloid disease. Am J Med 44:955, 1968.

16. Braunsteiner H, Oswald E, Pakesch F, Reimer E: Lymphoretikulosen mit Makroglobulinämie. Wien Z Inn Med 37:349, 1956.

17. Brouet JC, Clauvel JP, Danon F, Klein M, Seligmann M: Étude clinique et biologique des cryoglobulinémies. Actual Hématol 6:49, 1972.

18. Bryan CW, Healy JK: Acute renal failure in multiple myeloma. Am J Med 44:128, 1968.

19. Buxbaum J: Hyperviscosity syndrome in dysproteinemia. Am J Med Sci 264:123, 1972.

20. Caldwell JR, Ruddy S, Schur PH, Austen KF: Acquired CI inhibitor deficiency in lymphosarcoma. Clin Immunol Immunopathol 1:39, 1972.

21. Calkins E, Cohen AS: Diagnosis of amyloidosis. Bull Rheum Dis 10:215, 1960.

22. Capra JD, Kunkel HG: Aggregation of Gamma G_3 proteins: Relevance to the hyperviscosity syndrome. J Clin Invest 49:610, 1970.

23. Carr RE, Henkind P: Retinal findings associated with serum hyperviscosity. Am J Ophthalmol 56:23, 1963.

24. Carter PM, Hobbs JR: IgM in monoclonal IgM diseases. Br Med J 2:260, 1971.

25. Castaldi PA, Penny R: A macroglobulin with inhibitory activity against coagulation factor VIII. Blood 35:370, 1970.

26. Cathcart ES, Ritchie RF, Cohen AS, Brandt K: Immunoglobulins and amyloidosis. Am J Med 52:93, 1972.

27. Catovsky D, Ikoku NB, Pitney WR, Galton DAG: Thromboembolic complications in myelomatosis. Br Med J 3:438, 1970.

28. Cline MJ, Berlin NI: Studies of the anemia of multiple myeloma. Am J Med 33:510, 1962.

29. _____, Solomon A, Berlin NI, Fahey JL: Anemia in macroglobulinemia. Am J Med 34:213, 1963.

30. Cohen AS: Amyloidosis. N Engl J Med 277:522, 574, 628, 1967.

31. Cohen I, Yehuda B, Pick A, De Vries A: Plasma cell myeloma associated with an unusual myeloma protein causing impairment of fibrin aggregation and platelet function in a patient with multiple malignancies. Am J Med 48:766, 1970.

32. Cohen L, Blaisdell RK, Djordjevich J, Ormiste V, Dobrilovic L: Familial xanthomatosis and hyperlipidemia, and myelomatosis. Am J Med 40:299, 1966.

33. Cohen RJ, Bohannon RA, Wallerstein RO: Waldenström's macroglobulinemia: study of ten cases. Am J Med 41:274, 1966.

34. Coleman M, Vigliano EM, Weksler ME, Nachman RL: Inhibition of fibrin monomer polymerization by lambda myeloma globulins. Blood 39:210, 1972.

35. Cooke KB: Essential paraproteinaemia. Proc R Soc Med 62:777, 1969.

36. Cooper AG: Purification of cold agglutinins from patients with chronic cold haemagglutinin disease. Clin Exp Immunol 3:691, 1968.

37. _____, Hobbs JR: Immunoglobulins in chronic cold haemagglutinin disease. Br J Haematol 19:383, 1970.

38. Cooper DA, Penny R, Whitsed HM, Fiddes PJ, Warner NL, Whittingham S: Paraproteins with auto-antibody activity. Second Meeting, Asian-Pacific Congress of Haematology, Melbourne, 1971.

39. Cooper MD, Peterson RDA, South MA, Good RA: The functions of the thymus system and the bursa system in the chicken. J Exp Med 123:75, 1966.

40. Combined Staff Clinic: Plasma cell dyscrasias: Current clinical and biochemical concepts. Am J Med 44:256, 1968.

41. Cone L, Uhr JW: Immunological deficiency disorders associated with chronic lymphocytic leukemia and multiple myeloma. J Clin Invest 43:2241, 1964.

42. Costanzi JJ, Coltman CA: Kappa-chain cold-precipitable immunoglobulin G (IgG) associated with cold urticaria. Clin Exp Immunol 2:167, 1967.

43. ———, ———, Donaldson VH: Activation of complement by a monoclonal cryoglobulin associated with cold urticaria. J Lab Clin Med 74:902, 1969.

44. Craddock CG, Adams WS, Figueroa WG: Interference with fibrin formation in multiple myeloma by an unusual protein found in blood and urine. J Lab Clin Med 42:847, 1953.

45. ———, Longmire R, McMillan R: Lymphocytes and the immune response. N Engl J Med 285:324,378, 1971.

46. Curtain CC: Possible sites of macroglobulin synthesis—a study made with fluorescent antibody. Australas Ann Med 8:143, 1959.

47. Cwynarski MT, Cohen S: Polyclonal immunoglobulin deficiency in myelomatosis and macroglobulinaemia. Clin Exp Immunol 8:237, 1971.

48. Dameshek W, Schwartz R: Leukemia and autoimmunization—some possible relationships. Blood 14:1151, 1959.

49. Dartnall JA, Mundy GR, Baikie AG: Cytogenetic studies in myeloma. Blood 42:229, 1973.

50. Davies-Jones, GAB, Esiri MM: Neuropathy due to amyloid in myelomatosis. Br Med J 2:444, 1971.

51. Davis E, Landau J: Clinical capillary microscopy. Springfield, Ill., Thomas, 1966.

52. Delmas-Marsalet Y, Voisin D, Hennache G, Bauters F, Goudemand M: Étude clinique & biologique de la maladie des chaines lourdes gamma. A propos d'une nouvelle observation. Nouv Rev Fr Hématol 11:717, 1971.

53. Dintenfass L: Blood Microrheology-Viscosity Factors in Blood Flow, Ischaemia and Thrombosis. New York, Appleton-Century-Crofts, 1971.

54. Donnelly WJ, Grahn EP: Extraosseous manifestations of multiple myeloma. Med Clin N Am 49:229, 1965.

55. Doumenc J, Prost RJ, Somaina M, Bousser J: Anomalie de l'aggrégation plaquettaire au cours de la maladie de Waldenström. Nouv Rev Fr Hématol 6:734, 1966.

56. Drivsholm A: Myelomatosis: A clinical and biochemical study of 105 cases. Acta Med Scand 176:509, 1964.

57. Duggin GG, Penny R: Two cases of γD myeloma. Aust NZ J Med 1:72, 1971.

58. Editorial: Lymphoid stimulation and lymphoid neoplasia. Lancet 2:596, 1970.

59. Editorial: Hyperviscosity syndrome. Br Med J 2:184, 1971.

60. Editorial: Autoantibodies to serum lipoproteins. Br Med J 4:380, 1972.

61. Edwards GA, Zawadski ZA: Extraosseous lesions in plasma cell myeloma. Am J Med 43:194, 1967.

62. Eisen HN, Little JR, Osterland CK, Simms ES: A myeloma protein with antibody activity. Symp Quant Biol 32:75, 1967.

63. Ellman LL, Bloch KJ: Heavy chain disease: Report of a seventh case. N Engl J Med 278:1195, 1968.

64. Engle RL, Wallis LA: Para immunoglobulinopathies, in, Tice-Harvey Practice of Medicine, vol. 1. Springfield, Ill.: Thomas, 1965, p 301.

65. Evison G, Evans KT: Bone sclerosis in multiple myeloma. Br J Radiol 40:81, 1967.

66. Fahey JL: Serum protein disorders causing clinical symptoms in malignant neoplastic disease. J Chron Dis 16:703, 1967.

67. ———, Barth WF, Solomon A: Serum hyperviscosity syndrome. JAMA 192:464, 1965.

68. ———, Scoggins R, Utz FP, Szwed CF: Infection, antibody response and γ-globulin components in multiple myeloma and macroglobulinemia. Am J Med 35:698, 1963.

69. Farrow BRH, Penny R: Multiple myeloma in a cat. J Am Vet Med Assoc 158:606, 1971.

70. Favre-Gilly J, Greyssel R, Thouverez JP, Reval L, Croizat P: Antithrombine du type de l'héparine dans un gamma-myéloma; considerations sur les anticoagulants spontanés dans la maladie de Kahler. Hémostase 3:325, 1963.

71. Feinberg DH, Harlan WK: Amyloidosis of pituitary gland linked with multiple myeloma. Pa Med 64:761, 1961.

72. Feiwel M: Xanthomatosis in cryoglobulinaemia and other paraproteinaemias with report of a case. Br J Dermatol 80:719, 1968.

73. Fiddes P, Penny R, Castaldi P: Protein-induced bleeding. Med J Aust 2:667, 1971.

74. Fishkin BG, Orloff N, Scaduto LE, Borucki DT, Spiegelberg HL: IgE myeloma: A report of the third case. Blood 39:361, 1972.

75. Forget BG, Squires JW, Sheldon H: Waldenström's macroglobulinemia with generalised amyloidosis. Arch Intern Med 118:363, 1966.

76. Forte FA, Prelli F, Young WJ, Jerry LM, Kochwa S, Franklin EC, Kunkel HG: Heavy chain disease of the μ (γM) type: Report of the first case. Blood 38:137, 1970.

77. Franklin EC: Editorial: Heavy chain disease. N Engl J Med 282:1098, 1970.

78. ———: Some protein disorders associated with neoplasms of plasma cells and lymphocytes: Heavy chain diseases, in Amos B (ed): Progress in Immunology, vol. 1. New York, Academic Press, 1971, p 746.

79. ———, Lowenstein J, Byelow B, Meltzer M: Heavy chain disease—a new disorder of serum γ-globulins: Report of the first case. Am J Med 37:332, 1964.

80. Fredrickson DS, Levy RL, Rees RS: Fat transport in lipoproteins—an integrated approach to mechanisms and disorders. N Engl J Med 276:34, 1967.

81. Frick PG: Inhibition of conversion of fibrinogen to fibrin by abnormal proteins in multiple myeloma. Am J Clin Pathol 25:1263, 1955.

82. Fudenberg HH, Warner NL: Genetics of Immunoglobulin. Adv Genetics 1:131, 1970.

83. Gatti RA, Good RA: Aging, immunity and malignancy. Geriatrics 25:158, 1970.

84. Ginsberg DM: Circulating plasma cells in multiple myeloma. Ann Intern Med 57:843, 1962.

85. Glenner GG: The pathogenetic and therapeutic implications of the discovery of the immunoglobulin origin of amyloid fibrils. Hum Pathol 3:157, 1972.

86. ———, Ein D, Terry WD: The immunoglobulin origin of amyloid. Am J Med 52:141, 1972.

87. ———, Terry W, Harada M, Isersky C, Page D: Amyloid fibril proteins: Proof of homology with immunoglobulin light chains by sequence analysis. Science 171:1150, 1971.

88. Glovsky M, Fudenberg HH: Reduced complement activity in sera of patients with Waldenström's macroglobulinemia. J Immunol 104:1072, 1970.

89. Glueck HI, Hong R: A circulating anticoagulant in IgA multiple myeloma: its modification by penicillin. J Clin Invest 44:1866, 1965.

90. Godal HC, Borchgrevink CF: The effect of plasmapheresis on the hemostatic function in patients with macroglobulinemia Waldenström and multiple myeloma. Scand J Clin Lab Invest 17 (suppl 84):133, 1965.

91. Gordon RJ Jr: The preparation and properties of cold haemagglutinin. Immunology 71:220, 1953.

92. Grabar P, Burtin P: Immunoelectrophoretic analysis: Application to human biological fluids. Amsterdam, Elsevier, 1964.

93. Greaves MF, Hogg NM: Immunoglobulin determinants on the surface of antigen binding T- and B-lymphocytes in vivo, in Amos B (ed): Progress in Immunology, vol. 1. New York, Academic Press, 1971, p 111.

94. Grey HM, Kohler PF: A case of tetramer Bence Jones proteinaemia. Clin Exp Immunol 3:277, 1968.

95. ———, ———, Terry WD, Franklin EC: Human monoclonal G cryoglobulins with anti-γ globulin activity. J Clin Invest 47:1875, 1968.

96. Hällén J: Discrete gammaglobulin (M-) components in serum. Clinical study of 150 subjects without myelomatosis. Acta Med Scand Suppl. 462, 1966.

97. ———, Torsvik H: Protein abnormalities in the cold haemagglutinin syndrome. Scand J Haematol 6:416, 1969.

98. Harboe M, Van Furth R, Schubothe H, Lind K, Evans RS: Exclusive occurrence of k clones in isolated cold haemagglutinins. Scand J Haematol 2:259, 1965.

99. Harris JE, Alexanian R, Hersh EM, Migliore P: Immune function in multiple myeloma: impaired responsiveness to keyhole limpet hemocyanin. Can Med Assoc J 104:389, 1971.

100. Harris J, Bagai RC: Immune deficiency states associated with malignant disease in man. Med Clin N Am 56:501, 1972.

101. Harrison JF, Blainey JD: Adult Fanconi syndrome with monoclonal abnormality of immunoglobulin light chain. J Clin Pathol 20:42, 1967.

102. Heremans JF: A model for the development of immunocyte monoclones. Br Med J 2:319, 1971.

103. ———, Vaerman JP: Biological significance of IgA antibodies in serum and secretions, in Amos B (ed): Progress in Immunology, vol. 1. New York, Academic Press, 1971, p 875.

104. Herreman G, Piguet H, Zittoun R, Bilski-Pasquier G, Bousser J: L'Hypervolémie de la macroglobulinémie de Waldenström. Nouv Rev Fr Hématol 8:209, 1968.

105. Hirschboeck JS, and Woo M: A clinical evaluation of the "blood sludge" phenomenon. J Lab Clin Med 34:1609, 1949.

106. Hitzig WH: Clinical effects of anomalous serum globulins, in: Clinical Protein Chemistry, vol 1. New York, Karger, 1968, p 72.

107. Hobbs JR: Myelomatosis et al.—better understanding. Med News 10 November, 1967.

108. _____: Secondary antibody deficiency. Proc R Soc Med 61:883, 1968.

109. _____: Immunocytoma o' mice an' men. Br Med J 1:67, 1971.

110. _____: Immunoglobulins in clinical chemistry. Ann Rev Physical Chem 22:219, 1972.

111. _____, Corbett, AA: Younger age of presentation and extraosseous tumour in IgD myelomatosis. Br Med J 1:412, 1969.

112. _____, Jacobs A: Case Report—a half-molecule GK plasmacytoma. Clin Exp Immunol 5:199, 1969.

113. Hoffbrand AV, Hobbs JR, Kremenchuzky S, Mollin D: Incidence and pathogenesis of megaloblastic erythopoiesis in multiple myeloma. J Clin Pathol 20:699, 1967.

114. Holenberg CG, Hansson R: A case of granulocytopenia with cryoglobulinemia. Scand J Clin Lab Invest (suppl 69): 100, 1963.

115. Holt JM, Callendar STE, Robb-Smith AHT: Multiple myeloma: Development of alternative malignancy following successful chemotherapy. Br J Haematol 22:633, 1972.

116. Hollows FC: Retinal vascular throughput disorders. Trans Austr Coll Ophthalmol 2:20, 1970.

117. Hood LE: Two genes, one polypeptide chain—fact or fiction? Fed Proc 31:177, 1972.

118. Imhof JW, Baars H, Verloop MC: Clinical and haematological aspects of macroglobulinaemia of Waldenström. Acta Med Scand 163:349, 1959.

119. _____, Baillieux RE, Mul NAJ, Poen H: Monoclonal and diclonal gammopathies. Acta Med Scand (suppl. 445): 102, 1966.

120. Innes J, Newall J: Myelomatosis. Lancet 1:239, 1961.

121. Isersky C, Ein D, Page DL, Harada M, Glenner GG: Immunochemical cross reactions of human amyloid proteins with immunoglobulin light polypeptide chains. J Immunol 108:2,486, 1973.

122. Ishizaka K, Ishizaka T: Immunoglobulin E and homocytotropic properties, in Amos B (ed): Progress in Immunology, vol. 1. New York, Academic Press, 1971, p 859.

123. Issitt PD: I blood group system and its relation to other blood group systems. J Med Lab Technol 24:90, 1967.

124. Izam P, Paleirac G, Robinet M: La fonction thromboplastique plaquettaire au cours des dysglobulinémies. Nouv Rev Fr Hématol 6:729, 1966.

125. James TN, Monto RW, Rebuck JE: Thrombocytopenia and abnormal bleeding in multiple myeloma. Ann Intern Med 39:1281, 1953.

126. Jensen K, Jensen KB, Oleson H: Three M-components in serum from an apparently healthy person. Scand J Haematol 4:485, 1967.

127. Jerne NK: The somatic generation of immune recognition. Eur J Immunol 1:1, 1971.

128. Johansson BO: Prognostic factors in myelomatosis. Br Med J 2:327, 1971.

129. Josephson AS, Nicastri A, Price E, Biro L: Hμ chain fragment and monoclonal IgA in a lymphoproliferative disorder. Am J Med 54:127, 1973.

130. Kayden HT, Franklin EC, Rosenberg B: Interaction of myeloma gammaglobulin with human beta-lipoprotein. Circulation 26:639, 1962.

131. Kimball KG: Amyloidosis in association with neoplastic disease. Ann Intern Med 55:958, 1961.

132. Kissmeyer-Nielsen F, Jensen KB, Ersbak J: Severe haemolytic transfusion reactions caused by apparently compatible red cells. Br J Haematol 7:36, 1961.

133. Krick J A, Menache D: Anomalie de la polymérisation de la fibrine dans un cas de gamma-A myéloma. Nouv Rev Fr Hématol 6:744, 1966.

134. Krause RM, Haber E: Homogeneous antibody and myeloma proteins with antibody activity, in Amos B (ed.): Progress in Immunology, vol. 1. New York, Academic Press, 1971, p 1493.

135. Kritzman J, Kunkel HC, McCarthy J, Mellors RC: Studies of a Waldenström-type macroglobulin with rheumatoid factor properties. J Lab Clin Med 57:905, 1961.

136. Kyle RA, Pease GL, Richmond H, Sullivan L: Bone marrow aspiration in antemortem diagnosis of primary systemic amyloidosis. Am J Clin Pathol 45:252, 1966.

137. _____, Pierre RV, Bayrd ED: Multiple myeloma and acute myelomonocytic leukaemia. N Engl J Med 283:1121, 1970.

138. La Celle PL, Weed RI: The contribution of normal and pathologic erythrocytes to blood rheology. Prog Hematol 7:1, 1972.

139. Lachner H, Hunt V, Zucker MB, Pearson J: Abnormal fibrin ultrastructure polymerisation, and clot retraction in multiple myeloma. Br J Haematol 18:625, 1970.

140. Larrieu MJ, Beaumont JL, Caen J, Selig-
     mann M, Bernard J: Inhibition de la conver-
     sion du fibrinogène au cours d'un myélome.
     Rev. Fr Etude Clin Biol 3:617, 1958.

141. Lawson NS, Nosanchuk JS, Oberman HA,
     Meyers MC: Therapeutic plasmapheresis in
     treatment of patients with Waldenström's
     macroglobulinaemia. Transfusion 8:174,
     1968.

142. Lennard Jones JE: Myelomatosis with
     lipaemia and xanthomata. Br Med J 1:781,
     1960.

143. Levin WC, Ritzmann SE: Relation of ab-
     normal proteins to formed elements of
     blood: effects upon erythrocytes, leukocytes
     and platelets. Ann Rev Med 17:323, 1966.

144. Lewis LA, Page IH: Serum proteins and
     lipoproteins in multiple myelomatosis. Am
     J Med 17:670, 1954.

145. _____, _____: An unusual serum lipopro-
     tein-globulin complex in a patient with
     hyperlipemia. Am J Med 38:286, 1965.

146. Lynch PJ, Winkelmann RK: Generalized
     plane xanthoma and systemic disease. Arch
     Dermatol 93:639, 1966.

147. Mackenzie MR, Brown E, Fudenberg HH,
     Goodenday L: Waldenström's macroglobu-
     linemia: Correlation between expanded
     plasma volume and increased serum vis-
     cosity. Blood 35:394, 1970.

148. _____, Fudenberg HH: Macroglobu-
     linemia: An analysis of forty patients. Blood
     39:874, 1972.

149. McCallister BD, Bayrd ED, Harrison EG
     Jr, McGuckin WF: Primary macroglobu-
     linemia. Am J Med 43:394, 1967.

150. McGrath MA, Penny R: Haemorheological
     features of cryoproteinaemia (Abstract).
     Proc Austr Soc Med Res 3:55, 1972.

151. _____, _____: Hyperviscosity syndrome
     in paraproteinaemia (Abstract). Austr NZ J
     Med 3:2,223, 1973.

152. Magnus-Levy A: Amyloidosis in multiple
     myeloma. J Mt Sinai Hos 19:8, 1952.

153. Maldonado J, Bayrd ED, Brown AL: The
     flaming cell in multiple myeloma. A light
     and electron microscopy study. Am J Clin
     Pathol 44:605, 1965.

154. Mangalik A, Veliath AJ: Osteosclerotic
     myeloma and peripheral neuropathy: A case
     report. Cancer 28:1040, 1971.

155. Marmont AM, Fusco FA, Gay A, Mariotti
     L: Intravascular erythrocyte aggregation
     "sludged blood" in multiple myeloma. Acta
     Haematol 18:49, 1957.

156. Martin WJ, Mathieson DR: Pyroglobu-
     linemia. An unusual presenting sign in mul-
     tiple myeloma. Proc Staff Meet Mayo Clin
     28:545, 1953.

157. _____, _____, Eigler JDC: Pyroglobu-
     linemia. Further observations and review of
     20 cases. Proc Staff Meet Mayo Clin 34:95,
     1959.

158. Merrill EW: Rheology of blood. Physiol
     Rev 49:863, 1969.

159. Metzger H: Myeloma proteins and anti-
     bodies. Am J Med 47:837, 1969.

160. Meyers BR, Hirschman SZ, Axelrod JA:
     Current pattern of infection in multiple
     myeloma. Am J Med 52:87, 1972.

161. Miller JFAP, Osaba D: Current concepts of
     the immunological function of the thymus.
     Physiol Rev 47:437, 1967.

162. Mohler ER, Kennedy JN, Brakman P:
     Blood coagulation and fibrinolysis in mul-
     tiple myeloma. Am J Med Sci 253:325,
     1967.

163. Moossy J, Wilson CB: Solitary intracranial
     plasmacytoma. Arch Neurol 16:212, 1967.

164. Morris JC, Fudenberg HH: Impaired renal
     acidification in patients with hypergamma-
     globulinemia. Medicine 46:57, 1967.

165. Morris JC: Renal tubular acidosis
     mechanisms: Classification and implica-
     tions. N Engl J Med 281:1405, 1969.

166. Morel-Maroger L, Basch A, Danon F, Ver-
     roust P, Richet G: Pathology of the kidney
     in Waldenstrom's macroglobulinaemia. N
     Engl J Med 283:123, 1970.

167. Moulinier J, Leger H: Apparition d'un an-
     ticoagulant circulant au stade de générali-
     sation d'un plasmocytome initialement lo-
     calisé aux vois aéro-digestives supérieures.
     Nouv Rev Fr Hématol 6:749, 1966.

168. Mundy GR: DNA values in myeloma.
     Cancer, 32:61, 1973.

169. _____, Baikie AG: Myeloma treated with
     cyclophosphamide and terminating in re-
     ticulum cell sarcoma. Med J Austr 1:1240–
     1241, 1973.

170. Nathanson L, Schiller A: Case records of
     the Massachusetts General Hospital. Pe-
     ripheral neuropathy with osteoblastic le-
     sions. N Engl J Med 287:138, 1972.

171. Niléhn JE: On symptomatic antihaemo-
     philic globulin (AHF) deficiency. Acta Med
     Scand 171:490, 1962.

172. _____, Nilsson IM: Coagulation studies in
     different types of myeloma. Acta Med
     Scand 179 (suppl 445):194, 1966.

173. Nisonoff A, Wilson SK, Wang AC, Fuden-
     berg HH, Hopper JE: Genetic control of the
     biosynthesis of IgG and IgM, in Amos B
     (ed): Progress in Immunology, vol. 1. New
     York, Academic Press, 1971, p 61.

174. Norgaard O: Three cases of multiple myeloma in which the preclinical asymptomatic phases persisted throughout 15 to 24 years. Br J Cancer 25:417, 1971.

175. Nutter DD, Kramer NC: Macrocryogelglobulinemia. Am J Med 38:462, 1965.

176. Ogawa M, Kochwa S, Smith C, Ishizaka K, McIntyre OR: Clinical aspects of IgE myeloma. N Engl J Med 281:1217, 1969.

177. Oksala A: Intravascular aggregation of erythrocytes in some eye diseases. Acta Ophthalmol 35:393, 1957.

178. Osserman EF: Plasma cell myeloma. II. Clinical aspects. N Engl J Med 261:952, 1006, 1959.

179. _____: Multiple myeloma and related plasma cell dyscrasias, in Samter M (ed): Immunological Diseases (2nd Edition). Boston, Little, Brown, 1971, p 520.

180. _____: Clinical patterns of the plasma cell dyscrasias, in Beeson, PB, McDermott W (eds.): Cecil-Loeb Textbook of Medicine (ed 13). Philadelphia, Saunders, 1971, p 1581.

181. _____, Takatsuki K: Plasma cell myeloma. Medicine 42:357, 1963.

182. _____, _____: Clinical and immunochemical studies of four cases of heavy (Hγ2) chain disease. Am J Med 37:351, 1964.

183. _____, _____, Talal N: The pathogenesis of "amyloidosis": Studies on the role of abnormal gamma globulins and gamma globulin fragments of the Bence Jones (1-polypeptide) type in the pathogenesis of "primary" and "secondary amyloidosis" and the "amyloidosis" associated with plasma cell myeloma. Sem Hematol 1:3, 1964.

184. Ouchterlony O: Handbook of Immunodiffusion and Immunoelectrophoresis. Ann Arbor: Ann Arbor–Humphrey, 1968.

185. Pachter MR, Johnson SA, Basinski DH: The effect of macroglobulins and their dissociation units on release of platelet factor 3. Thromb Diath Haemorrh 3:501, 1959.

186. _____, _____, Neblett TR, Truaur JP: Bleeding, platelets and macroglobulinemia. Am J Clin Pathol 31:467, 1959.

187. Patterson, R, Nelson VL, Pruzansky JJ: Pyroglobulinemia: Some characteristics of a heat labile protein. Immunology 9:477, 1965.

188. _____, Roberts M, Pruzansky JJ: Studies of heat precipitable immunoglobulins. Clin Exp Immunol 7:657, 1970.

189. _____, Weiszer I, Rambach W, Roberts M, Suszko IM: Comparative cellular and immunochemical studies of two cases of pyroglobulinemia. Am J Med 44:147, 1968.

190. Pear BL: The plasma cell in radiology. Am J Roentgenol. Radium Ther Nucl Med 102:908, 1968.

191. Penn I, Halgrimson CG, Starzl TE: De Novo malignant tumors in organ transplant recipients. Transplant Proc 3:773, 1971.

192. Penny R: Functional aspects of disordered immunoglobulins. Med J Austr 2:515, 1969.

193. _____: Paraprotein patterns in Australia. Australas Ann Med 18:251, 1969.

194. _____: A study of neutrophil function in health and disease. M.D. Thesis, Sydney University, Sydney, Australia.

195. _____, Castaldi PA: Correlative studies on effects of M-protein, in Proceedings of the Twelfth Congress of the International Society of Hematology, 1968, p 133.

196. _____, _____, Whitsed HM: Inflammation and haemostasis in paraproteinaemias. Br J Haematol 20:35, 1971.

197. _____, Galton DAG: Studies on neutrophil function: II. Pathological aspects. Br J Haematol 12:633, 1966.

198. _____, Hughes S: Repeated stimulation of the reticuloendothelial system and the development of plasma cell dyscrasias. Lancet 1:77, 1970.

199. Perkins HA, Mackenzie MR, Fudenberg HH: Hemostatic defects in dysproteinemias. Blood 35:695, 1970.

200. Perry S: Coagulation factors in patients with plasma protein disorders. J Lab Clin Med 61:411, 1963.

201. Pick AI, Osserman EF: Amyloidosis associated with plasma cell dyscrasias, in Mondema E, Ruinen L, Scholten JH, Cohen AS, (eds.): Amyloidosis. Amsterdam; Excerpta Medica, 1968, p 100.

202. Pink R, Wang AC, Fudenberg HH: Antibody variability. Ann Rev Med 22:145, 1971.

203. Pitts NC, McDuffie FC: Defective synthesis of IgM antibodies in macroglobulinaemia. Blood 30:767, 1967.

204. Porter RR: The antigen binding sites of immunoglobulins, in Inman FP (ed.): Contemporary Topics in Immunochemistry, vol. 1. New York–London, Plenum Press, 1972.

205. Porush JG, Grishman E, Alter A, Mandelbaum H, Churg J: Paraproteinemia and cryoglobulinemia associated with atypical glomerulonephritis and the nephrotic syndrome. Am J Med 47:957, 1969.

206. Potter M: Myeloma proteins (M-

components) with antibody-like activity. N Engl J Med 284:831, 1971.

207. _____: Plasma cell tumour-formation and antigen-binding myeloma proteins in mice. Br Med J 2:319, 1971.

208. _____: Immunoglobulin-producing tumours and myeloma proteins of mice. Physiol Rev 52:631, 1972.

209. Powles R, Smith C, Kohn J, Fairley GH: Method of removing abnormal protein rapidly from patients with malignant paraproteinaemias. Br Med J 2:664, 1971.

210. Preston FE, Lee D: Fibrinolysis in myelomatosis. Acta Haematol 47:65, 1972.

211. _____, Milford-Ward A: Acute renal failure in myelomatosis from intravascular coagulation. Br Med J 1:604, 1972.

212. Preud'homme JL, Seligmann M: Surface-bound immunoglobulins as a cell marker in human lymphoproliferative diseases. Blood 50:777, 1972.

213. Proga C, Jean G, Cartellaro M: Anomalie de la formation du caillot dans un cas de IgG myélome. Nouv Rev Fr Hématol 7:353, 1967.

214. Pruzanski W, Ogryzlo M: The changing pattern of disease associated with M components. Med Clin N Am 56:371, 1972.

215. _____, Platts ME, Ogryzlo M: Leukemic form of immunocytic dyscrasia (plasma cell leukemia). Am J Med 47:60, 1969.

216. _____, Watt JG: Serum viscosity and hyperviscosity syndrome in IgG multiple myeloma. Ann Intern Med 77:853, 1972.

217. Pudlák P, Vorlová Z, Farská I, Deimlová E: Coagulation changes in multiple myeloma. Folia Haematol (Leipz) 82:400, 1965.

218. Ranlov P, Elling Nielson P: Systemic (primary) amyloidosis associated with IgM (β_2M) paraproteinemia: Biochemical, histochemical, and immunohistochemical investigations. Acta Pathol Microbiol Scand 66:154, 1966.

219. Rebuck JW, Crowley JH: A method of studying leukocytic functions in vivo. Ann NY Acad Sci 39:757, 1955.

220. Ritzmann SE, Levin WC: Cryopathies: A review. Arch Intern Med 107:186, 1961.

221. _____, _____: Polyclonal and monoclonal gammopathies, in Dettelbach HR, Ritzmann SE, (eds.): Laboratory Synopsis. Kansas City, Missouri, Hoechst, 1967, p 9.

222. Robbins R: Familial multiple myeloma: The tenth reported occurrence. Am J Med Sci 254:848, 1967.

223. Roge J, Druet P, Marche C: Lymphome meditérranéen avec maladie des chaines alpha. Triple rémission clinique, anat-

omique et immunologique. Pathol Biol 18:851, 1970.

224. Roitt IM, Greaves MF, Torrigiani G, Brostoff J, Playfair JHL: The cellular basis of immunological responses. Lancet 2:367, 1969.

225. Rowlands S, Skibo L: The morphology of red cell aggregates. Thromb Res 1:47, 1972.

226. Rozenberg MC, Dintenfass L: Platelet aggregation in Waldenström's macroglobulinaemia. Thromb Diath Haemorrh 14:202, 1965.

227. Salmon SE: Immunoglobulin synthesis and tumour cell number and the natural history of multiple myeloma. Br Med J 2:319, 1971.

228. _____, Fudenberg HH: Abnormal nucleic acid metabolism of lymphocytes in plasma cell myeloma and macroglobulinaemia. Blood 33:300, 1969.

229. _____, McIntyre OR, Ogawa M: IgE myeloma: total body tumour cell number and synthesis of IgE and DNA. Blood 37:696, 1971.

230. Saunders TE, Podos SM, Rosenbaum LJ: Intraocular manifestations of multiple myeloma. Arch Ophthalmol 77:789, 1967.

231. Scamps RA, O'Neill BJ, Newland RC: A case of multiple myeloma terminating with acute myelomonocytic leukaemia. Med J Austr 2:1129, 1971.

232. Schubothe H: Serologische und klinische befunde bei patienten mit Kryogelproteinämie. Schweiz Med Wochenschr 88:1035, 1958.

233. _____: The cold haemagglutinin disease. Sem Haematol 3:1, 1966.

234. Schur PH: Human Gamma-G subclasses, in Schwartz RS (ed.): Progress in Clinical Immunology, vol. 1. New York, Grune & Stratton, 1972, p 71.

235. Schwab PJ, Fahey JL: Treatment of Waldenström's macroglobulinemia by plasmapheresis. N Engl J Med 263:574, 1960.

236. _____, Okun E, Fahey JL: Reversal of retinopathy in Waldenström's macroglobulinemia by plasmapheresis. Arch Ophthalmol 64:67, 1960.

237. Seitanidis BA, Schulman G, Hobbs JR: Low serum cholesterol with IgA myelomatosis. Clin Chim Acta 29:93, 1970.

238. Seligmann M, Danon F, Basch A, Bernard J: IgG myeloma cryoglobulin with antistreptolysin activity. Nature 220:711, 1968.

239. _____, _____, Hurez D, Mihaesco E, Preud'homme, JL: Alpha-chain disease: A new immunoglobulin abnormality. Science 162:1396, 1968.

240. _____, Mihaesco E, Hurez D, Mihaesco C, Preud'homme JL, Rambaud JC: Immunochemical studies in 4 cases of α chain disease. J Clin Invest 48:2374, 1969.

241. Senchez-Avalos J, Soong BCF, Miller SP: Coagulation disorders in cancer. II. Multiple myeloma. Cancer 23:1388, 1969.

242. Sharma KD, Shrivastav JD: Extramedullary plasmacytoma of the gastrointestinal tract. Arch Pathol 71:229, 1961.

243. Silverstein A, Doniger DE: Neurologic complications of myelomatosis. Arch Neurol 9:534, 1963.

244. Simmons P, Penny R, Goller I: Plasma proteins— A review. Med J Austr 2:494, 1969.

245. Sirridge MS, Bowman KS, Garber PE: Fibrinolysis and changes in fibrinogen in multiple myeloma. Arch Intern Med 101:630, 1958.

246. Solomon A, Fahey JL: Plasmapheresis therapy in macroglobulinemia. Ann Intern Med 58:789, 1963.

247. _____, Waldmann TA, Fahey JL: Metabolism of normal 6.6 γ-globulin in normal subjects and in patients with macroglobulinemia and multiple myeloma. J Lab Clin Med 62:1, 1963.

248. Somer T: The viscosity of blood, plasma and serum in dys- and para-proteinaemias. Acta Med Scand 180 (suppl 456):1, 1966.

249. Spain DM, Greenblatt IJ, Snapper I, Cohn T: Degree of coronary and aortic atherosclerosis in necropsied cases of multiple myeloma. Am J Med Sci 231:165, 1956.

250. Spalter HF: Abnormal serum proteins and retinal vein thrombosis. Arch Ophthalmol 62:868, 1959.

251. Spiegelberg HL: γD immunoglobulin, in Inman FP (ed.): Current Topics in Immunochemistry, vol. 1. New York-London, Plenum Press, 1972, p 165.

252. Spikes JL, Cohen L, Djordjevich J: The identification of a myeloma serum factor which alters serum beta lipoproteins. Clin Chim Acta 20:413, 1968.

253. Stefanini M, McDonnell E, Andracki E, Swansbro WJ, Durr P: Macropyroglobulinemia: Immunochemical studies in three cases. Am J Clin Pathol 54:94, 1970.

254. Stevenson GT: Detection in normal urine of protein resembling Bence Jones protein. J Clin Invest 39:1192, 1960.

255. Strisower EH, Galleto AT: Waldenström's macroglobulinemia. Am J Med 32:304, 1962.

256. Stoop JW, Ballieux RE, Hijmans W, Zegers BJM: Alpha-chain disease with involvement of the respiratory tract in a Dutch child. Clin Exp Immunol 9:625, 1971.

257. Terry WD, Boyd MM, Rea JS, Stein R: Human M-proteins with antibody activity for nitrophenyl ligands. J Immunol 104:256, 1970.

258. Thorling EB: Dilution anaemia. Acta Pathol Microbiol Scand (Sect. A) 78:231, 1970.

259. Viala JJ, Thouverez JP, Belleville J, Revol L Croizat P: Étude de la coagulation du sang au cours des dysglobulinémies myélomes et maladie de Waldenström a propos de 48 observations. Hémostase 3:303, 1963.

260. Vigliano EM, Horowitz HI: Bleeding syndrome in a patient with IgA myeloma: Interaction of protein and connective tissue. Blood 29:823, 1967.

261. Wager O, Räsänen JA, Haltia K, Wasastjerna C: M components with antibody activity: Antismooth muscle, antithyroglobulin and antistreptolysin O activity in 5 M component sera. Ann Clin Res 3:86, 1971.

262. _____, _____, Lindeberg GL, Mäkelä V: Two cases of IgG heavy chain disease. Acta Pathol Microbiol Scand 75:350, 1969.

263. Waldenström J: Macroglobulinaemia. Adv Metab Disord 2:115, 1965.

264. Waldmann TA, Strober W, Blease RM: Metabolism of immunoglobulins, in Amos B (ed.): Progress in Immunology, vol. 1. New York, Academic Press, 1971, p 891.

265. Walsh JC: The neuropathy of multiple myeloma. Arch Neurol 25:404, 1971.

266. Weiner LP, Anderson PN, Allen JC: Cerebral plasmacytoma with myeloma protein in the cerebrospinal fluid. Neurology 16:615, 1966.

267. Weintraub LR, Galdabini JJ: Case records of the Massachusett's General Hospital. Monoclonal gammopathy and hyperviscosity. N Engl J Med 287:243, 1972.

268. Weiss HJ, Kochwa S: Antihaemophilic globulin (AHG) in multiple myeloma and macroglobulinaemia. Br J Haematol 14:205, 1968.

269. Weitzel RA: Carcinoma coexistent with malignant disorders of plasma cells—an autopsy survey. Cancer 11:546, 1958.

270. Wells JV: The nature and metabolism of serum immunoglobulins in clinical syndromes. M.D. Thesis, University of New South Wales, Sydney, Australia, 1969.

271. Wells R: Syndromes of hyperviscosity. N Engl J Med 283:183, 1970.

272. Wells RE: Rheology of blood in the microvasculature. N Engl J Med 270:832, 1964.

273. Welton J, Walker SR, Sharp GC, Herzenberg LA, Wistar R Jr, Creger WP: Macroglobulinemia with bone destruction. Am J Med 44:280, 1968.

274. Whitmore RL: Rheology of The Circulation. London, Pergamon Press, 1968.

275. Whitsed HM, Penny R: IgA/IgG cryoglobulinaemia with vasculitis. Clin Exp Immunol 9:183, 1971.

276. Williams RC: Editorial: Hyperviscosity syndromes. Circulation 38:450, 1968.

277. Williamson AR: Biosynthesis of antibodies. Nature 231:359, 1971.

278. Wiltshaw E: Extramedullary plasmacytoma. Myeloma Workshop. Br Med J 2:327, 1971.

279. Wintrobe MM: Clinical Hematology (ed 6). London, Kimpton, 1967.

280. Wolf RE, Alperin JB, Ritzmann SE, Levin WC: IgG–K–multiple myeloma with hyperviscosity syndrome—response to plasmapheresis. Arch Intern Med 129:114, 1972.

281. Young VH: Transient paraproteins. Proc R Soc Med 62:30, 1969.

282. Zawadski ZA, Benedek TG, Eid D, Easton JM: Rheumatoid arthritis terminating in heavy chain disease. Ann Intern Med 70:335, 1969.

283. _____, Edwards GA: Nonmyelomatous monoclonal immunoglobulinemia, in Schwartz RS (ed.): Progress in Clinical Immunology, vol. 1. New York, Grune & Stratton, 1972, p 105.

284. Zettervall O, Sjöquist J, Waldenström J, Winblad S: Serological activity in myeloma-type globulins. Clin Exp Immunol 1:213, 1966.

285. Ziegler JB, Penny R, Hansen P: Unpublished observations.

286. Zinneman HH, Hall WH: Recurrent pneumonia in multiple myeloma and some observations on immunological response. Ann Intern Med 41:1152, 1954.

287. Zlotnick A, Robinson E: Chronic lymphatic leukaemia associated with macroglobulinaemia. Israel J Med Sci 16:365, 1970.

14

Special Clinical and Laboratory Features
of Leukemia

ANEMIA

In time, every patient with leukemia develops anemia. Often anemia is the symptom which first brings him to medical attention; at this stage, leukemic changes are usually, but not invariably, present in the blood. If they are not, the underlying cause of the anemia may be overlooked, and, even if it is suspected, the diagnosis of leukemia may be difficult to prove. Months or sometimes years may elapse before such *preleukemic*, perhaps better called *undiagnosable* cases reveal their true nature.

Another group of patients may show obvious clinical signs such as enlargement of the lymph nodes or the spleen, and these may be accompanied by a characteristic leukemic leukocyte count, but not by anemia. Anemia may occur early in the course of chronic granulocytic leukemia, but it does not usually become severe until the disease is far advanced. In chronic lymphocytic leukemia it is often a late symptom, but once it appears there is usually rapid progression. The anemia of acute leukemia usually appears early and worsens rapidly.

In this section, we are concerned with the question how the anemia is produced. The answer formerly given was that the proliferating leukocytes in the marrow displace or "crowd out" the nucleated red cells until eventually very little erythropoietic tissue is left. This beguilingly simple explanation must be viewed with some caution, for if it represented the whole truth, it would have to account for the very different types of anemia of early and late leukemia, and would need to be applicable whatever the form of leukemia or of the hematologic changes which occur. We have much evidence that the crowding-out mechanism is incapable of doing this.

There are at least five mechanisms which could theoretically be involved in the causation of the anemia of leukemia:

1. Displacement or crowding out of erythropoiesis by rapidly proliferating leukemic leukocytes.
2. Inhibition of erythropoiesis, or competition by leukocytes for metabolites essential for erythropoiesis.

3. Hemolysis or excessive destruction of mature red cells.
4. Hemorrhage as a result of clotting difficulties or from other causes.
5. Interference with erythropoiesis by agents used in the treatment of leukemia.

These various mechanisms could act singly or in combination. The evidence bearing on these points will now be briefly reviewed.

The Crowding Out of Erythroblasts

This is the most commonly used explanation for the anemia of leukemia. When leukemic marrow is examined, there is generally a gross increase in the type-specific leukocytes, while erythroblasts appear to be much diminished in numbers. This is particularly so in untreated cases of chronic granulocytic and in acute leukemia. In chronic lymphocytic leukemia, the erythroid cells are only slightly diminished in the early stages in which anemia is absent, but as leukemic infiltration increases, erythroblasts diminish, and anemia appears as the disease progresses.[230]

Although there are indeed cases in which the development of anemia appears to run parallel with the gradual disappearance of the erythroid precursors in the marrow, the microscopic picture does not necessarily present the full story. In the first place, in examining the marrow, one generalizes from inspection of only a tiny sample of an organ which is as bulky as the liver, even when normal, and reaches a much more formidable size in leukemia. Thus, it may be that although the relative *proportion* of erythroblasts is quite low in any individual slide, the total *aggregate* may be little, if at all, diminished. Moreover, in some marrow counts, the percentage of erythroid cells is not diminished but may be as high as, or even higher than in normal marrow (Fig. 14-1).[91,113] Microscopic inspection of the marrow may

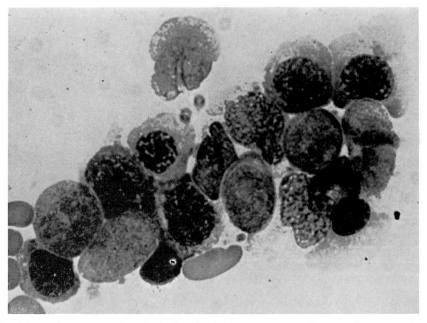

Fig. 14-1. Acute granulocytic leukemia. Marrow sample shows a large number of erythroblasts as well as myeloblasts ($\times$ 2000).

thus give an impression which either under- or overestimates the extent of erythropoiesis. This has been emphasized by Nathan and Berlin in their studies of the functional capacity of the marrow by determinations of plasma and red cell iron turnover.[157] By these means, it has been shown that in a number of cases of leukemia there is an actual increase in erythropoiesis; that in others, erythopoiesis, while very active, is ineffective in turning out a sufficient number of normal red cells; while in yet others, it is definitely decreased or even absent.[28,30,110,157,237] These and other studies indicate that the mechanism resulting in the anemia is by no means the same in all cases of leukemia.

Ineffective Erythropoiesis—Involvement of Red Cell Precursors in the Leukemic Process

Anemia occurs in some cases of leukemia, particularly the acute granulocytic type, although the marrow contains what appears to be normal or increased numbers of erythroblasts, and although excessive hemolysis cannot be demonstrated. *Ineffective erythropoiesis* is a concept invoked in such patients.[28] This is characterized by the combination of a normal or increased iron turnover, as measured by radioiron studies, and of a greatly decreased incorporation of iron into the mature red cells. Erythropoietin production is raised in such patients, but the marrow fails to respond normally to the hormone.[3] These findings are analogous to those in pernicious anemia and in some of the so-called refractory, sideroblastic, or sideroachrestic anemias.[54,99] According to a recent report there may be differences in erythropoietin production between the several types of acute leukemia.[244]

The mechanism causing the disturbance in ferrokinetics in these patients appears to be complex. There are abnormalities in the cell cycle of the dividing erythroblasts, especially a slowing of DNA synthesis, often with a partial arrest of cells before mitosis: these abnormalities, in turn, lead to difficulties in the process of mitosis itself.[147,240] Some of the erythroid cells may proceed to maturation with omission of concomitant cell divisions.[80] Finally, there may be an absolute shortage of stem cells committed to normal erythropoiesis. The long-held belief that granulocytic and erythroid cells are derived from a common stem cell has been confirmed in recent years by the demonstration, both by direct[181] and indirect[238] means, that the Philadelphia (Ph[1]) chromosome in chronic granulocytic leukemia is contained in the erythroid, as well as the granulocytic precursors. This can only mean that the mutation which led to the formation of the Ph[1] must have occurred in a common ancestral cell. In acute leukemia, less evidence points in the same direction, that of a single stem cell which gives rise to both the red and white cell series.[116] Two consequences may be expected to follow: First, there may be competition among the red and white cell series for the limited common supply of multipotent stem cells[134]; and second, the red cell series may itself be involved in the leukemic process, both in chronic granulocytic and in at least some cases of acute granulocytic leukemia. Anemia may be expected to be produced by both mechanisms.

As discussed in Chapter 11, there is good evidence that the abnormal megaloblastoid erythroblasts found in the Di Guglielmo syndrome are neoplastic—that is, leukemic—cells. It seems likely however, that the same is true also of many of the morphologically less abnormal or seemingly normal erythroblasts which are found, sometimes in large numbers, in other forms of acute granulocytic leukemia in relapse. Further circumstantial evidence supporting this view has recently come from the discovery that the red cells in many cases of leukemia are abnormally sensitive to cold-antibody lysis.[43] It is, in fact, difficult to draw a clear distinction between the Di Guglielmo syndrome and other forms of acute granulocytic leukemia, and frequent transitions are found. The realization that there is probably a common leukemic stem cell has supplied a plausible explanation for these long-known facts.

The question whether sideroblastic anemia is itself a malignant condition akin to the Di Guglielmo syndrome has been previously discussed.[57] (see Chapter 11). While the transition from sideroblastic anemia to overt acute leukemia is rare, there are a number of patients on record in whom it undoubtedly took place.[8,24,206] Moreover, abnormal clones have been found by cytogenetic methods in the marrow in cases of refractory sideroblastic anemia in which the transition to leukemia had not yet occurred, as judged by the usual criteria (Fig. 14-2).[63] It seems evident that there is a close relationship between the sideroblastic anemias and acute leukemias, especially the Di Guglielmo type: clearly, too, the mechanism of the anemia must be similar.

Finally, it is possible that paroxysmal nocturnal hemoglobinuria (PNH) may also fall into the same group as pointed out by Dameshek.[58,59] This rare condition, which spans the gap between the refractory and the hemolytic anemias, has been found at times to precede acute granulocytic leukemia[108,115,121] or the Di Guglielmo syndrome.[41] Paroxysmal nocturnal hemoglobinuria, too, is a panmyelopathy rather

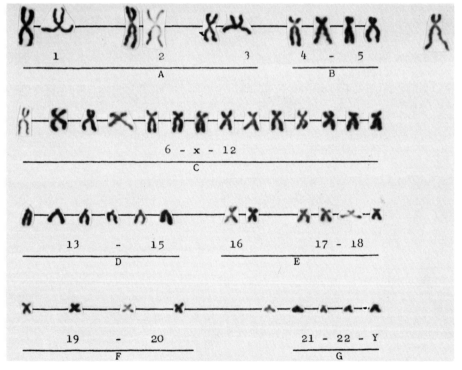

Fig. 14-2. Karyotype from patient with refractory sideroblastic anemia shows an abnormal marker chromosome. This chromosome characterized an abnormal clone which was known to be present for 18 months before this patient's death.

than a pure red cell dyscrasia. Of all the mechanisms concerned in the production of anemia in the leukemias, that succinctly classified as *ineffective erythropoiesis* is certainly the most interesting, for it raises questions of fundamental import in many areas of hematology.

Hemolysis

The possibility that excessive blood destruction might be the cause of the anemia in some or all cases of leukemia has been considered for many years, but the first case in which leukemia appeared to be definitely accompanied by a hemolytic anemia was not described until 1906 by Hirschfeld in *Folia Haematologica*.[105] This article appeared with an accompanying cautionary note from Pappenheim, the editor of the journal,[163] who pointed out that although hemolysis might have been a factor contributing to the anemia in the case under discussion, this was the exception rather than the rule in leukemia.

This position remained unchanged for nearly 30 years except for occasional reports on single patients who showed such indications of hemolysis as an increased fecal urobilinogen output, jaundice, or pronounced reticulocytosis.[9,99,164] In 1933 Whipple and Robscheit-Robbins,[239] having analyzed the liver iron content in 14 leukemic patients, found "little or no evidence for blood destruction," and concluded that the anemia in leukemia "would seem to depend upon marrow insufficiency due to encroachment of the white cells on the red cell chain." About the same time, however, the first determined advocates of hemolysis as a cause of anemia in leukemia made themselves heard. Thus, Jaffe found postmortem evidence of increased, rather than decreased, erythropoiesis, together with signs of erythrophagocytosis and hemosiderosis which he regarded as indicators of excessive hemolysis.[113,114] Support for this view came from Kress.[130] Klima,[123] while denying that hemolytic anemia was present in his cases of chronic granulocytic leukemia, found three patients with chronic lymphocytic leukemia who showed evidence of increased blood destruction. The question was reviewed by Watson,[232,233] who admitted that occasional leukemic patients showed a hemolytic anemia but stated that this must be exceptional. He pointed out further that some of the signs such as hemosiderosis, which had in the past been interpreted as indicating hemolysis, could equally well be evidence for an inability on the part of the bone marrow to use the available iron for erythropoiesis. Collins and Rose, who analyzed the anemia in 50 consecutive cases of leukemia, came to similar conclusions.[47]

In the early studies, only indirect evidence for or against excessive hemolysis could be obtained, for example, the presence or absence of reticulocytosis or hyperbilirubinemia. Rarely, the fecal urobilinogen was estimated. Only when the life span of the red cells could be measured directly was it realized how often this was shortened in leukemia.[15-18,28,36,65,75,112,157,194,222,223,234,237]

There are two groups of patients with a distinctly increased red cell destruction, those showing overt hemolytic anemia and those with an occult hemolysis.

Overt type. Those showing an overt type of hemolytic anemia, exhibit all the usual signs indicating rapid hemolysis, such as jaundice, marked reticulocytosis, spherocytosis, increased osmotic red cell fragility, a greatly increased fecal urobilinogen content, a low serum haptoglobin concentration, and, usually, a positive direct Coombs' (antiglobulin) test. As we have demonstrated,[189] the bone marrow generally shows a double abnormality: marked erythroblastosis and the leukemic proliferation, which is almost invariably lymphocytic. Granulocytic leukemia with an overt type of hemolysis is rare.

Occult type. For those with an occult type of hemolysis, there is a strikingly increased transfusion requirement, but with few hematologic signs pointing to blood destruction; little, if any, icterus; only a slight reticulocytosis; no spherocytosis; a normal osmotic fragility; and, generally, a negative direct Coombs' test; only the fecal urobilinogen output is increased, the serum haptoglobin concentration is lowered, and the ^{51}Cr red cell survival time is shortened.

The *overt* type of hemolytic anemia is most often seen in the lymphoproliferative group (chronic lymphocytic leukemia, disseminated lymphosarcoma). It is less common in Hodgkin's disease and rare in chronic granulocytic (2 of 27 patients in Videbaek's series[227]) and in acute forms. Hemolytic anemia may be found when the patient is first diagnosed, and may indeed be the presenting sign (see Chapters 10 and 12) or it may develop at a later stage of the disease (Figs. 14-3 and 14-4). It is generally associated with the development of an autoimmune state,[61] as shown by the common occurrence of a positive direct Coombs' test and often of circulating autoantibodies, usually of the warm IgG type, although both warm- and cold-reacting IgM may occur. In some patients, there is considerable splenic enlarge-

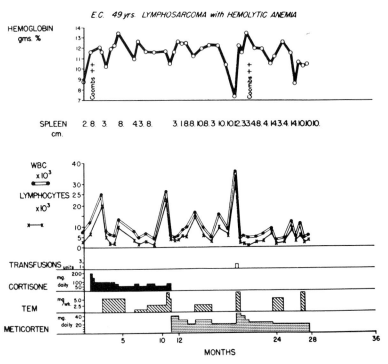

Fig. 14-3. Lymphosarcoma with splenomegaly and a marked degree of hemolytic anemia in a 49-year-old female who was treated by steroids. The neoplastic process was treated with TEM.

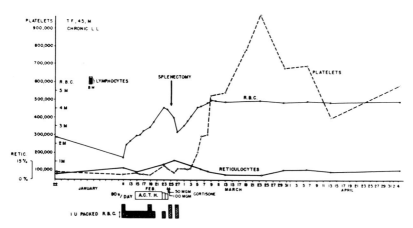

Fig. 14-4. A 44-year-old male with chronic lymphocytic leukemia who was treated with TEM. Hemolytic anemia and thrombocytopenia supervened. Splenectomy resulted in complete reversion of hemolysis and thrombocytopenia.

ment, and transfused cells are apparently sequestered and preferentially destroyed in that organ (Fig. 14-5). In many others, however, splenomegaly is not striking. The red cell survival time is grossly diminished. Treatment with large doses of steroids usually has the effect of restoring the survival time to more normal values, although in some patients anemia may be but slightly affected.[138] In these patients, splenectomy may be considered, but has only occasionally been of value in our hands (Figs. 14-4 and 14-6).

The hemolytic anemia may be the presenting symptom which brings the patient to the physician, the persistent and absolute lymphocytosis leading eventually to the diagnosis of chronic lymphocytic leukemia. Such cases may be quite mild, both with respect to the hemolytic anemia and to the leukemia. More often, hemolysis develops after the diagnosis of the leukemia. In Pirofsky's series, hemolysis was diagnosed simultaneously with chronic lymphocytic leukemia in 35 percent and subsequent to the clinical onset of chronic lymphocytic leukemia in 65 percent of

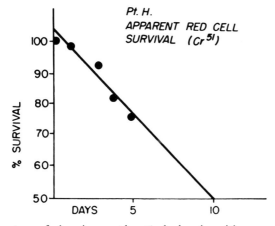

Fig. 14-5. Late stage of chronic granulocytic leukemia, with gross splenomegaly. Apparent 50 percent red cell survival (^{51}Cr) reduced to 10 days (normal 26 ± 2 days). Marked hemolytic anemia with increase in transfusion requirement.

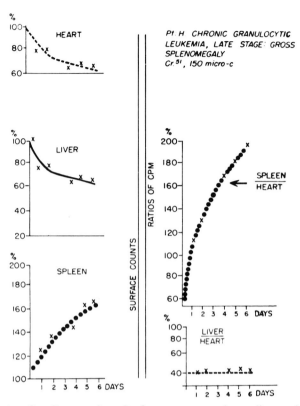

Fig. 14-5 (*Continued*).   Same patient. Surface counts over heart, liver and spleen following injection of 150 μc of ^{51}Cr. Left of diagram: actual CPM expressed as percentage of initial counts. Note fall in counts over the heart (apparent 50 percent survival 10 days) and liver, steep rise of counts over spleen. Right of diagram: ratio of liver and spleen to heart counts. Note that the ratio of liver:heart is practically constant, while ratio of spleen:heart rises very steeply. Result shows marked sequestration of red cells by spleen, leading to their excessive destruction.

patients.[170] The sudden development of anemia should always make one suspect the onset of a hemolytic episode, which can be readily confirmed by inspection of a blood smear (spherocytosis and increased polychromasia) and the presence of reticulocytosis, a positive Coombs' antiglobulin test, and slight bilirubinemia. There may be several hemolytic phases in the same patient.[227] We have noted the possibility that some cases of autoimmune hemolytic anemia occurring in the course of chronic lymphocytic leukemia have apparently been triggered by such factors as x-ray therapy (particularly of the total-body or spray types) or large doses of alkylating agents, including triethylenemelamine, cyclophosphamide, and chlorambucil.

It is conceivable, as we have postulated,[56] that a mass of lymphoid tissue borne by the patient with chronic lymphocytic leukemia is like a graft, which may be said to live in "peaceful coexistence" with the host patient for a lengthy period, but one which eventually becomes intolerant of the host, thus setting off a graft-versus-host reaction in which hemolytic anemia, wasting, and other systemic manifestations are prominent. More likely, in the course of leukemia, there is a gradual overgrowth of clones of lymphocytes with the power to form red cell antibodies. Small clones of

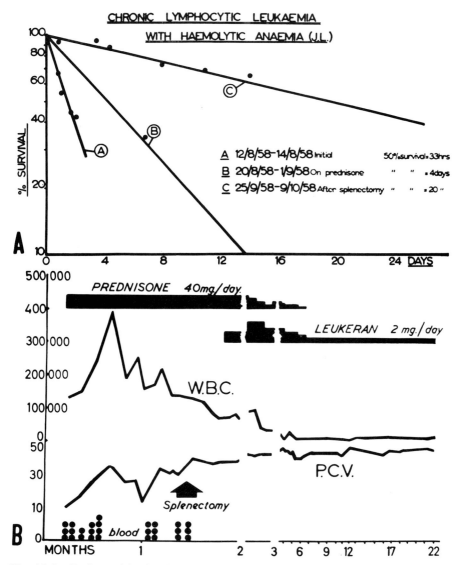

Fig. 14-6. Patient with chronic lymphocytic leukemia and sudden onset of hemolytic anemia. A. Red cell survival times (^{51}Cr) before and after splenectomy. B. Clinical course. (Reproduced by permission from Gunz FW, NZ Med J 60:441, 1961.)

such cells probably arise from time to time in the normal organism but are rapidly suppressed; in leukemia, the homeostatic mechanism fails, with an unhindered proliferation of the antibody-producing cells.[55] Different abnormal clones, each producing its own antibody, may flourish at different stages of the disease, thus accounting for those cases in which several hemolytic phases occur.

The *occult* type of hemolysis is always much more difficult to diagnose than the overt type, because there are so few hematologic signs pointing to it. An alert observer will often pick up an increasing need for transfusions while the leukemic process appears to be under reasonable control. In such patients, the fecal urobilinogen content is found to be increased and a determination of the red cell survival time will show a moderate reduction. Such cases are difficult to distinguish from others in which an enlarged spleen merely traps, rather than destroys, red cells. It has been shown that in chronic granulocytic leukemia as many as 30 percent of all the body's red cells may be in the spleen.[169]

In the occult hemolytic anemia associated with the leukemias, there may be little evidence of excessive hemolysis. The reduction in red cell life may be relatively slight: 70–83 days in one study compared with a normal average of 120 days.[15, 16] Using the Ashby method, some reduction in red cell survival was found in 12 of 15 patients with chronic granulocytic leukemia and in 6 of 9 with chronic lymphocytic leukemia.[18] From these results it may be concluded that in the majority of patients with the chronic leukemias, whether anemic or not, there is excessive hemolysis.

The question arises as to what part, if any, the latent hemolytic syndrome plays in the establishment of the common anemia of leukemia. In most of these patients the red cell survival is reduced only moderately. Although the normal marrow is capable of compensating for much greater reductions in red cell survival,[53] it is likely that the partially injured and infiltrated marrow of leukemia cannot respond nearly as well. Thus, if anemia exists with the red cell survival time reduced by only one-third or one-half, it must be concluded that a depression of erythropoiesis is present which makes the marrow incapable of responding normally to the increased regenerative demands. If, therefore, increased hemolysis is found in cases of leukemia, it should not be assumed that this is necessarily the only cause of the anemia or even a major contributory cause.[75, 222]

The mechanism leading to the development of occult hemolysis is by no means clear. There are generally no antibodies demonstrable, although this does not rule out an immunologic mechanism. Serum complement levels fluctuate but are mostly within normal limits.[153, 243] It is conceivable that the leukemic tissue, like neoplasms in general, may react with the normal tissues of the "host" patient as do the grafted spleen cells in experimentally induced runt disease. In line with this speculation are the following findings: In some rats with lymphomas, it has been shown that labeled red cells are rapidly disposed of in the tumors,[88] while some patients with large abdominal lymphosarcomas were found at autopsy to have "huge hemorrhagic areas laden with red cells, hemoglobin, hemosiderin and macrophages carrying hemosiderin in the tumors, sufficient to account for the anemia."[82]

Except in the Di Guglielmo syndrome, no evidence has been found by cross-transfusion studies for an intrinsic defect in the leukemic red cells which could explain their shortened survival.[112] The role of the spleen is variable; only sometimes can it be shown to destroy the red cells excessively.[224] For this reason, the results of splenectomy are uncertain.[93, 117] Vascular defects in leukemic organs might lead to extravasation of red cells and their subsequent destruction. In this sense, the so-called occult hemolytic anemia would be at least partially posthemorrhagic; and by measuring the red cell survival time, it would not be possible to distinguish between this type of anemia and one purely hemolytic in character.

To summarize, hemolysis occurs in leukemia under various conditions, and as the result of a variety of mechanisms, some better understood than others. Except in severe cases of autoimmune hemolysis, abnormal red cell destruction, wherever it may take place in the body, is not usually rapid enough to cause by itself anemia of a severe and intractable kind. The importance of investigating every case of presumed

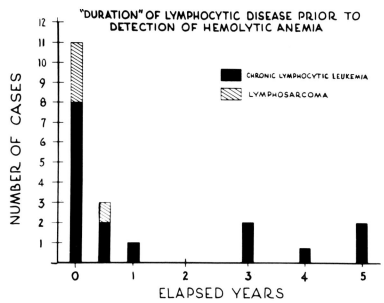

Fig. 14-7. Lymphocytic proliferative disorders, the development of autoimmune hemolytic anemia and its relation to the time the fundamental disease was discovered.

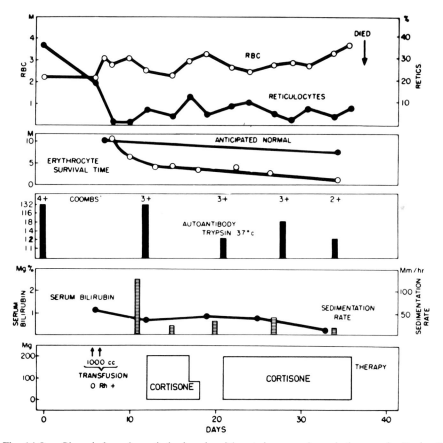

Fig. 14-8. Chronic lymphocytic leukemia with autoimmune hemolytic anemia. Reduction in all the parameters of increased blood destruction with cortisone therapy. Patient died suddenly of cerebrovascular accident.

511

hemolytic anemia as carefully as possible before therapy is instituted can scarcely be overemphasized (Figs. 14-7–14-11).

Posthemorrhagic Anemia

Hemorrhage is common in acute leukemia though it may also occur in the chronic granulocytic form, even in the early stages. It is rare in chronic lymphocytic leukemia, but we have seen several cases of apparently typical "idiopathic" thrombocytopenic purpura in the chronic lymphocytic disorder.[69] This may be one of the autoimmune abnormalities so commonly seen in the lymphoproliferative disorders.

There are relatively few instances in which hemorrhage alone accounts for anemia in chronic leukemia. When it does, there is usually a long history of slow bleeding. However, not every leukemic patient who bleeds persistently does so primarily because of the leukemia, and the possibility of associated disease must always be borne in mind, especially if the bleeding comes from a single site such as the alimentary tract. Peptic ulceration is common during corticosteroid therapy, and chronic lymphocytic leukemia may be associated with carcinoma of the large bowel;

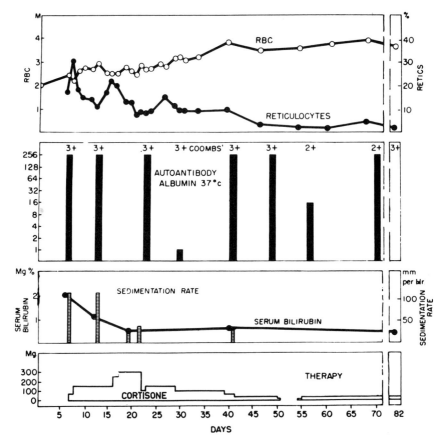

Fig. 14-9. Chronic lymphocytic leukemia with autoimmune hemolytic anemia. Therapy with cortisone resulted in improvement in red cell count and other indices of increased blood destruction, although autoantibody persisted.

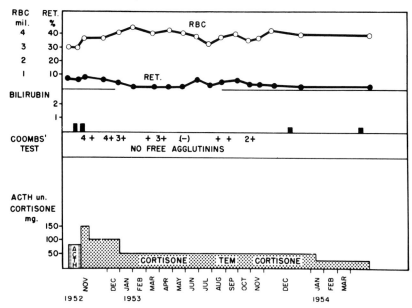

Fig. 14-10. Chronic lymphocytic leukemia with autoimmune hemolytic anemia. There was a striking response to cortisone therapy in this mild case.

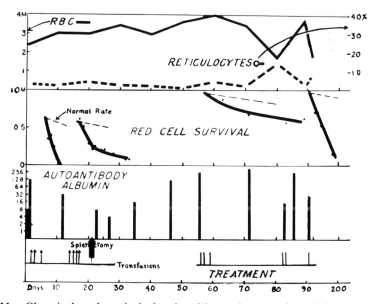

Fig. 14-11. Chronic lymphocytic leukemia with autoimmune hemolytic anemia. Splenectomy was performed on twenty-first hospital day. Red cell survival time (Ashby technique) temporarily improved, followed by a striking reduction in red cell survival and by death.

513

both are more likely causes of hemorrhage from the gastrointestinal tract than leukemic infiltration.

Anemia Caused by Therapeutic Agents

Practically all the agents used in the treatment of the leukemias, with the probable exception of the steroid group, act by virtue of their cytostatic effect. It is obvious, however, that leukemic cells are by no means the only cells affected. Thus, all other body cells capable of proliferating, particularly the most rapidly dividing ones, are attacked. Among these are the erythroid precursors. There may also be a more specific effect exerted by substances such as the folic acid antagonists and antimetabolites like cytosine arabinoside, and to a lesser extent 6-mercaptopurine, which can produce an actual megaloblastic change in the marrow.[217] It is therefore clear that, especially during periods of intense treatment, the administration of these active and toxic agents will often result in anemia, or in the aggravation of a preexisting anemia. It has also been shown that, even during periods of complete remissions in the acute leukemia of children and while maintenance therapy is in progress,[111] the hemoglobin level is on an average below the optimum for the age. The disturbances in the B_{12} and folate metabolism which are found in untreated leukemia are discussed below.

In summary, anemia probably occurs from a combination of many causes. Mechanical interference with erythropoiesis, marrow hypoplasia, excessive hemolysis, splenic pooling, drugs, and hemorrhages all play a part, and sometimes combine to producing anemia. Taken over the whole range of the leukemias, the most common cause of the anemia is probably diminished erythropoiesis, either from mechanical causes or because the erythroid series is itself involved in the leukemic process. This is so particularly in the chronic granulocytic and the acute leukemias. Although a latent form of hemolysis may also be operative in some of these patients, this may be of only moderate importance. The anemia is ordinarily relieved as soon as the leukemic process has been brought under temporary control, and this may be seen as an argument against the significance of latent hemolysis as a major factor contributing to the anemia.

On the other hand, there can be no question regarding those cases of leukemia, almost invariably of the chronic lymphocytic type, in which there is overt hemolytic anemia with all the usual signs indicating excessive red cell destruction and a very short life span of the erythrocytes.[16, 189] In these patients there appears to be a definite dichotomy in the clinical and hematologic picture, for the hemolysis may persist while the leukemia itself has been brought under control by means of radiation or chemotherapy. On the other hand, it is possible to combat the anemia with corticosteroid treatment, even though leukemic changes may persist. It is therefore of considerable importance to pinpoint the diagnosis of the anemia as accurately as possible.

THE HEMORRHAGIC STATE

Under the term *hemorrhagic state* we include bleeding from the body orifices and into the body organs and cavities, as well as cutaneous hemorrhages which may range from petechiae to large ecchymoses. Bleeding occurs most commonly in the uncontrolled leukemic process and is therefore much more prevalent in the acute than in the chronic forms. Although, at first glance, the mechanism of this hemorrhagic state appears to be rather simple, centering around the reduced platelet count, analysis indicates a rather complex problem. Thus, as in all problems related to hemorrhagic disorders, one must consider vascular and coagulation factors, the fibrinolytic system, as well as the platelets with their quantitative and, possibly, qualitative abnormalities.

The frequency of undue bleeding in various types of leukemia is discussed in Chapter 10. Hemorrhagic problems are particularly important in the acute leukemias, and they have to be faced at all stages of the disease process. In chronic granulocytic leukemia, bleeding is most troublesome in the terminal blastic phase, but not uncommonly it may be one of the early signs which attract attention. Chevallier reports that in one-third of 32 patients with chronic granulocytic leukemia and early bleeding, the hemorrhage occurred after surgical operations, especially dental extractions, in another third after minor trauma, and spontaneously in the remainder.[46] In all types of leukemia, serious and intractable bleeding nearly always indicates a worsening of the pathologic process, especially when there is also fever.

Platelets

Thrombocytopenia is by far the most important cause of bleeding in leukemia. Nearly always it is associated with a gross reduction of the megakaryocytes in the marrow, although a few cases resembling "idiopathic" thrombocytopenic purpura with normal or raised numbers of megakaryocytes have been described in chronic lymphocytic leukemia (Fig. 14-12).[69] These are probably of immunologic origin.

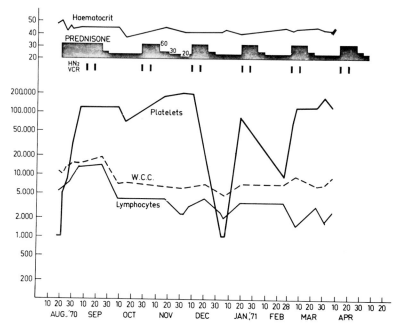

Fig. 14-12. A 64-year-old male with lymphosarcoma cell leukemia. The first symptom was sudden purpura due to "idiopathic" thrombocytopenia. The patient responded rapidly to corticosteroid therapy.

The relationship between thrombocytopenia and bleeding is complex.[81,189] A very high proportion of patients with acute leukemia have thrombocytopenia (95% in Rosenthal's series[190]), but by no means all have active bleeding. Bleeding is rare with platelet counts above 50,000 per cubic millimeter, and though more common below that figure, it is not inevitable even then. We have often had patients with fewer than 20,000 platelets per cubic millimeter and no sign of hemorrhagic phenomena. In many patients, the administration of small doses of steroids may control bleeding while leaving the low platelet count unaltered. In such situations the vascular component is probably important, as indicated by a negative tourniquet test. Again, other patients may bleed with relatively high platelet counts, and where this occurs functional platelet abnormalities are usually invoked though rarely is this proved.[64,77,168,192] Certainly, platelets in leukemia are often morphologically abnormal, having bizarre shapes, giant forms, large hyalomere, etc. Indeed, in chronic granulocytic leukemia, the presence of the Ph[1] chromosome in megakaryocytes (see Chapter 6) suggests that the megakaryocytes themselves may be involved in the leukemic process, and although the evidence is still scanty, the same may hold true for some acute granulocytic leukemias, especially those of the Di Guglielmo type (see Chapters 6 and 11). Studies on platelet function in leukemia, however, have produced contradictory results, and this uncertainty extends even to conditions like hemorrhagic thrombocythemia, in which, paradoxically, vast numbers of platelets go together with persistent bleeding. Here, extensive work on the mechanism of the hemorrhagic state has given many discordant results, and the only constant finding is the cessation of bleeding as treatment reduces the platelet count to less than 1.0 million per cubic millimeter.[90,182] This strange syndrome is discussed in Chapter 11.

Other Factors

It has been generally assumed that thrombocytopenia alone is not enough to cause undue bleeding and that there must be at least one other factor before it occurs. *Trauma*, either surgical or accidental, is certainly such a factor; thus, thrombocytopenic patients bleed excessively when injured. Spontaneous bleeding is more difficult to explain. A number of abnormalities referable to the complex coagulation process have been found. Whether these are of any particular significance is another matter. Some years ago, among 21 cases of acute leukemia, Soulier and Dausset found the bleeding time prolonged in 11, and the clotting time in 2 of 14 tests, the capillary resistance diminished in two, the prothrombin time (Quick) prolonged in one-third, and the prothrombin consumption diminished.[209] These abnormalities, except for the prolonged prothrombin time, could be accounted for by the thrombocytopenia. Moreover, the prothrombin time was never severely diminished, the average prothrombin concentration being 52 percent of normal. Similar figures were found by Chevallier in cases of chronic granulocytic leukemia with excessive bleeding.[46] Samama and Colombani made detailed investigations of the clotting factors known to be capable of altering the Quick prothrombin time and obtained the following results: a slight or moderate prolongation of the prothrombin time was almost invariably present in acute leukemia, fairly frequent in the chronic granulocytic type, but exceptional in chronic lymphocytic leukemia.[201] It was most likely to occur in relapse and might disappear in remissions, but it was never found to reach critical levels low enough to explain spontaneous bleeding without the inter-

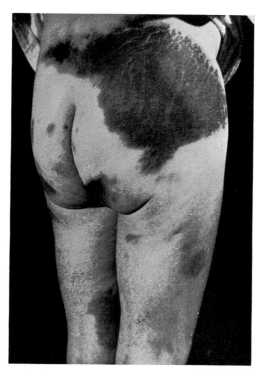

Fig. 14-13. Acute promyelocytic leukemia. Note widespread ecchymoses, associated with the presence of fibrinolysis.

vention of other factors. The most common reason for the prolongation was a deficit of labile factor (Factor V), a finding which was confirmed by Lewis et al.[137]

A good deal of interest has recently been taken in abnormalities of the fibrinogen content of the blood in leukemia.[52,211] In early acute leukemia in one of our own patients (Fig. 14-13), sudden and catastrophic hemorrhage developed in conjunction with the appearance of a fibrinolysin, possibly as the result of infection. Here, and in a second, more recent patient, extensive purpura was the first clinical sign, before leukemia was diagnosed: autopsy showed the presence of acute granulocytic leukemia with chloromatous tumors. The same mode of presentation has been seen in chronic granulocytic leukemia. A low serum fibrinogen concentration could be the result of any one of three mechanisms: deficient production by the liver, excessive destruction by means of rapid fibrinolysis, or excessive consumption. While in leukemia there is usually no sign of the liver function being sufficiently abnormal to lead to subnormal fibrinogen production, both of the other mechanisms have been responsible for fibrinogenopenic hemorrhage.

Low serum fibrinogen levels have generally been reported to be rare in leukemia and to be almost entirely confined to certain of the acute granulocytic types, but systematic study has shown that at times they are found among the other types of leukemia as well.

On the other hand, raised fibrinogen levels are not uncommon and are probably related to infection.[159] Early workers reported cases of acute granulocytic leukemia in which hemorrhage was believed to be due to excessive fibrinolysis,[49,171] and in

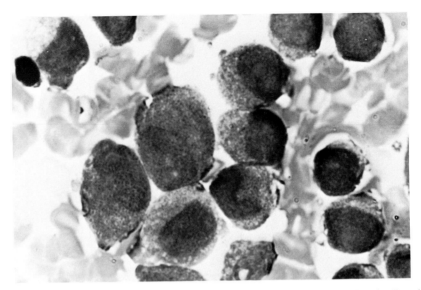

Fig. 14-14. Bone marrow from a patient with acute promyelocytic leukemia. Death occurred from hemorrhage associated with excessive fibrinolysis.

1957, Hillestad noted an apparent association between fibrinolytic hemorrhage and the predominance of promyelocytes, many of them atypical, in some acute leukemias (Figs. 14-14 and 14-15).[103] Nilsson et al. used huge doses of ε-aminocaproic acid in a similar case, and temporarily controlled the bleeding.[158] Activators of fibrinolysis (plasminogen activators) have been shown to be contained in the lysosomal fraction of promyelocytes,[44] and this may explain the association between fibrinolysis and what has been termed *promyelocytic leukemia*. However, although there is ample confirmation of the presence of fibrinogenopenia in some of these

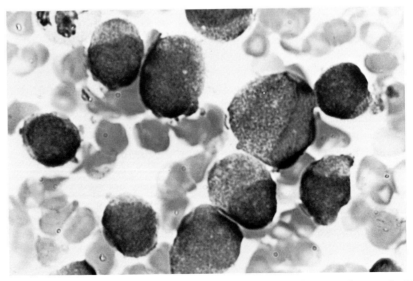

Fig. 14-15. Acute promyelocytic leukemia, bone marrow. Same patient as in Figure 14-14.

leukemias, the mechanism by which it is produced is still unsettled. Most of the evidence for fibrinolysis adduced by earlier observers is indirect or indecisive. Thus, a rapid disappearance of plasma clots could be caused by their poor quality because of a deficiency in fibrinogen, as well as by the activation of the fibrinolytic mechanism. Similarly, a low plasminogen level can also follow excessive fibrinogen consumption. Direct evidence in favor of fibrinolysis such as increased lysis of fibrin plates has often been lacking in published work.[106] A number of authors believe that a low fibrinogen level associated with hemorrhage in leukemia, as in other conditions, results from excessive consumption, probably in local thrombi. This is the syndrome of diffuse intravascular coagulation.[6,66,106,173,191,192] Although thrombi have rarely been found to be extensive in postmortem examination of patients with acute leukemia who died from hemorrhage, this does not negate the theory, for such clots may be only short-lived. Indeed, increased fibrinolysis itself may be a consequence of thrombosis, and thus add to the consequences of increased fibrinogen consumption. However, most of the evidence in favor of a consumption coagulopathy in leukemia is only indirect, and it is probable that the mechanism leading to fibrinogenopenic hemorrhage is not uniform.[48,85,179] Moreover, such hemorrhages nearly always occur in thrombocytopenic individuals, which makes both their precise diagnosis and their treatment unusually difficult.

Deficiencies in some of the other coagulation factors, especially Factors V, VIII, and X, occur in a number of cases of leukemia but may be secondary to increased consumption. An anticoagulant has been shown to be contained in the lysosomes of granulocytes[197] and found to be apparently responsible for bleeding in one patient with acute granulocytic leukemia,[96] probably by interference with the action of phospholipid during the formation of tissue thromboplastin. Earlier reports of frequent heparin-like anticoagulants have not been confirmed.[4] Characteristically, bleeding is controlled in acute leukemia, even in the presence of fibrinogenopenia, if a remission occurs and the leukemic cells disappear. This may be presumptive evidence that factors contained in the abnormal leukocytes, possibly plasminogen activators and anticoagulants, are concerned in the causation of the hemorrhage.

Clotting abnormalities sufficient to cause major bleeding may result from dysproteinemic states, including hyperglobulinemia and macrogobulinemia. This has been explained by "complexing" of the clotting factors, either by the excessive amounts of 7S gamma globulin or of the very viscid 17-19S macroglobulin (see Chapter 13).

In summarizing this brief discussion, we may say that thrombocytopenia is by far the most important cause of hemorrhage in leukemia. In many instances, the bleeding can be promptly controlled by the transfusion of fresh platelets.[104] There is no doubt that fresh blood, containing viable platelets, is more effective than bank blood.[7,74,211] The prophylactic use of platelet concentrates has become extremely important as an ancillary to increasingly potent chemotherapeutic regimens for the treatment of acute leukemia. The development of platelet antibodies, however, represents a problem which may not be overcome, until it becomes possible to use only material from donors who are tissue-type compatible.

Precisely how platelets exert their antihemorrhagic function in vivo is not yet clear, although there can be no question as to their importance in almost every stage of the clotting function. If the platelets are not concerned in the hemorrhagic disorder, pinpointing of the actual abnormality may require careful survey of all possible disturbances, including vascular and coagulation factors, and fibrinopenic mechanisms. The vascular factor may be important in those patients in whom there is extensive leukemic infiltration of the walls of small blood vessels, especially in the central nervous system.[78]

In most patients, hemorrhage is likely to result from a summation of abnormalities, none of which, other than severe thrombocytopenia, is sufficient by itself to lead to frank bleeding.

PURINE METABOLISM

The presence of deposits of uric acid in the renal pelvis and ureters was one of the first of the abnormal findings which were noticed in patients succumbing to the newly discovered disease, leukemia. Virchow, in 1853, mentions that he found it in 2 of his own patients and records that 13 similar patients had by then been described by others.[228] Salkowski, in 1870, determined the urinary uric acid excretion no less than thirty-one times in a single case of chronic granulocytic leukemia, and found it on an average to be twice as high as that in normal people.[198] Detailed investigations on the urinary uric acid excretion in three cases of acute and two of chronic leukemia were reported in 1898 by Magnus-Levy,[142] who established that there was a great increase in the output in the acute form, but a much less pronounced one in both chronic granulocytic and chronic lymphocytic leukemia. This author first suggested that his findings were probably produced by a great increase in tissue breakdown, but he was unable to establish a good correlation between the height of the leukocyte count and that of the uric acid output, a fact which he did not find altogether surprising, for, as he shrewdly observed, "It is doing the leukocytes of the blood too much honor if we attribute to them alone the remarkable changes in the metabolism, considering that there are so many more of these elements in the liver, spleen, etc."

Soon after the demonstration that many leukemic patients excrete increased quantities of uric acid, reports began to appear about increased serum concentrations of uric acid; also a number of clinical articles recorded the coexistence of leukemia and gout. Duckworth,[67] in 1889, reported the coexistence of gout and "splenic" leukemia in two patients. Brochner-Mortensen,[33] in a monograph published in 1940, quoted nine reports of increased serum uric acid and eleven of gout in leukemia. He himself was, however, unable to decide whether the simultaneous occurrence of the two diseases was more fréquent than might be expected from fortuitous coincidence. The relationship between leukemia, uric acid excess, and gout was extensively reviewed by Talbott, who showed unequivocally that there was a casual relationship between the two conditions, that it extended to other blood diseases besides the leukemias, and that as high a proportion as 10 percent of all cases of clinical gout were secondary to blood dyscrasias.[216] The increased incidence of urinary calculi in leukemia has been frequently reported. Thus, among 189 cases of leukemia, calculi were found in 9 (4.76 percent), whereas no instances of calculi were proved among 100 control patients suffering from miscellaneous metastatic malignant tumors, and the incidence of calculi among a general hospital population was 0.07 percent.[236]

Differences in the uric acid excretion within the various types of leukemia have been frequently noted, but the results have been variable. A reexamination of the problem produced the following findings in 38 leukemic patients[202]: there was a very pronounced rise in uric acid excretion in all patients with acute lymphocytic leukemia (all of whom, except one, were children); in acute and chronic granulocytic leukemia, an increased excretion was also found, but it was much less striking; the uric acid excretion was normal in chronic lymphocytic leukemia, a fact which had already been noted previously.[118] It was also established that a good correlation existed with the height of the leukocyte count in acute lymphocytic leukemia but in no other forms. Whether this was more than a coincidence seems doubtful for, as the authors pointed out, and as Magnus-Levy had already stressed nearly 60 years earlier,[142] the leukocyte count is a poor index of the total number of leukocytes in the body. Krakoff et al.[127] similarly found an increased uric acid excretion in acute and in chronic granulocytic leukemia, but could not correlate it with the cellular type or the level of the leukocyte count. The uric acid output is increased in all the chronic myeloproliferative disorders—chronic granulocytic leukemia, polycythemia vera, and myelosclerosis with myeloid metaplasia, but the highest values by far are attained in the latter condition. Here, blood uric acid values of two or three times normal may be found, gout is common, and the passage of uric acid stones in the urine may be a distressing symptom. Hickling has pointed out that the blood uric acid level in the myeloproliferative group of disorders is closely associated with the presence of large numbers of "megakaryocytelike giant cells" in the bone marrow

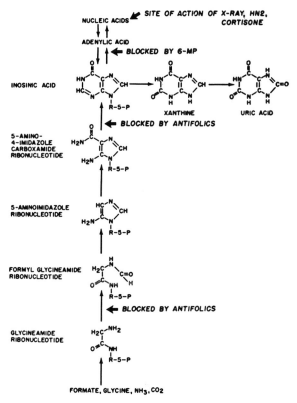

Fig. 14-16. Schema of purine metabolism (From Krakoff et al.,[127] reproduced by permission of the authors and the publisher.)

and spleen[102]; these cells are most numerous in myelosclerosis with myeloid metaplasia. It is likely that this correlation indicates no more than a particularly high
cellular turnover in those conditions which also have many megakaryocytes. Certainly, there can be no question of the enormous mass of granulocytic and
erythropoietic cells in the myeloproliferative syndromes, even where there is
myelofibrosis. In such patients, the myeloid metaplasia of spleen and liver alone is
massive, although erythropoiesis may be ineffective.

Figure 14-16 shows a greatly simplified scheme of the anabolism and catabolism of the purines.[126,127] Uric acid is formed in both metabolic phases, and
anything increasing the rate of purine metabolism must increase that of uric acid
formation. Since the purines are important constituents of the cellular nucleic acids,
the urinary uric acid output may be expected to measure the turnover of nucleic
acid, which, in leukemia, will be contained in both normal and leukemic cells. It is
reasonable to assume that any increase over normal figures will be largely a measure
of the nucleic acid metabolism of leukemic cells. As has been seen, there is always an
increased uric acid output in acute and in chronic granulocytic leukemia. This can be
very great and lead to various clinical symptoms in acute leukemia.[207] It reflects the
increased mass of leukocytes in the blood, hematopoietic and other organs.
However, such increases become much more marked as the results of effective
therapy when huge quantities of leukemic cells are destroyed (Fig. 14-17). Very large
amounts of uric acid are excreted during treatment with x-rays,[83,130] urethane,[79]
steroids and antimetabolites.[125,127,202,231] When patients enter remission, uric acid
output returns to normal. As Figure 14-16 shows, however, not all antimetabolites
will be expected to cause a rise in uric acid excretion; folic acid antagonists block
purine synthesis at a stage prior to that of uric acid formation, and their administration is followed by a fall, rather than a rise, in urinary uric acid.[127] No consistent
changes have been found following therapy in the excretion of purines other than
uric acid, or in pyrimidines[1,127] or amino acids.[19]

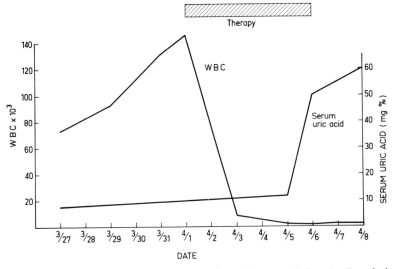

Fig. 14-17. Acute myelomonocytic leukemia in a 75-year-old female. Renal shutdown
with an extremely high serum uric acid concentration immediately following inception of
chemotherapy.

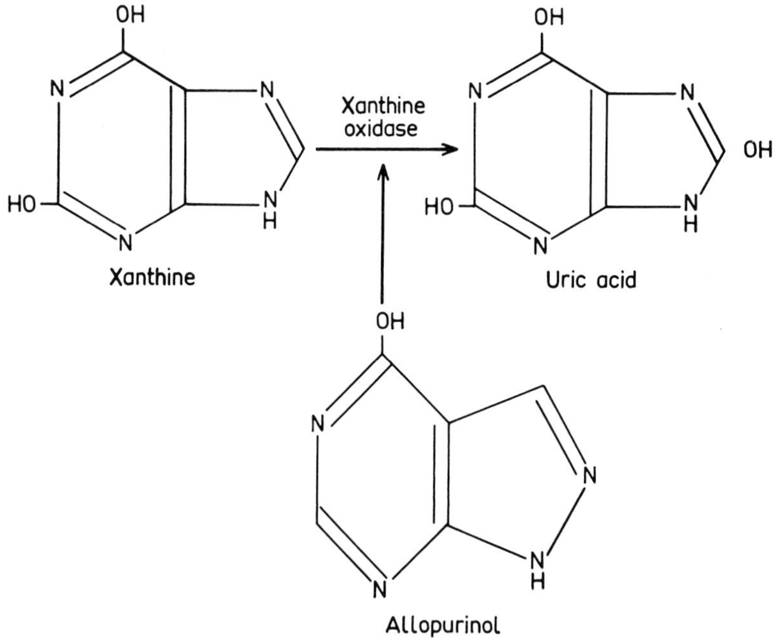

Fig. 14-18. Mode of action of allopurinol in purine catabolism.

The increase in uric acid excretion, which takes place as a result of the therapy of leukemia, may occur with such rapidity as to lead to renal shutdown caused by obstruction of the urinary tract. Renal failure and even death may occur.[129,131,135,236] Some of the most striking examples of hyperuricemia in our patients have occurred after large doses of corticosteroids had been given, particularly in acute leukemia, but also in other forms, including chronic lymphocytic leukemia. Serum uric acid concentrations of 20–25 mg per 100 ml or more have been noted, and temporary renal shutdown has occasionally had to be treated by hemodialysis.[92] These serious reactions should be anticipated whenever treatment, particularly with corticosteroids, is given to patients with a serum uric acid level at or above the upper limit of the normal range. The administration of allopurinol, an isomer of hypoxanthine, blocks the activity of xanthine oxidase, the enzyme which converts xanthine and hypoxanthine to uric acid in the course of purine catabolism (see Chapter 17 and Fig. 14-18). The relatively insoluble uric acid is thereby prevented from being formed and renal damage due to uric acid precipitation is avoided. Although neither xanthine nor hypoxanthine are more soluble than uric acid, their renal clearance occurs by a different mechanism. This accounts for the fact that they do not damage the kidney, even if excreted in the very large quantities which follow the administration of allopurinol in leukemia.[128]

INDICES OF LEUKOCYTE TURNOVER

The excretion of uric acid provides an indication of the turnover of leukemic leukocytes, but because of many uncertainties about catabolic pathways and especially about the possible reutilization of purines,[1,72] it cannot be regarded as a quantitative measure of cellular breakdown. Uric acid output is also greatly influenced by renal function: with any degree of renal failure the output is diminished. Other chemical parameters have therefore been investigated as possible indicators of leukocyte turnover in leukemia.

Among the earliest of these was the excretion of phosphorus and potassium which was noted to rise in the course of leukemia therapy,[37,156,231] a finding which was taken to indicate cellular breakdown of a nonspecific nature. More specific is the serum level of lactic acid dehydrogenase (LDH), an enzyme which is contained in many different cell systems. A rise in the serum concentration is generally regarded as an index of the excessive breakdown of cells containing it.

LDH exists in higher animals in the form of five isoenzymes, LDH 1-5, which can be separated and distinguished by means of electrophoresis. Different isoenzyme patterns are found in fetal and mature cells, and in the enzymes contained in various tissues. Among hematopoietic tissues, immature granulocytes are characterized by a predominance of isoenzymes 1-3, whereas mature granulocytes have more LDH-5. In the granulocytic leukemias, both acute and chronic, LDH-2, -3 and -4 tend to dominate the picture.[174,210] The serum LDH is only partly derived from disintegrated leukocytes. In the normal marrow plasma, the concentration of the enzyme much exceeds that in blood plasma.[97] In the leukemias there is frequently a conspicuous increase in serum LDH and the isoenzyme pattern usually suggests that this is derived from immature leukocytes. There may be striking correlations

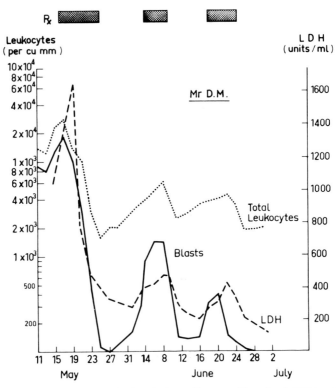

Fig. 14-19. Acute granulocytic leukemia in a 33-year-old male. LDH levels show close correlation with the number of circulating blasts. A *rise* in LDH levels follows the beginning of each course of therapy.

between the numbers of leukemic leukocytes and the serum LDH (Fig. 14-19). However, the concentration of the enzyme may also be very high in subleukemic cases, reflecting the greatly increased total mass of leukemic cells. Increased breakdown of leukemic cells following therapy will lead to rising levels of serum LDH, as shown in Fig. 14-19.

Muramidase (lysozyme). This is a hydrolytic enzyme found in the lysosomes of many tissues, including the bone marrow and blood, and in some exudates and secretions. Among the blood cells, monocytes and members of the granulocyte series are the sole sources of the enzyme. In the granulocytes, it is contained in the neutrophil granules, from the promyelocytes to mature neutrophils, its activity increasing with cellular maturity. Traces are present in eosinophils, but blasts have no muramidase; neither have red cells, lymphocytes, basophils, platelets, or megakaryocytes.[31] Although muramidase diffuses out of the cells containing it—at least in vitro—most of the enzyme in the plasma or serum is derived from the breaking down of leukocytes,[73] and thus provides some indication of leukocytic turnover. In normal marrow plasma, the muramidase concentration is two or three times as high as in blood plasma, probably because of intramedullary cell death.[98] Muramidase is found in the urine, its concentration increasing if there is renal failure, probably because of diminished tubular reabsorption.[241]

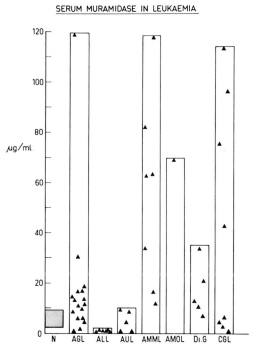

Fig. 14-20. Serum muramidase concentration in various types of leukemia. N, normal; AGL, acute granulocytic; ALL, acute lymphocytic; AUL, acute undifferentiated; AMML, acute myelomonocytic; AMOL, acute promyelocytic, DiG, Di Guglielmo; and CGL, chronic granulocytic.

In leukemia, the serum muramidase concentration is highly variable but strongly correlated with the cellular type.[5] Thus, it is normal in chronic lymphocytic leukemia but usually raised—often greatly—in chronic granulocytic leukemia,[167] and other myeloproliferative conditions.[42] Among the acute leukemias, the highest values are found in the myelomonocytic and monocytic forms.[161,167,203,246] Readings vary from normal to high in myeloblastic leukemia, but in the acute lymphocytic type the concentration is subnormal (Fig. 14-20).

It has been maintained that there is a close correlation between the serum muramidase concentration in the acute granulocytic and monocytic leukemias and the clinical activity of the disease,[241] and that the discovery of a high concentration in an untreated case of acute myeloblastic leukemia is a bad prognostic sign. We have confirmed that in some cases of the acute granulocytic types, therapy which reduces the leukocyte count and the proportion of leukemic cells also lowers the serum muramidase concentration concurrently, while the enzyme level rises with relapse (Fig.

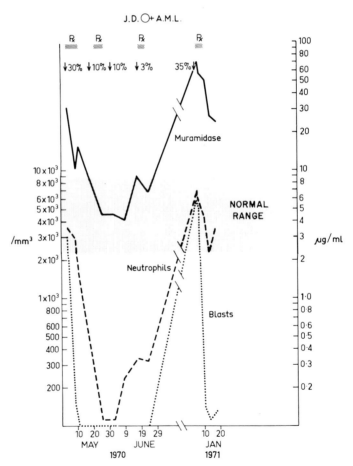

Fig. 14-21. Correlation between the serum muramidase level and leukemic leukocyte count in a patient with acute granulocytic leukemia. Percentages at top refer to blasts in marrow. The muramidase level falls with onset of remission, and rises in relapse.

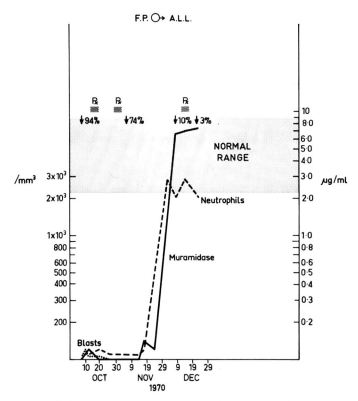

Fig. 14-22. Correlation between serum muramidase level and neutrophil count in a patient with acute lymphocytic leukemia. Percentages at top refer to blasts in marrow. The muramidase level is subnormal in relapse, and rises to the normal range as remission occurs.

14-21); in acute lymphocytic leukemia, on the other hand, an initially low serum muramidase level may rise to normal with successful therapy (Fig. 14-22).[136] However, neither we nor other workers[246] have found such changes sufficiently constant to permit us to dispense with other investigations such as serial marrow studies, in order to assess the precise effects of therapy and the presence or absence of early relapse.

In general, changes in the serum concentration of LDH and muramidase tend to run in parallel in the leukemias, but there are many exceptions. These are probably explained by the fact that LDH is contained chiefly in the less mature, and muramidase in the more mature granulocytic cells. In addition, LDH has a wide distribution among the hematopoietic cells while muramidase is confined to granulocytes and monocytes. High serum concentrations of both enzymes may safely be interpreted as valid indications of a relatively large total pool and, perhaps, a high turnover of leukemic (or normal) leukocytes, but low values do not exclude such a possibility. It should be remembered that a third parameter, that of serum vitamin B_{12}-binding protein, has also been found to fluctuate with the leukocyte count, for this protein too is contained in cells of the granulocytic series and released as they are destroyed.[40, 42] This substance is discussed in greater detail in a subsequent section.

THE BASAL METABOLIC RATE

The relationship of the basal metabolic rate (BMR) to the activity of the leukemic process was much discussed in the past. The BMR is readily measured and was in considerable use from the 1920s to the 1950s. Since it was often abnormally high, it provided a parameter, other than the blood itself, whose changes could be followed in individuals or groups of patients. It cannot, however, be claimed that much more is known today about the reasons for these changes than in 1893 when Bohland first described an increased BMR in one patient with chronic lymphocytic leukemia and in two with the chronic granulocytic variety.[27]

The basic fact is clear enough: namely, that a great many patients with leukemia have an increased BMR. The figures in the literature vary, probably because of differences in the technique of the test and the views of what constitutes a normal BMR. A rise was found in almost all of 33 patients by Riddle and Sturgis,[186] in 30 of 35 by Middleton et al.,[150] and in all of 40 patients with acute leukemia seen by Kaufmann and Lowenstein.[120] Our own experience does not suggest that an increased BMR is nearly as frequent in leukemia as would appear from these papers, and Griffiths et al.,[89] in a more recent survey, found the BMR usually normal or subnormal in acute leukemia, but tending to be raised in the chronic types. The actual rise when found is often moderate, but may be considerable, with figures in excess of 60 percent greater than normal being repeatedly reported. Patients with such high rates may have pronounced symptoms such as feelings of excessive warmth, hot flushes, increased tolerance to cold, and warm, moist skin and hands. At first glance, this might suggest a diagnosis of hyperthyroidism, but the nervousness, irritability, insomnia, tremor, and other symptoms which are so characteristic of the latter disease are usually lacking in leukemia.[154] Modern methods of investigating the thyroid gland have shown that it is functioning quite normally in leukemia despite an increased BMR (normal radioiodine uptake[2]; normal protein-bound iodine[145]). There is, therefore, no longer a rationale for attempting to treat leukemia by means of interference with the thyroid, as was done some time ago.[60,76]

It seems almost certain that the increased BMR is in some way a result of the leukemic process itself, and in some measure an indication of the mass of leukemic tissue, but unfortunately it is a highly variable indicator. The difficulties of explaining the mechanism of the phenomenon probably result from the fact that attempts have been largely restricted to correlating metabolic changes with the leukocyte count, anemia having been excluded as a major factor altering the BMR. However, in leukemia the circulating and marginated leukocytes form only a small fraction of all those in the body. Once practical means have been found for estimating the size of the *total-body leukocyte pool* under varying conditions, significant correlations between it and the height of the BMR may well be established. In that case, the use of the BMR as an index of the total activity of the leukemic process may become a rational procedure.

BLOOD GROUPS AND LEUKEMIA

The distribution of blood groups in a population of leukemia patients has been found by most observers not to be significantly different from normal. Thus, among 590 patients investigated by us in New Zealand (Gunz, unpublished observations), there were no deviations from the normal pattern in the ABH, Rh, MNS, Kell, Lewis, and Lutheran systems. Similar findings were obtained by others.[21,122,139,141,219] However, a few authors found an excess of Group A among children with acute leukemia,[29] as well as in patients of all ages with all types of leukemia,[205] while others claimed a slight deficiency of Group A in childhood leukemia[101] and an increased incidence of Rh-negative type in young children and patients over 50.[62] These aberrant results need further study.

While blood groups, taken over a series of leukemia cases, are normal or nearly so, there are many reports of individuals whose blood groups appeared to change in the course of the disease. Most of these had acute leukemia, usually granulocytic, but occasional instances of blood group changes have also been described in acute lymphocytic and the chronic leukemias. Most of the changes occurred in the ABH system, with a very few reports of losses of the $D(Rh_0)$ and, possibly, other Rh receptors on the red cells.[143,221] Furthermore there are some claims of the loss of the I antigen[140,242] though these have been denied.[71]

Two types of changes have been repeatedly found in the ABH system: first, a weakening or loss of reaction to anti-A in patients of Groups A or AB,[20,86,183,199] or rarely to anti-B in Group B patients[185]; and second, a loss of H antigen in Group O patients, and to a lesser extent in other groups.[144,200]

Losses or weakening of A antigen led to difficulties in determining the true ABH groups, Group A patients being mistakenly grouped as belonging to Group O or, if more detailed studies were made, to A_2, A_3, A , or A . "New" antigens were not found; thus, an AB patient might be grouped as B, and an A patient as O, but not as B. However, an apparently secondary change in the properties of Group B *antibody* has been found in patients in whom there were losses of A antigen in the course of leukemia.[20] Blood group changes have been shown not to be caused by therapy. They have at times been reversed during remission.

The mechanism causing changes in blood group antigens during leukemia is unclear. The most obvious possibility is a genetic change, and some reports cite chromosomal abnormalities in patients whose blood group underwent alterations.[68,178] It seems unlikely that these were more than coincidental, especially since the chromosomal abnormalities were variable. Somatic point mutation would more likely be a genetic cause. If blood groups are indeed altered because the genes controlling their expression have undergone modification, this would indicate rather strongly a connection with the basic leukemic changes. There is no fundamental obstacle to such a concept since it is now accepted that leukocytes and erythrocytes have a common stem cell. Moreover, it is known that the ABH factors are found in all leukocytes and can be modified in the various forms of leukemia.[35,119]

An alternative to the genetic interpretation of blood group changes in leukemia is the possibility that these are secondary to changes in the cell membrane. Shifts in the spatial position of the surface sites of blood group antigens might lead to alterations in their expression. Alternatively, abnormal substances such as sialomucins might block antigen sites.[119]

In contrast to the blood group antigens, far less extensive studies have revealed no losses of HL-A antigens in leukemia.[219] Moreover, most surveys have indicated a normal distribution of HL-A groups among leukemia patients,[124,133,219,225] even though irregularities have been found by some authors.[166,229] It is possible that these irregularities may be associated with the development of new "leukemia antigens."

Table 14-1

Titers of Anti-B and Anti-A Isoagglutinins in Lymphoma and Various Controls

	Anti-B Isoagglutinin Titers			Anti-A Isoagglutinin Titers		
Diagnosis	*No. of Patients*	*Geometric Mean Titer*	*95% Confidence Limits of the Mean*	*No. of Patients*	*Geometric Mean Titer*	*95% Confidence Limits of the Mean*
Controls	148	24	20–29	85	42	33–54
Malignant diseases of lymphocytes and plasma cells	125	6	4.5–7	71	13	9–19
Other reticuloses	117	15	12–17	85	42	33–53

1. The mean titers were calculated on a geometric scale $< 1 = 1, 1 = 2, 2 = 3, 4 = 4, 8 = 5$, etc., and then converted back to the actual titer. The confidence limits are also expressed in the original units.

2. Comparing controls with malignant diseases of lymphocytes and plasma cells, $t = 10.5$, d.f. = 271, $P < 0.001$, $t = 5.5$, d.f. = 154, $P < 0.001$ for anti-A.

3. Comparing malignant diseases of lymphocytes and plasma cells with other reticuloses, $t = 5.8$, d.f. = 240, $P < 0.001$ for anti-B.

4. There is no difference between the controls and patients with other reticuloses.

Data from Fairley and Akers.[70]

Or that they signify an increased sensitivity of leukemic cells, especially lymphocytes, to weak HL-A antibodies which are not recognized by normal cells.[160] In regard to blood group *antibodies,* these tend to be reduced in titer in the lymphoproliferative diseases and myelomatosis, in which there is a general defect in antibody production, but not in other forms of leukemia (Table 14-1). Alterations in serum groups (Gm, Inv) have been described by some,[194] but not others.[187] Similarly, there have been reports of changes in the distribution of the haptoglobin types.[165,226]

THE AUSTRALIA ANTIGEN

In 1965, Blumberg et al. recorded the discovery of a "new" antigen contained in the sera of "some normal individuals from foreign populations," but absent from those of normal U.S. subjects.[25] This antigen reacted with the sera of a number of people who had had numerous blood transfusions, and because one of the original two sera containing it had come from an Australian aborigine, the antigen itself was christened the Australia antigen [later Au(1)]. Despite this evocative name, it soon became apparent that neither geographic nor ethnic factors were responsible for the antigen's presence in any one individual.

In Blumberg's original material from patients with a variety of diseases,[25] Au(1) was present in much the highest proportion (11.4 percent) in leukemic sera, and the authors speculated that either persons with Au(1) had an increased susceptibility to leukemia, or that the antigen was itself a manifestation of the leukemic process, or that Au(1) might be related to the virus which had been suggested as a cause of leukemia. The relationship to leukemia became more intriguing when Au(1) was discovered in a high proportion of mongols who, of course, had a strong predisposition to developing leukemia (see Chapter 5). Moreover, family clusters of people with Au(1) were discovered, and these were consistent with an autosomal recessive inheritance of the antigen.[26] It appeared that there was a genetic predisposition both to leukemia and the development of Au(1).

However, this was not the whole story, for there was also a strong and consistent correlation between the presence of Au(1) and exposure to blood transfusions, and this suggested an external source of the antigen. Very extensive work in many laboratories established that the correlation was, in fact, with serum hepatitis, and alternative names such as *SH* or *hepatitis antigen* were introduced. The antigen could be shown to be present, after an incubation period, in most recipients of infected blood and to persist for a period of a few days or weeks, after which it disappeared. However, in a small proportion it persisted for much longer or indefinitely.[132,215] Infection, rather than genetic factors, accounted for the high incidence among mongols, for the antigen could be found only in patients kept in institutions but not in those at home.[132] The distribution of Au(1) could, in fact, be clearly seen as that of an agent either itself infective or associated with infection, and there is now no doubt about its importance in transfusion work, as an indicator of hepatitis virus.[247] Its occasional persistence may indicate anything from a carrier state to chronic active hepatitis.[204]

The realization that Au(1) is acquired through transfusions is at least a partial explanation of its high prevalence in leukemia. Table 14-2 shows that when patients with leukemia were considered according to the form of treatment they had received, there was a correlation between Au(1) and blood transfusion but not chemo- or radiotherapy.

However, patients with leukemia appear unduly prone to the *persistence* of Au(1), for the frequency of the antigen is much higher than in the general population or even in other individuals who have received multiple transfusions, such as hemophilics or those with thalassemia.[214] This raised susceptibility is largely confined to patients with acute and chronic lymphocytic leukemia, the former being mostly children and, hence, particularly easily infected and the latter often immunologically incompetent. Patients with acute or chronic granulocytic leukemia have the same in-

Table 14-2
Influence of Blood Transfusion on Au (1) in Leukemia

Therapy	No. of Patients	Au (1) (%)	X^2	p
Transfusion alone	48	5 (10.4)	5.3108	0.0212
No therapy	102	1 (1)		
Transfusion and chemotherapy	183	21 (11.5)	7.6210	0.0058
Chemotherapy alone	92	1 (1.1)		
Transfusion and chemotherapy and radiotherapy	61	11 (18)	1.6931	0.1930
Chemotherapy and radiotherapy	14	0		

From Sutnick et al.[213] (With permission.)

cidence of Au(1) as multitransfused hemophilics.[214,215] Whether there is also a genetic susceptibility to the acquisition of Au(1) is still uncertain. Family clusters of Au(1)-positive carriers have been described in some Asian and Oceanic populations,[27] but these are in need of confirmation.

It is by now almost certain that the Australia antigen is not related to any organism causing leukemia, but its high incidence in certain leukemias, with hints of the combined operation of infective, immunologic, and genetic factors, is of much interest and should be further investigated.

FOLIC ACID AND VITAMIN B$_{12}$

Since folic acid is known to be essential for the formation of nucleoproteins, and since there is an increased nucleoprotein turnover in leukemic cells, it might be expected that disturbances in the folic acid content of these cells occur. This is indeed the case. Whereas the folic acid content of 1 ml of packed normal leukocytes was found to have a mean value of 80 μg, that in chronic lymphocytic leukemia was 108 μg; in chronic granulocytic leukemia, 146 μg; and in acute leukemia, 460 μg.[22] There was a direct correlation between the folic acid level and the degree of immaturity of the leukocytes. Following irradiation treatment of chronic granulocytic leukemia, the folic acid content of the leukocytes fell. These findings have been repeatedly confirmed.[193] Although the increased figures in the leukemias could theoretically be produced either because of excessive folic acid requirements or an inability of the cells to utilize the vitamin, the reputed acceleration of the leukemic process by the administration of folic or folinic acids and its undoubted slowing in some cases by folic acid antagonists[208] suggests that leukemic leukocytes contain more folic acid because they require more of it for their growth. It has been shown that in at least some patients with chronic granulocytic leukemia the leukocytes contain a macromolecular factor which binds folic acid and which is not present in normal cells.[195] This may have some relationship—either physiologic or pathologic—to DNA synthesis.

In contrast to the generally increased folate levels of leukemic white cells, the serum folate is often low.[45,107,109,180,188] This is especially so during the active phases of acute and chronic granulocytic leukemia, while in remissions, varying folate levels are found. Many patients with low serum folate in leukemia also have a high urinary excretion of formiminoglutamic acid (FIGLU).[45] The low serum levels are not accounted for by inadequate intake or poor absorption, but in view of the fact that a low serum folate is often associated in the same patient with high levels in the leukocytes, it is most likely that both result from increased demands for the vitamin. Moreover, it is possible that the disease has to be active for some time before depletion of the stores of folate takes place and the serum level falls.[109] The folate content of the cerebrospinal fluid (CSF) is normally about three times higher than that of the serum, and the same ratio is found in uncomplicated acute leukemia. With the onset of meningeal leukemic infiltration, however, the CSF folate concentration falls, and the CSF:serum ratio becomes characteristically low (Table 14-3).[23]

Like the level of folic acid in the white cells, that of ascorbic acid, which is also indirectly concerned in the synthesis of nucleoproteins, is considerably increased in the chronic leukemias.[38,39]

Table 14-3
Relationships Between Serum, Red Cell, and CSF Folate Concentrations

	Controls	Acute Leukemia	
		Without Meningeal Involvement	*With Meningeal Involvement*
Number	27	61	11
Serum folate	6,87 (±0,3)	5,64 (±0,76)	4,71 (±2,3)
RBC folate	315 (±48)	326	381 (±180)
CSF folate	20,2 (±1,5)	19,02 (±1,8)	5,72 (±1,24)
CSF: serum folate	2,9	3,4	1,2
Correlation coefficient CSF/serum folate	0,67 (P0,02)	0,57 (P0,05)	0,74 (P0,01)

Data from Beuzard et al.[23]

In chronic granulocytic leukemia the serum level of vitamin B_{12} is greatly increased.[13,14] Lesser elevations are found in some cases of acute granulocytic leukemia, in polycythemia vera and myelosclerosis (Table 14-4),[84] but not in chronic lymphocytic leukemia. Vitamin B_{12} is normally bound to two serum proteins (Transcobalamin I and II),[94,95] one traveling with the alpha- and the other with the beta-globulin fraction on electrophoresis. Of these the beta globulin may be mainly a transport protein which is normally unsaturated and takes up B_{12} as it becomes available, prior to its delivery to the tissues, while the alpha protein is normally almost fully saturated and retains its B_{12} tenaciously, perhaps as a reserve.[100] In chronic granulocytic leukemia, the alpha globulin (transcobalamin I) is very greatly raised and largely unsaturated, in spite of a much increased amount of B_{12} bound to it,[10,12,148,172,177,184] although it is not yet certain if the increase occurs in the normal fraction or is due to an additional abnormal transcobalamin.[146,151,152,235] The high serum B_{12} in chronic granulocytic leukemia, acute leukemia,[176] and other myeloproliferative disorders is explained by excessive binding of B_{12} by the greatly increased

Table 14-4
Distribution of Serum B_{12} and Unsaturated B_{12}-Binding Capacity in Myeloproliferative Conditions

Diagnosis	No. of Subjects	Serum B_{12} Level Mean (Range)	Unsaturated Alpha Globulin Mean (Range)	Unsaturated Beta Globulin Mean (Range)
Normal	5	387 (258–584)	216 (119–301)	933 (731–1,093)
Polycythemia vera active	9	1,341 (376–4,528)	1,142 (412–2,557)	2,337 (1,114–3,675)
Polycythemia vera controlled	6	625 (418–1,339)	697 (298–1,570)	1,362 (634–2,494)
Myeloid metaplasia	8	861 (247–1,727)	587 (243–1,490)	1,481 (370–4,026)
Chronic granulocytic leukemia	5	4,484 (2,097–8,810)	10,902 (6,760–17,170)	2,346 (745–5,964)

Data from Gilbert et al.[84]

alpha binder. It is interesting that this bound fraction is abnormally slowly cleared from the serum,[34,155] and is not apparently available for ordinary B_{12} metabolism, for in two cases in which chronic granulocytic leukemia and pernicious anemia coexisted, the serum B_{12} concentration was found to be normal, in spite of clear evidence of B_{12} deficiency.[32,51] Chemotherapy reduces the binding capacity of Transcobalamin I when it produces remissions in chronic granulocytic leukemia.[175] Obviously, serum assay of B_{12} cannot be relied upon as a diagnostic finding in a patient with chronic granulocytic leukemia in whom pernicious anemia is suspected.

There is some correlation between the height of the granulocyte count and the concentration of B_{12} binders,[87] although exceptions occur.[212] Mature granulocytes have a high B_{12}-binding capacity, whereas immature members of the granulocytic series have much less.[149] Suggestions that the increased B_{12}-binding capacity of CGL serum is derived from granulocytes, either intact or disintegrated ones, have been made by many workers.[149,184,218,245] Beal[11] has shown that granulocyte-rich plasma binds more B_{12} in the alpha-globulin fraction than leukocyte-poor or lymphocyte-rich plasma, and recent work by Corcino et al. has produced evidence that intact, living, intravascular granulocytes synthesize and release B_{12}-binding protein.[50] It therefore seems clear that both the raised serum B_{12} and B_{12} binder in chronic granulocytic leukemia are consequences of the greatly increased numbers of granulocytes. First principles would indicate that serum concentrations of both factors depend on the total-body leukocyte mass and the rapidity of its turnover, and that, therefore, no simple relationship between the granulocyte count and serum B_{12} or binders need be expected. Nevertheless, in individual cases of leukemia, surprisingly close correlations between changes in the leukocyte counts under treatment and the B_{12} binding capacity have been reported.[40]

REFERENCES

1. Adams WS, Davis F, Nakatani M: Purine and pyrimidine excretion in normal and leukemic subjects. Am J Med 28:726, 1960.

2. Albright EC, Middleton WS: The uptake of radioactive iodine by the thyroid gland of leukemic patients. Blood 5:764, 1950.

3. Alexanian R, Alfrey C: Erythropoiesis in the anemia of bone marrow failure. J Clin Invest 49:1986, 1970.

4. Allen JG, Bogardus G, Jacobson LO, Spurr CL: Some observations on bleeding tendency in thrombocytopenic purpura. Ann Intern Med 27:382, 1947.

5. Asamer H, Schmalzl F, Braunsteiner H: Immunocytological demonstration of lysozyme (muramidase) in human leukaemic cells. Br J Haematol 20:571, 1971.

6. Baker WG, Bang NU, Nachman RL, Raafat F, Horowitz HI: Hypofibrinogenemic hemorrhage in acute myelogenous leukemia treated with heparin. Ann Intern Med 61:116, 1964.

7. Baldini M, Costea N, Dameshek W: The viability of stored human platelets. Blood 16:1669, 1960.

8. Barry WE, Day HJ: Refractory sideroblastic anemia. Clinical and hematologic study of ten cases. Ann Intern Med 61:1029, 1964.

9. Bauman L: The chemistry and clinical significance of urobilin. Arch Intern Med 28:475, 1921.

10. Beal RW: Preferential in vitro binding of radioactive Vitamin B_{12} by an abnormal serum protein in chronic myeloid leukaemia. Nature 213:81, 1967.

11. ———, Read WMF: Relationship of granulocytes to binding capacity. In: Studies on the plasma protein binding of (^{58}Co)-vitamin B_{12}. Austr J Exp Biol Med Sci 47:387, 1969.

12. ———, ———: Binding capacity of separated protein fractions. In: Studies on the plasma protein binding of (^{58}Co)-vitamin B_{12}. Austr J Exp Biol Med Sci 47:393, 1969.

13. Beard MF, Pitney WR, Sanneman EH: Serum concentrations of vitamin B_{12} in patients suffering from leukemia. Blood 9:789, 1954.

14. _____, _____, _____, Sakol MJ, Moorhead HH: Serum concentration of vitamin B_{12} in acute leukemia. Ann Intern Med 41:323, 1954.

15. Berlin NI, Lawrence JH, Lee HC: The life span of the red blood cell in chronic leukemia and polycythemia. Science 114:385, 1951.

16. _____, _____, _____: The pathogenesis of the anemia of chronic leukemia: measurement of the life span of the red blood cell with glycine-2-C^{14}. J Lab Clin Med 44:860, 1954.

17. Berlin R: The latent hemolytic syndrome in cases of leukemia with splenomegaly, in Proceedings of the Third Congress of the International Society of Hematology. New York, Grune & Stratton, 1951, p 99.

18. _____: Red cell survival studies in normal and leukemic subjects. Acta Med Scand Suppl 252, 1951.

19. Bernard J, Bourdon R, Caen J, Ardaillou R, Ranisteano S, Pays M: Étude des acides aminés urinaires et plasmatiques au cours de diverses hémopathies. Sang 30:32, 1959.

20. _____, Bessis M, Bussard A, Ducos J, De Grouchy J, Lejeune J, Salmon Ch, Seligmann M, Wurmser R: Changements de groupes sanguines dans les leucemies. Nouv Rev Fr Hématol 5:291, 1965.

21. Best WR, Limarzi LR, Ponder HG: Distribution of blood types in the leukemias. J Lab Clin Med 34:1587, 1949.

22. Bethell FH, Swendseid ME: The folic acid content of leukocytes: observations on normal subjects and persons with leukemia. J Clin Invest 25:917, 1946.

23. Beuzard Y, Saporta I, Schuller E, Dreyfus B: Serum and cerebrospinal fluid folates during the course of leukemic meningitis. Nouv Rev Fr Hématol 11:203, 1971.

24. Bjorkman SE: Chronic refractory anemia with sideroblastic bone marrow. Study of four cases. Blood 11:250, 1956.

25. Blumberg BS, Alter HJ, Visnich S: A "new" antigen in leukemia sera. JAMA 191:541, 1965.

26. _____, Gerstley BJS, Hungerford DA, London WT, Sutnick AI: A serum antigen (Australia antigen) in Down's syndrome, leukemia, and hepatitis. Ann Intern Med 66:924, 1967.

27. _____, Melartin L, Guinto RA, Werner B: Family studies of a human serum isoantigen system (Australia antigen). Am J Hum Genet 18:594, 1966.

27a. Bohland K: Ueber den respiratorischen Gaswechsel bei verschiedenen Formen der Anämie. Berl Klin Wochenschr 30:417, 1893.

28. Boiron M, Paoletti C, Tubiana M, Schapira G, Dausset J, Bernard J: L'anémie des leucoses aiguës. Sem Hôp Paris 31:1123, 1955.

29. Bonvini E: Relation between blood groups and acute leukemia in children. Minerva Pediatr 13:757, 1961.

30. Bothwell TH, Hurtado AV, Donohue DM, Finch CA: Erythrokinetics. IV. The plasma iron turnover as a measure of erythropoiesis. Blood 12:409, 1957.

31. Briggs RS, Perillie P, Finch C: Lysozyme in bone marrow and peripheral blood cells. J Histochem Cytochem 14:167, 1966.

32. Britt RP, Rose DP: Pernicious anemia with a normal serum vitamin B_{12} level in a case of chronic granulocytic leukemia. Arch Intern Med 117:32, 1966.

33. Brøchner-Mortensen K: The uric acid content in blood and urine in health and disease. Medicine 19:161, 1940.

34. Brody EA, Estren S, Wasserman LR: The kinetics of intravenously injected radioactive vitamin B_{12}: Studies on normal subjects and patients with chronic myelocytic leukemia and pernicious anemia. Blood 15:646, 1960.

35. Brody JI, Beizer LH: Alteration of blood group antigens in leukemic lymphocytes. J Clin Invest. 44:1582, 1965.

36. Brown GM, Elliott SM, Young WA: The hemolytic factor in the anemia of lymphatic leukemia. J Clin Invest 30:130, 1951.

37. Buckman TE, Daland CA, Weld M: The blood phosphorus in chronic myelogenous leukemia, especially as influenced by roentgen-ray therapy. Arch Intern Med 35:389, 1925.

38. Butler AM, Cushman M: Distribution of ascorbic acid in the blood and its nutritional significance. J Clin Invest 19:459, 1940.

39. _____, _____: An ascorbic acid-like reducing substance in the buffy layer of centrifuged oxalated blood. J Biol Chem 139:219, 1941.

40. Carmel R, Coltman CA Jr: Serum vitamin B_{12}-binding capacity and muramidase changes with cyclic neutropenia induced by cytosine arabinoside. Blood 37:31, 1971.

41. _____, _____, Yatteau RF, Costanzi JJ:

Association of paroxysmal nocturnal hemoglobinuria with erythroleukemia. N Engl J
Med 283:1329, 1970.

42. Catovsky D, Galton DAG, Griffin C,
Hoffbrand AV, Szur L: Serum lysozyme
and vitamin B_{12} binding capacity in
myeloproliferative disorders. Br J Haematol 21:661, 1971.

43. ——, Lewis SM, Sherman J: Erythrocyte
sensitivity to in-vitro lysis in leukaemia. Br J
Haematol 21:541, 1971.

44. Cattan A, Schwarzenberg L, Amiel J–L,
Schneider M, Schlumberger JR, Mathé G:
Fibrinogenopenic syndrome in the course of
acute leukemias and the decisive part played
in the onset by leucocytes. A study in vitro
of the leucocytes' fibrinolytic power. Rev Fr
Étud Clin Biol 11:155, 1966.

45. Chanarin I: Folate deficiency in the
myeloproliferative disorders. Am J Clin
Nutr 23:855, 1970.

46. Chevallier P: Les hémorragies des leucemies
myeloides Bull Acad Natl Méd 137:528,
1953.

47. Collins DH, Rose WM: The nature of
anaemia in leukaemia. J Pathol Bacteriol
60:63, 1948.

48. Cooperberg AA: Acute promyelocytic
leukemia. Can Med Assoc J 97:57, 1967.

49. ——, Neiman GMA: Fibrinogenopenia
and fibrinolysis in acute myelogenous
leukemia. Ann Intern Med 46:706, 1955.

50. Corcino J, Krauss S, Waxman S, Herbert
V: Release of vitamin B_{12}-binding protein by
human leukocytes in vitro. J Clin Invest
49:2250, 1970.

51. ——, Zalusky R, Greenberg M, Herbert
V: Coexistence of pernicious anaemia and
chronic myeloid leukaemia: An experiment
of nature involving vitamin B_{12} metabolism.
Br J Haematol 20:511, 1971.

52. Croizat P, Favre-Gilly J: Les aspects du
syndrome hémorragique des leucemies. A
propos de 12 cas de thrombocytopénie et
d'un cas de fibrinopénie. Sang 20:417, 1949.

53. Crosby WH, Akeroyd JH: The limit of hemoglobin synthesis in hereditary hemolytic
anemia. Its relation to the excretion of bile
pigment. Am J Med 13:273, 1952.

54. Dacie JV, Smith MD, White JC, Mollin
DL: Refractory normoblastic anaemia: A
clinical and haematological study of seven
cases. Br J Haematol 5:56, 1959.

55. ——, Worlledge SM: Auto-immune
hemolytic anemias, in Brown EB, Moore
CV (eds.): Progress in Hematology, vol. 6.
New York, Grune & Stratton, 1969, p 82.

56. Dameshek W: Theories of autoimmuniza-

tion. M.D. Anderson Hospital Symposium,
Houston, Texas, March 1–3, 1962, in Con-
ceptual Advances in Immunology and
Oncology. New York, Hoeber, 1963.

57. ——: Sideroblastic anaemia: Is this a malignancy? Br J Haematol 11:52, 1965.

58. ——: Riddle: What do aplastic anemia,
paroxysmal nocturnal hemoglobinuria
(PNH) and "hypoplastic" leukemia have in
common? Blood 30:251, 1967.

59. ——: PNH. A "candidate" myeloproliferative disorder? Blood 33:263, 1969.

60. ——, Berlin DD, Blumgart HL: Complete ablation of the thyroid gland in a case
of chronic lymphatic leukemia with hypermetabolism. N Engl J Med 210:723,
1934.

61. ——, Schwartz RS: Leukemia and
autoimmunization—some possible relationships. Blood 14:1151, 1959.

62. De George FV: Differences in Rh type between age groups of leukaemia patients.
Nature 228:168, 1970.

63. De Grouchy J, De Nava C, Zittoun R,
Bousser J: Analyses chromosomiques dans
l'anémie sidéroblastique idiopathique acquise. Une étude de six cas. Nouv Rev Fr
Hématol 6:367, 1966.

64. De Nicola P, Di Gugliemo L, Timossi G:
Study of the hemostatic and coagulation defect in patients during roentgen therapy with
particular reference to leukemias and malignancies. Am J Roentgenol Radium Ther
Nucl Med 79:142, 1958.

65. Desforges JF, Ross JD, Moloney WC:
Mechanisms of anemia in leukemia and malignant lymphoma. Am J Med 28:69, 1960.

66. Didisheim P, Thormbold JS, Vandervoort
RLE, Mibashan RS: Acute promyelocytic
leukemia with fibrinogen and factor V
deficiencies. Blood 23:717, 1964.

67. Duckworth D: A treatise on gout. London,
Griffin, 1889. Quoted by Talbott.

68. Ducos J, Ruffié J, Marty Y, Salles-Mourlan
AM, Colombies' P: Does a connexion exist
between blood group modifications observed in leukaemia and certain chromosomal alterations? Nature 203:432,
1964.

69. Ebbe S, Wittels B, Dameshek W: Autoimmune thrombocytopenic purpura ("ITP"
type) with chronic lymphocytic leukemia.
Blood 19:23, 1962.

70. Fairley GH, Akers RJ: Antibodies to blood
group A and B substances in reticuloses. Br
J Haematol 8:375, 1962.

71. Feizi T, Hardisty RM: I antigen in
leukaemic patients. Nature 210:1066, 1966.

72. Fenninger LD, Waterhouse C, Keutmann EH: The interrelationship of nitrogen and phosphorus in patients with certain neoplastic diseases. Cancer 6:930, 1953.

73. Fink ME, Finch SC: Serum muramidase and granulocyte turnover. Proc Soc Exp Biol Med 127:365, 1968.

74. Freireich EJ, Schmidt, PJ, Schneiderman MA, Frei E III: A comparative study of the effect of transfusion of fresh and preserved whole blood on bleeding in patients with acute leukemia. N Engl J Med 260:6, 1959.

75. Freymann JG, Burrell SB, Marler EA: Role of hemolysis in anemia secondary to chronic lymphocytic leukemia and certain malignant lymphomas. N Engl J Med 259:847, 1958.

76. Friedgood HB: The effect of Lugol's solution on chronic lymphatic leukemia and its bearing upon the pathogenesis of exophthalmic goiter. Am J Med Sci 183:515, 1932.

77. Friedman IA, Schwartz SO, Leithold SL: Platelet function defects with bleeding. Arch Intern Med 113:177, 1964.

78. Fritz RD, Forkner CE Jr, Freireich EJ, Frei E III, Thomas LB: The association of fatal intracranial hemorrhage and "blastic crisis" in patients with acute leukemia. N Engl J Med 261:59, 1959.

79. Fritze E: Der Purinstoffwechsel bei Leukämien unter Urethanbehandlung. Klin Wochenschr 27:366, 1949.

80. Gavosto F, Gabutti V, Masera P, Pileri A: The problem of anaemia in the acute leukaemias. Kinetic study. Eur J Cancer 6:33, 1970.

81. Gaydos LA, Freireich EJ, Mantel N: The quantitative relation between platelet count and hemorrhage in patients with acute leukemia. N Engl J Med 266:905, 1962.

82. Gellhorn A, Friend C, Ultmann JE, Feigelson P: The lymphomas: Combined clinic at the College of Physicians and Surgeons, Columbia University, New York, N.Y. Ann Intern Med 52:201, 1960.

83. Gerbrandy J, Hellendoorn HB, Lokkerbol H: The urinary excretion of metabolites during radiological cell-destruction in leukaemic patients. Br J Cancer 12:275, 1958.

84. Gilbert HS, Krauss S, Pasternack B, Herbert V, Wasserman LR: Serum vitamin B_{12} content and unsaturated vitamin B_{12}-binding capacity in myeloproliferative disease. Ann Intern Med 71:719, 1969.

85. Girolami A, Mootse G, Cliffton EE: Blood plasminogen (profibrinolysin) levels in patients with leukemia and lymphoma. Am J Med Sci 254:334, 1967.

86. Gold ER, Hollander L: Blood groups and leukemia. Blut 9:188, 1963.

87. Gottlieb CW, Retief FP, Pratt PW, Herbert V: Correlation of B_{12}-binding proteins with disorders of B_{12} metabolism: Relation to hypo- and hyper-leukocytic states and leukocyte turnover (Abstract) J Clin Invest 45:1016.

88. Greenfield RE, Sterling WR, Price VE: Studies on the anemia of tumor-bearing animals. II. The mechanism of erythrocyte destruction. J Natl Cancer Inst 21:1099, 1958.

89. Griffiths WJ, Wetherley-Mein G, Cottam DG: Metabolic studies in leukemia, with special reference to the B.M.R. and serum creatine, in: Proceedings of Sixth Congress of the International Society of Hematology. New York, Grune & Stratton, 1958.

90. Gunz FW: Hemorrhagic thrombocythemia: A critical review. Blood 15:706, 1960.

91. ———, Hough RF: Benign cryoglobulinaemic purpura. Br J Haematol 2:95, 1956.

92. ———, Ravich RBM, Vincent PC, Stewart JM, Crossen PE, Mellor J: A case of acute leukemia with a rapidly changing chromosome constitution. Ann Génét 13:79, 1970.

93. Hagen PS, Watson CJ: Hypersplenism and hemolytic anemia in leukemia: results of splenectomy, in Proceedings of the Third Congress of the International Society of Hematology. New York, Grune & Stratton, 1951, p 95.

94. Hall CA: Vitamin B_{12}-binding proteins of man. Ann Intern Med 75:297, 1971.

95. ———, Finkler AE: Abnormal transport of vitamin B_{12} in plasma in chronic myelogenous leukemia. Nature 204:1207, 1964.

96. Hampton JW: Leukocyte anticoagulant with myelogenous leukemia. Am J Med 48:408, 1970.

97. Hansen NE, Andersen V: Lactate dehydrogenase of human bone marrow in the study of haemopoiesis. Acta Med Scand 183:581, 1968.

98. ———, Karle H, Andersen V: Muramidase activity of bone marrow plasma. Acta Med Scand 185:387, 1969.

99. Heilmeyer L: Blutfarbstoffwechselstudien. B. Mitteilung: Der Farbstoffwechsel beim hämolytischen Ikterus und einigen hämolytischen Anämien verschiedener Genese. Wirkungen des Leberstoffs und pe-

roraler Milzverabreichung. Dtsch Arch
Klin Med 172:628, 1932.

100. Herbert V: Diagnostic and prognostic
values of measurement of serum vitamin
B_{12}-binding protein. Blood 32:305, 1968.

101. Hewitt D, Spiers PS: Low prevalence of A-
antigen in children with acute myeloid
leukaemia. Lancet 2:93, 1964.

102. Hickling RA: Leukaemia and related conditions and the blood uric-acid. Lancet 1:175,
1958.

103. Hillestad LK: Acute promyelocytic
leukemia. Acta Med Scand 159:189, 1957.

104. Hirsch EO, Gardner FH: The transfusion of
human blood platelets. With a note on the
transfusion of granulocytes. J Lab Clin Med
39:556, 1952.

105. Hirschfeld H: Ueber Leukanamie. Folia
Haematol 3:332, 1906.

106. Hirsh J, Buchanan JG, De Gruchy GC,
Baikie AG: Hypofibrinogenaemia without
increased fibrinolysis in leukaemia. Lancet
1:418, 1967.

107. Hoffbrand AV, Newcombe BFA: Leucocyte folate in vitamin B_{12} and folate
deficiency and in leukaemia. Br J Haematol
13:954, 1967.

108. Holden D, Lichtman H: Paroxysmal
nocturnal hemoglobinuria with acute
leukemia. Blood 33:283, 1969.

109. Hoogstraten B, Baker H, Gilbert HS:
Serum folate and serum vitamin B_{12} in
patients with malignant hematologic
diseases. Cancer Res 25:1933, 1965.

110. Huff RL, Hennessy TG, Austin RE, Garcia
JF, Roberts BM, Lawrence JH: Plasma and
red cell iron turnover in normal subjects and
in patients having various hematopoietic
disorders. J Clin Invest 29:1041, 1950.

111. Hyman CB, Borda E, Digumarthi G: What
are normal blood values for leukemia in remission? Blood 14:369, 1959.

112. Hyman GA, Gellhorn A, Harvey JL:
Studies on the anemia of disseminated malignant neoplastic disease. II. Study of the
life span of the erythrocyte. Blood 11:618,
1956.

113. Jaffé RH: Erythropoiesis in leukemia. Folia
Haematol 49:51, 1933.

114. _____: The nature of anemia in acute
leukemia. Arch Pathol 20:725, 1935.

115. Jenkins DE Jr, Hartmann RC: Paroxysmal
nocturnal hemoglobinuria terminating in
acute myeloblastic leukemia. Blood 33:274,
1969.

116. Jensen MK, Killmann S–A: Chromosome
studies in acute leukaemia. Acta Med Scand
181:47, 1967.

117. Jonsson U, Hansen–Pruss OC, Rundles

RW: Hemolytic anemia in myelogenous
leukemia with splenectomy. Blood 5:920,
1950.

118. Jugenberg A, Tschotschia K: Neue Ergebnisse zum Verständnis des Leukämie-
verlaufes. Strahlentherapie 41:86, 1931.

119. Kassulke JT, Hallgren HM, Yunis EJ:
Studies of red cell isoantigens on peripheral
leukocytes from normal and leukemic individuals. Am J Pathol 56:333, 1969.

120. Kaufmann J, Lowenstein L: A study of the
acute leukoses. Ann Intern Med 14:903,
1940.

121. Kaufmann RW, Schechter GP, McFarland
W: Paroxysmal nocturnal hemoglobinuria
terminating in acute granulocytic leukemia.
Blood 33:287, 1969.

122. Kay HEM, Shorter RG: Blood groups in
leukaemia and the reticuloses. Vox Sang
1:255, 1956.

123. Klima R: Uber Anämien und Erythropoese
bei leukämischen Erkrankungen. Wien
Arch Inn Med 26:277, 391, 1935.

124. Kourilsky FM, Dausset J, Feingold N,
Dupuy JM, Bernard J: Etude de la répar-
tition des antigenes leucocytaires chez las
malades atteints de leucémie aiguë en rémission, in Dausset J, Hamburger J, Mathe
G (eds.): Advances in Transplantation.
Copenhagen, Munksgaard, 1968, p 515.

125. Krakoff IH: Urinary uric acid excretion in
leukemia, in Rebuck JW, Bethell FH,
Monto RW, (eds.): The Leukemias:
Etiology, Pathophysiology and Treatment.
New York, Academic Press, 1957, p 401.

126. _____: Mechanisms of drug action in
leukemia. Am J Med 28:735, 1960.

127. _____, Balis ME, Magill JW, Nary, D:
Studies of purine metabolism in neoplastic
disease. Med Clin N Am 45:521, 1961.

128. _____, Meyer RL: Hyperuricemia in
leukemia and lymphoma. JAMA 193:1,
1965.

129. Kravitz SC, Diamond HD, Craver LF:
Uremia complicating leukemia chemotherapy. Report of a case treated with
triethylene melamine. JAMA 146:1595,
1951.

130. Kress H von: Die Leukämien im Rahmen
allgemein pathologischer Probleme. Dtsch
Arch Klin Med 176:359, 1934.

131. Kritzler RA: Anuria complicating the
treatment of leukemia. Am J Med 25:532,
1958.

132. Krugman S, Giles JP: Viral hepatitis. New
light on an old disease. JAMA 212:1019,
1970.

133. Lawler SD, Klouda PT, Hardisty RM, Till
MM: The HL-A system in lymphoblastic

leukaemia. A study of patients and their families. Br J Haematol 21:595, 1971.

134. Lawrence JC, Craddock CG: Stem cell competition—the response to anti-neutrophilic serum as affected by hemorrhage. J Lab Clin Med 72:731, 1968.

135. Lear H, Oppenheimer GD: Anuria following radiation therapy in leukemia. JAMA 143:806, 1950.

136. Levi JA, Speden JB, Vincent PC, Gunz FW: Studies on muramidase in hematologic disorders. I. Serum muramidase and serum lactic dehydrogenase in leukemia. Cancer, 31:939, 1973.

137. Lewis JH, Burchenal JH, Ellison RR, Ferguson JH, Palmer JH, Murphy ML, Zucker MB: Studies of hemostatic mechanisms in leukemia and thrombocytopenia. Am J Clin Pathol 28:433, 1957.

138. Linsk JA, Girsh S: Fatal auto-immune hemolytic anemia complicating lymphoma. Ohio State Med J 67:1088, 1971.

139. Lucia SP, Hunt MC: The significance of blood groups in the hematopoietic disorders, in Proceedings of the Third Congress of the International Society of Hematology. New York, Grune & Stratton, 1951, p 221.

140. McGinnis MH, Schmidt PJ, Carbone PP: Close association of I group and disease. Nature 202:606, 1964.

141. MacMahon B, Folusiak JC: Leukemia and ABO blood group. Am J Hum Genet 10:287, 1958.

142. Magnus-Levy A von: Ueber den Stoffwechsel bei acuter und chronischer Leukämie. Arch pathol Anat 152:107, 1898.

143. Majsky A: Some cases of leukaemia with modifications of the D (Rh$_o$)-receptor. Neoplasma 14:335, 1967.

144. _____: Modifikationen des H-Erythrozyten-Antigens bei Kranken mit Leukämien. Folia Haematol 87:17, 1967.

145. Meckstroth CV, Rapport RL, Curtis GM, Simcox SJ: The laboratory diagnosis of extrathyroidal hypermetabolism. J Clin Endocrinol 12:1373, 1952.

146. Mendelsohn RS, Warkin DM, Horbett AP, Fahey JL: Identification of the vitamin B_{12}-binding protein in the serum of normals and of patients with chronic myelocytic leukemia. Blood 13:740, 1958.

147. Menzies RC, Crossen PE, Fitzgerald PH, Gunz FW: Cytogenetic and cytochemical studies on marrow cells in B_{12} and folate deficiency. Blood 28:581, 1966.

148. Meyer LM, Bertcher RW, Cronkite EP, Suarez RM, Miller IF, Mulzac CW, Olivarreta ST: Co^{60} vitamin B_{12}-binding capacity of serum in persons with hematologic disor-

ders, various medical diseases and neoplasms. Acta Med Scand 169:557, 1961.

149. _____, Cronkite EP, Miller IF, Mulzac CW, Jones I: Co^{60} vitamin B_{12}-binding capacity of human leukocytes. Blood 19:229, 1962.

150. Middleton WS, Meyer OO, Pohle EA: The influence of roentgen therapy upon the basal metabolism in leukemia. Radiology 26:586, 1936.

151. Miller A, Sullivan JF: The in vitro binding of cobalt^{60}-labeled vitamin B_{12} by normal and leukemic sera. J Clin Invest 37:556, 1958.

152. _____, _____: Some physicochemical properties of the vitamin B_{12}-binding substances of normal and chronic myelogenous leukemic sera. J Lab Clin Med 53:607, 1959.

153. Miller JN, Meyers RL, Carpenter CM: Serum complement levels in children with acute lymphocytic leukemia. J Pediatr 64:134, 1964.

154. Minot GR, Means JH: The metabolism-pulse ratio in exophthalmic goiter and in leukemia. With remarks on certain similarities in the symptomatology of these diseases. Arch Intern Med 33:576, 1924.

155. Mollin DL, Pitney WR, Baker SJ, Bradley JE: The plasma clearance and urinary excretion of parenterally administered Co^{58} B_{12}. Blood 11:31, 1956.

156. Musser JH, Edsall DL: A study of metabolism in leukemia, under the influence of x-ray. With a consideration of the manner of action of the x-ray and of some precautions desirable in its therapeutic use. Trans Assoc Am Physicians 20:294, 1905.

157. Nathan DG, Berlin NI: Studies of the rate of production and life span of erythrocytes in acute leukemia. Blood 14:935, 1959.

158. Nilsson IM, Sjoerdsma A, Waldenstroüm J: Antifibrinolytic activity and metabolism of ε-amino-caproic acid in man. Lancet 1:1322, 1960.

159. Ogston D, McAndrew GM, Ogston CM: Fibrinolysis in leukaemia. J Clin Pathol 21:136, 1968.

160. Ohayon E, Ducos J, Goret P, Salmon H, Toma B: Cytotoxicity of ALS and anti-HL-A antibodies in human leukaemia. Lancet 1:39, 1972.

161. Osserman EF, Lawlor DP: Abnormal serum and urine proteins in 35 cases of multiple myeloma as studied by filter paper electrophoresis. Am J Med 18:462, 1955.

162. _____, _____: Serum and urinary lysozyme (muramidase) in monocytic and

monomyelocytic leukemia. J Exp Med 124:921, 1966.

163. Pappenheim A: Bemerkungen über Leukanämie in Anschluss an vorstehende Mitteilung von Hans Hirschfeld. Folia Haematol 3:339, 1906.

164. Paschkis K: Ueber atypische hämolytische Anämien. Z Klin Med 105:301, 1927.

165. Peacock AC: Serum haptoglobin type and leukemia: An association with possible etiological significance. J Natl Cancer Inst 36:631, 1966.

166. Pegrum GD, Balfour IC, Evans CA, Middleton VL: HL-A antigens on leukaemic cells. Br J Haematol 19:493, 1970.

167. Perillie PE, Kaplan SS, Lefkowitz E, Rogaway W, Kitch SC: Studies of muramidase (lysozyme) in leukemia. JAMA 203:317, 1968.

168. Perry S: Coagulation defects in leukemia. J Lab Clin Med 50:229, 1957.

169. Pettit JE, Williams ED, Glass HI, Lewis SM, Szur K. Wicks CJ: Studies of splenic function in the myeloproliferative disorders and generalized malignant lymphomas. Br J Haematol 20:575, 1971.

170. Pirofsky B: Autoimmune hemolytic anemia and neoplasia of the reticuloendothelium. Ann Intern Med 68:109, 1968.

171. Pisciotta AV, Schulz EJ: Fibrinolytic purpura in acute leukemia. Am J Med 19:824, 1955.

172. Pitney WR, Beard MF, Van Loon EJ: Observations on the bound form of vitamin B_{12} in human serum. J Biol Chem 207:143, 1954.

173. Polliack A: Acute promyelocytic leukemia with disseminated intravascular coagulation. Am J Clin Pathol 56:155, 1971.

174. Rabinowitz Y, Dietz AA: Malic and lactic dehydrogenase isozymes of normal and leukemic leukocytes separated on glass bead columns. Blood 29:182, 1967.

175. Rachmilewitz B, Rachmilewitz M: Chemotherapy—induced changes in serum vitamin B_{12}-binding proteins in myeloid leukemia. Israel J Med Sci 7:1140, 1971.

176. Rachmilewitz D, Rachmilewitz EA, Polliack A, Hershko Ch: Acute promyelocytic leukaemia: A report of five cases on the diagnostic significance of serum vitamin B_{12} determination. Br J Haematol 22:87, 1972.

177. Raccuglia G, Sacks MS: Vitamin B_{12}-binding capacity of normal and leukemic sera. J Lab Clin Med 50:69, 1957.

178. Ragen PA, McGuire P, Antonius JI: Decreased formation of erythrocyte antigen A and a consistent chromosome abnormality in a patient with myelomonocytic leukemia. Acta Haematol 39:309, 1968.

179. Rand JJ, Moloney WC, Sise HS: Coagulation defects in acute promyelocytic leukemia. Arch Intern Med 123:39, 1969.

180. Rao PBR, Lagerlöf B, Einhorn J, Reizenstein PG: Folic acid activity in leukemia and cancer. Cancer Res 25:221, 1965.

181. Rastrick JM, Fitzgerald PH, Gunz FW: Direct evidence for presence of Ph^1 chromosome in erythroid cells. Br Med J 1:69, 1968.

182. Ravich RBM, Gunz FW, Reed CS, Thompson IL: The danger of surgery in uncontrolled haemorrhagic thrombocythaemia Med J Aust 1:704, 1970.

183. Renton PH, Stratton F, Gunson HH, Hancock JA: Red cells of all four ABO groups in a case of leukaemia. Br Med J 1:294, 1962.

184. Retief FP, Gottlieb CW, Kochwa S, Pratt PW, Herbert V: Separation of vitamin B_{12}-binding proteins of serum, gastric juice and saliva by rapid DEAE cellulose chromatography. Blood 29:501, 1967.

185. Richards AG: Loss of blood-group-B antigen in chronic lymphatic leukaemia. Lancet 2:178, 1962.

186. Riddle MC, Sturgis CC: Basal metabolism in chronic myelogenous leukemia. Arch Intern Med 39:255, 1927.

187. Ropartz C, Audran R, Rivat L, Rousseau P-Y, Fine JM; Leucoses et groupes de gamma-globulines Gm et Inv. Vox Sang 8:627, 1963.

188. Rose DP: Folic acid deficiency in leukaemia and lymphomas. J Clin Pathol 19:29, 1966.

189. Rosenthal MC, Pisciotta AF, Komnios ZD, Goldenberg H, Dameshek W: The autoimmune hemolytic anemia of malignant lymphocytic disease. Blood 10:197, 1955.

190. Rosenthal N: in Proceedings of the second Conference on folic acid antagonists in leukemia treatment. Blood 7:152, 1952.

191. Rosenthal RL: Acute promyelocytic leukemia associated with hypofibrinogenemia. Blood 21:495, 1963.

192. Rosner F, Dobbs JV, Ritz ND, Lee SL: Disturbances of hemostasis in acute myeloblastic leukemia. Acta Haematol 43:65, 1970.

193. _____, Gabriel FD: Leukocytic folate activity in patients with leukemia. NY State J Med 71:2292, 1971.

194. Ross JF, Crockett CL Jr, Emerson CP: The mechanism of anemia in leukemia and ma-

lignant lymphoma. J Clin Invest 30:668, 1951.

195. Rothenberg SP, Da Costa M: Further observations on the folate-binding factor in some leukemic cells. J Clin Invest 50:719, 1971.

196. Ruffié J, Ducos J, Varsi M, Colombies P: Etude de la modification des facteurs Gm au cours des leucoses. Nouv Rev Fr Hématol 4:599, 1964.

197. Saba HI, Roberts HR, Herion JC: The anticoagulant activity of lysosomal cationic protein from polymorphonuclear leukocytes. J Clin Invest 46:580, 1967.

198. Salkowski E: Beiträge zur Kenntniss der Leukämie. Arch Pathol Anat 50:174, 1870.

199. Salmon C: Quantitative and thermodynamic data related to modifications of ABO blood groups in leukemia. Bibl Haematol 23:337, 1965.

200. _____, Salmon D: H antigen deficiency in certain subjects of blood group O with acute leukemia. Rev Fr Etud Clin Biol 10:212, 1965.

201. Samama M, Colombani J: Le temps de Quick et ses facteurs au cours des leucoses. Sang 27:304, 1956.

202. Sandberg AA, Cartwright GE, Wintrobe MM: Studies on leukemia. I. Uric acid excretion. Blood 11:154, 1956.

203. Senn HJ, Rhomberg WU: Muramidaseaktivität in Serum und Urin bei akuten und chronischen Leukämien. Schweiz Med Wochenschr 100:1993, 1970.

204. Sherlock S, Fox RA, Niazi SP, Scheuer PJ; Chronic liver disease and primary liver-cell cancer with hepatitis-associated (Australia) antigen in serum. Lancet 1:1243, 1970.

205. Shirley R, Desai RG: Association of leukaemia, and blood groups. J Med Genet 2:189, 1965.

206. Silberman S, Krmpotic E: Refractory anemia with leukemic transformation and chromosomal change. Acta Haematol 41:186, 1969.

207. Sinks LF, Newton WA, Nagi NA, Stevenson TD: A syndrome associated with extreme hyperuricemia in leukemia. J Pediatr 68:578, 1966.

208. Skipper HE, Chapman JB, Bell MJ: Studies on the role of folic acid in the leukemic process. Cancer 3:871, 1950.

209. Soulier JP, Dausset J: Les troubles de la crase sanguine dans les leucémies aiguës. Etude biologique et thérapeutique. Sang 21:602, 1950.

210. Starkweather WH, Spencer HH, Schoch HK: The lactate dehydrogenases of hemopoietic cells. Blood 28:860, 1966.

211. Stefanini M, Dameshek W: The hemorrhagic disorders. A clinical and therapeutic approach. New York, Grune & Stratton, 1955, p 192.

212. Stevenson TD, Beard MF: The effect of antimetabolites on the serum vitamin B_{12} level in leukemia, in Proceedings of the Sixth Congress of the International Society of Hematology. New York, Grune & Stratton, 1958, p 173.

213. Sutnick AI, Levine PH, London WT, Blumberg BS: Frequency of Australia antigen in patients with leukaemia in different countries. Lancet 1:1200, 1971.

214. _____, London WT, Blumberg BS, Yankee RA, Gerstley BJS, Millman I: Australia antigen (a hepatitis-associated antigen) in leukemia. J Natl Cancer Inst 44:1241, 1970.

215. _____, _____, Gerstley BJ, Crosslund MM, Blumberg BS: Anicteric hepatitis associated with Australia antigen. Occurrence in patients with Down's syndrome. JAMA 205:670, 1968.

216. Talbott JH; Gout and blood dyscrasias. Medicine 38:173, 1959.

217. Thiersch JB, Philips FS: Effects of 4-aminopteroylglutamic acid in dogs with special reference to megaloblastosis. Proc Soc Exp Biol Med 71:484, 1949.

218. Thomas JW, Anderson BB: Vitamin B_{12} content of normal and leukaemic leucocytes. Br J Haematol 2:41, 1956.

219. Thorsby E, Bratlie A, Lie SO: HL-A genotypes of children with acute leukaemia. A family study. Scand J Haematol 6:409, 1969.

220. Tinney WS, Watkins CH: Blood groups and the blood dyscrasias. Proc Staff Meet Mayo Clin 16:613, 1941.

221. Tovey GH, Lockyer JW, Tierney RBH: Changes in Rh grouping reactions in a case of leukaemia. Vox Sang 6:628, 1961.

222. Troup SB, Swisher SN, Young LE: The anemia of leukemia. Am J Med 28:751, 1960.

223. Tudhope GR: The survival of red cells and the causation of anaemia in leukaemia. Scot Med J 4:342, 1959.

224. Ultmann JE: The role of the spleen in the hemolytic anemia of cancer patients. Cancer Res 18:959, 1958.

225. Van Rood JJ, Van Leeuwen A, Schippers A, Balner H: Human histocompatibility antigen in normal and neoplastic tissues. Cancer Res 28:1415, 1968.

226. Veale AMO, Gunz FW: Haptoglobin and leukaemia. Proc Univ Otago Med Sch 45:36, 1967.

227. Videbaek A: Auto-immune haemolytic anaemia in some malignant systemic diseases. Acta Med Scand 171:463, 1962.

228. Virchow R: Zur pathologischen Physiologie des Bluts. Arch Pathol Anat 5:43, 1853.

229. Walford RL, Finkelstein S, Neerhout R, Konrad P, Shanbrom E: Acute childhood leukaemia in relation to the HL-A human transplantation genes. Nature 225:461, 1970.

230. Wasi P, Block M: The mechanism of the development of anemia in untreated chronic lymphatic leukemia. Blood 17:597, 1961.

231. Watkin DM, Silver RT: Nitrogen, mineral, uric acid and basal metabolism studies in a case of adult acute leukemia with extensive osteolytic bone disease. Am J Med 24:638, 1958.

232. Watson CJ: Studies of urobilinogen. II. Urobilinogen in the urine and feces of subjects without evidence of diseases of the liver or biliary tract. Arch Intern Med 59:196, 1937.

233. _____: The pyrrol pigments with particular reference to normal and pathologic hemoglobin metabolism, in H Downey (ed.): Handbook of Hematology, vol 4. New York, Hoeber, 1938, p 2445.

234. Weinstein IM, Le Roy GV: Radioactive sodium chromate for the study of survival of red blood cells. II. The rate of hemolysis in certain hematologic disorders. J Lab Clin Med 42:368, 1953.

235. _____, Weissman SM, Watkin DM: The plasma vitamin B_{12}-binding substance: I. Its detection in the seromucoid fraction of plasma from normal subjects and patients with chronic myelocytic leukemia. J Clin Invest 38:1904, 1959.

236. Weisberger AS, Persky L: Renal calculi and uremia as complications of lymphoma. Am J Med Sci 225:669, 1953.

237. Wetherley-Mein G, Epstein IS, Foster WD, Grimes AJ: Mechanisms of anaemia in leukaemia. Br J Haematol 4:281, 1958.

238. Whang J, Frei E III, Tjio JH, Carbone PP, Brecher G: The distribution of the Philadelphia chromosome in patients with chronic myelogenous leukemia. Blood 22:664, 1963.

239. Whipple GH, Robscheit-Robbins FS: Hemoglobin production factors in the human liver. III. Anemias—primary, aplastic and secondary—leukemias. J Exp Med 57:671, 1933.

240. Wickramsinghe SN, Cooper EH, Chalmers DG: A study of erythropoiesis by combined morphologic, cytochemical and autoradiographic methods. Blood 31:304, 1968.

241. Wiernik PH, Serpick AA: Clinical significance of serum and urinary muramidase activity in leukemia and other hematologic malignancies. Am J Med 46:330, 1969.

242. Yokoyama M: Suppression of A and I antigens in a case of chronic myelogenous leukemia. Blut 18:193, 1969.

243. Yoshikawa S, Yamada K, Yoshida TO: Serum complement level in patients with leukemia. Cancer 4:845, 1969.

244. Zaizov R, Matoth Y: The pathogenesis of anemia in acute leukemia. Israel J Med Sci 7:1025, 1971.

245. Zittoun J, Zittoun R, Guernet M, Bilski-Pasquier G, Bousser J: B_{12} hypervitaminaemia in leukaemia and myeloproliferative syndromes. Rev Fr Etud Clin Biol 13:684, 1968.

246. Zucker S, Hanes DJ, Vogler WR, Eanes RZ: Plasma muramidase: A study of methods and clinical applications. J Lab Clin Med 75:83, 1970.

247. Zuckerman AJ: The nature and significance of the Australia antigen. Proc R Soc Med 64:273, 1971.

15

Differential Diagnosis

In most cases of leukemia the diagnosis is first suspected on the grounds of clinical symptoms or signs and confirmed by means of laboratory investigation. The differential diagnosis will thus include two groups of conditions, that is, those that mimic leukemia either clinically or hematologically. Because of the many ways in which the different types of leukemia can present, there is a rather formidable list of alternatives which may have to be excluded.

CLINICAL FINDINGS

The onset of leukemia may be sudden or insidious, and the differential diagnoses to be considered differ in these two groups. Most chronic leukemias have an insidious onset, but the symptoms of acute leukemia may appear quite suddenly or as slowly as those of the chronic type.

Sudden Onset

Fever, hemorrhages, infections, and bone pain are common initial symptoms. In children, and at times in adults, acute leukemia is apt to present in the guise of an acute infection and the symptoms may not differ from those of influenza, an upper respiratory tract infection, or the prodromal stages of the exanthemata. Nonspecific rashes may resemble those of measles, rubella, or drug reactions, especially those caused by penicillin. When the rash becomes purpuric, the various septicemias—staphylococcal, meningococcal, etc.—must be excluded. If purpura is prominent, the list of alternatives embraces a large number of other causes such as idiopathic thrombocytopenic purpura, allergic (Henoch-Schönlein type) purpura, marrow aplasia, liver disease, and, occasionally, vitamin K deficiency and scurvy. The most important distinction to be made is between acute leukemia, idiopathic thrombocytopenic purpura, and aplastic anemia, all of which are characterized by thrombocytopenia. Since the leukocyte picture may not of itself be decisive, a bone marrow examination usually becomes an essential procedure at an early stage. In idiopathic thrombocytopenic purpura, the marrow shows adequate numbers of megakaryocytes in an otherwise normal marrow; in acute leukemia, when the blood is thrombocytopenic, the megakaryocytes are greatly reduced. The distinction between leukemia and aplastic anemia—both of which may present similar symptoms—can be a most difficult one, and even the bone marrow study may be inconclusive, since hypocellularity of the marrow is found in some cases of acute leukemia. Primitive leukocytes (myeloblasts, lymphoblasts, and others) are usually the determining feature between the two conditions; if 10 percent or more blast forms are present, the probability of primitive cell leukemia is great. Repeat specimens and, in some patients, trephine biopsies may be required to settle the question, which at times is only resolved by repeated observation over lengthy periods.

Bone pain often dominates the clinical picture of acute leukemia in children, and if this is the case, acute rheumatic fever, osteomyelitis, rickets, bone tumors, and syphilis must be excluded. Since the pains are often referred to the joints and there may be articular swelling, rheumatic fever, rheumatoid arthritis and Still's disease can be closely simulated. Quite often the lack of response to salicylates in supposed cases of rheumatic fever first raises the suspicion that there may be a different underlying pathology. Acute nephritis is another condition which is sometimes thought of in the early stages, especially when there is hematuria which may occur as part of the bleeding tendency of acute leukemia.

Leukemia may first show itself in the guise of tonsillitis or pharyngitis which is usually associated with some swelling of the cervical and, possibly, of other lymph nodes. Here, the diagnosis must be separated from septic tonsillitis, Vincent's angina, and from infectious mononucleosis which may give clinical and hematologic pictures extraordinarily similar to those of acute leukemia. This is further discussed below. Not infrequently, especially in myelomonocytic leukemia, gingival hyperplasia and painful gums are prominent, leading to the diagnosis of an infectious form of gingivitis or of dental caries. Indolent ulcers in the mouth and continued swelling of gums should always make one suspect the diagnosis of acute leukemia or such other forms of hematologic disorder as agranulocytosis or aplastic anemia in which the granulocytes are greatly reduced. We have seen several cases of leukemia diagnosed by dentists. Sepsis in other areas may be an early sign of leukemia; boils, pyodermia, and ischiorectal abscesses are also quite common.

The onset of leukemia may be indicated by hemorrhages from one of the mucous membranes, or following minor surgery, especially dental extractions, and, occasionally, tonsillectomy. Intractable menorrhagia may be an early sign, as in one of our patients who actually underwent a hysterectomy before the diagnosis was established. In all such patients, local and other general causes of bleeding will have to be considered, and this may involve extensive examinations if the blood picture is not immediately diagnostic. Elaborate investigations of the clotting mechanism may be undertaken, and any abnormalities found may be incorrectly interpreted as the expression of a *primary* clotting defect unless the possibility of leukemia is always borne in mind.

An acute onset of symptoms is much more common in young children than in adults, and it is instructive to examine some of the conditions which can be mistaken for leukemia in such patients. Mills collected a series of 44 children under 5 years of age, all of whom were initially suspected of having leukemia, but who were later found to be suffering from other diseases.[9] There were 26 acute infections, including 4 of pertussis and others of respiratory, intestinal, urinary, and septic infections; 4 with chronic conditions (rheumatoid arthritis, infantile cortical hyperostosis, eczema, urticaria pigmentosa); 6 with nutritional anemia; 2 with hepatoma; and 1 each with acquired hemolytic anemia, bleeding from the bowel for unknown reasons, drug reaction, brain tumor, and bleeding from an injection site. It is also interesting to remember that many of the babies with "congenital" leukemia reported upon in earlier years were undoubtedly suffering from erythroblastosis fetalis. The blood picture in these two conditions can be quite startlingly similar, but with the advent of the newer serological tests, confusion should rarely occur. A picture closely resembling that of congenital leukemia, but regressing spontaneously toward a normal blood count has been found in some infants with the features of mongolism.[12] We have seen diagnoses of acute leukemia made in neonates with cytomegalic inclusion disease, and in older children with disseminated neuroblastoma, and even in aregenerative crises of hereditary spherocytosis. In disseminated neuroblastoma, tumor cells may occur in marrow and peripheral blood, which may be readily mistaken for leukemic blast cells. In hereditary spherocytosis there may be fever and pancytopenia, and the marrow may show a large proportion of primitive nucleated red cells, at times mistaken for blast cells.

Gradual Onset

Patients may complain mainly of general symptoms, usually those of anemia; they may be found to have enlargement of the spleen, liver, or lymph nodes, or other sites such as the skin, bones, or central nervous system may be the first to show abnormalities. The differential diagnosis varies according to the mode of presentation.

"Pyrexia of unknown origin," continuing for weeks and at times of an intermittent character, is an occasional mode of onset in chronic leukemia. Alternative diagnoses here are autoimmune disorders, especially systemic lupus erythematosus or polyarteritis nodosa, chronic infections like tuberculosis, especially the generalized form; syphilis; brucellosis; systemic fungal infections; occult urinary lesions; and foremost perhaps, bacterial endocarditis. The last disorder, complete with splenomegaly and purpuric rashes, as well as with anemia and changes in the leukocyte count, may mimic leukemia quite closely. Hodgkin's disease and other generalized forms of lymphoma must be considered, to be ruled in or out by lymph node and bone marrow biopsies. Typhoid fever is still a possibility, and malaria can be very confusing where it is endemic.

The patient presenting with anemia but no other obvious clinical findings may pose a formidable diagnostic problem. Obvious causes of anemia such as iron deficiency or chronic bleeding can usually be readily excluded by hypochromia and other features of the red cells, as can most cases of frank hemolytic anemia; although here the existence of a primary cause, especially chronic lymphocytic leukemia, must always be suspected. The main difficulty lies in the rather amorphous group of "refractory" anemias which include the aplastic, hypoplastic, and sideroblastic varieties. The blood picture here is often confusing, and even the marrow findings may be far from clear-cut. This is so because in many of the acute leukemias the marrow may be hypoplastic for part of the course or, if hyperplastic, may show few of the characteristic neoplastic cells. If megaloblastic erythropoiesis is present, the chances of B_{12} or folic acid deficiency are high and the diagnosis can be confirmed by vitamin assays and absorption tests; however, the often bizarre megaloblastoid erythropoiesis of the Di Guglielmo syndrome and other cases of both acute and chronic granulocytic leukemia can be quite similar. Another diagnostic difficulty is presented by the fact that many patients are first seen after they have been treated—often ineffectively—before they can be properly investigated. After an injection of vitamin B_{12} or a transfusion, an originally megaloblastic marrow may have become normoblastic while the anemia is still severe and the need for an unequivocal diagnosis remains urgent. Many of the anemias which fall into the refractory group are secondary to renal, hepatic, or, more rarely, thyroid disease. Marrow involvement in carcinomatosis, and myelofibrosis with or without myeloid metaplasia of the spleen are considered below.

Splenomegaly as the leading symptom of leukemia raises its own diagnostic problems. If the size of the spleen is extreme, as in chronic granulocytic leukemia, the odds are heavily in favor of that diagnosis, or of myelosclerosis with myeloid metaplasia, even before the blood is examined.[3] In cases of moderate splenic enlargement, however, such other conditions as lymphosarcoma, or a splenic form of chronic lymphocytic leukemia, cirrhosis of the liver with the Banti syndrome, Gaucher's disease, Felty's syndrome, and other causes of hypersplenism, including sarcoidosis, tuberculosis, and tumors such as hemangiomas must all be considered. Examination of the blood, marrow and splenic aspirate, and lymphangiography may all be required before the precise pathology has been clarified, and in difficult cases, surgical biopsy of the marrow or even a laparotomy may eventually be found necessary. The distinction between chronic granulocytic leukemia and myeloid metaplasia of the spleen can usually be made by demonstration of the Philadelphia chromosome (as was discussed in Chapter 11). Hepatomegaly usually accompanies splenomegaly, but is sometimes relatively more prominent, in which case it is especially important to exclude conditions like cirrhosis, carcinomatous involvement, congestive heart failure, and amyloidosis.

Patients may show osseous lesions as the initial finding of leukemia, and their character has been described in Chapters 9 and 10. According to their type, they must be distinguished from carcinomatous and other tumor deposits; in children especially, neuroblastoma—which can give not only bone lesions, but also abnormal marrow findings—may be readily mistaken for leukemia. Chloroma, myelomatosis, eosinophilic granuloma; tuberculosis, particularly of the spine; the lesions of other blood diseases like thalassemia and sickle cell anemia; chronic pyogenic osteomyelitis; and hyperparathyroidism may all enter into the differential diagnosis in a particular patient.

The skin lesions of leukemia may resemble or imitate almost any other dermatologic disturbance. They may be the first indication (for example, lymphosarcoma, lymphoma, leukemia cutis, mycosis fungoides, erythrodermia, exfoliative dermatitis) of a future generalized, that is, leukemic disturbance. Histologic examination of the skin lesions will nearly always be required, but even this may not give an absolute distinction between a leukemic and other lesion, since the picture may not be entirely characteristic of the particular underlying disease process and may, in fact, change in appearance at different stages of the same disease. General carcinomatosis causes skin lesions much like those of some leukemias. The general, *leukemoid* (nonspecific) rashes can be difficult to distinguish from such conditions as psoriasis, the various eczemas, neurodermatitis, as well as nonleukemic forms of erythrodermia and exfoliative dermatitis.

The neurologic symptoms of leukemia which occasionally usher in the disease may simulate a large variety of other conditions of the central nervous system, notably Bell's palsy, trigeminal neuralgia, neoplastic and vascular lesions of the brain and, less commonly, the spinal cord or nerve roots, with or without meningeal irritation. An examination of the cerebrospinal fluid may reveal in these patients abnormalities such as high pressure, increased protein content, and pleocytosis, none of which are, however, specific.[13] Leukemic cells may, on the other hand, be found in some instances,[14] and are regularly present in the later stages during which CNS involvement becomes prominent.

LABORATORY FINDINGS

No diagnosis of leukemia can be considered established until it has been confirmed by means of a blood count and such other laboratory examinations as may be necessary to corroborate doubtful blood findings. In the majority of patients, the blood is by itself diagnostic; but quite often it is not, and suspicions raised by blood abnormalities may lead to extensive further investigations. The following sections discuss other conditions which may have to be excluded and in which the blood findings are not in themselves diagnostic.

Anemia

Anemia is sometimes the principal abnormality in the blood, and there may be only nonspecific changes in the leukocytes. The diagnosis of leukemia should be considered if the anemia is normocytic and normochromic, and especially if there is an associated thrombocytopenia. A macrocytic type of anemia does not exclude this possibility, but a definitely microcytic or hypochromic anemia makes it unlikely. Reticulocytosis of slight to moderate degree is often present in leukemia, and, if marked, may indicate an associated hemolytic element which occurs particularly in the chronic lymphocytic variety. The occasional difficulty of excluding pernicious anemia has already been mentioned.

Other types of anemia which may produce very similar blood findings are the aplastic and the various so-called refractory anemias. These may be particularly difficult to separate from the leukemias of the aleukemic or subleukemic types; in fact, sometimes the differentiation is impossible, not only in life but even at postmortem examination. These patients ordinarily present with pancytopenia, although the cytopenias may be of varying degree since not all marrow constituents may be equally involved. It is essential to search the blood carefully for the presence of abnormal white cells. This may be facilitated by the use of buffy coat preparations. Reticulocytosis usually speaks against marrow aplasia, though it does not exclude it completely, especially in children. There are all degrees of marrow damage, ranging from slight hypoplasia to complete aplasia, and the incomplete forms may be difficult to distinguish from leukemia, especially if the brunt of the damage should have fallen on the erythroid system, thus giving a relative myeloid preponderance in the marrow. We have seen several patients in whom the diagnosis of aplastic anemia was made by well-qualified observers but where the careful study of the peripheral blood revealed the presence of 2–4 percent of unequivocal blast forms, thus leading to the diagnosis of leukemia. It is evident that study of the blood smear is still the most important single means of diagnosis; too often the blood smear is passed over in favor of the undoubtedly important, but often nondiagnostic, bone marrow aspirate.

Hypoplastic anemia and hypoplastic leukemia may conceivably be variants of one and the same disorder, thus making differentiation difficult, if not impossible in a given patient. An interesting recent development in this field is the addition of paroxysmal nocturnal hemoglobinuria to the group of hypoplastic and conceivably preleukemic anemias.[4,5] It is conceivable that myelotoxic factors, such as drugs,[2] chemicals, ionizing radiation, or infection may injure the marrow severely, resulting in marked hypoplasia. The subsequent growth pattern may be a modified one, perhaps due to the development of a mutation. This may result in a leukemic type of proliferation, in which the cells in the bone marrow, though reduced in number, are abnormal or leukemic in type. The resultant blood picture is similar, if not identical, to that of hypoplastic anemia, except that in some patients a few primitive leukocytes are seen in the blood. The diagnosis is made on the basis of the bone marrow findings which show, in addition to hypocellularity, groups or clusters of primitive leukocytes, often with indentation or folding of the nuclei, prominent nucleoli, bizarre forms, asynchrony of nuclear-cytoplasmic differentiation, etc. Although the bone marrow findings seem unequivocal, one may hesitate even here to make a final diagnosis of leukemia, with the hopeless connotation of the term. Unusually careful search for primitive cells in the blood should be made in such patients, both in direct smears and those from the buffy coat. If primitive cells are seen, even in small numbers, the diagnosis of leukemia is much more likely than that of hypoplastic anemia. Occasionally, the transformation to a leukemic blood picture takes place suddenly and spontaneously. In other patients the diagnosis of leukemia seems quite obvious from the bone marrow picture, perhaps to a lesser extent from the blood, but at postmortem examination the pathologist may fail to find any indication of leukemia and may therefore conclude that the diagnosis of aplastic anemia is the correct one. Whether he is right or is simply seeing one stage in a "moving picture" of alternating hypoplastic leukemia and hypoplastic anemia is not certain. The uncertainty in differentiating aleukemic leukemia from hypoplastic anemia may make a therapeutic decision difficult. Should one attempt in a particular patient to use one of the chemotherapeutic agents or should corticosteroids alone be used, perhaps followed by other more radical measures such as splenectomy? Usually one compromises, at least for a given period, and gives the patient corticosteroid therapy, meanwhile awaiting more definite indications of one disease or the other. Eventually, a decision must be made, and it is to be remembered that whatever one does may be followed by worsening of the situation.

In many of the refractory and sideroblastic anemias the marrow is hyperplastic rather than hypoplastic and the resemblance to acute granulocytic leukemia may then be particularly close.

As noted above, we have seen occasional instances of very acute hemolytic anemias or the crisis of hereditary spherocytosis in which there was such extreme hyperplasia of the primitive erythroid cells in the marrow that the diagnosis of acute leukemia was mistakenly made. The differentiation of myelofibrosis is only mentioned here, being fully discussed elsewhere (Chapter 11). It may be among the most difficult ones to diagnose by laboratory methods. Rather akin to it are those cases of generalized tuberculosis which show involvement of the marrow. Here the resemblance to leukemia can be very striking, or perhaps the two conditions are present concurrently. Carcinomatous myelofibrosis may be difficult to differentiate from leukemia without a surgical or needle marrow biopsy. The differentiation of myelomatosis may also give rise to difficulty but in this condition bone marrow findings, abnormality of plasma and urinary proteins, and radiologic features may be diagnostic.

Leukocytosis: Leukemoid Reactions

A marked degree of leukocytosis (50,000–100,000 white cells per cubic millimeter of blood) does not necessarily indicate that leukemia is present; it may indicate a *leukemoid* reaction. Thus, in whooping cough, extreme degrees of lymphocytosis are occasionally found (130,000 per cubic millimeter[9]) and counts of 50,000 lymphocytes or more per cubic millimeter are seen in acute benign lymphocytosis. As a rule, children develop higher leukocyte figures than adults in response to comparatively slight stimuli. Not infrequently, they develop granulocyte counts in excess of 50,000 per cubic millimeter in acute infections, and in the acute hemolysis induced by certain drugs such as the sulfonamides. Where such high figures are found there is an increase, not only of mature neutrophil polymorphs, but also a shift to the left with a higher than normal proportion of band forms and, generally, the appearance of moderate numbers of metamyelocytes and even myelocytes. The finding of an occasional blast cell in children does not necessarily indicate that leukemia is present. However, in any patient with more than 2–3 percent of blasts in the blood, the diagnosis of leukemia must be seriously considered.[5] In adults, extremely high leukocyte counts not due to leukemia are much more rarely encountered. Occasionally, they occur in tuberculosis, disseminated carcinomatosis, carcinoma of the lung, liver, or pancreas, and in Hodgkin's disease, and polyarteritis nodosa. Here they may be reactive or associated with myeloid metaplasia (see Chapters 10 and 11). In adults, the appearance of even an occasional blast form should suggest the diagnosis of leukemia, although it is not always possible to identify isolated blasts with certainty. In doubtful cases a marrow examination is mandatory.

When we try to differentiate between leukemia and a leukemoid reaction, it becomes again readily apparent how little we actually know about the nature of leukemia. Is a given case of extreme leukocytosis leukemia, or does it look like leukemia but is not? Mostly there is no way of telling except by the course. If a case of severe lymphocytosis returns to normal blood levels in 1 or 2 months, this is an infectious state, but if it continues unremittingly, with associated anemia and thrombocytopenia, it is leukemia. If a polymorphonuclear leukocytosis with the presence of some myelocytes improves within 2–4 months, it is a leukemoid reaction; should it persist, it is chronic granulocytic leukemia. If a myeloblastosis is found in conjunction with miliary tuberculosis, is this acute granulocytic leukemia or is it a leukemoid reaction of a severe degree in response to the tuberculous infection?

These ever-recurrent problems indicate once again that as yet we do not have a definitive label that will allow us to state unequivocally in certain doubtful cases that this is or is not an example of leukemia. Exceptionally, help may be obtained from cytogenetic studies. The discovery of the Philadelphia chromosome in the marrow establishes the diagnosis of chronic granulocytic leukemia. Definite aneuploidy with a clonal distribution makes a questionable diagnosis of acute leukemia practically certain.[10] However, one-half or more of all patients with acute leukemia have normal chromosomes throughout their course and cannot thus be diagnosed by cytogenetic means.

INFECTIOUS MONONUCLEOSIS

This can give rise to serious diagnostic difficulties because of the high degree of abnormality exhibited by the leukocytes in the condition. As a matter of fact, this disorder may be classified as a *leukemoid* condition, or even as an atypical form of acute leukemia with a self-limited course, in which reversal to the previously normal status always takes place. In full-blown cases, the leukocytes are often highly immature, and large cells with deep cytoplasmic basophilia, nuclei with a fine chromatin pattern, and sometimes nucleoli may occur in large numbers. There is then an absolute, as well as a relative, increase of these cells. From what has been said, the close resemblance of some of these cells to leukemic blasts will be appreciated. The most important distinguishing feature is the marked variability in morphology of the lymphocytes, with every conceivable type, normal and abnormal, being found. In acute leukemia, there is usually a deadly monotony of the leukocytes with primitive cells predominating, although here, too, there can be a great deal of pleomorphism. While no single cell in mononucleosis may be clearly distinguished from a true blast, the aggregate of abnormalities present makes possible a ready distinction from leukemia in most cases. The most difficult problems arise on the rare occasions when mononucleosis is associated either with thrombocytopenia or hemolytic anemia. The three decisive diagnostic parameters are the heterophil antibody reaction, the more recently described finding of antibody against the Epstein-Barr herpes-type virus, and the examination of the marrow. Although the heterophil agglutination test is positive at some stage in infectious mononucleosis, it may not be so in the early and most difficult phase, and may have to be repeated several times before diagnostic titers are developed. The Henle test for Epstein-Barr viral antibody appears to be specific, provided that the individual can be shown to have been negative before the mononucleosis appeared. The marrow in infectious mononucleosis shows only minor abnormalities, whereas the findings in acute leukemia are usually striking.

LEUKOPENIA

While most cases of leukemia which show leukocytosis are readily diagnosed, those with peripheral leukopenia are apt to present much more difficulty. Here the diagnosis may not suggest itself unless careful search is made for abnormal leukocytes which are, however, nearly always discovered in leukemia; cases of complete aleukemic leukemia are rare. Once the suspicion of leukemia has been aroused, it is often helpful to make films of the buffy coat of the blood, since the abnormal cells will be highly concentrated by these means. Care should be taken regarding the presence of atypical mononuclear cells not obviously blast cells, which are common in many buffy coat preparations of normal blood. Marrow puncture is of the utmost importance in these difficult cases.

The conditions most easily confused with the subleukemic types of leukemia are toxic leukopenias, caused either by infections, or by drugs such as chloramphenicol, phenylbutazone, chlorpromazine, the sulfonamides, thiouracil, etc.; hypo- or aplastic conditions of the marrow; the group of "hypersplenic" neutropenias; autoimmune disorders; and a mixed group of leukopenias of varying etiology. Some of these have already been discussed. The syndrome of *hypersplenism* may be a source of difficulty since the marrow here is usually hypercellular, and there may also be a predominance of early myeloid cells, thus giving a superficial similarity to leukemia. Again the autoimmune disorders, which have been much investigated in recent years, can simulate leukemia with rather similar marrow appearances; this is particularly true of systemic lupus erythematosus, which often has many features in common with acute leukemia. In all doubtful cases, the LE cell test should be performed and in some cases repeated until the diagnosis of systemic lupus has been more or less definitely excluded.

Acute agranulocytosis, as first described in the 1920s in individuals addicted to amidopyrine, is still a problem, though the fashions in marrow depressants have changed. Such cases may resemble acute leukemia both clinically and hematologically. If the marrow is examined at an early stage, it may show merely a lack of mature leukocytes with a predominance of early myeloid cells and a striking similarity to leukemia. The later hypoplastic phase, sometimes with lymphocytosis, is more easily distinguished. Transitions from apparent pure marrow damage to leukemia have been described and are discussed more fully elsewhere (see Chapters 5 and 10).[2] Recovery from drug-induced agranulocytosis is often associated with a marrow "overshoot" which may be quite difficult to distinguish from leukemia.[8]

THROMBOCYTOPENIA

In almost all individuals with acute leukemia, *thrombocytopenia* is a prominent feature; these patients usually present clinically with purpura, and may be diagnosed as having purpura hemorrhagica. Since anemia can exist in all types of purpura and the leukocyte count may be nondiagnostic, the separation of leukemia from the benign condition can at times be made only by means of a bone marrow examination. The presence of normal or increased numbers of megakaryocytes in the marrow is strong evidence against a diagnosis of acute leukemia; but purpuras caused by toxic damage to the megakaryocytes are more difficult to distinguish from it. The autoimmune disorders must again be considered in this context, since they, and particularly lupus erythematosus, often present with thrombocytopenia.

THROMBOCYTOSIS

The condition of thrombocytosis is much less frequently found than its opposite number, but occurs in some early cases of chronic granulocytic leukemia. It does not often give rise to diagnostic difficulties, for when it exists in leukemia, the other findings tend to be quite clear. However, in occasional patients thrombocytosis is the leading feature in the blood picture, and the diagnosis may then lie between chronic granulocytic leukemia, polycythemia vera, and myelofibrosis with myeloid metaplasia. Here, the marrow picture may be difficult to interpret, for in each of the first two conditions it may show a gross hyperplasia of all the cell systems, while the dry tap of myelofibrosis is sometimes found in chronic granulocytic leukemia.[7] Splenic aspirations (see Chapter 10), blood volume estimations and other tests may be necessary to settle the question—if it *can* be settled, at all, since some of the chronic myeloproliferative disorders are difficult, if not impossible, to classify diagnostically, as has been pointed out in Chapter 11.

Conclusion

In nearly all cases in which the diagnosis of leukemia must be considered, the bone marrow will provide decisive evidence for or against it. There are, however, exceptions, some of which have already been mentioned, in which single or even repeated aspirations of the marrow may be inconclusive and other investigations such as marrow trephine biopsy or splenic puncture may be required. In Hodgkin's disease, there may be a marked marrow hyperplasia, especially of the myeloid series, and this can be striking enough to resemble granulocytic leukemia. Various degrees of lymphocytic infiltration may be found in the lymphocytic neoplasms, but the distinguishing line between these and chronic lymphocytic leukemia is at no time sharp, and it may be argued that lymphosarcoma becomes leukemia once it becomes disseminated and invades the marrow. A slight to moderate degree of lymphocytosis of the bone marrow occurs in a variety of nonmalignant conditions such as rheumatoid arthritis and some of the autoimmune diseases, and this should be remembered before a diagnosis of chronic lymphocytic leukemia is made on the strength of the marrow picture alone. Furthermore, lymphoid follicles may be found in normal marrow, and if one is by chance aspirated, the unwary observer may conclude that he has discovered a case of leukemia. If generalization is warranted in this difficult field, it may be said that the greatest weight in diagnosis is given to the laboratory findings, and of these, the blood film appearances are the most important. The bone marrow appearances and the clinical features are usually of secondary importance but should be weighed carefully for evidence, either confirmatory or contradictory, of the peripheral blood findings.

REFERENCES

1. Bernard J: Les aplasies pré-leucémiques. Nouv Rev Fr Hématol 9:41, 1969.
2. Brauer MJ, Dameshek W: Hypoplastic anemia and myeloblastic leukemia following chloramphenicol therapy. Report of three cases. N Engl J Med 277:1003, 1967.
3. Dameshek W: Splenomegaly—a problem in differential diagnosis. Med Clin North Am 41:1357, 1957.
4. _____: Riddle: What do aplastic anemia, paroxysmal nocturnal hemoglobinuria (PNH) and "hypoplastic" leukemia have in common? Blood 30:251, 1967.
5. _____: Foreword: PNH a "candidate" myeloproliferative disorder? Blood 33:263, 1969.
6. Diamond LK: Clinical Pathological Conference, Children's Medical Center, Boston. J Pediatr 48:647, 1956.
7. Gralnick HR, Harbor J, Vogel C: Myelofibrosis in chronic granulocytic leukemia. Blood 37:152, 1971.
8. Levine PH, Weintraub LR: Pseudoleukemia during recovery from dapsone-induced agranulocytosis. Ann Intern Med 68:1060, 1968.
9. Mills SD: Conditions mistaken for leukemia in children. Minn Med 37:444, 1954.
10. Nowell PC: Chromosome abnormalities in human leukemia and lymphoma, in Zarafonetis CJD (ed.): Proceedings of the International Conference on Leukemia–Lymphoma. Philadelphia, Lea & Febiger, 1968, p 47.
11. Pitney WR: Problems in the diagnosis of leukaemia. J Roy Coll Physicians 3:223, 1969.
12. Ross JD, Moloney WC, Desforges JF: Ineffective regulation of granulopoiesis masquerading as congenital leukemia in a mongoloid child. J. Pediatr., 63:1, 1963.
13. Schwab RS, Weiss S: The neurologic aspect of leukemia. Am J Med Sci 189:766, 1935.
14. Spriggs AI, Boddington MM: Leukaemic cells in cerebrospinal fluid. Br J Haematol 5:83, 1959.

IV

Treatment

16

Treatment: Introductory Principles

The history of leukemia therapy is almost as long as that of the disease itself. It encompasses a series of efforts to overcome a problem whose extent and difficulty were only slowly realized. From the outset, agents found to improve—however minimally—the clinical or hematologic condition of patients with leukemia were hailed as potential cures; from the outset, too, such hopes were repeatedly and inevitably dashed against the solid reality of an ill-understood, but clearly refractory, disease process. Only in recent years have some of the reasons for this resistance come to be appreciated, and with this insight came a spirit of defeatism or resignation: A profound doubt whether cure of leukemia would ever become possible or whether, instead, the most that could be hoped for might not be temporary control, with a possibility of extending survival by improved therapeutic techniques. Such, at any rate, was the position at the time the Second Edition of this work was published.

In the 10 years since then considerable progress has been made, not because of the discovery of fundamentally new means of attacking the neoplastic process leading to leukemia but by virtue of a progressive refinement in dealing with its results. Strangely enough, this progress has occurred in acute leukemia which had for many years appeared to be the least promising of all the types. Children with acute leukemia are now surviving in good health for increasingly long periods, and once again the word *cure* is abroad. Whether the cautious hopes that are now being voiced are destined to be borne out remains yet to be seen.

Attempts to influence the course of leukemia were made soon after the disease was first discovered. At first, the ubiquitous Fowler's solution was used, and it appeared to have some effect, particularly in chronic granulocytic leukemia. About 1910, shortly after the discovery that benzene was destructive to blood cells, this material was used fairly extensively for about a decade, but its often unpredictable toxic effects, together with the emergence of x-ray therapy, led to its discontinuance, perhaps prematurely so. The discovery of the roentgen rays toward the end of the nineteenth century and of their destructive effects on various tissues led to their use in the treatment of leukemia, and soon this modality became the standard form of

treatment in the disease. It is interesting to note that radiotherapy replaced splenectomy, which earlier had seemed to have a real place in the treatment of chronic
granulocytic leukemia.[2] Recently, however, splenectomy, early rather than late in
the course of that disease, has enjoyed a revival of interest. During the period of
preeminence of radiotherapy in the treatment of the chronic leukemias, radium and
other radioactive elements, including thorium X, mesothorium, radium emanation,
and thorotrast were used to some extent. Zadek made many studies of the use of
radiothorium and attempted to popularize its use.[11,12] Later, when radioactive
isotopes became available, radioactive phosphorus was used with considerable success, particularly in chronic granulocytic leukemia. That the isotopes might represent the final word in the treatment of leukemia was hoped for, but, unfortunately,
this was not borne out by further experience. In the same way, techniques of extracorporeal irradiation have proved disappointing as methods of treatment while, at
the same time, yielding valuable information about bone marrow activity and lymphoid cell kinetics.[7]

Thus, circa 1940, x-ray therapy for leukemia was almost the sole method of
treating the disease and certainly the standard one. Some individuals, like Forkner,
were emphasizing the value of carefully controlled arsenical therapy, and a few
adherents of benzene therapy were still faintly heard. The period of the radioactive
isotopes was just beginning. At about this time, during the early years of World War
II, experimental work with nitrogen mustard, the analog of a "poison gas," was in
progress in a number of pharmacology laboratories, including that of Goodman and
Gilman at Yale University School of Medicine.[5] The striking effects of this material
in causing severe leukopenia led to its therapeutic trial in apparently terminal cases
of lymphoma (Hodgkin's disease and lymphosarcoma), first at New Haven and
later in Dameshek's clinic in Boston. When it was seen that startling effects often
occurred, particularly in apparently hopeless cases, the use of the chemical was extended to cases of leukemia, where its value was found to be limited. However,
nitrogen mustard was soon found to be of particular value in certain cases of
disseminated lymphosarcoma. Studies of the pharmacology of nitrogen mustard by
Gilman and Philips indicated that its effects resembled those of x-rays, at least in
some measure.[5] The demonstration that a chemical could have what were then
believed to be radiomimetic effects was a powerful stimulus to the development of
other chemotherapeutic agents, and thus the introduction of nitrogen mustard may
be considered as the beginning of a new era in the treatment of leukemia and related
disease. Later, other nitrogen mustard derivatives, together with mustardlike agents
(termed generically, *alkylating agents*) were synthesized: triethylene melamine,
busulfan, and chlorambucil. Since they could be given orally, they proved to be particularly valuable for continued therapy. These agents, like x-rays, appeared to act
by killing the proliferating cell (cytocidal agents); the small margin between this
killing effect on the abnormal cells and those of the bone marrow was often strained.
Thus, myelotoxic effects with some pancytopenia were often prominent.

By 1948 no headway had been made in the treatment of acute leukemia. At the
Lederle Laboratories in Pearl River, New Jersey, SubbaRow had synthesized
pteroyl glutamic acid (folic acid), a potent growth factor for bacteria, cells in tissue
culture, and for the total animal as well.[1] An analog of folic acid—aminopteroylglu-
tamic acid or aminopterin—proved to be antagonistic to growth and was accordingly tried in animal and later in human leukemia. Farber showed that folic acid
possibly accelerated human leukemia but that its antagonist aminopterin brought

about striking remissions in about one-half the cases of acute leukemia in child-hood.[4] This demonstration, that an apparently irreversible and hopeless disease could be reversed and normalized, even temporarily, naturally led to a great burst of optimism and enthusiasm on the part of workers in the field, and to a concerted drive to control leukemia. It was soon found that the chances of success were much greater in the lymphocytic form of acute childhood leukemia than in adults in whom the great majority of cases belonged to one of the granulocytic types. The reasons for this difference are still uncertain, but one at least (as will be described in some detail in Chapter 18) could be the fact that acute lymphocytic leukemia resembles rather closely the experimental L 1210 model in the mouse whose kinetics are now well understood and which can be cured by means of therapy based on kinetic princi-ples.[9] Even though there must be considerable differences between mouse and human leukemias, the application of therapeutic methods derived from the murine model has been found to be fruitful in attempts to improve treatment of the human disease.

It appears that the time may be at hand when one-half of all children with acute lymphocytic leukemia who are treated by today's optimal methods can be promised long-term and, possibly, indefinite survival. This startling statistic is not matched by our foresight in individuals, for it is still virtually impossible to predict success or failure in any given case. The reasons for primary cellular resistance to che-motherapy have not been explained, and much remains to be learned about the mechanism by which leukemia relapses in successfully treated patients. Recent in-terest has been concentrated on leukemic cells in the central nervous system, not only as a form of residual disease, but also as a site of progressive cytogenetic change and a possible reserve of leukemic cells from which marrow may be repopu-lated.[3] One of the most alarming possibilities is that of a second induction of the disease in the same patient by a persistent leukemogenic agent, as suggested by the experiences of Thomas and his colleagues.[10]

Progress in the treatment of acute leukemia of adults has been much slower than that in children, but the advent of a number of new chemotherapeutic agents and, in particular, of combinations of agents with synergistic activities has begun to increase the proportion of remissions and the length of survival of those patients who obtain remissions. Perhaps the best hope for further advances in this difficult field lies in the exploitation of inherent kinetic or metabolic weaknesses of leukemic cell strains, especially if these should differ from the properties of surviving normal hematopoietic cells. The successful use of methods for synchronizing leukemic cells or for causing the reentry of dormant (G_0) cells into the synthetic cycle (see Chapter 8), would be major advances, for they might make possible a much more efficient destruction of neoplastic populations than is now possible in most instances. The in-troduction of L-asparaginase may foreshadow that of other and more specific agents capable of inhibiting the growth of leukemic cells by depriving them of essential me-tabolites.

In the general preoccupation with acute leukemia, research on the treatment of the chronic varieties has been largely neglected during the past decade, and, indeed, there has been little if any progress in therapeutic methods. Perhaps unfortunately, the realization that in chronic granulocytic leukemia all hematopoietic cells in the bone marrow carry the Philadelphia (Ph[1]) chromosome has dampened hopes of suc-cessfully suppressing a specifically leukemic cell-line in that disease. Only in a few exceptional cases of chronic granulocytic leukemia, has evidence emerged of the existence of normal cell-lines which may replace the leukemic cells in the bone marrow. As stated in Chapter 18, remissions, in the strict sense, have not been achieved in chronic granulocytic leukemia, and there are doubts if they can be. The situation is rather similar in the case of chronic lymphocytic leukemia, although the two diseases differ in many important respects.

The basic principle of all antileukemic therapies which have yet been employed is a quest for the complete elimination of neoplastic cells, so that the normal hematopoietic precursors may have the opportunity of repopulating the blood-forming organs and of fulfilling their functions in those sites. It is a simple philosophy based on the double premise that leukemic cells are sensitive to the therapy employed and that normal cells can survive to fight another day. That this is true at least in some cases has been shown by the successes in the treatment of acute leukemia in childhood, and, on a more theoretical basis, by the insights gained from cytogenetic studies (see Chapter 6). However, the validity of the concept of a double cell population is open to doubt in most cases of chronic granulocytic leukemia and in some of the acute leukemias. Moreover, there is little evidence to show that leukemic cells are more sensitive than normal ones to the activity of cytotoxic agents, and the danger of complete and permanent iatrogenic eradication of normal, as well as leukemic populations, thus imposes limitations on the intensity of chemotherapy, even when advanced supportive measures are available. If heterologous marrow could be transplanted to treated patients so as to replace normal hematopoietic cells destroyed along with leukemic ones, a major therapeutic advance might be achieved. Unfortunately, after prolonged efforts in many laboratories, there is as yet no sign that marrow transplantation can be successfully accomplished in patients with leukemia.

It has been the hope of those who could see the limitations of cytotoxic therapy in leukemia that eventually a deeper understanding of the leukemic process would lead to the discovery of the essential abnormalities in the cells or in the mechanism of their control. As Skipper et al. wrote, "There must be important biochemical differences between neoplastic cells and their normal counterparts. Accordingly, in suitable circumstances, these postulated differences might be exploited selectively to the disadvantage of malignant growth."[8] In spite of the huge effort to delineate the specific biochemical lesions of leukemic and other neoplastic cells, we are clearly a long way from the point at which they can be exploited. It is particularly disappointing that no specific biochemical abnormality has been associated with the highly specific deletion or translocation represented by the Ph^1 chromosome. Nor have the studies on the growth of leukemic cells in artificial media as yet produced any clear notion on specific disturbances in hematopoietic control mechanisms, although some claims to this effect have been made.[6] In the meantime, perhaps the most rational approach to the problem of supplementing cytotoxic therapy is the attempted stimulation of the body's own resistance to neoplastic invasion. Unfortunately, although there can be little doubt of the existence of immune responses to neoplastic cells, our knowledge of these responses is fragmentary. As a consequence, immunotherapeutic methods in leukemia are not as yet soundly based, but they would certainly appear to deserve intensive study.

How long one should persist in the treatment of leukemia, notably of acute cases in adults, is often the subject of debate. Modern therapy of leukemia involves the use of highly potent agents which have the power, in many cases, of producing a dramatic improvement in health, but are also capable of giving rise to unpleasant, dangerous, and even intolerable symptoms in the course of their employment. Moreover, some are slow to produce improvement. It seems entirely reasonable to accept the difficulties and risks of administering an agent when there is a good chance that worthwhile benefits will follow. We know, for instance, that some gastrointestinal disturbances can scarcely be avoided when nitrogen mustard is given to a patient with lymphosarcoma; however, in a disseminated example of this disorder, the chances of marked improvement occurring either with nitrogen mustard alone or in combination with other agents are so great as to outweigh this disadvantage. The same objection applies in acute leukemia regarding agents likely to produce side effects such as mucosal ulcerations, infections, or hemorrhages. Few would deny a patient with early lymphoma or leukemia the possible benefit of prolonged remissions on the grounds of temporary discomfort and inconvenience. It is much harder to know what to do in late cases. Is it still justifiable to worry a patient with a disagreeable or even dangerous treatment when there seems no likelihood of his being benefited by its use? Is it justifiable to employ desperate measures in desperate circumstances? Should we continue to treat a patient for complications of leukemia such as infections, hemorrhage, or severe anemia, when we know that the disease itself is no longer amenable to treatment? By means of antibiotics, by transfusions, by careful adjustment of their fluid and electrolyte balances, and by other similar measures, it is possible today to keep alive for considerable periods many patients who would have otherwise succumbed to their disease, and even to revive the almost dead. The question which has often arisen in our minds on watching such patients under treatment is how much we increase their happiness by thus enabling their kidneys, liver, heart, and brain to function a little while longer; or when by heroic measures, we bring back from the very brink of death, a patient with acute leukemia or one in the terminal phases of chronic leukemia. These are questions which should perhaps be more frequently considered, even in these days of aggressive optimism in the treatment of leukemia.

The future of the therapy of leukemia may lie in several directions: either in the development of newer and more potent chemicals or of better methods of employing them; or in immunologic or other methods of attacking the agents or the abnormal metabolic factors responsible for the leukemic aberration. It is also conceivable that prophylaxis may some day be applied: either by careful attention to various possible etiologic factors such as radiation exposure (as has already been done in the case of prenatal x-ray examinations) or, should a viral etiology be confirmed, by the development of vaccines against oncogenic viruses. Nevertheless, it should be remembered how limited has been our success in the control of nononcogenic viral diseases. It is well to reflect that, in spite of the plethora of therapeutic agents and methods presently available to us, our therapeutic programs, however good they may seem to us now, are undoubtedly in their infancy and that many new and better methods will almost surely be developed in the years to come.

REFERENCES

1. Angier RB, Boothe JH, Hutchings BL, Mowat JH, Semb J, Stokstad ELR, SubbaRow Y, Waller CW, Cosulich DB, Fahrenback MJ, Hultquist ME, Kuh E, Northey EH, Seegers DR, Sickels JP, Smith JM Jr: Structure and synthesis of liver L. casei factor. Science 103:667, 1946.

2. Baikie AG: The place of splenectomy in the

treatment of chronic granulocytic leukaemia: Some random observations, a review of the earlier literature and a plea for its proper study in a cooperative therapeutic trial. Australas Ann Med 17:175, 1968.

3. _____: What is a leukaemic remission? The evidence from cytogenetic studies, in Vincent PC (ed.): The Nature of Leukaemia, Proceedings International Cancer Conference, Sydney, New South Wales Government Printer, 1972, p 231.

4. Farber S, in Rebuck JW, Bethell FH, Monto RW (eds): The Leukemias: Etiology, Pathophysiology and Treatment. New York, Academic Press, 1957, p 617.

5. Gilman A, Philips FS: The biological actions and therapeutic applications of the B-chloroethyl amines and sulfides. Science 103:409, 1946.

6. Metcalf D: Human leukaemia: Recent tissue culture studies on the nature of myeloid leukaemia. Br J Cancer 27:191, 1973.

7. Schiffer LM, Atkins HL, Chanana AD, Cronkite EP, Greenberg ML, Stryckmans PA: Extracorporeal irradiation of blood (ECIB) in man. II. Treatment of acute myelocytic leukemia. Blood 31:17, 1968.

8. Skipper HE, Heidelberger L, Welch AD: Some biochemical problems of cancer chemotherapy. Nature 179:1159, 1957.

9. Skipper HE, Schabel FM, Wilcox WS: Experimental evaluation of potential anticancer agents. XIII. On the criteria and kinetics associated with "curability" of experimental leukemia. Cancer Chemother Rep 35:1, 1964.

10. Thomas ED, Bryant JI, Buckner CD, Cliff RA, Fefer A, Johnson FL, Neiman P, Ramberg RE, Storb R: Leukaemic transformation of human marrow cells in vivo. Lancet 1:1310, 1972.

11. Zadek I: Radiothorium bei leukamischer Lymphadenose. Folia Haematol 48:39, 1932.

12. _____: Tierexperimentelle Ergebnisse mit dem zur Behandlung der Leukamie verwendeten Radiothorium. Folia Haematol 47:418; 48:210, 1932.

Alexander S. D. Spiers

17

Mode of Action and Clinical Uses
of Therapeutic Agents in Leukemia

Knowledge of the pathogenesis and pathophysiology of leukemia, and of the physiology of normal and leukemic cells, is incomplete and, in some areas, fragmentary. Not surprisingly, current knowledge of the modes of action of therapeutic agents in leukemia is similarly inadequate. Advances in biochemistry have suggested how some agents exert their effects and have pointed the way to development of new and sometimes successful therapeutic approaches, but even in these instances it would be naïve to assume a genuine understanding of their mechanism of action. Moreover, such an assumption could impede further progress: the history of medicine has many examples of developmental retardation due to false impressions of omniscience. Elucidation of the biochemical mechanisms by which an agent may act within the leukemic cell supplies only part of the necessary information. The effect of a drug upon the overall leukemic process in a patient depends, not only on cellular biochemistry, but also on pharmacodynamic and pharmacokinetic factors, as well as the size and proliferative activity of leukemic and other cell populations present in the body. Most of this information is either lacking or available only in unrefined form, and it is doubtful whether the mode of action has been fully documented for any of the currently used antileukemic agents. The imperfection of our knowledge seems to be reflected in the limitations and inadequacies of even the most modern treatments for leukemia. It seems highly significant that our most consistent therapeutic success is in treating and curing certain transplanted murine leukemias, where the kinetics of the leukemic cells, and the dose-response curves of the drugs, are best known.[574,582] The following discussion of the modes of action of therapeutic agents in leukemia should be viewed with the reservation that it can give only part of a very complex and unfinished story. The principal types of therapy used in the leukemias are drugs and ionizing radiations.

IONIZING RADIATIONS

X-rays were among the first agents shown to be capable of influencing beneficially the course of certain leukemias. Only 7 years after their discovery by Roentgen in 1895, they were used by Pusey to treat a patient successfully,[507] and

Table 17-1

Methods of Applying Ionizing Radiations for the Treatment of Leukemia*

Sources	Target	References
External		
Radium, thorium, and other naturally occurring radioactive materials	Localized masses (e.g., lymph nodes); spleen; abdominal bath; whole-body irradiation; extracorporeal	223, 262
X-ray apparatus: ortho-voltage and supervoltage (linear accelerator)	irradiation of the blood (ECIB)	339, 481
Cobalt-60 machines		379, 473, 540,
ECIB apparatus		541, 589, 629
Internal		
Radionuclides administered orally or intravenously: ^3H, ^{90}Y, ^{32}P, ^{24}Na, ^{76}As, ^{198}Au	Necessarily whole-body application, but variable degrees of selective concentration occur in hemato-poietic tissues.	254 (^3H) 41 (^{90}Y) 41, 59, 476, 477 (^{32}P) 201, 632 (^{24}Na) 60 (^{76}As) 270, 511(^{198}Au)

*Only x-ray apparatus, cobalt machines, and radiophosphorus are in general clinical use.

similar good results were obtained by Senn,[561,562] and several other workers. Early papers hailed the treatment as a cure,[398] but doubts presently made their appearance with the publication of autopsy findings on some of the reportedly cured patients.[659] Soon the effects of x-rays were generally recognized as only palliative,[660] and statistical studies of large groups of treated and untreated patients suggested that life was not significantly prolonged by their use.[308,447,448] A radioactive isotope (^{32}P) was first used by Lawrence in 1936 for the treatment of leukemia,[394] although previously (1931–1932) Zadek had described the use of radioactive thorium.[690] The principal methods available for the application of ionizing radiations in the treatment of leukemia are summarized in Table 17-1.

MECHANISM OF ACTION

The application of x-rays, or other ionizing radiations, produces a characteristic series of changes in the blood of experimental animals and man. Following a single exposure, there is an almost immediate reduction in the number of lymphocytes, reaching a nadir within 4 days. After large doses, lymphopenia may be almost total. The granulocytes may show a brief rise lasting a day or so, and then decline. After heavy irradiation, granulocytopenia becomes very marked early in the second week, while in less severe cases the granulocyte count levels off about the eighth day and may even show a secondary rise lasting about 10–12 days. The count falls again, and in accidentally irradiated men who had survived, a critical phase of maximum granulocytopenia was reported during the fourth and fifth week.[70,292] In such cases, the platelet count begins to fall a few days after exposure, reaching a minimum at 28–32 days, more or less paralleling the changes in the granulocyte count. The effect of radiation on the red cell count is different from that on the leukocytes. There is an early diminution in the reticulocyte count, with a recovery after varying time intervals. The red cell count itself declines much more slowly, and anemia, if it occurs at all, is not detected until 2 weeks or longer after irradiation, and it is transient unless the radiation dose was very large. A different pattern of anemia may be seen if bleeding has occurred because of thrombocytopenia.

In contrast to the ease with which the blood count can be depressed by irradiating the intact organism, most normal blood cells are highly resistant when irradiated in vitro, and many thousands of rad (1 rad equals radiation equivalent to 100 ergs per gram of tissue) are necessary before changes in the morphology or functional activity of leukocytes or erythrocytes can be observed.[256,333,340,378,411,439,463,474,598] This is not merely because blood cells in vitro are not subjected to the mechanical stresses normal in the circulation: blood can be irradiated in an extracorporeal shunt and returned to the circulation without serious hemolysis unless a 60,000-rad dose is exceeded.[473] The only mature cell type whose survival in vitro is shortened by x-rays in the *therapeutic* range is the lymphocyte.[479,544,545,640] Doses as small as 5–20 rad produce a significant decrease in the survival of both normal and leukemic lymphocytes in vitro,[546,547] although the lymphocytes of chronic lymphocytic leukemia show an abnormally wide range of radiosensitivities, with some cells being resistant.[548]

These different effects produced on blood cells in vivo and in vitro are a consequence of the mechanisms by which radiation affects living cells. Most cells, with the exception of lymphocytes and developing gametes at certain stages of development, are relatively resistant to radiations during the resting (G_0, or interphase) stage of the cell cycle, and highly sensitive, only during the synthetic (S), premitotic (G_2), and mitotic phases. x-rays, gamma rays, and the particulate radiations—alpha particles, neutrons and π-mesons—all produce qualitatively similar effects, although their relative biological efficiencies and linear energy-transfer characteristics vary considerably.[69,658] The effect on mitosis is a double one: mitotic inhibition, presumably by interference with the function of the nuclear spindle, together with damage to the cellular DNA, which is particularly vulnerable when in its condensed form in mitotic chromosomes. A variety of chromosomal aberrations, including fragmentation, stickiness, anaphase lag, chromatid and chromosome breaks, interchanges, and the production of ring and dicentric forms, has been observed following therapeutic,[72,99,145,634] or even diagnostic,[62,600] irradiation.

It was commonly assumed that x-rays produced effects such as chromosome breakage by direct action on key molecules in the chromosome structure—the direct action or target theory.[397] There is, however, good evidence that much of the effect is due to an indirect mechanism, the result of ionization of the intracellular water, with production of active radicals ($2H_2O \rightarrow H_3^+O + OH^-$). The chances of a given cell being hit will depend on the intensity (dose-rate) and the total dose of radiation.[311] As an x-ray passes through the cell, it dissipates its energy by ionizing molecules along its path. A single cell having a volume of 1000 cu μ, exposed to 500 rad, experiences about 6.6 million ionizations: since the cell is about 75 percent water, some 5 million ionizations will be of water molecules. The active radicals produced can cause chemical changes in organic molecules in their vicinity[570] and significantly damage nuclear and cytoplasmic structures. How much of the total effect of radiation is due to direct action and how much to ionization is uncertain; the process is a complex one, affected by other factors such as the availability of oxygen to the cell at the time of irradiation.[165] Mitotic abnormalities may cause cell death directly, or may be visible evidence of a more widespread, underlying chemical lesion.[3] Radiation interferes with cellular synthesis of DNA,[237,380] but similar effects on other cellular constituents, including enzymes, may be important, and it is probably an oversimplification to attribute mitotic inhibition and damage to the cellular genetic apparatus solely to direct effects on DNA metabolism. Such a mechanism does not, for example, adequately explain the marked sensitivity of lymphocytes to irradiation during interphase, when DNA metabolism is apparently at a low level of activity.

Since dividing cells are injured by doses of radiation well within the therapeutic range, whereas very large doses are required to cause damage to most resting cells, it is evident that the changes in the blood count observed after irradiation of the whole organism must be produced by interference with mitotically active precursor cells in the marrow, spleen, and other hematopoietic organs, rather than with nondividing mature cells in the peripheral blood. The radiosensitivity of such precursor cells as the myelocyte has been shown directly by irradiation in vitro,[260,475,478,508] and contrasts strongly with the marked resistance of mature blood cells under similar conditions.

The injury to hematopoietic organs which follows irradiation of living organisms was first described over 60 years ago in dogs and rodents.[289-291] Destruction of lymphocytes was observed as early as $2\frac{1}{2}$ hours after irradiation, reaching a maximum in 12 hours, by which time myeloid cells were affected. With nonfatal doses, regeneration began about the sixth day and was complete within 17–21 days. These findings have been widely confirmed and extended.[16,36,121,122,176,403,441,521,556,641] More recently, the investigations undertaken in connection with nuclear energy research during and after World War II have defined quantitatively the effects of various radiations in numerous laboratory species and have clarified the order of radiosensitivity of the several classes of hematopoietic cells.[63] Lymphocytes are the most sensitive cells, closely followed by erythroblasts, which had previously been regarded as radioresistant,[64,328] and then by granulocytic precursors and megakaryocytes. As an outcome of nuclear warfare and of accidents with atomic reactors, it has been possible to describe in detail the alterations in human bone marrow which follow heavy radiation exposure.[10,292,515]

The changes observed in the hematopoietic organs following irradiation explain the pattern of alterations seen in the blood count. Interference with the multiplication of the radiosensitive hematopoietic cells produces a shortage of mature cells whose severity depends on the length of time during which no new cells are produced, and also on the rapidity with which the existing circulating cells perish in the course of their normal life cycle. Thus, arrested production of the comparatively short-lived granulocytes will express itself rapidly as a falling leukocyte count. On the other hand, although erythroblasts are very radiosensitive, mature red cells normally survive for up to 4 months, so that even complete and permanent inhibition of erythropoiesis will not produce significant anemia for some weeks. Moreover, despite its radiosensitivity, erythropoiesis recovers relatively fast after irradiation[63] and functional impairment of red cell production is less readily demonstrable than structural damage.[645,646] Lymphocytes are exceptional, in being radiosensitive during interphase, and the very rapid fall in the lymphocyte count following irradiation is the result of destruction of circulating cells, although mitotic inhibition of their precursors probably plays a part. Changes in the peripheral blood lymphocyte count are a delicate index of the amount of radiation received during a recent therapeutic or accidental exposure.[487] Estimation of the radiation dose received at some time in the more distant past is possible by studying the incidence of chromosomal aberrations in peripheral blood lymphocytes which were damaged but not destroyed during that exposure.[98]

THERAPEUTIC EFFECTS ON LEUKEMIA

A typical favorable response to radiotherapy in chronic granulocytic leukemia or chronic lymphocytic leukemia consists of a lowered leukocyte count, occasionally preceded by a transient rise; in an increased erythrocyte count and hemoglobin concentration; in the involution of pathologically enlarged organs; and an increase in the patient's general well-being. This complex chain of events has been attributed to the same mechanism which brings about destruction of normal hematopoietic tissue in experimental animals, that is, a direct interference with mitosis, affecting proliferating leukemic cells. This simple explanation is inadequate for several reasons. The doses of radiation required to control the leukemia are, in many patients, much smaller than those required to destroy normal hematopoietic cells. Control of the leukemia, at least in previously untreated patients, usually lasts much longer than the time required for recovery of experimentally irradiated normal marrow. Most puzzling of all, closely similar responses are obtained by irradiation of the whole body from external sources or with radionuclides such as ^{32}P systemically administered, or by external irradiation of single organs such as the spleen. It appears that leukemic cells may be more susceptible to irradiation than are normal hematopoietic cells, that they recover more slowly, and that the body burden of leukemic cells can be controlled by radiation, even when only a fraction of the leukemic cells are in the path of the beam.

Reports on morphologic changes in the blood-forming organs following therapeutic irradiation for leukemia are sparse and difficult to interpret. Some studies of bone marrow appearances before and after irradiation have been described,[41,52,76,195,356,449,599] but are contradictory, some authors finding changes after treatment and others denying them; information on dosages, dose fractionation, and irradiation ports has generally been inadequate. There are two reports of larger groups of patients with chronic granulocytic leukemia followed by means of sternal marrow punctures before and after splenic irradiation.[262,484] Both reports described definite though variable changes in the marrow following treatment. Cellularity was often decreased and there was increased maturation in the granulocytic series, or an increased percentage of erythroid cells, or both. Though inconstant in incidence and variable in degree, these changes were highly significant when the whole series of patients was considered. On the other hand, cytogenetic studies of the bone marrow have shown that splenic irradiation does not affect the occurrence of the Philadelphia chromosome (Ph¹) in the marrow,[636] although it reduces its incidence in cultures of the peripheral blood,[635] by clearing the blood of leukemic cells still capable of mitosis. Figures 17-1 and 17-2 show the sequence of events in a patient with chronic granulocytic leukemia, treated by splenic irradiation. In chronic lymphocytic leukemia, whole-body irradiation is frequently followed by diminution of the percentage of lymphocytes in the bone marrow, although clinical improvement is sometimes seen without definite evidence of such a change.[339]

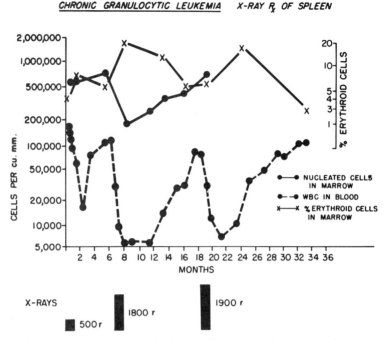

Fig. 17-1. Chronic granulocytic leukemia. Changes in the blood and marrow under x-ray treatment applied to the spleen.

Careful studies have been made of the histology of hematopoietic organs in patients treated for leukemia with local irradiation and the radioisotopes ^{32}P and [76]As.[59,60] The changes produced by local or whole-body irradiation were comparatively modest and did not correlate well with the clinical effects. Pronounced leukemic features sometimes persisted despite clinical remission, and identical histologic changes were seen in association with both clinical failure of therapy and clinical remission. It was suggested that radiation effects were prolonged, producing continuing slight damage which, though insufficiently severe to be seen in sections, might, nevertheless, result in decreased production of leukemic cells. The isotopes ^{32}P and [76]As are preferentially concentrated in hematopoietic organs, and the interference with cellular multiplication, which must follow their administration, should be maximal at these sites. Apparently histologic methods are too insensitive to detect the changes produced by therapeutic doses, presumably because histology provides only a static picture of what is in reality a dynamic situation. The anatomic effects of irradiation are not yet securely established, and, in any case, these are but the reflection of earlier and much more subtle radiochemical changes.[23] More delicate methods for investigating the effects of irradiation are available by the study of leukemic cellular kinetics (see Chapter 8).

It has already been noted that local as well as general irradiation can cause clinical remissions in chronic granulocytic leukemia and chronic lymphocytic leukemia, and clinicians have long known that x-rays can cause effects at distant, nonirradiated sites. Thus, treatment of the spleen may be followed by the disappearance of enlarged lymph nodes or skin infiltrates,[257,461,500] or the subsidence of priapism in chronic granulocytic leukemia.[148] It is obvious that irradiation can cause

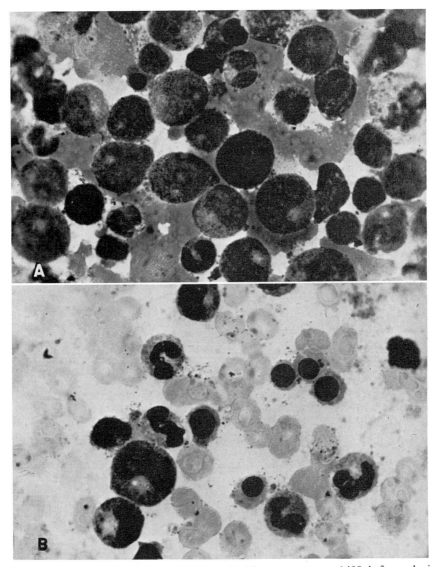

Fig. 17-2. A. Chronic granulocytic leukemia. Marrow smear, × 1400, before splenic irradiation. B. Chronic granulocytic leukemia. Marrow smear, × 1400, after splenic irradiation.

remote effects, but the underlying mechanism is not clear. Early investigators postulated that substances called *leukotoxins* were released by irradiated cells and affected the activity of cells at distant sites,[116,411,442,483,607] but the presence of such substances has not been conclusively demonstrated.[27,395] It has been shown that irradiation of experimental animals can cause impaired DNA synthesis at distant, nonirradiated sites,[295,312,350] but a leukotoxin mediating this effect has not been demonstrated.

The remote effects of radiation may be compared to another radiobiologic phenomenon which was at first attributed to humoral factors. This is the protective effect which the shielded spleen[326] or bone marrow[142,605] exerts in animals given whole-body irradiation. Mice in which the surgically exteriorized spleen is shielded with lead can withstand doses of radiation which are uniformly fatal to unprotected animals. Similarly, injections of homologous[418,419] or even heterologous bone marrow[417] into mice or guinea pigs after whole-body irradiation have a strong protective effect. It was believed that the unirradiated hematopoietic cells in the spleen or marrow liberated humoral substances which caused recovery of the irradiated bone marrow,[326,327] but this view now seems to be incorrect, since it has been shown conclusively that the protective effect of injected marrow is due to colonization of the irradiated marrow by unirradiated homologous or heterologous hematopoietic cells[216,408,465]: presumably the hematopoietic cells in the shielded spleen protect by the same means. Thus, the hematopoietic system is labile and cells can migrate from one site to colonize others; it is also possible that this cellular traffic between sites of hematopoiesis occurs under normal circumstances as well as under the stimulus of disease or radiation injury.

The treatment of chronic granulocytic or lymphocytic leukemias by localized irradiation of the spleen is a situation analogous to that intended to show the protective effect of splenic shielding, but with precisely opposite effects. Irradiation of a leukemic spleen inflicts damage, not only upon the cells which are more or less permanently contained in it, but also upon large numbers of leukemic cells which are circulating through the spleen and spending variable periods in the splenic pulp. Many of these leukemic cells possess proliferative potential, and are destined to settle in the bone marrow or lymph nodes and produce more leukemic cells. Through irradiation in transit, their proliferation would be prevented, and thus destruction of circulating cells could lead to depletion of leukemic cells in organs which had not been directly irradiated. Repeated doses of splenic irradiation could produce additive effects sufficient to explain the fall in the leukocyte count and the involution of organs previously infiltrated with leukemic cells. If normal hematopoietic cells such as erythroblasts do not enter into the circulation, they will be unaffected by splenic irradiation; alternatively, they may circulate, and suffer irradiation, but recover more rapidly than leukemic cells. Depletion of leukemic cells in the bone marrow is followed by proliferation of normal elements with improved hemoglobin and platelet levels.

The mode of action of ionizing radiations in leukemia is still imperfectly understood. There is little doubt that their major effects are destruction of leukemic cells and suppression of their reproduction, or that these effects are exerted directly upon cells in the irradiated area. Irradiation also has remote effects which are not entirely explained; a humoral mechanism has not been excluded. However, it appears likely that most of the remote effects of splenic irradiation are caused by the irradiation of circulating, immature leukocytes, and the same mechanism seems certain to underlie the effects of extracorporeal irradiation of the blood.[379]

Clinical Uses

Ionizing radiations from x-ray apparatus or naturally occurring radioactive materials were available for therapeutic use long before any potent antileukemic drugs were developed, and radiation therapy found a place in the treatment of leukemia 70 years ago. Despite the later development of improved x-ray apparatus and many synthetic radionuclides, the application of radiotherapy has decreased, and its importance lessened, owing to the significant advances in drug therapy for leukemia, which have taken place over the past 25 years. The relative importance of radiotherapy has declined noticeably since the Second Edition of this book was written, and further change may be expected. However, certain definite indications for radiation therapy in the patient with leukemia still apply, and further progress in radiotherapeutic techniques may lead to fresh applications of radiation treatment in this disease.

METHODS OF IRRADIATION

These have been summarized in Table 17-1. At present, external irradiation is most often administered using orthovoltage x-ray machines, usually delivering 250 kV. Supervoltage machines, delivering 1000 kV or more, and radioactive cobalt (^{60}Co) apparatus are also used, but have little advantage over orthovoltage machines, in view of the low total doses given. The very short wavelengths emitted by supervoltage machines, and the consequently reduced skin doses, may be important if an area such as the mediastinum has to be irradiated repeatedly. Radiophosphorus (^{32}P) is the only radioactive isotope commonly used in the treatment of leukemia, and its popularity has waned, although it undoubtedly produces good results in expert hands. Extracorporeal irradiation of the blood[379,473,541,629] and the use of radionuclides other than ^{32}P,[60,201,254,270,511,632] while of great research interest, have not yet become accepted in the therapy of the leukemias.

RADIATION THERAPY IN ACUTE LEUKEMIAS

Treatment of acute leukemia with x-rays was tried in the early years of this century, but it was soon found that patients did not respond favorably. Often they were made worse and died from a pancytopenia more severe than that already produced by their disease. For many years, acute leukemia has been regarded as a relative contraindication to radiotherapy, ionizing radiations being applied for only two groups of conditions, viz:

1. Localized lesions in the skeleton or soft tissues, such as the chloromas or myeloblastomas occasionally seen in acute granulocytic leukemia. Usually, such lesions were treated only if symptomatic.
2. Leukemia involving the meninges or other sites in the central nervous system. Radiation was applied to the skull, or to the skull and spinal cord, and was sometimes combined with treatment by antileukemic drugs administered intrathecally.[83,278,612]

Recently, radiation therapy has found a new role in the treatment of acute leukemia, particularly in acute lymphocytic leukemia in children. Improved chemotherapy for this disease has increased the median survival to over 3 years and it appears possible that a significant proportion of patients may eventually be cured.[594] However, in many patients, the prospect of cure is blighted by the occurrence of meningeal leukemia while the systemic disease is still in remission.[22] A series of controlled clinical studies,[21,22,235,502,503] recently summarized after 9 years' experience,[504] has demonstrated that prophylactic irradiation of the whole CNS to 2400 rad total dose, or irradiation of the skull to 2400 rad, together with intrathecal therapy with methotrexate, substantially reduces the incidence of meningeal leukemia and increases the proportion of children with long-term survival and possible eventual cure. In the past, prophylactic irradiation against meningeal leukemia was not acceptable because it caused severe alopecia and its value had not been proved, but now the role of prophylactic CNS irradiation in children with acute lymphocytic leukemia is securely established.

Renewed attempts have been made to treat the systemic manifestations of acute leukemia by ionizing radiations. Animal experiments have shown that mice could be cured of a transplanted leukemia by heavy doses of whole-body irradiation followed by transplantation of homologous bone marrow.[26] Unfortunately, the hope that a similar approach might cure human acute leukemias by destroying the entire body load of leukemic cells and repopulating the bone marrow with normal hematopoietic cells has not been realized in practice. In the past few years, many reports have described the treatment of patients with acute leukemia by high-dose radiation treatment and marrow transplantation.[15,33,248,250,422,431,432,443,493,627,630,631] Whole-body irradiation in doses up to 2000 rad has been given by means of x-rays or gamma rays from ^{60}Co sources. Marrow for transplantation has been obtained from identical twins (isologous), normal donors, or cadavers (homologous), and from fetal tissues. The best results have been obtained with identical twins, several patients achieving remission, but these remissions were not particularly lengthy and there was no suggestion that the leukemia had been cured. Results following administration of homologous bone marrow were much poorer and rejection of the engrafted marrow was frequent. The use of donors compatible for the major histocompatibility (HL-A) antigens[627] has improved the results of homologous marrow transplantation, but several major hazards remain.

1. The recipient may succumb because the transplant does not take, due to inadequate number of cells or poor technique in handling the cells prior to administration.
2. The graft may be rejected because its antigens evoke an immune response in the recipient. This may occur even when HL-A matching appears satisfactory,[628] but does not occur with transplants between identical twins.
3. The graft may be successful, but the immunocytes transplanted with the hematopoietic cells may set up a graft-versus-host reaction which may be fatal.[249,432,628] This secondary syndrome, which also occurs in successfully engrafted experimental animals,[472,639] may be controlled by immunosuppressive therapy.[430,626,628] A newer and promising approach is the attempted fractionation of the donor marrow prior to its administration in order to remove immunocytes and leave only the hematopoietic cells.
4. Despite successful transplantation, the recipient may succumb from a recrudescence of his acute leukemia, indicating that this was not eradicated by the radiation and/or chemotherapy administered before transplantation.
5. Most disturbing of all are reports[211,626] of patients dying some time after transplantation from recurrent acute leukemia, occurring in *donor* cells. The identity of the "new" leukemic cells was studied by cytogenetic techniques and it was established conclusively in one case,[626] and with a high degree of probability in the other,[211] that they were of donor origin. Conceivably, some factor in the recipient (leukemia virus?) persists after whole-body irradiation and can induce leukemic change in cells from another individual.

6. Bone marrow transplantation does not protect from all the consequences of heavy irradiation or drastic chemotherapy, and patients treated very vigorously with the object of eradicating their leukemia may later die, despite successful transplantation, from the effects of radiation upon the gut or other vital organs.

In summary, patients with leukemia can survive heavy whole-body irradiation and/or massive doses of cytotoxic drugs when supported with transplanted bone marrow. Most of the technical problems of obtaining sufficient marrow from donors and administering it in a viable state have been surmounted. The transplant regularly survives if obtained from an identical twin, but with lesser degrees of histocompatibility, rejection of the graft by the recipient, or graft-versus-host disease (rejection of the recipient by the graft) remain serious problems. There is no evidence that this approach has cured any patients with acute leukemia: Relapse of the original leukemia usually occurs after a variable interval, and on rare occasions the leukemic process has involved the previously normal donor cells. Increasing the dose of whole-body irradiation in an attempt to eradicate leukemic cells beyond all doubt presents a major risk to the patient from those radiation effects which are not circumvented by marrow transplantation. Moreover, it is uncertain whether even supralethal doses of radiation will, in fact, destroy all leukemic cells: Some leukemic lymphocytes can survive 4000 rad administered in vitro,[549] and 2500-rad doses failed to cure mouse leukemias in vivo, or even make them nontransplantable.[112,296] Earlier success in curing a mouse leukemia by irradiation[26] may have been due to the adjuvant effects of immunologic processes in a host genetically different from the inoculated leukemic cells.[296] In any case, these mouse experiments are not strictly comparable with marrow transplantation as carried out in leukemic patients.

Although present results in treating human acute leukemia by whole-body irradiation and bone marrow transplantation are not very encouraging, it must be remembered that the procedure is still relatively new and is probably capable of development and refinement. Because transplantation is an investigative, rather than an established, mode of therapy, it has been attempted only in terminal cases of acute leukemia resistant to conventional drug therapy. The characteristics of the leukemic cells in such patients, and the severe immunodeficiency which may follow extensive chemotherapy, might render these patients particularly poor subjects for this or any other treatment. Whole-body irradiation followed by marrow transplantation might give better results if it became ethically acceptable to administer such treatment to patients with acute leukemia that was less advanced or in remission.

RADIATION THERAPY IN CHRONIC LYMPHOCYTIC LEUKEMIA

The role of radiation in the management of chronic lymphocytic leukemia has diminished since cytotoxic agents, particularly chlorambucil, and adrenocortical steroid hormones became available. Local radiation therapy may be given for lymph node masses which are unsightly or causing pressure symptoms or obstruction, for example, in the mediastinum. If the patient is receiving systemic chemotherapy for his disease, localized node masses usually are irradiated, only if they do not involute satisfactorily with the systemic treatment, or if they are causing urgent symptoms. Doses of 800 to 1600 rad are generally sufficient to cause substantial regression of enlarged nodes: It may be unwise to exceed the dose which produces adequate regression, since the systemic disease remains and it is sometimes necessary to ir-radiate the same area again, months or years later. Radical irradiation on the first occasion does not guarantee that there will be no recurrence, and may make it difficult to give further irradiation to the same site, particularly if a vital structure such as the trachea is in the field to be treated. Spinal cord compression or osteolytic lesions are rare in chronic lymphocytic leukemia, but are indications for local radiotherapy.

Systemic treatment by irradiation is controversial. Radiotherapy may be ap-plied externally, either to the spleen or to the whole body,[338,339] or internally by the administration of radionuclides, usually ^{32}P.[300,476] Although all these techniques give satisfactory results in skilled hands, irradiation is used less widely than che-motherapy for chronic lymphocytic leukemia. However, there are no systematic prospective studies which indicate the superiority of chemotherapy over radio-therapy or vice versa. The good results obtained with ^{32}P at one center[476,477] may well be attributable to the high standard of general clinical care exercised by the group which used the isotope, rather than to the therapeutic technique per se.[571] Since this group[477] had diagnostic criteria which were slightly different from those generally adopted, it is also possible that the diagnosis in their patients was es-tablished somewhat earlier than at some other centers. This would lead to an auto-matic improvement in the median survival from time of diagnosis, even if no therapy were given. These considerations emphasize the need for comparative studies in which patients are randomly admitted to one of several arms of the therapeutic trial.

Recent uncontrolled studies of the effects of externally applied whole-body ir-radiation suggested a high response rate in symptomatic cases of chronic lymphocytic leukemia, with improvement in symptoms, physical signs, peripheral blood count, and bone marrow appearance.[338,339] In those patients achieving a good response according to carefully defined criteria, the median duration of unmain-tained remission was 19 months.[339] This seems encouraging since all those treated had active chronic lymphocytic leukemia with symptoms, but a controlled trial would be necessary to establish if this regimen can produce more prolonged survival, or survival in better health than other forms of therapy. The possible benefits of prophylactic treatment for inactive asymptomatic cases should also be evaluated.

Extracorporeal irradiation of the blood has been used in the treatment of chronic lymphocytic leukemia, but treatment usually has to be prolonged and the benefit has not been very striking, so this remains an experimental, not an es-tablished, procedure.[379,541,629] External irradiation of the spleen may be used when splenomegaly is very marked or causes symptoms, or in patients who respond poorly to chemotherapy. Treatment must be cautious, using dose fractions as small as 25 rads, since marked pancytopenia may occur, especially if splenomegaly is initially very gross. Splenic irradiation produces involution of the spleen and, fre-quently, shrinkage of lymph nodes at distant sites, while the peripheral blood lymphocyte count falls. Successful treatment is followed by improvement in the pe-ripheral blood levels of hemoglobin, platelets, and neutrophils. Hyperuricemia is sometimes seen when involution of CLL tissue is very rapid, and prophylactic treatment with allopurinol is advisable,[164] particularly in elderly patients with im-paired renal function. Splenic irradiation produces results less consistently successful than are obtained when the same therapy is used in chronic granulocytic leukemia.

RADIATION THERAPY IN CHRONIC GRANULOCYTIC LEUKEMIA

Because it was the first effective therapy for chronic granulocytic leukemia and produced very satisfactory results in a short time, radiation was for many years the standard treatment for this disease. Although splenic irradiation became the most common method, good clinical results were also seen with "abdominal bath" techniques or spray radiotherapy, where the whole body was treated, usually with cautious dose fractions of 25 rad or less.[481] The latter methods had no clear-cut advantage. Splenic irradiation continued to be popular, even after the introduction of chemotherapy with busulfan, and is still in use today. However, a controlled trial suggested that busulfan yields better results than irradiation.[437] In this trial, 54 previously untreated patients received intermittent splenic irradiation and 48 untreated patients received busulfan, initially, in 4-mg daily doses, and later at very low doses on a nearly continuous basis. The median survival of the irradiated group was 120 weeks while that of the busulfan-treated group was 170 weeks ($p < 0.03$). Treatment was altered if a patient's disease ceased to respond satisfactorily: 32 of the 54 irradiated patients eventually received busulfan, but only 4 of the 48 busulfan-treated patients received splenic irradiation. As well as longer survival, the patients treated with busulfan had a less fluctuant clinical course and better maintenance of hemoglobin levels. Control of splenomegaly was equally satisfactory and many patients who became refractory to radiotherapy responded to busulfan. The onset of metamorphosis of the chronic granulocytic leukemia occurred earlier in the group treated by irradiation; others have also suggested that irradiation favors earlier onset of blastic change in chronic granulocytic leukemia, as in polycythemia vera.[363] The trial has been criticized on several counts, but principally because it compared busulfan administered on a near-continuous basis with irradiation administered at long intervals: thus, the leukocyte counts of the irradiated patients were allowed to fluctuate much more widely than those of the patients treated with busulfan. For this reason, the trial was not a valid comparison of the two therapeutic agents per se, but a comparison of busulfan therapy versus radiotherapy *in the manner in which each is usually given*. It is possible that irradiation administered in frequent, small increments might be as effective as busulfan; unfortunately, no trial has been conducted to investigate this question.

The use of radiotherapy continues to decline in favor of busulfan therapy, but results by either method remain essentially unsatisfactory in the long run, and it is to be hoped that both types of treatment will become obsolete as therapy improves. At present, splenic irradiation may be indicated in chronic granulocytic leukemia when a particularly rapid reduction of the leukocyte count is required (for example, when the leukocrit is such that blood viscosity problems and retinal hemorrhages arise), or for symptomatic relief of painful splenomegaly in a patient whose disease has undergone metamorphosis and become refractory to chemotherapy. In the latter case, irradiation must be very cautious since severe thrombocytopenia is likely. A rare indication for radiotherapy may be the occurrence of chronic granulocytic leukemia in early pregnancy, when splenic irradiation with shielding of the uterus controls the disease without exposing the fetus to the effects of cytotoxic drugs:

many would prefer to treat such patients by transfusion alone because the hazard of radiation effects on the fetus cannot be altogether eliminated.

When chronic granulocytic leukemia has undergone metamorphosis to an acute phase, extramedullary leukemic deposits may occur in the orbit, spinal canal, paranasal sinuses, long bones, or soft tissues. Solitary lesions of this type are often best alleviated by local irradiation.

CHEMOTHERAPY

The chemotherapy of leukemia antedates such treatment for other forms of cancer. In 1865, on the suggestion of Rosencrantz, Lissauer first used arsenic in the form of potassium arsenite, the famous Fowler's solution, for the treatment of chronic leukemias, with apparent success.[412] The improvement produced by arsenic was modest and temporary, and the advent of radiation therapy later overshadowed drug treatment. Radiotherapy remained supreme for nearly 50 years and chemotherapy was largely neglected despite the skilled advocacy of Forkner and others.[217] In the early twentieth century, Ehrlich laid down the basic principles which apply to both antimicrobial and antineoplastic chemotherapy, and began a new era of medical progress with his cure for trypanosomiasis.[180] Unfortunately, his attempts to treat neoplastic disease with synthetic compounds were unsuccessful, and development of effective anticancer drugs was postponed until the combined results of primarily military research and of chance observations led to the first clinical use of nitrogen mustard during World War II.[244] Wartime security measures delayed the publication of results until 1946,[236,245] and were also responsible for the intentionally uninformative code name, *HN2*, which nitrogen mustard has borne ever since.

Since its rebirth in 1946, the chemotherapy of cancer has become a vast and complex field, distinguished by a great expenditure of time, money, and effort. Returns have not as yet been spectacular in the chemotherapy of most solid tumors, but very significant progress has been made in some of the less common tumors, especially the leukemias. Much of the discipline of cancer chemotherapy is outside the scope of this book but has been the subject of numerous reviews[274,593,688,689] and monographs[84,137,384,633] to which the reader is referred. Only a brief account directed toward the leukemias can be given here.

Development of Chemotherapeutic Agents

The use of arsenic in the nineteenth century for the treatment of leukemia had no real scientific basis but produced some benefit. Eighty years later, the use of nitrogen mustard and urethane in human leukemias and lymphomas was almost as empirical, arising initially from the observation that these compounds depressed the leukocyte count in animals. Although the evidence which prompted their use was so slender, the original clinical experiments were highly successful. The empirical approach has persisted ever since, with the refinement that screening of compounds in experimental animals and tumor systems has become highly developed, and new agents are not administered to patients until a considerable knowledge of their pharmacology has been acquired in vitro and in animals. The manufacture and screening of new compounds is a major endeavor: one institution alone tested 16,000 substances for possible antitumor activity,[35] and about 300,000 compounds had been tested in various centers up to 1959[234]; that number has now been more than doubled.

The empirical screening of synthetic compounds and natural products for antitumor activity has been supplemented by newer and less haphazard approaches. Compounds found to be effective by the former technique have been intensively studied in the attempt to elucidate their mode of action; further compounds have then been deliberately synthesized in a search for agents with enhanced activity and less undesirable toxicity. Even when the mode of action cannot be determined, a range of chemical derivatives of a useful agent can be prepared and tested; frequently, one of these second-generation compounds is better than the original. Some new antitumor compounds have been developed on the basis of knowledge of tumor cell metabolism; thus, cognizance of the high turnover of purines by many tumor cells was utilized when purine analogs were synthesized as antitumor agents.[305] The so-called rational approach to cancer chemotherapy—accumulating knowledge about the cancer cell and then devising agents which will exploit its weaknesses—is more attractive scientifically than the purely empirical approach, but it must be admitted that rationally developed drugs have often proved ineffective, while many useful compounds have been developed empirically. Pure chance has continued to provide valuable drugs, such as the observation that guinea pig serum inhibits certain transplanted murine lymphomas,[353] which eventually led to the successful clinical use of the enzyme L-asparaginase in human leukemia.[301]

The statement is still occasionally made that effective drug treatments for cancer will become available only when the essential nature and causes of neoplasia are known. This view is no longer tenable as a general rule: choriocarcinoma can certainly be cured by drug therapy, although its etiology and pathogenesis remain obscure, and the same is apparently true of some acute childhood leukemias.[504,594] While improved knowledge of the fundamental nature of neoplasms will almost certainly aid in devising better therapies, therapeutic advances also continue to occur independently of this quest.

Systems for Drug Screening

One of the greatest difficulties in the development of new antitumor agents has been the lack of suitable test systems. Drugs have been tested in plants and microorganisms, in animal tumors and leukemias, but it has repeatedly been found that some agents which produced dramatic results in animals or in vitro had little or no effect in human disease. It is also possible that agents which could be valuable in man have been denied clinical trials because they possessed no activity against the animal tumors used for screening. Pioneer work in animal screening,[602] with egg chorioallantoic membranes[345] and tissue culture methods[56,57] has helped to establish improved methods for the rapid effective screening of new compounds for possible antitumor activity. The Cancer Chemotherapy National Service Center of the U.S. Public Health Service has established standard screening methods and channels of technical communication[196] which expedite the evaluation of new compounds, but, at best, the models in use are only approximations to human tumors. Although laborious and costly, screening of large numbers of compounds must continue until features which enable preselection of the most suitable substances on the basis of their chemical structure are elucidated more clearly than at present. Screening programs have yielded several useful drugs, such as busulfan,[268] triethylene melamine,[406,520] and vincristine.[336]

Terminology

There is an unfortunate abundance of overlapping terms used to describe chemical agents employed in the treatment of neoplastic disease. Some of these terms, like *oncolytic* or *carcinostatic* are not without emotional overtones. It has been said that *cancer chemotherapy* is an unduly optimistic term, because it suggests the specificity and lack of host toxicity associated with antimicrobial chemotherapy, while *cytotoxic treatment* is an *anti* term, emphasizing the undesirable features of the drugs.

Cancer chemotherapeutic agent is used to describe any drug which inhibits or destroys cancer cells while having a margin of safety sufficient to permit its use. The term *cytotoxic agent* is commonly used to refer to any cancer chemotherapeutic agent *except* hormones: The distinction is somewhat unreal, since some hormones are quite toxic to cells—for example, adrenal corticosteroids commonly bring about lysis of lymphocytes and lymphoblasts.

Antileukemic agent are drugs which are clinically valuable in the treatment of leukemia and not merely toxic to leukemic cells, for example, 5-fluorouracil is a cancer chemotherapeutic agent but is not classified as an antileukemic agent. Antileukemic agents may be further subdivided into *cycle-active* (or *cycle-sensitive*) agents, and *cycle-insensitive* agents. *Cycle-active agents* affect cells which are about to enter, or are in, the DNA-synthetic, or S, phase of the cell cycle, and have little effect on resting cells (see Chapter 8). *Cycle-insensitive* agents appear to attack cycling cells or resting cells without discrimination. Although most drugs fall roughly into one or other category, there are overlaps, for example, alkylating agents can destroy resting cells, but cells in cycle are probably more susceptible. Knowledge of cycle sensitivity, or the lack of it, can be valuable in planning a therapeutic approach: thus, agents which are principally cycle-active are generally ineffective against neoplasms whose cellular turnover is slow, for example, mercaptopurine is valueless in the treatment of chronic lymphocytic leukemia.

A further classification of antileukemic agents, and of cancer chemotherapeutic drugs in general, is by their *mode of action,* into antimetabolites, alkylating agents, and so on. Inevitably this classification is incomplete, since the mode of action of some drugs is uncertain. Within a particular category—for example, the alkylating agents—drugs may be further classified according to their *chemical structure,* that is, as aliphatic, aromatic, or heterocyclic compounds.

Mode of Action

Although several ways in which antileukemic agents might affect leukemic cells were suggested many years ago,[343] and sophisticated therapeutic approaches have been based on the known principal effects of these drugs,[133] the finer details of their actions upon normal and neoplastic cells are mostly uncertain. The major recognized types of antineoplastic mechanism are outlined in Table 17-2 and Figure 17-3.

Table 17-2
Modes of Action of Cancer Chemotherapeutic Agents

Action	Cycle activity		Examples	
	Marked	*Slight*	*Class of Agent*	*Specific Drug*
Interference with DNA synthesis by deprivation of essential metabolites	+		Antimetabolites	Methotrexate
Incorporation into the structure of DNA with distortion of the genetic message	+		Antimetabolites	Thioguanine
Interference with readout of RNA from the DNA molecule		+	Antibiotics	Actinomycin D
Destruction of formed DNA; cross-linking of DNA helices		+	Alkylating agents	Nitrogen mustard
Derangement of the mitotic spindle apparatus and the mechanics of mitosis	+		Plant alkaloids	Vincristine
Interference with readout from mRNA to ribosomes in the cytoplasm		+	Antibiotics	Puromycin
Specific inhibition of cellular metabolic processes		+	Antimetabolites	2-Deoxyglucose
Nonspecific cytoplasmic poisoning		+	Metals	Arsenic
Interference with subcellular organelles, e.g., lysosomes		+	Hormones	Adrenal corticosteroids
Immunologic damage to the cell structure		+	Immunoglobulins	Antilymphocyte globulin
Deprivation of essential metabolites by action outside the cell		+	Enzymes	L-Asparaginase (colospase)

Note: It is not implied that the drugs quoted above as examples exert effects *only* in the way cited—for example, nitrogen mustard does not only damage formed DNA, it also disrupts mitosis and is a nonspecific cytoplasmic poison.

The antileukemic drugs in clinical use exert their beneficial effects by lessening the proportion of leukemic cells. This is achieved by destroying resting cells, by destroying cells which are in cycle and would otherwise reproduce, and by inhibiting cells from entering into cycle, thereby allowing natural wastage to overtake the leukemic cell mass. Those drugs which affect cells in cycle may affect DNA synthesis prior to mitosis, or may abort the mitotic process itself; however, it is incorrect to regard all antileukemic drugs as simply antimitotic agents although this view was once held.[177,179] Many chemotherapeutic agents fulfil several roles; thus, most alkylating agents will destroy resting cells,[420] inhibit or disrupt DNA synthesis, and kill cells in mitosis: Some alkylating agents are particularly active against dividing cells, while others, for example, busulfan, appear indifferent to the state of activity of the cell. Although exceptions occur, it is broadly true that cycle-active drugs such as the antimetabolites are most useful in the acute leukemias, while cycle-insensitive drugs, such as the alkylating agents, are more effective against the chronic leukemias and myeloma. The activity displayed in different parts of the cell cycle by the

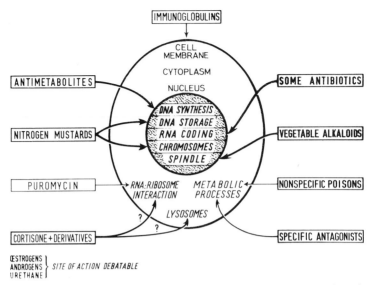

Fig. 17-3.   Major sites and processes within the cell which are affected by drugs used in cancer chemotherapy. The oversimplification is deliberate.

drugs of major importance in the treatment of the acute leukemias is summarized in Table 17-3.

Knowledge of these relationships is limited by the imperfections of present methods for studying leukemic cell kinetics (see Chapter 8). However, attempts are being made to improve the treatment of leukemia by exploiting the actions of different drugs upon different parts of the cell cycle. Thus, destruction of resting cells by alkylating agents or ionizing radiations may be followed by increased mitotic activity among the surviving leukemic cells: These cells will then be particularly vulnerable to an antileukemic drug which affects cells in mitosis. Administration of an agent which prevents cells entering mitosis will cause accumulation of cells in a premitotic stage of the cell cycle. At this time, the effects of a drug which aborts mitosis, for example, vincristine, would be minimized. However, if the first drug is discontinued some hours before the vincristine is given, a wave of "synchronized" mitoses will occur and the effects of vincristine given at the correct time will be enhanced. Thus, a knowledge of the mode of action of drugs in relation to the cell cycle can help the therapist to avoid drug antagonism and to take advantage of the synergistic effects of drugs by administering them in the optimal sequence and timing. Attempts to recruit cells from the nonproliferating to the proliferating pool, or to produce synchronous mitoses among the proliferating cells, are the subject of much current research (see Chapter 8) and it seems possible that this approach may greatly improve the clinical management of the acute leukemias.

Many antileukemic drugs produce chromosomal anomalies and mitotic aberrations which superficially resemble the effects of ionizing radiations[19] and they have been termed *radiomimetic;* however, this analogy should not be pushed too far, since their mechanism of action differs from that of irradiation.[361] The beneficial effect of antileukemic drugs in leukemia is not achieved without cost. Agents which destroy resting leukemic cells will also destroy normal cells and there is little evidence that the former are more sensitive to the drugs. Antimetabolic agents inhibit DNA synthesis in leukemic cells and prevent successful division, but are equally—and some-

Table 17-3
The Activity in Different Phases of the Cell Cycle of the Major Drugs used in the Acute Leukemias

Drug	Cycle-activity*		Cycle-phase Independent Activity	Cycle-phase Specific Activity
	Marked	*Slight*		
Prednisolone		+	Cell destruction (?effect on lysosomes)	Blocks passage of cells from G_1 to S
Vincristine	+		Disrupts cytoplasmic microtubular structures	Inhibits mitosis; inhibits G_0 to G_1 transition
Mercaptopurine	+		RNA inhibition	Inhibits DNA synthesis
Thioguanine	+		RNA inhibition	Formation of abnormal DNA
Methotrexate	+		RNA and protein inhibition	Inhibits DNA synthesis
Hydroxyurea	+			Inhibits DNA synthesis
Cytarabine	+			Inhibits DNA synthesis
Cyclophosphamide		+	Disruption and cross-linking of DNA helices	Blocks passage of cells from G_2
Daunorubicin		+	Forms complexes with DNA and distorts the helices	Blocks passage of cells from G_2
Asparaginase		+	Deprives leukemic cells of extracellular asparagine essential for metabolism	

*Most of the drugs have both cycle-dependent and cycle-independent activities. Those classified as showing marked cycle activity appear to have little or no *clinically important* effect upon resting cells, and can be expected to have little application in the treatment of neoplasms with very low cell turnover, such as chronic lymphocytic leukemia. (See also Skipper HE, et al: Cancer Chemother Rep 56:493, 1972.)

times more—potent against normal hematopoietic cells. Because normal cells appear to possess chemical processes which are qualitatively, and sometimes even
quantitatively, identical to those of leukemic cells, the available antileukemic drugs
always damage the normal marrow as well as the leukemic tissues. Although
prednisolone and vincristine have little or no toxic effects upon normal bone marrow, these drugs damage normal lymphoid and nervous tissues, respectively. The
most significant exception to the rule that antileukemic drugs damage normal marrow cells is the high requirement of some leukemic cells for asparagine and their
resultant susceptibility to the action of the enzyme L-asparaginase[149]: normal bone
marrow cells are not so affected and L-asparaginase has, therefore, the highest
therapeutic index* of any antileukemic drug. While it is hoped that other metabolic
differences between normal and leukemic cells can be detected and exploited, most
antileukemic drugs in use today have a low therapeutic index.

The success of antileukemic chemotherapy does not, therefore, depend on the
specificity of the drugs used, nor in most instances upon any special vulnerability of
the leukemic cell. At one time it was believed that leukemic cells were specially liable
to damage by so-called antimitotic agents because their rate of reproduction was
very high. In fact, although some leukemic cells divide relatively frequently, they
rarely do so faster than normal hematopoietic cells,[14] and usually their rate of
turnover is much slower than normal (see Chapter 8). This appears to be their real
weakness: because leukemic cells divide less often than normal hematopoietic cells
do, a given leukemic cell mass is replaced more slowly after chemotherapeutic insult
than is a corresponding mass of normal marrow cells. Convincing experiments with
the transplanted murine leukemia, L1210, have shown how the leukemic cell mass
can be progressively eroded by a series of treatments until all leukemic cells have
been destroyed: during such treatment the normal hematopoietic cells are able to
survive because of their superior capacity to restore their own numbers.[582] As a result of this work, attempts have been made to devise treatment schedules in which
successive doses of antileukemic agents are timed so as to take the maximum
possible advantage of the slow turnover of leukemic cells. Although the cytokinetics
of individual human acute leukemias must differ from those of L1210, such approaches have led to significant clinical advances. Relatively intensive therapy,
administered at intervals which permit recovery or even improvement of the normal
hematopoietic cell population, can be repeated on many occasions; if the treatments
are too close together to permit full recovery of the leukemic cells, the latter can be
progressively eliminated. Less intensive treatment, given continuously, allows both
cell populations to reach an equilibrium which is almost always eventually upset because the leukemic cells develop resistance to the drugs used. Used in this way, the
drugs produce a period of control, usually termed remission, which is terminated by
a recrudescence of the neoplastic cells which will never again respond to that particular therapy.

Careful timing of treatment makes possible the use of very large doses of some
antileukemic drugs, particularly the antimetabolites. While normal hematopoietic
cells and cells of the gastrointestinal mucosa can tolerate very large single doses of
antimetabolites,[139] leukemic cells are more vulnerable; furthermore, the use of large

---

*In man, the therapeutic index of a drug is the ratio between the median toxic dose and the median
effective dose (TD50/ED50). In laboratory animals the median lethal dose is often used, so the therapeutic index is LD50/ED50. For obvious reasons this is less helpful in clinical practice!

doses may overcome partial drug resistance or prevent resistance arising. In this connection it should be remembered that while the dose-response curves for some antileukemic drugs (for example, alkylating agents) are approximately linear, the corresponding curves for antimetabolic drugs are usually hyperbolic.[37] Thus "high" doses of drugs such as methotrexate may seem excessive but are not as high biologically as they appear; for example, a twofold increase in dose may increase a given cell "kill" from 50 to only 66 percent.

All successful chemotherapy so far devised for the leukemias is based upon destroying leukemic cells, thus resembling antimicrobial chemotherapy. These disciplines share many problems, such as finding agents without excessive host toxicity, and circumventing the development of resistance by the cells to be destroyed. Both disciplines employ drug combinations, and measures to enhance the immunologic defenses of the host organism, but at almost all points antimicrobial chemotherapy has been much more successful than cancer chemotherapy. However, a fundamentally different approach might be applicable in the leukemias. The uncontrolled proliferation and failure to undergo differentiation, which are characteristic of leukemic cells, may result from deficiency of cellular constituents due to the action of unknown leukemogens.[39] What may be needed is substitution therapy, or "a healing of the biochemical lesion, rather than a destruction of the cell which carries it" as Haddow put it.[264] The possibility of inducing differentiation in leukemic cells and thereby rendering them susceptible to normal homeostatic control is an exciting one: such therapy seems unlikely to be harmful to normal body cells and might offer permanent control of the disease, in the way that endocrine deficiencies are controlled by substitution therapy. Research on this approach has been neglected in the past, due perhaps to the enthusiasm evoked by the initial successes of antileukemic chemotherapy, when it was felt that a chemical cure for leukemia was imminent. A renewal of interest in substitution therapy is certainly in order, since conventional chemotherapy today still faces many unsolved problems which were pointed out over 20 years ago.[676,677,678]

The Alkylating Agents

Over 800 alkylating agents are known to the chemist; many of these have been screened in animal tumor systems for possible use in human cancer, and a few have won a place in clinical practice. Some of the latter are of value in the management of the leukemias.

Alkylating agents are organic chemicals which in solution liberate active alkyl radicals—organic cations—capable of combining with active sites, such as hydrogen bonds or sulfhydryl groups, on other molecules. In biological molecules, the occupation of such sites by alkyl groups frequently disturbs their physiologic function. More serious disturbance may occur when an alkylating agent with two reactive groups attaches to two sites, thus cross-linking two molecules or adjacent parts of a single large molecule. Alkylating agents are often classified as mono-, bi-, or polyfunctional, according to the number of reactive groups available, and it is significant that the former have low biological activity while the agents of clinical importance are all bi- or polyfunctional. Although alkylating agents were known to the chemists in the nineteenth century and were used as cross-linking agents in the dyestuffs industry, their introduction into medicine was an indirect outcome of research dating from World War I, when mustard gas was used extensively in the

Table 17-4
Alkylating Agents Commonly Used in Current Clinical Practice

Class	Subclass	Chemical Name	Official Name	Other Names	Uses in Leukemia*
Nitrogen mustards	Aliphatic	bis (2-chloroethyl) methylamine hydrochloride	mustine hydrochloride	HN2	
	Aromatic	4 (p-(bis (chloroethyl) amino)-phenyl) butyric acid	chlorambucil	Leukeran	CLL
		3 (p-(bis (chloroethyl) amino)-phenyl) α-alanine HCl	melphalan	Alkeran	MY
	Cyclic	1-bis (2-chloroethyl) amino-1-oxo-2-aza-5-oxaphosphoridin	cyclophosphamide	Cytoxan Endoxana Endoxan	AL, CLL, MY
Sulfonic acid esters	Dimethane-sulfonoxyalkanes	1, 4-dimethanesulfonoxybutane	busulfan	Myleran	CGL
Ethyleneimines	Triethyleneimines	triethyleneiminothio-phosphoramide	thio-TEPA		
	Ethyleneimino-quinones	2, 3, 5-triethyleneimino-1, 4-benzoquinone	triaziquone	Trenimon	
Nitrosoureas†	Ethylnitrosoureas	1, 3-bis (2-chloroethyl)-1-nitrosourea	carmustine	BCNU	AL
Halogenated carbohydrates‡	Brominated poly-hydric compounds	1, 6-dibromo-1, 6-dideoxy-D-mannitol	mitobronitol	Myelobromol; dibromannitol	CGL

*The letters AL, CGL, CLL, or MY signify that a drug is commonly used in the treatment of acute leukemias, chronic granulocytic leukemia, chronic lymphocytic leukemia, or myeloma, respectively.

†It is uncertain whether BCNU and related compounds are purely alkylating agents, but they do possess such activity,[675] and it is convenient to classify them with the alkylating agents.

‡Mitobronitol has alkylating activity in vitro, but it has been suggested that this drug may also have antimetabolic effects.[322,559]

582

field. The vesicant action of mustard gas (β,β' dichlorodiethyl sulfide) had been attributed to intracellular release of hydrochloric acid, and depression of the bone
marrow following exposure to the gas had been described.[244] During World War II,
nitrogen analogs of mustard gas were investigated for possible military use, and it
was rediscovered that both sulfur and nitrogen mustard, in addition to their local
vesicant action, had pronounced systemic effects. Tissues which proliferate actively,
notably the hematopoietic tissues and the gastrointestinal mucosa, were particularly
susceptible. A great deal of secret work was carried on during the war on the mode
of action of the mustards, and the first therapeutic trials were made during that period. Goodman and Gilman, then at Yale University, used nitrogen mustard in
patients with malignant lymphomas, and the late William Dameshek was consulted
regarding its effects on the hematopoietic organs. Striking palliation was obtained in
some patients with advanced leukemia, lymphosarcoma, and Hodgkin's disease.
The results of these investigations began to appear in the medical press in 1946[245]
and research has proceeded steadily since. This interesting early history is recounted
more fully elsewhere.[244] Alkylating agents commonly used in clinical practice at the
present time are listed in Table 17-4.

MECHANISM OF ACTION

The structural formulae of mustard gas and nitrogen mustard are shown in
Figure 17-4. Both compounds owe their great reactivity to their alkyl groups, which
in polar solvents lead to a molecular rearrangement which is depicted for nitrogen
mustard in Figure 17-5. An intramolecular cyclization leads to the formation of two
ethylenimonium cations with the release of chloride anions. The ethylenimonium
groups react with water, as shown in Figure 17-5, and also with many organic
radicals, including alpha amino, imidazole, sulfhydryl, sulfide, phenolic, and imino
groups of amino acids and peptides; with inorganic phosphate as well as glycero-
phosphate and hexosephosphates; the amino groups of adenosine and thiamine, hydrogen bonds, and the pyridino-N of nicotinic acid and pyridoxine.[244]

Although the biological activity of the alkylating agents is the subject of an extensive literature,[682] there is as yet no complete explanation for their physiologic
effects. Like other reactive chemicals they may poison cellular enzymes and inhibit
tissue respiration,[29] but although many enzymes are sensitive to their action,[526] only
choline oxidase is affected by the concentrations of alkylating agents encountered in
clinical practice.[28] Of much greater importance is the interaction of alkylating
agents and nucleic acids.[619] In vitro, both sulfur and nitrogen mustards react with
nucleoproteins,[38, 125] characteristically with conversion of nucleic acid solutions to a
gel consisting of denatured DNA.[3,4] Denaturation is produced by combination of the
mustard with the phosphate groups forming part of the main chain of the DNA

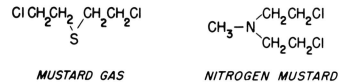

MUSTARD GAS   NITROGEN MUSTARD

Fig. 17-4. Structure of a sulfur mustard (β,β'-dichlorodiethyl-sulfide) and a nitrogen
mustard (bis [2-chloroethyl] methylamine).

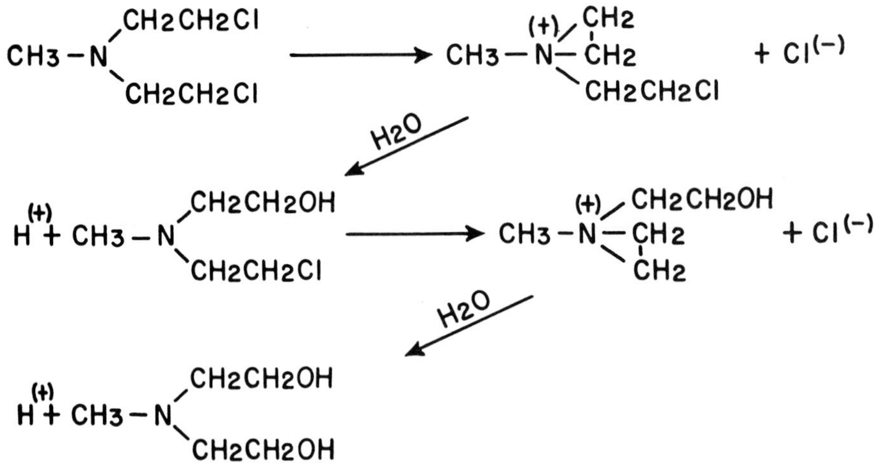

Fig. 17-5.   Intramolecular cyclization of nitrogen mustard.

molecule, with cross-linking of adjacent chains through the esterified phosphate moieties. Cross-linking requires the presence of two active sites in the alkylating agent, and experimental and clinical observations that bifunctional alkylating agents are much more active than monofunctional ones have been regarded as powerful supporting evidence for the hypothesis that cross-linking is a major mode of action of the alkylating agent.[239,266,420] Many experimental compounds have been designed on the basis of the cross-linking hypothesis. Additional mechanisms of action are also likely[58,264]: thus, many monofunctional agents are as effective as bifunctional compounds in the induction of mutations,[17] and some bifunctional agents, for example, sulfonates, react with nucleoprotein in vitro only at concentrations much greater than those attainable in vivo.[3] Alkylating agents react directly with the purines and pyrimidines of nucleic acid, especially guanine, and produce irreversible changes in the DNA molecule which must impair its functions.[3,85,513,654] Alkylating agents may possess other biologic effects not primarily connected with DNA.[637,638]

Biologically, the alkylating agents resemble ionizing radiations in their ability to produce point mutations,[17,19,20] growth inhibition associated with chromosome damage, and carcinogenesis.[657] Although for these reasons they have been termed *radiomimetic,* this is not entirely appropriate since comparison of genetic[18-20] and cytologic[361,362] effects discloses differences, suggesting fundamental disparities, in their mode of action. Radiations act on the nucleus in the late resting (G_2) or early mitotic phase, when the reduplication of DNA necessary for cell division has been completed.[397] Alkylating agents were thought to combine with DNA during the early resting (S) phase, thus preventing further DNA synthesis and mitosis.[362,572] Recent studies suggest that matters are more complex, with some alkylating agents resembling ionizing radiations more than others.[92] Nitrogen mustard and gamma radiation can kill cells in all portions of the cell generation cycle, and sensitivity is not a marked function of the proliferative state of the cells, whereas cyclophosphamide can also kill cells at all stages of activity, but the sensitivity of the cell population depends strongly on the fraction which are actually proliferating. The initial effect of exposure to radiation or an alkylating agent is temporary mitotic inhibition; as recovery proceeds, abnormal mitoses are frequent, notably fragmentation and abnormal stickiness of the chromosomes, leading to unequal segregation at anaphase. Many abnormal daughter cells are formed, a large proportion of them incapable of further division or even survival.[210,265,486,517] The production of chromosome damage, disturbed mitosis, and abnormal daughter cells is a more important effect of alkylating agents than is the initial mitotic inhibition.

Alkylating agents have marked effects upon the hematopoietic tissues. In rabbits and dogs, a progressive necrosis of the germinal centers of the lymph nodes and spleen is observed as early as 3 hours after injection of nitrogen mustard. There is congestion of the marrow sinusoids followed by depletion of the myeloid tissue from 1–3 days after injection, and recovery of cellularity—though not necessarily of functional capacity—in about 1 week.[115,246,347,348] Neutrophilia occurs in the blood during the first 24 hours and is followed by neutropenia. A fall of lymphocytes, basophils, and eosinophils begins within a few hours, reaching a nadir on the third or fourth day, with a return to normal at 5–7 days if the animal survives. The red cells are little affected by a single dose, but repeated doses for 4 weeks cause progressive anemia. Exposure of marrow cells in vitro to concentrations of nitrogen mustard comparable to those used therapeutically causes mitotic inhibition[260] and death of immature cells.[480] The observed hematologic changes after nitrogen mustard administration are best explained by a direct action upon dividing or potentially dividing cells.[347,348,462]

Experimental evidence indicates partial selectivity of various alkylating agents for different hematopoietic cell types. These agents cause at least three kinds of cell injury: First, the rapid destruction of mature lymphocytes occurs, which is an effect of many mustards; second, the rapid death of proliferating cells ensues, associated with the production of chromosomal abnormalities, which follows the administration of mustards such as chlorambucil; third, a slow decline in the numbers of erythropoietic and granulopoietic cells and megakaryocytes takes place, without visible evidence of cell damage and characteristic of the action of busulfan.[192–194,225] The net result of these differences is that the short-term effects of the mustard group fall chiefly on the lymphocytes, while busulfan affects the granulocyte precursors. In experimental animals, both agents administered concurrently give results closely resembling those seen with irradiation and this suggests that x-rays may have a dual action on hematopoietic tissues.[225] Large doses of any alkylating agent will destroy all kinds of hematopoietic cells, thus showing little or no selectivity; in fact, selectivity of action may be more apparent than real.[368,444] The action of mustards upon hematopoietic cells can be partially counteracted by the administration of sulfur-containing compounds such as L-cysteine,[669] although this has found little or no therapeutic use.

In leukemias and lymphomas, the alkylating agents act by mechanisms similar to those in experimental animals and in vitro. Proliferating cells, both normal and abnormal, in the bone marrow, spleen, and lymph nodes are destroyed, with changes in the blood reflecting those in the hematopoietic organs. Lymphopenia develops within 1–5 days of the administration of nitrogen mustard; neutropenia and thrombocytopenia are less constant or prolonged.[89,596] Hematopoietic cells in the marrow are destroyed, with a decrease in cellularity, regeneration beginning in the third week with apparent recovery by the sixth week. In the leukemias, the long-term effects of alkylating agents on the marrow resemble those of x-rays.[5,6] Increasing the dose of an alkylating agent, or repeating the same dosage at short intervals, leads to increased depression of the normal hematopoietic cells in the marrow. Even when doses are so spaced (for example, at 6-week intervals) that marrow cellularity appears fully recovered, cumulative effects of alkylating agents may be seen. Mere assessment of cellularity is an imperfect guide to the actual functional capacity of the marrow. Recovery of the peripheral blood count to normal suggests functional recovery of the marrow, but gives no clue to the functional *reserve* capacity of the hematopoietic system. If reserve capacity is seriously impaired by repeated doses of alkylating agents, a seemingly normal marrow may become grossly hypoplastic after a dose of the agent which formerly was well tolerated. Despite this long-term limitation, which applies particularly to busulfan, spacing of doses to enable partial hematopoietic recovery frequently makes possible the administration of larger total quantities of alkylating agents with improved clinical results in sensitive tumors.[382]

NITROGEN MUSTARD

Nitrogen mustard (mustine hydrochloride) (Fig. 17–4) is the oldest of the alkylating agents still in clinical use. Because of its chemical structure it is very soluble in water, hydrolyses rapidly, and is highly reactive, nearly all directly exposed cells being very susceptible.[619] Because the compound hydrolyses, solutions must be prepared immediately before use, and its high reactivity makes nitrogen mustard vesicant and corrosive, so it must be administered well-diluted into a large vein, with precautions taken to protect both doctor and patient. Clinically, these properties are disadvantageous but an advantage is the rapid onset and brief duration of its action; unfortunately, such activity is coupled with the almost invariable side effects of nausea and vomiting.

MUSTARD DERIVATIVES

From the early days of chemotherapy, attempts have been made to overcome the disadvantages of nitrogen mustard by structural alteration of its molecule. Small molecular changes were found to affect profoundly the character of the resulting compounds.[163] Preservation of the two chloroethyl groups is essential for retention of antitumor and antileukemic activity. A close relative of nitrogen mustard, the N-oxide, Nitromin, is more stable in solution and can be given orally as well as by injection. Its spectrum of activity resembles that of the parent compound,[365,376,604] but the availability of other alkylating agents which can be administered orally with lesser gastrointestinal side effects has limited the use of Nitromin outside Japan where it was developed.

Replacement of the aliphatic methyl group in the nitrogen mustard molecule by an aromatic (for example, phenyl) group leads to reduced solubility and decreased local irritant effects. Aromatic nitrogen mustards (see Table 17-4) can be given by mouth and have a milder and more prolonged action. An early derivative, naphthylamine mustard or R48, was used in chronic lymphocytic leukemia and lymphosarcoma,[516] and a related compound, R151, was combined with urethane in the treatment of myeloma.[321]

Chlorambucil (Leukeran).   Modification of the basic aromatic nitrogen mustard molecule by addition of a butyric acid chain produces chlorambucil (Fig. 17-6). This compound is the most widely used of the aromatic nitrogen mustards. Exten-

CHLORAMBUCIL

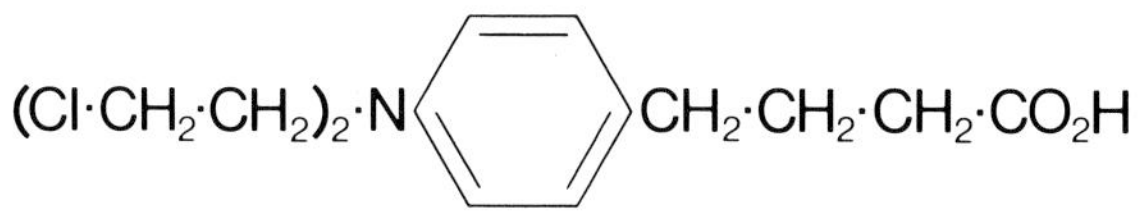

$$(Cl \cdot CH_2 \cdot CH_2)_2 \cdot N \langle \quad \rangle CH_2 \cdot CH_2 \cdot CH_2 \cdot CO_2H$$

Fig. 17-6.   Structural formula of chlorambucil (Leukeran).

sive laboratory and clinical tests[265] showed chlorambucil to be less toxic than most alkylating agents despite its powerful antitumor effects in experimental animals and favorable effect on human lymphomas. It is given orally and seldom causes gastrointestinal disturbance in conventional doses. A congener, aminochlorambucil, has similar properties and may be given parenterally; it is seldom used nowadays.[230]

Melphalan (Alkeran).   Although melphalan is classed as an aromatic nitrogen mustard in Table 17-4, it is also a member of the class of *metabolite-linked mustards,* compounds in which a nitrogen mustard moiety is linked with a natural metabolite such as an amino acid or a small peptide. In melphalan, a nitrogen mustard grouping is attached to L-phenylalanine (Fig. 17-7). The compound was synthesized by British[40] and Russian[385] workers and has been used clinically in its L-form, melphalan or L-phenylalanine mustard,[482] and in the racemic (DL) form, Sarcolysine (Fig. 17-8).[61,284] Only the L-form is widely used now. Melphalan can be administered orally or intravenously; its gastrointestinal side effects are more marked than those of chlorambucil, but much less severe than those produced by nitrogen mustard.

The rationale behind the development of the metabolite-linked mustards was that association of the alkylating radicals with a "carrier" of physiologic importance might lead to their rapid incorporation into tumor cells, with a resultant concentration of their alkylating effect in the target tissue, thereby producing a striking antitumor effect with little systemic toxicity. Besides phenylalanine, carrier molecules which have been combined with the dichloroethyl radical include pyrimidine, pyridine, thiazole, benzimidazole,[382,383] and uracil (see Fig. 17-8).[351,563] Substitution of the sugar mannitol for the methyl group of nitrogen mustard produces mannomustine (Degranol; see Fig. 17-8).[25,560,647] Most of these compounds have some effect in human leukemias and lymphomas. Unfortunately, the metabolite-linked mustards have not lived up to expectations. Although the carrier molecules produce interesting and sometimes useful variations in stability, absorption, distribution within the body, and excretion, the desired tumor selectivity

MELPHALAN

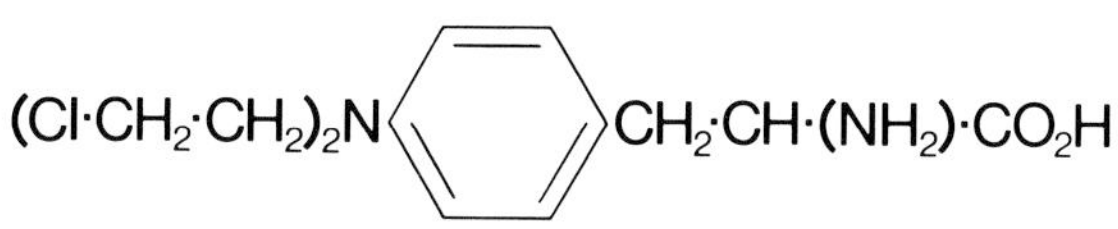

$$(Cl \cdot CH_2 \cdot CH_2)_2 N \langle \quad \rangle CH_2 \cdot CH \cdot (NH_2) \cdot CO_2H$$

Fig. 17-7.   Structural formula of melphalan (Alkeran).

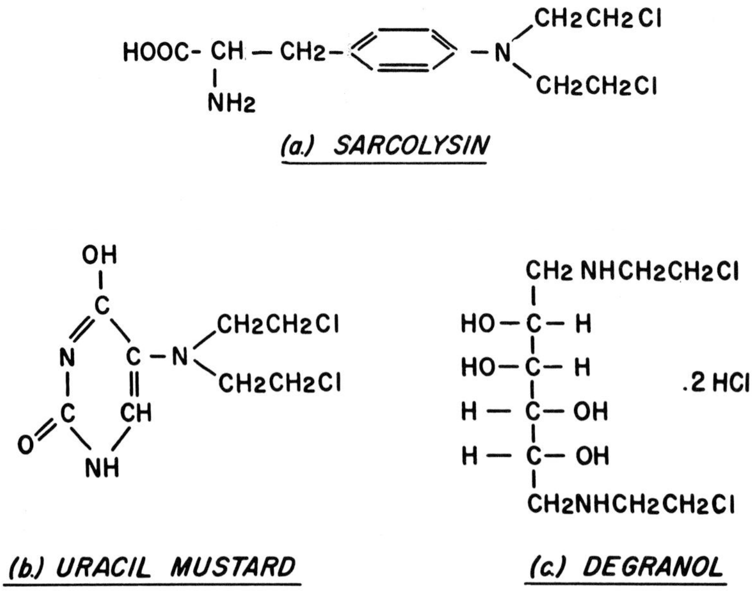
HOOC- CH — CH2-
NH2
N
CH2CH2Cl
CH2CH2Cl
(a.) SARCOLYSIN
(b.) URACIL MUSTARD
CH2 NHCH2CH2Cl
HO—C— H
HO—C— H
H — C— OH
H — C— OH
CH2NHCH2CH2Cl
.2 HCl
(c.) DEGRANOL

Fig. 17-8. Further nitrogen mustard derivatives.

has not been achieved. Melphalan, for example, might be expected to have an affinity for melanoma cells, since these cells require phenylalanine and might concentrate melphalan which would then destroy them. In fact, melphalan destroys hematopoietic cells much more rapidly than melanoma cells and is not an effective systemic treatment for malignant melanoma.

Cyclophosphamide (Cytoxan, Endoxana, Endoxan). Cyclophosphamide is a nitrogen mustard in which the dichloroethyl grouping is carried by a cyclic phosphamide ester (see Table 17-4 and Fig. 17-9).[11,12] It is inactive and stable in vitro and can be administered orally or intravenously. Activation was thought to occur within cells, enzymatic cleavage of the cyclic part of the molecule uncovering its alkylating potential. It is uncertain whether the molecule is split at the phosphorus–oxygen linkage by a phosphatase or at the phosphorus–nitrogen linkage by a phosphamidase.[215] Since tumor cells are commonly rich in both these enzymes, and megakaryocytes are not, it seemed possible that cyclophosphamide might possess

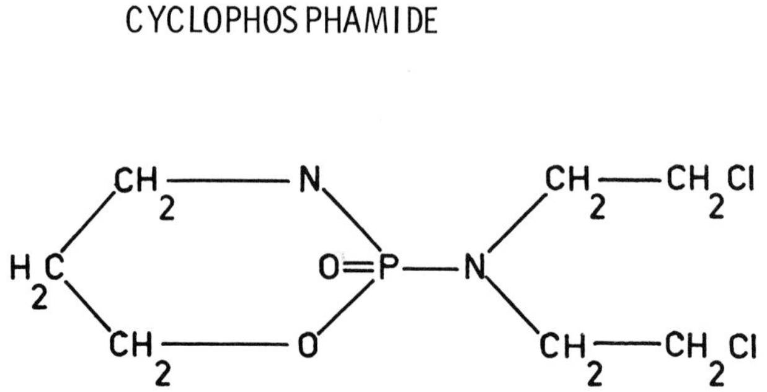
CYCLOPHOSPHAMIDE

Fig. 17-9. Structural formula of cyclophosphamide (Cytoxan, Endoxana).

some selective antitumor activity and might also have less tendency to cause thrombocytopenia than other alkylating agents. In fact, cyclophosphamide does appear to depress the platelet count less than equivalent doses of some other agents (for example, melphalan), but its selectivity against tumor cells is less than was hoped for, probably because activation of the molecule also occurs in plasma and in the liver.[244] Although not as tumor-specific as was originally hoped, cyclophosphamide is an effective and convenient drug with activity against a wide range of leukemias, lymphomas, and solid tumors,[203] and it is the most widely used alkylating agent in current clinical practice.

Sulfonic Acid Esters

The belief that antitumor and antileukemic activity requires a drug molecule with a minimum of two alkylating groups prompted a search for other types of compound with this basic feature. Some sulfonic esters with the functional group ($-OSO_2CH_3$) appeared likely candidates, and a series was prepared in which two such groups were joined by a chain of CH_2 groups whose length could be altered at will (Fig. 17-10). Animal experiments showed that the compound with four CH_2 groups (that is, the butane derivative) was active against the usual test tumor, Walker carcinoma 256, and also produced marked neutropenia in rats.[268] For this reason, the compound (now known as busulfan) was tested against human chronic granulocytic leukemia and found to be highly effective.[224,228,495] Busulfan is highly insoluble, and administration is restricted to the oral route. In animals, it inhibits DNA synthesis and probably mitosis[407]; studies in L1210 cells suggest that busulfan inhibits the incorporation of several nucleic acid precursors, apparently acting at a number of different sites.[638] In human leukemia, busulfan in conventional dosage acts relatively slowly, causing a gradual fall in the granulocyte count and decreasing cellularity of the bone marrow. In the usual therapeutic doses, the action of busulfan is almost specifically directed against myeloid cells,[192,193] making it particularly useful for treating chronic granulocytic leukemia and, to a lesser extent, polycythemia vera and myelofibrosis with myeloid metaplasia. The soluble analog of busulfan, dimethylmyleran (Fig. 17-10B) has similar hematologic effects[55] but is seldom used.

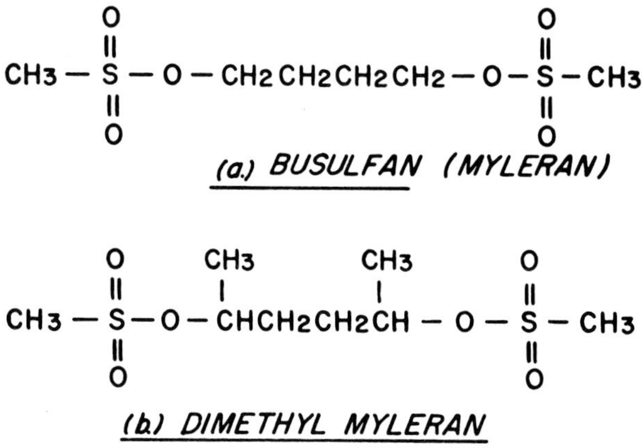

(a) BUSULFAN (MYLERAN)

(b) DIMETHYL MYLERAN

Fig. 17-10.   Structural formulae of busulfan (Myleran) and Dimethyl Myleran.

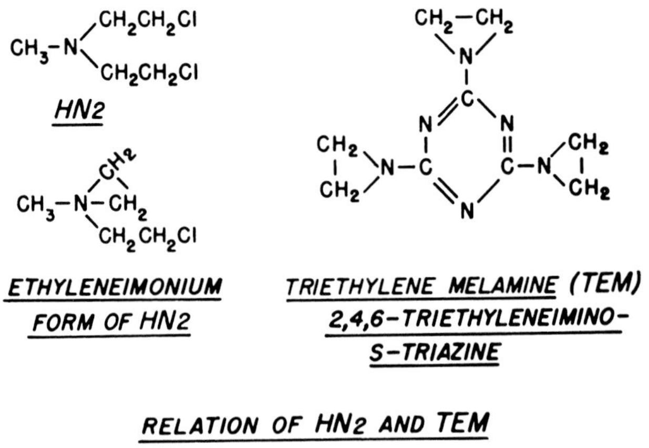

ETHYLENEIMONIUM
FORM OF HN2

TRIETHYLENE MELAMINE (TEM)
2,4,6-TRIETHYLENEIMINO-
S-TRIAZINE

RELATION OF HN2 AND TEM

Fig. 17-11.   Relation of nitrogen mustard and triethylene melamine.

Ethyleneimines

In solution, the nitrogen mustards undergo an intramolecular cyclization with formation of reactive ethyleneimonium groups (see Fig. 17-5). Realization of the biologic importance of ethyleneimino groups—the tertiary amine form which is nonreactive except in acid media—prompted the trial of compounds containing them. Such substances were already in use in the textile industry as cross-linking agents.[106] A triazine containing three ethyleneimino groups was found to have powerful antitumor effects[109,406,520] and came into clinical use as triethylene melamine (TEM). Its structure and relationship to nitrogen mustard are shown in Fig. 17-11.

Triethylene melamine is highly soluble and is two and a half times more active than nitrogen mustard on a weight basis[344]; its reactivity is due to the ethyleneimino groups rather than the triazine moiety.[106] It can be given intravenously, or by mouth with an alkali to retard its activation. TEM is rapidly cleared from the blood and broken down, metabolites of the ethyleneimino groups being excreted in the urine.[459] The drug is a potent depressant of all hematopoietic cells and has caused many deaths from the complications of marrow hypoplasia, principally because the effect of a standard dose is rather unpredictable. This variability persists, even when possible vagaries of absorption are avoided by intravenous administration of the drug, and it has been suggested that the erratic behavior of TEM may be due to self-polymerization.[274] This poor safety record, together with the availability of alternative drugs, have led to a steady decline in the clinical use of TEM.

A series of benzoquinone derivatives of the ethyleneimines has been synthesized[173] and several have been tested clinically.[45,50,332] Triethyleneiminobenzoquinone (triaziquone, Trenimon, Fig. 17-12) has been used quite extensively in Europe but has no special advantage over other alkylating agents.[409,410] A sulfonamide compound, 1,3-bis (ethyleneiminosulfonyl) propane has been tested in human leukemia,[486] but has not found a place in therapy.

Phosphoramide derivatives of the ethyleneimines have been used in the leukemias: the best-known member of the group, triethylenethiophosphoramide (thio-TEPA) is still used in treating some solid tumors, but these compounds no longer have a place in the treatment of leukemia.[32,207,423,565,618,692]

(a.)

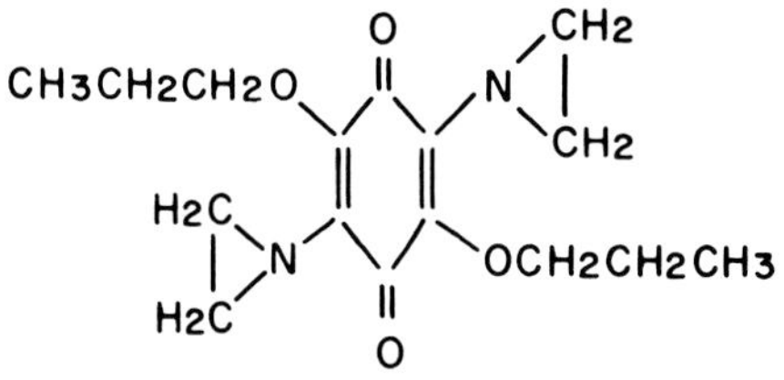

E-39

(b.)

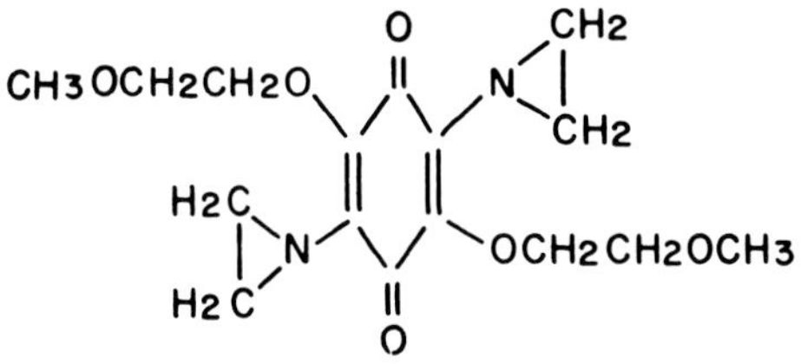

A-139

(c.)

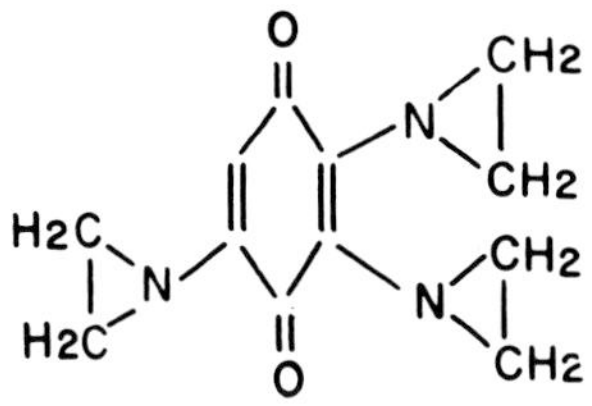

TRENIMON

Fig. 17-12. Ethylenimino benzoquinones.

BASIC EPOXIDES

This series of bifunctional alkylating agents is exemplified by epoxybutane (Fig. 17-13). They are very active against animal tumors and have been used in human leukemias and myeloma but with disappointing results.[370,445] Both epoxides and melamines are now more familiar in plastics technology than in hematology for, although the chemical activity of these compounds proved less than ideal for treating leukemias, they continue to be valuable in fabricating synthetic materials.

Nitrosoureas

The best-known of this series of compounds is an ethylnitrosourea, 1,3-bis(2-chloroethyl)-1-nitrosourea, BCNU or carmustine (Table 17-4). It is uncertain whether BCNU and related compounds are purely alkylating agents. Although they

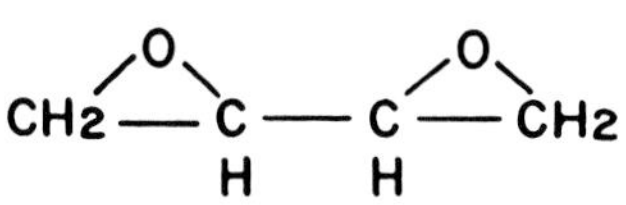

Fig. 17-13. Structural formula of epoxybutane.

DIBROMANNITOL

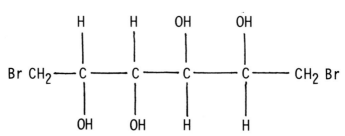

Fig. 17-14. Structural formula of dibromannitol (dibromomannitol, mitobronitol, Myelobromol).

possess alkylating activity[675] and produce chromosomal defects similar to those seen with alkylating drugs,[279] much of their biologic effect may be due to antimetabolite-like actions.[253,674] Unlike most other antileukemic drugs, BCNU is lipid soluble and consequently passes the blood-brain barrier, entering the brain and CSF. Although BCNU has activity against the systemic manifestations of the leukemias, its principal use is in the treatment of acute leukemia involving the CNS.[83] Two cyclohexyl congeners of BCNU, CCNU and methyl-CCNU, resemble the older compound but can be administered orally as well as intravenously, whereas BCNU can only be given by the intravenous route. Studies of CCNU and methyl-CCNU in leukemia are at a relatively early stage.[81,82] Intravenous BCNU lowers the leukocyte count in acute leukemia but the drug is very myelotoxic and seldom induces remission of the leukemia. BCNU is of value in malignant lymphomas, especially Hodgkin's disease, and in the chemotherapy of some solid tumors.

Halogenated Carbohydrates

A series of brominated polyhydric compounds has been synthesized by Hungarian workers, and 1,6-dibromo-1,6-di-deoxy-D-mannitol (dibromomannitol, dibromannitol, mitobronitol, Myelobromol) (Fig. 17-14) received extensive trials in human leukemia. Mitobronitol has alkylating activity in vitro, but, like BCNU, may also have antimetabolitelike effects.[322,559]

Target Tissues

Cancer chemotherapeutic agents may be classified according to their target tissue into three types[656]: (1) those active against all dividing cells, normal or neoplastic; (2) those selectively active against cells arising from one or more specific tissues; (3) those active against neoplastic cells as such. The enzyme L-asparaginase, together with certain tumor-specific antibodies and immunocytes, are the only agents with any claim to being members of the third class. Most antitumor drugs fall into the first class, and it is this fact which limits their usefulness so much. Many drugs are, in fact, pancytotoxic and damage nondividing cells, as well as dividing cells, with almost impartial severity. A very few agents, among them busulfan and chlorambucil, appear to belong to the second class, having some selectivity for myeloid and lymphoid cell-lines, respectively. Whether this apparent selectivity is a chemical one or has a cytokinetic basis is at present uncertain; that it can be valuable in clinical practice is well-established.

Clinical Uses of the Alkylating Agents

The usefulness of some of the alkylating agents in the leukemias is indicated in Table 17-4, and details of their mode of employment are given in Chapter 18.

NITROGEN MUSTARD

Nitrogen mustard and its close relatives have a wide spectrum of antineoplastic activity which includes chronic leukemias and polycythemia vera[346]; for some time it was advocated as a routine treatment for chronic granulocytic leukemia.[683,684] However, nitrogen mustard must be given intravenously and its rapidity of action is offset by a high incidence of nausea and vomiting. The availability of newer agents which are administered orally and have less violent effects has displaced nitrogen mustard from the field of leukemia therapy. Its commonest single use today is in the treatment of Hodgkin's disease as part of the MOPP (mustine-vincristine-procarbazine-prednisone) combination.[167]

CHLORAMBUCIL

This aromatic nitrogen mustard has particular value in the treatment of chronic lymphocytic leukemia and well-differentiated (lymphocytic) lymphosarcoma.[7,71,226,230] Chlorambucil is also effective in Hodgkin's disease[172,324,642] when given in doses higher than those used in chronic lymphocytic leukemia. Because it is taken by mouth and seldom causes gastrointestinal side effects, chlorambucil is suitable for long-term treatment of nonhospitalized patients with chronic lymphocytic leukemia. Although chlorambucil is thought to be specially effective in lymphoid neoplasms and to have a relatively specific action on lymphocytes,[193] it also beneficially affects chronic granulocytic leukemia[368,444] and polycythemia vera. In patients without leukemia, chlorambucil has produced lymphopenia and sometimes thrombocytopenia, apparently having less effect on granulocytes.[499] A cooperative study has shown that chlorambucil is more effective than busulfan in chronic lymphocytic leukemia, and less effective than busulfan in chronic granulocytic leukemia[532]: thus, the results of animal experiments with these two agents are borne out in clinical practice, each drug appearing to possess some target-specificity.

MELPHALAN

Melphalan has a wide spectrum of activity, including chronic leukemias, polycythemia vera, and malignant lymphomas. When taken by mouth it causes gastrointestinal disturbance only in high doses. It is widely used for the treatment of myeloma,[78,128,314,383,590,653] but is seldom employed in the leukemias.

CYCLOPHOSPHAMIDE

This drug is administered orally or parenterally and causes nausea and vomiting only in high doses. Despite the disagreeable side effects of alopecia and occasional hemorrhagic cystitis,[77,591] cyclophosphamide is widely used in leukemias, malignant lymphomas, and solid tumors.[203] Its activity resembles that of chlorambucil,[258,364,434,655] but the availability of a parenteral form makes possible the intermittent administration of very large doses, which is difficult to achieve with the former drug. Its tendency to spare the platelets makes cyclophosphamide useful in conditions complicated by thrombocytopenia. Apart from its activity in myeloma and macroglobulinemia, cyclophosphamide is also the only alkylating agent of proved value in the acute leukemias,[293] and is effective in both chronic granulocytic and chronic lymphocytic leukemias. Thus, it is the only drug which can be used with benefit in all the hematologic neoplasms.

BUSULFAN

This orally administered alkylating agent appears to affect selectively granulocytic proliferations of chronic type.[228,268,280,281,644] The selectivity of busulfan has been questioned[444]: relatively small doses may act principally on granulocytic cells,[229] but larger doses affect all hematopoietic cell lines. Thus, chronic *lymphocytic* leukemia can be controlled with busulfan,[617] but large doses are necessary; good results are less common than with chlorambucil; and control of the lymphocyte count is frequently associated with thrombocytopenia.[532] Busulfan in cautious dosage will control polycythemia vera and myeloid metaplasia.[158,358,470] For short-term therapy, busulfan is the most convenient and consistently effective drug for chronic granulocytic leukemia, but it has serious long-term disadvantages. Although the quality of life is improved, its length is increased but slightly; median survival in untreated CGL is about 31 months[447] and increases to only 40 months with busulfan therapy.[437] Busulfan can produce serious marrow toxicity, particularly in inexperienced hands, and the risks associated with long-term busulfan treatment are formidable.[74,123,166,169,194,224,227,286,325,377,457] They include pigmentation, interstitial pulmonary fibrosis, amenorrhea, infertility, teratogenesis, an Addisonianlike syndrome of weakness and pigmentation, cervical epithelial dysplasia, and the possible induction of skin and breast cancers. The control of chronic granulocytic leukemia in its chronic phase is relatively simple with busulfan and the early results of treatment are highly satisfactory. This success has engendered an unwarranted satisfaction with currently available treatment. If busulfan had proved less effective in the palliation of chronic granulocytic leukemia, therapeutic research in this disease might have progressed further.

ETHYLENEIMINES

These compounds were once widely used for treatment of the leukemias. Triethylene melamine was found to be effective in Hodgkin's disease, lymphosarcoma, chronic lymphocytic leukemia, and chronic granulocytic leukemia.[53,168,529] In the acute leukemias, TEM produces severe myelosuppression and frequently harms the patient, while benefit is rare. Chlorambucil, busulfan, and cyclophosphamide, being more reliable, less toxic, and at least as effective as TEM, have completely replaced it in the treatment of leukemias. Although the ethyleneiminoquinones are effective in lymphosarcoma and chronic granulocytic leukemia,[50,410] they have never been widely employed and there seems to be no special indication for their use in any type of leukemia.

BCNU

BCNU and related nitrosourea compounds possess some activity against the systemic manifestations of the acute leukemias, but their main application has been in therapy of meningeal leukemia.[83] However, the convenience of administering BCNU intravenously, instead of other drugs by lumbar puncture, is outweighed by its inferiority against meningeal leukemia when compared to intrathecal methotrexate.[611] The combination of BCNU with cytosine arabinoside has produced occasional remissions in acute granulocytic leukemia, and in chronic granulocytic leukemia after acute transformation,[283] but the principal value of BCNU appears to be in Hodgkin's disease and not in the leukemias.

DIBROMOMANNITOL

This drug is effective in chronic granulocytic leukemia in its chronic phase, and may occasionally control the disease when relative resistance to busulfan has arisen[124,509]: it is ineffective when acute transformation has occurred. It has no obvious superiority over busulfan and is usually reserved for relatively uncommon indications such as busulfan resistance, or pulmonary fibrosis or excessive pigmentation after long-term busulfan therapy.

Antimetabolites

These compounds are structurally similar but biologically antagonistic to vitamins or metabolites of physiologic importance. Because of their structural similarity to normal metabolites, antimetabolic drugs tend to replace them in biologic systems, thus causing a functional deficiency of the metabolite.[243] Antimetabolites compete with the naturally occurring substance for essential enzyme systems. Once accepted into the enzyme system, the drug either cannot be processed by the system, or can be altered only to a metabolically useless end-product. In either case, a deficiency of the normal product of that enzymatic pathway will develop. The property of inactivating enzyme systems is common to many cellular poisons, but the true antimetabolites are distinguished by their close structural relationship to the metabolite and the potential prevention or reversal of their action by an excess of the normal substance.[494] Usually the antimetabolite is competitive and its action is reversed over a wide range of concentrations, although some antimetabolites are so potent that their reaction kinetics are pseudo-irreversible and they almost qualify as enzyme poisons. Antimetabolites are often effective against the same enzyme in a range of animal species, although their potency varies in different species; thus, trimethoprim is a potent antifolate compound in bacteria but a weak one in man.[304] Closely related analogs of the same metabolite vary in activity from full metabolic potency to strong antimetabolic effects, while some analogs may be inert. Furthermore, a single analog may be active as a metabolite in some species and as an antimetabolite in others.[687]

The antimetabolites used in the treatment of the leukemias are all designed to compete with substances essential for the synthesis of DNA. An active search for such compounds was prompted by Farber's demonstration in 1949 of the value of folic acid antagonists in acute leukemia.[206] Crude folic acid antagonists had pre-

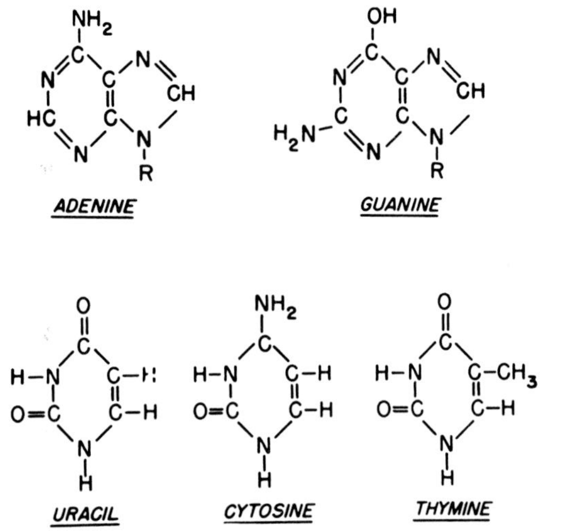

ADENINE GUANINE

URACIL CYTOSINE THYMINE

Fig. 17-15.   Purines and pyrimidines of nucleic acids.

viously been used in the treatment of the leukemias,[440] but Farber was the first to show that definite remissions could be obtained.

Nucleic acids are complex molecules composed of many nucleotides, each of which consists of a purine or pyrimidine heterocycle (Fig. 17-15) in combination with a pentose sugar and a phosphate group. The nucleotides are named after the purines or pyrimidines which they contain; thus, adenylic acid contains adenine and guanylic acid contains guanine (both purines), while uridylic, cytidylic, and thymidylic acids contain, respectively, the pyrimidines uracil, cytosine, and thymine. The two nucleic

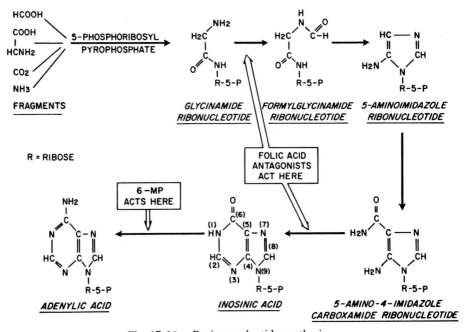

Fig. 17-16.   Purine nucleotide synthesis.

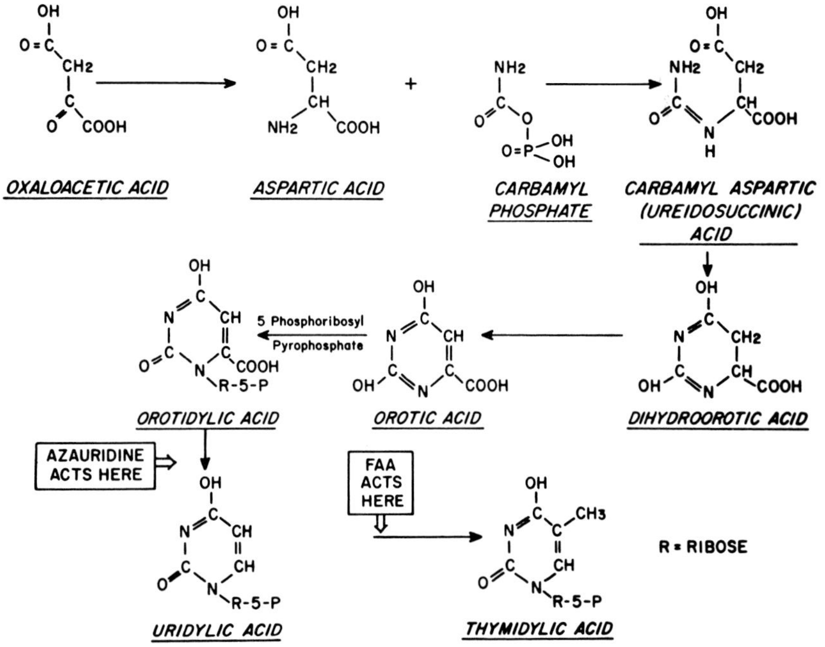

Fig. 17-17. Pyrimidine nucleotide synthesis.

acids, deoxyribose (DNA) and ribose (RNA) nucleic acids, differ in the nature of their constituent pentose sugars and also in their pyrimidine bases. Whereas both contain the same purines, as well as cytosine, RNA has uracil and DNA thymine as its second pyrimidine base.

The normal synthesis of nucleic acids may be exemplified by that of DNA. The building-up of purine and pyrimidine nucleotides is shown in Figures 17-16 and 17-17. Purine synthesis is better understood than that of the pyrimidines, and both pathways have been simplified in the diagrams. The nucleotides are built up as units in which sugar and phosphate groups are attached to the purine skeleton before ring closure. The precursors of the purines and pyrimidines are assembled from simple fragments such as glycine, formate, CO_2 and NH_3. Each synthetic step requires the presence of one or more enzymes and coenzymes, and it is at such points that antimetabolite drugs exert their inhibitory effects. The nucleotides are further built up into polynucleotides and these, in turn, into nucleic acids (Fig. 17-18). The Watson-Crick model of DNA consists of two polynucleotide chains arranged as counterwound helices around a common core.[663] The links of these chains are phosphate and deoxyribose groups, while the core is formed of the purine and pyrimidine bases which lie at right angles to the chains, one base from each chain pairing, by means of hydrogen bonding, with one from the opposite chain. Physicochemical factors determine that each purine must pair with a pyrimidine, and that only the adenine-thymine and guanine-cytosine bonds are possible. Alkylating agents interfere with the structure and function of DNA by breaking the polynucleotide chains and by producing irregular cross-linking between the bases. Moreover, the ionic bonds formed between the bases by alkylating agents differ from the normal hydrogen bonds by being relatively irreversible and preventing the temporary

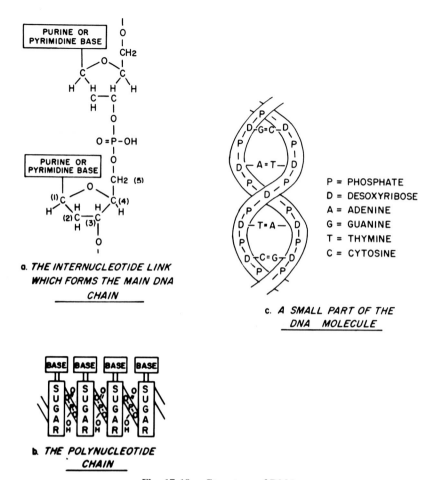

a. THE INTERNUCLEOTIDE LINK
WHICH FORMS THE MAIN DNA
CHAIN

c. A SMALL PART OF THE
DNA MOLECULE

P = PHOSPHATE
D = DESOXYRIBOSE
A = ADENINE
G = GUANINE
T = THYMINE
C = CYTOSINE

b. THE POLYNUCLEOTIDE
CHAIN

Fig. 17-18.   Structure of DNA.

separation of the helices which is essential for the replication of new DNA molecules.

FOLIC ACID ANTAGONISTS

These were the first antimetabolite drugs effective in leukemia and an extensive literature has grown up.[309,318] Folic acid or pteroylglutamic acid (Fig. 17-19) consists of pteridyl, p-aminobenzyl, and glutamyl moieties. Folinic acid or citrovorum factor, its active derivative, is a formyl compound of tetrahydrofolic acid (Fig. 17-19). Both substances occur naturally as conjugates (for example, polyglutamates) from which they are liberated by enzyme action. The conversion of folic to folinic acid requires the presence of folic acid reductase. This enzyme produces tetra-hydrofolic acid both directly from folic acid and also by regeneration from dihydrofolic acid that is formed as a by-product in the conversion of deoxyuridylic to thymidylic acid.[175] Folinic acid or other forms of tetrahydrofolic acid are essential in methylation reactions. These are concerned in several steps of purine synthesis and at least one step of pyrimidine synthesis which is itself a rate-limiting step in the synthesis of DNA.[307]

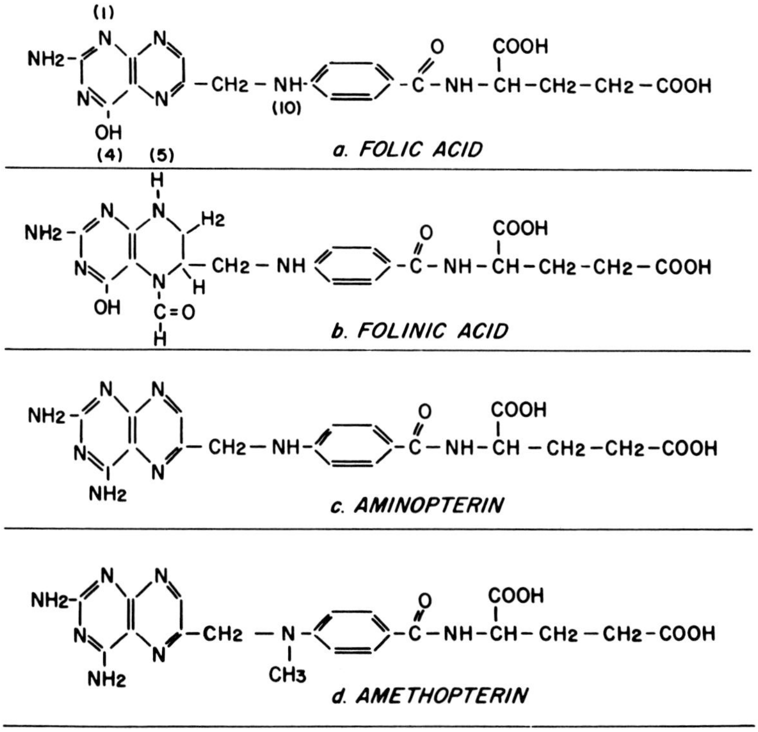

Fig. 17-19. Folic and folinic acids and their antagonists.

In experimental animals, dietary folate deficiency produces a syndrome of marked anemia, granulocytopenia, and severe diarrhea leading to death. A similar train of events is induced by continued administration of folic acid antagonists, of which 4-aminopteroylglutamic acid (aminopterin) is the prototype.[220,471,616] The most convenient objects for testing the activity of folic acid and its antagonists are folate-dependent bacteria like *Streptococcus faecalis* and *Lactobacillus casei*.[307,557] An important difference exists in the effect which antifolic drugs like aminopterin exert on bacteria and on higher organisms. Whereas in the former, their action can be prevented or reversed by folic acid, only partial or no reversal is obtained in mammals,[220,471] birds,[413-415] man,[206] or with human cells in vitro.[261] This discrepancy proved puzzling until the demonstration that although folic acid cannot reverse the effects of aminopterin, folinic acid can do so.[103,147,464,543,587] It is now recognized that aminopterin has multiple effects,[309] competing with folinic acid for enzymes necessary for nucleotide synthesis[255] and also inhibiting the conversion of folic to folinic acid by combining with folic reductase whose affinity for the antagonist is very much greater than that for folic acid.[671,672] Important differences between the folate reductases of different species greatly affect their response to antifolic drugs.[304]

Folic acid antagonists interfere with nucleic acid synthesis and the effect is more marked when this is in preparation for mitotic division.[30] Not all antifolic drugs act like aminopterin, but only those with an amino group in the (4) position— for example, amethopterin (methotrexate). Folic acid antagonists have been classified[101] into five groups according to the systems which they inhibit and the vitamin (folic or folinic acid) which reverses their action. The only antagonists of practical value in leukemia therapy are the 4-amino derivatives of folic acid; these possess sufficient selectivity to produce remissions without prohibitive toxicity.[101]

The first clinical use of folic acid antagonists by Farber grew out of his observation that the administration of folic acid or its conjugates appeared to accelerate the course of acute leukemia. The evidence that folic acid actually has a detrimental effect on acute leukemia is not entirely satisfactory, but there is no doubt that folic acid antagonists can exert striking beneficial effects. Farber's report[209] of remissions in acute leukemia in children was speedily confirmed and extended to adults by many others[43, 110, 153–155, 157, 506, 534, 601, 685] who established clearly the changes in the blood and marrow which follow therapy with antifolic drugs. In responsive patients, the leukocyte count returned to normal and the red cell and platelet counts rose. The bone marrow showed a decrease in the proportion of blast cells and an increase in normal erythroid and granulocytic cells and megakaryocytes. All degrees of remission were observed, that is, clinical only, incomplete, and complete. Complete remission was defined differently by different observers, but the most acceptable definition was a complete clinical response, with the patient looking and feeling well, a normal peripheral blood picture, and no excess of primitive cells in the bone marrow. Disappearance of blast cells from the blood did not necessarily indicate a similar occurrence in the marrow, and it was soon recognized that examination of the bone marrow was essential for the proper specification of the remission status attained. Prolonged administration of folic acid antagonists produces a folic acid deficiency syndrome with megaloblastic changes in the bone marrow, as first shown in animals[497, 625] and also repeatedly described in patients.[42, 323, 601] Large doses of folic acid antagonists immediately inhibit erythropoiesis[140, 514] as well as leukopoiesis.[139] This may progress to severe marrow hypoplasia,[583] which is an indication for interrupting treatment. Modern practice is to administer folic acid antagonists in short, intermittent courses at high dosage, and marrow hypoplasia is relatively uncommon with such regimens. Folinic (but not folic) acid is capable of preventing the toxicity of the folate antagonists; it cannot reverse established damage and is ineffective if administered too late, when marrow depression is already severe.[255, 543, 614, 615]

The mechanism of action of folate antagonists in leukemia is still under investigation. They inhibit incorporation of formate into nucleic acid purines of leukemic leukocytes[578, 579, 686]: this effect is due to inhibition of folate reductase, thus restricting the availability of tetrahydrofolic acid to cells[51, 672] and thereby critically limiting the metabolic transfer of one-carbon fragments in a variety of biochemical reactions. The activity of folate antagonists varies in different cell strains, and the sensitivity of human cell strains in vitro does not always parallel that in the patient.[686] Leukemic cells have been reported to contain more folic acid than normal leukocytes,[613] the highest levels occurring in acute leukemia, but the increased "folate" activity is at least partly due to metabolites such as thymidine as well as folic acid.[188] Displacement of folate by its antagonist has been observed in vivo[615] and this, combined with a lack of renal tubular reabsorption,[141] leads to excessive folate excretion. At the cellular level there is inhibition of mitosis both in vitro and in vivo.[2, 261, 329, 330, 355]

The mechanisms whereby leukemic cells may develop resistance to folic acid antagonists are partially elucidated. In human as in animal leukemias,[105] resistance may be of two types, primary and acquired. Primary resistance exists in patients who, without previous exposure to folate antagonists, fail to respond to their administration. Acquired resistance develops during the course of antifolate therapy, after an initial response. Both phenomena are of great importance since primary resistance limits the proportion of patients who can achieve a remission with antifolate drugs, while acquired resistance limits the duration of remissions when these are maintained by antifolate therapy. It is surprising that an agent which powerfully inhibits nucleoprotein synthesis and, with it, cell development and division, can produce improvement in only less than half the children with acute leukemia and in less than a quarter of adult patients. Neither clinical findings nor cytologic features successfully predict which patients will respond to antifolate therapy, although early studies seemed to point the way to more informative in vitro tests of cellular responsiveness.[113]

Information regarding the mechanisms underlying acquired resistance to folic acid antagonists is more extensive and much of it has been available for many years.[390] Thus, microorganisms which acquire resistance to folic acid antagonists may become dependent upon them or upon preformed purines. While unable to synthesize purines in the normal way, these organisms have acquired the ability to utilize preformed purines, bypassing the metabolic steps which are blocked by antifolate drugs. Similar dependence has been found in strains of mouse leukemia treated with amethopterin and the change is permanent and heritable.[391] The incorporation of formate into nucleic acids, which is inhibited by folic acid antagonists in the viscera and leukemic tumors of sensitive animals, is much less affected by these agents in resistant ones.[355] Transformation to resistance or dependence in mouse leukemias may occur by spontaneous mutation: by destroying the sensitive cells, the therapeutic agent exerts a selective effect, favoring the survival and eventual predominance of the resistant mutants.[389] The biochemical mechanisms of resistance may be multiple. Development of augmented levels of folate reductase within the cell may negate the enzyme-inhibitory effects of antifolate compounds, and resistant strains of mouse leukemia as well as other animal tumor cells have been found to contain greatly increased amounts of folate reductase.[213,272] The drug entering the cell may become bound to the enzyme with an excess of enzyme remaining which is sufficient for continuing folic-folinic acid conversions and, hence, cell multiplication. Such a highly specific mechanism would explain why resistance to folic acid antagonists is usually not associated with resistance to other antimetabolites such as antipurine compounds.[272,319,498,648] A further mechanism of resistance may be related to impaired cellular uptake of folate antagonists; in resistant cells, the rate of methotrexate uptake may be less than the rate of folate reductase synthesis.[271] In tumor-bearing mice the rate of methotrexate uptake by the tumor cells shows a positive correlation with the drug's ability to prolong the life of the host.[242]

Although aminopterin (4-aminopteroylglutamic acid) was the first folate antagonist to be used successfully in leukemia, the 10-methylated derivative, amethopterin (see Fig. 17-19) is now much more commonly used; it is generally known by its alternative name, methotrexate.

PURINE ANTAGONISTS

Although nucleic acids contain as much pyrimidine as purine, clinically useful purine antagonists were developed several years before any pyrimidine antagonists proved efficacious in leukemia. Analogs of adenine are more easily incorporated into

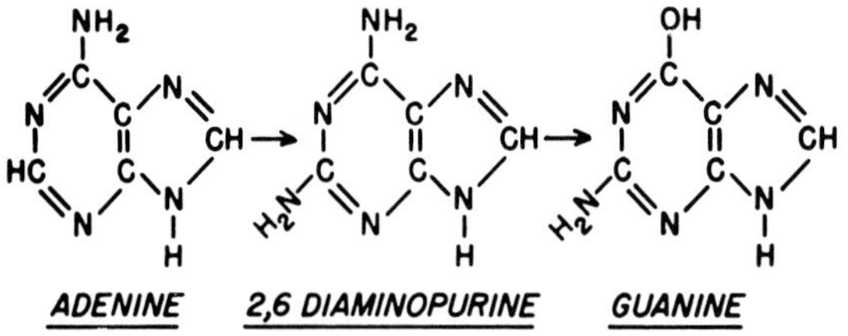

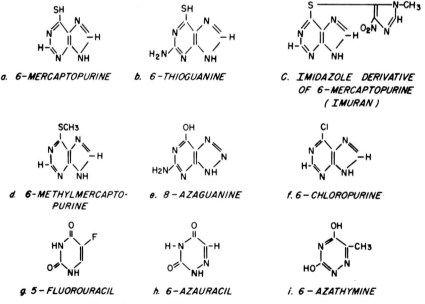

ADENINE   2,6 DIAMINOPURINE   GUANINE

Fig. 17-20.   Possible conversion of adenine to guanine.

nucleotides than are those of guanine, but interconversion occurs in vivo: radioactivity from isotopically labeled adenine can be recovered from the guanine fraction after administration[91, 275] and vice versa if labeled guanine is administered.[564] The transformation takes place via the intermediary 2,6-diaminopurine (Fig. 17-20).[90] This compound is easily incorporated into nucleic acid and has some antileukemic effect,[104, 576] probably by inhibiting the incorporation of guanine into nucleotides and its conversion to adenine.[564]

Substitution of a mercapto group in the (6) position of the purine ring was found to produce substances inhibitory to microbial growth whose action was reversed by the administration of purines.[184] Both 6-mercaptopurine (6-MP) and 6-thioguanine (Fig. 17-21) were synthesized and tested in animals: 6-MP was considered less toxic[496] and was effective against animal tumors,[130, 131] rendering the majority of murine tumor cells no longer transplantable. Clinical tests of 6-MP in leukemias and allied diseases soon confirmed its potency and relative lack of toxic effects.[111]

Mercaptopurine (6-mercaptopurine, 6-MP, Purinethol). The major importance of this drug (Fig. 17-22) and the interest it aroused is reflected in the large

a. 6-MERCAPTOPURINE   *b. 6-THIOGUANINE*   *C. IMIDAZOLE DERIVATIVE OF 6-MERCAPTOPURINE (IMURAN)*

d. 6-METHYLMERCAPTO-PURINE   *e. 8-AZAGUANINE*   *f. 6-CHLOROPURINE*

g. 5-FLUOROURACIL   *h. 6-AZAURACIL*   *i. 6-AZATHYMINE*

Fig. 17-21.   Purine and pyrimidine antagonists.

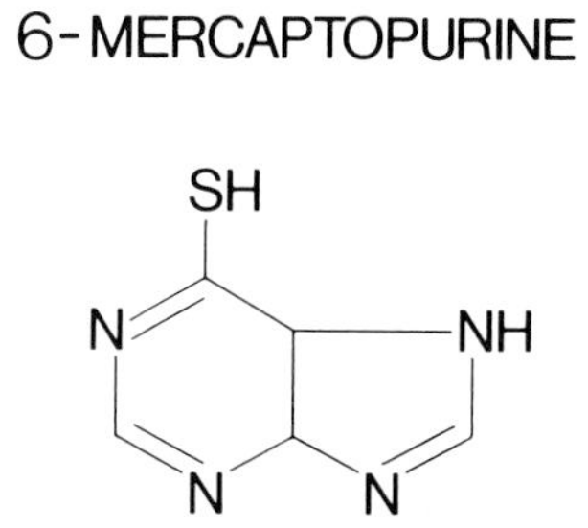

6-MERCAPTOPURINE

SH

N———NH

N   N

Fig. 17-22. Structural formula of mercaptopurine (6-mercaptopurine, 6-MP, Purinethol).

body of literature relating to its use, which accumulated in a very brief period after its introduction.[446] It inhibits mitosis in low concentrations.[57] When 6-MP labeled with radioactive sulfur is administered, much of the radioactivity becomes incorporated into nucleic acid, particularly DNA[276]: however, the deoxyribonucleotide of 6-MP has not been isolated and consequently there is no direct evidence that 6-MP itself is incorporated into DNA.[175] The biochemical actions of 6-MP are complex and include competition with inosinic acid, preventing its conversion to adenylsuccinic acid on the pathway to adenylic acid (see Fig. 17-16).[273] To exert this effect, 6-MP must first be converted to its ribonucleotide by the action of ribonucleotide pyrophosphorylase. One mechanism whereby cells become resistant to 6-MP is a failure to metabolize the drug to its active form: resistant cells contain abnormally small amounts of ribonucleotide pyrophosphorylase.[79,80] Other biochemical effects of 6-MP include inhibition of the conversion of inosinic acid to xanthylic acid, the immediate precursor of guanylic acid, and inhibition of nicotinamide-adenine dinucleotide synthesis. The latter action, by a feedback mechanism, may inhibit the formation of the purine precursor phosphoribosylamine.[175] The actions of 6-MP which inhibit DNA synthesis are specific for the S phase of the cell cycle, but the drug also has some cycle-phase independent activity, as it inhibits RNA.

Although interference with nucleic acid synthesis is an important mechanism by which antipurine compounds produce their cytotoxic effects, other actions are probably also important.[573] Nucleotides form part of a number of important coenzymes, and purine analogs may enter these. Experiments on the mode of reversal of the action of 6-MP, in which purines, nucleosides, nucleotides, and other substances were used, disclosed a complicated relationship, and a nonnucleic acid compound, coenzyme A, was found to be most effective in relieving the mitotic suppression caused by 6-MP.[57] Several antipurines, including 6-MP, are antagonists of vitamin B_{12} despite their lack of structural analogy, and part of their cytotoxic effect may be due to this antagonism,[198] which may also explain the occasional production by 6-MP of megaloblastic changes in the bone marrow. Synergy has been observed between 6-MP and some folic acid antagonists,[241,393] as well as with the serine analog azaserine.[241] Resistance to 6-MP develops readily in both human and animal leukemias, and, when induced, extends to other antipurine compounds. For this reason, little clinical use was made of other purine antimetabolites once 6-MP became an established drug, since the other analogs seemed to offer nothing to patients whose leukemia had already become resistant to 6-MP. Resistance to purine antagonists carries no cross-resistance to folic acid antagonists and some resistant mouse leukemias have actually developed increased sensitivity to metho-trexate.[393] The suggestion in 1955[303] that the combination of several classes of antileukemic agents might produce potentiation of their action was of much theoretical interest and, within a short time, clinical study[221] suggested that this ap-proach was of practical value. Combination chemotherapy with antimetabolites and other drugs has now assumed such importance in the management of the acute leukemias that single-drug therapy of the type used some years ago has become obsolete (see Chapter 18).

Mercaptopurine is usually administered by the oral route although an intravenous preparation (sodium 6-MP) can be used on the rare occasions when it is impossible for the patient to swallow tablets. The drug is well absorbed from the gastrointestinal tract and the half-life of the pure compound in the circulation is about 90 minutes.[496] The principal route of excretion is in the urine, both as 6-MP and as 6-thiouric acid; very large doses of 6-MP can lead to the formation of 6-thiouric acid calculi. The principal toxic effect of 6-MP is bone marrow depression, with its attendant risks of hemorrhage and infection. Nausea, vomiting, diarrhea, and mucous membrane ulceration are rare when 6-MP is administered in conven-tional doses, but cholestatic jaundice is occasionally encountered.

Thioguanine (6-thioguanine, 6-TG, Lanvis).   As mentioned above, 6-TG (Fig. 17-23) underwent initial testing at the same time as 6-MP.[458] It appeared to possess no special advantages over 6-MP and the latter drug received more extensive clinical trial, was marketed, and for over 15 years was the principal purine antagonist in clinical use. Recently, 6-TG has become widely used and seems likely to replace 6-MP in routine practice; this change is due to two factors.

First, one of the hazards encountered in the leukemias, particularly during the early stages of treatment of patients with acute leukemia, is excessive uric acid production with hyperuricemia, uricosuria, urate nephropathy, and nephrolithi-asis.[374] This sometimes fatal complication can be averted by the administration of the purine isomer, 4-hydroxypyrazolo(3,4-*d*)pyrimidine (allopurinol, Zyloprim, Zyloric), which inhibits in vivo the enzyme xanthine oxidase, essential for uric acid production.[531] The effectiveness of allopurinol prophylaxis against hyperuricemia in leukemia[164,369] has been widely confirmed and its use has become generally accepted. Since 6-MP is partly metabolized by xanthine oxidase, concurrent administration of allopurinol with 6-MP tends to potentiate the effects of the 6-MP by retarding its elimination; such potentiation can lead to excessive bone marrow depression.

THIOGUANINE

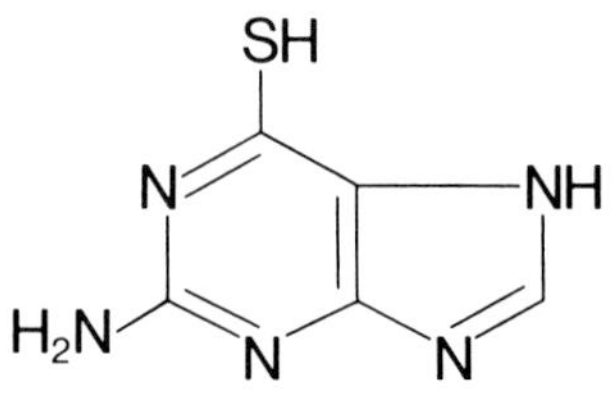

Fig. 17-23. Structural formula of thioguanine (6-thioguanine, 6-TG, 6-mercaptogua-nine, Lanvis).

Reducing the dose of 6-MP is not an entirely satisfactory answer since the degree of potentiation which the allopurinol produces is not predictable from one patient to another: thus, dose modification was arbitrary and therapy less precise than desirable. Since 6-TG does not depend upon xanthine oxidase for its metabolism, its therapeutic effects are unaltered by the concurrent administration of allopurinol or by the discontinuation of the latter during the course of thioguanine treatment. Thus, the practice of using prophylactic allopurinol has prompted more widespread use of 6-TG.

Second, a study of the treatment of acute granulocytic leukemia with the pyrimidine antagonist cytosine arabinoside—either alone or in combination with 6-MP or 6-TG—showed, not only that the combinations were superior to cytosine arabinoside alone, but also suggested that the combination incorporating 6-TG might be more effective than that using 6-MP.[119] This apparently superior synergy with cytosine arabinoside seemed a sound reason for preferring thioguanine to 6-MP, and the combination of 6-TG with the pyrimidine antagonist is now used very widely (see Chapter 18).

Thioguanine is administered by mouth, and its clinical effects resemble those of 6-MP; bone marrow depression and, rarely, cholestatic jaundice are the only major toxic effects seen with conventional doses of 6-TG. At the cellular biochemical level, 6-TG differs from 6-MP in at least one major respect. It is incorporated into both DNA and RNA and it has been postulated that 6-TG may act by producing an abnormal DNA rather than by inhibiting DNA synthesis. In resistant cells, less 6-TG may become incorporated into DNA.[401]

Other purine antagonists. Mercaptopurine has been the purine antagonist most widely used in the past and thioguanine seems likely to become the most widely used in the future. Very large numbers of other purine antagonists have been tested in animals and some of them in human leukemia. Among these are 6-methylmercaptopurine,[623] 8-azaguanine,[138] 6-chloropurine,[189,190] thioguanosine,[367] and 6-methylmercaptopurine riboside.[222] While some of these compounds remain of considerable experimental interest, none has found a permanent place in clinical practice.

Immunodepressant effects. Mercaptopurine and other purine antagonists possess striking antiimmune effects,[553,555] and have been termed *immunosuppressant* drugs, although *immunodepressant* is a more accurate description of their effects. The immunodepressant properties of purine antagonists are in no sense specific—they are also possessed by ionizing radiations, alkylating agents, and antitumor antibiotics—and simply reflect the general toxicity of these agents toward actively dividing cells. The immunologic reaction is a proliferative response of one of the white cell groups, and is vulnerable to the same agents as leukemia. Most immunologic reactions are self-limited, but autoimmune reactions are usually self-perpetuating. Mercaptopurine depresses autoimmune reactions[161] and also transplantation reactions to homografts.[554] The apparent correlation between the antileukemic and antiimmune effects of drugs[160] implies only that the cytokinetics of leukemias and of immune reactions may be similar, but the development of abnormal drug-resistant immunoblasts during experimental immunodepression in ani-

AZATHIOPRINE

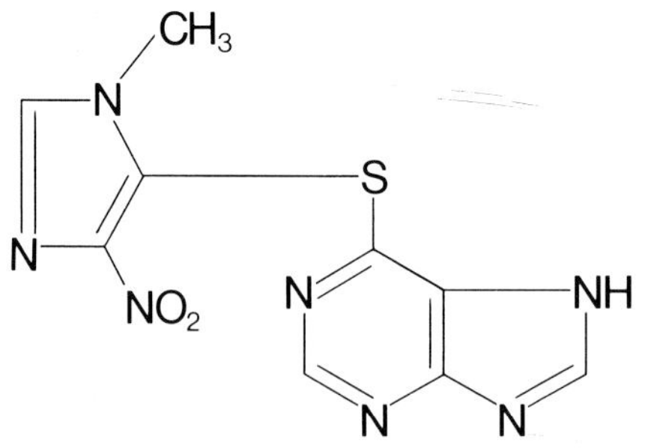

Fig. 17-24.   Structural formula of azathioprine (Imuran).

mals[8,9] bears an interesting analogy to the drug resistance commonly seen in the leukemias.

One of the principal immunodepressant drugs in current use is azathioprine (Imuran), an analog of mercaptopurine (Fig. 17-24). This compound is metabolized to 6-mercaptopurine in vivo[182] and has immunodepressant and antileukemic effects resembling those of mercaptopurine. As would be expected, azathioprine, like mercaptopurine, is potentiated by the concurrent administration of allopurinol. The antileukemic activity of azathioprine is not greater than that of 6-MP[183,606] and the drug appears to possess no special advantages; in particular, there is no evidence that leukemias which have become resistant to thioguanine or mercaptopurine will respond to azathioprine.

PYRIMIDINE ANTAGONISTS

Numerous pyrimidine analogs have been developed and tested against animal and human leukemias. These include 5-fluorouracil,[238] 5-fluorodeoxycytidine,[108] 6-azauracil,[569] 6-azauridine,[204] and 6-azathymine.[191] Although 5-fluorouracil has useful activity against some gastrointestinal carcinomas, none of these drugs proved valuable in human leukemias; severe toxicity was common but remissions were not achieved. The first pyrimidine antimetabolite shown to be useful in human leukemia was *cytosine arabinoside* (ara-C, arabinosylcytosine, cytarabine), a synthetic nucleoside which differs from the normal nucleosides cytidine and deoxycytidine in that the sugar moiety is arabinose rather than ribose or deoxyribose (Fig. 17-25). Whereas 6-azauridine acts by blocking the transformation of orotidylic to uridylic acid,[205] cytarabine appears to act further along the pyrimidine metabolic pathway, by interfering with the reduction of ribonucleotides to their deoxy form.[126] As a powerful inhibitor of DNA synthesis, cytarabine has antiviral,[643] antibacterial,[505] antiimmune,[342] and antileukemic[200] effects and also induces chromosomal abnormalities in human leukocytes.[357] Its depressant effects upon DNA viruses are sufficiently great for cytarabine to have a place in the treatment of severe viral infections, including herpes simplex,[643] zostervaricella,[424] and smallpox.[315]

Cytosine arabinoside is effective against both acute lymphocytic and acute granulocytic leukemia.[187,294,317] The drug is administered by intravenous, subcutaneous, or intramuscular injection: since its plasma half-life is only a few minutes after rapid intravenous injection, it is sometimes administered as a con-

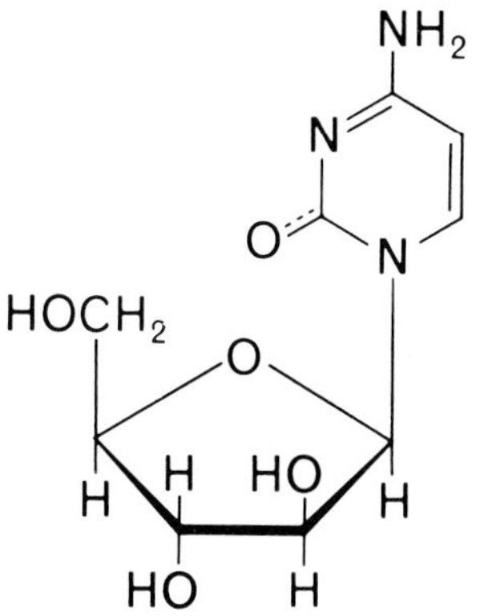

Fig. 17-25. Structural formula of cytosine arabinoside (arabinosylcytosine, ara-C, cytarabine, Cytosar).

tinuous intravenous infusion for periods up to 5 days or more, which usually augments both its therapeutic and toxic effects. The principal adverse effects of cytarabine are depression of the bone marrow, which may be severe and accompanied by gross megaloblastic changes, nausea and vomiting, and ulceration of mucous membranes when dosage is high or administration prolonged. Used as a single therapeutic agent, cytarabine produces a relatively low response rate, and secondary resistance of the leukemic cells is common; therefore, the drug is almost always used in combination with another antileukemic agent, for example, daunorubicin or thioguanine (see Chapter 18).

AMINO ACID ANALOGS

It is theoretically possible to influence cell division, not only by changes in the nucleic acid fraction of nucleoproteins, but also by altering the protein moiety of these substances or the proteins of the cytoplasm. Analogs of natural amino acids might cause such a change in nucleoprotein and might also alter the composition and metabolism of the cytoplasm, inhibiting cellular reproduction. Early results of research along these lines have not been promising. The best-known amino acid analog, azaserine, was discovered accidentally during screening of antibiotics for antitumor activity. A crude filtrate from a *Streptomyces* was found to have such activity and when purified the active principle was identified as a substituted L-serine (Fig. 17-26). This was effective against the Crocker mouse sarcoma,[603] and was tested extensively in human leukemia.[102] Unfortunately, azaserine has little activity when administered alone in man, and though in animals it appears to have a synergistic effect when given with 6-MP, no similar effect has been consistently obtained in human leukemia.[297] The same is true of another amino acid antagonist, 6-diazo-5-oxo-L-norleucine (DON, Fig. 17-26).[107, 132, 425, 609] Although no amino acid analog has so far been found of value in human leukemia, depriving leukemic cells of asparagine by use of the enzyme L-asparaginase (see below) is very effective in many cases of acute lymphocytic leukemia. Thus, it is possible to influence leukemic cells by altering their amino acid metabolism, and clinically useful amino acid antagonists may yet be developed.

The special importance of cysteine and cystine in the metabolism of leukocytes is referred to in Chapter 6. The rapid and preferential incorporation of L-cystine into

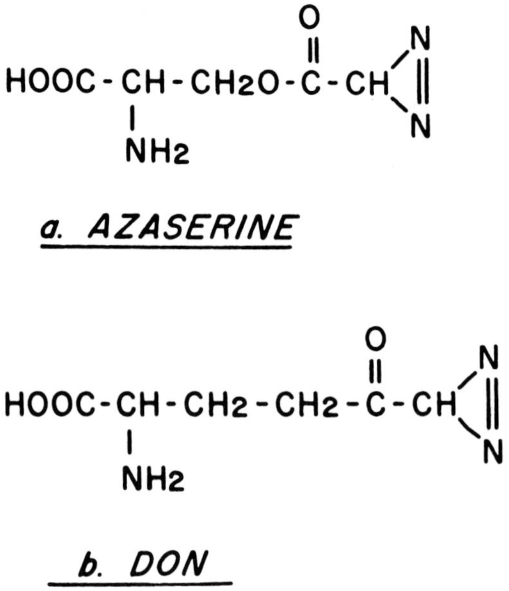

$$HOOC-\underset{\underset{NH_2}{|}}{CH}-CH_2O-\overset{\overset{O}{\|}}{C}-CH\diagdown\overset{N}{\underset{N}{\|}}$$

a. AZASERINE

$$HOOC-\underset{\underset{NH_2}{|}}{CH}-CH_2-CH_2-\overset{\overset{O}{\|}}{C}-CH\diagdown\overset{N}{\underset{N}{\|}}$$

b. DON

Fig. 17-26. Amino acid antagonists.

leukemic leukocytes both in vitro and in vivo[664,666,667] suggested the possible value of analogs which might prevent this incorporation and possibly inhibit leukemic cell proliferation. Of the analogs tested, only selenium cystine and phenyl selenium cystine prevented the incorporation of radioactive L-cystine in vitro.[669] When selenium cystine was given to patients with acute or chronic granulocytic leukemia, a prompt and pronounced decline in the leukocyte count and spleen size was observed, but toxic effects were very severe and the compound could not be tolerated except for brief periods.[668] This approach to leukemia therapy may well produce important results with continued research. It is of interest that certain sulfhydryl compounds protect the bone marrow of animals against the effects of ionizing radiation. This may be of considerable importance if such protection can be shown to benefit normal marrow elements more than neoplastic cells.

The observation that chronic administration of a racemic mixture of D,L-dopa to patients with Parkinsonism can produce granulocytopenia with bone marrow changes resembling those seen in phenylalanine deficiency[144] suggested that D-dopa might be an antagonist to phenylalanine, since granulocytopenia was not observed in patients treated with pure L-dopa.[114] However, the administration of pure D-dopa in doses of 8 gm daily to patients with chronic granulocytic leukemia for periods of up to 1 month produced no fall in leukocyte counts[595] and this agent now seems unlikely to be of value in leukemia therapy.

Vegetable Alkaloids

Several species of plants produce alkaloids which are potent inhibitors of the later stages of mitosis. Possibly the biologic function of these substances is to avert the partition of chromosomes seen in normal mitoses, and thus enable certain plant cells to achieve a tetraploid or octoploid chromosomal constitution, advantageous

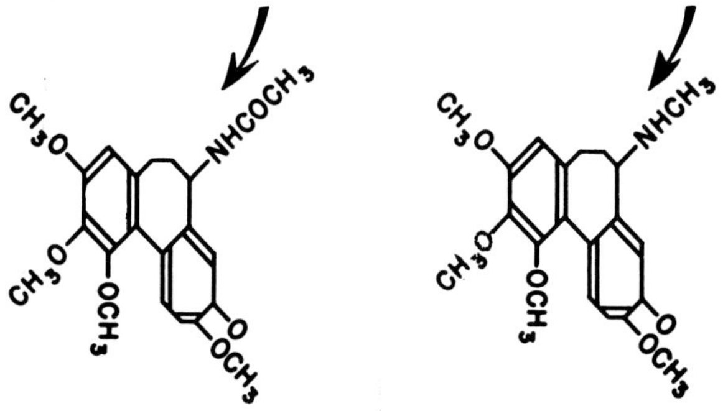

Fig. 17-27.   Colchicine—deacetylmethylcolchicine.

for some plant activities. This power to interfere with mitosis makes some plant alkaloids valuable in the treatment of leukemia.

THE COLCHICINE GROUP

Colchicine (Fig. 17-27), an alkaloid extracted from *Colchicum autumnale*, the autumn crocus, has been known for many years as a mitotic poison of exceptional power and interest. It arrests mitosis in metaphase, an effect produced by interference with the formation of the mitotic spindle. Under certain conditions the nucleus may revert to the interphase state after metaphase arrest, the cell therefore becoming tetraploid,[95,96] a phenomenon which has been widely exploited in agriculture and horticulture. Because of its antimitotic property, the trial of colchicine as a chemotherapeutic agent in leukemia and other neoplasms was of obvious interest. Equivocal results were, however, obtained,[93,381] probably because the toxic effects of colchicine, particularly vomiting and diarrhea, severely limit the doses which can be tolerated. This line of research was therefore not pursued.

With the isolation of pure alkaloids from the mixture contained in *C. autumnale*,[537] it was possible to study congeners of colchicine. Deacetylmethylcolchicine (demecolcine, Colcemid) proved of special interest. Experiments in vitro[438,539] and on animals[452] showed an antimitotic activity similar to that of colchicine, but accompanied by thirty to forty times less gastrointestinal toxicity. In rabbits and cats, demecolcine appeared to depress granulocytic cells strikingly while leaving other hematopoietic cells relatively unaffected.[452] Clinical trials gave promising results in chronic granulocytic leukemia, with gradual return of the blood and marrow toward normal, usually without severe side effects,[334,400,402] although occasional toxic reactions have been reported.[567] Some beneficial effects also occurred in patients with chronic granulocytic leukemia which had undergone acute transformation.[402,451,452] Although we have not been able to achieve remissions with demecolcine in chronic granulocytic leukemia after acute transformation, the drug will often reduce the leukocyte count and relieve severe constitutional symptoms of malaise, fever, and night sweats. As the leukocyte count sometimes falls precipitously there is a risk of hyperuricemia and concurrent administration of allopurinol is advisable.

Demecolcine is of little value in neoplasms other than chronic granulocytic leukemia, and the good quality and high degree of consistency of results when busulfan is used have discouraged the widespread use of demecolcine. However, with the realization that the benefits of busulfan therapy in chronic granulocytic leukemia are purely temporary and that busulfan is not without long-term adverse effects, it is apparent that demecolcine merits further evaluation, perhaps as one component of a cyclical drug regimen (see Chapter 18).

THE VINCA ALKALOIDS

These important compounds are extracted from the Madagascar periwinkle, a flowering plant which until recently was classified as *Vinca rosea* (Linn.). In fact, the Madagascar periwinkle does not belong to the genus *Vinca* at all and is correctly classified as *Catharanthus roseus* (G.Don.) although the former misclassification may well endure in the medical, if not the botanical, literature! Extensive data on the antitumor effects of these alkaloids in a wide variety of neoplasms have been summarized elsewhere.[231,335,337,566]

VINBLASTINE

This substance and its congener, vincristine, are closely related (Fig. 17-28). Vinblastine (also Velbe or Velban; vincaleukoblastine is an obsolete name) was discovered in the course of pharmacologic research on periwinkle extract seeking a postulated hypoglycemic principle. Vinblastine did not lower the blood sugar of experimental animals but had a potent effect on their bone marrow[152] and also on some animal tumors.[337] The drug had a pronounced colchicinelike effect, arresting cells in the metaphase of mitosis.[118,151] Vinblastine was tried in human neoplasia and produced occasional regressions in solid tumors, more frequent benefit in lympho- and reticulum-cell sarcoma, and a high incidence of substantial regressions in Hodgkin's disease. A few remissions occurred in acute leukemia but these were unpredictable while myelotoxicity was common.[298] Hodgkin's disease is usually very responsive to vinblastine, even after resistance has developed to alkylating agents, and the drug probably has its greatest usefulness in this condition,[306,661,662,681] although combination chemotherapy has become more important in Hodgkin's disease than the use of vinblastine alone.[167] Vinblastine no longer has any place in the chemotherapy of leukemia.

VINCRISTINE

Although demecolcine, vinblastine, and vincristine possess similar visible effects at the cellular level, namely, inhibition of the mitotic spindle and the production of metaphase arrest, their clinical spectra are very different. Vincristine is virtually inactive in chronic granulocytic leukemia in the chronic phase and has less activity in Hodgkin's disease than vinblastine, but has potent activity in acute leukemia. Apart from producing mitotic arrest,[335,428] apparently by spindle inhibition,[426] vincristine inhibits soluble RNA production in at least some cell-lines[136] and is clearly most active against dividing cells.[92,538] Vincristine has little depressant effect on normal hematopoietic cells and its major dose-limiting toxicity is nervous system damage, particularly peripheral neuritis.[536] This property may be attributable to the fact that neuronal tissue contains large amounts of microtubular structures similar in composition to mitotic spindles.[558] Despite frequent toxic

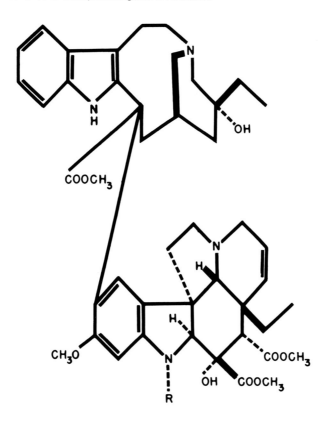

$$R= \begin{array}{ll} CH_3 & VINBLASTINE \\ CHO & VINCRISTINE \end{array}$$

Fig. 17-28.   Structural formulae of vinblastine (Velbe) and vincristine (Oncovin).

effects on the peripheral nervous system and occasional CNS toxicity, vincristine does not enter the CSF in sufficient concentration to influence the course of CNS leukemia.[349] Vincristine causes alopecia in most patients, and the severity of hair loss is related to the length of time for which the drug is administered, more than four injections at weekly intervals usually causing significant loss. Fine silky hair, which is sometimes curly, will regrow even while vincristine therapy is continued.

Vincristine is a most valuable drug in acute lymphocytic leukemia, since it induces remission rapidly, without significant marrow depression, and in a high proportion of patients even when administered alone.[269,293,349] It will induce repeated remissions in the same patient if restricted to this function[316,335] and, given intermittently, it will significantly prolong the duration of remissions which are being maintained with antimetabolites.[44,310] Because it lacks myelotoxicity, vincristine can safely be combined with marrow-depressant drugs such as mercaptopurine, methotrexate, cytarabine, and cyclophosphamide.

Although it is highly effective in acute lymphocytic leukemia, vincristine has little activity in acute granulocytic leukemia: the majority of cases are completely unresponsive,[136,199,349] and it may be speculated that this lack of effect is linked to the lack of myelotoxicity which makes vincristine so valuable in acute lymphocytic leukemia. One form of combination chemotherapy, which is effective in many cases of acute granulocytic leukemia, incorporates vincristine,[679] but also contains prednisolone, cyclophosphamide, and cytarabine; in the presence of three other antileukemic drugs it is impossible to assess how much is contributed by the vincristine.

Antitumor Antibiotics

Antibiotics are substances elaborated by microorganisms which inhibit the multiplication of competitor organisms, thereby conferring a survival advantage upon the antibiotic-producing organism. All antibiotics are cellular poisons, but those which are useful clinically for the treatment of infection are distinguished by their potent effects against bacterial cells and negligible effects on mammalian cells. An antibiotic may, for example, affect a process which does not occur at all in mammals—for example, cell wall formation—or it may affect a process common to mammals and bacteria such as DNA synthesis, but its effects may be of little importance in the higher species because of differences in metabolic pathways as compared to bacteria. Certain antibiotics, however, affect mammalian cells profoundly, exerting cytostatic or cytocidal effects. Such compounds are unsuitable for the treatment of infections, no matter how great their antibacterial activity, but they are sometimes useful antitumor agents. Many of the antitumor antibiotics in clinical use were originally screened in animals as antibacterial substances and later rescreened as possible antitumor agents when they were found to destroy the animals' bone marrow or other tissues.

DAUNORUBICIN

Daunorubicin (daunomycin, rubidomycin, Cerubidin) is an antibiotic derived from *Streptomyces ceruleorubidus* or *S. peucetius* and consists of a red aglycone, daunomycinone, in glycoside linkage with an amino sugar, daunosamine (Fig. 17-29). The antibiotic has profound effects upon both leukemic and normal marrow cells and is believed to inhibit DNA synthesis by complexing with preformed DNA.[170,533] Daunorubicin appears unique among antileukemic drugs in being equally effective against both acute lymphocytic and acute granulocytic leukemia.[46,622] About 40 percent of patients having either of the principal varieties of acute leukemia can be expected to respond to daunorubicin[293] and higher response rates have been achieved when the drug was combined with prednisone, or prednisone plus vincristine.[44,46,313,433] Thus, daunorubicin has a wide spectrum of usefulness in the treatment of the acute leukemias.

Unfortunately, daunorubicin has serious drawbacks. It must be administered by intravenous injection and, unless well-diluted, can cause thrombophlebitis. Extravasation of the injection causes painful tissue necrosis which in at least one patient necessitated amputation of a limb. Vomiting is often severe after daunorubicin, and alopecia and mucous membrane ulceration occur frequently. The most consistent toxic manifestation of daunorubicin is gross bone marrow depression with marked hypoplasia and peripheral blood pancytopenia and its attendant hazards of hemorrhage and infection. Such serious risks might not be acceptable in

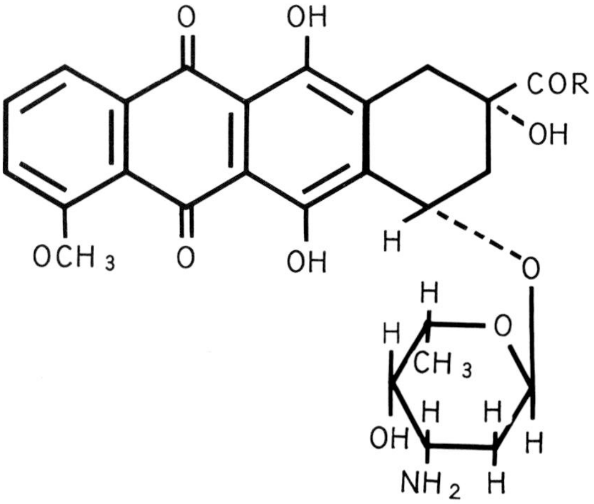

R = CH₃   DAUNORUBICIN

R = CH₂OH   DOXORUBICIN

Fig. 17-29. Structural formulae of daunorubicin (daunomycin, rubidomycin, Ceru-bidin) and doxorubicin (Adriamycin).

the treatment of a new case of acute lymphocytic leukemia, where other therapies will almost certainly induce remission with less hazard, but in acute granulocytic leukemia, where gentler therapy has much less to offer, daunorubicin is frequently the agent of choice, either alone or in combination with other drugs. Indeed, some feel that severe marrow hypoplasia is an unavoidable prelude to the induction of re-mission in acute granulocytic leukemia.[49] Daunorubicin also possesses serious myocardial toxicity, causing arrhythmias, electrocardiographic abnormalities, and, occasionally, sudden death.[49] Irreversible cardiac failure is an uncommon but some-times fatal complication of daunorubicin therapy[46]; it occurs principally in patients who have received a total dose exceeding 20 mg per kilogram of body weight over periods of only a few weeks. We have not seen this complication in patients who have received considerably larger total doses spread over periods of many months.

DOXORUBICIN

Doxorubicin (Adriamycin) is closely related to daunorubicin (Fig. 17-29), but appeared superior to that drug in experimental mouse leukemias.[535] In man, it is effective in acute lymphocytic leukemia,[68,680] and also in a number of lymphomas and solid tumors,[65,68] but early experience suggests that doxorubicin may be inferior to daunorubicin in acute granulocytic leukemia.[49,65] There is no good evidence that leukemias which have become resistant to daunorubicin will respond to doxorubicin at equivalent dosage. The cardiotoxic effects of doxorubicin occur at dosage levels similar to those reported for daunorubicin, but in terms of hematologic effects, doxorubicin has a milligram potency approximately twice that of daunorubicin; thus, a dosage which imperils cardiac function is less likely to be attained in a given time interval when doxorubicin is administered. Against this advantage must be set

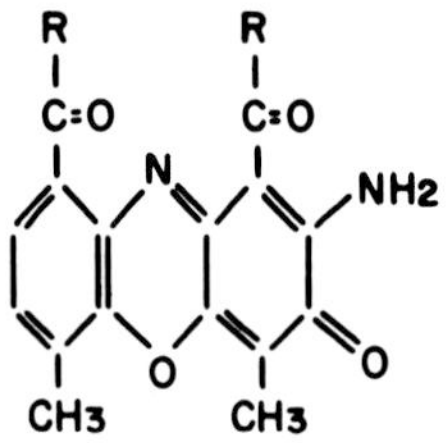

(a) ACTINOCYN (CHROMOPHORIC PORTION OF MOLECULE)

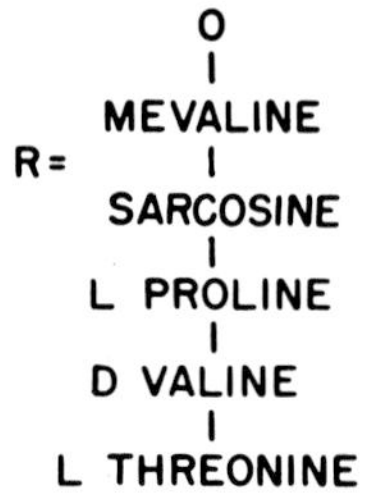

R =

O
|
MEVALINE
|
SARCOSINE
|
L PROLINE
|
D VALINE
|
L THREONINE

(b.) PEPTIDE PORTION

Fig. 17-30.   Actinomycin D.

the drawbacks of alopecia and stomatitis, both of which are commoner and more severe with doxorubicin than with daunorubicin. An extensive literature on doxorubicin has recently been reviewed.[120]

THE ACTINOMYCINS

The actinomycins are a group of antibiotics originally obtained from *Streptomyces* by Waksman.[652] They are closely related polypeptides linked to a chromophoric quinenoid group (Fig. 17-30). The most widely used member of the group is *actinomycin D* (dactinomycin, Cosmegen). This drug has produced some remissions in Hodgkin's disease and lymphosarcoma but none in acute leukemia. Actinomycin D is of limited value in malignant lymphomas but is effective against some solid neoplasms, particularly Wilms' tumor.[171,501,621] It appears to have a potentiating effect on ionizing radiations, and combined therapy with radiation and actinomycin D is valuable in certain childhood tumors.[208] Although the administration of actinomycin D to children with acute lymphocytic leukemia in remission produces some prolongation of remission,[399] the drug has not been widely used. Administration of actinomycin D in acute lymphocytic leukemia when the disease is in relapse is apt to produce catastrophic pancytopenia.

Mitomycin C, an antibiotic isolated from *S. caespitesus*, has a wide spectrum of activity against experimental tumors.[608,610] Some promising results were obtained in human disease,[219] but the drug has considerable marrow toxicity[341] which limits its use. Chronic granulocytic and chronic lymphocytic leukemia respond to mitomycin C but acute leukemia does not.[219] Further work on the mitomycins may produce less toxic and more effective agents[651]; a derivative, methyl-mitomycin C, is currently undergoing clinical trials.

ACTH and the Corticosteroids

The use of ACTH, cortisone, and the synthetic adrenocortical steroid hormones in the treatment of leukemia is an indirect outcome of much earlier work on the effect of pituitary adrenocorticotropic hormone (ACTH) on lymphoid tissue. Injections of ACTH into normal mice produced involution in the axillary, inguinal, and mesenteric lymph nodes and thymus but not in the spleen,[174] and, similarly, cortisone caused atrophy of rat lymph nodes and thymus.[320,670] In 1942, Heilman and Kendall discovered that cortisone—then termed Compound E—inhibited the growth of a transplanted lymphosarcoma and produced rapid regression of established tumors in mice.[288] Cortisone and ACTH were found by Murphy and Sturm[454] to prevent the growth of a transplanted mouse leukemia and to induce regression of enlarged lymphoid organs in mice affected with a spontaneous lymphocytic leukemia.[392] Both Heilman and Kendall[288] and Murphy and Sturm[454] warned against a premature application of their experimental results to therapeutic purposes, and it was partly to avoid raising unjustified hopes that the former authors delayed the publication of their 1942 studies until 1944.

Human leukemias were first treated with ACTH and cortisone 5 years later.[159,488–492,510] Since the hormones were known to affect chiefly lymphoid tissue, they were first employed in cases of chronic lymphocytic leukemia and lymphosarcoma. Rapid involution of the enlarged organs occurred but there were few striking hematologic remissions. No success was achieved in acute monocytic or myelomonocytic leukemia or in chronic granulocytic leukemia, but the best remissions, rather surprisingly, ensued in acute lymphocytic and acute granulocytic leukemia. At that time no difference in the response was noted between these two leukemias, although later studies have demonstrated that the frequency of response to steroid therapy in acute lymphocytic leukemia is about three times that seen in acute granulocytic leukemia.[293] Although remissions proved to be temporary and resistance arose rapidly,[498] the advent of the hormones had opened a distinct new phase in the chemotherapy of leukemia. Whereas previously most therapeutic agents had been merely toxic substances which damaged particularly cells in mitosis, ACTH and cortisone were normally produced in the body, or closely related to normally occurring metabolic products, and, furthermore, were not myelotoxic—in fact, they were possibly myelostimulatory. Although many facts are known about the physiologic effects of these substances, the precise mode of their action in leukemia has not been elucidated. The effectiveness of corticosteroids in chronic lymphocytic leukemia strongly suggests that they suppress nondividing cells, thus differing from the synthetic antimetabolite drugs.

Corticosteroid drugs cause a neutrophil leukocytosis in normal individuals. An elevation of the lymphocyte count is seen frequently after their first administration to patients with chronic lymphocytic leukemia, while in acute granulocytic leukemia there may be a rise in the cells of the granulocyte series. The suggestion has been made that ACTH and the corticosteroids actually accelerate the course of acute granulocytic leukemia.[281,523] This now seems to be untrue, since corticosteroids in massive doses can cause remissions in acute granulocytic leukemia with improved survival,[247] and, in a large-scale cooperative trial, steroid alone was found to be more effective than mercaptopurine alone.[436] The apparent worsening of the disease in some patients after the beginning of steroid therapy is probably due to misinterpretation of the increased leukocytosis, which is not necessarily a genuine index of deterioration. When the leukemia is not responsive to steroids, it may well worsen, not because of steroid therapy but as part of its natural progression with time. The condition of some patients worsens because of the complications of steroid therapy, particularly infection, which are especially likely when the leukemia does not respond favorably to the steroid treatment.

Remissions following cortisone or ACTH administration may be complete or incomplete, the former comprising restoration of the blood and marrow to normal appearances. Quantitative studies of the marrow during treatment have shown that the first change is a striking diminution of mitoses in the blast cells.[146,232,427] No definite alteration in cellular distribution occurs in the first week, after which there is an increase in the numbers of normal erythroid and myeloid precursors and in their mitotic rate, which rises to a peak. Findings such as these, together with the reticulocytosis and rise in platelets as remission occurs,[522] led to the suggestion that steroid hormones, while inhibiting leukemic, and especially lymphocytic leukemic cells, may stimulate normal marrow cells to proliferate.[232,551] This view is difficult to test experimentally, but the known facts about the mode of action of the hormones do not suggest that they stimulate cellular proliferation: thus, normal human marrow shows no change in cellularity, morphology, or cell distribution during steroid therapy,[523] and steroids have not been demonstrated to improve the rate of recovery from aplastic anemia. Prolonged administration of ACTH to rats actually leads to diminished cellularity and mitotic activity in the marrow, spleen, and thymus.[518] Stress, with attendant adrenocortical hyperfunction, produces a pronounced fall in mitotic activity,[100] and while certain transplanted animal neoplasms may show unusually rapid proliferation under cortisone treatment, this has been attributed to inhibition of the host's immunologic defenses rather than to tumor growth stimulation.[251] In vitro, cortisone has a direct destructive effect on lymphocytes,[287] but not on normal human marrow or the granulocytes of chronic granulocytic leukemia.[373] It appears likely that the reticulocytosis and rapid recovery of marrow function and peripheral blood values seen when remission in acute leukemia is induced by the use of steroid hormones alone is caused, not by a hypothetical marrow-stimulatory effect of the hormones but to their lack of myelotoxicity as compared to most other antileukemic drugs. Thus, patients whose leukemia is responsive to steroids may achieve remission without any preliminary aggravation of their initial pancytopenia; an eminently satisfactory state of affairs.

The changes observed in the hematopoietic organs and blood following steroid administration in vivo are probably an expression of the more general metabolic alterations produced by these drugs. Loss of weight is common initially unless there is marked fluid retention, and muscle wasting is sometimes prominent. A pronounced negative phosphorus and nitrogen balance accompanies the fall in the leukocyte count and improvement in the patient's condition. As steroids are withdrawn, retention of phosphorus occurs.[1] Uric acid excretion is high while the leukocyte count is falling,[588] and it is advisable to begin treatment with allopurinol when steroids are begun, to avoid the risk of hyperuricemia and urate nephropathy. The uricosuria is followed by creatinuria, which appears to accompany the disappearance of blast cells from the marrow. These findings might be interpreted as being the result of the antianabolic action of the steroid hormones, leukemic cells being destroyed when substances essential for their proliferation and survival are restricted. Why normal marrow cells should be immune from such effects, or nearly so, is unexplained.

ACTH is now seldom used in leukemia therapy, since it must be administered by injection and sometimes causes allergic reactions to the foreign protein it contains: furthermore, the effects of ACTH therapy are mediated through, and limited by, the patient's own adrenals, whose function may be in doubt. Cortisone is rarely used, since it has pronounced androgenic effects leading to hirsutism, and mineralocorticoid effects producing fluid and electrolyte retention. Modern, synthetic steroid hormones, given in equivalent antileukemic doses, have lesser adverse effects of the androgenic and mineralocorticoid type compared to cortisone or hydrocortisone. Unfortunately, steroid compounds which lack the glucocorticoid effects of cortisone, such as hyperglycemia and other metabolic changes, also lack antileukemic effect, so that muscle wasting, hyperglycemia, and iatrogenic diabetes mellitus must be accepted as presently unavoidable hazards of steroid therapy for leukemia. Even with modern steroid preparations, virilization and fluid retention are apt to occur with high doses or prolonged administration.

Many steroid drugs are now available for leukemia therapy. Prednisone (Δ^1-cortisone) has been the most widely used,[293] partly because it became available relatively early and is less costly than several other preparations. Prednisone must be activated in the body by conversion to prednisolone (Δ^1-hydrocortisone); the liver is the principal site of this conversion. Since prednisolone itself (Fig. 17-31) is now readily available and is not more expensive than prednisone, it seems more logical to use this compound rather than its metabolic precursor, prednisone.

Other steroid drugs such as triamcinolone, methylprednisolone, betamethasone, and dexamethasone have differing potencies and different degrees of mineralocorticoid activity compared to prednisolone, but there is no good evidence pointing to a significant difference in their antileukemic effects.

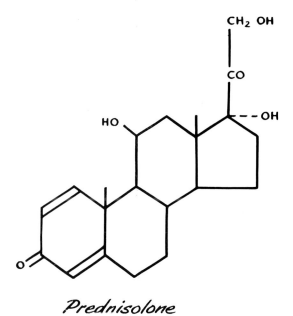

Prednisolone

Fig. 17-31. Structural formula of prednisolone (delta-1-hydrocortisone).

Clinical Uses

Prednisolone and related compounds are of great value in leukemia therapy. When administered for only brief periods they rarely have serious side effects: instead of the anorexia and nausea sometimes produced by other antileukemic drugs, steroids often lead to improved appetite and an increased sense of well-being; the patient may gain weight and undergo mood elevation or even euphoria, which is seldom a disadvantage. When the leukemia is responsive, the beneficial effects of steroids are rapidly exerted. Most important, improvement in the leukemia is effected without inflicting further damage upon a bone marrow which is already impaired by the leukemia itself. Against these merits must be set a relatively low response rate: in untreated acute leukemias, about one-half of patients with acute lymphocytic leukemia and only about one-sixth of patients with acute granulocytic leukemia can be expected to achieve complete remission with steroid therapy alone.[293,436] Remission rates are lower in patients previously treated with corticosteroids. So long as the drugs available for treating leukemia were few and the therapeutic aim was exclusively palliation, steroid therapy was used quite freely, particularly when there was doubt as to the correct course of action. Now that more antileukemic agents are available and the therapeutic aim in many patients is long-term survival, or even eradication of the leukemia, the indiscriminate use of steroids is to be discouraged.

Prednisolone and related compounds appear to possess the following effects in the leukemias:

1. Stimulation of appetite and psyche.
2. Inhibitory or lytic effects upon lymphoid, splenic, thymic, and plasmacytic tissues, which tends to affect beneficially the course of acute and chronic lymphocytic leukemias and, to a much lesser extent, lymphosarcoma and myelomatosis.
3. Some tendency to improve cytopenia caused by leukemia or by myelotoxic drugs, although the evidence that this is due to direct myelostimulation is inadequate.
4. Antagonism toward the autoimmune hemolytic processes found in chronic lymphocytic leukemia and lymphosarcoma, occasionally also benefiting autoimmune thrombocytopenia, in both disorders, even when direct evidence of autoimmunity may be lacking.
5. Improvement of the bleeding tendency in thrombocytopenia, possibly by an effect upon capillary fragility.

Unfortunately, the mechanisms whereby these effects are produced are very poorly understood. The *myelostimulatory* effects of steroids already mentioned may be caused by mobilization, not by increased production, of the formed elements of the blood. The effect of steroids upon the bleeding tendency in thrombocytopenia is difficult to quantitate and has even been denied by some workers. Similarly, though it has been stated that steroids may reduce the myelotoxic effects of alkylating agents and folic acid antagonists, there is no convincing evidence for this. Certainly, the availability of steroids should not encourage overenthusiastic administration of myelotoxic drugs.

The use of adrenocortical steroids in different forms of leukemia is discussed in detail in Chapter 18; general indications for their use are

1. Leukemias with a relatively predictable responsiveness to these drugs—acute lymphocytic leukemia and chronic lymphocytic leukemia.
2. Pancytopenia due to leukemia, so severe that initial treatment with marrow-depressant agents is not favored—even in this situation, steroids are a poor choice if the leukemia is of a type unlikely to be responsive.
3. Bleeding due to thrombocytopenia. Here the use of steroids should be a strictly temporary expedient: generally, platelet transfusions are a much better measure (see Chapter 18).
4. Transient cytopenia resulting from therapy, but the value of treatment must be offset against an augmented risk of infection.
5. Autoimmune complications, commonly encountered in chronic lymphocytic leukemia and rarely in other leukemias.
6. Occasionally, to produce symptomatic improvement in the terminal patient.
7. As a component of combination chemotherapies for leukemia (Chapter 18).

In the past there was a tendency to make excessive use of steroids in the leukemias, partly because of the lack of other agents. It is now felt that these valuable and important drugs should be restricted to situations where a definite indication exists. They should be used in adequate doses, preferably for brief periods, and their value should always be weighed against the risks inherent in their use. The adverse effects of adrenocortical steroids are listed in Table 17-5.

Table 17-5
Adverse Effects of Adrenocortical Steroid Hormones

Type of Effect	Manifestations
Psychic	Euphoria, mania, irritability, depression, suicide, insomnia, raised intracranial pressure, convulsions, fever
Ocular	Glaucoma, posterior subcapsular lens cataract
Androgenic	Acne, hirsutism, voice changes, menstrual disorders
Mineralocorticoid	Sodium retention, hypokalemia, water retention, edema, cardiac failure, hypertension, cerebral hemorrhage
Glucocorticoid	Hyperphagia, weight gain, obesity, hyperglycemia, diabetes mellitus, hypercatabolism, negative nitrogen balance, muscle wasting, hyperuricemia, uricosuria, nephrolithiasis, osteoporosis, delayed wound healing, blood hypercoagulability, Cushingoid features: moon face, supraclavicular and nuchal fat pads, striae, bruising
Immunodepressant	Lymphoid atrophy, impaired humoral and cellular immune processes
Gastrointestinal	Promotion of peptic ulceration, hematemesis, melena
Anti-inflammatory	Increased susceptibility to infections, particularly tuberculosis, superficial and systemic mycoses, and septicemias: impaired tissue responses to infection, suppression, or modification of clinical signs of infection
Endocrine	Adrenal cortical suppression and atrophy

Note: The relative prominence of a given effect varies with the particular steroid drug administered, but all the preparations available possess some or most of the effects listed.

ʟ-Asparaginase

ʟ-Asparaginase (asparaginase, colospase, Crasnitin) represents a new class of antitumor agents. It is an enzyme which inhibits and destroys tumor cells by depriving them of an exogenous supply of asparagine, which is an essential metabolite for some neoplastic cells. At first thought to be specific for leukemic cells,[467] asparaginase is the first enzyme to be introduced therapeutically in leukemia, and its purification and production on a large scale from special strains of bacteria represents a remarkable technological achievement.

Asparaginase is an enzyme widely distributed in nature. Its application in the treatment of leukemia was prompted by the observation[353,354] that injection of normal guinea pig serum produced striking regression of transplanted lymphomas in mice and rats. Sera from horse, rabbit, and man did not cause tumor regression. Broome[86–88] provided good evidence that ʟ-asparaginase was responsible for the antilymphoma effects of guinea pig serum after finding an early paper[135] which described the distribution of amino acid-degrading enzymes in different animal species. ʟ-asparaginase was present in the liver and kidney of many species, but in the blood of only one of the animals studied—the guinea pig. Sera lacking the enzyme have no antilymphoma properties. The action of ʟ-asparaginase is thought to depend on depletion of the available body pool of asparagine. Normal cells can synthesize asparagine except in critical situations in which their capacity for synthesis is inadequate for their requirement; asparagine is an essential nutrient for the blasts of many strains of mouse leukemia which are unable to synthesize it.[467] Susceptible strains of murine leukemia are curable by ʟ-asparaginase without any toxic effects in the host. Unfortunately, in human leukemia asparaginases from several sources have proved to be far less effective than in murine leukemia, and many toxic effects have been recorded.[34,117,468] Toxicity varies somewhat with the source of the enzyme, but anorexia, nausea, vomiting, weight loss, hypoproteinemia, hypofibrinogenemia, abnormal liver function tests and allergic reactions are common with most preparations.

Asparaginase is nevertheless a useful addition to the drugs available for the treatment of leukemia, being effective in acute lymphocytic leukemia, but of very little value in acute granulocytic leukemia.[34,48,134,149,299,429] The blast cells of acute granulocytic leukemia resemble many normal cells in being initially susceptible to asparagine deprivation, but able rapidly to activate a mechanism for synthesizing it. The reason why susceptible cells die rapidly when deprived of asparagine is unknown: some cultured human leukemic cells grow normally in the log phase in the absence of ʟ-asparagine and the growth rate is not increased by its addition; yet growth is suppressed by the addition of ʟ-asparaginase.[396] Such anomalies may perhaps be explained by the presence, in many preparations, of other enzymes, such as glutaminase. Most ʟ-asparaginase for use in the treatment of human leukemia is derived from *Escherichia coli,* but a clinically effective preparation has also been obtained from *Erwinia carotovora.*

In acute lymphocytic leukemia, ʟ-asparaginase will induce remissions in about 30 percent of patients who have become refractory to other drugs; if treatment is continued by daily intravenous injections the patients eventually become resistant to ʟ-asparaginase also, although sometimes not for several months. Patients who achieve remission after a course of 28 days may respond again, sometimes more than once, to later courses,[202] and those who develop prohibitive allergic complications may tolerate asparaginase derived from a different source. Apart from its lack of cross-resistance with other antileukemic drugs, L-asparaginase has the advantage of very little myelotoxicity: Pancytopenia rarely develops as a result of L-asparaginase therapy, and preexisting pancytopenia is not usually worsened by its administration. Thus, L-asparaginase is an excellent drug for the treatment of pancytopenic patients with acute lymphocytic leukemia and also in combination with myelotoxic agents, since it contributes no important myelotoxicity of its own.

L-asparaginase may be only the first of a series of enzymes which will prove valuable in leukemia therapy, and studies continue on the effects of depriving leukemic cells of amino acids other than asparagine by the use of different deaminating enzymes.

Hydroxyurea

Hydroxyurea was first synthesized in 1869. When introduced into cancer chemotherapy screening programs 90 years later, it was found to have activity against L1210 leukemia and a variety of other rodent neoplasms.[597] Hydroxyurea, classed as an antimetabolite, inhibits DNA synthesis by blocking the formation of deoxyribonucleotides from ribonucleotides.[366] It causes a marked and rapid fall in the peripheral blood leukocyte and platelet counts in experimental animals and man. This is rapidly reversible upon cessation of the drug. Ulceration of the buccal and gastrointestinal mucosa occurs with high doses; whereas folic acid antagonists cause ulceration of the palate and the inner surfaces of the lips, hydroxyurea rather characteristically causes reddened painful areas on the margins of the tongue. The drug can be taken by mouth and causes few side effects in doses not exceeding 1 gm daily. Hydroxyurea is effective in chronic granulocytic leukemia,[352,371] but has no clear advantage over busulfan, except that toxicity is so rapidly reversible. The drug has been used experimentally in acute leukemia in attempts to produce synchronization of the mitoses of leukemic cells prior to therapy with cycle-active agents (see chapters 8 and 18).

Methylglyoxal-bis-guanylhydrazone

Methylglyoxal-bis-guanylhydrazone (methyl-GAG) is a synthetic compound with an uncertain mode of action. It has profound effects on bone marrow cells, mucosal surfaces, and connective tissues. Although methyl-GAG is active in acute granulocytic leukemia,[404,512] severe side effects have limited its use. The drug must be given parenterally, and excretion is incomplete and protracted over 2–3 weeks[293]; this suggests prolonged storage within the body and may account for the slowly developing clinical toxicity seen with daily dose schedules.[404] The distressing toxic effects of methyl-GAG therapy include pharyngeal and anal ulceration, myelosuppression with thrombocytopenia and hemorrhage, polyneuropathy, arthritis, episcleritis, desquamation of the palms and soles, and diffuse vasculitis. Although as many as 45 percent of patients with acute granulocytic leukemia may achieve remission with methyl-GAG, the remissions are usually of short duration.[404] Combinations of methyl-GAG with mercaptopurine,[66] or with mercaptopurine and cytosine arabinoside[44] have produced good results in acute granulocytic leukemia. Despite its undoubted activity in acute leukemia, the combination of extremely unpleasant and dangerous toxic effects with a narrow therapeutic margin of safety has prevented methyl-GAG being widely used in clinical practice.

Miscellaneous Agents with Uncertain Modes of Action

A group of agents exists which are of known or disputed efficacy in the leukemias and lymphomas but whose modes of action have not been satisfactorily explained. These include the oldest chemotherapeutic drugs, arsenic and benzol, and more recently discovered ones such as urethane and procarbazine. These substances have been regarded as antimitotic agents and, without doubt, some of them are capable of preventing cell division. However, the events observed in experimental cell systems in vitro may well differ from those which follow therapeutic administration of these substances to patients, since the doses employed in some experiments were one hundred times greater than those given therapeutically. Even though mitotic inhibition has been observed in vitro, this need not be the means by which effects are produced on human leukemias in vivo.

ARSENIC

Arsenic in the form of arsenious oxide is the oldest chemotherapeutic substance known to be effective in leukemia. Its reappraisal by Forkner and Scott[218] temporarily renewed interest in it, but as the authors pointed out, the mechanism of its action in chronic granulocytic leukemia, the disease in which it was chiefly employed, is not clear. It is known that arsenic inhibits certain enzymes, particularly those containing sulfhydryl groups, and that it is concentrated in blood cells and bone marrow,[93] but since other organs, including bone and skin, accumulate equally large amounts, the predilection of arsenic for myeloid cells remains something of a mystery. Arsenic, in common with other cytostatic agents, prevents the incorporation of radioactively labeled formate into the nucleic acid purines of experimental animals and is therefore presumed to inhibit nucleic acid synthesis,[580] but not enough work has been done to clarify the significance of this finding. The advent of ionizing radiations and later the alkylating agents, particularly busulfan, has displaced arsenic from the therapy of chronic granulocytic leukemia.

BENZENE

Benzene possesses pronounced myelotoxic effects, readily giving rise to irreversible marrow aplasia, and has been implicated as a possible etiologic agent in leukemia (see Chapter 5). As the myelotoxicity of benzene was known early in this century, trials were soon made in leukemia and considerable numbers of patients were treated with it. The voluminous older literature was reviewed by Forkner,[217] who concluded that benzene might well be valuable in the treatment of leukemia, and that in spite of widespread warning concerning its dangers, there was insufficient evidence in the literature to incriminate benzene as a useless or a dangerous drug. Some research on its action has been carried out, even in comparatively recent times, and its use in both chronic granulocytic and chronic lymphocytic leukemia was advocated as late as 1953.[75] Several animal leukemias are sensitive to benzene, among them a strain of murine myeloid chloroleukemia, on which the chemical has a potent action leading to degeneration of many of the cells.[214] It appears likely that benzene, like arsenic, acts by damaging vital intracellular enzymes. It is no longer used clinically.

URETHANE

Urethane (ethyl carbamate) was among the earliest of the drugs which ushered in the renaissance of chemotherapy in the treatment of leukemia. Because of its emergence in a virtually clear field, it attracted a great deal of attention, and more experimental work on urethane has been reported than seems justified by its clinical usefulness, which became confined to suppressing plasma cell growth in the treatment of myeloma: even this use is becoming very uncommon with the introduction of the newer alkylating agents, BCNU, and refinements in radiotherapy.

Urethane had been in common use for many years as an anesthetic for laboratory animals, when in the 1940s a study was made of the effects of a variety of chemicals upon cell division in plants in a search for selective weed killers.[624] It was found that very low concentrations of several carbamates blocked mitosis in cereal seedlings and arrested their growth, and when carbamic esters were tested on animal tissues and experimental tumors,[267] it was found that the common urethane, ethyl carbamate, was the most active. Urethane tested in patients with advanced malignant disease caused sporadic tumor regressions[485] as well as leukopenia, a property which had already been noted 20 years earlier.[282] These findings prompted the use of urethane in leukemia and the effects proved comparable to those of irradiation.[485]

In chronic granulocytic leukemia, urethane caused reduction in leukocytosis, improvement in hemoglobin levels, and reduction of splenomegaly with decreased mitoses in the myeloid cells and increased mitoses in the erythroid cells of the bone marrow.[450] Urethane causes abnormal mitoses in leukemic cells,[552] and cell destruction in leukemia[42] and myeloma.[416,530] The marked activity of urethane in animal leukemias[197,359,360,388,455,456] may be mediated by mitotic depression,[177,178,263] production of mitotic abnormalities,[252,524,525] promotion of cellular differentiation,[267] or cell-surface effects related to its anesthetic properties.[386] Urethane in vitro is frequently active only at concentrations exceeding those attained in vivo.[31,96,97,212,233,260,421,453,460]

Urethane enters the nuclei of dividing cells[143,575] while closely related urethane analogs are inactive.[577] The drug may inhibit pyrimidine metabolism[73,181,185]; the structurally related compounds formamide and N-methylformamide have similar biologic effects but are extremely hepatotoxic.[129,581] For a short time urethane was used in the treatment of chronic granulocytic leukemia,[568] but was replaced by busulfan. Although urethane is moderately effective in multiple myeloma,[530] it is now very seldom used because better drugs are available. Urethane causes nausea and vomiting, even when administered rectally, and centrilobular hepatic necrosis has been reported.[469] Tumor induction has been described in animals but not in man.[519] Although urethane no longer has any clinical importance, its hitherto unexplained mode of action and simple molecular structure remain of pharmacologic interest.

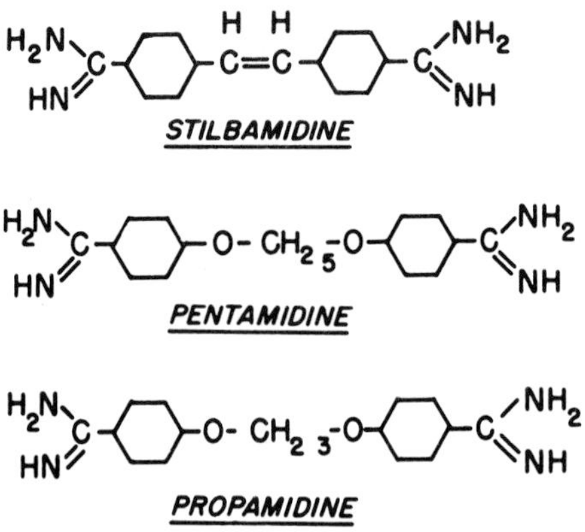

Fig. 17-32. Some aromatic diamidines.

AROMATIC DIAMIDINES

Stilbamidine (Fig. 17-32) is the best-known member of this group of drugs. Stilbamidine was tested in myeloma because this disease, like kala-azar, is characterized by marked hyperglobulinemia, and because the drug is an effective remedy in kala-azar.[586] It causes only limited and temporary improvement in myeloma but its action is of interest because it causes unusual morphologic changes in myeloma cells. Tumor growth was not inhibited, but marrow examination showed large basophil cytoplasmic granules in many of the myeloma cells and these tended to become confluent. The granules were pyronin-positive and ribonuclease-soluble and were concluded to be complexes of RNA and stilbamidine.[584,585] Although stilbamidine treatment caused no diminution in numbers of myeloma cells, the evidence that this drug and the related pentamidine and 2-hydroxystilbamidine could produce morphologic changes in tumor cells correlated well with the demonstration that aromatic diamidines can inhibit the growth of experimental tumors, probably by means of denaturation of cellular proteins.[542] Stilbamidine is now seldom used in myeloma since its only clinically useful effect is relief of bone pain. Conceivably this is due to a slightly diminished rate of tumor cell proliferation, but it is also possible that the benefit is due to sensory neuropathy, a recognized side effect of the drug.

The only use of the aromatic diamidines in leukemia therapy today is an indirect one, in that pentamidine isethionate is an effective treatment for infections with the protozoon *Pneumocystis carinii*, which occur occasionally in neutropenic, immunodepressed patients.[405,673]

PROCARBAZINE

Procarbazine (ibenzmethyzin, Natulan) belongs to a group of chemical compounds which incorporate methylhydrazine in their molecules and possess tumor-inhibitory properties.[67] It is thought to behave as an alkylating agent but may also possess antimetabolic properties, inhibiting transmethylation.[372] Procarbazine is administered orally or intravenously and is principally useful in the therapy of Hodgkin's disease.[94,167] It has been used in the palliative treatment of terminal acute leukemia with only limited success,[592] but the occasional production of euphoria, which may be due to its known monoamine oxidase (MAO) inhibitory effects, can be a welcome side effect of the drug.

OTHER AGENTS

These compounds are mainly of historic interest, although elucidation of their mechanisms of action would necessarily throw more light upon the biochemistry of tumor cells. Among them is *antimony,* advocated for the treatment of myeloma on the same grounds as stilbamidine, namely, that it is effective in kala-azar.[527,528] Most known myelotoxic agents have at some time been tried in the treatment of leukemia, among them thiouracil.[47,277] Para-aminobenzoic acid has been used in chronic granulocytic leukemia and both increases[13,54] and reductions[435,691] in the leukocyte count have been reported according to the doses given, but no useful results have been observed. With the development of antileukemic drugs of proved efficacy, ethical barriers to the clinical trial of apparently nonspecific, myelotoxic substances in the leukemias have become very great: thus, some of these early studies are of value because they provide toxicologic data which could not now be sought by deliberate studies in man.

Clinical Uses of Antileukemic Agents

Details of the use of antileukemic drugs in the treatment of various forms of leukemia are given in Chapter 18. A few general principles regarding the clinical employment of these compounds can however be listed here.

FOLIC ACID ANTAGONISTS

The different antifolic compounds appear to work in closely similar or identical fashion; there seems little to choose between various analogs, and methotrexate is by far the most commonly used member of the group. Antifolic drugs were originally employed in acute lymphocytic leukemia in children and their most striking beneficial effects are still seen in this condition. Although less than one-third of children achieve complete remission with methotrexate given as a single agent,[293] the combination of methotrexate with a corticosteroid drug induces remission in about 80 percent of cases.[162,375] Folic acid antagonists are much less effective in acute granulocytic leukemia of adults; complete remission rates as low as 3 percent have been reported.[221] A widespread feeling exists that purine antagonists are more effective than folic acid antagonists in acute granulocytic leukemia of adults, but, in fact, both are almost equally bad, remission rates being low with either type of compound when it is given as a single agent.[650] However, the toxic effects of folic acid antagonists, particularly mucosal ulceration, are more obvious and cause more severe symptoms than the toxic effects of antipurine drugs; thus there is a natural reluctance to use methotrexate in varieties of leukemia which are unlikely to respond, since adverse effects can be anticipated almost with certainty. A series of halogenated folic acid antagonists, notably 3'5'dichloroamethopterin, was found to have a greater therapeutic effect and less myelotoxicity in mice than did methotrexate,[240,319,649] but results in human patients were less promising.[550] While extremely valuable in acute lymphocytic leukemia of childhood and in meningeal leukemia of any cell type,[24,83] the folic acid antagonists are unsatisfactory as single-agent therapy in adult acute granulocytic leukemia. They do not appear valuable in chronic lymphocytic leukemia or lymphosarcoma, and, although effective in chronic granulocytic leukemia in its chronic phase, are seldom used in that disease because better and more convenient drugs exist.

PURINE ANTAGONISTS

Mercaptopurine (6-MP) is the most widely used purine antagonist but thioguanine is finding an increasing place in leukemia therapy. The major use of these drugs is in the treatment of the acute leukemias, although they are also useful in chronic granulocytic leukemia in its chronic phase and, to a much lesser extent, after metamorphosis. Purine antagonists have not been shown to be useful in chronic lymphocytic leukemia.

When used as a single agent in acute lymphocytic leukemia of childhood, mercaptopurine induces complete remission in about one-third of patients.[111,221] In acute granulocytic leukemia in adults, the remission rate when mercaptopurine is used alone varies from 10–20 percent in different series.[111,186,285,436] Purine antagonists and folic acid antagonists do not exhibit cross-resistance and patients whose leukemia has become refractory to either may respond to the alternate agent. Attempts to predict the clinical usefulness of antipurine compounds by studies of their effects on leukocyte metabolism in vitro[113,387] have been partially successful, and this is a field of continuing research.

VINCRISTINE, L-ASPARAGINASE, AND CORTICOSTEROIDS

Although these agents have been employed in many varieties of leukemia, they are highly effective as single agents only in acute lymphocytic leukemia, especially in childhood.[227,293] Vincristine and L-asparaginase share with corticosteroids the advantages of a relatively high response rate in acute lymphocytic leukemia, coupled with negligible toxicity to normal bone marrow. It is no longer accepted practice to administer any of these agents alone in the treatment of acute leukemia, and their lack of myelotoxicity makes them very suitable for inclusion in combinations with drugs which are myelotoxic, such as mercaptopurine or cyclophosphamide.

DAUNORUBICIN

This drug is effective in both acute lymphocytic and acute granulocytic leukemia, but has the drawback of pronounced marrow toxicity. The tendency to use daunorubicin infrequently, or only in late stages, of acute lymphocytic leukemia does not reflect on its therapeutic efficacy, but merely signifies that there is a relatively wide selection of equally effective and less toxic drugs from which the therapist may choose when managing the disease. However, the combination of daunorubicin with vincristine and steroid is extremely potent, yielding remission rates as high as 97 percent[46] and it is thus far too good a drug to overlook. Daunorubicin, alone or in combination, is one of the few agents effective in a relatively high proportion of cases of acute granulocytic leukemia.

CYTOSINE ARABINOSIDE

Like daunorubicin, cytosine arabinoside is effective in both major forms of acute leukemia, and, similarly, it has significant myelotoxicity. It causes nausea and vomiting, but does so less frequently than does daunorubicin. When administered intrathecally, cytosine arabinoside is effective against meningeal leukemia.[83] When it is used systemically, resistance to cytosine arabinoside arises readily and the tendency is to use it in combination with another agent, such as thioguanine[119] or daunorubicin,[150] or both.[594] Such combinations are theoretically less likely to lead to the emergence of drug-resistant leukemic cell-lines; they are highly myelotoxic, but perhaps because of this, more effective than any single agent against acute granulocytic leukemia.

THE ADVERSE EFFECTS

In common with other drugs, antileukemic agents have two main types of adverse effect. *Idiosyncratic reactions* occur sporadically and unpredictably and are unrelated to the usual pharmacologic effects of the drug: They represent an interaction between the drug and an individual patients—for example, allergic drug rashes fall into this category. *Pharmacologic* adverse effects are predictable consequences of the known actions of the drug; for example, myelosuppression, megaloblastosis, and buccal ulceration are adverse effects of methotrexate from the clinician's viewpoint, but are inherent properties of an effective folic acid antagonist.

The majority of antileukemic drugs are myelotoxic, and their administration damages, not only leukemic cells, but also the remaining normal marrow elements. When the leukemia is first diagnosed, or is in relapse, the normal hematopoietic cells are already much reduced, and the depressant effects of the antileukemic drugs are all the more serious. The drugs appear to injure normal and abnormal cells with little selectivity: improvement of the hematologic picture seems to depend on the normal elements possessing powers of recovery (that is, proliferative capacity) exceeding those of the leukemic cells. When remission has been achieved and leukemic cells are few in number, and when normal hematopoietic cells predominate, patients will tolerate aggressive antileukemic therapy, which would have had fatal results if given during relapse. Thus, it is reasonable to treat the patient with acute leukemia in remission more vigorously than before, using larger doses of antileukemic drugs in an attempt to avert the emergence of drug resistance and conceivably to extirpate the residual leukemic cells altogether. However, attempts to destroy the entire leukemic cell population must always be cautious, since the myelotoxic agents can produce anemia, thrombocytopenia with hemorrhage, and neutropenia with infection, and thereby bring about a death not unlike that caused by acute leukemia itself.[466]

Serious or even fatal toxic effects may be produced in organs other than the bone marrow. Thus, mercaptopurine[127] and methotrexate[620] may produce liver damage and jaundice, and many of the experimental antimetabolites have found little clinical application because of their propensity for producing hepatotoxicity[191] or neurotoxicity.[569] The myocardial toxicity of daunorubicin[46] undoubtedly has caused some deaths, though these are less common now that its adverse effect is widely recognized. The commoner adverse effects of the drugs most important in the treatment of the acute leukemias are summarized in Table 17-6. It can be seen that only prednisolone, vincristine, and L-asparaginase are without significant myelotoxicity. These drugs should be ideal for the initial treatment of acute leukemia at the time of diagnosis or during a relapse, when marrow function is impaired and further marrow damage is to be avoided. Although the combination of prednisolone, vincristine, and L-asparaginase is highly effective in acute lymphocytic leukemia, unfortunately, none of these drugs is very potent in adults with acute granulocytic leukemia; nor is their combination.

Inspection of Table 17-6 shows that, by judicious selection of drugs, combinations of several agents may be used without excessive overlap of toxic effects. Thus,

Table 17-6
Adverse Effects of Antileukemic Drugs in Common Use

Drug	Bone Marrow Toxicity	Vomiting, Other G-I Disturbances	G-I Mucosal Damage	Bone Marrow Megaloblastosis	Neurotoxicity	Alopecia	Metabolic Effects	Allergic Reactions	Immunosuppression	Hemorrhagic Cystitis	Altered Protein Synthesis	Hepatotoxicity	Cardiotoxicity
Prednisolone	0	±	+	0	0	0	++	0	++	0	++	0	0
Vincristine	0	++	0	0	++	++	0	0	+	0	0	0	0
Mercaptopurine	++	±	±	±	0	0	0	±	++	0	0	+	0
Methotrexate	++	±	++	++	0	±	0	±	++	0	0	+	0
Cyclophosphamide	++	±	0	0	0	++	0	±	++	++	0	0	0
Daunorubicin	++	++	+	0	0	+	0	0	+	0	0	0	++
Cytarabine	++	++	++	++	±	0	0	0	+	0	0	0	0
Asparaginase	0	++	0	0	±	0	++	++	+	0	++	±	0

++, Effect common and/or severe; +, effect relatively common; ±, effect rare; 0, no clinically significant effect.

methotrexate and mercaptopurine, which are both myelotoxic, may be used together although some modification of the dose of each may be necessary. However, prednisolone and vincristine may then be added to this combination without any dose modification, since neither drug is myelotoxic and their principal toxicities differ from each other, vincristine being neurotoxic and prednisolone having mainly metabolic side effects. It is apparent that all the drugs used in acute leukemia are to some degree immunosuppressive, and this type of overlap in toxicity, therefore, cannot be avoided, although its effects may be minimized by employing intermittent, rather than continuous, drug administration.

SYMPTOMATIC MEASURES

Symptoms may occur in patients with leukemia when the disease is uncontrolled, or at any time as a result of antileukemic therapy itself. One of the less desirable results of advances in leukemia therapy is that patients frequently suffer from the adverse effects of drugs, and combinations such as alopecia, peripheral neuritis, chemical cystitis, and buccal ulceration, or other symptom complexes may disable a patient seriously, even if only temporarily. Against such drawbacks must be set the fact that well-treated patients seldom suffer from symptoms of the leukemia itself, and live much longer and in better health than untreated patients. In managing acute leukemia, it is extremely difficult to avoid drug-induced symptoms altogether; so much so that if such symptoms never occur it must be suspected that the patient is being undertreated! This is particularly true of the folic acid antagonists; a patient who never develops a mouth ulcer is unlikely to be receiving optimal antifolic therapy.

Drug-induced symptoms may be minimized by the skill and experience of the therapist and may also be relieved by judicious use of appropriate drugs, for example, antiemetics, sedatives, mucosal anesthetics, and laxatives. Symptoms caused by the leukemia itself are best relieved by bringing the disease under good control: meanwhile, symptoms from anemia or thrombocytopenia are alleviated by blood or platelet transfusion as appropriate. Even when there is no prospect of securing a remission of the leukemia, much can be done to relieve symptoms. Pain may be treated with simple or narcotic analgesics, by local irradiation, or palliative chemotherapy. Anxiety or depression may respond to psychotropic drugs, and, in the terminal patient, the physician may employ drugs of addiction, such as narcotics and amphetamines, to good advantage, since the problem of long-term drug dependence is irrelevant in such patients. In the severely depressed, dying patient, antidepressant drugs such as amitriptyline and its analogs are often ineffective, but morphine, cocaine, and dextroamphetamine are often excellent euphoriants in this brief but distressing phase. The meticulous and understanding care of the patient with terminal neoplastic disease, securing a dignified end to life with minimal discomfort, is an underemphasized but extremely important part of the physician's art.[302]

SUPPORTIVE THERAPY

Supportive therapy, including the transfusion of blood, platelets, granulocytes, and blood products, the use of antimicrobial agents, and protected environments for the patient, is required to a very variable extent, because the need for supportive measures varies with the type of leukemia, the age of the patients, and other factors peculiar to individual cases. Supportive therapy is discussed in detail in Chapter 18.

SUMMARY

Only 30 years ago, the available treatments for leukemia were ionizing radiations, a few highly toxic and unreliable drugs of dubious value, and blood transfusion. Today, many potent antileukemic agents are available, and the choice of possible drug combinations and therapeutic programs is bewilderingly wide. There is no *correct* therapy for any form of leukemia, for such a term implies a 100 percent cure rate and zero percent iatrogenic morbidity. Nor is there an established treatment for any of the leukemias since, fortunately, the scene is one of continual improvement. It is even difficult to define a "best available" therapy, since at any one time numerous, well-designed regimens are under study, and their relative merits may take several years to demonstrate conclusively. A regimen thought to be the best available, and thus to be recommended, may be rendered obsolete at any time by further advances. Thus, the development of new drugs and improved approaches to therapy in the leukemias has in some ways made the physician's task more difficult, though more rewarding.

Because in all the forms of leukemia there now exist several acceptable methods of treatment, it is possible to vary the therapeutic approach in each patient according to the needs of the situation. Thus, in chronic lymphocytic leukemia, an alkylating agent may be indicated for control of widespread disease without pancytopenia, but a corticosteroid drug may be more appropriate if marrow insufficiency or autoimmune hemolytic anemia later comes to dominate the picture. Uncontrollable hemolysis or thrombocytopenia may require splenectomy, while localized symptomatic lymphadenopathy is best treated by local irradiation. Treatment programs must remain flexible because the patient's needs may change during the course of the disease.

Although some of the therapeutic advances of recent years have come from the development of new and better antileukemic drugs, the stage where specific forms of leukemia are treated by specific chemicals[156] has not yet been reached. Some of the most significant recent advances are, in fact, due to the discovery of improved ways of using existing drugs, particularly in combinations. This approach has had its greatest impact in acute lymphocytic leukemia of childhood, but is also improving the outlook for adults with acute granulocytic leukemia: it remains to be seen whether combined drug therapy will prove valuable in the chronic leukemias, where little therapeutic progress has been made in the past 10 years.

REFERENCES

1. Adams WS, Valentine WN, Bassett SH, Lawrence JS: The effect of cortisone and ACTH in leukemia. J Lab Clin Med 39:570, 1952.
2. Albrecht M, Boll I: Die Einwirkung von Aminopterin auf menschliches Knochenmark in vitro. Z Krebsforsch 57:496, 1951.
3. Alexander P: Mechanism of the cytotoxic action of the radiomimetic agents, in Radiobiology. London, Butterworth, 1961, p 287.
4. _____, Stacey KA: Comparison of the changes produced by ionizing radiations and by the alkylating agents: evidence for a similar mechanism at the molecular level. Ann NY Acad Sci 68:1225, 1958.
5. Algenstaedt D: Quantitätive Veränderungen des Zellgehaltes von Blut und Knochenmark unter der Chemotherapie

menschlicher Leukämien. Ärztl Wschr 14:461, 1959.

6. _____: Der Einfluss der Chemotherapie auf das Knochenmarkzellbild der Leukosen. Verh Dtsch Ges Inn Med 66:961, 1961.

7. Altman SJ, Haut A, Cartwright GE, Wintrobe MM: Early experience with p-(N,N-di-2-chloroethyl)-aminophenylbutyric acid (CB1348), a new chemotherapeutic agent effective in the treatment of chronic lymphocytic leukemia. Cancer 9:512, 1956.

8. André J, Schwartz RS, Mitus WJ, Dameshek W: Morphologic responses of the lymphoid system to homografts: I. First and second set responses in normal rabbits. Blood 19:313, 1962.

9. _____, _____, _____, _____: Morphologic responses of the lymphoid system to homografts: II. The effects of antimetabolites. Blood 19:334, 1962.

10. Andrews GA: Criticality accidents in Vinca, Yugoslavia, and Oak Ridge, Tennessee. JAMA 179:191, 1962.

11. Arnold H, Bourseaux F: Neuartige Krebs-chemotherapeutica aus der Gruppe der zyklischen N-Lost Phosphamidester. Naturwissenschaften 45:64, 1958.

12. _____, _____, Brock N: Chemotherapeutic action of a cyclic nitrogen mustard phosphamide ester (B518-ASTA) in experimental tumours of the rat. Nature 181:931, 1958.

13. Astaldi G, Baldini M: L'aumento leucocitario provocato dall'acido p-aminobenzoico nella leucemia acuta. Acta Vitaminol Enzymol 2:82, 1948.

14. _____, Mauri C: Recherches sur l'activité proliférative de l'hemocytoblaste de la leucémie aiguë. Rev Belge Pathol 23:69, 1953.

15. Atkinson JB, Mahoney FJ, Schwartz IR, Hesch JA: Therapy of acute leukemia by whole-body irradiation and bone-marrow transplantation from an identical normal twin. Blood 14:228, 1959.

16. Aubertin C, Beaujard E: Action des rayons X sur le sang et les organes hématopoïétiques. CR Soc Biol 58:217, 1905.

17. Auerbach C: The induction by mustard gas of chromosomal instabilities in drosophila melanogaster. Proc R Soc Edinburgh 62:307, 1947.

18. _____: Mutagenic effects of alkylating agents. Ann NY Acad Sci 68:731, 1958.

19. _____, Robson JM: Production of mutations by alkyl isothiocyanate. Nature 154:81, 1944.

20. _____, _____, Carr JG: The chemical production of mutations. Science 105:243, 1947.

21. Aur RJA, Simone J, Hustu HO, Vergosa M: A comparative study of central nervous system irradiation and intensive chemotherapy early in remission of childhood acute lymphocytic leukemia. Cancer 29:381, 1972.

22. _____, _____, _____, Walters T, Borella L, Pratt C, Pinkel D: Central nervous system therapy and combination chemotherapy of childhood lymphocytic leukemia. Blood 37:272, 1971.

23. Bacq ZM, Alexander P: Fundamentals of Radiobiology (ed.2). London, Pergamon Press, 1963.

24. Baikie AG, Spiers ASD: Methotrexate in meningeal leukaemia. Lancet 2:259, 1967.

25. Barlow AM, Leeming JT, Wilkinson JF: Mannomustine in treatment of leukaemias, polycythaemia, and malignant disorders. Br Med J 2:208, 1959.

26. Barnes DWH, Corp MJ, Loutit JF, Neal FE: Treatment of murine leukaemia with X-rays and homologous bone marrow. Preliminary communication. Br Med J 2:626, 1956.

27. Barnes WA, Furth OB: Studies on the indirect effect of roentgen rays in single and parabiotic mice. Am J Roentgenol Radium Ther Nucl Med 49:662, 1943.

28. Barron ESG, Bartlett GR, Miller ZB: The effect of nitrogen mustards on enzymes and tissue metabolism. I. The effect on enzymes. J Exp Med 87:489, 1948.

29. _____, _____, _____, Meyer J, Seegmiller JE: The effect of nitrogen mustards on enzymes and tissue metabolism. II. The effect on tissue metabolism. J Exp Med 87:503, 1948.

30. Barton AD, Laird AK: Effects of amethopterin on nucleic acid metabolism in mitotic and non-mitotic growth. J Biol Chem 227:795, 1957.

31. Bastrup-Madsen P: Action of mitotic poisons in vitro: effect of urethane on division of fibroblasts. Acta Pathol Microbiol Scandinav 26:93, 1959.

32. Bateman JC: Palliation of cancer in human patients by maintenance therapy with NN'N''-triethylene thiophosphoramide and N-(3-oxapentamethylene)-N'N''-diethylene phosphoramide. Ann NY Acad Sci 68:1057, 1958.

33. Beard AG, Barnhard HJ, Ross SW, Conlin FD: Acute leukemia treated by irradiation

and marrow transplant. J Pediatr 55:42, 1959.

34. Beard MEJ, Crowther D, Galton DAG, Guyer RJ, Fairley GH, Kay HEM, Knapton PJ, Malpas JS, Scott RB: L-asparaginase in treatment of acute leukaemia and lymphosarcoma. Br Med J 1:191, 1970.

35. Bendich A: Structure activity relationships. Symposium on antitumour agents. Proc R Soc Med 50:6, 1957.

36. Benjamin E, von Reuss H, Sluka E, Schwartz G: Beiträge zur Frage der Einwirkung der Röntgenstrahlen auf das Blut. Wien Klin Wochenschr 19:788, 1906.

37. Berenbaum MC: Immunosuppressive agents: generation and consequences of differing dose-response curves. Proc R Soc Med 65:255, 1972.

38. Berenblum I, Schoental R: Action of mustard gas (B,B¹-dichlorodiethylsulphide) on nucleoproteins. Nature 159:727, 1947

39. Bergel F: New developments in carcinochemo-therapy. Br Med J 2:399, 1961.

40. _____, Stock JA: Cyto-active amino-acid and peptide derivatives. I. Substituted phenylalanines. J Chem Soc 157:2409, 1954.

41. Berlin NI, Lawrence JH: The changes in the bone marrow differential in chronic leukemia treated with P³² and Y⁹⁰. Acta Med Scand 140:99, 1951.

42. Berman L, Axelrod AR: Effect of urethane on malignant diseases. Am J Clin Pathol 18:104, 1948.

43. _____, _____, Von der Heide EC, Sharp EA: Use of a folic acid antagonist in chronic leukemia. Am J CLin Pathol 19:127, 1949.

44. Bernard J: Acute leukemia treatment. Cancer Res 27:2565, 1967.

45. _____, Boiron M, Jacquillat C: Étude comparée sur les affections tumorales malignes humaines de l'activité thérapeutique de deux nouveaux dérivées de l'éthyléneimino-quinone. Bull Assoc Fr Cancer 46:34, 1959.

46. _____, _____, _____, Weil M: Rubidomycin in 400 patients with leukemia and other malignancies, in: Abstracts of the XII Congress of the International Society of Hematology. 1968, p 5.

47. _____, Deltour G, Velez E, Christol D: Étude de l'éffet du thiouracile dans quelques cas de leucémie. Sang 23:629, 1952.

48. _____, Jacquillat C, Boiron M, Weil M, Bussel A, Larrieu MJ, Delobel J, Goguel A, Levy D, Tanzer J: Treatment of acute leukemia with L-asparaginase: Preliminary results in 84 cases. Presse Méd 78:161, 1970.

49. _____, _____, Weil M; Treatment of the acute leukemias. Sem Hématol 9:181, 1972.

50. _____, Mathé G, Weil M: Traitement par le E39 des hémopathies malignes chroniques et d'autres affections tumorales. Sangre 23:629, 1957.

51. Bertino J: The mechanism of action of the folate antagonists in man. Cancer Res 23:1286, 1963.

52. Bertola A, Ravetto M, Zelaschi C: Roentgen-irradiazone dei tessuti emopoietici in soggetti normali ed emopatici (modificazioni del midollo osseo); nota preventiva. Gazz Osp Clin 59:1255, 1938.

53. Bethell FH: Myleran and triethylene melamine in the treatment of chronic granulocytic leukemia. Ann NY Acad Sci 68:996, 1958.

54. Bichel J: Effect of p-aminobenzoic acid on leucocyte count in leukaemia. Nature 161:353, 1948.

55. Bierman HR, Kelly KH, Knudson AG, Maekawa T, Timmis GM: The influence of 1,4-dimethylsulfonoxy-1,4-dimethylbutane (CB2348, Dimethyl Myleran) in neoplastic disease. Ann NY Acad Sci 68:1112, 1958.

56. Biesele JJ: Some negative screening results with miscellaneous compounds in tissue cultures of several tumors. Cancer Res (suppl) 1:1, 1953.

57. _____: Effects of 6-mercaptopurine on experimental tumors in tissue culture. Ann NY Acad Sci 60:228, 1954.

58. _____, Philips FS, Thiersch JB, Burchenal JH, Buckley SM, Stock CC: Chromosome alteration and tumour inhibition by nitrogen mustards: the hypothesis of cross-linking alkylation. Nature 166:1112, 1950.

59. Block M: Histopathologic effects of x-rays, radiophosphorus, nitrogen mustard, urethane, and steroids upon the spleen in leukemias and lymphomas. Radiology 71:477, 1958.

60. _____, Jacobson LO, Neal W: Biological studies with arsenic 76. IV. The histopathologic effect of arsenic 76 upon the hematopoietic tissues of patients with leukemia. J Lab Clin Med 41:499, 1953.

61. Blokhin N, Larionov L, Perevodchikova N, Chebotareva L, Merkulova N: Clinical experiences with sarcolysin in neoplastic disease. Ann NY Acad Sci 68:1128, 1958.

62. Bloom AD, Tjio JH: In vivo effects of diagnostic x-irradiation on human chromosomes. N Engl J Med 270:1341, 1964.

63. Bloom MA: Bone marrow, in Bloom W (ed.): Histopathology of Irradiation from

External and Internal Sources. New York, McGraw-Hill, 1948, p 162.

64. ———, Bloom W: The radiosensitivity of erythroblasts. J Lab Clin Med 32:654, 1947.

65. Blum RH, Friedman MA, Carter SK: Adriamycin NSC-123127: Clinical brochure. Bethesda, National Cancer Institute, 1972.

66. Boiron M, Jacquillat C, Weil M, Bernard J: Combination of methylglyoxal-bis-guanyl-hydrazone (NSC32946) and 6-mercapto-purine (NSC755) in acute granulocytic leukemia. Cancer Chemother Rep 45:69, 1965.

67. Bollag W, Grunberg E: Tumor inhibitory effects of a new class of cytotoxic agents: methylhydrazine derivatives. Experientia 19:130, 1963.

68. Bonadonna G, Monfardini S, de Lena M, Fossati-Bellani F: Clinical evaluation of adriamycin, a new antitumour antibiotic. Br Med J 3:503, 1969.

69. Bond VP: Negative pions: Their possible use in radiotherapy. Am J Roentgenol Radium Ther Nucl Med 111:9, 1971.

70. ———, Fliedner T, Archambeau JO: Mammalian Radiation Lethality, a Disturbance in Cellular Kinetics. New York, Academic Press, 1965.

71. Bouroncle BA, Doan CA, Wiseman BK, Frajola WJ: Evaluation of CB1348 in Hodgkin's disease and allied disorders. Arch Intern Med 97:703, 1956.

72. Boyd E, Buchanan WW, Lennox B: Damage to chromosomes by therapeutic doses of radioiodine. Lancet 1:977, 1961.

73. Boyland E, Koller PC: Effects of urethane on mitosis in Walker rat carcinoma. Br J Cancer 8:677, 1954.

74. Boyles PW: Interstitial pulmonary fibrosis after long-term busulphan therapy. Clin Med 76:11, 1969.

75. Braier L: Traitement des leucoses chroniques par le benzène et ses homologues: Le rôle des donneurs de méthyles. Sang 24:603, 1953.

76. Brauner R, Gottlieb F: Les modifications du myélogramme au cours de la roentgenthérapie. Sang 13:963, 1939.

77. British Medical Journal (Leading Article): Cyclophosphamide and the bladder. Br Med J 2:726, 1971.

78. Broad AF, Emery EW, Godlee JN, Prankerd TAJ: The management of myelomatosis. Postgrad Med J 44:803, 1968.

79. Brockman RW: A mechanism of resistance to 6-mercaptopurine: metabolism of hypoxanthine and 6-mercaptopurine by

80. ———, Sparks C, Simpson MS, Skipper HE: Decreased ribonucleotide pyrophosphorylase activity of Streptococcus faecalis and L.1210 leukemia resistant to purine antagonists. Biochem Pharmacol 2:77, 1959.

81. Broder LE, Carter SK: CCNU clinical brochure. Bethesda, National Cancer Institute, 1971.

82. ———, ———: Methyl CCNU brochure. Bethesda, National Cancer Institute, 1971.

83. ———, ———: Meningeal Leukemia. New York, Plenum Press, 1972.

84. Brodsky I, Kahn SB, Moyer JH: Cancer Chemotherapy. Basic and Clinical Applications. New York, Grune & Stratton, 1967.

85. Brookes P, Lawley PD: The reaction of mustard gas with nucleic acids in vitro and in vivo. Biochem J 77:478, 1960.

86. Broome JD: Evidence that the L-asparaginase activity of guinea pig serum is responsible for its antilymphoma effects. Nature 191:1114, 1961.

87. ———: Evidence that the L-asparaginase of guinea pig serum is responsible for its antilymphoma effects. I. Properties of the L-asparaginase of guinea pig serum in relation to those of the antilymphoma substance. J Exp Med 118:99, 1963.

88. ———: Evidence that the L-asparaginase of guinea pig serum is responsible for its antilymphoma effects. II. Lymphoma 6C3HED cells cultured in a medium devoid of L-asparagine lose their susceptibility to the effects of guinea pig serum. J Exp Med 118:121, 1963.

89. Brown A, Davis LJ: The haematological effects of nitrogen mustard therapy with special reference to the cytology of the sternal bone marrow. Glasgow Med J 31:93, 1950.

90. Brown GB: The biosynthesis of nucleic acids as a basis for an approach to chemotherapy. Ann NY Acad Sci 60:185, 1954.

91. ———, Roll PM, Plentl AA, Cavalieri LF: The utilization of adenine for nucleic acid synthesis and as a precursor of guanine. J Biol Chem 172:469, 1948.

92. Bruce WR, Meeker BE, Valeriote FA: Comparison of the sensitivity of normal hematopoietic and transplanted lymphoma colony-forming cells to chemotherapeutic agents administered in vivo. J Natl Cancer Inst 37:233, 1966.

93. Brues AM, Jacobson LO: Comparative therapeutic effects of radioactive and chemical agents in neoplastic disease of the

hemopoietic system. Am J Roentgenol Radium Ther Nucl Med 58:774, 1947.

94. Brunner KW, Young CW: A methylhydrazine derivative in Hodgkin's disease and other malignant neoplasms. Ann Intern Med 63:69, 1965.

95. Bucher O: Divisions nucléaires amitotiques dans des cultures de fibrocytes après l'administration de colchicine. Acta Anat 4:60, 1947.

96. _____: Zur Wirkung von Urethan auf Gewebekulturen in vitro; vorläufige Mitteilung. Schweiz Med Wochenschr 77:1229, 1947.

97. _____: Die Wirkung von Äthylurethan auf die mitotische Zellteilung, untersucht an Gewebekulturen in vitro. Helv Physiol Pharmacol Acta 7:37, 1949.

98. Buckton KE, Dolphin GW, McLean AS: Human Radiation Cytogenetics. Amsterdam, North-Holland, 1967, p 174.

99. _____, Jacobs PA, Court Brown WM, Doll R: A study of the chromosome damage persisting after x-ray therapy for ankylosing spondylitis. Lancet 2:849, 1962.

100. Bullough WS: Stress and epidermal mitotic activity. I. The effects of the adrenal hormones. J Endocrinol 8:265, 1952.

101. Burchenal JH: Folic acid antagonists. Am J Clin Nutr 3:311, 1955.

102. _____: in Rebuck JW, Bethell FH, Monto RW (eds): The Leukemias: Etiology, Pathophysiology and Treatment. New York, Academic Press, 1957, p 625.

103. _____, Babcock GM, Broquist HP, Jukes TH: Prevention of chemotherapeutic effects of 4-amino-N^{10}-methyl-pteroylglutamic acid on mouse leukemia by citrovorum factor. Proc Soc Exp Biol Med 74:735, 1950.

104. _____, Bendich A, Brown GB, Elion GB, Hitchings GH, Rhoads CP, Stock CC: Preliminary studies on the effect of 2,6-diaminopurine on transplanted mouse leukemia. Cancer 2:119, 1949.

105. _____, Burchenal JR, Kushida MN, Johnston SF, Williams BS: Studies on the chemotherapy of leukemia. II. The effect of 4-aminopteroylglutamic acid and 4-amino-N^{10}-methyl-pteroylglutamic acid on transplanted mouse leukemia. Cancer 2:113, 1949.

106. _____, Crossley ML, Stock CC, Rhoads CP: The action of certain ethylenimine (aziridine) derivatives on mouse leukemia. Arch Biochem 26:321, 1950.

107. _____, Dagg MK: Effects of 6-diazo-5-oxo-L-norleucine and 2-ethylamino-thiadiazole on strains of transplanted mouse leukemia. Proc Am Assoc Cancer Res 2:97, 1956.

108. _____, Holmberg EA, Fox JJ, Hemphill SC, Reppert JA: The effects of 5-fluorodeoxycytidine, 5-fluorodeoxyuridine, and related compounds on transplanted mouse leukemias. Cancer Res 19:494, 1959.

109. _____, Johnston SF, Cremer MA, Webber LF, Stock CC: Chemotherapy of leukemia. V. Effects of 2,4,6-triethylenimino-S-triazine and related compounds on transplanted mouse leukemia. Proc Soc Exp Biol Med 74:708, 1950.

110. _____, Karnofsky DA, Kingsley-Pillers EM, Southam CM, Myers WPL, Escher GC, Craver LF, Dargeon HW, Rhoads CP: The effects of the folic acid antagonists and 2,6-diaminopurine on neoplastic disease. With special reference to acute leukemia. Cancer 4:549, 1951.

111. _____, Murphy ML, Ellison RR, Sykes MP, Tan TC, Leone LA, Karnofsky DA, Craver LF, Dargeon HW, Rhoads CP: Clinical evaluation of a new antimetabolite, 6-mercaptopurine, in the treatment of leukemia and allied diseases. Blood 8:965, 1953.

112. _____, Oettgen HF, Holmberg EA, Hemphill SC, Reppert JA: Effect of total-body irradiation on the transplantability of mouse leukemias. Cancer Res 20:425, 1960.

113. Burk D, Laszlo J, Hunter J, Wight K, Woods M: Differential metabolic responses of susceptible and resistant mouse leukemia cells to 8-azaguanine. J Natl Cancer Inst 25:57, 1960.

114. Calne DB, Spiers ASD, Stern GM, Laurence DR, Armitage P: L-Dopa in idiopathic Parkinsonism. Lancet 2:973, 1969.

115. Cameron GR, Courtice FC, Jones RP: The effects of β, β^1-dichlorodiethyl methylamine hydrochloride on the blood-forming tissues. J Pathol Bacteriol 59:425, 1947.

116. Capps JA, Smith JF: Experiments on the leukolytic action of the blood serum of X-rayed cases of leukemia and the injection of human leukolytic serum in a case of leukemia. J Exp Med 9:51, 1907.

117. Carbone PP, Haskell CM, Canellos GP, Leventhal BG, Block J, Serpick AA, Selawry OS: Asparaginase: Early clinical and toxicology studies, in Mathé G (ed.): Advances in the Treatment of Acute (Blastic) Leukemias. New York, Springer-Verlag, 1970, p 46.

118. Cardinali G, Cardinali G, Blair J: Stathmokinetic effect of vincaleukoblastine on

normal bone marrow and leukemic cells. Cancer Res 21:1542, 1961.

119. Carey RW: Comparative study of cytosine arabinoside therapy alone and combined with thioguanine, mercaptopurine or daunomycin in acute myelocytic leukemia. Proc Am Assoc Cancer Res 11:15, 1970.

120. Carter SK, Di Marco A, Ghione M, Krakoff IH, Mathé G (eds.): International Symposium on Adriamycin. New York, Springer-Verlag, 1972.

121. Casati A: Experimentelle Untersuchungen über die Röntgenwirkung auf das Knochenmark. Strahlentherapie 32:721, 1929.

122. ———: Experimentelle Untersuchungen über die Röntgenwirkung auf das Knochenmark. II. Mitteilung. Strahlentherapie 38:315, 1930.

123. Case Records of Massachusetts General Hospital: Case No.3, 1965. New Engl J Med 272:95, 1965.

124. Cerny V, Ujhazy V, Sandor L: Clinical application of myelobromol in chronic myeloses. Neoplasma 13:177, 1966.

125. Chanutin A, Gjessing EC: The effect of nitrogen mustards upon the ultraviolet absorption spectrum of thymonucleate, uracil and purines. Cancer Res., 6, 599, 1946.

126. Chu MY, Fischer GA: A proposed mechanism of action of 1-β-arabino-furanosyl-cytosine as an inhibitor of the growth of leukemic cells. Biochem Pharmacol 11:423, 1962.

127. Clark PA, Hsia YE, Huntsman RG: Toxic complications of treatment with 6-mercaptopurine. Two cases with hepatic necrosis and intestinal ulceration. Br Med J 1:393, 1960.

128. Clark RL Jr (ed): Multiple myeloma, in: Cancer Chemotherapy, Springfield, Ill., Thomas, 1961, p 126.

129. Clarke DA, Barclay RK, Stock CC: Effects of N-methyl-formamide and related compounds in mouse sarcoma 180. Proc Soc Exp Biol Med 84:203, 1953.

130. ———, Philips FS, Sternberg SS, Stock CC, Elion GB, Hitchings GH: 6-Mercaptopurine: Effects in mouse sarcoma 180 and in normal animals. Cancer Res 13:593, 1953.

131. ———, ———, ———, ———: Effects of 6-mercaptopurine and analogs on experimental tumors. Ann NY Acad Sci 60:235, 1954.

132. ———, Reilly C, Stock CC: A comparative study of 6-diazo-5-oxo-L-norleucine and 0-

133. diazoacetyl-L-serine on sarcoma 180. Proc Amer Assoc Cancer Res 2:100, 1956.

133. Clarkson BD, Fried J: Changing concepts of treatment in acute leukemia. Med Clin N Am 55:561, 1971.

134. ———, Krakoff I, Burchenal JH, Karnofsky DA, Golbey R, Dowling M, Oettgen H, Lipton A: Clinical results of treatment with E. coli L-asparaginase in adults with leukemia, lymphoma and solid tumors. Cancer 25:279, 1970.

135. Clementi A: Désamidation enzymatique de l'asparagine. Arch Intern Physiol 19:369, 1922.

136. Cline MJ, Rosenbaum E: Prediction of in vivo cytotoxicity of chemotherapeutic agents by their in vitro effect on leukocytes from patients with acute leukemia. Cancer Res 28:2516, 1968.

137. Cole WH: Chemotherapy of Cancer (ed 1). Philadelphia, Lea & Febiger, 1970.

138. Colsky J, Meiselas LE, Rosen SJ, Schulman J: Response of patients with leukemia to 8-azaguanine. Blood 10:482, 1955.

139. Condit PT: Studies on the folic acid vitamins. II. The acute toxicity of amethopterin in man. Cancer 13:222, 1960.

140. ———, Berlin NI, Nathan DG: Studies on the folic acid vitamins. VI. The effect of amethopterin on erythropoiesis in man. Cancer 13:245, 1960.

141. ———, Grob D: Studies on the folic acid vitamins. I. Observations on the metabolism of folic acid in man and on the effect of aminopterin. Cancer 11:525, 1958.

142. Congdon CC, Uphoff D, Lorenz E: Modification of acute irradiation injury in mice and guinea pigs by injection of bone marrow: A histopathologic study. J Natl Cancer Inst 13:73, 1952.

143. Cornman I, Skipper HE, Mitchell JH: The fixation of urethan carbon atoms in sperm and in resting and rapidly dividing cells. Cancer Res 11:195, 1951.

144. Cotzias GC, Van Woert MH, Schiffer LM: Aromatic amino acids and modification of Parkinsonism. N Engl J Med 276:374, 1967.

145. Court Brown WM, Buckton KE, McLean AS: Quantitative studies of chromosome aberrations in man following acute and chronic exposure to x-rays and gamma rays. Lancet 1:1239, 1965.

146. Cramer R: Mitoseverhältnisse bei mit Cortison behandelten Leukämien des Kindesalters. Acta Haematol 8:209, 1952.

147. Cravens WW, Snell EE: Reversal of aminopterin inhibition in the chick embryo

with the *Leuconostoc citrovorum* factor. Proc Soc Exp Biol Med 75:43, 1950.

148.   Craver LF: Priapism in leukemia. Surg Clin N Am 13:472, 1933.

149.   Crowther D: L-Asparaginase and human malignant disease. Nature 229:168, 1971.

150.   _____, Powles RL, Bateman CJT, Beard MEJ, Gauci CL, Wrigley PFM, Malpas JS, Fairley GH, Scott RB: Management of adult acute myelogenous leukaemia. Brit Med J 1:131, 1973.

151.   Cutts JH: The effect of vincaleukoblastine on dividing cells in vivo. Cancer Res 21:168, 1961.

152.   _____, Beer CT, Noble RL: Biological properties of vincaleukoblastine, an alkaloid in *Vinca rosea* Linn., with reference to its antitumor action. Cancer Res 20:1023, 1960.

153.   Dacie JV, Dresner E, Mollin DL, White JC: Aminopterin in the treatment of acute leukaemia. Br Med J 1:1447, 1950.

154.   Dameshek W: Editorial. Blood 3:1057, 1948.

155.   _____: The use of folic acid antagonists in the treatment of acute and subacute leukemia. Blood 4:168, 1949.

156.   _____: The outlook for the eventual control of leukemia. N Engl J Med 250:131, 1954.

157.   _____, Freedman MH, Steinberg L: Folic acid antagonists in the treatment of acute and subacute leukemia. Blood 5:898, 1950.

158.   _____, Granville NB, Rubio F: Therapy of the myeloproliferative disorders with Myleran. Ann NY Acad Sci 68:1001, 1958.

159.   _____, Saunders RH, Zannos L: The use of ACTH in the treatment of acute and subacute leukemia. Bull N Engl Med Center 12:11, 1950.

160.   _____, Schwartz R: Leukemia and autoimmunization—some possible relationships. Blood 14:1151, 1959.

161.   _____, _____: Treatment of certain "autoimmune" diseases with antimetabolites: a preliminary report. Trans Assoc Am Physicians 73:113, 1960.

162.   Dargeon HW: Leukemia in childhood. Current therapeutic considerations. NY J Med 56:2079, 1956.

163.   Davis W: Chemical structure and biological activity of the cytostatic (alkylating) agents. Symposium on anti-tumour agents. Proc Roy Soc Med 50:1, 1957.

164.   De Conti RC, Calabresi P: Use of allopurinol for prevention and control of hyperuricemia in patients with neoplastic disease. N Engl J Med 274:481, 1966.

165.   Deeley TJ, Wood CAP (eds.): Modern Trends in Radiotherapy. London, Butterworth, 1967.

166.   Desai RG: Treatment of chronic granulocytic and lymphocytic leukemia and allied disorders with Myleran and Leukeran in Indian subjects. Acta Haematol Jap 22:160, 1959.

167.   De Vita VT, Serpick AA, Carbone PP: Combination chemotherapy in the treatment of advanced Hodgkin's disease. Ann Intern Med 73:881, 1970.

168.   Diamond HD: Clinical indications for the use of nitrogen mustard and triethylene melamine in malignant lymphomas and leukemias. Ann NY Acad Sci 68:974, 1958.

169.   Diamond I: Transplacental transmission of busulfan (Myleran) in a mother with leukemia. Production of fetal malformation and cytomegaly. Pediatrics 25:85, 1960.

170.   Di Marco A: Mechanism of action of daunomycin. Acta Genet Med Roma 17:102, 1968.

171.   Di Paolo JA, Moore GE, Niedbala TF: The influence of Actinomycin D on animal and human tumors. Proc Amer Assoc Cancer Res 2:195, 1957.

172.   Doan CA, Wiseman BK, Bouroncle BA: Clinical evaluation of CB 1348 in leukemias and lymphomas. Ann NY Acad Sci 68:979, 1958.

173.   Domagk G: Chemotherapy of cancer by ethylenimino quinones: Its foundations and problems. Ann NY Acad Sci 68:1197, 1958.

174.   Dougherty TF, White A: Effect of pituitary adrenotropic hormone on lymphoid tissue. Proc Soc Exp Biol Med 53:132, 1943.

175.   Dowling MD, Krakoff IH, Karnofsky DA: Mechanism of action of anti-cancer drugs, in Cole WH (ed.): Chemotherapy of Cancer. Philadelphia, Lea & Febiger, 1970.

176.   Dunlap CE: Effects of radiation on normal tissue. III. Effects of radiation on the blood and the hemopoietic tissues, including the spleen, the thymus and the lymph nodes. Arch Pathol 34:562, 1942.

177.   Dustin P: Some new aspects of mitotic poisoning. Nature 159:794, 1947.

178.   _____: The cytological action of ethylcarbamate (urethane) and other carbamic esters in normal and leukaemic mice, and in rabbits. Br J Cancer 1:48, 1947.

179.   _____: The growth-inhibiting action of mitotic poisons in experimental and human leukaemias, in Ciba Symposium on Leukaemia Research. London, Churchill, 1954, p 244.

180.   Ehrlich P: in Himmelweit F (ed.): The

Collected Papers: Including a Complete Bibliography. New York, Pergamon, 1956–1957.

181. Elion GB, Bieber S, Nathan HC, Hitchings GH: Uracil antagonism and inhibition of mammary adenocarcinoma 755. Cancer Res 18:802, 1958.

182. ———, Callahan SW, Hitchings GH, Rundles RW: The metabolism of 2-amino-6((1-methyl-4-nitro-5-imidazolyl) thio) purine (B.W.57–322) in man. Cancer Chemother Rep 8:36, 1960.

183. ———, Hitchings GH, Rundles RW: The antitumor effects of 2-amino-6-(1-methyl-4 nitro-5 imidazolyl) thiopurine. Proc Am Assoc Cancer Res 3:18, 1959.

184. ———, ———, Vanderwerff H: Antagonists of nucleic acid derivatives. VI. Purines. J Biol Chem 192:505, 1951.

185. ———, Nathan HC: The effects of metabolites on the antitumor activity of the combination of 6-azauracil and urethane. Proc Am Assoc Cancer Res 2:294, 1958.

186. Ellison RR: Management of acute leukemia in adults. Med Clin N Am 40:743, 1956.

187. ———, Holland JF, Weil M, et al: Arabinosyl cytosine: a useful agent in the treatment of acute leukemia in adults. Blood 32:507, 1968.

188. ———, Hutchison DJ: Metabolism of folic acid and citrovorum factor in leukemic cells, in: Rebuck JW, Bethell FH, Monto RW (eds): The Leukemias. New York, Academic Press, 1957, p 467.

189. ———, Karnofsky DA, Burchenal JH: Clinical evaluation of 6-chloropurine in leukemia of adults. Blood 13:705, 1958.

190. ———, Silver RT, Engle RL: Comparative study of 6-chloropurine and 6-mercaptopurine in acute leukemia in adults. Ann Intern Med 51:322, 1959.

191. ———, Tan CTC, Murphy ML, Krakoff IH: Clinical investigations of 6-azathymine, a thymine analog. Cancer Res 20:435, 1960.

192. Elson LA: A comparison of the effects of radiation and radiomimetic chemicals on the blood. Br J Haematol 1:104, 1955.

193. ———: Hematological effects of the alkylating agents. Ann NY Acad Sci 68:826, 1958.

194. ———, Galton DAG, Till M: The action of chlorambucil (CB1348) and busulfan (Myleran) on the haemopoietic organs of the rat. Br J Haematol 4:355, 1958.

195. Emile-Weil P, Perlès S: Un cas de leucémie myélogène étudié régulièrement par les ponctions couplées des centres hématopoiétiques. Sang 14:161, 1940.

196. Endicott KM: National cancer chemotherapy program. J Chron Dis 8:171, 1958.

197. Engstrom RM, Kirschbaum A, Mixer HW: Effect of urethane on mouse myelogenous leukemia. Science 105:255, 1947.

198. Epstein SS, Timmis GM: "Simple" vitamin B_{12} antimetabolites. Proc Assoc Adv Cancer Res 3:223, 1961.

199. Evans AE, Farber S, Brunet S, Marians PJ: Vincristine in the treatment of acute leukemia in children. Cancer 16:1302, 1963.

200. Evans JS, Musser EA, Mengel GD, Forsblad KR, Hunter JH: Antitumor activity of 1-β-D-arabinofuranosylcytosine hydrochloride (26355). Proc Soc Exp Biol Med 106:350, 1961.

201. Evans TC, Quimby EH: Studies on the effects of radioactive sodium and of roentgen rays on normal and leukemic mice. Am J Roentgenol Radium Ther Nucl Med 55:55, 1946.

202. Fairley GH, Malpas JS, Galton DAG: Clinical experience with L-asparaginase, in: Grundmann E, Oettgen HF (eds.): Recent Results in Cancer Research, vol. 33. London, Heinemann, 1970, p 257.

203. ———, Simister JM (eds.): Cyclophosphamide. Bristol, Wright, 1964.

204. Fallon HJ, Frei E: Clinical and biochemical effect of 6-azauridine in leukemia. Proc Am Assoc Cancer Res 3:224, 1961.

205. ———, ———, Block J Seegmiller JE: The uricosuria and orotic aciduria induced by 6-azauridine. J Clin Invest 40:1906, 1961.

206. Farber S: Some observations on the effect of folic acid antagonists on acute leukemia and other forms of incurable cancer. Blood 4:160, 1949.

207. ———, Appleton R, Downing V, Heald F, King J, Toch R: Clinical studies on the carcinolytic action of triethylenephosphoramide. Cancer 6:135, 1953.

208. ———, D'Angio G, Evans A, Mitus A: Clinical studies on actinomycin D with special reference to Wilms' tumor in children. Ann NY Acad Sci 89:421, 1960.

209. ———, Diamond LK, Mercer RD, Sylvester RF, Wolff JW: Temporary remissions in acute leukemia in children produced by folic acid antagonist, 4-aminopteroyl-glutamic acid (aminopterin). N Engl J Med 238:787, 1948.

210. Fell HB, Allsopp CB: The action of mustard gas (β, β^1-dichlorodiethylsulfide) on living cells in vitro. Cancer Res 8:145, 1948.

211. Fialkow PJ, Thomas ED, Bryant JI, Neiman PE: Leukaemic transformation of

engrafted human marrow cells in vivo. Lancet 1:251, 1971.

212. Fischer A, Laser H: Studien über Sarkomzellen in vitro V. Über Phagozytose von Zellen des Rous' Sarkom und von Fibroblasten in vitro. Arch exp Zellforsch 3:363, 1927.

213. Fischer G: Increased levels of folic acid reductase as a mechanism of resistance to amethopterin in leukemic cells. Biochem Pharmacol 7:75, 1961.

214. Flory CM, Steinhardt ID, Furth J: Further observations on the effect of benzene on a strain of myeloid chloroleukemia in mice and on changes produced in the leukemic cells by the chemical. Blood 1:367, 1946.

215. Foley GE, Friedman OM, Drolet BP: Studies on the mechanism of action of Cytoxan. Evidence of activation in vivo and in vitro. Cancer Res 21:57, 1961.

216. Ford CE, Hamerton JL, Barnes DWH, Loutit JF: Cytological identification of radiation-chimaeras. Nature 177:452, 1956.

217. Forkner CE: Leukemia and Allied Disorders. New York; Macmillan, 1938.

218. _____, Scott TFM: Arsenic as a therapeutic agent in chronic myelogenous leukemia. Preliminary report. JAMA, 97:3, 1931.

219. Frank W, Osterberg AE: Mitomycin C (NSC-26980)—an evaluation of the Japanese reports. Cancer Chemother Rep 9:114, 1960.

220. Franklin AL, Stokstad, ELR, Jukes TH: Observations on the effect of 4-aminopteroylglutamic acid on mice. Proc Soc Exp Biol Med 67:398, 1948.

221. Frei E, III et al: Studies of sequential and combination antimetabolite therapy in acute leukemia: 6-mercaptopurine and methotrexate. Blood 18:431, 1961.

222. Freireich EJ, Bodey GP, Harris JE, Hart JS: Therapy for acute granulocytic leukemia. Cancer Res 27:2573, 1967.

223. Galbraith PR: Mechanism of action of splenic irradiation in chronic myelogenous leukemia. Canad Med Assoc J 96:1636, 1967.

224. Galton DAG: Myleran in chronic myeloid leukaemia. Lancet 1:208, 1953.

225. _____: A comparison of the effects of radiomimetic drugs and radiation on haemopoiesis in the rat, in Ilbery PLT (ed): Radiobiology. London, Butterworth, 1961, p 298.

226. _____: Israels LG, Nabarro JDN, Till M: Clinical trials of p-(di-2-chloroethylamino)-

phenylbutyric acid (CB1348) in malignant lymphoma. Br Med J 2:1172, 1955.

227. _____, Spiers ASD: Progress in the leukemias. In Brown EB, Moore CV (eds): Progress in Hematology, Vol 7. New York, Grune & Stratton, 1971, p 343.

228. _____, Till, M: Myleran in chronic myeloid leukaemia. Lancet 1:425, 1955.

229. _____, _____, Wiltshaw E: Busulfan (1-4-dimethanesulfonyloxybutane, Myleran): Summary of clinical results. Ann NY Acad Sci 68:967, 1958.

230. _____, Wiltshaw E, Szur L, Dacie JV: The use of chlorambucil and steroids in the treatment of chronic lymphocytic leukaemia. Br J Haematol 7:73, 1961.

231. Garrattini S, Sproston EM (eds.): Antitumoral Effects of Vinca Rosea Alkaloids. Amsterdam, Excerpta Medica, 1966.

232. Gasser C, Cramer R: Leukämie im Kindesalter unter Cortisone und Aminopterin. Helvet Paediatr Acta 8:10, 1953.

233. Geiersbach U: Über den Einfluss der Narkose (Urethan) auf Gewebekulturen. Arch Exp Zellforsch 23:210, 1939.

234. Gellhorn A: Invited remarks on the current status of research in clinical cancer chemotherapy. Cancer Chemother Rep 5:1, 1959.

235. George P, Hernandez K, Hustu O, Borella L, Holton C, Pinkel D: A study of "total therapy" of acute lymphocytic leukemia in children. J Pediatr 72:399, 1968.

236. Gilman A, Philips FS: The biologic actions and therapeutic applications of the β-chloroethyl amines and sulfides. Science 103:409, 1946.

237. Gitlin D, Commerford SL, Amsterdam E, Hughes WL: X-rays affect the incorporation of 5-iododeoxyuridine into deoxyribonucleic acid. Science 133:1074, 1961.

238. Gold GL, Hall TC, Shnider BI, Selawry O, Colsky J, Owens AH, Dederick MM, Holland JF, Brindley CO, Jones R: A clinical study of 5-fluorouracil. Cancer Res 19:935, 1959.

239. Goldacre RJ, Loveless A, Ross WCJ: Mode of production of chromosome abnormalities by the nitrogen mustards: the possible role of cross-linking. Nature 163:667, 1949.

240. Goldin A, Humphreys SR, Chapman GO, Chirigas MA, Venditti JM: Immunity of mice surviving systemic leukemia (L1210) to antifolic resistant variations of the disease. Nature 185:219, 1960.

241. _____, Venditti JM, Humphreys SR, Dennis D, Mantel N, Greenhouse SW: Studies on the toxicity and antileukemic action of 6-mercaptopurine in mice. Ann NY Acad Sci 60:251,1954.

242. _____, _____, _____, Mantel N: Modification of treatment schedules in the management of advanced mouse leukemia with amethopterin. J Natl Cancer Inst 17:203, 1956.

243. Goodhart RS: Introduction to symposium on the antimetabolites. Am J Clin Nutr 3:271, 1955.

244. Goodman LS, Gilman A: The Pharmacological Basis of Therapeutics ed 4 London, Macmillan, 1970.

245. _____, Wintrobe MM, Dameshek W, Goodman MJ, Gilman A, McLennan M: Nitrogen mustard therapy: Use of methylbis (β-chloroethyl) amino hydrochloride for Hodgkin's disease, lymphosarcoma, leukemia and certain allied and miscellaneous disorders. JAMA 132:126, 1946.

246. Graef I, Karnofsky DA, Jager VB, Krichesky B, Smith HW: The clinical and pathologic effects of the nitrogen and sulfur mustards in laboratory animals. Am J Pathol 24:1, 1948.

247. Granville NB, Rubio F, Unugur A, Schulman E, Dameshek W: The treatment of acute leukemia in adults with massive doses of prednisone and prednisolone. N Engl J Med 259:207, 1958.

248. Graw RG, Brown JA, Yankee RA, Leventhal BG, Whang-Peng J, Rogentine GN, Henderson ES: Transplantation of HL-A identical allogeneic bone marrow to a patient with acute lymphocytic leukemia. Blood 36:736, 1970.

249. _____, Herzig GP, Rogentine GN, Yankee RA, Leventhal BG, Whang-Peng J, Halterman RH, Krüger G, Berard C, Henderson ES: Graft versus host reactions complicating HL-A matched bone marrow transplantation. Lancet 2:1053, 1970.

250. _____, Leventhal BG, Yankee RA, Rogentine GN, Whang-Peng J, Ginnif MH, Herzig GP, Halterman RH, Henderson ES: HL-A and MLC matched allogeneic bone marrow transplantation in patients with acute leukemia. Transplantation Proc 3:405, 1971.

251. Green HM, Whiteley HJ: Cortisone and tumour growth. Br Med J 2:538, 1952.

252. Green JW, Lushbaugh CC: Histopathologic study of the mode of inhibition of cellular proliferation by urethane: Effect of urethane on Walker rat carcinoma 256. Cancer Res 9:199, 1949.

253. Green S, Bodansky O: A relationship between NADase activity, NAD+ content and the proliferation of Ehrlich ascites cells. Proc Am Assoc Cancer Res 8:23, 1967.

254. Greenberg ML, Chanana AD, Cronkite E, Schiffer LM, Stryckmans PA: Tritiated thymidine as a cytocidal agent in human leukemia. Blood 28:851, 1966.

255. Greenspan EM: Some theoretical and practical aspects of the use of folic acid antagonists in human neoplasia. J Mt Sinai Hos 19:583, 1952.

256. Gregori A: Wirkung von Röntgenstrahlen auf das Knochenmark "in vivo" und "in vitro." Strahlentherapie 65:163, 1939.

257. Grilli A: Rendiconto statistico di un quinquennio die roentgenterapia; considerazioni in merito alla roentgenterapia delle flogasi oculari e delle leucemie. Arch Radiol 14:463, 1938.

258. Gross R, Lambers K: Erste Erfahrungen in der Behandlung maligner Tumoren mit einem neuen N-Lost-Phosphamidester. Dtsch Med Wochenschr 83:458, 1958.

259. Gunz FW: Culture of human leukaemic blood cells in vitro; some effects of X-rays. Br J Cancer 3:330, 1949.

260. _____: Studies of leukaemic blood in vitro with special reference to the effect of some therapeutic agents. Ph.D. Thesis, Cambridge, 1949.

261. _____: Effect of 4-amino-pteroylglutamic acid (aminopterin) on human leukemic leukocytes in vitro. Blood 5:161, 1950.

262. _____: Bone marrow changes in patients with chronic leukemia treated by splenic x-irradiation. Blood 8:687, 1953.

263. Guyer MF, Claus PE: Effects of urethane (ethyl carbamate) on mitosis. Proc Soc Exp Biol Med 64:3, 1947.

264. Haddow A: Discussion, in Ciba Symposium on Leukaemia Research. London, Churchill, 1954, p 212.

265. _____: Experimental and clinical aspects of the action of various carboxylic acid derivatives in the aromatic nitrogen mustard series, in Ciba Symposium on Leukaemia Research. London, Churchill, 1954, p 196.

266. _____, Kon GAR, Ross WCJ: Effects upon tumours of various haloalkylarylamines. Nature 162:824, 1948.

267. _____, Sexton WA: Influence of carbamic esters (urethanes) on experimental animal tumours. Nature 157:500, 1946.

268. _____, Timmis GM: Myleran in chronic

myeloid leukaemia. Chemical constitution and biological action. Lancet 1:207, 1953.

269. Haggard ME, Fernbach DJ, Holcomb TM, Sutow WW, Vietti TJ, Windmiller J: Vincristine in acute leukemia of childhood. Cancer 22:438, 1968.

270. Hahn PF, Lareau DG, Feaster BL, Carothers EL, Gollan F, Meneely GR, Sherman D: Intravenous radioactive gold in the treatment of chronic leukemia. Acta Radiol 50:565, 1958.

271. Hakala M: On the role of drug penetration in amethopterin resistance of sarcoma-180 cells in vitro. Biochem Biophys Acta 102:198, 1965.

272. _____, Lakrzewski S, Nichol C: Relation of folic acid reductase to amethopterin resistance in cultured mammalian cells. J Biol Chem 236:952, 1961.

273. _____, Nichol CA: Studies on the mode of action of 6-mercaptopurine and its ribonucleoside on mammalian cells in culture. J Biol Chem 234:3224, 1959.

274. Hall TC: Chemotherapy of cancer. N Engl J Med 266:129, 1962.

275. Hamilton L: Utilization of purines for nucleic acid synthesis in man. Nature 172:457, 1953.

276. _____, Elion GB: The fate of 6-mercaptopurine in man. Ann NY Acad Sci 60:304, 1954.

277. Hansen-Pruss OC: Thiouracil in the treatment of leukemia. Proc Soc Exp Biol Med 64:496, 1947.

278. Hardisty RM, Norman PM: Meningeal leukaemia. Arch Dis Child 42:411, 1967.

279. Harrod EK, Cortner JA: Prolonged survival of lymphocytes with chromosomal defects in children treated with 1,3-bis(2-chloroethyl)-1-nitrosourea. J Nat Cancer Inst 40:269, 1968.

280. Haut A, Abbott WS, Wintrobe MM, Cartwright GE: Busulfan in the treatment of chronic myelocytic leukemia. The effect of long-term intermittent therapy. Blood 17:1, 1961.

281. _____, Altman SJ, Cartwright GE, Wintrobe MM: The influence of chemotherapy on survival in acute leukemia. Blood 10:875, 1955.

282. Hawkins JA, Murphy JB: The effect of ethyl urethane anesthesia on the acid-base equilibrium and cell contents of the blood. J Exp Med 42:609, 1925.

283. Hayes DM, Ellison RR: Production of remissions in blastic phase of chronic myelocytic leukemia (CML) and acute myelocytic leukemia (AML) by arabinosyl cytosine (ara-C) plus 1,3 bis-β(2-chloro-

ethyl)-1-nitrosourea (BCNU). Blood 34:840, 1969.

284. _____, Spurr CL, Schroeder LR, Freireich EJ: A clinical trial of sarcolysin in acute leukemia. Cancer Chemother Rep 12:153, 1961.

285. Hayhoe FGJ: 6-Mercaptopurine in acute leukaemia. Lancet 2:903, 1955.

286. Heard BE, Cooke RA: Busulphan lung. Thorax 23:187, 1968.

287. Heilman DH: The effect of 11-dehydro-17-hydroxycorticosterone and 11-dehydrocorticosterone on lymphocytes in tissue culture. Proc Staff Meet Mayo Clin 20:310, 1945.

288. Heilman FR, Kendall EC: The influence of 11-dehydro-17-hydroxycorticosterone (compound E) on the growth of a malignant tumor in the mouse. Endocrinology 34:416, 1944.

289. Heineke H: Über die Einwirkung der Röntgenstrahlen auf innere Organe. Münch Med Wochenschr 51:785, 1904.

290. _____: Experimentelle Untersuchungen über die Einwirkung der Röntgenstrahlen auf innere Organe. Mitt Grenzgeb Med Chir 14:21, 1905.

291. _____: Experimentelle Untersuchungen über die Einwirkung der Röntgenstrahlen auf das Knochenmark, nebst einigen Bemerkungen über die Röntgentherapie der Leukämie und Pseudoleukämie und des Sarkoms. Dtsch Z Chir 78:196, 1905.

292. Hempelmann LH, Lisco H, Hoffman JG: The acute radiation syndrome—A report of nine cases and a review of the problem. Ann Intern Med 36:279, 1952.

293. Henderson ES: Treatment of acute leukemia. Sem Hematol 6:271, 1969.

294. _____, Serpick A, Leventhal B, Henry P: Cytosine arabinoside infusions in adult and childhood acute myelocytic leukemia. Proc Am Assoc Cancer Res 9:29, 1968.

295. Hevesy G: The application of radioactive indicators in biochemistry. J Chem Soc 2:1618, 1951.

296. Hewitt HB, Wilson CW: A survival curve for mammalian leukaemia cells irradiated in vivo (implications for the treatment of mouse leukaemia by whole-body irradiation). Br J Cancer 13:69, 1959.

297. Heyn RM, Brubaker CA, Burchenal JH, Cramblett HG, Wolff JA: The comparison of 6-mercaptopurine with the combination of 6-mercaptopurine and azaserine in the treatment of acute leukemia in children: results of a co-operative study. Blood 15:350, 1960.

298. Hill JM, Loeb E: Treatment of leukemia,

lymphoma, and other malignant neoplasms with vinblastine. Cancer Chemother Rep 15:41, 1961.

299. _____, _____, MacLellan A, Khan A, Roberts J, Shields WF, Hill NO: Response to highly purified L-asparaginase during therapy of acute leukemia. Cancer Res 29:1574, 1969.

300. _____, _____, Speer RJ: Colloidal zirconyl phosphate P^{32} in lymphomas. JAMA 187:106, 1964.

301. _____, Roberts J, Loeb E, Khan A, MacLellan A, Hill RW: L-asparaginase therapy for leukemia and other malignant neoplasms. JAMA 202:882, 1967.

302. Hilton J: Dying. Baltimore, Penguin Books, 1967.

303. Hitchings GH: Purine and pyrimidine antagonists. Amer J Clin Nutr 3:321, 1955.

304. _____: Species differences among dihydrofolate reductases as a basis for chemotherapy. Postgrad Med J 45 (suppl): 7, 1969.

305. _____ and Elion GB: Chemistry and biochemistry of purine analogs. Ann NY Acad Sci 60:195, 1954.

306. Hodes ME, Rohn RJ, Bond WH: Vincaleukoblastine, preliminary clinical studies. Cancer Res 20:1041, 1961.

307. Hoffbrand AV: Megaloblastic anaemias, in Hoffbrand AV, Lewis SM (eds.): Tutorials in Postgraduate Medicine: Haematology. London, Heinemann, 1972.

308. Hoffman WJ, Craver LF: Chronic myelogenous leukemia; value of irradiation and its effect on duration of life. JAMA 97:836, 1011, 1931.

309. Holland JF: Folic acid antagonists. Clin Pharmacol Ther 2:374, 1961.

310. _____: Progress in the treatment of acute leukemia, in Dameshek W, Dutcher RM (eds): Perspectives in Leukemia. New York, Grune & Stratton, 1968, p 217.

311. Hollcroft J, Lorenz E, Congdon CC, Jacobson LO: Factors influencing the irradiation treatment of experimental lymphoid tumors. Rev Mex Radiol 7:115, 1953.

312. Holmes BE: The indirect effect of x-rays on the synthesis of nucleic acid in vivo. Br J Radiol 22:487, 1949.

313. Holton CP, Vietti TJ, Nora AH, Donaldson MH, Stuckey WJ, Watkins WL, Lane DM: Daunomycin and prednisone for induction of remission in advanced leukemia. N Engl J Med 280:171, 1969.

314. Hoogstraten B, Sheehe PR, Cuttner J, Cooper T, Kyle RA, Oberfield RA, Townsend SR, Harley JB, Hayes D, Costa G, Holland JF: Melphalan in multiple myeloma. Blood 30:74, 1967.

315. Hossain MS, Foerster J, Hryniuk W, Israels LG, Chowdhury AS, Biswas MK: Treatment of smallpox with cytosine arabinoside. Lancet 2:1230, 1972.

316. Howard JP: Response of acute leukemia in children to repeated courses of vincristine (NSC 67574). Cancer Chemother Rep 51:465, 1967.

317. _____, Albo V, Newton WA: Cytosine arabinoside. Results of a co-operative study in acute childhood leukemia. Cancer 21:341, 1968.

318. Huennekens FM, Osborn MJ, Whiteley HR: Folic acid coenzymes. Science 128:120, 1958.

319. Humphreys SR, Goldin A: Investigation of tumor variants recovered from mice with systemic leukemia (L1210) after extensive therapy with 3^15^1-dichloroamethopterin and 3^1-bromo-5^1-chloroamethopterin. J Nat Cancer Inst 23:633, 1959.

320. Ingle DJ, Mason HL: Subcutaneous administration of cortin compounds in solid form to the rat. Proc Soc Exp Biol Med 39:154, 1938.

321. Innes J, Rider WD: Multiple myelomatosis treated with a combination of urethane and oral nitrogen mustard. Blood 10:252, 1955.

322. Institoris L, Eckhardt S, Horvath IP, Sellei C: Comparative data on the action mechanism of 1,6-dibromo-1,6-dideoxy-D-mannitol and 1,4-dimethane-sulfonyloxy-n-butane. Arzneim Forsch 16:45, 1966.

323. Isaacs R, Trimmer RW: Blood cell changes in leukemia during aminopterin therapy. Ann Intern Med 35:236, 1951.

324. Israels LG, Galton DAG, Till M, Wiltshaw E: Clinical evaluation of CB 1348 in malignant lymphoma and related diseases. Ann NY Acad Sci 68:915, 1958.

325. Jackson H: The effects of alkylating agents on fertility. Br Med Bull 20:107, 1964.

326. Jacobson LO: Modification of radiation injury. Bull NY Acad Med 30:675, 1954.

327. _____: Hematopoietic responses to radiation injury. Ann Rev Med 7:345, 1956.

328. _____, Marks EK, Gaston EO, Simmons EL, Block MH: Studies on radiosensitivity of cells. Science 107:248, 1948.

329. Jacobson W: The role of the *Leuconostoc citrovorum* factor (LCF) in cell division and the mode of action of folic acid antagonists on normal and leukaemic cells. J Pathol Bacteriol 64:245, 1952.

330. _____: The mode of action of folic acid antagonists on cells. J Physiol 123:603, 1954.

331. _____: The function of the Leuconostoc ci-

trovorum factor in cell division and the inactivation of aminopterin. J Physiol 123:618, 1954.

332. Jansen L: Zur Behandlung chronischer Leukosen mit Ethyleneimidobenzoquinones. Ärztl Wochenschr 13:361, 1958.

333. Jansson G: Die Einwirkung der Röntgenstrahlen auf das Zellprotoplasma. Acta Radiol 8:427, 1927.

334. Jelliffe AM, MacIver JE: Desacetylmethylcolchicine in the treatment of myeloid leukaemia. Br J Cancer 10:634, 1956.

335. Johnson IS, Armstrong JG, Gorman M, Burnett JP: The vinca alkaloids: A new class of oncolytic agents. Cancer Res 23:1390, 1963.

336. _____, Wright HF, Svoboda GH: Experimental basis for clinical evaluation of antitumor principles derived from *Vinca rosea* Linn. J Lab Clin Med 54:830, 1959.

337. _____, Wright HF, Svoboda GH, Vlantis J: Antitumor principles derived from *Vinca rosea* Linn. I. Vincaleukoblastine and leurosine. Cancer Res 20:1016, 1960.

338. Johnson RE: Modern approaches to the radiotherapy of lymphoma. Sem Hematol 6:357, 1969.

339. _____: Total body irradiation of chronic lymphocytic leukemia: Incidence and duration of remission. Cancer 25:523, 1970.

340. Jolly J, Lacassagne A: De la résistance des leucocytes du sang vis-à-vis les rayons X. CR Soc Biol 89:379, 1923.

341. Jones R: Mitomycin C. A preliminary report of studies of human pharmacology and initial therapeutic trial. Cancer Chemother Rep 2:3, 1959.

342. Kaplan S, Calabresi P: Suppression of delayed hypersensitivity in vivo and in vitro by cytosine arabinoside. Clin Res 13:543, 1965.

343. Karnofsky DA: Chemotherapy of neoplastic disease. N Engl J Med 239:226, 260, 299, 1948.

344. _____: Triethylene melamine in the treatment of lymphomas and leukemias. Med Clin N Am 38:541, 1954.

345. _____: Assay of chemotherapeutic agents on developing chick embryo. Cancer Res (Suppl) 3:83, 1955.

346. _____: Summary of results obtained with nitrogen mustard in the treatment of neoplastic disease. Ann NY Acad Sci 68:899, 1958.

347. _____, Graef I, Smith HW: Studies on the mechanism of production of systemic injury by di-β-chloroethylmethylamine hydrochloride. Fed Proc 5:224, 1946.

348. _____, _____, _____: Studies on the mechanism of action of the nitrogen and sulfur mustards in vivo. Am J Pathol 24:275, 1948.

349. Karon M et al: The role of vincristine in the treatment of childhood acute leukemia. Clin Pharmacol Ther 7:332, 1966.

350. Kelly LS, Jones HB: Effects of irradiation on nucleic acid formation. Proc Soc Exp Biol Med 74:493, 1950.

351. Kennedy BJ, Theologides A: Uracil mustard, a new alkylating agent for oral administration in the management of patients with leukemia and lymphoma. N Engl J Med 264:790, 1961.

352. _____, Yarbro JW: Metabolic and therapeutic effects of hydroxyurea in chronic myeloid leukemia. JAMA 195:1038, 1966.

353. Kidd JG: Regression of transplanted lymphomas induced in vivo by means of normal guinea pig serum: I. Course of transplanted cancers of various kinds in mice and rats given guinea pig serum, horse serum, or rabbit serum. J Exp Med 98:565, 1953.

354. _____: Regression of transplanted lymphomas induced in vivo by means of normal guinea pig serum. II. Studies on the nature of the active serum constituent: histological mechanism of the regression: tests for the effects of guinea pig serum on lymphoma cells in vitro: discussion. J Exp. Med 98:583, 1953.

355. Kieler J, Kieler E: The effect of A-methopterin on sensitive and resistant leukemic cells in vitro. Cancer Res 14:428, 1954.

356. Kienle F: Die Sternalpunktion in der Diagnostik. Leipzig, Thieme, 1943.

357. Kihlman BA, Nichols WW, Levan A: The effect of deoxyadenosine and cytosine arabinoside on the chromosomes of human leukocytes in vitro. Hereditas 50:139, 1963.

358. Killman S-Å, Cronkite EP: Treatment of polycythemia vera with Myleran. Amer J Med Sci, 241:218, 1961.

359. Kirschbaum A, Judd T, Lu CS, Engstrom RM, Mixer H: Effect of urethane, x-rays, potassium arsenite, benzol on survival time in transplanted mouse leukemia. Proc Soc Exp Biol Med 68:377, 1948.

360. _____, Lu CS: Effect of urethane on maturation of leukocytes of mouse myelogenous leukemia. Proc Soc Exp Biol Med 65:62, 1947.

361. Koller PC: Comparison of the biological effects of x-rays and radiomimetic chemical agents, in Ilbery PLT (ed): Radiobiology. London, Butterworth, 1961, p 281.

362. _____, Casarini A: Comparison of cytological effects induced by X-rays and nitrogen mustard. Br J Cancer 6:173, 1952.

363. Korbitz BC, Reiquam CW: Radiation

therapy in chronic granulocytic leukaemia. Lancet 1:794,1967.

364. Korst DR, Johnson FD, Frenkel EP, Challenger WL: Preliminary evaluation of the effect of cyclophosphamide on the course of human neoplasms. Cancer Chemother Rep 7:1, 1960.

365. Koyama Y, Tokuyama H: Clinical experience with Nitromin. Ann NY Acad Sci 68:1105, 1958.

366. Krakoff IH, Brown NC, Reichard P: Inhibition of ribonucleoside diphosphate reductase by hydroxyurea. Cancer Res 28:1559, 1968.

367. _____, Ellison RR, Tan CT: Clinical evaluation of thioguanosine. Cancer Res 21:1015, 1961.

368. _____, Karnofsky DA, Burchenal JH: Remission induced by CB1348 in chronic granulocytic leukemia. JAMA 166:629, 1958.

369. _____, Meyer RL: Prevention of hyperuricemia in leukemia and lymphoma: use of allopurinol, xanthine oxidase inhibitor. JAMA 193:1, 1965.

370. _____, Miller DG, Karnofsky DA, Diamond HD, Burchenal JH, Craver LF: Clinical observations of 1,4-bis (2,3-epoxypropyl)-piperazine, one of a new class of alkylating agents. Acta Un Int Cancer 16:867, 1960.

371. _____, Savel H, Murphy ML: Phase II studies of hydroxyurea in adults: Clinical evaluation. Cancer Chemother Rep 40:53, 1964.

372. Kreis W, Burchenal JH, Hutchison D: Influence of a methylhydrazine derivative on the in vivo transmethylation of the S-methyl group of methionine onto purine and pyrimidine bases of RNA. Proc Am Assoc Cancer Res 9:38, 1968.

373. Krippaehne ML, Osgood EE: Studies of the influence of cortisone and hydrocortisone on human leukocytes in culture and in eosinophilic leukemia. Acta Haematol 13:145, 1955.

374. Kritzler RA: Anuria complicating treatment of leukemia. Am J Med 25:532, 1958.

375. Krivit W, Brubaker C, Thatcher LG, Pierce M, Perrin E, Hartmann JR: Maintenance therapy in acute leukemia of childhood. Comparison of cyclic vs. sequential methods. Cancer 21:352, 1968.

376. Kurokawa T: Clinical experience about the Nitromin treatment of malignant new growths. Chiryo Clin Mag 39, no. 10, 1952.

377. Kyle RA, Schwartz RS, Oliner HL, Dameshek W: A syndrome resembling adrenal

cortical insufficiency associated with long-term busulfan (Myleran) therapy. Blood 18:497, 1961.

378. Lacassagne A, Gricouroff G: Au sujet de l'action directe ou indirecte des rayons X. Recherches sur les tissus lymphoïdes en survie. CR Soc Biol 96:862, 1927.

379. Lajtha LG, Lewis CL, Oliver R, Gunning AJ, Sharp AA, Callender ST: Extracorporeal irradiation of the blood. A possible therapeutic measure. Lancet 1:353, 1962.

380. _____, Oliver R, Kumatori T, Ellis F: On the mechanics of radiation effect on DNA synthesis. Radiat Res 8:1, 1958.

381. Landolt RF: Über die Wirkung des Colchicins auf das normale und leukämische Blutbild und Knochenmark. Dtsch Arch Klin Med 191:378, 1943.

382. Larionov LF: Some biological and clinical results from the investigations of the chloroethylamines as anti-tumour drugs. Br J Cancer 10:26, 1956.

383. _____: Peptides, amides and esters of chloroethylamino derivatives of amino acids and of phenylalkancarboxylic acids. A new class of antitumor compounds. Cancer Res 21:99, 1961.

384. _____: Cancer Chemotherapy. Oxford, Pergamon, 1965.

385. _____, Shkodinskaja EN, Troosheikina VI, Khoklov AS, Vasina OS, Novikova MA: Studies on the anti-tumour activity of p-di-(2-chloroethyl)-amino-phenylalanine (sarcolysine). Lancet 2:169, 1955.

386. Lasnitzki I: Some effects of urethane on the growth and mitosis of normal and malignant cells in vitro. Br J Cancer 3:501, 1949.

387. Laszlo J, Stengle J, Wight K, Burk D: Effects of chemotherapeutic agents on metabolism of human acute leukemia cells in vitro. Proc Soc Exp Biol Med 97:127, 1958.

388. Law LW: Effect of urethane on a transplantable acute lymphoid leukemia. Proc Soc Exp Biol Med 66:158, 1947.

389. _____: Origin of the resistance of leukemic cells to folic acid antagonists. Nature 169:628, 1952.

390. _____: The phenomena of resistance and dependence in leukaemic cells, in: Ciba Symposium on Leukaemia Research. London, Churchill, 1954, p 105.

391. _____, Boyle PJ: Development of resistance to folic acid antagonists in transplantable lymphoid leukemia. Proc Soc Exp Biol Med 74:599, 1950.

392. _____, Speirs R: Response of spontaneous lymphoid leukemias in mice to injection of

adrenal cortical extracts. Proc Soc Exp Biol Med 66:226, 1947.

393. _____, Taormina V, Boyle PJ: Response of acute lymphocytic leukemias to the purine antagonist 6-mercaptopurine. Ann NY Acad Sci 60:244, 1954.

394. Lawrence JH: The treatment of chronic leukemia. Med Clin N Am 38:525, 1954.

395. Lawrence JS, Dowdy AH, Valentine WN: Effect of radiation on hemopoiesis. Radiology 51:400, 1948.

396. Lazarus H, McCoy TA, Farber S, Barcell EF, Foley GE: Nutritional requirements of human leukemic cells. Asparagine requirements and the effect of L-asparaginase. Exp Cell Res 57:134, 1969.

397. Lea DH: Actions of Radiations on Living Cells. Cambridge University Press, 1946.

398. Ledingham JCG, McKerron RG: The x-ray treatment of leukaemia. Lancet 1:71, 1905.

399. Leikin S, Brubaker C, Hartmann J, Murphy ML, Wolff J: The use of combination therapy in leukemia remission. Cancer 24:427, 1969.

400. Leonard BJ, Wilkinson JF: Desacetyl-methylcolchicine in treatment of myeloid leukaemia. Br Med J 1:874, 1955.

401. Le Page GA, Jones M: Further studies on the mechanism of action of 6-thioguanine. Cancer Res 21:1590, 1961.

402. Lessmann EM, Sokal JE: A colchicine derivative in therapy of chronic myelocytic leukemia. JAMA 175:741, 1961.

403. Levin I: Action of radium and the x-rays on the blood and blood-forming organs. Am J Roentgenol Radium Ther Nucl Med 9:112, 1922.

404. Levin RH, Henderson E, Karon M, Freireich EJ: Treatment of acute leukemia with methylglyoxal-bis-guanylhydrazone (methyl-GAG). Clin Pharmacol Ther 6:31, 1965.

405. Levine AS, Graw RG, Young RC: Management of infections in patients with leukemia and lymphoma: Current concepts and experimental approaches. Sem Hematol 9:141, 1972.

406. Lewis MR, Crossley ML: Retardation of tumour growth in mice by oral administration of ethylenimine derivatives. Arch Biochem 26:319, 1950.

407. Li JG, Leonard ME, Harrison G: Effect of myleran treatment on the P^{32} uptake of leukocytic deoxyribonucleic acid in chronic granulocytic leukemia. Cancer 9:963, 1956.

408. Lindsley DL, Odell TT, Tausche FG: Implantation of functional erythropoietic elements following total-body irradiation. Proc Soc Exp Biol Med 90:512, 1955.

409. Linke A: Die Behandlung der Hämo-blastosen und malignen Tumoren mit Trisäthyleniminobenzochinon. Dtsch Med Wochenschr 85:1928, 1960.

410. _____, Freudenberger B: Über die Chemotherapie der Hamoblastosen und malignen Tumoren, in: Symposien aktueller therapeutischer Probleme, No. 3. Stuttgart: Enke, 1960, p 38.

411. Linser P, Helber E: Experimentelle Untersuchungen über die Einwirkung der Röntgenstrahlen auf das Blut und Bemerkungen über die Einwirkung von Radium und ultraviolettem Lichte. Dtsch Arch Klin Med 83:479, 1905.

412. Lissauer: Zwei Fälle von Leucaemie. Berl Klin Wochenschr 2:403, 1865.

413. Little PA, Oleson JJ, SubbaRow Y: The effect of nutrition on the tumor response in Rous chicken sarcoma. J Lab Clin Med 33:1139, 1948.

414. _____, Sampath A, Paganelli V, Locke E, and SubbaRow, Y: The effect of folic acid and its antagonists on Rous chicken sarcoma. Trans NY Acad Sci. [Series II] 10:91, 1948.

415. _____, _____, SubbaRow Y: The use of antagonists of pteroylglutamic acid in controlling Rous chicken sarcoma. J Lab Clin Med 33:1144, 1948.

416. Loge JP, Rundles RW: Urethane (ethyl carbamate) therapy in multiple myeloma. Blood 4:201, 1949.

417. Lorenz E, Congdon CC: Modification of lethal irradiation injury in mice by injection of homologous or heterologous bone marrow. J Natl Cancer Inst 14:955, 1954.

418. _____, _____, Uphoff D: Modification of acute irradiation injury in mice and guinea pigs by bone marrow injections. Radiology 58:863, 1952.

419. _____, Uphoff D, Reid TR, Shelton B: Modification of irradiation injury in mice and guinea pigs by bone marrow injections. J Natl Cancer Inst 12:197, 1951.

420. Loveless A, Revell S: New evidence on the mode of action of "mitotic poisons". Nature 164:938, 1949.

421. Ludford RJ: The action of toxic substances upon the division of normal and malignant cells in vitro and in vivo. Arch Exp Zellforsch 18:411, 1936.

422. McGovern JJ, Russell PS, Atkins L, Webster EW: Treatment of terminal leukemic relapse by total-body irradiation and intravenous infusion of stored autologous bone marrow obtained during remission. N Engl J Med 260:675, 1959.

423. McIver FA, Curreri AR, Russo FR, Hogle

GS, Schilling RF, Jaesche WH: Oxa-pentamethylenediethylene thiophosphor-amide (OPSPA) in the treatment of human cancer. Ann NY Acad Sci 68:1183, 1958.

424. McKelvey EM, Kwaan HC: Cytosine arabinoside therapy for disseminated herpes zoster in a patient with IgG pyroglobu-linemia. Blood 34:706, 1969.

425. Magill GB, Myers WPL, Reilly HG, Putnam RC, Magill JW, Sykes MP, Escher GC, Karnofsky DA, Burchenal JH: Pharmacological and initial therapeutic ob-servations on 6-diazo-5-oxo-L-norleucine (DON) in human neoplastic disease. Cancer 10:1138, 1957.

426. Malawista SE, Sato H, Bensch KG: Vin-blastine and griseofulvin reversibly disrupt the living mitotic spindle. Science 160:770, 1968.

427. Marmont A: Il cortisone come anti-mitotico, e le sue associazioni con gli antimitotici, nel trattamento delle emolinfoblastosi, in: Proceedings of the first Symposium on Antimitotics, San Remo, Italy, 1955.

428. _____, Damasio E: The effects of two al-kaloids derived from *vinca rosea* on the ma-lignant cells of Hodgkin's disease, lympho-sarcoma and acute leukemia *in vivo*. Blood 29:1, 1967.

429. Mathé G: Advances in the Treatment of Acute (Blastic) Leukemias. London, Heine-mann, 1970.

430. _____, Amiel JL, Schwarzenberg L, Cat-tan A, Schneider M: Haematopoietic chimera in man after allogeneic homolo-gous bone marrow transplantation. Control of the secondary syndrome. Specific tolerance due to chimerism. Br Med J 2:1666, 1963.

431. _____, Bernard J: Essai de traitement des leucémies expérimentales par la greffe de cellules hématopoiétiques normales. Sang 30:789, 1959.

432. _____, _____, de Vries MJ, Schwarzen-berg L, Larrieu MJ, Lalanne CM, Dutreix A, Amiel JL, Surmont J: Nouveaux essais de greffe de moelle osseuse homologue après irradiation totale chez des enfants at-teints de leucémie aiguë en rémission. Le problème du syndrome secondaire chez l'homme. Rev Hématol 15:115, 1960.

433. _____, Hayat M, Schwarzenberg L, Amiel JL, Schneider M, Cattan A, Schlumberger JR, Jasmin C: Acute lymphoblastic leukaemia treated with a combination of prednisone, vincristine, and rubidomycin. Value of pathogen-free rooms. Lancet 2:380, 1967.

434. Matthias JQ, Misiewicz JJ, Scott RB: Cy-clophosphamide in Hodgkin's disease and related disorders. Br Med J 2:1837, 1960.

435. May HB, Vallance-Owen J: Para-aminobenzoic acid in leukaemia. Effect on the leucocyte count. Lancet 2:607, 1948.

436. Medical Research Council's Working Party on the Evaluation of Different Methods of Therapy in Leukaemia: Treatment of acute leukaemia in adults: Comparison of steroid and mercaptopurine therapy alone and in conjunction. Br Med J 1:1383, 1966.

437. Medical Research Council's Working Party for Therapeutic Trials in Leukaemia: Chronic granulocytic leukaemia: Com-parison of radiotherapy and busulphan therapy. Br Med J 1:201, 1968.

438. Meier R, Schär B, Neipp L: Die Wirkung von Demecolceinamiden an Zellen in vitro. Experientia 10:74, 1954.

439. Meldolesi G, Giusti M: Azione del radon sulle culture in vitro di tessuto mieloide. Pathologica 26:235, 1934.

440. Meyer LM: Use of folic acid derivatives in the treatment of human leukemia. Trans NY Acad Sci 10:99, 1948.

441. Milchner R, Mosse M: Zur Frage der Be-handlung der Blutkrankheiten mit Röntgenstrahlen. Berl Klin Wochenschr 41:1267, 1904.

442. _____, Wolff W: Bemerkungen zur Frage der Leukotoxinbildung durch Röntgenbes-trahlung. Berl Klin Wochenschr 43:747, 1906.

443. Miller DG, Diamond HD: The biological basis and clinical application of bone mar-row transplantation. Med Clin N Am 45:711, 1961.

444. _____, _____, Craver LF: The clinical use of chlorambucil; a clinical study. N Engl J Med 261:525, 1959.

445. _____, _____, _____: The clinical use of epoxypiperazine, a new alkylating agent, in the treatment of lymphomas and other neo-plasms. Cancer Res 19:1204, 1959.

446. Miner RW: 6-mercaptopurine. Ann NY Acad Sci 60: 183, 1954.

447. Minot GR, Buckman TE, Isaacs R: Chronic myelogenous leukemia: age inci-dence, duration and benefit derived from ir-radiation. JAMA 82:1489, 1924.

448. _____, Isaacs R: Lymphatic leukemia: age incidence, duration and benefit derived from irradiation. Boston Med Surg J 191:1, 1924.

449. Moeschlin S: Die Milzpunktion. Basel, Schwabe, 1947.

450. _____: Zum Wirkungsmechanismus des Urethans bei Leukämien. Helvet Med Acta 14:279, 1947.

451. _____: Phase contrast microscopy of leukocytes, in: Rebuck JW, Bethell FH, Monto RW (eds): The Leukemias, Etiology, Pathophysiology and Treatment. New York, Academic Press, 1957, p 646.

452. _____, Meyer H, Lichtman A: A new colchicine derivative (demecolcin Ciba) as a cytostatic agent in myelogenous leukaemia, in: Ciba Symposium on Leukaemia Research. London, Churchill, 1954, p 216.

453. Mollendorff W von: Zur Kenntnis der Mitose: über regulierbare Einwirkungen auf die Zahl und den Ablauf der Mitosen in Gewebekulturen. Arch Exp Zellforsch 21:1, 1938.

454. Murphy JB, Sturm E: The effect of adrenal cortical and pituitary adrenotropic hormones on transplanted leukemia in rats. Science 99:303, 1944.

455. _____, _____: The effect of urethane on lymphatic leukemia in rats. Science 104:427, 1946.

456. _____, _____: The inhibiting effect of ethyl urethane on the development of lymphatic leukemia in rats. Cancer Res 7:417, 1947.

457. Murphy ML, Del Moro A, Lacon C: The comparative effects of five polyfunctional alkylating agents on the rat fetus, with additional notes on the chick embryo. Ann NY Acad Sci 68:762, 1958.

458. _____, Tan TC, Ellison RR, Karnofsky DA, Burchenal JH: Clinical evaluation of chloropurine and thioguanine. Proc Am Assoc Cancer Res 2:36, 1955.

459. Nadkarni MV, Trams EG, Smith PK: Preliminary studies on the distribution and fate of TEM, TEPA and Myleran in the human. Cancer Res 19:713, 1959.

460. Nagel A: Ueber die Wirkung verschiedener Faktoren, inbesondere narkotisierender Substanzen auf die vitale Methylenblaufärbung bei in vitro gezüchteten Fibrocyten. Z. Zellforsch Mikrosk Anat 13:405, 1931.

461. Napier LE, Sen Gupta PC, Chaudhuri RN: Myeloid leukaemia: The treatment by deep x-rays. Indian Med Gaz 72:329, 1937.

462. Needham DM, Cohen JA, Barrett AM: The mechanism of damage to the bone marrow in systemic poisoning with mustard gas. Biochem J 41:631, 1947.

463. Neumann A: Über die Wirkung der Röntgenstrahlen auf die Leukocyten in vitro. Strahlentherapie 18:74, 1924.

464. Nichol CA, Welch AD: On the mechanism of action of aminopterin. Proc Soc Exp Biol Med 74:403, 1950.

465. Nowell PC, Cole LJ, Habelmeyer JG, Roan PL: Growth and continued function of rat marrow cells in X-irradiated mice. Cancer Res 16:258, 1956.

466. Oehme J: Nebenwirkungen von Cytostatica im Kindesalter, in: Klinik und Therapie der Nebenwirkungen. Stuttgart, Thieme, 1960, p 1099.

467. Oettgen HF, Old LJ, Boyse EA, Campbell HA, Philips FS, Clarkson BD, Tallal L, Leeper RD, Schwartz MK, Kim JH: Inhibition of leukemia in man by L-asparaginase. Cancer 27:2619, 1967.

468. _____, et al: Toxicity of E. coli L-asparaginase in man. Cancer 25:253, 1970.

469. Ohler RL, Houghton JD, Moloney WC: Urethane toxicity. N Engl J Med 243:984, 1950.

470. Oishi N, Swisher SN, Troup SB: Busulfan therapy in myeloid metaplasia. Blood 15:863, 1960.

471. Oleson JJ, Hutchings BL, SubbaRow Y: Studies on the inhibitory nature of 5-aminopteroylglutamic acid. J Biol Chem 175:359, 1948.

472. Oliner H, Schwartz R, Dameshek W: Studies in experimental autoimmune disorders. I. Clinical and laboratory features of autoimmunization (runt disease) in the mouse. Blood 17:20, 1961.

473. Oliver R, Shepstone BJ: Extracorporeal irradiation of the blood: the mathematical problem of dosimetry. Br J Haematol 10:181, 1964.

474. Ono J: Studies on the survival length of leucocytes in vitro, tested by their amoeboid movements. III. The influence of various radiant energies thereon. Trans Jap Pathol Soc 19:172, 1929.

475. Osgood EE: Effects of irradiation on leukemic cells in marrow cultures. Proc Soc Exp Biol Med 45:131, 1940.

476. _____: The results of a 15-year program of treatment of the chronic leukemias with titrated, regularly spaced total-body irradiation with P^{32} or x-rays, in: Proceedings of the Sixth Congress of the International Society of Hematology. New York, Grune & Stratton, 1956.

477. _____: Treatment of the chronic leukemias. J Nucl Med 5:139, 1964.

478. _____, Aebersold PC, Erf LA, Packham EA: Studies of the effects of million volt roentgen rays, 200 kilovolt roentgen rays, radioactive phosphorus, and neutron rays by the marrow culture technique. Am J Med Sci 204:372, 1942.

479. _____, Bracher GJ: Culture of human

marrow. Studies of the effects of roentgen rays. Ann Intern Med 13:563, 1939.

480. _____, Chu IT: The effect of nitrogen mustard on granulocytic cells as observed by the marrow culture technic. Cancer Res 10:98, 1950.

481. _____, Seaman AJ: Treatment of chronic leukemias. Results of therapy by titrated, regularly-spaced total body radioactive phosphorus, or roentgen irradiation. JAMA 150:1372, 1952.

482. Papac R, Galton DAG, Till M, Wiltshaw E: Preliminary clinical trial of p-di-2-chloroethyl-amino-L-phenylalanine (CB-3025, melphalan) and of di-2-chloroethyl methane-sulfonate (CB1506). Ann NY Acad Sci 68:1126, 1958.

483. Pappenheim A: Experimentelle Beiträge zur neueren Leukämie-Therapie. Z Exp Pathol Therap 15:39, 1914.

484. Parsons WB, Watkins CH, Pease GL, Childs DS: Changes in sternal marrow following roentgen-ray therapy to the spleen in chronic granulocytic leukemia. Cancer 7:179, 1954.

485. Paterson E, Haddow A, ApThomas I, Watkinson JM: Leukaemia treated with urethane compared with deep x-ray therapy. Lancet 1:677, 1946.

486. _____, Kunkler PB: The effect of 1:3 bis(ethyleneimino sulphonyl) propane in animal tumours and human leukaemia, in: Ciba Symposium on Leukaemia Research. London, Churchill, 1954, p 231.

487. Patt HM: Factors in the radiosensitivity of mammalian cells. Ann NY Acad Sci 59:649, 1955.

488. Pearson OH, Eliel LP: Use of pituitary adrenocorticotropic hormone (ACTH) and cortisone in lymphomas and leukemias. JAMA 144:1349, 1950.

489. _____, _____: Experimental studies with ACTH and cortisone in patients with neoplastic disease. Recent Prog Hormone Res 6:373, 1951.

490. _____, _____, Rawson RW: Regression of lymphoid tumors in man induced by ACTH and cortisone, in Mote, JR (ed.): Proceedings of the First Clinical ACTH Conference, vol 1. Philadelphia, Blakiston, 1950, p 381.

491. _____, _____, _____, Dobriner K, Rhoads CP: ACTH and cortisone-induced regression of lymphoid tumors in man. A preliminary report. Cancer 2:943, 1949.

492. _____, _____, Talbot TR, Burchenal JH, Petro AT, Poppel JW, Craver LF: The use of ACTH and cortisone in acute leukemia. Blood 5:786, 1950.

493. Pegg DE: Bone Marrow Transplantation. London, Lloyd-Luke, 1966.

494. Petering HG: Folic acid antagonists. Physiol Rev 32:197, 1952.

495. Petrakis NL, Bierman HR, Kelly KH, White LP, Shimkin MB: The effect of 1,4-dimethanesulfonoxybutane (GT-41 or Myleran) upon leukemia. Cancer 7:383, 1954.

496. Philips FS, Sternberg SS, Hamilton L, Clarke DA: The toxic effects of 6-mercaptopurine and related compounds. Ann NY Acad Sci 60:283, 1954.

497. _____, Thiersch JB, Ferguson FC: Studies of the action of 4-aminopteroyl-glutamic acid and its congeners in mammals. Ann NY Acad Sci 52:1349, 1950.

498. Pillers EMK, Burchenal JH, Eliel LP, Pearson OH: Resistance to corticotropin, cortisone and folic acid antagonists in leukemia. JAMA 148:987, 1952.

499. _____, Magalini SI: Hematological changes following treatment with p(di-2-chloroethylamino)-phenylbutyric acid (CB1348) in cancer. I. Effect on lymphocytes and platelets. Cancer 11:410, 1958.

500. Piney A, Riach JS: The treatment of chronic myeloid leukaemia. Br J Radiol 5:393, 1932.

501. Pinkel D: Actinomycin D in childhood cancer. A preliminary report. Pediatrics 23:342, 1959.

502. _____: Five year follow-up of "total therapy" of childhood lymphocytic leukemia. JAMA 216:648, 1971.

503. _____, Hernandez K, Borella L, Holton C, Aur R, Samoy G, Pratt C: Drug dosage and remission duration in childhood lymphocytic leukemia. Cancer 27:247, 1971.

504. _____, Simone J, Hustu HO, Aur RJA: Nine years' experience with "total therapy" of childhood acute lymphocytic leukemia. Pediatrics 50:246, 1972.

505. Pizer LI, Cohen SS: Metabolism of pyrimidine arabinonucleosides and cyclonucleosides in Escherichia coli. J Biol Chem 235:2387, 1960.

506. Poncher HG, Waisman HA, Richmond JB, Horak OA, Limarzi LR: Treatment of acute leukemia in children with and without folic acid antagonists. J Pediatr 41:377, 1952.

507. Pusey WA: Report of cases treated with roentgen rays. JAMA 38:911, 1902.

508. Rachmilewitz M, Rosin A, Goldhaber G,

Doljanski L: Studies on bone marrow in vitro. IV. The effect of roentgen rays on explanted bone marrow. Am J Roentgenol Radium Ther Nucl Med 58:464, 1947.

509. Ramanan SV, Israëls MCG: Treatment of chronic myeloid leukaemia with dibromannitol. Lancet 2:125, 1969.

510. Rambert P: Action d'une cortine extractive sur un cas de leucémie lymphoïde splénomégalique. Bull Mém Soc Méd Hôp Paris 66:302, 1950.

511. Reboul J, Delorme G, Tavernier J, Geindre M: Essai thérapeutique à l'or radioactif dans les leucémies chroniques. Ann Radiol 4:11, 1961.

512. Regelson W, Holland JF: Clinical experience with methylglyoxal bis (guanylhydrazone) dihydrochloride: A new agent with clinical activity in acute myelocytic leukemia and the lymphomas. Cancer Chemother Rep 27:15, 1963.

513. Reiner B, Zamenhof S: Studies on the chemically reactive groups of deoxyribonucleic acids. J Biol Chem 228:475, 1957.

514. Reizenstein PG: Cytochemical changes in bone marrow cells from rats affected by aminopterin. A microspectrophotometric study of individual cells. Acta Haematol 23:65, 1960.

515. Report of the United Nations Scientific Committee on the Effects of Atomic Radiation. Supplement no. 14 (A/5814). New York, United Nations, 1964.

516. Rider WD, Warwick OH: Clinical experience with the use of R-48 (NN-di-2¹-chloroethyl-2¹-naphthylamine). Ann NY Acad Sci 68:1116, 1958.

517. Rinaldini LM: The antimitotic action of an aromatic nitrogen mustard on tissue cultures. Br J Cancer 6:186, 1952.

518. Robbins GP, Cooper JAD, Alt L: Effect of corticotropin on cellularity and mitosis in the rat bone marrow, spleen and thymus. Endocrinology 56:161, 1955.

519. Rogers S: Studies of the mechanisms of action of urethane in initiating pulmonary adenomas in mice. J Exp Med 105:279, 1957.

520. Rose FL, Hendry JA, Walpole AL: New cytotoxic agents with tumour-inhibitory activity. Nature 165:993, 1950.

521. Rosenow G: Ueber die Resistenz der einzelnen Leukocytenarten des Blutes gegen Thorium X. Z Gesamte Exp Med 3:385, 1914.

522. Rosenthal MC: In Proceedings of the Second Clinical ACTH Conference, vol. II. Philadelphia, Blakiston, 1951, p 259.

523. _____, Saunders RH, Schwartz LI, Zannos L, Perez-Santiago E, Dameshek W: The use of adrenocorticotropic hormones and cortisone in the treatment of leukemia and leukosarcoma. Blood 6:804, 1951.

524. Rosin A: Effect of urethane (ethyl carbamate) on the mitotic activity in the bone marrow of normal mice. Blood 6:652, 1951.

525. _____, Goldhaber G: The effect of repeated doses of urethane (ethyl carbamate) on the mitotic activity and cellular composition of the bone marrow of normal mice. Blood 11:1032, 1956.

526. Ross WCJ: In vitro reactions of biological alkylating agents. Ann NY Acad Sci 68:669, 1958.

527. Rubinstein MA: Chemotherapy of multiple myeloma; the use of antimony; a preliminary report. Blood 2:555, 1947.

528. _____: Use of antimony in multiple myeloma. Blood 4:1068, 1949.

529. Rundles RW, Coonrad EV, Willard NL: Summary of results obtained with TEM. Ann NY Acad Sci 68:926, 1958.

530. _____, Dillon ML, Dillon ES: Multiple myeloma. III. Effect or urethane therapy on plasma cell growth, abnormal serum protein components and Bence Jones proteinuria. J Clin Invest 29:1243, 1950.

531. _____, Wyngaarden JB, Hitchings GH, Elion GB, Silberman HR: Effects of xanthine oxidase inhibitor on thiopurine metabolism, hyperuricemia and gout. Trans Assoc Am Physicians 76:126, 1963.

532. _____, et al: Comparison of chlorambucil and Myleran in chronic lymphocytic and granulocytic leukemia. Am J Med 27:424, 1959.

533. Rusconi A, Calendi E: Action of daunomycin on nucleic acid metabolism in HeLa cells. Biochem Biophys Acta 119:413, 1966.

534. Sacks MS, Bradford GT, Schoenbach EB: The response of acute leukemia to the administration of the folic acid antagonists, aminopterin and amethopterin. Report of 14 cases. Ann Intern Med 32:80, 1950.

535. Sandberg JS, Howsden FL, Di Marco A, Goldin A: Comparison of the antileukemic effect in mice of adriamycin (NSC-123127) with daunomycin (NSC-82151). Cancer Chemother Rep 54:1, 1970.

536. Sandler SG, Tobin W, Henderson ES: Vincristine-induced neuropathy: A clinical study of fifty leukemia patients. Neurology 19:367, 1969.

537. Santavy F, Reichstein T: Isolierung neuer Stoffe aus den Samen der Herbstzeitlose

Colchicum autumnale L. Substanzen der Herbstzeitlose und ihre Derivate. Helvet Chim Acta 33:1606, 1950.

538. Schabel FM, Skipper HE, Trader MW, Wilcox WS: Experimental evaluation of potential anticancer agents XIX. Sensitivity of nondividing leukemic cell populations to certain classes of drugs in vivo. Cancer Chemother Rep 48:17, 1965.

539. Schär B, Loustalot P, Gross F: Demecolcin (Substanz F) ein neues, aus Colchicum autumnale isoliertes Alkaloid mit starker antimitotischer Wirkung. Klin Wochenschr 32:49, 1954.

540. Schiffer LM, Atkins HL, Chanana AD, Cronkite EP, Greenberg ML, Stryckmans PA: Extracorporeal irradiation of blood (ECIB) in man. II. Treatment of acute myelocytic leukemia. Blood 31:17, 1968.

541. _____, Chanana AD, Cronkite EP, Greenberg ML, Joel DD, Schnappauf HP, Stryckmans PA: Extracorporeal irradiation of the blood. Sem Hematol 3:154, 1966.

542. Schoenbach EB, Greenspan EM: The pharmacology, mode of action, and therapeutic potentialities of stilbamidine, pentamidine, propamidine and other aromatic diamidines—a review. Medicine 27:327, 1948.

543. _____, _____, Colsky J: Reversal of aminopterin and amethopterin toxicity by citrovorum factor. JAMA 144:1558, 1950.

544. Schrek R: Studies in vitro on cellular physiology. The effect of x-rays on the survival of cells. Radiology 46:395, 1946.

545. _____: Studies in vitro on the physiology of cells. Factors affecting the delayed cytocidal action of x-rays. J Cell Comp Physiol 28:277, 1946.

546. _____: Dual morphologic reactions of rabbit lymphocytes to x-rays. Arch Pathol 63:252, 1957.

547. _____: In vitro sensitivity of normal human lymphocytes to x-rays and radiomimetic agents. J Lab Clin Med 51:904, 1958.

548. _____, Friedman IA, Leithold SL: Variability of the in vitro sensitivity of human leukemic lymphocytes to x-rays and chemotherapeutic agents. J Natl Cancer Inst 20:1037, 1958.

549. _____, Leithold SL, Friedman IA: In vitro sensitivity of human leukemic cells to x-rays. Proc Soc Exp Biol Med 94:250, 1957.

550. Schroeder LR: Clinical trial of 3'5' dichloromethotrexate. Proc Am Assoc Cancer Res 3:267, 1961.

551. Schulman I: In: Proceedings of the Second

Clinical ACTH Conference, vol. II. Philadelphia, Blakiston, 1951, p 281.

552. Schulze E, Fritze E, Müller HH: Die Wirkung des Urethans bei Leukämien. Dtsch Med Wochenschr 72:371, 1947.

553. Schwartz R, Dameshek W: Drug-induced immunological tolerance. Nature 183:1682, 1959.

554. _____, _____: Effects of 6-mercaptopurine on homograft rejection. J Clin Invest 39:952, 1960.

555. _____, Stack J, Dameshek W: Effect of 6-mercaptopurine on antibody production. Proc Soc Exp Biol Med 99:164, 1958.

556. Schwarz G: Die Röntgenbehandlung einiger Erkrankungen des Blutes und der blutbildenden Organe (Leukämie und Lymphogranulomatose). Wien Med Wochenschr 11:1275, 1927.

557. Seeger DR, Smith JM, Hultquist ME: Antagonist for pteroylglutamic acid. J Am Chem Soc 69:2567, 1947.

558. Seil FJ, Lampert PW: Neurofibrillary tangles induced by vincristine and vinblastine sulfate in central and peripheral neurons in vitro. Exp Neurol 21:219, 1968.

559. Sellei C: Treatment of myeloproliferative diseases. Ther Hung 14:135, 1966.

560. _____, Eckhardt S: Clinical observations with 1,6-bis (β-chloroethylamino)-1,6-deoxy-D-mannitol dihydrochloride (BCM) in malignant diseases. Ann NY Acad Sci 68:1164, 1958.

561. Senn N: The therapeutic value of the roentgen ray in the treatment of pseudoleucaemia. N.Y. Med J 77:65; 1903.

562. _____: Case of splenomedullary leukemia successfully treated by the use of the Roentgen ray. Med Rec 64:281, 1903.

563. Shanbrom E, Miller S, Haar H, Opfell R: Therapeutic spectrum of uracil mustard, a new oral antitumor drug: with special reference to effects of small dosage in lymphomas, chronic leukemias and ovarian carcinoma. JAMA 174:1702, 1960.

564. Shapira J, Cornstein I, Wells W, Winzler RJ: Metabolism of human leukocytes in vitro. IV. Incorporation and interconversion of adenine and guanine. Cancer Res 21:265, 1961.

565. Shay H, Zarafonetis C, Smith N, Woldow I, Sun DCH: Treatment of leukemia with triethylene thiophosphoramide (thioTEPA). Preliminary results in experimental and clinical leukemia. Arch Intern Med 92:628, 1953.

566. Shedden WIH (ed.): The Vinca Alkaloids in

the Chemotherapy of Malignant Disease, vol. 2. London, Lilly Industries Ltd, 1971.

567. Sheehy TW, Ransome JW: Demecolcine (Colcemid) toxicity. Arch Intern Med 100:85, 1957.

568. Sherwood F: Use of urethane in treatment of leukemia (review of literature). Acta Haematol 1:253, 1948.

569. Shnider BI, Frei E, Tuohy JH, Gorman J, Freireich EJ, Brindley CO, Clements J: Clinical studies of 6-azauracil. Cancer Res 20:28, 1960.

570. Silk MH, Hawtrey AO, Macintosh IJC: Indirect effects during x-radiation of malignant tumors. Cancer Res 18:1257, 1958.

571. Silver RT: The treatment of chronic lymphocytic leukemia. Sem Hematol 6:344, 1969.

572. Skipper HE: A review: On the mechanism of action of certain temporary anti-cancer agents. Cancer Res 13:545, 1953.

573. _____: On the mechanism of action of 6-mercaptopurine. Ann NY Acad Sci 60:315, 1954.

574. _____: Cellular kinetics associated with "curability" of experimental leukemia, in Dameshek W, Dutcher RM (eds): Perspectives in Leukemia. New York, Grune & Stratton, 1968.

575. _____, Bennett LL, Bryan CE, White L, Newton MA, Simpson L: Carbamates in the chemotherapy of leukemia. VIII. Overall tracer studies on carbonyl-labeled urethan, methylene-labeled urethan and methylene-labeled ethyl alcohol. Cancer Res 10:166, 1951.

576. _____, _____, Edwards PC, Bryan CE, Hutchison OS, Chapman JB, Bell M: Antileukemic assays on certain pyrimidines, purines, benzimidazoles, and related compounds. Cancer Res 10:166, 1950.

577. _____, Bryan CE, Riser WH, Welty M, Stelzenmuller A: Carbamates in the chemotherapy of leukemia. II. The relationship between chemical structure, leukopenic action and acute toxicity of a group of urethan derivatives. J Natl Cancer Inst 9:77, 1948.

578. _____, Burchenal JH: The nucleic acid inhibiting action of 4-amino-N^{10}-methyl-pteroylglutamic acid in mice with a sensitive and resistant strain of leukemia. Cancer Res 11:229, 1951.

579. _____, Mitchell JH, Bennett LL: Inhibition of nucleic acid synthesis by folic acid antagonists. Cancer Res 10:510, 1950.

580. _____, _____, _____, Newton MA, Simpson L, Eidson M: Observations on in-hibition of nucleic acid synthesis resulting from administration of nitrogen mustard, urethan, colchicine, 2,6-diaminopurine, 8-azaguanine, potassium arsenite, and cortisone. Cancer Res 11:145, 1951.

581. _____, Schabel FM, Binns V, Thomson JR, Wheeler GP: Studies on the mechanism of action and anticancer activity of N-methylformamide. Cancer Res 15:143, 1955.

582. _____, _____, Wilcox WS: Experimental evaluation of anticancer agents. XIII. On the criteria and kinetics associated with "curability" of experimental leukemia. Cancer Chemother Rep 35:1, 1964.

583. Smith CH: Discussion in: Proc. 2nd. Conf. Folic Acid Antagonists in the Treatment of Leukemia. Blood 7:140, 1952.

584. Snapper I: Stilbamidine and pentamidine in multiple myeloma. JAMA 133:157, 1947.

585. _____, Mirsky AE, Ris H, Schneid B, Rosenthal M: Development of inclusion bodies containing ribose nucleic acid in myeloma cells after injections of stilbamidine. Determination of stilbamidine in myeloma tissue. Blood 2:311, 1947.

586. _____, Schneid B: On the influence of stilbamidine upon myeloma cells. Blood 1:534, 1946.

587. Snell EE, Cravens WW: Reversal of aminopterin inhibition in the chick embryo with desoxyribosides. Proc Soc Exp Biol Med 74:87, 1950.

588. Snelling CE, Donohue WL, Laski B, Jackson SH: Pituitary adrenocorticotropic hormone (ACTH) and 11-dehydro-17-hydroxycorticosterone (cortisone) therapy in the leukemias and lymphomas of children. Pediatrics 8:22, 1951.

589. Souhami RS, Clifton JS, Emery EW, Godlee JN, Prankerd TAJ, Provan JL: Extracorporeal irradiation in the treatment of acute leukaemia. Lancet 2:13, 1969.

590. Speed DR, Galton DAG, Swan A: Melphalan in the treatment of myelomatosis. Br Med J 1:1664, 1964.

591. Spiers ASD: Haemorrhagic cystitis and cyclophosphamide. Lancet 2:1282, 1963.

592. _____: Experience with procarbazine in the treatment of acute leukaemia and other neoplasms. Med J Aust 2:732, 1967.

593. _____: Chemotherapy of cancer: its application in general practice. Clin Med 76:22, 1969.

594. _____: Cure as the aim in therapy for the acute leukaemias. Lancet 2:473, 1972.

595. _____: In preparation.

596. Spurr CL, Smith TR, Jacobson LO: Che-

motherapy in human lymphomas, leukemias, and allied disorders of the hemopoietic system. Radiology 50:387, 1948.

597. Stearns B, Losee KA, Bernstein J: Hydroxyurea: A new type of potential antitumour agent. J Med Chem 6:201, 1963.

598. Stenstrom W, King JT: Effects of radiation on tissue cultures of lymph nodes. Proc Soc Exp Biol Med 31:909, 1934.

599. Stephens DJ: Chronic myelogenous leukemia. Observations before and during remissions induced by solution of potassium arsenate and by roentgen therapy with particular reference to bone marrow. Am J Med Sci 194:25, 1937.

600. Stewart JSS, Sanderson AR: Chromosomal aberration after diagnostic x-irradiation. Lancet 1:978, 1961.

601. Stickney JM, Mills SD, Hagedorn AB, Cooper T: The treatment of acute leukemia with folic acid antagonists. Mayo Clin Proc 24:525, 1949.

602. Stock CC: Aspects of approaches in experimental cancer chemotherapy, Am J Med 8:658, 1950.

603. _____, Reilly HC, Buckley SM, Clarke DA, Rhoads CP: Azaserine, a new tumour-inhibitory substance; studies with Crocker mouse sarcoma 180. Nature 173:71, 1954.

604. Stoll BA: Advanced cancer treated with Nitromin. Med J Aust 2:882, 1956.

605. Storer JB, Lushbaugh CC, Furchner JE: The protective effect of shielded ectopic bone marrow against total body x-irradiation. J Lab Clin Med 40:355, 1952.

606. Storti E: Clinical studies on the effect of imuran and vincristine in the treatment of leukaemia. Acta Genet Med 17:220, 1968.

607. Strumia MM: On the generalized effect of radiations in myelogenous leukemia. Am J Med Sci 177:676, 1929.

608. Sugiura K: Antitumor activity of mitomycin C. Cancer Chemother Rep 13:51, 1961.

609. _____, Schmid MS: Effects of antibiotics on the growth of a variety of mouse and rat tumors. Proc Am Assoc Cancer Res 2:151, 1956.

610. _____, Stock CC: The effect of Mitomycin on a spectrum of tumors. Proc Am Assoc Cancer Res 2:350, 1958.

611. Sullivan MP, Haggard ME, Donaldson MH, Krall J: Comparison of the prolongation of remission in meningeal leukemia with maintenance intrathecal methotrexate (IT MTX) and intravenous bis-nitrosourea (BCNU). Proc Am Assoc Cancer Res 11:77, 1970.

612. _____, Vietti TJ, Fernbach DJ, Griffith KM, Haddy TB, Watkins WL: Clinical investigations in the treatment of meningeal leukemia: radiation therapy regimens vs conventional intrathecal methotrexate. Blood 34:301, 1969.

613. Swendseid ME, Bethell FH, Bird OD: The concentration of folic acid in leukocytes. Observations on normal subjects and persons with leukemia. Cancer Res 11:864, 1951.

614. _____, Swanson AL, Meyers MC, Bethell FH: The nutritional status of folic acid in persons with leukemia and its possible relation to effects of aminopterin therapy. Blood 7:307, 1952.

615. _____, _____, Miller S, Bethell FH: The metabolic displacement of folic acid by aminopterin. Studies in leukemia patients. Blood 7:302, 1952.

616. _____, Wittle EL, Moersch GW, Bird OD, Brown RA: Studies in the rat of inhibitors of pteroylglutamic acid structurally related to this vitamin. Fed Proc 7:299, 1948.

617. Sykes MP: Myleran in the treatment of lymphomas. Ann NY Acad Sci 68:1035, 1958.

618. _____ Karnofsky DA, Philips FS, Burchenal JH: Clinical studies on triethylenephosphoramide and diethylenephosphoramide, compounds with nitrogen mustard-like activity. Cancer 6:142, 1953.

619. _____, Philips FS, Karnofsky DA: Comparative therapeutic activity of the nitrogen mustards and allied compounds. Med Clin N Am 40:837, 1956.

620. Taft LI: Methotrexate induced hepatitis in childhood leukemia. Israel J Med Sci 1:823, 1965.

621. Tan CTC, Dargeon HW, Burchenal JH: The effect of actinomycin D on cancer in childhood. Pediatrics 24:544, 1959.

622. _____, Tasaka H, Yu KP, Murphy ML, Karnofsky D: Daunomycin, an antitumor antibiotic, in the treatment of neoplastic disease. Cancer 20:333, 1967.

623. Tarnowski GS, Stock CC: Chemotherapy studies on the RC and S790 mouse mammary carcinomas. In: Cancer Res., 18, Cancer Chemotherapy Screening Data, I, 1.

624. Templeman WA, Sexton WA: Effect of some arylcarbamic esters and related compounds upon cereals and other plant species. Nature 156:630, 1945.

625. Thiersch JB, Philips FS: Effects of 4-aminopteroylglutamic acid in dogs with special reference to megaloblastosis. Proc Soc Exp Biol Med 71:484, 1949.

626. Thomas ED, Bryant JI, Buckner CD, Clift
      RA, Fefer A, Johnson FL, Neiman P,
      Ramberg RE, Storb R: Leukaemic
      transformation of engrafted human marrow
      cells in vivo. Lancet 1:1310, 1972.

627. ———, Buckner CD, Rudolph RH, Fefer
      A, Storb R, Neiman PE, Bryant JI, Chard
      RL, Clift RA, Epstein RB, Fialkow PJ,
      Funk DD, Giblett ER, Lerner KG,
      Reynolds FA, Slichter S: Allogeneic mar-
      row grafting for hematologic malignancy
      using HL-A matched donor-recipient sibling
      pairs. Blood 38:267, 1971.

628. ———, ———, Storb R, Neiman PE,
      Fefer A, Clift RA, Slichter SJ, Funk DD,
      Bryant JI, Lerner KE: Aplastic anaemia
      treated by marrow transplantation. Lancet
      1:284, 1972.

629. ———, Epstein RB, Eschbach JW, Prager
      D, Buckner CD, Marsaglia G: Treatment of
      leukemia by extracorporeal irradiation. N
      Engl J Med 273:6, 1965.

630. ———, Lochte HL, Cannon JH, Sahler
      OD, Ferrebee JW: Supralethal whole-body
      irradiation and isologous marrow trans-
      plantation in man. J Clin Invest 38:1709,
      1959.

631. ———, ———, Ferrebee JW: Irradiation
      of the entire body and marrow trans-
      plantation: Some observations and com-
      ments. Blood 14:1, 1959.

632. Thygesen JE, Videbaek A, Villaume I:
      Treatment of leukaemia with artificial
      radio-active sodium. Acta Radiol 25:305,
      1944.

633. Timmis GM, Williams DC: Chemotherapy
      of Cancer. The Antimetabolite Approach.
      London, Butterworth, 1967.

634. Tough IM, Buckton KE, Baikie AG, Court
      Brown WM: X-ray induced chromosome
      damage in man. Lancet 2:849, 1960.

635. ———, Court Brown WM, Baikie AG,
      Buckton KE, Harnden DG, Jacobs PA,
      Williams JA: Chronic myeloid leukaemia:
      Cytogenetic studies before and after splenic
      irradiation. Lancet 2:115, 1962.

636. ———, Jacobs PA, Court Brown WM,
      Baikie AG, Williamson ERD: Cytogenetic
      studies on bone-marrow in chronic myeloid
      leukaemia. Lancet 1:844, 1963.

637. Trams EG, Nadkarni MV, Smith PK: On
      the mechanism of action of the alkylating
      agents. I. Interaction of alkylating agents
      with nucleic acids. Cancer Res 21:560, 1961.

638. ———, ———, ———: On the
      mechanism of action of alkylating agents.
      II. Effects of nitrogen mustard, Myleran
      and x-radiation on nucleic acid biosynthesis.
      Cancer Res 21:567, 1961.

639. Trentin JJ: Transplantation of bone mar-
      row. Blood 13:266, 1958.

640. Trowell OA: The sensitivity of lymphocytes
      to ionizing radiation. J Pathol Bacteriol
      64:687, 1952.

641. Tsuzuki M: Experimental studies on the bio-
      logical action of hard roentgen rays. Am J
      Roentgenol Radium Ther Nucl Med 10:134,
      1926.

642. Ultmann JE, Hyman GA, Gellhorn A:
      Chlorambucil and triethylene thiophos-
      phoramide in the treatment of neoplastic
      disease. Ann NY Acad Sci 68:1007, 1958.

643. Underwood GE: Activity of 1-β-D-
      arabinofuranosyl cytosine hydrochloride
      against herpes simplex keratitis. Proc Soc
      Exp Biol Med 111:660, 1962.

644. Unugur A, Schulman E, Dameshek W:
      Treatment of chronic granulocytic leukemia
      with Myleran. N Engl J Med 256:727, 1957.

645. Valentine WN, Pearce ML: Studies on the
      radiosensitivity of bone marrow. I. The
      relative sensitivity of erythroid and myeloid
      elements. Blood 7:1, 1952.

646. ———, ———, Lawrence JS: Studies on
      the radiosensitivity of bone marrow. II. The
      effect of large, repeated whole-body irradia-
      tion exposure on hematopoiesis. Blood 7:14,
      1952.

647. Vargha L: Über neue Zuckerderivate mit
      zytostatischer Wirksamkeit. Naturwissen-
      schaften 42:582, 1955.

648. Venditti JM, Humphreys SR, Mantel N,
      Kline I, Goldin A: Evaluation of
      antileukemic agents employing advanced
      leukemia L1210 in mice. III. Congeners of
      folic acid. Cancer Res 20: 698, 1960.

649. Vogel AW: Tumor and marrow damage oc-
      curring from methotrexate, monofluo-
      romethotrexate, and dichloromethotrexate.
      Cancer Res 21:743, 1961.

650. Vogler WR, Huguley CM, Rundles RW:
      Comparison of methotrexate with 6-
      mercaptopurine-prednisone in treatment of
      acute leukemia in adults. Cancer 20:1221,
      1967.

651. Wakaki S: Recent advance in research on
      antitumor mitomycins. Cancer Chemother
      Rep 13:79, 1961.

652. Waksman S: Actinomycin. Antibiot Che-
      mother 4:502, 1954.

653. Waldenström J: Melphalan therapy in my-
      elomatosis. Br Med J 1:859, 1964.

654. Walker IG, Watson WJ: The reaction of
      mustard gas with the purine portion of
      deoxyribonucleic acid. Can J Biochem
      39:365, 1961.

655. Wall RL, Conrad FG: Cyclophosphamide
      therapy. Its use in leukemia, lymphoma and

solid tumors. Arch Intern Med 108:456, 1961.

656. Walpole AL: In: Symposium on Anti-Tumour Agents. Proc Roy Soc Med 50:4, 1957.

657. _____: Carcinogenic action of alkylating agents. Ann NY Acad Sci 68:750, 1958.

658. Warren S: Mechanism of radiation effects against malignant tumors. JAMA 133:462, 1947.

659. Warthin AS: An experimental study of the effects of roentgen rays upon the blood-forming organs, with special reference to the treatment of leukemia. Int Clin 4:243, 1906.

660. _____: The minute changes produced in leukemic tissues by exposure to Roentgen rays. Amer J Med Sci 147:72, 1914.

661. Warwick OH, Alison RE, Darte JMM: Clinical experience with vinblastine sulfate. Can Med Assoc J 85:579, 1961.

662. _____, Darte JMM, Brown TC: Some biological effects of vincaleukoblastine, an alkaloid in *Vinca rosea* Linn., in patients with malignant disease. Cancer Res 20:1032, 1961.

663. Watson JD, Crick FHC: Molecular structure of nucleic acids: A structure for deoxyribose nucleic acid. Nature 171:737, 1953.

664. Weisberger AS, Heinle RW: Protective effect of cysteine on leucopenia induced by nitrogen mustard. J Lab Clin Med 36:872, 1950.

665. _____, _____, Levine B: Some structural requirements for the prevention of leukopenia induced by nitrogen mustard. J Clin Invest 31:217, 1952.

666. _____, _____: Incorporation of radioactive L-cystine by normal and leukemic leukocytes in vivo. Blood 9:1082, 1954.

667. _____, Suhrland LG: Comparative incorporation of S^{35} L-cystine and S^{35} sodium sulfate by normal and leukemic leukocytes. Blood 10:458, 1955.

668. _____, _____: Studies on analogues of L-cysteine and L-cystine. II. The effect of selenium cystine on leukemia. Blood 11:19, 1956.

669. _____, _____, Seiffer J: Studies on analogues of L-cysteine and L-cystine. I. Some structural requirements for inhibiting the incorporation of radioactive L-cystine by leukemic leukocytes. Blood 11:1, 1956.

670. Wells BB, Kendall EC: The influence of corticosterone and C17 hydroxydehydrocorticosterone (Compound E) on somatic growth. Proc Staff Meet Mayo Clin 15:324, 1940.

671. Werkheiser WC: Specific binding of 4-amino folic acid analogues by folic acid reductase. J Biol Chem 236:888, 1961.

672. _____: The biochemical, cellular, and pharmacological action and effects of the folic acid antagonists. Cancer Res 23:1277, 1963.

673. Western KA, Perera DR, Schultz MG: Pentamidine isethionate in the treatment of *Pneumocystis carinii* pneumonia. Ann Intern Med 73:695, 1970.

674. Wheeler GP, Bowdon BJ: Effects of 1,3-bis(2-chloroethyl)-*1*-nitrosourea and related compounds upon the synthesis of DNA by cell-free systems. Cancer Res 28:52, 1968.

675. _____, Chumley S: Alkylating activity of 1,3 bis-(2-chloroethyl)-*1*-nitrosourea and related compounds. J Med Chem 10:259, 1967.

676. Whitby L: Whither clinical pathology? Trends and opportunities. J Clin Pathol 4:129, 1951.

677. _____: The present-day treatment of acute leukemia. in: Proceedings of the Sixth Congress of the International Society of Hematology. New York, Grune & Stratton, 1956.

678. _____: The concept of leukaemia. Austr Ann Med 5:237, 1956.

679. Whitecar JP, Bodey GP, Freireich EJ: Combination chemotherapy (COAP) of adult acute leukemia. Proc Am Assoc Cancer Res 11:83, 1970.

680. Whitehouse JMA, Crowther D, Bateman CJT, Beard MEJ, Malpas JS: Adriamycin in the treatment of acute leukaemia. Br Med J 1:482, 1972.

681. Whitelaw DM, Teasdale JM: Vincaleukoblastine in the treatment of malignant disease. Can Med Assoc J 85:584, 1961.

682. Whitelock O v. St, Furness FN, Cameron MP, Stahl FS, Karnofsky DA: Comparative clinical and biological effects of alkylating agents. Ann NY Acad Sci 68:657, 1958.

683. Wilkinson JF: Chemotherapy of the reticuloses. Proc Roy Soc Med 46:685, 1953.

684. _____, Fletcher F: Effect of B-chlorethylamine hydrochlorides in leukaemia, Hodgkin's disease and polycythaemia vera. Lancet 2:540, 1947.

685. Wilson SJ: Platelet regeneration during therapy of acute leukemia with folic acid antagonists. Proc Soc Exp Biol Med 73:620, 1950.

686. Winzler RJ, Williams AD, Best WR: Metabolism of human leukocytes in vitro. I. Effects of A-methopterin on formate-C^{14} incorporation. Cancer Res 17:108, 1957.

687. Woolley DW: Recent advances in the study of biological competition between structurally related compounds. Physiol Rev 27:308, 1947.

688. World Health Organization: Chemotherapy of cancer. First Report of an expert committee. WHO Tech Rep Ser 272: 1972.

689. _____: Drug Therapy of Cancer. Geneva: WHO, 1973.

690. Zadek I: Radiothorium bei leukämischer Lymphadenose. Tierexperimentelle Ergebnisse mit dem zur Behandlung der Leukämie verwendeten Radiothorium. Folia Haematol 48:39, 210, 1932.

691. Zarafonetis CJD, Andrews GA, Meyers MC, Bethell FH: Para-aminobenzoic acid in leukemia. Blood 3:780, 1948.

692. _____, Shay H, Sun DCH: Triethylenethiophosphoramide in the treatment of chronic leukemia. Cancer 8:512, 1955.

Alexander S. D. Spiers

18

Management of the Different Forms
of Leukemia

The treatment of chronic lymphocytic leukemia and chronic granulocytic leukemia by organized medicine has a long history, beginning with the use of arsenic in 1865.[203] This toxic and relatively inefficient treatment was replaced by more potent therapy after ionizing radiations were first used in 1902.[268] Many technical refinements were introduced to facilitate the application of radiotherapy, which continues to be widely employed in the chronic leukemias after 70 years, although advances in antileukemic chemotherapy in the last 20 years have lessened its importance.

In contrast, effective treatment for any form of acute leukemia has been available for only a quarter of a century. In 1948, Farber[104] reported remissions in acute leukemia in children after treatment with the folic acid antagonist, aminopterin. Although these remissions proved only temporary, and all the patients eventually relapsed and died, a new era had begun. For the first time, it was possible by administration of a chemical agent to affect the course of a hitherto inexorably fatal disease so that the patient was restored to good health and apparent clinical and hematologic normality. The years since this initial limited success have seen remarkable progress as a result of the efforts of thousands of workers in scores of centers. It is not possible here to consider in detail the many small steps by which this major progress has been achieved, but it is summarized in numerous reviews.[25,28,66,91,114,117,118,127,152,159,160,213,232,242,306,307,357] Study of such reviews in the order of their publication reveals both an evolution of methodology and a basic alteration of approach with the passage of time. The method of leukemia therapy 20 years ago was by today's standards an uninformed empiricism. A small number of drugs were used in a relatively haphazard fashion and often in a way now known to be suboptimal; therapy with one agent at a time was the rule, and combination therapy was exceptional and sometimes strongly criticized as being reckless. The present methodology of treatment for the acute leukemias, though very imperfect, is much more sophisticated and takes into account the clinical pharmacology of the antileukemic drugs, their activity in the different phases of the cell cycle, and some basic knowledge of the reproductive kinetics of leukemic cells. Combination drug therapies for acute leukemia are becoming the rule rather than the exception, and with the increasing use of such treatment, more attention is now being paid to possible synergistic and antagonistic effects between different antileukemic agents when they are administered together. Without doubt these advances have greatly improved the treatment of acute leukemia; with equal certainty they have made the practice of leukemia therapy more difficult and complex.

As treatment has improved and prognosis has lengthened, the basic approach to the patient with acute leukemia has altered. It used to be felt—with excellent reason—that all acute leukemias were inevitably fatal, and few physicians would employ hazardous or unpleasant therapy in order to secure a short postponement of this unavoidable outcome. Therapeutic programs rightly laid much emphasis on the quality of life rather than its duration alone, and this attitude was reinforced by the usually disastrous results of heroic therapy applied to the near-terminal patient. However, acceptance of the idea that some acute leukemias might be eradicated, or their course greatly prolonged by aggressive chemotherapy appropriately applied, led to programs where the heroic measures were used on well patients early in their disease, rather than on ill patients near to death. It is not surprising that this approach has yielded much better results in terms of survival and possible eradication of the disease in some patients. Because the advantages of this type of program are now becoming apparent, this altered approach to the patient is now becoming widely accepted. Twenty years ago the physician's attitude could fairly have been described as a compassionate fatalism, whereas today it is an aggressive optimism.

THE ACUTE LEUKEMIAS

When to Treat Acute Leukemia

Acute leukemia does not always require treatment at the time of diagnosis. Virtually all patients require some supportive measures such as the correction of anemia by transfusion, but a few patients require no more than this. Although the number of patients who should not receive antileukemic chemotherapy from the outset is small, it is important to recognize them. Acute lymphocytic leukemia should almost always be treated at once, because its course is uniformly one of fairly rapid deterioration, while the available therapy is highly effective and relatively nontoxic, inducing remission in over 90 percent of patients in 3–6 weeks with little myelosuppression.

Not all patients with acute granulocytic leukemia should be treated immediately. It has been suggested[72] that some varieties of acute granulocytic leukemia should not receive intensive chemotherapy because they usually respond poorly: most physicians concerned with leukemia do not accept this view, but it did draw attention to the fact that the risks of chemotherapy for acute granulocytic leukemia must be balanced against the possible benefits and the possible outcome of employing supportive measures alone. Certain groups of patients may be recognized in whom aggressive therapy may be withheld, at least until the benefits of conservative measures have been assessed:

1. Patients over the age of 60 or those with multiple pathology not related to their leukemia
2. Patients with smoldering acute leukemia
3. Patients with refractory acute leukemias

The older patient.   The aged or those with serious cardiac, respiratory, renal, or hepatic disease are very prone to develop serious multiple complications when antileukemic chemotherapy is administered. For example, neutropenia and infection are common in the early stages of treatment of any patient with acute leukemia: in the elderly patient, such infections are not infrequently further complicated by the onset of cardiac and renal failure, often with a fatal outcome. The greatly enhanced risks of therapy in these patients must decrease the likelihood of a beneficial result. Transfusion of blood and platelets will sometimes maintain such patients in reasonable health for weeks or even months, whereas aggressive chemotherapy not uncommonly leads to their early demise.

Smoldering acute leukemia.   This variant of acute leukemia is difficult to diagnose without a period of observation and conservative treatment. Smoldering acute leukemia may account for about 5 percent of acute leukemia in adults,[184,271] but is insufficiently characterized to be classified as a disease entity. There is usually a pancytopenia in the peripheral blood and the bone marrow is cellular, with the morphologic features of an acute granulocytic leukemia, but the picture does not progress, even though no specific therapy is given. The patients are usually over 50 years old and may survive for months or years, with more or less static hematologic features, when treated by transfusion alone. Antileukemic chemotherapy does not usually benefit smoldering leukemia, and if this diagnosis is suspected, usually in an elderly patient, it may be advisable to administer only supportive therapy until observation over a period has established whether the leukemia is, indeed, nonprogressive. However, it must be emphasized that even in the elderly, most acute granulocytic leukemias are not of the smoldering type, and in progressive acute leukemia, excessive therapeutic procrastination may do harm.

Refractory acute leukemias.   Certain acute leukemias, including a high proportion of cases of erythroleukemia, the metamorphosis of chronic granulocytic leukemia, and the acute leukemias which occasionally terminate the course of polycythemia vera, myelofibrosis, or aplastic anemia are recognized as exceptionally refractory to treatment. Complete hematologic remission is very rare, while serious complications of the aggressive chemotherapy usually required are very common. Occasionally, such leukemias respond to a more conservative approach, and this may be tried before committing the patient to aggressive chemotherapy with small hope of benefit. In special centers this conservative attitude must be balanced against a very great need to pursue research into the treatment of these refractory conditions.

Apart from the above small groups, the majority of patients with acute leukemia should receive specific antileukemic chemotherapy from the time of diagnosis.

Remission in Acute Leukemia

Remission in acute leukemia has nowadays become sufficiently commonplace as to excite little comment, yet it is a remarkable phenomenon. The untreated patient usually has florid manifestations of a lethal condition, with symptoms, clinical signs, and gross abnormalities in the peripheral blood and the bone marrow (see Chapter 10). With the successful induction of remission, all these findings be-

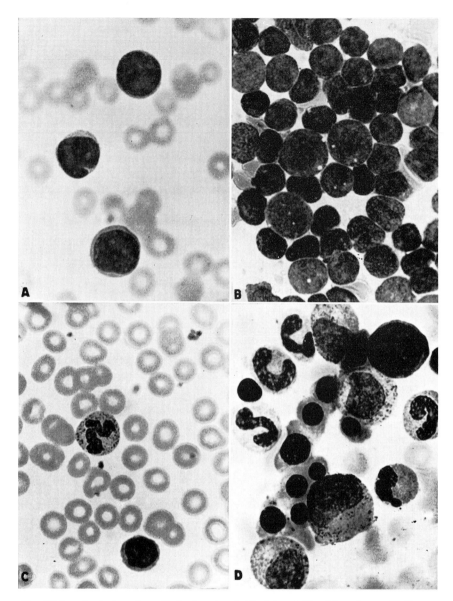

Fig. 18-1. Acute lymphocytic leukemia. A. Peripheral blood in relapse. B. Bone marrow in relapse. C. Peripheral blood in remission. D. Bone marrow in remission. All, × 1100.

come, for a time, both clinically and pathologically undetectable and the patient is restored to his previous state of health (Fig. 18-1). This change is so dramatic that understandably some of the earliest remissions were mistaken for cures, but this misapprehension was short-lived. After a variable interval the disease always reappeared, usually in identical form, and progressed to a fatal termination. This seemingly inevitable recrudescence of the illness reflects the inadequacy of current hematologic techniques for demonstrating residual leukemia after remission has been induced. Extensive histologic studies of 31 patients with acute leukemia in remission, involving biopsy of the kidneys, liver, and testes, multiple bone marrow aspirations, and lumbar puncture demonstrated foci of leukemic cells in 12 patients.[216]

Even studies of this type, which are too extensive for routine clinical use, are clearly inadequate since there was no reason to suppose that the 19 patients in whom no evidence of residual leukemia was found had actually been cured. Thus, the attainment of complete clinical and hematologic remission must be regarded as only one step along the road toward eradication of the patient's leukemia.

To compare the results of treatment by different programs and at different institutions, it is necessary to have specific criteria for the definition of remission. One set of criteria is set out in Table 18-1, but is no longer entirely acceptable. First, the normal blood values for leukemia in remission are not really definable[160]: with many

Table 18-1
Criteria for Evaluation of Response to Therapy in Acute Leukemia

A. Bone marrow (differential on 200 cells)
   1. Reduction in the number of blasts to less than 10 percent with lymphocytes to less than 20 percent; essentially normal-appearing granulopoiesis, erythropoiesis, and thrombopoiesis
   2. Improvement as evidenced by an increase in normal myelopoiesis to more than 30 percent of total nucleated cells, and a reduction in number of blasts and lymphocytes to less than 70 percent
   3. No improvement, or less than that sufficient to qualify for A2
B. Peripheral blood
   1. Return to and maintenance for more than one month of:
      a. Hemoglobin greater than 11 gm per 100 ml for children under 15 years or 10 gm per 100 ml for infants under 2 years of age
      b. Granulocyte levels in excess of 1500 per cubic millimeter
      c. Platelet counts greater than 100,000 per cubic millimeter
      d. Absence of leukemic cells
   2. Improvement as evidenced by an increase in normal granulocytes to levels as in B-1b, and maintenance of hemoglobin at levels of 9 gm per 100 ml or better for more than 1 month
   3. No change, or less than that shown in B-2
C. Physical findings
   1. Subsidence of all evidence of leukemic infiltration
   2. Fifty percent or more reduction in physical measurement of organ with greatest leukemic infiltration
   3. No change
D. Clinical symptoms
   1. No symptoms ascribable to leukemia
   2. Definite improvement though still symptomatic
   3. No change

Complete remission: A-1, B-1, C-1, D-1
Partial remission: A-1 or A-2, B-1 or B-2, C-1 or C-2, D-1 or D-2
Relapse: Complete remission shall be terminated when:
   1. Leukemic cells in marrow increase to 20 percent or more, or the total number of leukemic cells and lymphocytes exceeds 50 percent
   2. In the peripheral blood the leukemic cells appear in excess of 10 percent of the differential count, or the total number of leukemic cells and lymphocytes exceeds 70 percent
   3. Definite evidence of leukemic infiltration (other than CNS) occurs
   4. Symptoms definitely ascribable to leukemia appear

From Bisel.[30]

of the programs of intensive antileukemic chemotherapy in use today, patients in hematologic remission at times have anemia, neutropenia, and thrombocytopenia and would fail to meet the criteria cited in Table 18-1. In acute lymphocytic leukemia of childhood, some centers now use the remission criteria laid down at the St. Jude's Children's Research Hospital, Memphis, Tennessee.[252] In remission, bone marrow is cellular with satisfactory hematopoiesis and contains 5 percent or less lymphoblasts plus stem cells and 40 percent or less lymphocytes plus lymphoblasts plus stem cells. The peripheral blood count shows not less than 500 granulocytes per cubic millimeter of blood and 75,000 or more platelets per cubic millimeter. A *hematologic remission* signifies that the peripheral blood and the bone marrow satisfy these criteria. However, the St. Jude's workers define *complete remission* as hematologic remission *plus* no evidence of leukemia in the central nervous system (CNS) or elsewhere. The duration of hematologic remission may thus exceed that of complete remission if leukemic involvement occurs in the CNS while the bone marrow still shows no evidence of the disease. This special subdivision of remission status is useful in acute lymphocytic leukemia of childhood because CNS involvement is so common.

In acute granulocytic leukemia, the quality of completeness of remission is harder to assess. Maintenance of normal or near-normal peripheral blood parameters, with a cellular bone marrow containing no excess of myeloblasts and no frankly abnormal cells is usually accepted as remission, but it is not at present possible to determine whether primitive cells in the marrow are leukemic, or represent regeneration of normal marrow. Cytologic changes induced by drugs such as daunorubicin and cytarabine make interpretation of marrow preparations more difficult, and both erythroid and granulocytic hyperplasia may occur, apparently as a result of the stresses imposed by continuing treatment with myelotoxic drugs.

The inability to reliably detect residual leukemic cells in the bone marrow or elsewhere hampers the treatment of acute leukemia, since the response to treatment cannot be directly assessed once the marrow has assumed the appearance of remission status. Neither morphologic nor cytogenetic study enables detection of minute numbers of neoplastic cells, and some more refined—possibly immunologic—method would be of great value.

Cytologic Diagnosis and Therapeutic Policy

In the acute leukemias, the cytologic diagnosis (see Chapters 3 and 10) in an individual case has some effect on both the choice of therapy and the physician's expectations as to its likely outcome. For example, when any of the major antileukemic drugs is used as a single agent, the probability of achieving a complete hematologic remission is always greater in acute lymphocytic leukemia than in acute granulocytic leukemia (Table 18-2). The same rule appears to apply to antileukemic drugs used in combinations.

Although the commonly used drugs are usually less effective in acute granulocytic leukemia, some—for example, daunorubicin, cytarabine—are significantly more so than others, and a firm cytologic diagnosis of acute granulocytic leukemia is, therefore, an indication for their use. Furthermore, once remission has been obtained in an acute leukemia, attempts to maintain the remission by continued drug therapy are conspicuously more successful when the leukemia is lymphocytic.

Table 18-2

Responsiveness to Drug Therapy of Acute Lymphocytic
and Acute Granulocytic Leukemia

Treatment	Percentage of Patients Achieving Complete Remission (Total No. Patients)		References
	Lymphocytic (Mostly children)	Granulocytic (Mostly adults)	
Single drugs			
Methotrexate	21 (48)	16 (44)	1, 330
Prednisone*	57 (72	15 (39)	109, 213
Mercaptopurine	27 (43)	10 (31)	1
Cyclophosphamide	18 (44)	4 (45)	75, 100
Vincristine	55 (119)	36 (14 children)	170, 171
		0 (7 adults)	62
Daunorubicin	33 (32)	43 (21)	21, 22
Cytarabine	30 (10)	44 (31)	148, 157
L-Asparaginase	67† (21)	Information inadequate but response seems rare.	240
Drug Combinations			
Prednisone + mercaptopurine	82 (154)	3 (77)	106, 319
Prednisone + vincristine	84 (63)	−	281
Prednisone + vincristine + methotrexate + mercaptopurine	94 (35)	29 (83)	143, 147

*Information for Prednisolone (delta-1-prednisone) is insufficient.

†This high response rate, in a small series of patients, has not been generally confirmed. A more realistic figure seems to be a complete remission rate of 45 percent. Similarly, the response rate of acute lymphocytic leukemia to cytarabine is unlikely to be accurate because of the very small numbers involved.

Therefore, the cytologic diagnosis can provide a useful guide to the choice of initial therapy, the likelihood of the patient's achieving a remission, and a very approximate estimate of the likely remission duration.

Careful examination of well-stained films of peripheral blood and bone marrow will establish the cytologic diagnosis in the majority of cases. Utilization of a few simple cytochemical tests[147] is of value in some doubtful cases, while more elaborate techniques, such as the quantitative estimation of cellular enzymes[321] and the examination of intracellular hydrogen transport mechanisms,[322] help to classify a few more. However, some 5–10 percent of acute leukemias are so undifferentiated as to be at present unclassifiable as either lymphocytic or granulocytic. One widely used approach is to treat undifferentiated acute leukemia as lymphocytic in patients below age 20 and as granulocytic in patients above this age. Some justification for this course is seen in Table 18-3, in which it is apparent that survival of children with acute granulocytic leukemia may be superior to that of adults considered to have acute lymphocytic leukemia. Thus, chronological age may be at least as good a guide to therapeutic response and prognosis as is the cytologic diagnosis. Furthermore, the patient's age is indisputable, where the finer points of morphologic diagnosis are often contentious, even with the most expert observers. In the past, considerable stress has been laid upon the importance of precise cytologic diagnosis in the acute leukemias. Although diagnostic precision is scientifically desirable, it is not always attainable, and, in any case, is considerably less crucial in the clinical

Table 18-3
Survival in Acute Leukemia, Optimally Treated, by Age and Cytologic Type

Cytologic Type	Age Group	Median Survival (Months from diagnosis)*	References
Lymphocytic	Children	33.0	145
Granulocytic	Children	13.0†	144
Lymphocytic	Adults	11.0†	144
Granulocytic	Adults	6.0	144

*In each category, the best median survival reported on the basis of a substantial series has been selected.

†Since children with acute granulocytic leukemia and adults with acute lymphocytic leukemia are both relatively uncommon, median survivals in these categories are based on smaller numbers and may be less accurate.

situation than is sometimes supposed. It is almost always possible to formulate an appropriate therapeutic approach to the patient's problem by applying the following rules:

1. When the cytologic diagnosis—acute lymphocytic or acute granulocytic leukemia—seems clear, therapeutic action and prognostic expectations are based on this information.
2. In the minority of patients whose leukemias cannot be classified as lymphocytic or granulocytic, patients younger than 20 years of age are treated initially as having acute lymphocytic leukemia.
3. If the cytology is equivocal and the patient is close to 20 years of age, genuine doubt may still exist and the second course may not commend itself, particularly if the patient is so ill with his leukemia that the risk of employing an initial therapy which may be ineffective is unacceptable. In this situation it is reasonable to employ one of the drug combinations known to be effective for acute granulocytic leukemia, since they are also very potent against acute lymphocytic leukemia. In contrast, regimens popular for remission induction in acute lymphocytic leukemia (for example, vincristine plus prednisolone) are relatively ineffective in acute granulocytic leukemia.

Thus, it is usually possible to differentiate acute lymphocytic from acute granulocytic leukemia, and to choose therapy with some discrimination, even in those cases which cannot be so classified. It is more difficult to subdivide accurately the various types of acute granulocytic leukemia; but from a clinical viewpoint this is not at present a great disadvantage, since therapy has not yet reached the stage of refinement where a different treatment can be advocated for each of these subtypes, nor is there incontestable evidence that the prognosis of any of them is significantly better or worse than that of any other.

Historical Perspectives in Treatment of Acute Leukemia

Historically, the therapy of the acute leukemias can be divided into four partially overlapping eras, each of which had its own philosophical outlook.

THE PERIOD PRIOR TO THE ANTILEUKEMIC CHEMOTHERAPY

No therapy other than blood transfusion and a limited number of antimicrobial agents was available, and these did not greatly affect the duration of life.[32] To establish the diagnosis of acute leukemia was to pass a death sentence, since the median survival from diagnosis was only about 2.2 months for both children and adults.[334] Occasional "spontaneous" remissions were reported following blood transfusion or viral infections,[119,302] but attempts to induce remission by transfusion[31,34,349] or the production of infection[33,351] were usually fruitless. Most inadvertent infections in acute leukemia patients caused rapid deterioration of their general condition. Treatment by ionizing radiations was of very limited value, serving only to relieve symptomatic organomegaly or bone pain and did not control the systemic disease.[273] The therapeutic outlook was relatively nihilistic; it was accepted that all the patients would die rapidly and the best that could be offered was limited palliation and sympathetic terminal care. In this era, it was uncommon to acquaint the patient with his diagnosis and sometimes even his relations were not told.

POSSIBLE INDUCTION OF DISEASE REMISSION

In 1948, Farber and his colleagues showed that treatment with the folic acid antagonist aminopterin could induce remissions in some patients, particularly children, with acute leukemia.[104] The pathophysiologic changes associated with successful remission induction were so striking and unprecedented that it almost appeared as if a cure had been effected, but this misapprehension was short-lived. Nevertheless, it has since been conclusively established that the induction of disease remission is associated with significant prolongation of survival in both children and adults and in both acute lymphocytic and acute granulocytic leukemias.[92,116,179,354] The second therapeutic era concerned itself with the development of more drugs and improved therapeutic schedules aimed at inducing remission in an ever-increasing proportion of patients with acute leukemia. Improved methods of drug administration, particularly the use of antileukemic drugs in combinations, have done more to increase the incidence of remission than the introduction of new agents per se, but both developments have played a part. The folic acid analogs were followed by the adrenal corticosteroids, the purine antagonists, and other valuable drugs (see Chapter 17). With the acquisition of these potent antileukemic agents, a nihilistic outlook upon leukemia therapy became indefensible, but the overall outlook was not greatly changed. Although it was now possible to help many of the patients positively, all could still be expected to succumb to their disease relatively soon.

THE EVOLUTION OF TECHNIQUES FOR REMISSION MAINTENANCE

The seemingly inevitable recrudescence of the leukemic process after the induction of remission—leukemic relapse—is a phenomenon no less remarkable than remission itself. The third phase in leukemia chemotherapy is the development of technics for remission maintenance, with the aim of postponing relapse and prolonging health and life. At first, remission maintenance therapy was viewed with reservations, since it was felt that the long-term administration of cytotoxic drugs might lead to irreversible bone marrow failure with fatal consequences. However, it has been shown convincingly that the use of remission maintenance therapy prolongs the duration of remission.[71,116,292] Furthermore, increased duration of remission is correlated with prolongation of survival. In acute lymphocytic leukemia this correlation is strong: almost all of the increased length of survival seen in successive therapeutic trials over the years is due to additional time spent in remission.[152] In acute granulocytic leukemia the relationship between remission duration and length of survival has not always been demonstrable[77] but in many series a positive correlation has been found.[92,119,152] When remission maintenance therapy in acute granulocytic leukemia becomes more effective this correlation will become stronger: at present, it is vitiated both by the relative inefficiency of available maintenance treatments and by the existence of some patients with acute granulocytic leukemia who survive for relatively long periods although their disease is not actually in remission.

The techniques for maintaining remission in acute leukemia have undergone an interesting evolution. At first there was no attempt at maintenance: drug therapy was ended once remission had been attained, and the same or another drug treatment was reinstituted at the earliest sign of relapse; now this approach is obsolete. The earliest maintenance technique was to administer during remission the drug which had been used to induce remission, usually at a lesser dose than before, until relapse occurred, when a different therapy was begun. This policy was less than optimal for several reasons. First, there is commonly an inverse correlation between the ability of a drug to induce and to maintain remission[118]: for example, steroid drugs will induce remission in over half the patients with acute lymphocytic leukemia, but steroid-maintained remissions in this disease are not significantly longer than unmaintained remissions. Second, some drugs useful for remission induction are not only ineffective for remission maintenance therapy but also have side effects which are both undesirable and cumulative—again, adrenocorticosteroid drugs are a good example. Third, the use of reduced dosage has no sound basis, since it is desirable to suppress the leukemic process as completely as possible, and full dosage is likely to do this more effectively. In fact, increased doses are often indicated, since during remission the bone marrow can tolerate considerably more cytotoxic insult than can be borne during the initial phase of treatment, when marrow failure is present. Acceptance of this fact led to maintenance therapy being administered, using full doses of antileukemic drugs and later, augmented doses. However, even using large doses, it is unwise to delay administering any differing agents until the leukemia has relapsed, since relapse is usually associated with ill health and is always attended by the risk of serious complications. The next evolutionary step in remission maintenance was the deliberate alteration of therapy, in predetermined fashion, before relapse was likely. Maintenance schedules thus evolved from reduced dosages to full and then to enhanced dosages. Regimens in which different drugs were administered in cyclic fashion, without waiting for relapse of the leukemia to occur, received extensive trial and yielded some improvements in survival and/or decrease in the mean number of relapses occurring during the period of survival.[14,50,356]

Since drug combinations are more effective than single drugs in producing remission in acute leukemia (see Table 18-2), similar or identical combinations have been tried for remission maintenance. Combination antileukemic chemotherapy may be given as reinduction (more correctly, pseudoreinduction) courses at intervals during continuous maintenance of remission with other drugs: this approach considerably prolongs survival in acute lymphocytic leukemia.[171] Alternatively, the doses and frequency of administration of the drug combinations may be increased and the continuous drug therapy omitted entirely, since it depresses the bone marrow and hampers or precludes the administration of repeated courses of drugs in combination. Treatment by drug combinations alone in acute lymphocytic leukemia produces a high incidence of remissions which are of long duration; if therapy is discontinued after 14 months, the median duration of subsequent *unmaintained* remission is 8 months,[150] but the relapse experience of these patients shows that their leukemia had not been eradicated at the time therapy was ceased.

In this latest phase of its evolution, so-called maintenance therapy for acute leukemia in some centers has become a prolonged and intensive program of pseudoreinductions, vastly different from the accepted practice of only a few years ago. With the ability to maintain many patients with acute leukemia in clinical and hematologic remission for extended periods came a further change of outlook. For example, practical concerns such as the schooling or employment—or marriage—of patients, formerly almost irrelevant, became common problems in leukemia practice. Elective surgical procedures—for example, hemorrhoidectomy—which previously would not have been considered in leukemia patients, had to be considered and often undertaken. Ethical and other problems also arose. Could remissions be maintained indefinitely, and was it justifiable to subject patients to hazardous and unpleasant therapeutic programs in order, perhaps, to secure long survival in a minority? Some patients had been on maintenance therapy for several years—was it safe to discontinue treatment? One study[189] suggested that in children with acute lymphocytic leukemia who had been in complete remission for 3 years, the eventual outcome was unaffected by the decision to continue or interrupt antileukemic chemotherapy. Some children were still in unbroken remission 2 years after all therapy had ceased and it seemed possible that their leukemia had been eradicated. The concept of cure in acute leukemia could be considered as a real possibility rather than a remote utopian objective.

THERAPEUTIC PROGRAMS AIMED AT CURE

In acute granulocytic leukemia of adults, cure in most cases seems a distant prospect because available therapy is very inadequate, but in acute lymphocytic leukemia of childhood the greatest remaining obstacle to cure in some patients seems only to be the lack of an acceptable definition of the term. Even 5 years without therapy with no sign of recrudescence of the disease may not be a sufficiently strict criterion of cure: experience with small numbers of patients who have attained this status suggests that it is not.

Prolonged survival with acute leukemia is not necessarily a result of the most recently developed, intensive therapeutic programs. Burchenal was able to collect from hematologists in many countries records of 157 patients with acute leukemia who had survived more than 5 years from diagnosis.[53] Some of these patients had been without therapy for several years and were still in continuous remission. He concluded from his data that relapse of the leukemia became less, rather than more, frequent with increasing duration of freedom from the disease: patients still in remission 5 years after diagnosis had a 50 percent chance of not relapsing, and after 10 years the chance of relapsing was negligible. It is difficult to deny that some of these patients are actually cured of their leukemia. However, analysis of their case histories showed no common feature: they included both children and adults, acute lymphocytic and acute granulocytic leukemias, and had received a wide variety of therapies. Significantly, many of the treatments would be considered quite inadequate by modern standards—for example, one patient was given a short course of a single drug which was never repeated. Since many other patients treated by similar, or more intensive, methods have relapsed and died, it may be concluded that these were "chance" cures, attributable to the characteristics of the leukemia in particular patients, rather than to any inherent virtues of the treatment administered. The size of the patient population covered by Burchenal's survey is unknown, but it appears that the 157 5-year survivors are unlikely to have been more than 1 percent of the total.

A more recent study of long-term survivors with acute leukemia showed similar results.[332] In 83 patients with acute lymphocytic leukemia who survived more than 4 years, the annual death rate fell from 25 percent in the fifth and sixth years to 6 percent thereafter; no patient died after the tenth year. Patients who survived for four years *without relapse* appeared to have a 70 percent chance of very long survival, compared with only about a 17 percent chance for those who reached four years after one or more relapses of their leukemia. Over the 15 years covered by the survey, the proportion of 4-year survivors approximately trebled (0.95–2.6 percent), but that of very long-term survivors only increased by about 50 percent (about 0.5–0.75 percent). These results suggest that very long survival with acute leukemia is usually dependent upon achieving a lengthy period of *unbroken* complete remission: long survival with several relapses of the disease carries no such favorable prognosis. The absence of relapses among the 10-year survivors in this study and that of Burchenal suggests that these patients are indeed cured.

Although the previously categoric statement that leukemia is incurable and always fatal can no longer be sustained, it must be emphasized that cures of this type are so rare that their occurrence has not altered the median survival figures or the overall prognosis of acute leukemia. However, the existence of cured patients has greatly altered medical thought on the treatment of acute leukemia: the cure of leukemia is no longer merely the province of the charlatan. As a necessary condition of their present status, none of the 10-year survivors with acute leukemia was initially treated with one of the modern intensive chemotherapy regimens: most of these patients represent exceptionally favorable results of standard therapeutic regimens which failed to produce long survival in many apparently similar patients.

Modern treatment programs now produce unbroken remissions of several years' duration in as many as 50 percent of patients[12] and it is uncertain whether these patients, when going without therapy, will have the same 10-year relapse experience as those who had long remissions with much less intensive therapy. It is certainly possible that many patients who experience long remissions with aggressive treatment are cured of their acute leukemia,[66] but definite evidence is not yet available because insufficient time has elapsed since the various intensive treatment regimens were instituted. The final proof will lie in the number of patients who live normal life spans without recurrence of disease, and this will require about 50 years' follow-up. Whether late complications will develop in the long-term survivors remains to be seen.

In this current phase of acute leukemia therapy there is an important change of outlook. Instead of administering palliative therapy, aimed at producing remission and prolonging comfortable survival while accepting eventual relapse and death as inevitable, therapeutic programs are devised from the outset with total eradication of the disease in mind.[260,306,307] Many of these programs aim at the early use of most or all of the first-line drugs for acute leukemia; no drug is reserved to treat relapse because the programs are cure-oriented, not relapse-oriented. Such treatment is often more unpleasant than the older palliative approaches, and because it is so intensive, has major risks: deaths from infection during complete remission are a recognized hazard.[13,260] The change of therapeutic outlook requires an acceptance of the increased risks and complications of therapy: this is not an easy decision but the chances of securing long-term survival are now sufficiently good to justify relatively drastic therapy. Regimens of this type do not sacrifice the interests of many patients for the benefit of a select few; on the contrary, the *median* survival of patients treated by intensive protocols is at least as good as that obtained with other methods, while the *long-term* survival rates are much superior.[133]

It must be emphasized that improvements in therapeutic programs and resultant lengthening of prognosis have affected the different types of acute leukemia unequally. The common acute leukemia of adults—acute granulocytic—is only in the second and third phases of therapeutic development: the major efforts are directed toward increasing the incidence of initial remission induction and to devising effective programs for remission maintenance, and cure is a more remote possibility. Although similar efforts are still directed toward acute lymphocytic leukemia in children, this disease has moved into the fourth therapeutic phase, where treatment programs are aimed at cure. Furthermore, deliberate therapeutic cure can now be expected to be achieved by treatment, and such cures will outnumber the fortuitous cures observed in former years.

The Cytokinetic Basis for Curative Therapy

Cell kinetics in human acute leukemia is described in Chapter 8. Much of the reasoning on which current treatment programs are based is, however, derived from the important studies of Skipper and his colleagues with the experimental mouse leukemia, L1210.[299] Although men are not mice, and L1210 is almost certainly a more homogeneous entity than any of the subtypes of human leukemia, it is reasonable to assume that many of the principles demonstrated by Skipper do, in fact, apply to human acute leukemias, particularly acute lymphocytic leukemia.

Before treatment, or during severe relapse, it is estimated that the average child with acute leukemia has about 10^{12} leukemic cells—1 kg of tumor tissue—in his body.[114] In a logarithmic sense, this figure is quite accurate, since 10^{13} cells (10 kg) is obviously too much, while 10^{11} cells (100 gm) is clearly an underestimate. Conventional treatment that produces a complete remission effects a reduction of 2–4 logs in the leukemic cell mass. Even a 2-log "kill" of leukemic cells is compatible with the conversion of the bone marrow population from 100 percent blast cells to 1 percent blast cells, acceptable as a complete bone marrow remission, although about 10^{10} leukemic cells remain in the body. In the L1210 model it has been shown that *the fractional kill of leukemic cells is the same for a given amount of treatment, regardless of the absolute number of cells present.* Therefore, it should be possible, in man as well as in mice, to destroy all the leukemic cells in the body by repeated or long-continued treatment, extirpating a fraction of the surviving leukemic cells on each occasion until only one cell remains, which will not survive the next course of antileukemic therapy.

In practice it is not possible to give very protracted courses of antileukemic drugs in high doses, since a large fraction of the normal hematopoietic cells and of the gut mucosal cells will also be destroyed, with fatal results. However, it is feasible to administer repeated short courses of therapy, with treatment-free intervals. During the latter, both leukemic and normal marrow cells will multiply, but so long as the rate of recovery of the normal tissue is faster than that of the leukemic cells a chemotherapeutic cure is possible, provided the treatment-free intervals are not too long. The fact that remission can be induced in acute lymphocytic leukemia, even using drugs that are myelotoxic, with eventual improvement in the peripheral blood levels of hemoglobin, platelets, and neutrophils, shows that the capacity for recovery of normal bone marrow cells exceeds that of the leukemic cells. By administering antileukemic drugs at frequent intervals (for example, for 5 days every 2 weeks) in doses that are just compatible with an acceptable peripheral blood count, that is, an asymptomatic slight pancytopenia, the eventual destruction of all leukemic cells seems assured. Unfortunately, this is not uniformly the case in practice, particularly in nonlymphocytic acute leukemias. Several reasons for the repeated failure of such therapies may be adduced:

1. Resistance of some leukemic cells to the drugs used may be present from the outset, or may arise during treatment. For this reason, in some programs three or more drugs are always given together, in the hope that resistance may be prevented, as in antituberculous chemotherapy.
2. Leukemic cells in certain situations may be protected from the antileukemic drugs; thus, the blood-CSF barrier may protect cells in the meninges, since most antileukemic agents, with the exception of adrenocortical steroids and BCNU, cross this barrier poorly. Similar protected environments may exist in the brain, the gonads, and the thyroid.
3. Some resting or out-of-cycle leukemic cells may exist, which are not vulnerable to the drugs but may later become active and repopulate the bone marrow after therapy has ceased.
4. Occasional patients relapse at very long intervals after cessation of therapy, and in these individuals the actual reinduction of the leukemic process by some unknown agent is not impossible.

There seems little doubt that the Skipper model does not apply exactly to human acute leukemia, even of the acute lymphocytic variety. Nevertheless, treatment programs based on this model are showing better results than earlier regimens, and it appears that these improved results are not attributable merely to newer drugs or better supportive therapy. The principles of therapy according to the L1210 model are summarized in Figure 18-2.

Therapeutic Fallacies

Fallacies about leukemia and its treatment abound in the popular press and, judging by the frequency with which leukemia patients present them to their doctors, do much harm by raising false hopes or giving rise to baseless fears. Unfortunately, misinformation is not confined to the lay press but is also to be found in

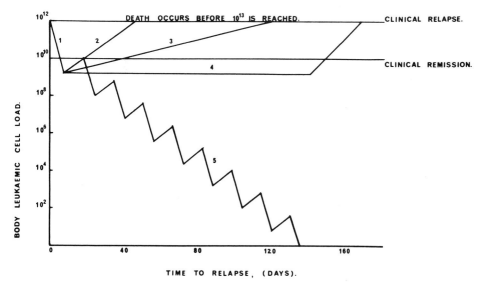

Fig. 18-2. The effect of treatment on the total-body load of leukemic cells, according to the Skipper model based on the mouse leukemia L1210. 1, The effect of remission induction therapy; about 10^9 leukemic cells remain; 2, No maintenance therapy, or ineffective maintenance: replacement of leukemic cells leads to relapse in about 40 days. 3, Effective maintenance therapy—relapse is significantly delayed but inevitably occurs, either because the rate of leukemic cell recovery exceeds the rate of cell killing by the maintenance drug, or because a primarily resistant cell strain is being selected by the therapy. 4, Maintenance therapy which has achieved an equilibrium—this has eventually broken down because a new and resistant cell clone has emerged. From the slope at the end of line 4, it is apparent that the new clone has a faster growth rate than the original leukemia. 5, The potentially curative effect of repeated reinduction treatments. Note that each treatment has destroyed the same fraction of leukemic cells and cell kill is much faster than cell recovery: the treatment is repeated before recovery of leukemic cells to their former level has occurred. In this example, no resistance to the drugs has arisen. Because the leukemia is undetectable when less than 10^{10} cells are present, any cytokinetic events below this threshold can only be inferred, not demonstrated directly. (From Spiers ASD: Clin. Hematol. 1:127, 1972. With permission.)

medical writings. Perhaps the most serious sources of apparently authoritative but spurious data are out-of-date textbooks of general medicine. In any rapidly developing subject, textbooks are inevitably outdated by the time of publication and this particularly applies to any highly specialized field when treated in a general textbook where it is necessarily condensed because it is of restricted interest. In the present era of meetings and workshops, even the medical journals lag well behind the latest practice in special fields. Some items of medical misinformation about the leukemias seem so firmly entrenched that it is worth examining them: numerous other examples could be quoted!

Precise cytologic classification is all-important in determining treatment and prognosis. As already discussed, the patient's age is a useful guide in itself; classification of acute leukemias into lymphocytic and granulocytic varieties is valuable, though not essential, in choosing therapy, and the detailed subclassification of the various types of acute granulocytic leukemia contributes very little to management at present.

Since no patient is ever cured it is pointless to treat acute leukemia actively. Although it may still be argued that "cure" in the sense of normal life span has not yet been demonstrated, the existence of 10-year survivors is indisputable. Furthermore, many patients experience months or years of useful life, which in itself justifies active treatment.

The treatment is worse than the disease and patients should be allowed to die comfortably. This is a double fallacy. Although the treatments used for the acute leukemias are sometimes decidedly unpleasant, they are rarely as distressing as the symptoms produced by active, untreated acute leukemia (see Chapter 10). An exception to this is smoldering acute leukemia, which is sometimes indolent and asymptomatic and may justifiably be treated conservatively. Secondly, patients with untreated acute leukemia rarely die comfortably unless they are so fortunate as to sustain an abrupt cataclysmic intracranial hemorrhage with sudden death. Before any antileukemic drugs were available, the terminal stages of acute leukemia were often accompanied by agonizing generalized bone pain, a symptom which cytotoxic drugs will nearly always alleviate, even when remission of the leukemia can no longer be induced.

Pancytopenia at presentation is a contraindication to treatment because drug therapy will make matters worse. In acute lymphocytic leukemia it is possible to induce disease remission in about 90 percent of patients by using drugs with no significant myelotoxicity, and the pancytopenia usually improves rapidly without preliminary deterioration. In acute granulocytic leukemia, myelotoxic drugs must be used to induce remission and the pancytopenia commonly is made worse. However, if treatment is withheld the leukemia itself will cause progression of the pancytopenia, accompanied by accumulation of a greater leukemic cell mass, making treatment increasingly less likely to succeed.

Pancytopenia occurring during drug treatment is always an indication for its interruption. This is a particularly widespread but nevertheless erroneous belief. It is based on a misconception—that treatment is directed toward control of the peripheral blood count—whereas the object of antileukemic therapy is control of the disease in the bone marrow and peripheral blood values are only important insofar as they reflect the status of the marrow and the need for supportive measures such as transfusion of blood or platelets. A more correct *modus operandi* is as follows: (1) persistence of leukemic cells in the peripheral blood is an indication for further therapy despite neutropenia and/or thrombocytopenia; (2) a pancytopenia without apparent leukemic cells is an indication for a further bone marrow examination; (3) a bone marrow with numerous blast cells indicates a need for further therapy despite pancytopenia; (4) a hypocellular bone marrow is sometimes an indication for interruption of therapy, observation, and reassessment of the marrow after an interval. A bone marrow with a high proportion of blast cells is often regarded as an indication for continuing therapy, even if it is quite hypocellular—some workers consider that in acute granulocytic leukemia, severe marrow hypoplasia is an almost invariable prelude to achieving remission.[28]

Results of treatment in acute leukemia are insufficiently good to justify referral of patients to special centers. It is disappointing that this view still exists: sometimes it is linked with the opinion that special centers serve the needs of research better than those of the patient. In fact, the survival of children with acute lymphocytic leukemia is significantly longer at special centers compared to similar children

Table 18-4

Common Abbreviations for Drugs and Therapeutic Programs

Drugs	
Methotrexate	MTX
Prednisone or prednisolone[1]	PRED
Mercaptopurine	MP[2]
Thioguanine	TG[3]
Cyclophosphamide	CY
Vincristine	VCR
Daunorubicin	DR
Cytarabine (cytosine arabinoside)	ara-C[4]
L-Asparaginase	L-ase
Drug Combinations[5]	
Prednisone-vincristine-methotrexate-mercaptopurine	POMP
Cyclophosphamide-vincristine-cytarabine-prednisone	COAP
Thioguanine-daunorubicin-cytarabine-prednisone	TRAP
Cytarabine-L-asparaginase-daunorubicin-thioguanine	CART

[1] There is no separate symbol for prednisolone.
[2,3] Sometimes written as "6MP" and "6TG" but this has no special advantage.
[4] Sometimes abbreviated as "CA" but this is less widely used.
[5] Abbreviations are made up by taking official or proprietary names, as appropriate, to make a readable word.

treated elsewhere,[223] while in adults with acute granulocytic leukemia, the remission rates achieved at some special centers are definitely superior to those generally encountered.[28,66,74] The concentration of trained personnel and special equipment required for the optimal management of patients with leukemia is such that only a specialized center can provide it.

Abbreviations Used in the Text

Like other disciplines—notably obstetrics—leukemia therapy has its own shorthand, which facilitates the setting down of information in concise form. Because of certain very widely circulated publications, such as *Leukemia Abstracts,* many of these abbreviations are internationally recognized and the trend is one to be encouraged. Table (18-4) sets out some standard abbreviations which hereafter are used in the text and subsequent tables.

Synergy and Antagonism Between Antileukemic Drugs

Combinations of two or more antileukemic drugs are often more effective than single agents for inducing remission in acute leukemia (for examples, see Table 18-2). In acute lymphocytic leukemia, sufficient data are available to express some drug interactions mathematically.[114] If it is assumed that drugs act independently, that is, the responsiveness of a patient with acute lymphocytic leukemia to a drug is unrelated to his responsiveness or resistance to any other antileukemic drug, then the complete remission rate, CRR, obtainable in a series of patients, using a combination of two drugs, A and B, should be given by the following formula:

$$CRR_{A+B} = CRR_A + CRR_B \times \frac{(100 - CRR_A)}{100}$$

Thus, if both drugs have a complete remission rate of 50 percent, half the patients will respond to drug A, and half the remainder will respond to drug B, the complete remission rate of the combination $A + B$ being 75 percent. If 100 patients are treated, 75 will enter complete remission—25 A-responders, 25 B-responders, and 25 who are responsive to both drugs. If the hypothesis of independent drug action is true, the use of three drugs, each with a complete remission rate of 50 percent, should produce 87.5 percent remissions, and so on. This would represent a purely additive effect of different drugs acting independently.

However, clinical results are actually somewhat better than the formula predicts. Thus, prednisone has a complete remission rate of 57 percent and vincristine has a complete remission rate of 55 percent in acute lymphocytic leukemia (Table 18-2). Their combination should have a complete remission rate of about 79 percent, whereas it is, in fact, 84 percent or better in clinical practice. Taking 84 percent as the complete remission rate obtainable with this combination, the addition of daunorubicin (with a complete remission rate of 33 percent) should raise the rate to about 89 percent, whereas it is actually 97 percent.[21] These results, which are based on relatively large numbers of cases, suggest that there is, in fact, true *synergy* in some drug combinations, that is, some cases of leukemia which are responsive to neither drug alone will respond to two or three agents given together. Thus, the theoretical advantages of using combination therapy for the induction of remission in acute leukemia are more than borne out in clinical practice, at least for acute lymphocytic leukemia.

It is easily seen that the remission rates obtained in acute granulocytic leukemia with single drugs and with combinations (Table 18-2) do not follow the above formula. Sometimes this may be explained by the fact that in acute granulocytic leukemia the dose schedules used in combination treatments are often different to those used in single-agent chemotherapy. Thus, in acute lymphocytic leukemia the doses of PRED and VCR are usually the same whether the drugs are used together or singly, whereas in acute granulocytic leukemia the combination of myelotoxic drugs such as DR, ara-C and MP into a single regimen entails some reduction in the dosage of each, together with alterations in the timing and duration of therapy. Nevertheless, it still appears that drug combinations are more successful in inducing remissions in acute granulocytic leukemia than most, or perhaps all, of the agents which might be used singly: for example, the combination (ara-C + TG) has produced a 50 percent remission rate in acute granulocytic leukemia, while (DR + ara-C) has induced remission in 60 percent of a small series.[74]

It seems likely that combined drug therapies will remain the preferred method for remission induction in the acute leukemias, since they offer enhanced response rates at the expense of small and acceptable increases in toxicity. They also possess the theoretical advantage that the use of multiple agents from the inception of therapy should delay or prevent the emergence of drug-resistant cell clones, an important concept if chemotherapeutic eradication of the leukemia is contemplated.

Antagonism between antileukemic drugs is also possible. This might not be absolute but dependent upon the time sequence in which drugs are administered. For example, administration of an agent which prevents cells from entering mitosis should antagonize the effects of a second agent which destroys cells only in mitosis, if the drugs were administered in that order. On the other hand, administration of the drug which affected cells in mitosis *first,* followed by the agent which inhibited entry of further cells into mitosis, would produce additive rather than antagonistic effects. Thus, the activity of drugs in the various phases of the cell cycle is an important factor in planning their administration with the aim of exploiting their possible synergy and avoiding antagonism (see Chapter 8). The interaction of antileukemic drugs to produce antagonistic effects can be demonstrated with experimental leukemias. For example, cells in culture which have been deprived of asparagine by prior exposure to L-ase are resistant to the cytotoxic action of MTX.[59] When MTX and ara-C are added to cell cultures simultaneously, or the MTX is added 6 hours before the ara-C, marked drug antagonism is demonstrable: only slight antagonism occurs when the ara-C is added before the MTX.[328] In mice with transplanted leukemia L1210, demecolcine and vinblastine, drugs which cause metaphase arrest in leukemic and normal cells, may antagonize or enhance the effects of ara-C depending upon the schedule of drug administration.[338] The temporary inhibition of mitotic activity is followed by a synchronization of the cycles of different cells when the drug effect decays. Thus, shortly after the administration of vinblastine, little DNA synthetic activity is present and the administration of ara-C has little effect, but if the administration of ara-C is delayed until a cohort of synchronized cells is entering S phase, its effects are enhanced.

Synergistic and antagonistic effects of drugs are more difficult to demonstrate in human leukemias in vivo. However, it has been shown that the administration of a single dose of ara-C leads to the progressive accumulation of cells in S phase: twenty-four hours after administration of ara-C, the effects of a dose of VCR should be minimal because very few cells are in mitosis, whereas at 72 hours its effects are possibly enhanced because a synchronized cell cohort is entering the mitotic phase.[191] It has been suggested[97] that treatment with PRED should not precede the administration of VCR or MTX, because PRED apparently prevents cells from passing from the G_1 to the S phase of the cell cycle: thus, methotrexate which acts in the S phase, and vincristine which acts upon cells in mitosis, might be antagonized by the corticosteroid. Some caution is necessary in applying the results of experimental studies to the clinical management of the acute leukemias. The animal leukemias are at best only analogs of the human disease and, in some respects, may be extremely atypical; for example, many animal leukemic cell-lines appear to be homogeneous, all the cells possessing similar biochemical and cytokinetic characteristics, whereas many human leukemias consist of two or more cell-lines from the time of diagnosis; cytogenetic studies sometimes demonstrate multiple cell clones (see Chapter 6). In a multiclonal neoplasm, the disadvantages of antagonism when several drugs are administered together may sometimes be outweighed by the advantage that a greater proportion of the neoplastic cells may be susceptible to a combination of cytotoxic agents, compared to the possibly small fraction of the cell population which may be sensitive to any one of the agents administered alone. Experiments on drug antagonism in human leukemias are perhaps more relevant, but have been performed on few patients so that generalizations cannot be made with safety. Experiments on leukemic cells in vitro may be misleading because the cell environment is artificially simplified—for example, the possible synergy between ara-C and L-ase in vivo[198] may occur from the effects of ara-C on *normal* cells in the marrow population: such effects might not be detectable in vitro. However, the possible effects of schedules of administration of drugs, their activity in different phases of the cell cycle, and antagonism and synergy between different agents, are already affecting the programs by which agents are screened for antitumor activity[339] and will increasingly affect therapeutic strategy in the clinical treatment of the acute leukemias.

ACUTE LEUKEMIA IN CHILDREN

Although acute leukemia is a rare disease at any age, it is of special importance in children. Because of the rarity of other neoplasms in children, acute leukemia is the commonest cancer of childhood and an important cause of death. Because of its dramatic clinical features and usually fatal outcome (see Chapter 10) it has always received much attention, both lay and medical, and there is a surprisingly widespread belief that leukemia is actually commoner in children than in adults. The majority of acute leukemias in children are of the lymphocytic variety (see Chapter 4).

Acute Lymphocytic Leukemia

In the past 20 years, medical attitudes toward acute lymphocytic leukemia in childhood have undergone a change comparable to that which occurred with pernicious anemia half a century earlier. Before the advent of specific antileukemic therapy, half of all children with acute lymphocytic leukemia were dead within 3 months of diagnosis and very few survived a year.[334] Now this form is regarded as the most treatable of all the leukemias and median survival in childhood is beginning to surpass that seen in the chronic leukemias. Therapeutic principles elucidated in the treatment of patients with acute lymphocytic leukemia, in particular, the advantages of combination chemotherapy, have since been applied to the management of malignant lymphomas with considerable benefit and are now under study in the therapy of solid tumors.

REVIEW OF THERAPY

It is neither possible nor necessary to consider all the steps by which the treatment of acute lymphocytic leukemia has evolved over the past 25 years. The major changes in thought and clinical practice which have occurred are based on several advances.

1. The realization that the period immediately following the diagnosis of acute lymphocytic leukemia is the time of greatest risk, and that the induction of disease remission is a matter of urgency.
2. The ability to induce remission more rapidly, with less toxicity, and in a higher proportion of children.
3. The introduction of more drugs with antileukemic activity and lacking mutual cross resistance.
4. The acceptance of the need for maintenance therapy to prolong remission.
5. The realization, based on experimental studies,[298] that treatment in acute lymphocytic leukemia should be aimed at cure and should be continued inten-

sively long after evidence of the persistence of leukemic cells is lacking. Coupled with this point is the principle that maintenance therapy must be more aggressive than are most forms of induction therapy.

Remission induction in childhood is usually straightforward, about half the patients responding to PRED alone. Once it was common to treat children with PRED initially, adding other drugs—MP, or in more recent times VCR—only if they did not respond. This approach is now considered reprehensible, since combinations of two drugs used from the outset will induce remission in over 80 percent of patients, while some combinations of four drugs are effective in almost 100 percent of children (Table 18-5). Use of the less effective, single-agent approach exposes the patient to a greater risk of not remitting promptly, with prolongation of the particularly dangerous period between diagnosis and the securing of remission. Even if the disease does respond to such therapy, exposure of a large population of leukemic cells to a single drug is an excellent way of selecting out a drug-resistant cell strain and compromising the long-term prognosis of the disease. The most widely used induction therapy for acute lymphocytic leukemia today is (VCR + PRED), although many prefer to use COAP or other quadruple combinations. Various dosages are used, often relating dose to body weight or body surface area, but, in fact, the antileukemic activity and toxicity of VCR and PRED do not correlate particularly well with these parameters. A simple and reliable formula is to administer VCR 1mg on days 1, 8, and 15 of treatment (using the same dose for *all* children) and PRED 2mg per kg body weight per day from days 1–21 inclusive, and discontinuing abruptly; tailing-off of the PRED is necessary only in the presence of infection or other physiologic stress. Continuation of the VCR beyond 4 weeks increases the incidence of toxic effects but improves the remission rate very little.[179] Since both

Table 18-5
Remission Induction by Chemotherapy in Children with Acute Lymphocytic Leukemia

Treatment	Number of Patients	% Complete Remission	References
Single Drugs			
MTX	48	21	2
PRED	72	57	116
MP	43	27	2
CY	44	18	107
VCR	119	55	178
DR	32	33	26
ara-C	10	30	165
L-ase	21	67	249
Drug Combinations			
PRED + MP	154	82	113
PRED + VCR	63	84	292
PRED + MTX	80	80	188
PRED + CY	58	76	106
PRED + DR	60	65	163
MP + MTX	39	43	2
PRED + VCR + DR	33	97	26
POMP	35	94	150
COAP	25	100	310

Table 18-6
Suitability of the Major Antileukemic Drugs for Remission Induction
and Remission Maintenance in Acute Lymphocytic Leukemia

Drug	Rapidity of Action	Toxicity to Marrow	Cumulative Side-Effects	Suitability for Remission Induction	Suitability for Maintenance
MTX	Intermediate	++	Uncommon	±	++
PRED	Fast	Nil	+++ (Metabolic)	+++	–
MP	Slow	++	Uncommon	±	++
CY	Slow	++	Cystitis fairly common	±	+
VCR	Fast	Slight	+++ (Neurotoxic)	+++	±
DR	Fast	++	Cardiotoxicity fairly common	+	+
ara-C	Fast	++	Uncommon	+	+
L-ase	Slow	Nil	Allergy common	+++	+

Note: These criteria apply to *continuous* use of the drugs but not to their intermittent use for pseudoreinduction.

drugs have long-term toxic effects, which are notably cumulative, their continuous use would be unacceptable for remission maintenance therapy. Furthermore, PRED is not very effective in maintaining remission, unmaintained remissions being approximately as long as those obtained when the PRED is continued after remission has been achieved.[167] It was claimed that VCR is ineffective in maintaining remission,[179] but other studies suggest that in some patients VCR can maintain remission for many months.[14]

From consideration of their speed of action, short-term and long-term side effects, and ability to maintain disease remission, antileukemic drugs can be classified as suitable for remission induction or better suited to remission maintenance (Table 18-6). In general, drugs with rapid action, little marrow toxicity, and cumulative side effects (for example, VCR, PRED) are best for remission induction, while drugs with a slower action, myelotoxic effects, but few cumulative side effects (for example, MP, MTX), are suitable for remission maintenance. These differences apply principally to drugs used *continuously;* when used *intermittently,* drugs such as PRED and VCR are valuable for remission maintenance in acute lymphocytic leukemia.

With the combination (VCR + PRED), which is simple and easy to use, an initial complete remission can be secured in over 80 percent of children with acute lymphocytic leukemia. Some patients succumb to infection or hemorrhage before remission can be achieved; a few simply do not respond—occasionally this is attributable to a mistaken original diagnosis, but in others it is unexplained. Once achieved, remission must be maintained, if possible without interruption, since there is increasing evidence that the occurrence of even a brief relapse is associated with a poor long-term prognosis. The proper maintenance of remission is a more difficult problem than its induction.

A selection of the many remission maintenance programs which have been used is shown in Table (18-7). By studying Table 18-7, it becomes apparent that if a simple induction therapy is followed by no maintenance, the duration of remission is

Table 18-7
Duration of Remission and Survival in Children with Acute Lymphocytic Leukemia Treated by Various Regimens

Workers and References	Remission-induction Therapy	Remission-maintenance Therapy	No. of Patients	% Complete Remission	Median C.R. Duration (months)*	Median H.R. Duration (months)*	Median Survival (months)	5-Year Survival (%)	5-Year Cure (%)*
Freireich et al. (1963)[116]	PRED	Nil	46	52		2.2	11		
	PRED	MP	46	52		8.2	12.5		
Zuelzer (1964)[356]	PRED + MP	Cyclic PRED, MTX, MP	175			11	17	4	
Selawry (1965)[292]	PRED + VCR	Intermittent high-dose parenterally administered MTX	22	84		11	27		3.4
Acute Leukemia Group B (1969)[1]	PRED + VCR	Intermittent high-dose oral MTX	20	96		10.4			
Australian Cancer Society's Childhood Leukaemia Study Group (1968)[14]	PRED + VCR	VCR,MP,CY,MTX—in cycles or sequentially	101	85			24		
Henderson & Samaha (1969)[153]	POMP	POMP	35	91		13.5	33	5.7	5.7
Pinkel (1971)[260]	PRED + VCR	MP—daily MTX + VCR + CY—weekly. Radiation (1200 rads) to cerebrospinal axis	26	92	15	22	35	23	19

*C.R. (complete remission) signifies that no manifestation of leukemia is detectable. H.R. (hematologic remission) denotes remission status of the bone marrow and peripheral blood; other manifestations of leukemia—most commonly meningeal involvement—may, however, be present. Five-year cure signifies that the patient is off all therapy and remains without evidence of leukemia.

brief, whereas even a single-drug maintenance regimen substantially extends the remission. Comparison of the next three studies shows that intermittent therapy with methotrexate in high dosage results in a median remission duration equal to that previously obtained with three drugs (PRED, MP and MTX in conventional daily dosage) used in a cyclical fashion. This result could be obtained with both orally[3] and parenterally[292] administered MTX. Thus, by a simple alteration of dosage and timing of administration, the usefulness of MTX could be greatly enhanced. Furthermore, children relapsing from the high-dose MTX schedule had become resistant to only one drug, whereas those relapsing from the cyclic regimen were usually resistant to all three of the maintenance agents, and this seems to be reflected in the 27-month median survival of the high-dose MTX group, as against only 17 months for the cyclic therapy group. As a result of these and other studies, it became widely accepted practice to administer methotrexate intermittently, usually twice a week by mouth, in high doses, about 20–30 mg per square meter of body surface area.

Much investigation has centered around the advantages or disadvantages of administering maintenance drugs in a cyclic or a sequential fashion. With a sequential regimen, one antileukemic drug is given until relapse occurs, then the next drug is begun, and so on. In cyclic programs, several drugs are given one at a time by a predetermined rotation—for example, 6 weeks on each agent in succession. Cyclical drug therapy might possess the advantage of alternately suppressing different strains of leukemic cells with different drug sensitivities. The good results obtained with a cyclic regimen[356] were however equalled by those of a similar but sequential therapeutic program.[284] The Australian Cancer Society's trial (see Table 18-7) compared the cyclic versus the sequential administration of four drugs (VCR, MP, CY, MTX): although patients in the cyclic group may have had about one relapse fewer than those in the sequential group, no advantage in terms of increased median survival was demonstrable. Studies have been performed comparing the efficacy of MTX and MP for remission maintenance in acute lymphocytic leukemia when these drugs are used sequentially, in cycles, and simultaneously.[1,2] None of these methods was significantly superior to the others, which suggests that only a certain "mileage" could be obtained from each drug, irrespective of the manner in which the drugs were used. In these studies, the MTX was given in conventional doses and administered daily, a method not used nowadays. MP appears to be less dose- and schedule-sensitive than MTX: the administration of MP in high doses may increase the speed of onset of its action,[169] but it leads to gastrointenstinal toxicity not usually seen with standard doses.

It appears that cyclic drug therapy has little advantage over sequential drug administration, although patients may have fewer relapses and may be less likely to suffer from the cumulative side effects of any particular drug, due to the rotation. The median survivals of patients treated by any type of single-agent therapy were short and could not be considered satisfactory. However, much better results are obtainable when remission is maintained with antimetabolite drugs (mercaptopurine and methotrexate), supplemented by reinductions (more correctly, psuedoreinductions) with PRED plus VCR and/or DR.[25,64,161]

Of particular interest are the two studies at the end of Table 18-7. Henderson and Samaha used a regimen of maintenance by reinduction alone, giving repeated courses of the same four agents (PRED, VCR, MTX, MP). The median duration of their patients' first remissions was 13.5 months, and the median survival a very creditable 33 months. The program described by Pinkel was based on continuous maintenance with MP and intensive reinduction therapy by the intravenous administration of VCR, MTX, and CY every week. This therapy produced a remarkable median duration of first hematologic remission—22 months. Pinkel rightly distinguishes hematologic remission from "complete remission," when no signs of nonhematologic disease, such as CNS leukemia, are present. The median duration of complete remission was 15 months and there was no evidence that the doses of radiation administered to the brain and spinal cord affected the incidence of CNS leukemia in this series.[260] The median survival of these patients was 35 months, which compares favorably with any other series and surpasses most. More important, 23 percent of the children were alive at 5 years, and 19 percent had no evidence of leukemia, being classifiable as 5-year "cures." These figures are much superior to any previously reported. The five patients considered to have a 5-year cure had been in complete remission for 66–76 months and off all antileukemic therapy for 42–43 months, so the term *cure* did not seem excessively optimistic. Two other findings, which seem highly significant, are that all patients in the study who remained in continuous complete remission for longer than 28 months had 5-year cures; and chemotherapy was discontinued for patients in continuous complete remission after 24–33 months, and none of these patients subsequently relapsed. Although based on a small series, these results are so impressive that they must affect the design of future therapeutic programs for acute lymphocytic leukemia. In a later series of patients studied by Pinkel and his colleagues,[13] a more effective prophylaxis for CNS leukemia reduced its incidence and the median duration of complete remission lengthened from 15–25 months. Because of the reduced incidence of CNS leukemia, if the hematologic remission pattern in these patients follows that of the earlier series,[260] a 50 percent leukemia-free 5-year survival is to be expected.[12]

Some tentative conclusions can therefore be drawn regarding maintenance therapy in children with acute lymphocytic leukemia:

1. It should aim to avoid relapse entirely, and at present the best means of doing this appears to be the use of multiple drugs.
2. Prophylactic measures against the development of CNS leukemia should be incorporated into the maintenance program (see below).
3. If continuous complete remission is maintained for a period between 2–3 years, further maintenance therapy may be unnecessary, and leukemia-free survival for several years after cessation of therapy seems probable.

Until these conclusions have been verified at other centers and in large series of patients they cannot, of course, be more than provisional.

RECOMMENDED THERAPY

It must always be contentious to recommend a particular therapy for acute lymphocytic leukemia of childhood, since no available treatment is perfect. Many different therapeutic programs are under study and their relative merits will not be apparent until the studies are completed. A particularly promising program may be selected and recommended, but may shortly become only second-rate therapy after further advances have been made. With all these reservations in mind, it is however reasonable to recommend two programs which aim to cure acute lymphocytic leukemia in children and which show promising results so far.

The St. Jude's Hospital "total therapy" program.   This program has been under study for 10 years and many successive modifications of the protocol have been described by its originators.[11,13,132,133,260-262,297] When the diagnosis of acute lymphocytic leukemia is established, evidence of CNS leukemia is sought by an early lumbar puncture. Remission is induced with VCR (1.5 mg per square meter of body surface area) and PRED (40 mg per square meter): 80 to 90 percent of patients remit with this therapy. Immediately following the induction of remission, a 7-day course of intensive chemotherapy (MTX + MP + CY) used to be given for the purpose of remission consolidation: this was later discarded because a controlled study showed that its omission made no difference to the long-term results while its toxic effects were considerable.[12]

After remission induction (and consolidation therapy if any), prophylactic therapy for CNS leukemia is given (details are discussed on page 697). The patients then receive maintenance therapy with MP (50 mg per square meter given per day by mouth), MTX (20 mg per square meter per week) and CY (200 mg per square meter per week): the last two agents were administered intravenously in the earlier protocols but are now given by mouth. In the original protocol, VCR was administered every week; later, 3-week pulses of VCR + PRED were given every 10 weeks, and in the most recent protocol these reinduction pulses have been omitted, apparently without deterioration in results. The maintenance therapy with these three agents is aggressive, and some patients have succumbed to overwhelming infection during complete remission of their leukemia. However, one study demonstrated that treatment with the same drugs at half-dosage, though less toxic, was significantly less effective for remission maintenance.[261]

The results of this program are good. Even the earlier series produced a substantial number of 5-year, leukemia-free survivors after ceasing therapy at about $2\frac{1}{2}$ years (see Table 18-7), while the projected 5-year, leukemia-free survival of the later programs with better CNS prophylaxis is around 50 percent. Thus, this type of treatment is too effective to be ignored. On the debit side, it is far from perfect: the valuable antileukemic drugs ara-C, DR, and L-ase are not used at all, and possibly because of this, about half the patients enter hematologic relapse at some time during the maintenance phase, thereby losing most of their chance of becoming long-term survivors. However, initial relapse in the nervous system is uncommon in these children. The daily administration of MP for $2\frac{1}{2}$ years continuously is certainly immunosuppressive, probably more so than the use of the same total amount of the drug in intermittent fashion, and mercaptopurine-induced immunosuppression may be an important cause of the infective deaths during remission seen in these studies. On the other hand, a small percentage of infective deaths in remission is less unacceptable than a much higher death rate in leukemic relapse due to inadequate therapy, and there can be little doubt that the St. Jude's program cures many children with acute lymphocytic leukemia.

The COAP-POMP-CART program of the Medical Research Council Leukemia Unit.   This program (for meaning of acronyms see Table 18-4) was devised in our unit but two of its components were first developed in the United States—the POMP combination by Frei and Freireich[114] and COAP (cyclophosphamide-vincristine-cytarabine-prednisone) by Freireich and his colleagues. The method of prophylaxis against CNS leukemia resembles that used in the St. Jude's program (see page 697). The program is a composite cyclic therapy and is shown schematically in Figure 18-3. In the first 12 weeks, remission is induced with

A.L.L. PROGRAM

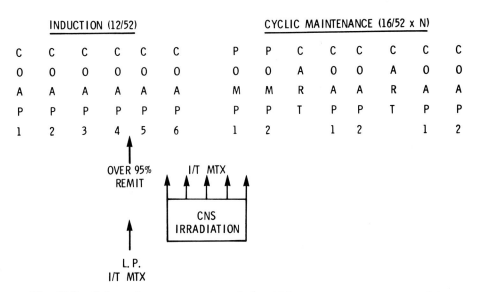

INDUCTION (12/52)   CYCLIC MAINTENANCE (16/52 x N)

C	C	C	C	C	C		P	P	C	C	C	C	C	C
O	O	O	O	O	O		O	O	A	O	O	A	O	O
A	A	A	A	A	A		M	M	R	A	A	R	A	A
P	P	P	P	P	P		P	P	T	P	P	T	P	P
1	2	3	4	5	6		1	2		1	2		1	2

OVER 95%   I/T MTX
REMIT

CNS
IRRADIATION

L.P.
I/T MTX

Fig. 18-3. Schematic representation of the ALL treatment program used by the Medical Research Council Leukaemia Unit. Six courses of the COAP are administered during a 12-week induction period: the complete remission rate exceeds 95 percent. One cycle of maintenance therapy takes 16 weeks and incorporates eight courses of the POMP, CART, and COAP combinations in the order shown. The 16-week cycle is then repeated until 130 weeks ($2\frac{1}{2}$ years) of continuous complete remission has been achieved, when therapy is discontinued. At the time when marrow remission is first demonstrated, a lumbar puncture is performed to obtain CSF for cytologic study. Methotrexate (7.5 mg/m²) is instilled into the spinal theca at the time of lumbar puncture. If examination of the CSF shows *no evidence* of leukemia, the prophylactic use of cranial irradiation and five additional injections of intrathecally administered methotrexate is begun. (Details are given in the text).

six cycles of COAP: over 95 percent of children enter complete remission. This induction therapy is followed by repeated 16-week cycles of intensive drug maintenance therapy. Each cycle of therapy incorporates four courses of COAP, two courses of POMP, and two of CART. The details of these four-drug combinations are given in Tables 18-8 through 18-10; the name of each combination is an acronym derived from the initial letters of the official or proprietary names of the drugs; these names are invaluable verbal shorthand in clinical practice. Nearly all patients will respond very rapidly to the COAP combination as shown by clearance of blast cells from the blood and bone marrow, but the hemoglobin, platelet, and neutrophil levels usually take longer to attain normal values than is the case if initial treatment has been with vincristine and prednisone alone. As a result, one or two blood transfusions are commonly necessary during the early phases of therapy, and special measures for protection against infection are sometimes required. The justification for this aggressive initial treatment, which incorporates two myelotoxic drugs, CY and ara-C, is both practical and theoretical. If only VCR and PRED are used at the outset, there is a 10 percent drop in the remission rate, to about 85 percent. Furthermore, the use of only two drugs when the total population of leukemic cells is at its highest would seem to incur a considerable risk of selecting resistant strains from

Table 18-8

Medical Research Council Leukaemia Unit Modification of the COAP Combination
for Acute Lymphocytic or Granulocytic Leukemia

Drug	Dose	Period of Time	Route
CY	100 mg/m^2/day	Days 1–5[1]	Oral[2]
Oncovin[3]	1 mg[4]	Day 1	Intravenous
Ara-C[5]	100 mg/m^2/day	Days 1–5[1]	Intravenous/intramuscular[2]
Prednisolone[6]	100 mg/day	Days 1–5	Oral

[1] Can be reduced to days 1–3 (first course), days 1–4 (second course), days 1–5 (third and later courses). After third course, a 20 percent dose increase in CY and ara-C is attempted at each successive course, until intolerance. The doses of VCR and PRED are not increased.

[2] Given intravenously in the original Houston study.

[3] Vincristine.

[4] It is pointless to relate the dose of VCR to surface area. Doses of 0.5 mg for infants and 2 mg for adults are appropriate; all children appear to tolerate 1-mg doses regardless of their weight or surface area.

[5] Cytosine arabinoside.

[6] Prednisone was used in the original Houston study.

[7] It is pointless to relate the dose of PRED to surface area. Doses of 50 mg for infants and 200 mg for adults are appropriate, and 100 mg for all children.

The original regimen was designed by E. J. Freireich and his associates at Houston.[352]

among the 10^{12} candidate cells present. However, an alternative induction therapy (VCR + PRED + L-ase) has recently been studied: the complete remission rate in children who have had no previous therapy approaches 100 percent.[10] Such a response rate is certainly acceptable and indicates that considerable synergy must exist between the drugs used. The leukemic cells are exposed to three drugs from the outset so that the possibility of selecting resistant strains is reduced. Because none

Table 18-9

M.R.C. Leukaemia Unit Modification of the POMP Combination for Acute Lymphocytic
or Granulocytic Leukemia

Drug	Dose	Period of Time	Route
Prednisolone[1]	100 mg/day[2]	Days 1–5	Oral[3]
Oncovin[4]	1 mg[5]	Day 1	Intravenous
MTX	7.5 mg/m^2/day	Days 1–5[6]	Intravenous/Intramuscular[3]
Purinethol[7]	300 mg/m^2/day	Days 1–5[8]	Oral[3]

[1] Prednisone in the original National Cancer Institute protocol.

[2] It is pointless to relate the dose of PRED to surface area. Doses of 50 mg for infants and 200 mg for adults are appropriate, and 100 mg for all children.

[3] Given intravenously in the original National Cancer Institute protocol.

[4] VCR.

[5] It is pointless to relate the dose of VCR to surface area. Doses of 0.5 mg for infants and 2 mg for adults are appropriate; all children appear to tolerate 1-mg doses regardless of weight or surface area.

[6] Can be reduced to days 1–3 (first course), days 1–4 (second course), days 1–5 (third and later courses). After third course, a 20 percent dose increase in MTX is attempted at each successive course, until intolerance. The doses of VCR and PRED are not increased.

[7] Mercaptopurine.

[8] Given by a sliding scale as for MTX, but MP is given on the *first* only of each *pair* of POMP treatments, otherwise cumulative myelotoxicity is common.

The original regimen was designed at the U.S. National Cancer Institute.[114]

Table 18-10

The CART Combination for Therapy of Acute Lymphocytic Leukemia in Children and Adults

Drug	Dose	Period of Time	Route
ara-C[1]	100 mg/m^2/day	Days 1–5[2]	Intravenous/intramuscular
L-ase[3]	30,000 IU/m^2	Days 1,4,7,10,13[4]	Intravenous/intramuscular
Rubidomycin[5]	40 mg/m^2 [6]	Day 1	Intravenous
TG	100 mg/m^2/day	Days 1–5[2]	Oral

This combination was designed in the M.R.C. Leukaemia Unit and utilizes both the synergy that exists between ara-C and TG[60] and that between DR and L-ase.[73]

[1] Cytosine arabinoside.

[2] Full dosage can usually be tolerated, but reduction can be made to days 1–3 (first course), days 1–4 (second course), days 1–5 (third and later courses). Thereafter, a 20 percent increase in the dosage of both ara-C and TG is attempted at each course.

[3] L-ase.

[4] A less convenient alternative is to give 6000 IU/m^2/day, days 1–14.

[5] DR.

[6] A 20 percent dosage increase is attempted on each successive course. This may take priority over increasing the dosages of ara-C or TG.

of the drugs used has significant myelotoxicity, recovery of marrow function is more rapid and less risk is incurred. The use of this combination (Table 18-11) as a 4-week initial therapy, followed immediately by the six COAP cycles, is currently under study. Children who are already in hematologic remission when COAP is initiated tolerate the quadruple therapy very well.

It is usually possible to begin a 5-day course of COAP, POMP, or CART

Table 8-11

Alternative Remission Induction Therapy for Use with the COAP/POMP/CART Program

Drug	Dose	Period of Time	Route
Prednisolone	50 mg/day[1]	Days 1–14[2]	Oral
VCR	1 mg[3]	Days 1, 8, and 15	Intravenous
L-ase*	8000 IU/day/m^2	Days 1–28 inclusive	Intravenous/intramuscular/subcutaneous[4]

The response rate to this treatment in previously untreated children with acute lymphocytic leukemia approaches 100 percent.[10] Unlike the COAP combination, none of the drugs used has significant myelotoxicity. Adequate peripheral blood values are therefore reached more rapidly and without a preliminary exacerbation of pancytopenia which sometimes occurs with COAP. The six cycles of COAP therapy follow immediately after this induction, that is, COAP (1) begins on day 29.

[1] It is pointless to relate the dose of prednisolone to surface area. Doses of 25 mg for infants and 100 mg for adults are appropriate with this regimen, and 50 mg for all children.

[2] The steroid is discontinued abruptly, without tapering off the dose.

[3] It is pointless to relate the dosage of VCR to surface area. Doses of 0.5 mg for infants, 2 mg for adults, and 1 mg for all children are appropriate.

[4] This dose can be dissolved in 2–3 ml of physiologic saline and administered by any of these three routes: there is much to be said for avoiding the use of veins whenever possible and thus conserving them. Adults usually develop much more severe anorexia and nausea during L-ase therapy than occurs in children; the reason for this is unknown.

*Recent studies suggest that L-asparaginase has greater myelosuppressive effects than was originally thought. It is safer to begin treatment with (VCR + PRED) and introduce asparaginase only after initial improvement has occurred. (See Brit. Med. J., 3:81, 1974.)

treatment every 14 days; the 9-day rest period is generally long enough for hematologic recovery. As the bone marrow population of normal hematopoietic cells increases, most children can tolerate this therapy every 14 days with enhanced doses. It is our practice to increase the doses in COAP, POMP, and CART to a level which maintains a persistent, asymptomatic, moderate pancytopenia: although all the children have mild anemia and intermittent neutropenia, some exhibit persistent slight thrombocytosis, and thrombocytopenia is relatively uncommon during the maintenance phase. Reticulocytosis is a common hematologic finding at the end of each 9-day period free from drug therapy. Rarely, adequate dose levels of the antileukemic drugs can be maintained only by administering 5-day courses at 21-day intervals, with 16-day rest periods: this is probably preferable to adhering strictly to 14-day intervals at the cost of seriously reduced dosages.

As maintenance therapy progresses and the child grows, drug doses may need to be further increased, although in the second year of therapy this effect is often offset by a decreased marrow tolerance to cytotoxic therapy; thus, the absolute doses may remain constant while the dose per square meter of surface area falls slightly. In this program, the children are receiving no drugs for almost two-thirds of the time, and, in consequence, side effects are reduced: for example, neuropathy due to VCR is uncommon in these children, and Cushingoid facies are seldom marked. The bone marrow is examined every 6 weeks for evidence of relapse, but the rarity of this occurrence (see page 685) suggests that this interval might be lengthened.

It must be stressed that this treatment program, though aggressive, is not particularly unpleasant; certainly it is not worse than the disease, as is occasionally alleged about all therapeutic programs by those with small experience of childhood acute leukemia. Once remission has been achieved, all treatment can be managed on an outpatient basis. Children attend the hospital every 2 weeks for a blood examination and their initial intravenous injections: the remaining injections are given at home by the family physician or, in many cases, a family member whom we have trained to administer them. Once the sensitivity of each patient to the drugs used has been established it is usually unnecessary to examine the peripheral blood more often than every 2 weeks. These children attend school full time; moreover, they usually progress through school at the same rate as their peers and some are at the head of their classes. We have not observed any morbid dread of doctors or of hospitals in any of these children, nor has there been hostility or emotional overreaction by their parents.

Since this program was begun in 1970, and only a few of the children are as yet off therapy, it is not possible to assess long-term results. However, of 25 children entered into the program, 25 attained complete remission and only 1 has had a relapse of his leukemia. Two children died of infection during remission (1 of pneumococcal septicemia; 1 of fulminant measles) and 22 remain in complete (hematologic and CNS) remission at intervals of 0.75–4 years from diagnosis. Thus, an 88 percent incidence of long-term survivors is theoretically possible, although it would be unduly optimistic to actually expect this figure. Infective deaths in remission may be the principal obstacle to long-term survival, since the one patient whose leukemia relapsed did so only 4 months from diagnosis: no late relapses have occurred so far. These preliminary results have led us to continue with the program and to recommend its use elsewhere, with the cautionary note that experience in leukemia therapy in general, and practice with this program in particular, are necessary for good results and low morbidity. In these respects, of course, the above program is no different from any of the more sophisticated therapies for acute lymphocytic leukemia of childhood.

FAILURES OF THERAPY

These may be primary or secondary. *Primary* failure of therapy, that is, the failure to induce remission with initial treatment, is rare in childhood acute lymphocytic leukemia when modern therapies are used. Thus, if the initial therapy was POMP, COAP, or PRED + VCR + DR, in which remission rates exceeding 90 percent are seen (see Table 18-6), failure of response calls first for review of the diagnosis. Has the child an undifferentiated acute granulocytic leukemia, or disseminated malignant lymphoma? If the diagnosis of acute granulocytic leukemia is sustained, alternative induction treatment must be selected (see Table 18-6) and the choice will, of course, depend on the nature of the treatment first given. Thus, a child who fails to respond to (VCR + PRED) may then be treated with, for example, (DR + ara-C + L-ase + TG).

Secondary failure of therapy, that is, the occurrence of relapse after an initial remission, used to be universal in children with acute lymphocytic leukemia. Most had several such relapses, and the usual practice was simply to proceed to the next antileukemic agent which had not previously been administered. In this way, the patient might survive long enough to have remissions with, and later relapse from, all the principal drugs available, and finally succumb, completely resistant to all therapy. Although secondary failures of therapy are less common with more aggressive treatment, they still occur and their management depends on the past treatment experience of the specific patient. Some general rules can be formulated:

1. Benefit is rarely seen as a result of merely increasing the dosage of a drug to which the leukemia has clearly become resistant. Altering the *schedule* (for example, from continuous oral administration to intermittent, high-dose intravenous infusions) is sometimes effective.
2. The best chance of obtaining a further remission is to use a drug never previously administered to the patient.
3. If the patient has apparently become resistant to all the standard drugs, they may be used in novel combinations which the patient has not received before.
4. Alternatively, recourse may be had to second-line drugs such as BCNU, methyl GAG, or actinomycin D (see Chapter 17), but the morbidity and mortality from their use must be weighed against the relatively small chances of substantial benefit.

The maintenance of second or later remissions is also a problem. Patients who have had even one relapse seldom make long-term survivors.[332] We have found that two or three consecutive courses of CART usually will reinduce remission in children who have relapsed off single-drug (for example, MP) therapy, but attempts to maintain remission with the COAP-POMP-CART program (see above) have seldom been effective for more than a year. Other children were treated with the eight-drug TRAMPCOL regimen (see Table 18-12),[308] and although all patients treated achieved another remission, most of these were brief, despite maintenance therapy with the same combination. While it appears reasonable to use aggressive

Table 8-12
The TRAMPCOL Combination,* Designed in the M.R.C. Leukaemia Unit
for the Treatment of Refractory Acute Leukemias

Drug	Dose	Period of Time	Route
TG	100 mg/m^2/day	Days 1–5[1]	Oral
Rubidomycin[2]	40 mg/m^2 [3]	Day 1	Intravenous
Ara-C[4]	100 mg/m^2/day	Days 1–5[1]	Intravenous
MTX	7.5 mg/m^2/day	Days 1–5	Intravenous
Prednisolone	100 mg/day[5]	Days 1–5	Oral
CY	100 mg/m^2/day	Days 1–5[1]	Intravenous
Oncovin[6]	1 mg[7]	Day 1	Intravenous
L-ase	8,000 IU/m^2/day	Days 1–28[8]	Intravenous

*In nonlymphocytic acute leukemias the L-ase is sometimes omitted and the combination is then referred to as TRAMPCO.

[1] TG, ara-C, MTX, and CY may be given days 1–3 (first course), days 1–4 (second course), days 1–5 (third and later courses), making the increments if tolerated. Doses may be increased independently—for example, that of MTX may be kept low if oral toxicity is marked.

[2] DR.

[3] Attempt a 20 percent dosage increase on each successive course.

[4] Cytosine arabinoside.

[5] Adults receive 200 mg/day and children 100 mg/day.

[6] VCR.

[7] Adults receive 2 mg and children 1 mg.

[8] Discontinue before 28 days if toxicity is severe or resistance of the leukemia is obvious—for example, rising blast cell count.

treatment for a child with acute lymphocytic leukemia who has relapsed once, it seems that long-term survival is unlikely for most patients. After more than one relapse, many would feel that the benefits likely to accrue from further aggressive treatment are outweighed by the morbidity which is certain to occur. At some stage it may be decided that only palliative measures should be adopted—for example, corticosteroids, analgesics, and tranquillizers. Painful bone lesions may be palliated by irradiation,[78] but generalized bone pain or painful organomegaly are better treated by daunorubicin or cyclophosphamide, which usually will destroy leukemic cells and relieve symptoms, even when remission cannot be reinduced.

Acute Granulocytic Leukemia in Children

Acute granulocytic leukemia is uncommon in children. From the morphologic viewpoint, some very undifferentiated acute leukemias of childhood might be classified as acute granulocytic or lymphocytic leukemia with equal uncertainty, but most such patients respond to treatment like those with morphologically typical acute lymphocytic leukemia, and are often classified as such on therapeutic response. Undoubted acute granulocytic leukemia in children is much less responsive to treatment than is acute lymphocytic leukemia of childhood, and this is reflected in a poor median survival (see Table 18-3).

Because acute granulocytic leukemia is uncommon in childhood it has been less well characterized than acute granulocytic leukemia in adults, and it is difficult to be certain whether there are major differences between the two age groups. Acute granulocytic leukemia in very young infants has a reputation of being poorly responsive to therapy, but whether this is a characteristic of the leukemia itself or merely reflects the fragility of this type of host is uncertain. Median survival of children with acute granulocytic leukemia appears better than that of adults (see Table 18-3), and may even surpass that of adults with acute lymphocytic leukemia, although some survival figures for adults may be affected by the accidental inclusion of cases which were not true acute lymphocytic leukemia. There is some evidence that children with acute granulocytic leukemia may achieve remission more frequently than adults treated by the same protocols[65,152]: in one study, 16 of 38 children and only 14 of 48 adults with acute granulocytic leukemia achieved complete remission when treated with (DR + VCR + PRED).[254] This increased remission rate may signify that childhood acute granulocytic leukemia differs intrinsically from the adult disease, but it might merely reflect the fact that, in adults, the clinical course is more often complicated by cardiac, renal, pulmonary, hepatic, and other diseases, contributing to early death and inevitably lowering the response rate. Evidence whether maintenance therapy is more effective in prolonging remission in childhood acute granulocytic leukemia than it is in adults is lacking; the better median survival of children may only be a consequence of a higher initial response rate. Certainly, many children who respond to initial therapy have only brief remissions and do not survive long: from a therapist's viewpoint, the childhood disease resembles adult acute granulocytic leukemia and has little in common with childhood acute lymphocytic leukemia.

There is no evidence that the treatment of acute granulocytic leukemia in children should be different to its management in adults. The physician may expect a greater likelihood of remission, and possibly a longer remission duration than obtained in most adult patients, but there seems no reason to use different drug regimens in those patients with acute granulocytic leukemia who happen also to be children. Accordingly, the management in children is not discussed separately here.

ACUTE LEUKEMIA IN ADULTS

Although the same broad principles apply, the details of treatment for acute leukemia, and its results, differ greatly between children and adults. Most important, the great majority of adults with acute leukemia have one of the granulocytic forms of the disease, all of which appear to be less responsive to chemotherapy. Initial remission rates are low and, because maintenance therapy is not very effective, remission duration is poor; these factors combine to produce a short median survival figure. Second, as referred to above, adults frequently suffer from multiple pathology. Preexisting disorders of the heart, lungs, kidneys, liver, or gastrointestinal tract are often exacerbated by the leukemia and also by its treatment. Anemia, infection, hemorrhage, and metabolic disturbances are poorly tolerated in older patients, and death early in the course of acute leukemia becomes increasingly common as the patient's age at diagnosis increases,[221] so much so that many physicians try to avoid aggressive therapy in patients over 60 years of age on the grounds that supportive therapy alone not infrequently produces survival for some months, while radical chemotherapy will kill the patient in a few days. Although it may be speculated that acute leukemia in elderly adults is a more malignant disease, perhaps because of impaired immunologic responses in the host, the poor survival of these patients can equally be explained by coexisting pathology which precludes their deriving benefit from antileukemic therapy.

Acute Granulocytic Leukemia in Adults

The acute granulocytic leukemias can be subdivided into myeloblastic, promyelocytic, myelomonocytic and apparently monocytic varieties (see Chapter 3), to which may be added erythroleukemia and the acute form of the Di Guglielmo syndrome. This subdivision is not always easy to accomplish, particularly when variations in terminology and in diagnostic criteria further complicate the issue. From the therapeutic viewpoint, such subdivision is not very important, because there is no good evidence that the treatment of the different subvarieties should be different, although with further refinements in therapy, precise cytologic classification might assume a new importance. At present, the only exception to the above statement is that the recognition of promyelocytic leukemia can be important, since some patients have a special predisposition to diffuse intravascular coagulation and may require special supportive measures at the outset of therapy (see Chapter 14).

It is doubtful whether the prognosis varies between the different subvarieties of acute granulocytic leukemia. Thus, acute myelomonocytic leukemia was said to have a particularly poor response to treatment,[72] but this view has been challenged.[200] The rarer varieties, such as monocytic leukemia and erythroleukemia, have been said to remit seldom or never, but inevitably therapeutic experience with these varieties is inadequate for proper assessment because of their relative uncommonness. Acute promyelocytic leukemia may carry a very unfavorable prognosis if the tendency to disseminated intravascular coagulation is unrecognized, but with proper supportive therapy the remission rate in these patients is not significantly different from that of patients with other types of acute granulocytic leukemia.[135] The age of patients probably affects their prognosis more than does the cytologic subvariety.

The poor response of acute granulocytic leukemia to chemotherapy is as unexplained as the relatively good response of acute lymphocytic leukemia. The average age of patients with acute granulocytic leukemia, most of whom are adults, exceeds that of patients with acute lymphocytic leukemia, but age is unlikely to be the sole explanation. Thus, children with the latter fare much better than children with the former, and one series of adults with acute lymphocytic leukemia, in which the diagnosis was established carefully and the therapy was modern, appeared to respond to treatment as well as a corresponding group of children.[65] It has been suggested that in the granulocytic leukemias there may be no population of normal hematopoietic cells remaining in the bone marrow, or that the disease itself may be a disorder of external factors which regulate hematopoiesis.[40,231] Such factors might explain the failure of some patients to achieve remission with any form of therapy, but seem unlikely to apply in the majority of patients.[65] However, partial explanations are available in chemotherapeutic terms. Since none of the available antileukemic agents is sufficiently selective in killing leukemic myeloblasts, induction therapy is, of necessity, myelotoxic and has a significant mortality, which decreases the possible remission rate. Because relatively few drugs are dependably lethal to leukemic myeloblasts, the effective consolidation of an established hematologic remission is difficult and this probably decreases the median remission duration.[65] These properties of the leukemic cells in acute granulocytic leukemia may explain the poor results of treatment, but the reason *why* such cells have these characteristics is as mysterious as that underlying the more exploitable properties of the cells in acute lymphocytic leukemia.

REVIEW OF THERAPY

Specific antileukemic drugs have been used in acute granulocytic leukemia for 25 years, as in acute lymphocytic leukemia. In the former, however, therapeutic progress has been slow: significant advances have occurred only in the past 10 years—dating from the introduction of daunorubicin—and, at present, the treatment of the former is far less satisfactory than that of the latter. The first major problem is that of inducing an initial remission of the disease, and from Table 18-13 it can be seen that the major antileukemic drugs induce relatively few remissions in acute granulocytic leukemia; only in recent times has the remission rate approached the 50 percent level with the introduction of various drug combinations. The remission rates shown should be regarded as only approximate since the criteria of evaluation are not necessarily the same in all series. Moreover, some reports are based on relatively small numbers of patients and variable results are sometimes reported by different groups employing the same therapy. The importance of the individual therapist's experience, expertise, and faith in the potential value of the

Table 18-13
Remission Induction by Chemotherapy in Acute Granulocytic Leukemia

Treatment	No. of Patients*	% Complete Remission	References
Single Drugs			
MTX	44	16	342
PRED	39	15	221
	29 children	14	354
MP	31	10	2
	11 children	9	2
CY	45	4	82
VCR	7	0	69
	14 children	36	179
DR	21	43	27
ara-C	31	44	155
L-ase	Transient fall in blast count not uncommon but hematologic remission rare.		
Drug Combinations			
PRED + MP	77	3	331
POMP	83	29	154
PRED + VCR + DR	48	29	254
	38 children	42	254
PRED + VCR + ara-C + CY	33	39	352
ara-C + TG	53	65 approx.	84
DR + ara-C	30	53	135
DR + ara-C (± L-ase)	23	61	74

*Patients were adults except where indicated.

therapeutic regimen should be emphasized. Life-threatening complications are frequent during attempted induction of remission, and their optimal management requires, not only skill, experience, and considerable material resources, but also confidence in the ability of the antileukemic therapy to eventually induce remission and secure an acceptable quality of life despite devastating complications; in the face of which less aggressive or less confident physicians might be inclined to let the patient die without further suffering. Thus, good results with a particular induction regimen at a specialized leukemia center may not be reproduced in a wider trial among cooperating, nonspecialized institutions: such disparity is more likely to occur when the regimen is complex. From a practical viewpoint, it may be claimed that therapy which only succeeds in a specialized environment is undesirable, but equally it may be said that the dissemination of expertise is one of the most practical methods of improving difficult therapeutic situations.

It appears that approximately one-half of adults with acute granulocytic leukemia may achieve complete remission of their disease with aggressive drug therapy when this is given expertly in a setting where facilities for supportive therapy are adequate. However, the maintenance of remission is unsatisfactory and survival is short compared with that of acute lymphocytic leukemia (Table 18-14). From Table 18-14 it can be seen that in 10 years the remission induction rate has risen from 7 to over 60 percent at some centers. Throughout the period surveyed, patients with acute granulocytic leukemia which is unresponsive to chemotherapy have had very short survival times, possibly shorter than might have been achieved by supportive therapy alone—a fact which must be considered before embarking upon aggressive therapy in elderly or other poor-risk patients with acute granulocytic leukemia. Patients who achieve complete hematologic remission survive significantly longer, but *all* the median survivals shown in Table 18-13 are close to 1 year, although one trial is "ongoing" since more than half the patients were alive when the results were published.

RECOMMENDED THERAPY

Most therapeutic programs claim a remission rate around 50 percent and a median survival around 12 months for those patients who remit—that is, about 25 percent of all patients will be alive 1 year from diagnosis. Clearly, all these programs are very imperfect and none can be recommended with enthusiasm. However, three programs may be cited as meriting further evaluation.

The "L6" protocol used at Memorial Hospital. This program has been reported extensively.[65,84,130] Remission is induced with ara-C (3 mg per kilogram of body weight, given intravenously every 12 hours) and TG (2.5 mg per kilogram of body weight, administered orally every 12 hours), the doses being spaced 12 hours apart in order to prevent any cells from completing their DNA-synthetic (S) phase without being exposed to possibly cytocidal concentrations of the agents.[66] It is aimed to destroy 90 percent of the leukemic cell population in the first course of treatment and the number of doses given varies from eleven to thirty-six. The length of each course of treatment can be judged roughly from the initial blast cell count in the bone marrow, but is modified by the rapidity and extent of the clinical and hematologic response and the general condition of the patient. Since maximum

Table 18-14
Duration of Survival in Adults with Acute Granulocytic Leukemia Treated by Various Regimens*

Workers and References	Remission-induction Therapy	Remission-maintenance Therapy	No. of Patients	% Complete Remission	Median Survivals (months)	
					C.R.[1]	N.R.[2]
Medical Research Council (1963)[220]	MP or MP + PRED	Same as induction.	86	7	13[3]	<2
Levi et al. (1972)[200]	ara-C + TG + hydroxyurea	Monthly ara-C + TG	22	41	8	<2
Clarkson (1972)[65]	ara-C + TG	Multiple drugs (ara-C, TG, VCR, DR, BCNU, CY, MTX, hydroxyurea) in cycles.	43	65	>10[4]	2
Crowther et al. (1973)[75]	DR + ara-C	MP + MTX or immunotherapy	40	57	11.5	<1
Pavlovsky et al. (1973)[254]	PRED + VCR + DR	MTX + MP or MTX alone; both with intermittent PRED + VCR + DR	86[5]	35	11.8	<1

*Median duration of remission is not ascertainable for all these series. Where given, it has some correlation with median survival.
[1] C.R. = complete hematologic remission.
[2] N.R. = nonresponders.
[3] This surprisingly good figure is based on only six patients and seems unlikely to be of real significance.
[4] Median survival was 10 months if all the patients died immediately after publication of the data.
[5] The 86 patients included 38 children, but survival was analyzed by pooling the groups.

hematologic depression occurs 10–14 days after interruption of treatment, the decision to stop must be partly anticipatory. After a rest period of about 3 weeks, a further course is administered. About 65 percent of previously untreated adults with acute granulocytic leukemia can be expected to achieve remission usually after two or three courses, but this high remission rate is unlikely if supportive facilities are not good. When marrow remission has been achieved, the remission is consolidated with three additional courses of ara-C + TG. Each course is carried to moderate marrow hypoplasia, with the aim of further reducing the body leukemic cell load. Remission maintenance in the L6 program is with a complex sequence of cytotoxic drugs: VCR, MTX + BCNU, TG + CY, hydroxyurea + DR, then repeating the maintenance cycle indefinitely as long as remission persists. The inherent drawback of a complex schedule such as this is that if one or two of the component drugs are contributing nothing to the therapy (that is, if the leukemic cells are resistant to their action) there is no way of ascertaining this: The administration of ineffective drugs is not unimportant, since their use limits the amounts of the *effective* drugs which can safely be given, particularly as most of these drugs have an overlapping myelotoxic potential. However, the results of this complex maintenance therapy are most promising.[65] Of 28 patients who achieved complete remission, only 8 had relapsed between 4 and 24 months from diagnosis; 2 had died in remission, and 18 were alive and in remission for periods between 2 and 24 months. Eight patients had survived more than 1 year, and 5 of these remained in complete remission. Further follow-up is required to assess the results of the L6 program properly, but it is obviously a good means of inducing disease remission, and may be better for maintenance of remission than are other programs.

The TRAP program of the Medical Research Council Leukemia Unit. This program was devised in our unit, but two combinations in the maintenance schedule were first developed in the United States—POMP by Frei and Freireich[114] and COAP by Freireich and his colleagues.[352] The program is a composite cyclic therapy and is shown schematically in Figure 18-4. The three drug combinations used, COAP, POMP, and TRAP are shown in Tables 18-8, 18-9, and 18-15, respectively. The TRAMPCO combination, used for patients whose leukemia is unresponsive to TRAP induction, is shown in Table 18-12.

The TRAP combination (TG + DR + ara-C + PRED) utilizes the synergies thought to exist between DR and ara-C and between ara-C and TG. PRED was included because it appeared to be the best single agent for use in acute granulocytic leukemia in earlier studies.[220,221] The combination thus incorporates two widely used two-drug treatments (see Table 18-13), adding another antileukemic drug which has no myelotoxic effects (PRED) and which increases the patients' sense of well-being. In a series of 26 adults, 5 of 17 previously untreated patients and 5 of 9 patients who had received prior therapy attained complete remission. The overall remission rate in this small series is 40 percent, and TRAP-induction therapy is at present being studied in a cooperative multicenter trial.

The maintenance regimen (see Fig. 18-4) utilizes the COAP and POMP combinations as well as TRAP. In this way, all the first-line drugs are used early in the clinical course, and, theoretically, this cyclic maintenance might avoid the emergence of drug-resistant leukemic cell-lines. Furthermore, the cyclic pattern

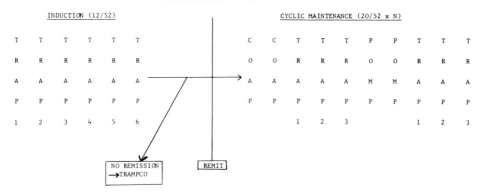

Fig. 18-4. Schematic representation of the TRAP program, one of the protocols used in the Medical Research Council Leukaemia Unit for treatment of acute granulocytic leukemia in adults and children. Six courses of the TRAP combination (see Table 18-15) are administered during the 12-week induction period: about 50 percent of patients achieve remission. Patients not in complete remission, but with continually improving appearances in the bone marrow, may have eight or more courses of TRAP before entering the maintenance phase. Patients whose progress is unsatisfactory are treated with the TRAMPCO combination (see Table 18-12), sometimes before the full six courses of TRAP have been administered. One cycle of maintenance therapy takes 20 weeks and incorporates ten courses of the COAP (see Table 18-8), TRAP, and POMP (see Table 18-9) combinations in the order shown. The 20-week cycle is then repeated. Therapy is discontinued when complete remission has been maintained for 130 weeks: unfortunately, most patients show evidence of relapse of their disease before this time is reached.

Table 18-15
The TRAP Combination, Designed in the M.R.C. Leukaemia Unit
for the Treatment of AGL in Adults and Children*

Drug	Dose	Period of Time	Route
TG[1]	100 mg/m^2/day	Days 1–5	Oral
Rubidomycin[2]	40 mg/m^2/day[3]	Day 1	Intravenous
Ara-C[4]	100 mg/m^2/day	Days 1–5[5]	Intravenous
Prednisolone[6]	30 mg/m^2/day	Days 1–5	Oral

*This regimen utilizes the synergies which exist between ara-C and TG, and between ara-C and DR.

[1] Thioguanine is used in preference to MP because there is evidence that the former compound displays more synergy with ara-C than does MP (55). In addition, the concurrent administration of allopurinol does not alter the dosimetry of TG.

[2] DR.

[3] If possible, a 20 percent dosage increment is made on each successive course.

[4] Cytosine arabinoside.

[5] Usually given on days 1–3 (first course), Days 1–4 (second course), Days 1–5 (third and later courses). Thereafter, a 20 percent dosage increase is attempted at each course, and the dose of TG is increased *pari passu* with that of ara-C.

[6] Used in preference to PRED because PRED must be metabolized (principally in the liver) before becoming active.

prevents cumulative toxicity: Cushingoid changes are uncommon, neurotoxicity from VCR is not seen, and cardiotoxicity from DR has not been observed, although some patients have now received a total of 2 gm of daunorubicin. The median remission duration in the 10 patients who entered the maintenance arm is 9 months, and the first patient to be treated by the TRAP program remains in remission some 37 months from diagnosis. Once remission has been obtained it is not difficult to continue maintenance therapy in the outpatient clinic, and most of our patients continue fulltime with their normal occupations. As with our acute lymphocytic leukemia therapy program, the patients are free of drug therapy for 9 days in every 14. Some adults develop undue pancytopenia if TRAP maintenance is administered every 14 days; they receive 5 days' therapy every 21 days. Obviously, the TRAP program is far from ideal, since at least half the patients do not achieve initial remission, but it merits further study and refinement.[255]

The immunotherapy program of St. Bartholomew's Hospital. Immunotherapy is an experimental, not an established, method of treatment in human leukemia. In acute lymphocytic leukemia, many workers would feel that the use of immunotherapy is inappropriate, because chemotherapy alone can produce long-term survival and possible cure. However, in acute granulocytic leukemia, chemotherapy at present has much less to offer, and immunotherapy should certainly be studied, particularly if this can be done without jeopardizing the modest benefits which might be expected from chemotherapy alone. The St. Bartholomew's program appears to achieve this end and its preliminary results are of considerable interest; so much so that a cooperative, multicenter study is now in progress.

Adult patients with acute granulocytic leukemia are treated initially with DR (1.5 mg per kilogram of body weight, given intravenously on day 1) and ara-C (2 mg per kilogram of body weight, given intravenously, on days 1–5).[75] These 5-day courses are repeated at 10-day intervals, that is, with 5-day rest periods between courses. The complete remission rate in 94 patients was 49 percent, which well illustrates the variability within a center, since in a smaller series treated by the same drugs, the same group found 61 percent of remissions (see Table 18-13).[74] After remission is achieved, one further course of ara-C + DR is given as consolidation. Thereafter, all patients receive 5 days of chemotherapy once a month, alternating between agents used in the same schedule for remission induction, and ara-C (2 mg per kilogram per day, given intravenously, on days 1–5) with TG (2 mg per kilogram per day, given by mouth, on days 1–5). Half the patients also receive immunotherapy with intradermal BCG vaccine plus subcutaneous, irradiated, allogeneic leukemic blast cells, administered every week.

Long-term follow-up on these patients is not yet available. The median remission duration in the chemotherapy-alone group is 8 months, that is, quite unremarkable. The median remission duration in the patients receiving immunotherapy in addition to their chemotherapy has not yet been reached but exceeds 10 months with 3 patients in continuous remission for 1–2 years. These preliminary results suggest that immunotherapy in acute granulocytic leukemia should be studied further, but its use cannot as yet be recommended outside the setting of a formal controlled trial.

Acute Lymphocytic Leukemia in Adults

Acute lymphocytic leukemia is relatively uncommon in adults. It has the reputation of being less responsive to therapy than the childhood form, but it seems likely that this apparent difference is due to the inclusion, among adult patients, of those with highly undifferentiated acute leukemia among the group. Many such cases behave like acute granulocytic leukemia in being relatively unresponsive to drugs. It is our policy to regard as having acute lymphocytic leukemia only those whose cytology and cytochemistry are unequivocally that of the childhood form: undifferentiated acute leukemias without definite features of acute lymphocytic leukemia are classified and treated as acute granulocytic leukemia.

Our policy is to treat adults with unequivocal acute lymphocytic leukemia by the COAP-POMP-CART program (see above), just as for children. We have not found any difference in response in the small number of adults studied. All have achieved complete remission with two or three courses of COAP and none has relapsed from the maintenance therapy; the patient we have followed for the longest period has been in continuous complete remission for 2 years. All these adults have had prophylactic therapy against CNS leukemia (see below) and none has as yet developed this complication. Our experience is similar to that of others who find that adults with undoubted acute lymphocytic leukemia respond just as well as childhood cases.[65,142]

REFRACTORY LEUKEMIA

Refractory acute granulocytic leukemia is common in adults and may be classified into several types.

Primary failures of remission induction.   About 50 percent of patients fail to remit with available primary treatments. If primary induction failure is not associated with a dead or moribund patient, as it frequently is, the problem arises what further therapy to try. It is our practice to attempt induction with the TRAMPCO regimen (see Table 18-12); among eight patients, we have seen one complete and four partial remissions. One patient who failed to achieve remission with TRAP later remitted with POMP. Patients who fail to remit when TRAP is the initial therapy have not, in our experience, remitted if later treated with COAP or ara-C + TG. Primary induction failure with any reasonable drug regimen may well signify a very refractory case which is unlikely to respond to any presently available alternative therapy.

Relapses after previous remissions.   It appears to be very uncommon to secure a second remission in acute granulocytic leukemia, unless relapse occurs when the patient is receiving no therapy or very inadequate therapy. We have observed a second complete remission in two patients who had discontinued their therapy: remission was obtained by restoring them to the same therapy. Ten patients who relapsed while on adequate therapy were treated with the TRAMPCO regimen with two complete second remissions. Patients who relapse while receiving very aggressive therapy (for example, the TRAP program) seem never to have another remission; leukemias which relapse despite such therapy may well be a selected particularly refractory group.

Secondary types of acute granulocytic leukemia. When acute granulocytic leukemia arises secondary to a preexisting bone marrow disorder, such as myelofibrosis, polycythemia vera, aplastic anemia, or chronic granulocytic leukemia, it is usually highly refractory to treatment and remission in the usual sense is exceedingly rare with any therapy. Frequently, this may reflect the fact that there is no surviving population of normal hematopoietic cells in the bone marrow. In such cases, inadequate therapy leaves persisting leukemia, and more aggressive therapy produces irreversible fatal marrow aplasia. Sometimes, particularly in chronic granulocyte leukemia, the secondary acute leukemia has a remarkable tendency to develop resistance to antileukemic drugs, so that even control of the total leukocyte count—seldom lost in other situations—becomes difficult. We have had no success in treating acute leukemia secondary to aplastic anemia, polycythemia vera, or myelofibrosis; such cases are of course uncommon. For chronic granulocytic leukemia which has undergone metamorphosis to a picture resembling acute granulocytic leukemia, we use the TRAMPCO regimen with moderate success (see below).

CNS Leukemia

Clinical involvement of the CNS, most commonly the meninges, by acute leukemia was something of a curiosity prior to the advent of effective chemotherapy for the systemic disease. Now that median survival has increased substantially, meningeal leukemia has become a common and serious clinical problem. An extensive literature on the epidemiology, prophylaxis and treatment of CNS leukemia has recently been summarized (see Chapter 10).[48,96] Involvement of the CNS is rare in chronic lymphocytic leukemia, and in chronic granulocytic leukemia is occasionally seen after the disease has undergone metamorphosis to an invasive neoplasm resembling acute granulocytic leukemia. In acute lymphocytic leukemia, CNS leukemia is common, in the acute granulocytic form considerably less so. Although in autopsy studies the brain is more often involved than the meninges,[199] meningeal leukemia is more often clinically manifest. The occurrence of meningeal leukemia in children with acute lymphocytic leukemia is the central problem of CNS leukemia and its presence seems to depend mainly on the duration of survival.[99,347] The relationship is, however, a complex one since the development of CNS leukemia has, in turn, an adverse effect on the subsequent survival of those so affected.[229] Apart from the immediate hazards, this is readily explained by the tendency of CNS leukemia to recur, however energetically it is treated.

CNS leukemia is not peculiar to acute lymphocytic leukemia in children although they account for 90 percent of cases, and the acute granulocytic and chronic granulocytic forms after metamorphosis for the remainder.[48] Survival, age, and cytological type seem to be inextricably linked: long survival is linked with acute lymphocytic leukemia of childhood, and short survival times are linked with acute granulocytic leukemia of adults in almost all cases.[48,313] Adults with acute lymphocytic leukemia, children with acute granulocytic leukemia, and long-surviving patients with acute granulocytic leukemia at all ages are relatively uncommon, so that generalizations based on a few cases are unjustified.

The factors in the pathogenesis of CNS leukemia have not all been assessed. Cytogenetic studies[212] indicate that leukemic cells in the cerebrospinal fluid are metastases from bone marrow, and that they commonly undergo cytogenetic evolution in the CNS.[20] The mechanism of leukemic seeding of the meninges is incompletely understood. Autopsy studies suggest direct extension from the diploic bone marrow,[340] but the findings at death may not reflect the effects at and before diagnosis when seeding is believed to occur. Other autopsy findings in children with acute lymphocytic leukemia[267] suggest that CNS invasion by leukemic cells occurs via the superficial arachnoid veins, into the arachnoid trabeculae. In contrast, a recent study from Britain[347] showed the occurrence of CNS leukemia in children to be inversely related to the platelet count at presentation and directly related to the total leukocyte count and lymph node enlargement. These observations are interpreted as evidence that seeding follows minute intracranial hemorrhages at or before diagnosis, effective seeding being associated with thrombocytopenia and marked leukocytosis.

CNS leukemia may obviously impair survival by the direct effects of leukemic infiltration considered as an intracranial neoplasm. In addition, it may adversely affect survival by providing a site of residual disease not readily accessible to systemic treatment. In this role, CNS leukemia may be likened to residual leukemia in kidney, liver, and testes, all of which have been demonstrated in cases in otherwise complete remission.[216,246]

Once CNS leukemia has become manifest, it is generally agreed that it is exceptionally difficult to eradicate permanently. Its occurrence frequently means that normal health and long survival can no longer be expected: moreover, the presence, or suspicion, of CNS leukemia may mean that systemic antileukemic therapy cannot be discontinued. Proper antileukemic therapy, carried on indefinitely, has an appreciable mortality and morbidity which any physician would wish to avoid.

PROPHYLACTIC THERAPY

Interest in prophylactic measures against CNS leukemia has increased as survival in acute lymphocytic leukemia has improved, making CNS disease more and more important. It should be pointed out that such therapy is never truly "prophylactic"—in patients with undetectable CNS leukemia, perhaps 75 percent of children with acute lymphocytic leukemia, the prophylaxis is actually therapeutic. In the other 25 percent, who have no CNS deposits of leukemic cells, the prophylaxis is worse than wasted therapy as it may cause undesirable side effects and therapeutic hazards without compensatory benefit. However, since there is no known way of detecting this minority of patients, it would be justifiable to give some form of prophylaxis to all.

It required some years of study to evolve an effective therapy for prevention of CNS leukemia. A single, intrathecal injection of MTX following the diagnosis of acute lymphocytic leukemia did not prevent the occurrence of CNS disease.[229] However, in patients whose initial leukocyte count was over 10,000 per cubic millimeter, the time of onset of CNS complications was 12.4 months in those given methotrexate intrathecally and 5.1 months in control children: this difference was statistically significant. In a group of patients given monthly intrathecal injections of MTX, the overall incidence of meningeal leukemia was only 10 percent,[305] but the median survival of the patients studied was only 18.5 months: with more modern systemic chemotherapy and a longer median survival, more cases of meningeal leukemia would be expected. The finding that MTX given intrathecally every 2 months is effective in maintaining remissions of treated meningeal leukemia,[323,325] while BCNU administered intravenously at the same intervals is ineffective, suggests that methotrexate might be a useful prophylaxis in patients who have never had overt meningeal leukemia, while BCNU might not be useful. However, remission maintenance in patients who have had meningeal leukemia may not exactly parallel the prophylaxis of meningeal leukemia in previously unaffected patients. Repeated intrathecal injections are troublesome to both patients and physicians, and there is some doubt whether this form of prophylaxis would affect leukemic deposits within the cerebral substance, so at many centers interest has been concentrated on the prophylactic use of ionizing irradiations.

Studies on prophylactic irradiation of the CNS shortly after the induction of remission in children with acute lymphocytic leukemia have been pursued for several years by Pinkel and his associates at Memphis. Initially, 500 rad of ^{60}Co teletherapy was administered to the entire craniospinal axis.[132,134] Later, a dose of 1200 rad was used, but neither dose appeared to be effective as prophylaxis against CNS leukemia.[133] However, in a later study where no prophylactic irradiation was administered,[261] the median time of onet of CNS disease was shorter, suggesting that low doses of craniospinal irradiation may delay the onset of meningeal leukemia although not preventing it entirely. In their next study,[13] these investigators administered 2400 rad of irradiation to the skull only, together with five doses of intrathecally administered methotrexate (12 mg per square meter per dose). In the next 2 years, only 3 out of 20 children who completed all phases of this therapy developed CNS leukemia, whereas 10 or more cases might have been expected. It was later shown that irradiation of the whole craniospinal axis to 2400 rad, without the administration of methotrexate, was also effective prophylaxis against meningeal leukemia.[11,12]

Irradiation of the spinal column to 2400 rad is not without risk. In most children, the systemic antileukemic therapy has to be curtailed during spinal irradiation; even so, serious pancytopenia is sometimes seen, and, in addition, irradiation of the spinal epiphyses in young children may lead to retardation of growth with eventual short stature—an important consideration if prolonged survival or cure of their leukemia is envisaged. Cranial irradiation combined with methotrexate injected intrathecally is rather more troublesome to administer but equally effective and less hazardous. In a recently completed, controlled trial[226] the CNS prophylaxis used was 2500 rad of cranial irradiation plus 1000 rad of spinal irradiation plus eleven doses of methotrexate spread over a 38-week period. The occurrence of meningeal leukemia in 26 of the 80 children who had no prophylaxis and in only 1 of the 75 children who received prophylactic therapy strongly supports the case for routine use of this therapy in acute lymphocytic leukemia of childhood. In this trial it was found that tolerance to further antileukemic chemotherapy was reduced in the patients who had received spinal irradiation: this effect was seen in the older (10–13 years) children, possibly because at this age the reserve of unirradiated bone marrow in the long bones of the limbs is smaller than in younger children.

Although there is a natural reluctance to administer to every patient a prophylactic therapy which involves temporary severe epilation and several lumbar punctures, the case for deferring such measures until meningeal leukemia actually develops is very weak indeed. Although prophylactic treatment of the CNS is highly effective, the administration of identical therapy to children with overt meningeal leukemia usually fails to eradicate the condition, and relapses of the CNS disease are frequent.[12] At present, it is our policy to administer prophylactic therapy to all children with acute lymphocytic leukemia shortly after remission has been induced (see Fig. 18-3). When an M1 marrow status has been demonstrated, a diagnostic lumbar puncture is performed. The CSF is examined cytologically, using a Shandon-Elliott cytocentrifuge and staining the preparations in the same manner as blood films. Periodic-acid-Schiff and Sudan black preparations can also be made from cytocentrifuge slides. Methotrexate in a 7.5-mg dose per square meter is instilled at the time of lumbar puncture. If the CSF shows no evidence of leukemia, 2400 rad of irradiation are delivered to the entire cranial contents, using a linear accelerator with two horizontally opposed fields and giving twelve doses of 200 rad in 19 days. During this period, five further intrathecal injections of MTX (7.5 mg per square meter) are given. It is rarely necessary to utilize systemic folinic acid with this regimen, but the systemic antileukemic chemotherapy may be modified or deferred during the period of CNS treatment. Mild nausea is not uncommon during irradiation and occasionally pyrexia and/or meningeal irritation are observed after the drug has been injected. Alopecia becomes nearly complete shortly after radiotherapy is finished and regrowth of hair does not begin for several weeks, but after 4 months or so the child has an adequate head of hair, which grows despite the continuing cytotoxic therapy and does not fall out thereafter unless the nature of the treatment is radically altered.

It is uncertain whether CNS prophylaxis should be administered to adults with acute lymphocytic leukemia or to patients of any age with acute granulocytic leukemia. It is our practice to give CNS prophylaxis to adults with the former but the relative rarity of such patients makes it difficult to carry out a controlled study to determine if this is a correct policy.

TREATMENT

The best treatment for CNS leukemia is "prophylaxis," but this is not always possible—occasional patients with acute lymphocytic or acute granulocytic leukemia have meningeal leukemia at presentation, and patients with the former, who for some reason have not had prophylactic therapy, have a high chance of developing meningeal leukemia. Occasional patients with acute granulocytic leukemia enjoy lengthy hematologic remissions and develop meningeal leukemia as a late complication; such patients are sufficiently rare so that routine CNS prophylaxis in patients with acute granulocytic leukemia would be hard to justify. Therefore, the physician still has to treat patients with meningeal leukemia, though it is hoped less often than formerly. An extensive literature on the therapy of CNS leukemia has recently been reviewed.[48]

Radiation. The external application of ionizing radiations for meningeal leukemia has been used for 20 years. Doses as low as 400 rad produced remission of meningeal leukemia in 49 of 50 children, with a mean remission duration of 2.8

months.[98] Pooled data[48] from 147 episodes of meningeal leukemia in 135 patients show an overall *subjective* response rate of 82 percent: doses up to 1400 rad do not increase the incidence or duration of remission. Even a 2400-rad dose often fails to eradicate leukemic deposits in the CNS.[12] Radiotherapy has the advantages of being painless and of reaching the interior of the brain as well as the meninges; the regular production of alopecia is a drawback but this is outweighed by the seriousness of the symptoms of meningeal leukemia.

Intrathecally administered methotrexate. There has been more experience with intrathecally administered methotrexate than with any other drug in meningeal leukemia: the first patients were treated 20 years ago.[283] Pooled data from 144 episodes of meningeal leukemia in 144 children showed objective and subjective response rates of 80 and 83 percent, respectively.[48] However, the median duration of remissions in different series never exceeded 5.4 months, and usually was less. Thus, intrathecally administered MTX has a relatively satisfactory response rate, but clearly does not eradicate meningeal leukemia in children; and the same appears to be true in adults.[21,48,313] Lumbar puncture is a procedure which neither physicians nor patients enjoy, and, as a result, the intrathecal treatment of meningeal leukemia is frequently inadequate, neither the intensity nor the duration corresponding to what would be used to treat systemic leukemia. In addition, lumbar puncture is not without risk; in the thrombocytopenic patient, hemorrhage may occur and subdural hematoma with spinal cord compression has been reported.[353] There is an increasing literature on adverse reactions to MTX intrathecally administered—cerebral necrosis,[293] sudden death,[15] paraparesis,[16] a meningitic syndrome,[241,243,278] and fibrinoid necrosis of cerebral blood vessels[181] have all been described. We have seen two cases of stroke and one of progressive dementia in patients treated with prolonged courses of intrathecally administered MTX. It has been postulated that the preservative parabens in the commercial drug may be responsible for these effects: the pH and osmolarity of methotrexate injections have also been incriminated,[87] but it remains likely that the drug itself is responsible. In our own experience, adverse reactions to MTX can occur in the absence of overt meningeal leukemia, in patients who are receiving extended intrathecal prophylactic treatment, for which reason we have abandoned long-term intrathecal prophylaxis. Despite the associated risks, intrathecally administered methotrexate is so effective in the treatment of meningeal leukemia that it remains widely used, and this appears reasonable considering the seriousness of the condition it is used to treat.

Other intrathecally administered drugs. Numerous other drugs have been administered intrathecally for the treatment of meningeal leukemia, although none has been used as widely as MTX. The other folic acid antagonist, aminopterin, is highly effective[274]; on a weight basis, it has a neurotoxicity equal to that of MTX, but five to ten times the antifolic activity. In view of the adverse effects which have been observed with MTX (see above), there is a case for further study of intrathecally administered aminopterin. L-asparaginase has been administered intrathecally[48] and a 50 percent response rate was observed in meningeal leukemia. Similar results have been observed using L-asparaginase intravenously: very little of the drug passes the blood-brain barrier, but the plasma asparagine falls to very low levels, and this may cause asparagine depletion within the CNS. Intrathecally administered hydrocortisone has been used occasionally and is effective against meningeal leukemia, but there is a risk of precipitating convulsions and, in any case, corticosteroid administered orally enters the CSF in adequate concentrations.[48] Quite extensive use has been made of cytarabine by the intrathecal route.[48,345] Adverse reactions other than nausea and vomiting have not been prominent, but experience with intrathecally administered ara-C is much less extensive than with MTX and it would be premature to assume that ara-C is entirely safe. We have used intrathecally administered ara-C for several years, both for therapy of meningeal leukemia and in some prophylactic programs, and have found a dose of 100 mg per square meter to be effective and free of complications, other than occasional nausea.[314] Cytarabine may be specially indicated if there is evidence of toxicity to methotrexate or of a case of meningeal leukemia being resistant to methotrexate. CNS involvement by acute granulocytic leukemia is not a special indication for the use of ara-C, since intrathecally administered methotrexate is fully effective in this condition.[48]

Systemic therapy. If they are administered systemically, most antileukemic drugs do not pass the blood-brain barrier in adequate concentrations to affect meningeal leukemia. Corticosteroids are an exception to this rule but should not be used as the *sole* treatment for meningeal leukemia since there is a risk of encouraging drug resistance: the effect of steroids in lowering raised intracranial pressure is valuable in the early stages of treatment. Systemic L-ase will affect meningeal leukemia but probably not by entering the CSF (see above). The lipid-soluble alkylating agents BCNU and CCNU enter the CNS when administered systemically; BCNU can induce remissions in meningeal leukemia, but these are brief[48] and the drug is very much inferior to methotrexate for maintaining remissions.[323,325] Published experience with CCNU in meningeal leukemia is insufficient to assess its possible role. The antimalarial drug, pyrimethamine, is a mild folic acid antagonist in man and is also lipid-soluble and enters the CNS. It has been used to treat meningeal leukemia in man,[131] but its success was only modest; the CSF never becoming free of leukemic cells and the patient developing thrombocytopenia from the high oral doses of pyrimethamine. If, for some reason, irradiation or intrathecal therapy is precluded, pyrimethamine given by mouth may provide useful palliation for meningeal leukemia, but in normal circumstances it is never the drug of choice for CNS leukemia.

Combined radiotherapy and chemotherapy. Since meningeal leukemia is notoriously hard to eradicate, combined therapy might offer better results. In a recent study,[324] irradiation of the skull alone was ineffective in producing objective remissions, whereas irradiation of the cerebrospinal axis to 1000 rad produced a 92 percent remission rate, although the median remission duration was only 1.75 months. Irradiation plus intrathecally administered methotrexate produced 100 percent remissions, but the median remission duration was only 3 months, similar to the remission duration seen with methotrexate therapy alone. This form of combined therapy obviously does not eradicate CNS leukemia.

Recommended therapy. Patients with CNS leukemia and a poor general prognosis (for example, those in hematologic relapse) are best treated by intrathecally administered methotrexate because the remission rate is high, response is rapid, and the patient is not distressed by radiation-induced epilation. When the general prognosis is good (for example, childhood acute lymphocytic leukemia in continuous hematologic remission), more vigorous therapy, aimed at eradication of the CNS disease, is indicated. Our program for therapy of CNS leukemia is shown in Figure 18-5. Since neither irradiation nor short courses of intrathecal therapy can be relied upon to eradicate leukemic cells in the CNS, we have combined initial aggressive radiotherapy and intrathecally administered methotrexate with a prolonged course of intrathecal maintenance therapy incorporating ara-C as well as MTX. To facilitate the long-continued intrathecal therapy, an Ommaya subcutaneous CSF reservoir is installed at the beginning of treatment (Fig. 18-6). These reservoirs have been in use for 10 years[251] and have proved valuable in the management of both neoplastic and infective intracranial lesions.[270] They have been used for purposes of extended *prophylactic* intrathecal therapy,[306,307,314] but proof that prophylaxis by

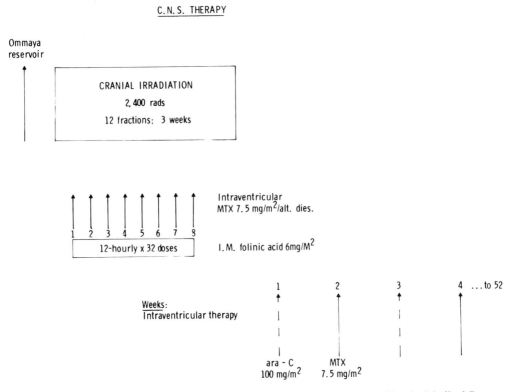

Fig. 18-5. Schematic representation of the treatment program used by the Medical Research Council Leukaemia Unit for established CNS leukemia. This aggressive program is not used in patients whose leukemia is in hematologic relapse and whose overall prognosis is therefore doubtful. An Ommaya subcutaneous CSF reservoir is inserted (see Fig. 18-6) and cranial irradiation is begun when the incision has healed. During the irradiation, eight intrathecal injections of methotrexate are administered over a 16-day period: to prevent systemic toxicity from methotrexate (total dose 60 mg/m²), intramuscular folinic acid is administered every 12 hours throughout this period. After irradiation is finished, maintenance intraventricular chemotherapy is administered once a week for 6–12 months, alternating between methotrexate (7.5 mg/m²) and cytarabine (100 mg/m²). An Ommaya reservoir is almost essential for this therapy since few patients would accept sixty lumbar punctures.

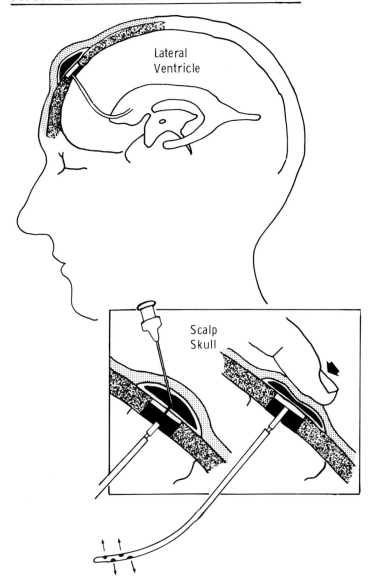

Fig. 18-6. Diagram of an Ommaya subcutaneous CSF reservoir in situ. Insertion is via a frontal burr hole into the anterior horn of the lateral ventricle of the nondominant cerebral hemisphere (usually the right). The incision is placed within the hairline and a small area is kept shaved, with the hair combed over it. Use of a denervating scalp incision makes puncture of the reservoir painless. The silicone rubber reservoir is self-sealing and withstands multiple punctures. The cannula has multiple ports at the distal end and is radio-opaque. After injection of drugs, the reservoir can be emptied and flushed by finger pressure (*inset*). CSF can be sampled from the reservoir—mononuclear cells are usually found, presumably as a reaction to the reservoir itself. CSF manometry can be performed via the reservoir just as through a lumbar puncture needle. The positioning of the cannula is always checked by limited air ventriculography before the patient leaves the operating theater.

irradiation and five doses of intrathecal MTX is highly effective[262] has made this particular use obsolete. Problems of infection or blockage of the reservoir,[81] and occasional problems due to the intraventricular administration of cytotoxic drugs have been reported,[293] but we, like others,[263] continue to use Ommaya reservoirs as part of the management of all patients with established meningeal leukemia, unless their general prognosis is very poor. Since adopting a frontal approach for insertion of the reservoirs[312] we have had no operative problems, and no patient has developed a relapse of meningeal leukemia while undergoing treatment. With the reservoirs, drugs can be instilled into the CSF easily and painlessly, and with a correctly positioned ventricular cannula there is certainty as to their location. Lumbar puncture has none of these advantages. Moreover, the distribution of the injected drug is superior; whereas drugs injected by lumbar puncture do not enter the cerebral ventricles,[272] drugs administered intraventricularly travel with the CSF flow and traverse the entire subarachnoid space.[185]

Supportive Treatment in the Acute Leukemias

In acute lymphocytic leukemia, the remission rate with all modern forms of therapy is high and remission is usually achieved rapidly. Thus, such patients spend little time in a state of severe bone marrow failure and, as a result, usually require relatively little supportive therapy. By contrast, patients with acute granulocytic leukemia frequently do not achieve complete remission, and when remission does occur it often takes many weeks of aggressive therapy to attain it. During this period bone marrow function is inadequate and supportive therapy is required. In children with acute lymphocytic leukemia, modern programs of intensive chemotherapy have led to very little increase in the need for blood components,[297] but in adults with acute granulocytic leukemia who receive modern chemotherapy the demand for blood components often imposes severe strains on even highly developed blood banking facilities.

BLOOD TRANSFUSION

This was the first treatment to affect beneficially the clinical course of acute leukemia. Although transfusion alone hardly ever causes remission in acute leukemia, it is sometimes the best treatment for elderly or frail patients with smoldering acute leukemia. Most patients with acute leukemia require transfusion at the beginning of therapy and usually this promptly increases their well-being. Children with acute lymphocytic leukemia frequently need only one transfusion because their marrow function is rapidly restored as their disease remits. Patients with acute granulocytic leukemia are slower to achieve remission and their drug therapy depresses erythropoiesis, so that repeated transfusions are frequently necessary. Packed red blood cells are usually given, both to avoid overexpanding the patient's blood volume and because donor plasma is required for numerous other purposes. Maintenance of a hemoglobin level between 10 and 12 gm per 100 ml is usually adequate for hospitalized patients, but a level of 14 gm per 100 ml may be desirable in the presence of infection. Severe anemia is debilitating and also increases the liability to retinal hemorrhage. Formerly it was common practice to use fresh whole blood for transfusing patients with leukemia, but it is preferable to replace components selectively: it is more efficient to use packed red cells for correcting anemia, platelet concentrates for thrombocytopenia, and so on.

PLATELET TRANSFUSION

The transfusion of platelet-rich plasma, prepared from fresh whole blood, effectively raises the platelet count in thrombocytopenic patients with acute leukemia.[115] Pathologic studies have suggested that intracranial and pulmonary hemorrhages are less common in patients with acute leukemia who receive platelet transfusions, and survival is prolonged slightly.[144] Clinically, it is repeatedly observed that hematuria or cutaneous purpura can be arrested by the transfusion of platelets, but it is more difficult to demonstrate the value of *prophylactic* platelet transfusion in patients who are not bleeding. In the presence of gross splenomegaly (for example, chronic granulocytic leukemia after metamorphosis), platelet transfusion usually fails to raise the platelet count or to confer any detectable benefit. In some leukemia centers it is standard practice to administer platelet concentrates prophylactically, maintaining the platelet count above 20,000 per cubic millimeter. Such prophylaxis is probably more important in the elderly, the hypertensive, and in patients with high leukocyte counts, because these patients are particularly prone to cerebral hemorrhage. Young children usually tolerate thrombocytopenia with equanimity, presumably because their blood vessels are healthy. The principal risks of platelet transfusion are allergic reactions, the formation of platelet antibodies which may negate the value of future platelet transfusions, and the transmission of serum hepatitis. It seems pointless to use platelets simply to prolong life slightly in patients with acute leukemia which is refractory to chemotherapy: their proper use is to support patients who may achieve remission if hemorrhage can be prevented for a finite period. The demands of leukemia centers for supplies of platelets customarily tax the powers of the most advanced blood transfusion services, and a leukemia treatment center can only be as effective as the blood banking facilities to which it has access.

LEUKOCYTE TRANSFUSION

It has long been possible to raise the hemoglobin level of leukemic patients, and platelet transfusion has been practicable for some years, but the effective supply of granulocytes for patients with granulocytopenia and infection is a recent development, made possible by the development of the closed, continuous-flow cell centrifuge by the U.S. National Cancer Institute and the IBM Corporation.[175] Patients with chronic granulocytic leukemia and greatly elevated neutrophil counts are particularly suitable for the collection of large quantities of neutrophils,[52] but normal donors can also be used.[205] Since chronic granulocytic leukemia is a rare disease, the use of normal relatives as leukocyte donors for patients with leukemia, neutropenia, and infection seems a more practical proposition. Transfused CGL neutrophils appear to function well in infected recipients, "homing in" on infective lesions in the same manner as normal neutrophils.[101] It has been claimed that neutrophil transfusions are highly effective in combating serious infections in neutropenic patients with leukemia,[138,289,290] but in some centers equally good results have been obtained by using antibiotics in high doses and no neutrophil transfusions.[316,329] It appears that to obtain optimal results in treating infection, neutrophils should be administered daily, in large doses (about 2×10^{10} normal leukocytes or 1×10^{11}

CGL leukocytes), and from HLA-compatible donors.[205] At present, the value of neutrophil transfusion cannot be regarded as proved, but it appears likely that it is indeed useful when used liberally and in conjunction with good antimicrobial drug therapy.

DISSEMINATED INTRAVASCULAR COAGULATION

This syndrome, which is accompanied by thrombocytopenia, hypofibrinogenemia, hemorrhage, and often renal failure, is encountered as a clinical problem in patients who do not have leukemia (see Chapter 14). Treatment with heparin arrests the progressive coagulation, and the platelet count and plasma fibrinogen level rise because their consumption has ceased—thus the use of an anticoagulant (heparin) results in arrest of hemorrhage. When disseminated intravascular coagulation occurs in a patient with acute leukemia, the use of heparin alone is dangerous, since the platelet count may not rise, particularly if cytotoxic therapy has recently been administered, and hemorrhage may simply be increased. Disseminated intravascular coagulation is particularly common in patients with acute promyelocytic leukemia[30,135]: a high risk of this complication is indicated by the appearance in the bone marrow of numerous promyelocytes packed with large abnormal granules and/or sheaves of reddish crystalline bodies resembling classic Auer rods but far more numerous.[326] Characteristically, leukemic patients with disseminated intravascular coagulation have hemorrhage from the oral mucous membranes, and its presence is confirmed by finding thrombocytopenia, hypofibrinogenemia, and an elevated titer of fibrin-degradation products in the serum. When antileukemic chemotherapy is begun, disseminated intravascular coagulation may suddenly increase and there is great risk of cerebral hemorrhage: this acceleration of the process may be due to rapid destruction of leukemic promyelocytes with release of substances with thrombin-like activity. Patients with acute promyelocytic leukemia are particularly important because if they survive the initial phases of therapy they have a greater chance of becoming long-term survivors than patients with other types of acute granulocytic leukemia.[30] Some success has been achieved by treating the disseminated intravascular coagulation and the leukemia simultaneously by platelet transfusions, heparin, and cytotoxin drugs.[35] Our policy is to administer the platelet concentrate from 15 units of blood (equal to three platelet packs) every 12 hours. As soon as platelet transfusion has begun, the patient is heparinized, aiming to keep the kaolin-activated, partial thromboplastin time (PTTK) at about twice normal. Treatment with ara-C and DR is begun once the patient is heparinized. The anticoagulant therapy is monitored by platelet counts, PTTK, plasma fibrinogen levels (which should rise) and the serum titer of fibrin-degradation products, which should fall. Like others,[135] we have found that if the initial antileukemic chemotherapy is intensive, the risk of disseminated intravascular coagulation is over in a few days and such vigorous supportive measures and monitoring are no longer necessary.

PROPHYLAXIS OF INFECTION

Patients with acute leukemia have a special liability to infection, principally because of neutropenia caused by both their disease and its treatment. The administration of adrenal corticosteroids, antimetabolites, and other immunodepressant drugs may further predispose them to infections, particularly from organisms which normally are of low pathogenicity. The incidence of infection in leukemia patients is inversely correlated with the absolute neutrophil count[36]; in some patients the functional capacity of neutrophils is impaired[201] so that the *effective* neutrophil count may be lower than the absolute count. The control of hemorrhage by platelet transfusion has increased the importance of infective mortality by decreasing the incidence of hemorrhagic deaths, and despite developments in antimicrobial therapy, infection is the leading cause of death in patients with leukemia.[156,201,287] This great liability to infection is particularly marked in patients with acute granulocytic leukemia, since their antileukemic therapy is usually very myelotoxic, and remission may take many weeks to achieve.

Numerous measures to prevent serious infections in leukemia patients have been studied. At some centers, *surgical treatment* of infective foci (for example, pilonidal sinus) or *dental treatment* of carious teeth or gingival disease precedes any aggressive antileukemic chemotherapy, and there is much to be said for this policy.[309] *Protected environments* for the leukemia patient have received much attention. Nursing in single rooms is the most elementary precaution of this nature. More sophisticated devices include laminar airflow rooms where bacterial counts are very low,[202] and plastic isolator tents which can be rendered completely sterile.[37,317] The use of such facilities has been combined with the application of antiseptics and/or antibiotics to the skin and the mucous membranes of the nose, mouth, pharynx, and vagina in an attempt to decontaminate the patient as much as possible. The administration of oral nonabsorbable antibiotics to produce *gastrointestinal sterilization* has been studied, with or without sterile food and protective isolation.[202,265] It appears that with suitable care, the bowel contents can be rendered virtually sterile,[137] the type of infections which occur in leukemia patients can be altered,[129] and the overall incidence of infections can be reduced, while cross-infection is almost eliminated.[37,172,202] Unfortunately, it has not been conclusively shown that these measures increase the remission rate in patients with acute granulocytic leukemia. In some studies the patients in protective isolation and the conventionally treated patients received identical chemotherapy: if more drastic treatment had been used in the isolated patients their remission rate might have been higher. Since infective deaths are rare in properly isolated and decontaminated patients,[202] it seems likely that more vigorous chemotherapy could be tolerated. If it is admitted that some patients who die of infection could achieve complete remission if they survived, a substantial reduction in infective deaths should improve the overall remission rate. How great this effect may be cannot be predicted. Elaborate and costly protective measures cannot, on present evidence, be recommended for general use in the management of leukemia, but research in this field remains of great importance, and several controlled studies now being conducted may delineate the future role of protective isolation and decontamination procedures.

TREATMENT OF INFECTION

Infection in neutropenic, immunodepressed patients with acute leukemia may be caused by a very wide range of viruses, bacteria, fungi, and protozoa (see Chapter 10).[9,95,201,238,244,259] Multiple organism septicemias are not uncommon and are usually fatal.[38] *Pseudomonas aeruginosa* is a particularly common cause of infection in leukemia patients, and it has been suggested that antileukemic drugs may encourage colonization by this organism, since *Pseudomonas* is resistant to most antileukemic agents, whereas many other gram-negative bacteria are not.[136] Infections in neutropenic patients are often fulminant, death occurring in 50 percent of patients within 72 hours—that is, often before bacteriologic identification and sensitivity testing of the causative organism is available.[286] A practical policy for treating febrile episodes in leukemia patients can be formulated:

1. Cultures of blood, urine, sputum and any infected lesions should be taken immediately.
2. Because of the high early death rate, antibiotic therapy usually must begin before bacteriologic results are established.
3. Antibiotic treatment must therefore be empiric, but it need not be unintelligent—in view of the wide range of possible organisms, the antibiotics chosen should cover a broad spectrum with special emphasis on the gram-negative organisms (*Pseudomonas* particularly) which are the predominant cause of infection in leukemia.
4. Antibiotic therapy will be modified as necessary in the light of subsequent bacteriologic results.
5. If there is no response to antibiotic therapy and bacteriology is negative, it is pointless to continue antibiotics for a fever that may well be viral or neoplastic in origin.
6. It is not reasonable to attempt to cover fungi, viruses, and mycobacteria in an initial course of empiric antibiotic therapy.

Several empiric antibiotic regimens have been described for the management of febrile episodes in neutropenic patients[186,277,286,329,330]: their success rate ranges up to 54 percent, which is reasonably good in such an unpromising group of patients.[316] If logistic problems are overcome, the use of regular neutrophil transfusions (see above) might substantially improve these results but a controlled study is necessary. The details of a regimen which provides cover with bactericidal antibiotics against all the common gram-positive and gram-negative bacteria, including most anaerobic organisms, are given in Table 18-16. This regimen has no useful activity against mycobacteria, fungi, protozoa, and viruses but these organisms seldom cause fulminating infections and rapid death in the manner of more common organisms. The treatment of the more exotic infections occasionally encountered in leukemia patients has recently been reviewed.[201]

COMPLICATIONS OF TREATMENT

The numerous adverse effects of the cytotoxic drugs used in the treatment of acute leukemia are discussed in Chapter 17. Although complications such as neurotoxicity from vincristine or myocardial toxicity from daunorubicin are occasionally encountered, they are seldom life-threatening. All the major complications of antileukemic therapy are most common in the middle-aged and elderly, most of whom have acute granulocytic rather than acute lymphocytic leukemia. The most notable complications are discussed below.

Myelodepression. In acute granulocytic leukemia this is a seemingly inevitable accompaniment of remission induction, and the patient requires blood and platelet transfusions and is at risk of infection, hemorrhage, and cardiac failure, or CNS symptoms from anemia.

Table 18-16

Antibiotic Combinations Used in the M.R.C. Leukaemia Unit for the Empiric Therapy of Febrile Episodes in Patients with Leukemia and Neutropenia*

Antibiotics	Dosage/m^2/24 hr
Carbenicillin	20 gm
Cephalothin	8 gm
Gentamicin	160 mg
Lincomycin	1.5 gm
For patients with significant penicillin allergy, omit carbenicillin and substitute polymyxin B	1.5 × 10^6 IU

*A 54 percent success rate has been obtained.[316]

Notes: 1. All the antibiotics are given as separate 6-hourly intravenous push injections.

2. The regimen without carbenicillin is inferior and only used for serious penicillin allergy.

3. Hypokalemia is very common with this regimen[327] and intravenously administered potassium supplements with repeated monitoring of the serum potassium are required.

4. Cephalothin plus gentamicin is probably nephrotoxic, particularly if frusemide is used as a diuretic;[108] intravenously administered mannitol appears to be safe and effective if diuresis is required.

Infection. The infections most often encountered are septicemias, pneumonias, oral sepsis (see below), and perianal lesions—fissures, fistulas, and abscesses. Whereas septicemias usually run a rapid course to recovery or death, pneumonia in neutropenic patients often has a protracted course and frequently is fatal despite vigorous therapy. At autopsy, pulmonary abscesses, carnification, and fibrosis seem commoner than classic pneumonic changes. Perianal infections are distressing, hard to eradicate, and a source of septicemia. Avoidance of constipation and frequent rectal examinations may lessen their incidence; the role of gastrointestinal sterilization with oral nonabsorbable antibiotics as prophylaxis against such lesions is uncertain (see above).

Mucous membrane lesions. Doxorubicin (Adriamycin), daunorubicin, cytarabine, methotrexate, and antipurine drugs in high doses all may cause oral and gastrointestinal ulceration. Colonization of such lesions by bacteria and *Candida* is common and leads to most distressing symptoms: esophageal candidiasis may lead to obstruction, perforation, or fungal septicemia. Liberal and frequent use of topical antiseptics and antifungal agents decreases both the incidence of mucous membrane ulcers and the frequency of their colonization.

Progressive system failure. This syndrome is most often seen in elderly patients. In its characteristic form the sequence is: myelodepression, septicemia (or pneumonia), congestive cardiac failure, renal failure (perhaps with hepatic failure), and death. This progression is extremely difficult to arrest, even with the best facilities and expertise, and it occurs sufficiently often that many physicians adopt a relatively conservative attitude toward the management of acute leukemia in elderly patients (for example, those whose chronologic age or apparent physiologic age exceeds 60 years). Progressive system failure is much less common in younger patients.

Destruction of the peripheral venous system. Cytotoxic agents and antibiotics are harmful to veins, and their prolonged or repeated administration over a few weeks can render all the patient's peripheral veins temporarily useless for further therapy. In leukemia patients (as in patients with hemophilia), every effort should be made to conserve veins, and intravenous therapy must never be administered by the inexpert. Central venous catheters inserted via a peripheral vein or by direct subclavian puncture will avoid the destruction of superficial veins, but occasionally these have fatal complications.[4] The alarming association between intravenous catheters and septic thrombophlebitis calls for the strictest asepsis in intravenous therapy for leukemia patients.[194]

The above are but a few of the many complications of modern therapy for the acute leukemias, but an awareness of these risks can lead to reduced morbidity and mortality, particularly among patients who are treated outside special centers.

GENERAL PRINCIPLES OF MANAGEMENT

Children. It is absolutely essential that children with acute leukemia are under the care of a physician who both likes and understands children. The physician need not necessarily be a pediatrician (frequently, he is a clinical oncologist), but he must be capable of establishing and maintaining close relationships with the child and his parents. Even when the outcome is successful, the treatment of acute lymphocytic leukemia in children is a long and uncomfortable process: the children suffer considerably and their parents a great deal more. Secure interpersonal relationships with the physician, and continuity of care, can do much to smooth the path, even when the disease leads to a fatal termination. Communication with the child's family doctor and the local education and health authorities must also be good. For example, it is not unusual for well-meaning educational authorities to offer to arrange home schooling for a child in the belief that a child with leukemia could not attend normal classes. On the contrary, children with their disease in remission should attend school full time and should in every way be treated as a normal child: present indications are that many of these children will indeed become healthy adults. Procedures such as bone marrow aspiration and lumbar puncture are terrifying to many children and extremely disturbing to their parents. Trauma of this kind is minimized by the use of intravenously administered diazepam, ketamine, or brief general anesthesia to cover such procedures.[100] The complexity of modern treatments for acute lymphocytic leukemia, and the better results obtained by specialist units,[223] mean that every child with acute leukemia should, if at all possible, be managed at a special center.

Adults. Many physicians acquaint adults having acute leukemia with their diagnosis, although some do not, the decision depending upon the opinion of the physician and his assessment of the individual patient (see Chapter 20). Clearly, good communication is essential in caring for an adult with acute leukemia, and this implies giving the patient excellent reasons for all the unpleasant therapy to which he is subjected. The most straightforward way of doing this is to explain the diagnosis and its implications in a manner appropriate to the patient's intelligence and background. In adults with acute granulocytic leukemia, the course of the illness is often distressing. Remission induction is protracted and often attended by complications; frequently, it is unsuccessful. Even if the patient survives and has a complete remission, all too often this is short and the maintenance therapy, whether effective or not, is generally unpleasant. Death within 2 years at most is the unfortunate lot of the majority of patients. Usually the patient himself, and some responsible relative always, should know that his life expectancy is restricted: the communication of this information does not necessarily preclude the physician from assuming an optimistic role. Adult patients frequently wish to return to their employment and, whenever possible, this should be encouraged; communication with employers to ensure the patient's return to whole- or part-time work may be necessary. The patient's possible fears that his condition may be transmitted to a spouse or children should be explored and allayed. Continuity of care by a physician who knows him well as an individual does much to help the adult with leukemia; this physician should, whenever possible, assume responsibility for the patient's terminal care and the follow-up care of his bereaved relatives. It cannot be claimed that the results obtained by special centers in treating adults with acute granulocytic leukemia are excellent, but the difficulties which beset their treatment and the extensive supportive measures which are often needed suggest that the care of adults with leukemia should be centralized as it is for children.

General considerations. Leukemia and its complications have no off-duty hours and no holidays. It is imperative that all patients with acute leukemia be able to contact a doctor who has personal knowledge of their case or direct access to their medical records, at any time. The provision of administrative machinery to supply this type of unceasing service is an essential part of the organization of any center where patients with leukemia are treated.

Patients with acute leukemia rapidly amass a bewildering collection of hematologic and biochemical results and records of drug therapy. For efficient utilization of such masses of data, proper record-keeping is essential. The maintenance of some type of flow-sheet, or of graphic hematologic charts[306,315] is a useful practice which has now been adopted by most leukemia physicians. Such charts are as valuable in treating leukemia as is the temperature chart in managing infections, and their usefulness as a teaching aid is also great.

CHRONIC GRANULOCYTIC LEUKEMIA

The Second Edition of this book noted that:

The treatment of chronic leukemia, in contrast with that of the acute types, is a relatively pleasant task. The patient's symptoms are at first not very severe, and he does not have the unhealthy, acutely ill appearance of the acute leukemic. There is, furthermore, the knowledge that although the disease is serious, therapy is by no means futile and a complete return to clinical and hematologic health, often for several years, is probable. As one continues with the treatment of the patient with chronic leukemia and notes his usually healthy vigor, the contrast between his optimism and lack of symptomatology with the pessimistic approach and the many complaints of the neurotic or neurasthenic patient becomes striking. The opportunity to learn to know such persons over a period of years, their usually sanguine temperaments, and the often beneficial effects of therapy make treatment of the patient with the chronic disease, *except towards the end,* a relatively pleasant task.

Ten years later, one may still concur that patients with chronic leukemia are often estimable characters and it is indeed a pleasure to know them well over a period of several years. There is considerable satisfaction in knowing that their health can be greatly improved, in the majority of cases, by relatively simple therapy. But the satisfaction ends—or should end—there. Although it has been possible to treat the chronic leukemias since the turn of the century, there is little evidence that their survival has been much increased, although the quality of life for such patients has been improved. In some centers the median survival of children with acute lymphocytic leukemia now surpasses that of adults with chronic granulocytic leukemia, and some of these children appear to be cured of their disease, while cure of the chronic form has not even been claimed, let alone substantiated. Patients with chronic granulocytic leukemia, so easy to treat at the outset, have a strong tendency for their disease to undergo metamorphosis to a refractory state—most often an acute leukemia which is exceptionally difficult to treat. Thus, in 10 years the picture has altered greatly: in acute lymphocytic leukemia the outlook has become hopeful, in acute granulocytic leukemia it has improved, whereas many physicians are now profoundly dissatisfied with the relative lack of progress in the chronic leukemias.

In chronic granulocytic leukemia, therapeutic stagnation may largely be attributed to the availability and efficacy—in the short-term period—of busulfan. The simplicity of busulfan therapy and its high success rate have discouraged research; furthermore, many such patients are never referred to special centers where new treatments might be tried. In chronic lymphocytic leukemia, it is difficult to plan therapeutic studies because some physicians would object to administering any therapy at all to patients who appear to have a very benign disease. The patients are frequently elderly, and the mortality from intercurrent unrelated diseases is sufficiently great to make difficult the assessment of the effects of antileukemic therapy upon survival. Because of these problems, the following remarks from the Second Edition unfortunately still apply: "No exact dogma regarding therapy can be given; almost every clinic seems to have its own favored methods. Whether the life span of a group treated with one method differs markedly from that treated by another is questionable. From statistics compiled several years ago by the American Cancer Society, some indication is present that the patients treated by physicians with experience in these cases have a longer life span than the average."

Review of Therapy

IONIZING RADIATIONS

Until a few years ago the standard therapy for chronic granulocytic leukemia was splenic irradiation. With leukocyte counts of 200,000–300,000 per cubic millimeter of blood, six to twelve treatments of 100 rad each, from an orthovoltage x-ray apparatus, were given as three to four treatments per week. With this regimen, slight anorexia and nausea may occur but reactions are usually mild. Regression of the enlarged spleen is often marked by the end of the first week and the leukocyte count begins to fall, often reaching 40,000 or 50,000 per cubic millimeter by the end of treatment and continuing to fall thereafter, while immature granulocytic cells in the peripheral blood become less numerous and then disappear (see Figs. 18-7 and 18-8). In 1–2 months the spleen is usually impalpable, while the leukocyte count is normal or slightly reduced. The differential blood count shows normal proportions of granulocytes and lymphocytes, and the platelet count is generally normal. Baso-philia of 6 to 12 percent or even higher is not uncommon at this time. The hemo-globin begins to rise and usually reaches normal levels, eventually. The patient's symptoms of abdominal discomfort, anorexia, and fatigue improve as the splenomegaly regresses and the hemoglobin rises.

If no further treatment is given, the hematologic manifestations of the leukemia reappear from 3–18 months later: physical signs and, finally, clinical symptoms ap-pear. It is incorrect to speak of chronic granulocytic leukemia as remitting with therapy or relapsing after therapy, since cytogenetic studies indicate that the bone marrow remains 100 percent leukemic, even when the disease has been treated, all the dividing cells possessing the characteristic Philadelphia (Ph[1]) chromosome (see Chapter 6). It is therefore preferable to speak of *hematologic control,* or the lack of it. As the leukocyte count rises, immature granulocytes reappear in the peripheral blood, the hemoglobin begins to fall, and the platelet count often becomes super-

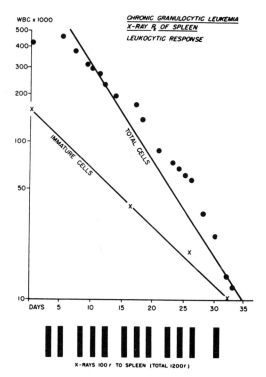

Fig. 18-7. Chronic granulocytic leukemia. Initial response of leukocyte count to splenic radiation.

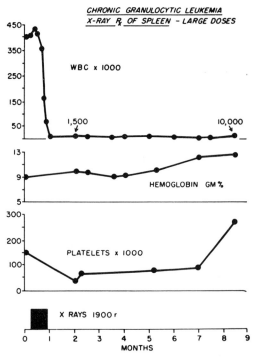

Fig. 18-8. Chronic granulocytic leukemia. This patient was treated with an unusually large dose of x-rays to the spleen and developed marked depression of all marrow elements which lasted about 7 months.

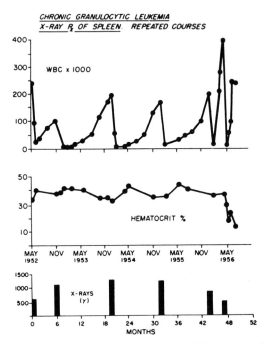

Fig. 18-9. Chronic granulocytic leukemia treated with a repeated course of x-rays to spleen over a period of 4 years. Four relapses occurred, with eventual radioresistance.

normal. Eventually, splenomegaly appears and progresses. Further radiotherapy is usually administered before severe anemia or clinical symptoms develop. A second period of control is generally achieved, and some patients are successfully treated on four or more occasions, but, characteristically, each successive period of control is shorter than the last, and more difficult to induce. Eventually, radiotherapy fails to secure further benefit, either because the chronic granulocytic leukemia has undergone metamorphosis to an accelerated phase, or because it has simply become refractory without evidence of other change (Fig. 18-9).

Other forms of external irradiation have been used, including an *abdominal bath* technique and total-body irradiation from a distance, using relatively low doses.[252] There appears to be no special advantage to these methods. In fact, the only merit that may nowadays be claimed for any of the external irradiation techniques is that they decrease the leukocyte count sharply and cause rapid regression of splenomegaly. In terms of duration of control of the disease, these techniques are inferior to drug therapy (see below).

Internal irradiation in the form of ^{32}P has been used extensively at some centers.[252] The ^{32}P may be administered intravenously or by mouth, and small titrated doses may be used. This is a convenient way to administer radiation, and something approximating maintenance therapy can be given, whereas with external irradiation the leukocyte count is usually allowed to increase to a relatively high level before treatment is reinstituted. There is no doubt that ^{32}P gives satisfactory results in experienced hands, but it has not been demonstrated to be superior to splenic irradiation. Maintenance therapy with small doses of radiophosphorus resembles maintenance with busulfan in that the total granulocyte mass is closely controlled. Since busulfan appears to be superior to splenic irradiation in chronic granulocytic leukemia, it would be of interest to know whether ^{32}P occupies an intermediate position.

BUSULFAN THERAPY

This agent has been used in the treatment of chronic granulocytic leukemia for over 20 years.[29, 141, 204, 318, 337] (Figs. 18-10, 18-11, 18-12). In a recent series,[255] 98 of 100 patients responded favorably to busulfan as their initial therapy: the response rate would have been lower if so-called atypical patients (that is, those who on strict criteria do not have chronic granulocytic leukemia at all) had been included. The extraordinarily high response rate, the simplicity and acceptable nature of busulfan therapy, and the satisfactory control which is achieved when the leukemia is in its chronic phase[123, 255] have led to its increasing use, while splenic irradiation has been employed much less frequently over recent years (Figs. 18-13 and 18-14).

Only one large-scale, controlled trial of busulfan versus radiotherapy has been reported.[222] The median survival of 54 patients treated by splenic irradiation was 120 weeks while the median survival of 48 patients treated with regular busulfan was 170 weeks. Of the 54 radiotherapy patients, 32 eventually had to be switched to busulfan therapy because of poor control of their disease, whereas only 4 of the 48 busulfan patients were switched to radiotherapy. The busulfan-treated patients had a less fluctuant clinical course and their hemoglobin levels were better maintained. Once their chronic granulocytic leukemia had undergone metamorphosis, patients in groups succumbed within a short time, and the increased survival of the busulfan

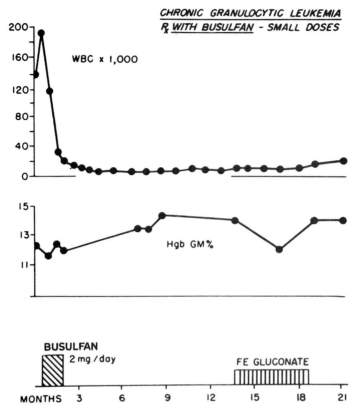

Fig. 18-10. Chronic granulocytic leukemia. A previously untreated patient who responded rapidly to daily doses of only 2 mg of busulfan with a remission sustained for nearly 2 years.

group appeared to be due to a later onset of metamorphosis. One possible explanation of this is that the closer control of the total granulocyte mass obtained with continuous busulfan therapy provides a lesser opportunity for the spontaneous emergence of mutant cell-lines which lead to metamorphosis: the smaller total granulocyte mass means that there are fewer candidate cells available for mutation. It is also possible that ionizing radiations are, in fact, more mutagenic than busulfan and actually cause metamorphosis: this, however, seems less likely, since the survival of patients treated with radiotherapy is not less than that of patients who received no specific therapy.[235] In a recent study,[239] no difference in survival could be found between patients treated by chemotherapy alone (principally busulfan) and those treated by both splenic irradiation and chemotherapy: However, this was a retrospective study and the use of chemotherapy in both groups of patients might be expected to minimize any differences between them.

Although busulfan therapy improves the quality of life in patients with chronic granulocytic leukemia and apparently prolongs it slightly beyond the duration observed with radiotherapy or no therapy, it has serious drawbacks. Treatment with busulfan appears to select in favor of aneuploid Ph¹-positive cells as against diploid

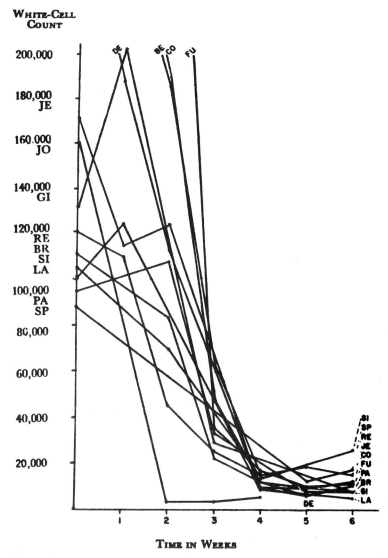

Fig. 18-11. Composite chart on 11 patients with chronic granulocytic leukemia treated with busulfan, demonstrating the uniform reduction in the white cell count, normal levels being achieved by the fourth week of therapy (Reproduced from Unugur et al.,[325] by courtesy of the authors and publisher).

Ph[1]-positive cells,[256] suggesting that the former are more resistant. Aneuploid Ph[1]-positive cells seem frequently to be involved in the occurrence of metamorphosis in chronic granulocytic leukemia,[350] so although busulfan effectively reduces the total granulocytic mass it may still select potentially anaplastic, leukemic-cell clones and thus be a fundamentally bad agent for long-term therapy. The numerous adverse effects of long-continued administration of busulfan are described in Chapters 10 and 17. Clinically the most important side effects are pulmonary fibrosis, which is

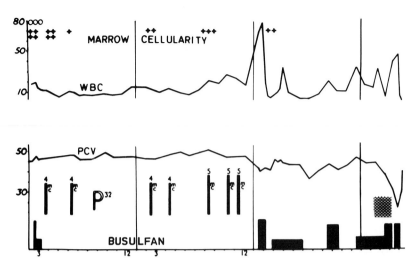

Fig. 18-12. Chronic granulocytic leukemia in a 37-year-old male treated continuously with ^{32}P and busulfan. Absence of symptoms except during terminal metamorphosis (symptoms indicated by cross-hatching).

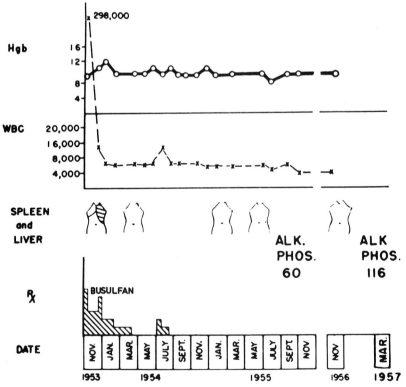

Fig. 18-13. Chronic granulocytic leukemia treated with busulfan.

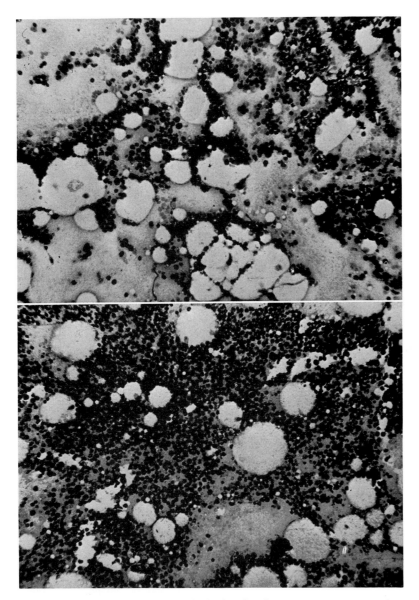

Fig. 18-14. A. Chronic granulocytic leukemia. Bone marrow smear. Appearance during remission induced by busulfan. B. Same patient. Bone marrow smear taken 2 years after last treatment shows incipient relapse. Both, × 140.

rare, and pigmentation, which is common (Figs. 18-15 and 18-16). Interstitial pulmonary fibrosis occurs in patients who have received busulfan for protracted periods[49,149,250]; occasionally, it becomes manifest a few months following the cessation of many months of busulfan therapy. Dyspnea and disability may be very severe and the suspicion of early pulmonary fibrosis is an indication to withdraw busulfan permanently. Treatment with corticosteroids may improve some cases, and there is sometimes gradual, spontaneous improvement following cessation of busulfan.

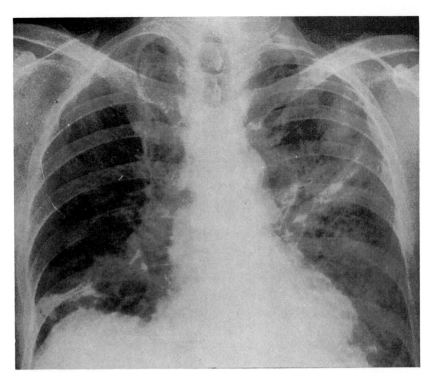

Fig. 18-15. Roentgenogram of the chest of a patient with chronic granulocytic leukemia treated with busulfan. Bilateral mottled densities and linear infiltrates are present. (From Oliner et al.[250])

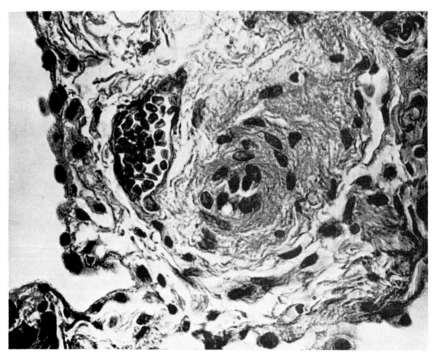

Fig. 18-16. Same patient as Fig. 18-15. Photomicrograph of a biopsy specimen of the lung demonstrates marked proliferative endarteritis without inflammation, × 440. (From Oliner et al.[250])

Busulfan pigmentation is much commoner; it is more marked in dark-skinned individuals and is exaggerated by exposure to sunlight,[79] and, like the pulmonary changes, is usually associated with prolonged ingestion of busulfan. More important is the development in some patients of a symptom complex which superficially resembles Addison's disease.[190] At first, there is increasing pigmentation of the skin of the entire body, followed by increasing debility, anorexia, nausea, and weight loss (Fig. 18-17). The hyperpigmentation of the skin is brownish, generalized, and most pronounced on the trunk, face, and hands (Fig. 18-18); it is indistinguishable from the melanosis of Addison's disease, except that scars, palmar creases, and mucous membranes are not ordinarily involved (Fig. 18-19). Skin biopsy reveals only melanosis. Anorexia and weight loss may be severe; two of five patients lost 40 pounds or more in 3 months. Marked distaste for meat, continued nausea, and other vague gastrointestinal symptoms may persist for 1–3 months after busulfan is discontinued. The blood pressure may be low and this, coupled with the wasting

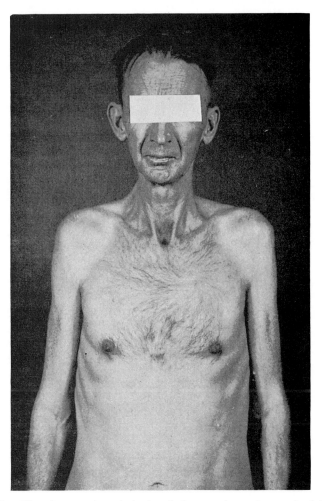

Fig. 18-17. Chronic granulocytic leukemia in a patient who received busulfan for 4 years. There was marked weakness, weight loss, and skin pigmentation. There was no evidence of myeloblastic crisis.

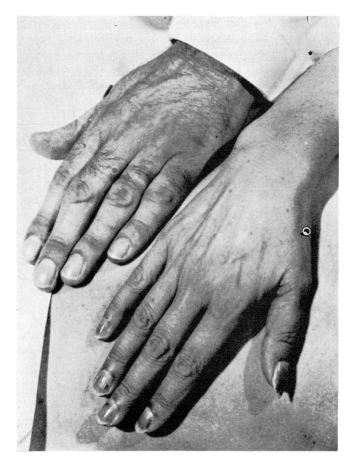

Fig. 18-18. Chronic granulocytic leukemia in a patient who received busulfan therapy for 4 years. Note marked pigmentation of the hand, especially the fingers on the right, as compared with the normal hand above.

and pigmentation, may suggest Addison's disease; however, the urinary 17-hydroxycorticosteroids and 17-corticosteroids are generally normal. It is important to recognize this syndrome early and discontinue busulfan before cachexia develops. The syndrome must be distinguished from metamorphosis of chronic granulocytic leukemia, when weakness and wasting are common and busulfan pigmentation may be present, but, in addition, there is generally splenomegaly and a marked increase in immature cells in the peripheral blood and/or bone marrow.

OTHER DRUG THERAPY

Busulfan was available before many other antileukemic drugs and rapidly proved itself a satisfactory and quite predictable agent in chronic granulocytic leukemia. As a result, there have been few extensive studies of other drugs in its chronic phase. Mercaptopurine was reported as unsatisfactory, failing to give the smooth control seen with busulfan.[303] In fact, this probably overstates the case—certainly, mercaptopurine is a useful agent when chronic granulocytic leukemia is accompanied by thrombocytopenia or when the chronicity of the disease is ques-

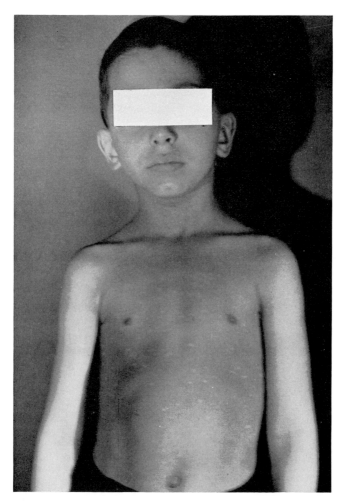

Fig. 18-19. Chronic granulocytic leukemia in a child who received busulfan therapy for 3 years. Note pigmentation of skin except in the scars of a previous attack of varicella.

tionable, since MP is not particularly depressant to platelets and, unlike busulfan, has some beneficial effect in both the chronic phase and in the early stages of metamorphosis. Desacetylmethylcolchicine has not been widely used in chronic granulocytic leukemia, but controls the disease satisfactorily in some patients despite great variation in individual responses; like MP it is sometimes effective for a short time after metamorphosis has occurred, and there is a need for further study of this drug.[44,120] Dibromomannitol is effective and occasionally will control the disease when busulfan resistance has arisen,[90,257,269] but not if metamorphosis has occurred. It has the advantages of not causing pigmentation or amenorrhea, and it also merits further evaluation. Hydroxyurea also will control chronic granulocytic leukemia, but some patients require doses which cause nausea or stomatitis[109,183,290]; the leukocyte count rises rapidly if treatment is stopped, which may be an advantage if the patient is a leukocyte donor.[290] Melphalan,[291] chlorambucil, and most other alkylating agents will control the disease but no special advantages to be obtained by their use have been demonstrated. Thus, chronic granulocytic leukemia is a rare disease in which many different drugs are effective, but only one drug—busulfan—has been adequately evaluated. It is unknown whether any of the other drugs has special advantages but several seem worth investigating. Unfortunately, none of the drugs has much useful activity in chronic granulocytic leukemia after metamorphosis.

Recommended Therapy

Only two forms of therapy have been adequately evaluated in chronic granulocytic leukemia: splenic irradiation and busulfan. Of these, busulfan is the better agent but neither should be regarded as satisfactory since they do not produce true remission, merely controlling the disease for a limited period.

It is safest to begin busulfan therapy cautiously, at a 4-mg dose given daily, or 0.0625 mg per kilogram of body weight, whichever is the less, and to increase the dose only if response is inadequate after 3 weeks' trial. Very occasionally, it is desirable to reduce the leukocyte count rapidly—for example, when leukocytosis is so great that there is hyperviscosity of the blood with retinal hemorrhages or priapism. In such cases, 1–2 mg of busulfan per kilogram of body weight may be administered as a single dose and no further busulfan given for about 4 weeks. With either form of treatment, but particularly the latter, prophylactic allopurinol therapy is advisable since a great mass of granulocytic tissue has to be lysed and hyperuricemia is not uncommon; frequently, it is present before therapy is begun.

When busulfan is given at conventional dosage, very little happens for 10–14 days when the leukocyte count begins to fall. Simultaneously, the more immature granulocytes become less numerous in the peripheral blood; characteristically, they disappear in the order of their immaturity until only mature neutrophils remain. The platelet count, often elevated at the start of therapy, falls more gradually, and the hemoglobin level begins to rise as the leukocyte count approaches normality. Regression of the enlarged spleen lags behind all these changes: 3 months or longer may be required for a large spleen to become impalpable, by which time several courses of intermittent busulfan therapy may have been given.

The characteristic delay in the onset of the effects of busulfan is mirrored when the drug is discontinued, for the leukocyte count usually continues to fall for 2–3 weeks. For this reason, busulfan is discontinued when the leukocyte count is around 20,000 per cubic millimeter, or at a higher level if the rate of fall has been very steep. The average patient requires 4–6 weeks of busulfan therapy initially, and it is always safest to cease busulfan therapy when in doubt and resume therapy if the leukocyte count levels off at too high a value. Overenthusiastic busulfan therapy can cause marrow aplasia which carries a mortality rate of about 50 percent. The judicious use of busulfan is greatly facilitated by the maintenance of a hematologic chart on semilogarithmic paper.[123,127,315]

Most physicians use busulfan maintenance therapy. This may be intermittent—for example, beginning the drug when the leukocyte count reaches 30,000 and ceasing when it reaches 7,000 per cubic millimeter. Others prefer to give busulfan continuously, keeping the leukocyte count between 7,000–12,000 per cubic millimeter by continuous small doses. The average requirement for this varies from

0.5–3 mg of busulfan daily, and tends to increase gradually in the individual patient with the passage of time. It is not known whether the survival of patients differs according to the type of regimen used: theoretically, continuous therapy might be more desirable since it provides very close control of the total granulocyte mass, but it requires more frequent blood counts and occasional patients suddenly develop severe marrow hypoplasia while on continuous maintenance busulfan. Some physicians follow the practical course of using intermittent busulfan therapy in those patients whose leukocyte count rises very slowly when therapy is discontinued, and continuous therapy in those who develop leukocytosis rapidly.

With busulfan therapy, almost all patients are restored to apparent hematologic normality. Rarely, busulfan therapy eliminates the intermediate granulocytic forms from the blood, leaving blast cells and neutrophils with a hiatus between. This simply means that the patient's chronic granulocytic leukemia has undergone metamorphosis before treatment was begun; this change is not always apparent when a very high count of more mature forms is present, and busulfan unmasks it. Apart from this fortunately rare event, patients are restored to health by busulfan therapy and this state continues for a period which varies from a few weeks to 7 years or more. At any time after diagnosis, but most often between 1–4 years, the chronic granulocytic leukemia undergoes metamorphosis (Chapter 10).[17,19] The best-recognized form of metamorphosis is the so-called blastic crisis with fever, rapidly enlarging splenomegaly, large numbers of blasts in the peripheral blood, and falling platelet and neutrophil counts and hemoglobin levels. It is important to realize that, although the median survival of busulfan-treated patients is about 170 weeks, the scatter of survivals is very broad; furthermore, although most hematologists have one or more 7-year survivors attending their clinic, such patients are, in fact, exceptional, as any large-scale study shows.[222,239] Metamorphosis may also assume the appearances of red cell aplasia, myelofibrosis, thrombocythemia, thrombocytopenia, or the development of extramyeloid tumors (chloromas). The one common factor in all these variants is a failure to respond to busulfan, and most of them fail to respond satisfactorily to any other form of treatment which may be tried. The more rapidly progressive forms of metamorphosis, particularly the blastic crisis are usually fatal within a few weeks and vigorous therapy sometimes hastens this outcome.

Treatment after Metamorphosis

When metamorphosis is a protracted occurrence, treatment may be largely symptomatic—that is, transfusions for anemia, cautious irradiation for painful splenomegaly, and trial of drugs such as MP or dibromomannitol to lower the leukocyte count and alleviate symptoms of night sweating or hypermetabolism. Thrombocytopenia is relieved only temporarily by platelet transfusions and often not at all if there is marked splenomegaly: in patients whose metamorphosis seems to be relatively chronic, splenectomy may be considered for the relief of thrombocytopenia with hemorrhage (see below).

However, when metamorphosis of chronic granulocytic leukemia is to an acute blastic leukemia, more vigorous therapy seems indicated. Unfortunately, the results of such treatment are exceptionally poor, much worse than the results of treating *de*

Table 18-17

Treatment of Chronic Granulocytic Leukemia in Metamorphosis of the "Acute Blastic" Variety[310]

Drug Administered with Prednisolone[1]	No. of Patients	Therapeutic Response (no. patients)[2]		
		Good	Some	Nil
MP	10	0	3	7
Demecolcine	7	0	2	5
CY	1	0	0	1
VCR	6	0	1	5
TOTALS	24	0	6[3]	18[4]

[1] All patients received oral prednisolone (1 mg/kg/day) plus a second drug.

[2] It is not possible to classify results as "remission" or otherwise. Good—patient well and active with an acceptable but not necessarily normal blood count. Some—patient and blood count both significantly improved by treatment. Nil—no improvement in patient's well-being, or patient is feeling worse, and blood count is not improved (for example, the leukocyte count is lower but the proportion of blast cells is unchanged or increased; hemoglobin and platelets are not improved—usually lower than before therapy).

[3] All six responses were short lived.

[4] Most of these 18 patients were apparently made worse by therapy.

Table 18-19

Some Published Results of Treatment of Chronic Granulocytic Leukemia in Metamorphosis of the "Acute Blastic" Variety

Drugs	No. of Patients	Therapeutic Response (no. patients)			References
		Good	Some	Nil	
POMP	13	1	3	9[1]	111
BCNU + ara-C	24	4	4	16[2]	146
PRED + VCR	30	9	0	21	56, 57
TOTAL	67	14	7	46	

[1] The nine failures included four drug-induced deaths.

[2] Toxicity with this regimen was very severe.

Table 18-18

Treatment* of Chronic Granulocytic Leukemia in Metamorphosis of the "Acute Blastic" Variety[310]

Drugs	No. of Patients	Therapeutic Response (no. patients)		
		Good	Some	Nil
PRED + VCR + MP	2	1	0	1
PRED + MP + DR + ara-C	2	0	1	1
PRED + TG + hydroxyurea	1	0	0	1
CY + Demecolcine + Dibromomannitol	1	0	0	1
PRED + DR + TG + ara-C + MTX	1	0	0	1
PRED + VCR + TG + DR + ara-C + CY + hydroxyurea	1	0	1	0
TOTALS	8	1	2	5

*Combinations of three or more drugs were administered simultaneously.

novo acute granulocytic leukemia. The outcome of therapy in blastic metamorphosis of chronic granulocytic leukemia is summarized in Tables 18-17 through 18-19. Several possible reasons for these depressing results may be adduced:

1. The leukemic cell mass in these patients with hyperplastic marrow, and often massive splenomegaly, is probably much greater than in ordinary acute granulocytic leukemia.
2. The leukemic cells have generally had much exposure to busulfan and may therefore be selected for a high degree of drug resistance.
3. There is cytogenetic evidence of multiple cell clones in some of these patients[311] and this may contribute to the rapid emergence of resistance to each new drug which is employed, due to selection from a preexisting heterogeneous population.
4. These patients probably have no normal bone marrow at all, the "best" cell population they possess being itself Ph[1]-positive and of chronic-phase chronic granulocytic leukemia type; this population may be very much reduced by the time resistance to busulfan has become clinically obvious, as shown by the rapid fall in mature granulocytes and platelets if busulfan is continued after metamorphosis has begun.

Treatment with PRED + VCR appears to produce clinical and cytogenetic remissions in about 30 percent of patients with chronic granulocytic leukemia after metamorphosis and a 3-week trial of this therapy for every patient seems justified,[56,57] since these drugs are unlikely to depress any residual functional marrow. Occasional responses have been obtained with BCNU + ara-C,[146] but this therapy is very myelotoxic, and severe pancytopenia is to be expected. In patients whose leukemia does not respond favorably to this combination, the marrow failure induced by BCNU and ara-C is unlikely to recover, so the treatment may hasten their deaths.

We have had some favorable responses when patients whose chronic granulocytic leukemia had undergone metamorphosis to an acute blastic picture were treated with the TRAMPCO regimen.[308] Eight patients were treated: five had a good response and were able to return to their normal occupations and receive maintenance TRAMPCO as outpatients; while three patients had some response, with improvement in their symptoms, physical signs, and hematologic parameters. No patient was entirely unresponsive, and one of the best responses lasted 14 months. Splenomegaly after metamorphosis is notoriously refractory to therapy, but usually regresses with remarkable rapidity with TRAMPCO therapy. Since the treatment proves to be far less toxic than the list of drugs (see Table 18-12) would suggest, we have continued to use it for all patients whose chronic granulocytic leukemia has undergone an aggressive type of metamorphosis.

Possible Advances in Therapy

Regrettably, the therapy of chronic granulocytic leukemia has improved very little in 70 years. The use of busulfan instead of radiotherapy might be accounted a small advance, and the slightly improved management of metamorphosis an even smaller one. If survival is to be substantially improved, however, this seems most likely to be achieved by methods which postpone the onset of metamorphosis. The patient with chronic granulocytic leukemia presents a unique therapeutic problem—here is an individual who has a 70 percent chance of developing a form of AGL in the next few years—what can be done to prevent it?

EARLY ELECTIVE SPLENECTOMY

Around the turn of the century, occasional splenectomies were performed in patients with chronic granulocytic leukemia who had received no specific antileukemic therapy. Since their spleens were very large and difficult to remove and the patients had uncontrolled leukemia, it is not surprising that operative mortality and morbidity were high. Understandably, the procedure never became popular, and the advent of radiotherapy tended to discourage the surgical approach. Now that the limitations of radiation therapy and conventional chemotherapy are well-known, the possible role of splenectomy needs reappraisal.[127,355]

Experience of, and opinions on, splenectomy vary widely. Early surgical series did not suggest that the operation held any great promise,[218,219] but the selection of these patients was less than ideal.[18] A recent review of the literature did not produce a good case for splenectomy in chronic granulocytic leukemia,[320] although most of the patients reviewed had undergone splenectomy for an *indication* such as hypersplenism or refractory splenomegaly and the results obtained might therefore be irrelevant to the question of the desirability of purely elective splenectomy.

There is evidence that splenectomy can modify the natural history of chronic granulocytic leukemia. In a previously untreated patient, splenectomy was followed by 8 months' hematologic control of the disease without cytotoxic therapy.[76] Splenectomy in a patient who had received busulfan 2 years earlier was followed by 3 years' apparent remission, with a 6-year survival from operation.[86] Since the median survival in chronic granulocytic leukemia is between 120 and 170 weeks, the achievement of 6 years' survival or more in a series of patients would represent a substantial gain. In a series of 15 patients with chronic granulocytic leukemia and hypersplenism or symptomatic splenomegaly,[228] there were 3 operative deaths and 8 patients improved hematologically after splenectomy: in 4 of these, prolonged hematologic control was achieved and 1 patient was alive 9 years after splenectomy. These workers later stressed that their high operative mortality and morbidity seemed attributable to the relatively advanced disease in their patients.[237] Since the splenectomies nevertheless conferred substantial benefits on some of their patients, they felt it should be considered earlier in the course of the disease. The relatively uncommon complication of thrombocytopenia, occurring while chronic granulocytic leukemia is still in its chronic phase, responds very well to splenectomy.[58]

Since most of the splenectomies performed in patients with chronic granulocytic leukemia and reported in the literature were done for a medical indication, usually connected with poor hematologic or clinical control, they cannot be used as a guide to the possible effects of the same operation performed electively. There is, in fact, a mythology (it appears to be no more than that) to the effect that splenectomy can accelerate the occurrence of metamorphosis in chronic granulocytic leukemia: this seems to be based upon the appearance of overt blastic change in patients who have had splenectomy for refractory splenomegaly. Since refractory splenomegaly is a common early sign that metamorphosis has occurred, the unmasking of this change by splenectomy is not surprising, but the operation cannot have caused an event which, in fact, preceded surgery.

Several purely empirical reasons for early elective splenectomy in chronic granulocytic leukemia may be cited:

1. Late in the disease, serious splenic problems occur in as many as 70 percent of patients. These include abdominal discomfort, anorexia, dyspepsia, wasting, splenic pain, infarction, rupture, intraabdominal hemorrhage, hypersplenism, and massive splenic blood pooling, with anemia almost unresponsive to transfusion.
2. Splenectomy at this time is hazardous, since the patient is ill and wasted, often with thrombocytopenia and neutropenia, and has a massive spleen which frequently has adhesions and is difficult to remove, even with a large thoracoabdominal incision.
3. Nevertheless, splenectomy late in the course of the disease, its hazards notwithstanding, can lead to significant clinical and hematologic improvement, with increased comfort, substantial weight gain, an improved blood picture, and decreased or nonexistent transfusion needs.
4. Chronic granulocytic leukemia which has undergone metamorphosis is less difficult to manage in the splenectomized patient, because symptoms and bleeding are lessened and transfused blood and platelets are effective for longer periods.
5. Although splenectomy is hazardous at late stages of chronic granulocytic leukemia, and particularly so after metamorphosis has occurred, it is a much simpler undertaking early in the course of the disease, when its manifestations are first controlled, because patients then have normal peripheral blood values, and the spleen is small and usually without adhesions, being easily removed through a small abdominal incision. At the cost of a 12–14-day hospital stay the patient is relieved of a 70 percent liability to future splenic complications of his chronic granulocytic leukemia.

Theoretical reasons may also be cited which favor early splenectomy. The spleen in chronic granulocytic leukemia contains a substantial proportion of the total granulocyte mass, and much chemotherapy is expended in controlling this mass of tumor tissue: the chemotherapy probably selects out drug-resistant, aneuploid leukemic cell clones.[256] Early splenectomy permits better control of the total granulocyte mass with relatively less exposure to potentially harmful chemotherapy, while close control of the total granulocyte mass would be expected to delay the onset of metamorphosis if this occurs as a random event in a susceptible cell population. Second, refractory splenomegaly is often the first sign of metamorphosis in chronic granulocytic leukemia, sometimes appearing when the peripheral blood and even the bone marrow show no evidence of the change which will occur in a few weeks and terminate fatally in a few more weeks. It is possible that the spleen is a "pharmacologic hideout" where new clones of drug-resistant Ph[1]-positive cells develop and lead to metamorphosis; its early removal might delay this process.[17]

In a series of eighteen splenectomies performed during the chronic phase of chronic granulocytic leukemia, no definite effect on the duration of the disease before metamorphosis could be demonstrated,[290] but the chemotherapy and other treatment of these patients was unconventional, and survival was marred by three postoperative deaths caused by hospital infections. However, it was shown that the splenectomized patients survived longer after the occurrence of metamorphosis than nonsplenectomized patients. We have performed splenectomy in 17 patients with chronic granulocytic leukemia with no postoperative mortality or morbidity.[316] Fourteen of these patients were in the chronic phase of their disease; 1 developed metamorphosis of an acute blastic type 52 weeks from diagnosis and 29 weeks postsplenectomy, but survived 61 weeks from the occurrence of metamorphosis, for most of this time remaining in good health and living at home. The remaining 13 patients are alive and well and in the chronic phase of their disease; their median survival time from splenectomy is 91 weeks and the median time from diagnosis is 120 weeks. The eventual median survival is, of course, unknown. On the basis of these pilot studies, a controlled cooperative trial has begun: patients are treated with busulfan until their disease is controlled and splenomegaly has become slight or no longer detectable. The patients are then screened for their fitness to undergo surgery, and those who pass this screening process are randomized to splenectomy or nonsplenectomy groups. Patients who do not pass the screening process cannot be used as controls since this would bias the nonsplenectomy group by the inclusion of an excess of elderly and unfit patients. Individuals in the splenectomy group are treated with busulfan so that their preoperative platelet count is less than 200,000 per cubic millimeter. Using this technique, we have not had problems with postoperative thrombocythemia or thromboembolic phenomena. In both splenectomy and nonsplenectomy groups, further maintenance chemotherapy is with busulfan in conventional dosage aiming at a leukocyte count between 7000–12,000 per cubic millimeter. Further experience of patients after splenectomy is, however, desirable before these criteria for busulfan therapy are accepted. Because of the relatively long course of chronic granulocytic leukemia, the results of this trial will not be established for several years.

Intensive Chemotherapy in the Chronic Phase

Some patients treated with busulfan develop bone marrow hypoplasia, sometimes because the drug has been administered injudiciously, and sometimes because their marrow is extremely sensitive to conventional or even small doses of the drug. The commonest outcome of severe busulfan hypoplasia is death from hemorrhage and infection, because the marrow depression is often protracted and sometimes irreversible. Other patients recover from the hypoplasia and redevelop the picture of chronic granulocytic leukemia. Of particular interest is a third group of patients who on recovery show a normal blood picture and a mixed population of Ph^1-positive and Ph^1-negative cells in the bone marrow (see Chapter 10).[127] These patients enjoy exceptionally long remissions from their disease—up to 14 years—during which time serial cytogenetic studies show gradual replacement of the bone marrow Ph^1-negative population until all the dividing cells are once more Ph^1-positive as at the time of diagnosis. The appearance of Ph^1-negative cells after hypoplasia suggests that such cells are present at the time of diagnosis but homeostatically suppressed by the mass of proliferating Ph^1-positive cells: if the total granulocyte mass is reduced drastically, as during hypoplasia, this homeostatic suppression is abrogated. It is probably significant that this type of outcome is observed most often in patients who became hypoplastic after *small* amounts of busulfan were administered—their Ph[1]-positive cells may possess an unusual sensitivity to the drug. Hypoplasia resulting from excessive doses of busulfan may actually eliminate the small population of Ph[1]-negative cells while the Ph[1]-positive population survives. The possibility of deliberately inducing busulfan hypoplasia has been considered,[122] but this maneuver is dangerous and in many cases might simply eliminate the sought-after Ph[1]-negative cells. Other less toxic drugs might be used, in particular cycle-active agents which would eliminate proliferating cells but leave a nonproliferating population of Ph[1]-negative cells unscathed. The presence of a chromosomal marker for the leukemic cells means that this type of therapy in chronic granulocytic leukemia could be monitored closely, in sharp contrast to the "blind" approach which has to be used in the acute leukemias once hematologic remission has been established and leukemic cells are undetectable.

"Prophylactic" Therapy for Metamorphosis

Metamorphosis in chronic granulocytic leukemia occurs because at some time, which varies widely among patients, a new and less differentiated clone of cells arises in the granulopoietic tissue. After an uncertain interval, this clone occupies enough of the bone marrow and spleen to alter the hematologic picture so that the features of chronic granulocytic leukemia in its chronic phase are no longer present. Clinical deterioration and death usually follow. Chemotherapy with the agents generally used for acute granulocytic leukemia is not very effective when metamorphosis has become overt, but there is a possibility that better results might be achieved at an earlier stage, when the undifferentiated clone is small and the amount of "chronic-phase" chronic granulocytic leukemia tissue is larger. Regular courses of chemotherapy suitable for acute granulocytic leukemia—such as, daunorubicin and cytarabine, or TRAP (see Table 18-15)—might prevent the further development of new clones by destroying them at an early stage. The dosage used in such prophylaxis could safely be large, because the high total granulocyte mass present can withstand a good deal of chemotherapy: if courses were reasonably close together it would be unnecessary to use other therapy to control the chronic-phase component of the disease. The chief drawback to this approach is that, compared to standard treatment with busulfan, it is troublesome to both patient and physician, and large numbers of patients would have to be studied for a lengthy period to establish its value or nonvalue. However, the present unsatisfactory state of therapy for chronic granulocytic leukemia indicates the need for some systematic study along these lines.

Cyclic Drug Therapy in the Chronic Phase

Although numerous drugs will control chronic granulocytic leukemia in its chronic phase, only busulfan has been fully exploited. An alternative approach currently under investigation is the sequential use of seven different drugs for 6-week periods each: at the end of 42 weeks the sequence is begun again.[310] The drug sequence is mercaptopurine, melphalan, hydroxyurea, dibromomannitol, demecolcine, busulfan, cyclophosphamide. With this therapy, the patient is unlikely to suffer from the cumulative side effects of any one of the drugs, and the alternation of drugs which depress the platelet count and drugs which do not is useful. Theoretically, the cycling of drugs could discourage the emergence of drug-resistant cell clones. The therapy is acceptable to patients and, after the first cycle, dosage adjustments are not particularly frequent; this treatment has also proved satisfactory in previously splenectomized patients. Whether survival will be prolonged will, as in all therapeutic studies in CGL, take time to determine.

CHRONIC LYMPHOCYTIC LEUKEMIA

A major problem in chronic lymphocytic leukemia is when to treat the disease and when to merely observe it. A secondary problem is what constitutes the optimal treatment. Neither of these questions has been definitely answered, although very strong opinions are quite unjustifiably held by many workers: frequently, these are diametrically opposed. One of the few respects in which chronic lymphocytic leukemia resembles chronic granulocytic leukemia is in the lack of any major advances in therapy in recent years. The age group of most CLL patients, the benign nature of the disease in many cases, the evident harm caused by treatment in some instances, and a strong tendency for these elderly patients to succumb to intercurrent unrelated diseases—often without ever having required treatment for their leukemia—have perhaps combined to retard research on the treatment of this disease.

It is widely believed that therapeutic restraint is in the best interests of the patient with chronic lymphocytic leukemia; mere diagnosis of the condition is not an indication for treatment. There is no strong evidence against this view, and currently accepted practice is merely to observe the majority of patients for at least a few months after diagnosis. Many times the disease is found to make no apparent progress in this period, and the policy of observation is extended, sometimes for many years, and often to the end of the patient's life. However, this practice should not be generally accepted. Although anecdotes abound of patients with chronic lymphocytic leukemia who were observed for 20 years and never treated, finally dying of unrelated disease at an advanced age, such patients really represent only one extreme of a continuous spectrum, and the prognosis is not really as good as this. Estimates of the median survival of patients with chronic lymphocytic leukemia vary quite widely. Figures of 2.77 years,[333] 1.53 years,[105] 6.3 years,[253] and 4.0 years[139] have been reported. Part of this variation stems from the varying ways of calculating survival time—from diagnosis, from onset of therapy, or from onset of disease, the latter being a dubious figure often obtained by backdating from the time of diagnosis to the time when symptoms were first noticed. For practical purposes, the median survival from diagnosis to death is the most useful, and a reasonable estimate of this figure is between 4–6 years (see also Chapter 19).[296] Thus, chronic lymphocytic leukemia is not as benign a condition as is sometimes implied; although some patients survive for one or two decades and suffer little disability from the disease, the majority do much less well. Differences in survival rates have been ascribed to the adverse effects of therapy on patients with a short survival, and not to its benefits in those with a long survival.[358] Certainly, many of the very long-term survivors are patients who never required any therapy for their disease, and, not uncommonly, such individuals have died of illnesses with no known relationship to their chronic lymphocytic leukemia. It is indeed difficult to conceive how any form of therapy could alter the prognosis of such cases (except unfavorably!), but they are a minority. At any center where patients receive treatment only if their disease appears to need it, it may well be found that treated patients have a shorter median survival than do untreated individuals. It does not necessarily follow that treatment shortens the prognosis since the patients in the treatment group are already a selected population with a more aggressive form of chronic lymphocytic leukemia.

Chronic lymphocytic leukemia has been subdivided on hematologic findings and trends over a period of observation into benign and malignant forms, and clinically too, chronic lymphocytic leukemia is not a homogeneous disease (see Chapter 10).[40,121] It is likely, however, that chronic lymphocytic leukemia is a spectrum rather than two discrete groups, and not every case will be readily classifiable into a prognostic category. Probably the most important factors affecting the survival of such a patient are the stage of the disease at diagnosis and its rate of evolution. Earlier diagnosis, even in the absence of any therapy, would consistently produce a dramatic and factitious improvement in survival.

Generally accepted indications for treatment in chronic lymphocytic leukemia are:

1. Evidence of bone marrow failure—anemia, neutropenia, or thrombocytopenia.
2. The development of autoimmune acquired hemolytic anemia.
3. The presence of splenomegaly which is symptomatic or accompanied by hypersplenism.
4. Troublesome involvement of lymph nodes, skin, or other tissues.

It is generally felt that the leukocytosis itself, if unaccompanied by any of the above, does not constitute an indication for therapy.

Although it is accepted practice to treat chronic lymphocytic leukemia only when specific indications are present, the evidence on which this is based is inconclusive. In two studies,[42,139] the survival rates of patients treated infrequently or symptomatically when compared with those treated regularly, regardless of the presence or absence of symptoms, were similar. However, in each report the cases treated conservatively belonged to the authors' institutions, whereas those treated more aggressively were culled from other reports, one of which included no untreated patients. Comparisons of this sort cannot be accorded the same weight as properly controlled trials. Even if the conclusions are correct, they only show that the treatments then current were not beneficial for chronic lymphocytic leukemia, not that the disease should not be treated. The value of active treatment in early chronic lymphocytic leukemia is still unknown. At present, the majority of centers treat chronic lymphocytic leukemia only when it appears necessary, and a few centers treat the condition from diagnosis, but neither has a control group managed in the opposite manner. There is a definite need for controlled therapeutic trials. For example, the established approach—offering treatment only when it is specifically indicated—might be compared with more active approaches: prolonged low-dose chemotherapy; long-term, intermittent, high-dose chemotherapy with single drugs or combinations; and radiotherapy. The indications from earlier studies—that therapy is not particularly successful—signify that more, not less, therapeutic research is required in this disease.

Review of Therapy

IONIZING RADIATIONS

Until about 1950, irradiation was the standard treatment for chronic lymphocytic leukemia at many centers. It was applied to the spleen and/or groups of enlarged lymph nodes, or as a spray to areas of the body. Dosage was usually gentle, since pancytopenia was readily produced in patients with compromised marrow function. Radiotherapy in chronic lymphocytic leukemia seldom produced the striking benefit seen in chronic granulocytic leukemia, and with advances in chemotherapy its use has declined at most centers.

Local irradiation is still the treatment of choice for troublesome lymph node masses in chronic lymphocytic leukemia. Such lesions require a good deal of chemotherapy for their complete resolution, and there is a risk of damaging the bone marrow, whereas with radiotherapy the masses rapidly melt away with quite low doses. Because the radiation is concentrated on a target area, exerting its maximum effect at that site, the therapeutic ratio is very much higher than with systemic chemotherapy. Irradiation may also be used in those patients who are receiving chemotherapy but have a leukemic mass—tonsillar, pharyngeal infiltrate, lymph nodes or even spleen—which is not responding satisfactorily. Rare instances of tracheal or spinal cord compression require urgent radiotherapy. In chronic lymphocytic leukemia, lymph node masses are apt to recur, presumably being repopulated by circulating lymphocytes, and repeated irradiation is sometimes required: after a period of some years, problems may arise because the radiation tolerance of adjacent normal tissues has been reached and further radiotherapy is not possible. Fortunately, this is an uncommon occurrence.

Systemic treatment of chronic lymphocytic leukemia by irradiation is more controversial. Radiotherapy may be applied externally, either to the spleen or to the whole body[173,174] or internally by the administration of radionuclides, usually ^{32}P. All these techniques give good results in skilled hands, but there have been no systematic prospective studies which directly compare radiotherapy with systemic chemotherapy. Good results have been obtained by some centers using carefully titrated radiotherapy (notably by Osgood[252,253]) but it has been suggested that these results may well be attributable to the overall high standard of clinical care exercised by this group, rather than to the irradiation technique per se.[296] Osgood[253] also had diagnostic criteria slightly different from those generally adopted,[253] and it is possible that the diagnosis in his patients was established somewhat earlier than at other centers. This would lead to an automatic improvement in median survival so long as the therapy given was not actively harmful, and emphasizes the need for studies in which each institution has patients in both treatment and control groups. Recent studies of the effects of externally applied, total-body irradiation in chronic lymphocytic leukemia have shown interesting but uncontrolled results that suggest a high response rate in symptomatic cases[173,174] with improvement in symptoms, physical signs, peripheral blood counts, and bone marrow appearances. In those patients achieving a good response, according to carefully defined criteria, the median duration of unmaintained remission was 19 months.[174] Since all the patients treated had active, symptomatic, chronic lymphocytic leukemia, it seems that this therapy may significantly prolong life as well as improving its quality. If a controlled study of total-body irradiation in chronic lymphocytic leukemia substantiates its efficacy in the active disease state, the possible benefits of prophylactic treatment in patients with inactive disease should be evaluated.

ADRENOCORTICOSTEROIDS

These agents have been used in chronic lymphocytic leukemia for over 15 years.[124, 128, 180, 294, 296] The late William Dameshek investigated the systematic use of steroids in this disease because of the similarities between the terminal wasting syndrome seen in chronic lymphocytic leukemia and the immunologic runt disease produced experimentally in mice.[177] Steroid therapy can produce striking benefit in chronic lymphocytic leukemia, even when the condition is very advanced and has become refractory to radiotherapy or alkylating agents (Figs. 18-20 and 18-21). The special virtue of steroids is their ability to cause lysis of lymphoid tissue without producing bone marrow depression: therefore, they are the safest method for effectively treating chronic lymphocytic leukemia when marrow failure is already present. Against this important advantage must be set an enhanced liability to infection: such patients are already at risk from infection by reason of neutropenia and defective antibody production, and any therapy which increases this risk is not to be undertaken without careful consideration. The metabolic effects of steroids are particularly unwelcome, since most patients are middle-aged or elderly and are prone to hypertension, fluid retention, diabetes mellitus, and osteoporosis even before steroids are prescribed. A reasonable policy in chronic lymphocytic leukemia is to use alkylating agents when one can and steroids when one must, and to avoid long-term, high-dose corticosteroid therapy whenever possible.

Currently accepted indications for steroid therapy are:

1. The presence of bone marrow failure with neutropenia and/or thrombocytopenia.
2. Autoimmune acquired hemolytic anemia.
3. Autoimmune thrombocytopenic purpura.
4. Resistance to alkylating agents used alone (see Fig. 18-21).
5. Thrombocytopenia with purpura, whether autoimmune or not, and whether or not the leukemia itself is responsive to steroids. Here, steroids are used for their nonspecific beneficial effect on thrombocytopenic bleeding.

Only item 1 is an indication for the use of steroids *alone;* in the remainder, the concurrent use of alkylating agents or radiotherapy will often be advisable.

Following the institution of therapy with prednisolone, the peripheral blood lymphocyte count commonly rises, but generally declines after the first 2 weeks of treatment[294] although it may remain raised for months; while the levels of platelets, neutrophils, and hemoglobin rise. Occasionally, there is a very rapid fall in lymphocyte count and rapid lysis of lymphoid tissue accompanied by hyperuricemia: since renal failure is readily precipitated in elderly patients, prophylactic allopurinol therapy is advisable to prevent hyperuricemia in the early stages of therapy.[187] Usually, regression of lymphadenopathy, splenomegaly, and hepatomegaly is gradual. An initially positive direct antiglobulin (Coombs') test may decrease in titer, and hemolytic anemia will abate. Concurrently, the side effects of prednisolone therapy emerge and become progressively more marked, eventually compelling a reduction in dosage. Although autoimmune phenomena in chronic lymphocytic leukemia may respond to long-term therapy with low doses of prednisolone, the

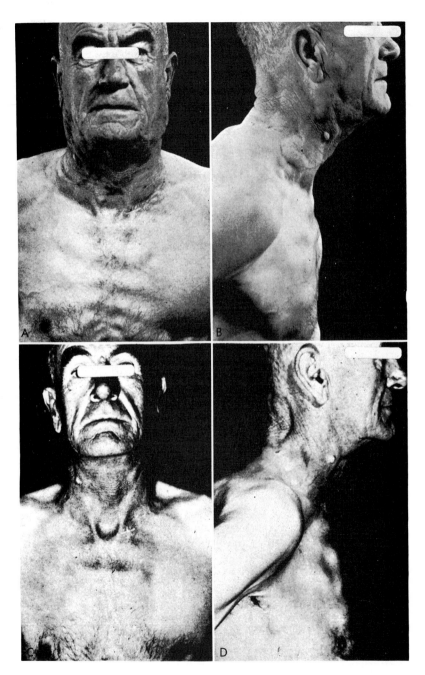

Fig. 18-20. Chronic lymphocytic leukemia. The patient, resistant to chlorambucil, was treated with 40 mg of prednisone daily at first. A and B, before treatment. C and D, six months later. The swelling in the left pectoral region is a lipoma. (Courtesy, Dr. A. J. Campbell.)

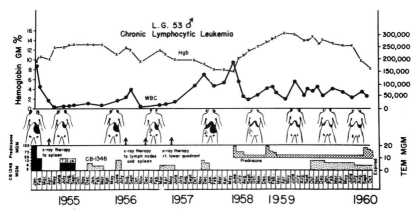

Fig. 18-21. Chronic lymphocytic leukemia in patient L.G. who had undergone treatment with various modalities (x-ray, alkylating agents) from 1955 to June 1958. At that time, the patient was seriously ill, unable to work, very anemic, and his leukemia was refractory to all therapy. Abdominal masses were present and spleen was huge. High-dose corticosteroid therapy (prednisone in a 125-mg daily dose) was instituted and followed by a rapid subsidence of lymphoid masses, and a quick improvement in the anemia (Coombs' negative) and thrombocytopenia. The patient was able to return to work and was in reasonably good health for more than 2 years on maintenance prednisone therapy (25 mg daily). Eventually, refractoriness developed and the patient died.

disease itself is seldom controlled by doses small enough to be acceptable on a long-term basis. Patients with advanced disease have been treated at first with high daily doses of steroids until improvement occurred, and then maintained with intermittent high doses of steroids.[54] A dose of 100 mg of prednisone given once or twice a week was effective in some patients, and steroid side effects were reduced. Further investigation of this technique is indicated.

There are other unresolved questions concerning optimal steroid therapy in chronic lymphocytic leukemia. It would be an advantage to know whether the use of steroids, either concurrently with alkylating agents or immediately before a course of an alkylating agent, can improve the therapeutic response or lessen the incidence of serious toxicity. One report suggests that the subsequent addition of chlorambucil in patients first treated with prednisolone does not significantly potentiate therapeutic response,[102] but another study has shown that the steroid plus chlorambucil is superior to chlorambucil alone.[143]

ALKYLATING AGENTS

Chronic lymphocytic leukemia will usually respond to almost any alkylating agent, but relatively few of the available agents are commonly used in this condition. Nitrogen mustard is inconvenient and causes vomiting, while triethylene melamine, once popular, has been discarded because of its unpredictability and tendency to cause serious thrombocytopenia. Busulfan is effective, but less so than chlorambucil, and is seldom used.[279] The treatment of chronic lymphocytic leukemia is usually carried out with alkylating agents given in low doses over prolonged periods; therefore, most experience has been gained with those agents which can be given orally on an outpatient basis, especially chlorambucil.[43, 102, 124, 126, 166, 180, 296, 336] Apart from its reliable absorption from the gastrointestinal tract and freedom from side effects such as vomiting, alopecia, or cystitis, chlorambucil appears to possess some selective cytotoxicity, in that lymphoid cells are more affected than cells of the myeloid series.[93,94]

Chlorambucil, usually administered in a daily dose of 0.1–0.2 mg per kilogram of body weight, reduces the peripheral blood lymphocytosis in at least 70 percent of patients with chronic lymphocytic leukemia. As with corticosteroids, allopurinol should be given concurrently. Lymphadenopathy is reduced in about 50 percent of chlorambucil-treated patients and splenomegaly in about 25 percent of patients.[128] Thus, the physical signs of the disease are favorably affected and symptoms may improve also. However, the treatment has serious limitations. Bone marrow infiltration responds slowly, variably, and sometimes not at all, while lymphocytosis and neutropenia may persist despite the reduction in total leukocyte count. It is important to remember that some of the apparent alterations in neutrophil count during chlorambucil therapy are factitious, and occur merely because the differential leukocyte count becomes more accurate as the lymphocytosis decreases: when the total leukocyte count is 100,000 and about 99 percent of the cells are lymphocytes, a differential leukocyte count is almost meaningless unless it is performed on 500–1,000 cells, which is not done as often as it should be. Unfortunately, anemia and thrombocytopenia are often not improved by chlorambucil therapy[42,128,296] while hypogammaglobulinemia rarely responds to chlorambucil or to any other alkylating agent.[41,124] During treatment with chlorambucil, neutropenia, thrombocytopenia, and anemia may all be aggravated, and serious infection may lead to death, an occurrence partially attributable to therapy. Thus, active treatment in chronic lymphocytic leukemia readily causes harm, while, at their best, results are rarely as dramatic as those which occur in the acute leukemias or chronic granulocytic leukemia. Cyclophosphamide has a lesser tendency to produce thrombocytopenia than do other alkylating agents and, for this reason, it may be preferred to chlorambucil in the presence of thrombocytopenia.[248]

It is common practice to administer chlorambucil in courses, discontinuing therapy when the desired result has been obtained. Two studies comparing the effects of continuous and intermittent therapy with an alkylating agent in chronic lymphocytic leukemia showed no difference in survival,[102,166] but the evidence is not conclusive. An inherent discouragement to instituting trials in chronic lymphocytic leukemia, and a difficulty in carrying them out, is the long natural history of the disease. Follow-up should be continued for a minimum of 5 years from the entry of the last patient into a trial.

OTHER CYTOTOXIC AGENTS

Drugs other than alkylating agents have been little used and not widely tested in chronic lymphocytic leukemia. The antimetabolite drugs MP[55] and MTX[88] and the mitotic inhibitor VCR[80] all appear to be ineffective, and the first two agents damage the bone marrow. Unlike the alkylating agents, these drugs do not damage small lymphocytes, and their ineffectiveness is further evidence that the cytokinetics of chronic lymphocytic leukemia differ greatly from those of more anaplastic neoplasms such as acute lymphocytic leukemia.

ANDROGENIC HORMONES

The use of testosterone enanthate or fluoxymesterone was originally intended to stimulate erythropoiesis and correct anemia;[182] results which were achieved in several patients. In others, the platelet count rose and leukocytosis increased, perhaps because steroids were administered concurrently with the androgen. A 2-month period of treatment was considered necessary for evaluation of the response. In another study, androgens were administered without corticosteroids and the hemoglobin, platelets, and neutrophil count rose, while in some patients a lympholytic effect was reported.[348] The above results, and a report that androgens increase the tolerance of bone marrow to cytotoxic agents,[49] suggest that the less virilizing androgens such as oxymetholone might have a place in therapy of chronic lymphocytic leukemia. Further investigation is indicated, since despite their occasional hepatotoxicity androgens are less potentially harmful therapy than either prednisolone or alkylating agents. Since androgens appear to have protective effects against osteoporosis, and to increase marrow tolerance to alkylating agents, they might advantageously be combined with steroids and/or alkylating drugs.

Recommended Therapy

From the foregoing discussion it will be apparent that it is not possible to recommend a scientifically based optimal therapy for chronic lymphocytic leukemia: there are too many unknown factors which have yet to be evaluated. Accordingly, it is possible only to advise what seems to be a reasonable approach, and to add that further studies may well show it to be less than optimal.

Patients with chronic lymphocytic leukemia should be carefully assessed at the time of diagnosis, with documentation of serum immunoglobulin levels, direct antiglobulin (Coombs') test, and evidence of bone marrow failure, including the degree of lymphocytic infiltration of the marrow. Measurements of hepatomegaly, splenomegaly, and of the principal lymph node masses are recorded and a chest radiograph is taken for evidence of mediastinal lymphadenopathy or pulmonary tuberculosis. Chest radiography should be repeated regularly as part of follow-up. It is wise to search for evidence of iron, folic acid, and vitamin B_{12} deficiencies, since these remediable causes of anemia are not uncommon in elderly patients. A minority of patients require treatment once the initial assessment has been completed, but most patients merely require observation at intervals of 3–6 months, with rechecking of the baseline observations previously established. Despite a gradually increasing leukocytosis, this period of observation may extend for many years without apparent deterioration in the patient's condition.

If, at some stage, one of the generally accepted indications for treating chronic lymphocytic leukemia (see above) arises, the most appropriate therapy for the particular indication is instituted. If systemic chemotherapy is indicated, therapy is begun with prednisolone in doses of 1 mg per kg daily, and for the first 4 weeks it is wise to prescribe, in addition, 5–7 mg of allopurinol per kg daily. Evidence of diabetes mellitus should be sought before and during steroid therapy. After 2–3 weeks of steroid therapy, the peripheral blood lymphocytosis is usually decreasing and platelet and neutrophil counts are improved. At this stage, chlorambucil may be added in a 0.1–0.2-mg dose per kilogram of body weight per day—in the presence of thrombocytopenia, 2 mg of cyclophosphamide per kilogram of body weight may be preferred. Therapy with chlorambucil is usually continued until the blood picture has been restored to as near normal as attainable and splenomegaly and lymphadenopathy have regressed. Steroid therapy is gradually discontinued between the fourth and sixth weeks of therapy but low-dose chlorambucil may be continued for several months. Decreased lymphocytic infiltration of the bone marrow, if it occurs, usually requires more than 3 months of therapy to achieve.

In most patients it is reasonable to discontinue chemotherapy once the desired result has been achieved, and to observe the patient once more. The need to resume therapy may not occur for months or years, but more active cases of chronic lymphocytic leukemia will require retreatment within a shorter period, and in cases which prove to be of this type, long-term maintenance therapy (see Fig. 18-22) is advisable. It is important to follow patients who are on long-term chlorambucil therapy quite closely, since insidious, drug-induced marrow hypoplasia may occur. Although the initial response to steroids and chlorambucil is usually satisfactory, resistance to both these agents is apt to occur. The situation is particularly awkward when resistance to chlorambucil has arisen, since the physician must choose between the dangers of long-term steroid therapy and those of uncontrolled chronic lymphocytic leukemia.

SPLENECTOMY

Splenectomy may not alter the natural history of chronic lymphocytic leukemia,[296] but acceptable indications for splenectomy are usually considered to be

1. Autoimmune hemolytic anemia which is unresponsive to steroids or immunodepressant drugs, or responsive only to doses which are too high to be acceptable.
2. Autoimmune thrombocytopenia, when similarly unresponsive to drug therapy.[89]
3. Hypersplenism, or apparent hypersplenism, which is uncontrolled by drugs and causing serious disability.

An alternative approach, cautious irradiation of the spleen, may be used in frail patients considered unfit for surgery, but it is quite hazardous in itself, and often is not very effective. Splenectomy may be recommended if hypersplenism is demonstrated, for example, by excessive sequestration of isotopically labeled red cells and/or platelets in the enlarged spleen. The case for splenectomy is stronger if studies of the bone marrow do not suggest advanced failure: for example, if morphologic preparations do not show total replacement by lymphocytes and isotopic methods demonstrate significant iron utilization. Splenectomy can be expected to benefit a majority of the patients who satisfy these criteria, and for uncertain reasons the operation sometimes benefits patients who do not. Thus, isotopic studies are a useful, but by no means infallible guide.[247]

Splenectomy has occasionally been performed in chronic lymphocytic leukemia for neutropenia or thrombocytopenia when these are manifestations of bone marrow failure rather than of hypersplenism, and, rarely, the operation has been performed for splenomegaly alone. The merit of this course is debatable. In the presence of severe marrow failure, splenectomy would seem to be unrewarding, but

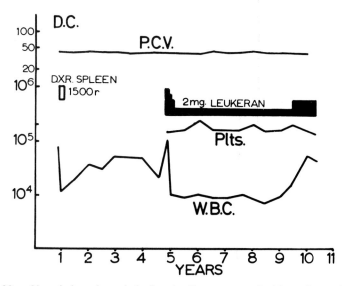

Fig. 18-22.   Chronic lymphocytic leukemia. Ten-year survival in male aged 54 at onset, who received continuous treatment with chlorambucil during the last 6 years.

improvement has followed the operation, permitting more active chemotherapy than was possible preoperatively, with consequent sustained improvement.[245] Although splenectomy for autoimmune hemolysis may succeed, even in the absence of significant splenic sequestration of isotopically labeled erythrocytes,[7] the outcome of the operation for other indications is more variable.[51,110,228] The consensus of opinion appears to be that splenectomy can be a valuable measure in chronic lymphocytic leukemia, but the patients must be carefully selected and the risks of surgery, considerable in this age group, must be weighed against the likelihood and probable extent of benefit.[127,162,236,245,320]

Blast Cell Leukemia Terminating Chronic Lymphocytic Leukemia

The manifestations of chronic lymphocytic leukemia commonly worsen with time, but it is doubtful whether chronic lymphocytic leukemia unlike chronic granulocytic leukemia undergoes transformation to a blastic phase (see Chapter 10). Although a recent review cites a number of instances of acute leukemia arising in chronic lymphocytic leukemia,[208] the incidence of acute leukemia in these patients was not demonstrably greater than in the general population. Since the rate of ascertainment of acute leukemia is likely to be particularly high in patients who are regularly observed by hematologists because they have chronic lymphocytic leukemia, the lack of demonstrable increase is very likely to be meaningful. A true *acute transformation* of chronic lymphocytic leukemia should take the form of an acute lymphocytic leukemia, or some morphologic variant related to the lymphoid cell series. In fact, most of the acute leukemias in such patients have been monocytic, myeloblastic,[208] or myelomonocytic.[61] These patients are exposed to both therapeutic and diagnostic irradiation and this may be responsible for the development of acute leukemia. Since prolonged exposure to alkylating agents has been followed by the appearance of acute leukemia,[196] prolonged courses of chlorambucil might lead to acute leukemia in occasional patients.

Chronic Lymphocytic Leukemia and Other Neoplastic Diseases

For a complete discussion, see Chapters 10 and 12 and references 22, 140, 319 at the end of this chapter.

Autoimmune Hemolytic Anemia in Chronic Lymphocytic Leukemia

Hemolytic anemia associated with a positive direct antiglobulin (Coombs') test may occur at any time in the course of chronic lymphocytic leukemia. It may even occur as the presenting symptom in some cases, the indications of the disease being relatively slight, for example, moderate lymphadenopathy, or slight leukocytosis and lymphocytosis. Once the diagnosis has been established, treatment with steroids—for example, prednisolone—should be begun: a large initial dose such as 1.5–2.0 mg per kilogram of body weight is advisable, particularly if hemolysis is severe. When the reticulocyte count begins to fall and the hemoglobin to rise, the dose of steroid is reduced stepwise, seeking the smallest dose which will control the hemolysis. Some patients are satisfactorily maintained by 5–10 mg of prednisolone daily, which is an acceptable dose for long-term use. Doses above 15 mg daily are potentially hazardous when administered for long periods in elderly patients, so that other measures should be sought to improve the control of hemolysis and enable reduction of the steroid dose. Cyclophosphamide is suitable for this purpose, since it is immunodepressant and also will control the chronic lymphocytic leukemia itself. Autoimmune hemolysis also responds to antimetabolite drugs such as mercaptopurine, thioguanine, and azathioprine,[7,288] but these drugs are less suitable since they depress the normal elements of the bone marrow without having beneficial effects on the leukemia. Severe and poorly controlled hemolysis is an indication for splenectomy (see above).

Infections

In general, the frequency of infection in chronic lymphocytic leukemia correlates well with the presence of hypogammaglobulinemia and impaired antibody response.[295] In patients with marrow depression caused by the leukemia or by the alkylating agents, neutropenia increases the liability to infection. Antibiotic prophylaxis has been claimed to be helpful in treatment of leukemia with hypogammaglobulinemia and recurrent serious infections,[234] but close follow-up and immediate vigorous therapy of infections as they arise is more easily justified: a good family physician who is well apprised of the patient's hematologic state is better prophylaxis than the use of antibiotics. Pooled human gamma globulin has been recommended for both prophylaxis and treatment of infections in chronic lymphocytic leukemia.[234] Its efficacy in either role is difficult to assess, but it is worth trying in the presence of serious infection which does not respond promptly to antibiotics alone. The intramuscular injections of gamma globulin required are bulky and painful and may cause hematomas in thrombocytopenic patients, but some gamma globulin preparations can be administered intravenously, diluted in physiologic saline, without serious untoward effects.[39] Quite large amounts of gamma globulin are routinely administered intravenously when a 4-unit transfusion of whole blood is given. The principal hazard of the repeated administration of pooled human immunoglobulins is the transmission of serum hepatitis. In patients with chronic lymphocytic leukemia, infections which appear minor and might be left untreated in normal individuals—for example, gastroenteritis or mild bronchitis—should be treated vigorously. Serious infections are apt to become fulminant and often require therapy before bacteriologic results are available. The possibility of less common infections, particularly tuberculosis, should always be borne in mind, because these patients are elderly, hypogammaglobulinemic, and often have received prolonged corticosteroid therapy.

Exfoliative Dermatitis

This distressing dermatologic manifestation is relatively resistant to treatment with irradiation and corticosteroid drugs. Control of the chronic lymphocytic leukemia with chlorambucil and prednisolone, together with topical corticosteroids such as fluocinolone acetonide with occlusive dressings to treat the dermatitis may all be tried, but the condition is sometimes very stubborn.

Herpes Zoster

This painful condition occurs frequently in patients with chronic lymphocytic leukemia, although, in one published series, only about one-third as commonly as in Hodgkin's disease, and about three times as often as it occurs in patients with carcinoma.[233] The zoster may become disseminated (zoster-varicella) and secondarily infected. Zoster-varicella is sometimes fatal in elderly debilitated patients. Prompt treatment with ara-C by continuous intravenous infusion can be highly effective in aborting the course of zoster, arresting the progression of the lesions with sometimes dramatic suddenness.[176,207] Treatment for 48–72 hours is often adequate, and prolonged infusion is to be avoided, since cytarabine depresses the bone marrow and does not affect the leukemia itself.

Possible Therapeutic Advances

IMPROVED CHEMOTHERAPY

Problems relating to the use of alkylating agents which merit further study by means of controlled clinical trials include:

1. Comparison of treatment only when indicated, with treatment upon diagnosis
2. Full evaluation of the effects of intermittent therapy versus continuous maintenance therapy, both at conventional doses, with special precautions to ensure initial comparability of the cases in the two groups
3. Investigation of the possible synergy between alkylating agents and corticosteroids
4. Comparison of the usual regimens in which alkylating agents are administered daily in low doses with the effects of intermittent high-dose parenteral therapy

For the last, cyclophosphamide would be a more suitable agent than chlorambucil for this type of study. A recent study of lymphocyte kinetics in chronic lymphocytic leukemia during treatment with an alkylating agent suggests that kinetic alterations in response to this therapy may vary considerably between patients.[69] If these results are confirmed, it will be important to establish correlations with the clinical behavior of the chronic lymphocytic leukemia and its response to different treatments. It appears clinically obvious that chronic lymphocytic leukemia is not a homogeneous disease, ranging as it does from extremely benign to relatively malignant disease, and this variability in character of the disorder is an additional hazard in assessing the merits of any therapy.

ANTILYMPHOCYTE GLOBULIN

The treatment of chronic lymphocytic leukemia with antilymphocyte serum (ALS) or antilymphocyte globulin (ALG) is theoretically attractive, since an immunologic approach promises a target specificity much greater than that of alkylating agents, or even corticosteroid hormones. In a recent study,[192] allogeneic ALS was prepared by immunizing normal volunteers with normal lymphocytes. Administration of the ALS to CLL patients caused a fall in the lymphocyte count and reduction in lymph node enlargement, but no change occurred in the differential leukocyte count. In another study,[335] xenogeneic ALS prepared in horses was administered. The resulting fall in the peripheral blood lymphocyte count was transient, and it was concluded that long-term treatment with ALS would be necessary. Such therapy carries the risk of serious allergic reactions to horse serum and also of complete immunosuppression with fatal infection. However, in one trial of intravenously administered, xenogeneic ALG,[258] the injections were continued without ill effect for 58 days. The lymphocyte count fell but there was no reduction of hepatomegaly, splenomegaly, or lymphadenopathy. In another study,[210] the administration of xenogeneic ALG for periods up to 31 days was accompanied by a fall in the lymphocyte count and a decrease in organomegaly. Isotopic studies suggested that the fall in lymphocyte count was caused, not by the cytotoxicity of ALG but to an altered distribution of leukemic lymphocytes.

Active immunotherapy—that is, the induction of immunity to a tumor within its possessor—is known to be effective, only after the maximum possible reduction in tumor cell mass has been effected by more conventional means.[5, 103] Similarly, the results of passive immunotherapy with ALG might be improved if the treatment were given to CLL patients whose leukemia had already been effectively treated by vigorous radiotherapy and/or chemotherapy.

In summary, the treatment of chronic lymphocytic leukemia cannot be described as either wholly satisfactory or as having been adequately studied. However, recent developments in radiotherapy, chemotherapy and in immunological approaches have indicated several promising lines for future therapeutic research in this disease.

IMMUNOTHERAPY FOR THE LEUKEMIAS

The concept of immunotherapy for cancer is over 70 years old. During this period, it initially passed through a phase of optimism, but repeated failures led to an outlook of pessimism and immunotherapy almost became equated with quackery.

Now, immunotherapy has reached a stage where controlled experiments, rather than uncontrolled opinions, are the order of the day.

Immunotherapy may be broadly subdivided into three types. *Passive* immunotherapy signifies the administration of antibodies preformed in a human or animal donor—for example, equine ALG. *Active* immunotherapy implies immunization of the patient bearing a tumor. Such immunization may be *nonspecific,* that is, with BCG vaccine, or *specific,* that is, with cells or fractions from the patient's own tumor or an allogeneic tumor of the same kind. *Adoptive* immunotherapy means the transfer of immunologically competent cells, which may previously have been activated against the tumor, from a donor to the patient. Experimental work in animals with leukemias and other tumors has shown that in many cases immunotherapy is effective, either in preventing the successful "take" of a transplanted tumor in an immunized animal, or even in causing the rejection of an established tumor. Results in man are much less definite, partly because experiments such as those in animals are ethically impossible. In human leukemias, immunotherapy must be considered an important and challenging field of research, but it could not be recommended as a method of treatment, except within the framework of a formal, controlled, therapeutic trial.

Immunotherapy in chronic lymphocytic leukemia has principally been passive, using ALS or ALG. The preliminary results are less than dramatic, but many refinements of the method are possible and these may greatly improve its effects. Since this form of leukemia is generally accompanied by a state of partial immunoincompetence, active immunotherapy in this disease might be difficult, but might make a highly significant difference to the course of the disease. Adoptive immunotherapy in chronic lymphocytic leukemia is also of great theoretical interest. In chronic granulocytic leukemia, one study reports the use of myeloblasts from a patient with acute granulocytic leukemia and of blast cells from a patient with chronic granulocytic leukemia which had undergone metamorphosis, to immunize patients whose chronic granulocytic leukemia was well controlled.[301] The blast cells were mixed with BCG vaccine as an adjuvant, and injected intradermally. The preliminary results suggest that such patients, whose disease is in the chronic phase and who are thus immunized, remain in the chronic phase longer than unimmunized patients, while patients whose disease is in metamorphosis, which has been controlled by chemotherapy, remain controlled for many months if treated with the blast cell preparation. If these results are confirmed they will have an important impact on the management of chronic granulocytic leukemia.

The principal effort has been in studying immunotherapy for the acute leukemias. Early studies concentrated particularly on acute lymphocytic leukemia, but recently immunotherapy for acute granulocytic leukemia has attracted much attention. The finding of leukemia-specific antigens on leukemic cells, and the evidence that some patients produce cellular immune reactions[340,341] and humoral antibodies[83] against them, suggested the possibility that the course and outcome of acute leukemia might be influenced by the host defences. Long-term survivors of acute lymphocytic leukemia have sometimes relapsed with blast cell tumors confined to the ovaries or testes, sites which may be less accessible to immunocytes, but there have been no hematologic relapses in such patients. A case of acute granulocytic leukemia has been reported which relapsed,[63] after a 10-year remission, by developing a localized encapsulated tumor in the median nerve sheath which was composed histologically and cytologically of myelomonocytic leukemic blast cells; the confinement of the blast cells to a portion of the nervous system might be attributable to host immunologic defenses.

The very extensive literature on the pioneering work in immunotherapy for acute lymphocytic leukemia has recently been reviewed.[214] Attempts have been made to reinforce the host defenses in this disease by specific stimulation with repeated injections of irradiated blast cells pooled from several patients, and by nonspecific stimulation with BCG vaccine.[215,217] The immunotherapy was given only to patients in complete remission and was started only after a long period of preliminary chemotherapy. The number of residual ALL cells would then be expected to be very small; only in this circumstance has immunotherapy in experimental animals been shown to be effective. The 30 patients in one study were allocated at random to one of four schedules: (1) no treatment (10 patients); (2) BCG vaccination (8 patients); (3) vaccination with leukemic cells (5 patients); and (4) vaccination with both BCG and leukemic cells (7 patients). All the schedule 1 patients relapsed between 20–130 days after chemotherapy was stopped, compared with only 9 of the 20 patients in schedules 2, 3, and 4. The difference in survival of the immunotherapy-treated and the control groups was highly significant. Because of these results, which were obtained in France, a larger trial was mounted in the United Kingdom.[224] In this trial, 191 patients with acute lymphocytic leukemia were treated by chemotherapy for 5 months; the treatment including consolidation therapy and intrathecally administered MTX. Complete remission was achieved in 177 patients (93 percent) and these were randomly allocated to intermittent MTX maintenance, no therapy, and BCG vaccine. At the time of analysis, 26 months from the beginning of the trial, 143 patients were still alive, including 70 in their first remission. The median remission durations after the cessation of intensive chemotherapy were 17 weeks (no therapy), 27 weeks (BCG), and 52 weeks MTX. There was no statistically significant difference between the BCG and no-therapy groups. The only observed effect of BCG was the production of lymphocytosis. Thus, this study failed to confirm the results of the earlier small-scale trial. The results of the French trial could be explained if the 10 patients in the no-therapy group had an unusually brief remission duration after their prolonged intensive chemotherapy, while the patients in the other groups had a more typical course and the immunotherapy had no influence for good or ill. Such findings readily occur in small groups of patients. It has, in fact, been pointed out[161] that the survival curve from the end of chemotherapy in a group of patients receiving no treatment after the completion of one regimen of chemotherapy in an Acute Leukemia Group B (ALGB) study (schedule "D" of Study 6601) is similar to that of the group of patients receiving immunotherapy in the French trial.

The evidence that immunotherapy with leukemic blast cells and/or BCG vaccine can affect the duration of remission in acute lymphocytic leukemia after chemotherapy has been discontinued is thus inconclusive. Since recent developments strongly indicate that this disease can be eradicated by chemotherapy alone in a high proportion of patients,[262,306,307] interest in immunotherapy has waned in many quarters. Many physicians would now find ethical difficulties in using this form of therapy for acute lymphocytic leukemia if its use involved any curtailment of antileukemic chemotherapy below the levels which appear to eradicate the disease.

In the management of acute granulocytic leukemia, on the other hand, no such confidence exists in the efficacy of available chemotherapy. There have been improvements in remission-induction techniques and in supportive measures, but therapy for maintaining remissions is unsatisfactory. Because of this unsatisfactory state, trials of immunotherapy are acceptable to many physicians. The St. Bartholomew's Hospital immunotherapy program for patients with acute granulocytic leukemia has been briefly described (see page 000). A preliminary report suggests that this treatment may prolong remissions in acute granulocytic leukemia, but the evidence is not yet conclusive.[75] The U.K. Medical Research Council is at present conducting a large-scale, cooperative controlled trial with the aim of ascertaining the effects of immunotherapy in a large group of patients with acute granulocytic leukemia. Even if immunotherapy of the type described is shown to be without effect, or to benefit only a small subpopulation of patients, the method is capable of much refinement. Thus, *autologous* blast cells, harvested from peripheral blood or bone marrow before chemotherapy is begun, might be more effective for immunotherapy because they carry the tumor antigens against which it is desired to stimulate an immune response. *Allogeneic* blast cells raise fewer logistic problems, since sufficient blast cells to treat five or more patients can be harvested from AGL patients who have a gross leukocytosis on presentation. The allogeneic blasts may possess immunologic advantages since they carry foreign antigens which may exert adjuvant effects upon the immunogenicity of any "leukemic" antigens they also carry. The use of nonspecific immune stimuli other than BCG needs to be investigated; some of the earlier work on *Corynebacterium parvum* vaccine might well be repeated in AGL patients.[214]

One major limitation of immunotherapy is that it is probably only applicable to patients whose acute granulocytic leukemia is already in hematologic remission; thus, until chemotherapy is improved, almost one-half of such patients will be ineligible for whatever benefits immunotherapy might confer. It must also be borne in mind that immunotherapy might sometimes be harmful; for example, the production of blocking antibodies which attach to leukemic cells and prevent the access of cytotoxic lymphocytes might negate any beneficial effects of the therapy and also any spontaneous cellular immune reaction mounted by the tumor host. Acceleration of the leukemia might result, and this would be particularly dangerous since it is difficult to detect with certainty in individual patients owing to the variable behavior of acute granulocytic leukemia.

TREATMENT OF MYELOMA

The management of myeloma has changed considerably in the past 10 years. Formerly, this was a disease in which neither patient nor physician derived much satisfaction from treatment. A variety of chemotherapeutic agents produced very occasional responses which were only partial; very often, chemotherapy made the patient significantly worse, aggravating a preexisting pancytopenia and adding anorexia, nausea, and vomiting to his problems. Localized irradiation relieved bone pain but caused pancytopenia if large areas had to be treated. Frequently, new painful areas became manifest during therapy, and the process of pursuing bone pain with radiotherapy depressed the patient and led to chronic hospitalization and

Table 18-20
Early Therapeutic Attempts in Myeloma

Agent	Comments
External irradiation	Useful in localized bone pain and in treating myelomatous tumors, particularly those compressing vital structures. Unsuitable for generalized pain—even local irradiation sometimes caused pancytopenia.
Radionuclides	^{32}P occasionally beneficial, but dangerous in presence of marrow failure.[198] Au sometimes helpful for pain relief.
Alkylating agents	Nitrogen mustard appeared both valueless and harmful. Chlorambucil was thought to be ineffective.
Antimetabolites	MP, MTX, 5-fluorouracil had no definite effects other than aggravation of immunodepression and marrow insufficiency.
Urethane	Nausea, vomiting, and myelodepression very common: occasionally relieved pain but did little else.
Stilbamidine	Sometimes relieved pain but did not affect tumor growth; interesting unexplained cytologic changes in myeloma cells (see Chapter 17).
Estrogens	Sometimes relieved bone pain; very occasional prolonged benefit
Androgens	Occasionally improved anemia and bone pain
Gamma globulin	Said to lessen the incidence of recurrent pneumonia but results mainly uncontrolled
Transfusions	Improved anemia, sometimes improved renal function.
Analgesics	Almost always necessary, particularly in terminal stages. Narcotics often required. Probably increased the liability to pneumonia.

immobility. The combination of bed rest and deficient immune responses, together with neutropenia caused by therapy or by the myeloma, itself, often resulted in hypostatic pneumonia and death. From Table 18-20 it is apparent that a large number of widely differing therapeutic agents were tried in this disease with very little success.

Review of Therapy

An extensive literature dealing with the therapy of multiple myeloma has been summarized on several occasions.[125,209,300] For the chemotherapist, multiple myeloma should be an ideal disorder to study, since so many parameters are available by which the effects of therapy can be evaluated quantitatively. As in the leukemias, the peripheral blood count and the extent of bone marrow infiltration with tumor cells can be followed. In addition, radiologic changes in the skeleton and the biochemical values which reflect function and calcium metabolism can be monitored. Most important, myeloma is one of the few human tumors in which the cells regularly produce measurable amounts of metabolites that give some indication of the amount of tumor present. These metabolites are the serum paraproteins, and from their study it has been possible to deduce the probable growth characteristics of human multiple myeloma, which appear to follow a Gompertzian, rather than an exponential, pattern.[281,282] Careful serial study of the paraproteins also enables the early detection of resistance to previously effective therapy, and even provides some indication of the cytokinetic alterations which underly the process of relapse in the individual patient.[157]

Despite these extraordinary possibilities for its study, myeloma is an obdurate tumor and reports of successful therapy have become frequent only in the past 10 years. Early studies with urethane,[280] and urethane combined with an alkylating agent,[170] yielded unimpressive results; although pain was sometimes relieved, there was rarely much alteration in paraproteinemia or Bence Jones proteinuria. Therapy with the alkylating agent melphalan (L-phenylalanine mustard), however, brought definite subjective and objective benefit to a majority of myeloma patients, resulting in an increased survival time[24, 164, 304, 343] as compared to patients who received radiotherapy alone.[47] Cyclophosphamide, another alkylating agent, is also effective in multiple myeloma[85, 344]; it has the advantage of causing less thrombocytopenia than melphalan, but alopecia and cystitis are decided drawbacks to its long-term use, although many patients escape these complications altogether. A comparative trial of melphalan and cyclophosphamide[285] in patients with myeloma has failed to show any significant difference between the two agents,[225] and it appears that cross-resistance between them is complete.[125]

Adrenocorticosteroid hormones must pose some hazards in patients with multiple myeloma, who are often elderly, are already partially immunoincompetent, and who frequently have numerous osteoporotic bony lesions before steroids are begun. However, steroid therapy can lower an elevated serum calcium and also retard the proliferation of plasma cells. The addition of prednisone to treatment with melphalan improves the response of multiple myeloma.[6] It also appears that treatment with intermittent courses of melphalan may be more effective than the continuous administration of low doses of the drug. At present a cooperative trial is comparing the intermittent administration of melphalan with and without concurrent steroid therapy.

The treatment of multiple myeloma which has become resistant to alkylating agents and steroids remains a problem. Radiotherapy will relieve localized bone pain but control of the systemic disease is unsatisfactory. Trials of BCNU, doxorubicin, and other drugs are in progress: we have found that these first-named agents will relieve bone pain in refractory myeloma, and modest reduction in the serum paraprotein level has been observed. It has been suggested that fractionated total-body irradiation to about 1000 rads could produce lengthy remissions,[23] because the rate of proliferation of the tumor cells is very slow. This dose of irradiation may only be administered in stages, with shielding of part of the bone marrow at each stage. Such a therapeutic approach might well be investigated in myeloma patients for whom systemic chemotherapy no longer has anything to offer.

Recommended Therapy

Most patients with myeloma have symptoms of anemia or bone pain or recurrent infections at the time of diagnosis and require immediate treatment. The worst overall prognosis attaches to patients who present because of renal failure: these patients are treated for their disease only if the renal failure can be controlled, and specific treatment for the tumor must be cautious because its toxic effects are enhanced in the presence of renal impairment. Some patients are asymptomatic and without evidence of renal or bone marrow failure; they may be diagnosed because of an unexpectedly high erythrocyte sedimentation rate, rouleaux formation on a routine blood film, or difficulties in crossmatching blood for an unrelated surgical operation. Whether symptomatic or not, it is usually best to treat patients with multiple myeloma from the time of diagnosis—in contrast to patients with chronic lymphocytic leukemia—because if therapy is delayed until complications arise, the tumor cell mass to be controlled by chemotherapy is correspondingly greater. Before treatment is begun, careful assessment of the patient's hematologic and biochemical status is made (Table 18-21). These investigations afford evidence as to the likely prognosis and the problems which require immediate attention, and also provide baselines by which the progress of therapy may be followed and incipient failure of therapy detected early.

Evidence of azotemia is of major prognostic importance. In a recent study of 276 patients with myeloma,[227] the relative death rate of patients whose BUN remained over 40 mg per 100 ml was five times greater than that of patients in whom the BUN was less than 20 mg per 100 ml, and the median survival times in these groups were 2 and 37 months, respectively. The concentration of high molecular weight protein in the urine was correlated with the BUN, but also with the median survival after allowing for the BUN: the relative death rate for patients with proteinuria of 40 mg per 100 ml or more was about twice that of patients with less proteinuria at all BUN levels. Bence Jones proteinuria was correlated with elevated BUN but did not appear to have an independent effect on prognosis. A low serum albumin or a hemoglobin concentration below 7.5 gm per 100 ml were correlated with a poor prognosis, but, curiously, the absolute concentration of paraprotein in

Table 18-21

Baseline Investigations Prior to Treatment in a Patient with Myeloma

Hematologic	Hemoglobin, hematocrit, reticulocyte count, platelet count, total leukocyte count, differential leukocyte count, erythrocyte sedimentation rate, estimation of plasma cells in bone marrow aspirate, (examination of marrow from several sites, ferrokinetic studies, serum B_{12} and folate levels)*
Radiologic	Chest radiograph, skeletal survey, (bone scintiscans)
Plasma proteins	Total serum protein, serum albumin, serum globulins, serum electrophoretic strip, serum immunoelectrophoresis, urinary Bence Jones and total protein, electrophoresis of concentrated urine, (gel diffusion for characterization of serum and urine paraproteins, plasma viscosity, immunofluorescent staining of marrow plasma cells).
Renal	BUN, serum creatinine, creatinine clearance, urine microscopy and culture, (renal biopsy; intravenous pyelography if BUN not grossly elevated—test performed *without* prior fluid restriction, which may precipitate anuria); (rectal biopsy for amyloid).
Other biochemistry	Serum calcium and phosphate, 24-hour urinary calcium output, serum uric acid, serum alkaline phosphatase (alkaline phosphatase isoenzyme determinations)

*Tests in parentheses are desirable and the other tests should be considered essential.

the plasma failed to show a significant correlation with survival. Presumably, an elevated BUN at presentation is less ominous if there is an obvious precipitating cause (for example, dehydration) and there is a prompt and satisfactory response to correction of this factor.

Chemotherapy

It is reasonable to begin with melphalan, unless thrombocytopenia is severe, when cyclophosphamide is preferred. In either case the alkylating agent is combined with an adrenocortical steroid, generally prednisolone. A suitable schedule is to administer 10 mg of melphalan daily, by mouth, for 7 days, and to accompany this with prednisolone 40 mg daily, by mouth, for 7 days. In the majority of patients in whom anemia is slight or absent, and the neutrophil and platelet counts are within the normal range, the first course of treatment is followed by a marked fall in the neutrophil and platelet counts, which usually reach their nadir between 10–28 days after the last dose of melphalan. The lowest neutrophil count is usually reached 7–14 days before the platelet nadir, and both counts usually return to their former level 4–6 weeks after the end of the first course. Experience has shown that, if courses are to be repeated indefinitely, the optimal gap between them is 6 weeks, even if the count has recovered before that time. In patients who respond to this treatment, the fall in neutrophil and platelet counts after the second and subsequent courses of therapy is negligible. The probable explanation, by analogy with the response to chemotherapy in leukemia, is that before treatment bone marrow function is grossly impaired as a result of plasma cell infiltration and is still further depressed by the treatment. After the first course, the myelotoxic effect of the melphalan is buffered by the improved marrow reserve and is less apparent.

Newly discovered patients with multiple myeloma, whose marrow function is more severely reduced, so that they have anemia, thrombocytopenia, or neutropenia before any therapy has been given, are specially vulnerable to the myelotoxic effects of melphalan and should be treated with great caution. Less harm is done by giving initial therapy which is too gentle than can be done by overdosing the patient and precipitating life-threatening pancytopenia. An initial course of melphalan, 10 mg daily for only 2–4 days, plus steroid for 7 days, is advisable. Two or more courses may be required before full dosage can be attained with safety. The myelotoxicity of melphalan is greatly enhanced in the presence of uremia, and dosage should be reduced by 50 or even 75 percent. If the uremia is due to a reversible cause such as dehydration, the full dosage of melphalan can be used once renal function has improved. If renal failure is severe and irreversible, the full dosage of melphalan is unlikely ever to be tolerated: however, the prognosis of these patients is so poor because of the renal failure itself that the chemotherapy of their myeloma is often of only secondary importance.

Radiotherapy

Generalized bone pains are often relieved by chemotherapy, but several weeks may elapse before relief is complete. In some patients, severe bone pain at a particular site—most often in the spine—is the major presenting feature, and in occasional patients, a severe localized pain develops during the course of chemotherapy, even when this is beneficial as measured by other parameters. Local irradiation is the treatment of choice for these localized pains since relief is nearly always obtained, often within a few days. The absence of a radiographically demonstrable bony lesion is no contraindication to irradiation, nor does it lessen the likelihood of pain relief but its presence is of value in planning radiotherapy fields. When bony destruction is far advanced, for example, with collapse of several vertebrae, pain relief with irradiation may be incomplete due to irreversible anatomic changes: radiotherapy may have to be supplemented with an appropriate orthopedic appliance. Bone pain leading to immobility is an indication for urgent radiotherapy since bed rest in multiple myeloma patients is hazardous, promoting further demineralization of bones, nephrocalcinosis, and hypostatic pneumonia. Paraplegia of sudden onset requires urgent decompression followed by irradiation. In all these situations the volumes of hematopoietic tissue irradiated are relatively small, and bone marrow depression, resulting from the radiotherapy, rarely necessitates the interruption of chemotherapy. Newly diagnosed patients, however, should receive radiotherapy first to secure relief of their localized pains as rapidly as possible; the special vulnerability of their bone marrow makes it unwise to administer their first course of melphalan during irradiation, while the neutropenia and thrombocytopenia which follow initial chemotherapy would require undue delay before radiotherapy can begin. The possible use of total-body irradiation for refractory disease has been mentioned above.

Management of Hypercalcemia

Chronic low-grade hypercalcemia is treated by a low-calcium diet (including distilled drinking water where local supplies are of high-calcium content), a high fluid intake, and by controlling the underlying disease by chemotherapy. In the early stages these measures may be supplemented by a small dose of prednisolone. Acute severe hypercalcemia, with thirst, drowsiness, mental confusion, and vomiting requires more urgent treatment and alkylating agents alone are too slow in their effects. Treatment should include: a high fluid intake, using the intravenous route until vomiting is controlled; dietary calcium restriction; melphalan or cyclophosphamide, in cautious dosage if the BUN is raised; adrenal corticosteroids, given parenterally and in large doses, for example, a daily increment of 1–2 mg of prednisolone per kilogram of body weight[230]; the administration of sodium phosphate, intravenously or by mouth, at a dose of 1–2 gm of inorganic phosphorus per day. Phosphate administration often causes diarrhea, whichever route is used, and the dose may have to be reduced to the maximum tolerated. Several other measures, such as the administration of calcitonin, have been used in the treatment of hypercalcemia but may be regarded as investigative, rather than established, procedures.[193,346]

Renal Failure

As described above, the presence of renal failure in myeloma at the time of presentation is an ominous prognostic sign. However, in some patients the renal failure is reversible because it has a remediable cause, in which case the prognosis is much better. An immediate search should be made for reversible causes of renal failure and these are treated appropriately:

1. Dehydration is corrected by the liberal administration of oral and/or intravenous fluids.
2. Anemia is treated by blood transfusion.
3. Hyperviscosity syndrome is treated by plasmapheresis (see below).
4. Hypercalcemia is treated by the measures already described, together with the administration of a potent diuretic such as frusemide and adequate replacement of urinary losses of electrolytes and water.[211]
5. Hyperuricemia is managed by alkalinizing the urine and administration of allopurinol.
6. Nephrolithiasis, sometimes seen in myeloma patients who have had chronic hypercalciuria, may require prompt surgical relief.
7. Pyelonephritis, relatively common in myeloma patients who have been bedridden, is treated with fluids and the appropriate antibacterial agent(s).

Patients who remain in renal failure after correction of all remediable parameters obviously have a poor outlook. A renal biopsy may establish the diagnosis of "myeloma kidney" with irreversible damage: chronic hemodialysis will maintain the patient, but in many centers their underlying neoplasm would disqualify them from entrance into overfull chronic dialysis facilities. Occasionally, acute renal failure in myeloma is associated with diffuse intravascular coagulation.[266]

Infections

Recurrent serious infections are common in myeloma patients and this may be attributed to bone marrow depression induced by therapy, as well as to the neutropenia and immunoglobulin deficiency produced by their primary disease. Pneumonia is very common and often is seen in association with bed rest enforced by skeletal pain, or with painful lesions of the ribs or sternum which impair respiratory function. As in chronic lymphocytic leukemia, it is wise to treat every infection in a myeloma patient as potentially serious and administer antibiotics promptly. The value of pooled human gamma globulin is hard to assess but it seems advisable to administer it if an infection does not respond rapidly to antibiotics alone. Long-term antibiotic therapy may be considered for chronic bronchitis or chronic urinary tract infections, but there seems to be no case for the administration of antibiotics prophylactically to myeloma patients. Regular injections of gamma globulin are claimed to be of value in the prophylaxis of infection in such patients but this is unproved.

Hemorrhage

Defective clot retraction, thrombocytopenia, and interference with platelets and clotting factors by high concentrations of paraprotein may all result in bleeding from the mucous membranes or into the skin. Epistaxes may be of extreme severity. Transfusion of platelets, fresh blood, and fresh plasma may all be of value. Plasmapheresis (see below) is occasionally useful. Steroid therapy sometimes helps, apparently through a nonspecific effect in decreasing the fragility of capillary walls. In the long run, control of the myeloma leads to improvement in the hemorrhagic tendency. *Thromboembolic disease* is also relatively common in patients with multiple myeloma and pulmonary embolism is a significant cause of death[62]: possibly a hypercoagulable state and the presence of secondary amyloidosis are important in the pathogenesis of this complication.

The Hyperviscosity Syndrome

This uncommon but serious syndrome is encountered in both multiple myeloma and macroglobulinemia (see Chapter 13).[197] In the long run the treatment of the hyperviscosity syndrome consists in attempts to control the underlying disease, but for the acute episode with CNS manifestations, plasmapheresis is recommended. Much paraprotein can be removed by combined venesection and transfusion, but the procedure can be performed more quickly and efficiently, with less disturbance of blood volume, by the use of a cell separator.[264] The patient's plasma is collected, while his red cells are returned to the circulation; the volume deficit is replaced by normal donor plasma, or donor whole blood if the patient is also anemic. It is possible to maintain the *total* blood volume constant throughout the operation. The effects of plasmapheresis last longer in patients with macroglobulinemia, because their excessive IgM is mostly intravascular. Patients with multiple myeloma, on the other hand, restore their excessive paraprotein levels in a few days from the extravascular fluid compartment (see also Chapter 13).

Fluoride Therapy

Osteolytic lesions in multiple myeloma are often arrested by chemotherapy but often fail to heal: even after local irradiation with extirpation of a plasma cell deposit, bony healing is commonly unsatisfactory. The administration of sodium fluoride, with or without androgen therapy, may promote new bone formation in multiple myeloma, but the value of this treatment has not been established.[70, 195] A recent study suggested that fluoride therapy was valueless and possibly harmful.[145]

Secondary Acute Granulocytic Leukemia

Recent improvements in management have been associated with longer survival of patients with multiple myeloma. This appears to have been accompanied by an increase in the number of patients who develop, and succumb to, acute granulocytic leukemia.[8, 196, 198, 284] Terminal acute granulocytic leukemia has also been reported in macroglobulinemia.[112] It is possible that prolonged exposure to melphalan or other alkylating agents, and to diagnostic and therapeutic irradiation, may be responsible for leukemogenesis in these patients. However, it is also possible that leukemia is a natural development of multiple myeloma, possibly because of the associated immunoincompetence, and that the increased incidence of leukemia is a result of the prolonged survival of patients with multiple myeloma. Most of the acute leukemias described in such patients have been monocytic or myelomonocytic and, therefore, presumably not derived from the neoplastic plasma cells themselves. While the possible leukemogenic potential of melphalan should be recognized, this is no contraindication to treating patients with multiple myeloma: as Holland pointed out, "late death from leukemia after a definite period of remission from myeloma is to be preferred to early death without remission" (see also Chapter 13).[158]

MACROGLOBULINEMIA

Waldenström's macroglobulinemia, although a neoplastic disorder based on the proliferation and accumulation of abnormal lymphoid cells and the production of excessive IgM by these cells, may follow a protracted and relatively benign course. In the most benign cases, in which the concentration of the macroglobulin remains below the threshold necessary for the production of the hyperviscosity syndrome, the bone marrow function keeps pace with the progressive lymphoid infiltration, and the lymphoid proliferation is slow, the disease may run a course like that of chronic lymphocytic leukemia, without deterioration for 10 years or more. In other patients, the disease is more aggressive, so that even patients who do not appear to require treatment at the time of presentation should be carefully followed up. When symptoms arise, they are generally due to the harmful effects of high concentrations of IgM in the plasma. If cryoglobulins are produced, patchy areas of cutaneous necrosis may be the presenting complaint, while occasional patients develop cold agglutinins and present with symptoms of anemia. Less common is presentation with infection or hemorrhage due to bone marrow failure secondary to lymphoid infiltration.

REVIEW OF THERAPY

Retardation or reversal of the lymphoproliferative process may be attempted with alkylating agents. Chlorambucil is the drug most commonly used for this purpose,[67] but cyclophosphamide or melphalan are also effective. The effect of treatment is to reduce the bone marrow infiltration with ensuing improvement in function and in the peripheral blood count. As the mass of abnormal lymphoid cells is reduced, the plasma IgM level gradually falls. These changes are slow and many months of continuous low-dose therapy may be necessary before the maximum benefit attainable is reached. The limitations of such alkylating agents are several. In patients with severe marrow infiltration, therapy must be very cautious and may have to be intermittent in the early stages. Eventually, resistance may arise and the plasma IgM gradually rises despite continued therapy. Occasionally, acute granulocytic leukemia may develop terminally[112] and this may be attributable to chronic administration of alkylating drugs.

The adrenocortical steroids are also effective against the lymphoid proliferation, just as they are in chronic lymphocytic leukemia, and are valuable when marrow function is impaired, but resistance to their action may arise and their long-term use leads to numerous side effects. Since treatment with chlorambucil and/or steroids produces benefit slowly, this therapy is not useful for hyperviscosity syndrome. A direct attack upon the abnormal globulin with agents which break up the large IgM molecule into smaller fragments is a logical way to reduce the plasma viscosity. Both penicillamine[276] and mercaptopyridoxin[275] are said to accomplish this by disrupting the disulfide bonds which unite the five pairs of heavy chains in the IgM molecule. These agents have never been widely used but may deserve reassessment, particularly in patients whose macroglobulinemia has become resistant to chlorambucil and steroids and whose plasma viscosity is rising.

RECOMMENDED THERAPY

Patients with symptomatic macroglobulinemia should be treated once the diagnosis has been established. Asymptomatic patients should be assessed, the important baselines being the peripheral blood values, degree of bone marrow infiltration, serum level of abnormal protein, and the plasma viscosity. These parameters should be carefully followed and treatment instituted if deterioration occurs, preferably before significant symptoms develop.

Initial therapy should be with daily doses of chlorambucil, 0.1 mg per kilogram of body weight, given by mouth. This dose may be increased if the patient tolerates it well, and the therapy should be continued for several months, monitoring the blood count, bone marrow appearances, and serum IgM level. When these have returned to normal, or ceased to improve, it is reasonable to discontinue therapy and observe the patient once more, since it may take months or years for significant deterioration to occur. Patients in whom the IgM rises relatively rapidly may be considered for continuous maintenance with chlorambucil. Probably because of the rarity of the condition, it has not been established whether continuous therapy is superior to intermittent treatment with chlorambucil, and in the United Kingdom a controlled multicenter trial is being conducted with the aim of providing this information. Cyclophosphamide may be preferred to chlorambucil in patients with marrow infiltration and thrombocytopenia. There is probably nothing to be gained by switching to cyclophosphamide or melphalan therapy if resistance arises to chlorambucil, but use of a different *schedule,* for example, intravenously administered cyclophosphamide every 3 weeks in doses of 10–30 mg per kilogram of body weight, may secure a further period of control of the disease.

Adrenocortical steroids, for example, prednisolone, may be used either alone or in combination with an alkylating agent if the response to chlorambucil alone is unsatisfactory. Courses of a few weeks' duration at a daily dose of 1 mg per kilogram of body weight are preferable to prolonged prednisolone therapy. Prednisolone may be used alone as initial therapy in patients with compromised marrow, just as in chronic lymphocytic leukemia, and chlorambucil introduced after an improvement has been effected. Blood transfusion is often necessary in the early stages of treatment, since chemotherapy improves the marrow function rather slowly. The hyperviscosity syndrome should be regarded as an emergency and treated promptly by plasmapheresis, preferably using a continuous-flow cell separator (see section entitled "The Hyperviscosity Syndrome").

When resistance to alkylating agents and steroids has arisen, chemotherapy becomes difficult. A successful result with the use of azathioprine, prednisone, and folic acid has been reported but requires confirmation.[148] Short courses of cyclophosphamide-vincristine-high-dose steroids may be tried, but any success obtained is usually short lived. Blood transfusion and the treatment of infection benefit the patient, and serum IgM levels can be controlled by repeated plasmapheresis. The effects of plasmapheresis last a relatively long time since most of the IgM is intravascular, readily removed, and replaced only slowly. Cryoglobulinemia is usually controlled when the macroglobulinemia is effectively treated, but when the response is unsatisfactory, environmental manipulation is sometimes very helpful—for example, improved domestic heating and the provision of electrically heated boots, jackets and gloves for outdoor wear can prevent painful skin necrosis.

REFERENCES

1. Acute Leukaemia Group B: Studies of sequential and combination antimetabolite therapy in acute leukemia: 6-mercaptopurine and methotrexate. Blood 18:431, 1961.
2. _____: The effectiveness of combinations of antileukemic agents in inducing and maintaining remission in children with acute leukemia. Blood 26:642, 1965.
3. _____: Acute lymphocytic leukemia in children. Maintenance therapy with methotrexate administered intermittently. JAMA 207:923, 1969.
4. Adar R, Mozes M: Fatal complications of central venous catheters. Br Med J 3:746, 1971.
5. Alexander P: Prospects for immunotherapy of cancer: experience in experimental systems. Br Med J 4:484, 1970.
6. Alexanian R, Haut A, Khan AU, Lane M, McKelvey EM, Migliore PJ, Stuckey WJ, Wilson HE: Treatment for multiple myeloma. Combination chemotherapy with different melphalan dose regimens. J Am Med Ass 208:1680, 1969.
7. Allgood J, Chaplin H: Idiopathic acquired autoimmune hemolytic anemia. Amer J Med 43:254, 1967.
8. Andersen E, Videbaek A: Stem cell leukaemia in myelomatosis. Scand J Haematol 7:201, 1970.
9. Aston DL, Cohen A, Spindler MA: Herpesvirus hominis infection in patients with myeloproliferative and lymphoproliferative disorders. Br Med J 4:462, 1972.
10. Aur RJA: Personal communication, 1973.
11. _____, Hustu HO, Verzosa M, Simone J: A comparative study of "prophylactic" craniospinal irradiation in 94 children with acute lymphocytic leukemia (ALL). Proc Am Assoc Cancer Res 12:19, 1971.
12. _____, Simone JV, Hustu HO, Verzosa M: A comparative study of central nervous system irradiation and intensive chemotherapy early in remission of childhood acute lymphocytic leukemia. Cancer 29:381, 1972.
13. _____, Simone J, Hustu HO, Walters T,

Borella L, Pratt C, Pinkel D: Central nervous system therapy and combination chemotherapy of childhood lymphocytic leukemia. Blood 37:272, 1971.
14. Australian Cancer Society's Childhood Leukaemia Study Group: Cyclic drug regimen for acute childhood leukaemia. Lancet 2:313, 1968.
15. Back EH: Death after intrathecal methotrexate. Lancet 2:1005, 1969.
16. Bagshawe KD, Magrath IT, Golding PR: Intrathecal methotrexate. Lancet 2:1258, 1969.
17. Baikie AG: Chromosomes and leukaemia. Acta Haemat 36:157, 1966.
18. _____: The place of splenectomy in the treatment of chronic granulocytic leukaemia: some random observations, a review of the earlier literature and a plea for its proper study in a cooperative therapeutic trial. Aust Ann Med 17:175, 1968.
19. _____: Chronic granulocytic leukaemia: the metamorphosis of a conditioned neoplasm to an autonomous one. Proceeding of Fourth Congress of Asian & Pacific Society of Haematology, 1969, p 197.
20. _____: What is a leukaemic remission? The evidence from cytogenetic studies, in Vincent PC (ed.): The Nature of Leukaemia, Proceedings of the International Cancer Conference, Sydney, 1972, p 231.
21. _____, Spiers ASD: Methotrexate in meningeal leukaemia. Lancet 2:1042, 1967.
22. Berg JW: The incidence of multiple primary cancers. I. The development of further cancers in patients with lymphomas, leukemia, and myeloma. J Natl Cancer Inst 38:741, 1967.
23. Bergsagel DE: Total body irradiation for myelomatosis. Br Med J 2:325, 1971.
24. _____, Migliore PJ, Griffith KM: Myeloma proteins and the clinical response to melphalan therapy. Science 148:376, 1965.
25. Bernard J, Boiron M: Current status: treatment of acute leukemia. Sem Hematol 7:427, 1970.
26. _____, _____, Jacquillat C, Weil M: Rubidomycin in 400 patients with leukemia and

other malignancies. Abstract Twelfth Congress International Society Hematology. New York, International Society of Hematology, 1968, p 5.

27. _____, Jacquillat C, Boiron M, Najean Y, Seligmann M, Tanzer J, Weil M, Lortholary P: Experimental treatment of acute lymphoblastic and myeloblastic leukaemias with a new antibiotic—rubidomycin. Presse Méd 75:951, 1967.

28. _____, _____, Weil M: Treatment of the acute leukemias. Sem Hematol 9:181, 1972.

29. _____, Mathé G, Najean Y: Traitement de 50 leucemies myéloïdes chroniques par le 1—4 diméthane-sulfonyl-oxybutane. Sem Hôp Paris, 31:3082, 1955.

30. _____, Weil M, Boiron M, Jacquillat C, Flandrin G, Gemon M: Acute promyelocytic leukemia: results of treatment by daunorubicin. Blood 41:489, 1973.

31. Bessis M: Use of replacement transfusion in diseases other than hemolytic disease of the newborn. Blood 4:324, 1949.

32. Bierman HR, Cohen P, McClelland JN, Shimkin MB: The effect of transfusions and antibiotics upon the duration of life in children with lymphogenous leukemia. J Pediatr 37:455, 1950.

33. _____, Crile DM, Dod KS, Kelly KH, Petrakis NL, White LP, Shimkin MB: Remissions in leukemia of childhood following acute infectious disease. Cancer 6:591, 1953.

34. _____, Kelly KH, Centero PA, Cordes FL: The influence of cellular fractions of whole blood on the course of acute lymphocytic leukemia: a preliminary report, in Rebuck JW, Bethell FH, Monto RW (eds.): The Leukemias. New York, Academic Press, 1957, p 301.

35. Bisel HF: Letter to the Editor. Blood 11:676, 1956.

36. Bodey GP, Buckley M, Sathe YS, Freireich EJ: Quantitative relationships between circulating leukocytes and infection in patients with acute leukemia. Ann Intern Med 64:328, 1966.

37. _____, Hart J, Freireich EJ, Frei E: Studies of a patient isolator unit and prophylactic antibiotics in cancer chemotherapy. Cancer 22:1018, 1968.

38. _____, Nies BA, Freireich EJ: Multiple organism septicemia in acute leukemia. Arch Intern Med 116:266, 1965.

39. _____, _____, Mohberg NR, Freireich EJ: Use of gamma globulin in infection in acute-leukemia patients. JAMA 190:1099, 1964.

40. Boggs DR: Data on the cause of leukemia. N Engl J Med 284:1267, 1971.

41. _____, Fahey JL: Serum protein changes in malignant disease. II. The chronic leukemias, Hodgkin's disease, and malignant melanoma. J Natl Cancer Inst 25:1381, 1960.

42. _____, Sofferman SA, Wintrobe MM, Cartwright GE: Factors influencing the duration of survival of patients with chronic lymphocytic leukemia. Am J Med 40:243, 1966.

43. Bouroncle BA, Doan CA, Wiseman BK, Frajola WJ: Evaluation of CB1348 in Hodgkin's disease and allied disorders. Arch Intern Med 97:703, 1956.

44. Bousser J, Christol D: Essais de chimiothérapie de la leucémie myéloïde par 3 corps nouveaux: démécolcine, thiocholchicine, myléran. Presse Méd 63:1229, 1955.

45. Boutis L, Obrecht P, Musshoff K, Jochmann P: The prognosis of chronic lymphatic leukaemia. Dtsch Med Wochenschr 93:2111, 1968.

46. Boyles PW: Interstitial pulmonary fibrosis after long-term busulfan therapy. Clin Med 76:11, 1969.

47. Broad AF, Emery EW, Godlee JN, Prankerd TAJ: The management of myelomatosis. Postgrad Med J 44:803, 1968.

48. Broder LE, Carter SK: Meningeal Leukemia. New York, Plenum Press, 1972.

49. Brodsky I, Dennis LH, Kahn SB: Testosterone enanthate as a bone marrow stimulant during cancer chemotherapy (preliminary report). Cancer Chemother Rep 34:59, 1964.

50. Brubaker CA, Wheeler HE, Sonley MJ, Hyman CB, Williams KO, Hammond D: Cyclic chemotherapy for acute leukemia in children. Blood 22:820, 1963.

51. Buchanan JG, de Gruchy GC: Splenectomy in chronic lymphatic leukaemia and lymphosarcoma. Med J Aust 2:6, 1967.

52. Buckner D, Graw RG, Eisel R, Henderson ES, Perry S: Leukapheresis by continuous flow centrifugation (CFC) in patients with chronic myelocytic leukemia (CML). Blood 33:353, 1969.

53. Burchenal JH: Long-term survivors in acute leukemia and Burkitt's lymphoma. Cancer 21:595, 1968.

54. Burningham RA, Restrepo A, Pugh RP, Brown EB, Schlossman SF, Khuri PD, Lessner HE, Harrington WJ: Weekly high dose glucocorticosteroid treatment of lymphocytic leukemias and lymphomas. N Engl J Med 270:1160, 1964.

55. Cancer Chemotherapy National Service Center: 6-Mercaptopurine: the clinical effect on tumors other than acute leukemia and chronic myelogenous leukemia. Cancer Chemother Rep 9:144, 1960.

56. Canellos GP, De Vita VT, Whang-Peng J, Carbone PP: Chronic granulocytic leukemia: clinical and cytogenetic correlations in: Proceedings of the Thirteenth Congress of the International Society of Hematology Munich, Lehmann 1970, p 320.

57. _____, _____, _____, _____: Hematologic and cytogenetic remission of blastic transformation in chronic granulocytic leukemia. Blood 38:671, 1971.

58. _____, Nordland J, Carbone PP: Splenectomy for thrombocytopenia in chronic granulocytic leukemia. Cancer 29:660, 1972.

59. Capizzi RL, Summers WP, Bertino JR: Antagonism of the antineoplastic effect of methotrexate (MTX) by L-asparaginase (ASN'ASE) or L-asparagine (ASN) deprivation. Proc Am Assoc Cancer Res 11:14, 1970.

60. Carey RW: Comparative study of cytosine arabinoside therapy alone and combined with thioguanine, mercaptopurine or daunomycin in acute myelocytic leukemia. Proc Am Assoc Cancer Res 11:15, 1970.

61. Catovsky D, Galton DAG: Myelomonocytic leukaemia supervening on chronic lymphocytic leukaemia. Lancet 1:478, 1971.

62. _____, Ikoku NB, Pitney WR, Galton DAG: Thromboembolic complications in myelomatosis. Br Med J 3:438, 1970.

63. Chan BWB, Hayhoe FGJ: Long-term remission in acute leukaemia. Lancet 2:728, 1970.

64. Chevalier L, Glidewell O: Schedule of 6-mercaptopurine and effect of inducer drugs in prolongation of remission maintenance in acute leukemia. Proc Am Assoc Cancer Res 8:10, 1967.

65. Clarkson BD: Acute myelocytic leukemia in adults. Cancer 30:1572, 1972.

66. _____, Fried J: Changing concepts of treatment in acute leukemia. Med Clin N Am 55:561, 1971.

67. Clatanoff DV, Meher OO: Response to chlorambucil in macroglobulinemia. J Am Med Assoc 183:40, 1963.

68. Cline MJ, Rosenbaum E: Prediction of in vivo cytotoxicity of chemotherapeutic agents by their in vitro effect on leukocytes from patients with acute leukemia. Cancer Res 28:2516, 1968.

69. Coco F, Merritt JA: Cyclophosphamide-induced changes in circulating lymphocyte kinetics in chronic lymphocytic leukemia. Cancer 25:721, 1970.

70. Cohen P, Gardner FH: Induction of subacute skeletal fluorosis in a case of multiple myeloma. N Engl J Med 271:1129, 1964.

71. Colebatch JH, Baikie AG, Clark ACL, Jones DL, Lee CWG, Lewis IC, Newman NM: Cyclic regimen for childhood leukaemia. Lancet 2:869, 1968.

72. Crosby WH: To treat or not to treat acute granulocytic leukemia? Arch Intern Med 122:79, 1968.

73. Crowther D: L-asparaginase and human malignant disease. Nature 229:168, 1971.

74. _____, Bateman CJT, Vartan CP, Whitehouse JMA, Malpas JS, Fairley GH, Scott RB: Combination chemotherapy using L-asparaginase, daunorubicin, and cytosine arabinoside in adults with acute myelogenous leukaemia. Br Med J 4:513, 1970.

75. _____, Powles RL, Bateman CJT, Beard MEJ, Gauci CL, Wrigley PFM, Malpas JS, Fairley GH, Scott RB: Management of adult acute myelogenous leukaemia. Br Med J 1:131, 1973.

76. Cutting HO: The effect of splenectomy in chronic granulocytic leukemia. Report of a case. Arch Intern Med 120:356, 1967.

77. Dameshek W, Necheles TF, Finkel HE: Survival in myeloblastic leukemia of adults. N Engl J Med 275:700, 1966.

78. D'Angio GJ, Evans AE, Mitus A: Roentgen therapy of certain complications of acute leukemia in childhood. Am J Roentgenol Radium Ther Nucl Med 82:541, 1959.

79. Desai RG: Treatment of chronic granulocytic and lymphocytic leukemia and allied disorders with Myleran and Leukeran in Indian subjects. Acta Haematol Jap 22:160, 1959.

80. Desai DV, Ezdinli EZ, Stutzman L: Vincristine therapy of lymphomas and chronic lymphocytic leukemia. Cancer 26:352, 1970.

81. Diamond RD, Bennett JE: A subcutaneous reservoir for intrathecal therapy of fungal meningitis. N Engl J Med 288:186, 1973.

82. Dick DAL: The response to cyclophosphamide—a review of a sample of the literature, in Fairley GH, Simister JM (eds.): Cyclophosphamide. Bristol, John Wright, 1964, p 131.

83. Doré JF, Marholer L, Ajuria E, Doré M, Painfrand M, Thé G, Mathé G: Serological evidence for immune reaction to leukaemia in man, in Proceedings of the Thirteenth Congress of the International Society of

Hematology. Munich, Lehmann, 1970, p 276.

84. Dowling MD, Gee TS, Lee BJ, Clarkson BD, Burchenal JH: Treatment of acute nonlymphoblastic leukemia with arabinosylcytosine (araC) and 6-thioguanine (TG) every 12 hours. Proc Am Assoc Cancer Res 13:21, 1972.

85. Dubois-Ferrière H: Experimental and clinical results obtained in the treatment of haematoblastoses and carcinomas with Endoxan alone or in combination with prednisone. Arzneim Forsch 11:202, 1961.

86. ———, Rudler JC: Seven-year-long survival time following splenectomy in a case of chronic myelocytic leukemia. Schweiz Med Wochenschr 97:182, 1967.

87. Duttera MJ, Gallelli JF, Kleinman LM, Tangrea JA, Wittgrove AC: Intrathecal methotrexate. Lancet 1:540, 1972.

88. Duvall LR: The clinical effect of methotrexate on tumors other than acute leukemia and choriocarcinoma. Cancer Chemother Rep 14:145, 1961.

89. Ebbe S, Wittels B, Dameshek W: Autoimmune thrombocytopenic purpura ("ITP" type) with chronic lymphocytic leukemia. Blood 19:23, 1962.

90. Eckhardt S, Sellei C, Horvath IP, Institoris J: Effect of 1,6-dibromo-1, 6-dideoxy-D-mannitol on chronic granulocytic leukemia. Cancer Chemother Rep 33:57, 1963.

91. Ellison RR: Management of acute leukemia in adults. Med Clin N Am 40:743, 1956.

92. ———, et al: Arabinosyl cytosine: a useful agent in the treatment of acute leukemia in adults. Blood 32:507, 1968.

93. Elson LA: Experimental approaches to the chemotherapy of leukaemia. Proc Roy Soc Med 56:631, 1963.

94. ———, Galton DAG, Till M: The action of chlorambucil (CB1348) on the haemopoietic organs of the rat. Br J Haematol 4:355, 1958.

95. Enders JF, McCarthy K, Mitus A, Cheatham WJ: Isolation of measles virus at autopsy in cases of giant-cell pneumonia without rash. N Engl J Med 261:875, 1959.

96. d'Eramo N, Levi M: Neurological Symptoms in Blood Diseases. London, Harvey Miller & Medcalf, 1972.

97. Ernst P, Killman S-A: Perturbation of generation cycle of human leukemic blast cells by cytostatic therapy in vivo: effect of corticosteroids. Blood 36:689, 1970.

98. Evans AE: Central nervous system involvement in children with acute leukemia. Cancer 17:256, 1963.

99. ———, Gilbert ES, Zandstra R: The increasing incidence of central nervous system leukemia in children. Cancer 17:404, 1970.

100. Evans DIK, Jones PM, Morris P, Shaw EA: Outpatient anaesthesia for a children's leukaemia clinic. Lancet 1:751, 1971.

101. Eyre, HJ, Goldstein IM, Perry S, Graw RC: Leukocyte transfusions: function of transfused granulocytes from donors with chronic myelocytic leukemia. Blood 36:432, 1970.

102. Ezdinli EZ, Stutzman L: Chlorambucil therapy for lymphomas and chronic lymphocytic leukemia. J Am Med Assoc 191:444, 1965.

103. Fairley GH: Evidence for antigenicity in human tumours with reference to both melanoma and acute leukaemia. Br Med J 4:483, 1970.

104. Farber S, Diamond LK, Mercer RD, Sylvester RF, Wolff JA: Temporary remissions in acute leukemia in children produced by folic acid antagonist, 4-aminopteroyl-glutamic acid (aminopterin). N Engl J Med 238:787, 1948.

105. Feinleib M, MacMahon B: Variation in the duration of survival of patients with the chronic leukemias. Blood 15:332, 1960.

106. Fernbach DJ, Griffith KM, Haggard ME, Holcomb TM, Sutow WW, Vietti JJ, Windmiller J: Chemotherapy of acute leukemia in childhood: comparison of cyclophosphamide and mercaptopurine. N Engl J Med 275:451, 1966.

107. ———, Sutow WW, Thurman G, Vietti TJ: Clinical evaluation of cyclophosphamide. A new agent for the treatment of children with acute leukemia. J Am Med Assoc 182:30, 1962.

108. Fillastre JP, Laumonier R, Humbert G, Dubois D, Metayer J, Delpech A, Leroy J, Robert M: Acute renal failure associated with combined gentamicin and cephalothin therapy. Br Med J 2:396, 1973.

109. Fishbein WN, Carbone PP, Freireich EJ: Clinical trials of hydroxyurea in patients with cancer and leukemia. Clin Pharmacol Ther 5:574, 1964.

110. Fisher JH, Welch CS, Dameshek W: Splenectomy in leukemia and leukosarcoma. N Engl J Med 246:477, 1952.

111. Foley HT, Bennett JM, Carbone PP: Combination chemotherapy in accelerated phase of chronic granulocytic leukemia. Arch Intern Med 123:166, 1969.

112. Forbes IJ: Development of acute leukaemia in Waldenström's macroglobulinaemia

after prolonged treatment with chlorambucil. Med J Aust 1:918, 1972.

113. Frei E, et al: The effectiveness of combinations of antileukemic agents in inducing and maintaining remission in children with acute leukemia. Blood 26:642, 1965.

114. ———, Freireich EJ: Progress and perspectives in the chemotherapy of acute leukemia, in Advances in Chemotherapy. New York, Academic Press, 1965, p269.

115. Freireich EJ: Effectiveness of platelet transfusion in leukemia and aplastic anemia. Transfusion 6:50, 1966.

116. ———, et al: The effect of 6-mercaptopurine on the duration of steroid-induced remissions in acute leukemia: a model for evaluation of other potentially useful therapy. Blood 21:699, 1963.

117. ———, Bodey GP, Hart JS, Whitecar JP, McCredie KB: Current status of therapy for acute leukemia. Recent Results Cancer Res 36:119, 1971.

118. ———, Frei E: Recent advances in acute leukemia, in Brown EB, Moore CV (eds): Progress in Hematology, vol IV. New York, Grune & Stratton, 1964, p 187.

119. ———, Gehan EA, Sulman D, Boggs DR, Frei E: The effect of chemotherapy on acute leukemia in the human. J Chron Dis 14:593, 1961.

120. Fromowicz KK: Observations on the therapeutic effect of demecolcin in chronic granulocytic leukemia. Pol Tyg Lek 10:602, 1955.

121. Galton DAG: The pathogenesis of chronic lymphocytic leukemia. Can Med Assoc J 94:1005, 1966.

122. ———: The possibility of radical chemotherapy in chronic myelocytic leukemia. Haematol Lat 12:703, 1969.

123. ———: The chemotherapy of chronic myelocytic leukemia. Sem Hematol 6:323, 1969.

124. ———: Management of the chronic leukaemias, in Ultmann JE, Griem ML, Kirsten WH, Wissler RW (eds.): Recent Results in Cancer Research. Berlin, Springer, 1971.

125. ———: Myelomatosis, in Hoffbrand AV, Lewis SM (eds.): Tutorials in Postgraduate Medicine: Haematology. London, Heinemann, 1972, p 515.

126. ———, Israels LG, Nabarro JDN, Till M: Clinical trials of p-(di-2-chlorethylamino)-phenylbutyric acid (CB1348) in malignant lymphoma. Br Med J 2:1172, 1955.

127. ———, Spiers ASD: Progress in the leukemias, in Brown EB and Moore CV (eds.):

Progress in Hematology, vol VII. New York, Grune & Stratton, 1971, p 343.

128. ———, Wiltshaw E, Szur L, Dacie JV: The use of chlorambucil and steroids in the treatment of chronic lymphocytic leukaemia. Br J Haematol 7:73, 1961.

129. Gaya H, Tattersall MHN, Hutchinson RM, Spiers ASD: Changing patterns of infection in cancer patients. Eur J Cancer 9:401, 1973.

130. Gee TS, Yu K-P, Clarkson BD: Treatment of adult acute leukemia with arabinosyl cytosine and thioguanine. Cancer 23:1019, 1969.

131. Geils GP, Scott CW, Baugh CM, Butterworth CE: Treatment of meningeal leukemia with pyrimethamine. Blood 38:131, 1971.

132. George P, Hernandez K, Borella L, Pinkel D: "Total therapy" of acute lymphocytic leukemia in children. Proc Am Assoc Cancer Res 7:23, 1966.

133. ———, ———, Hustu O, Borella L, Holton C, Pinkel D: A study of "total therapy" of acute lymphocytic leukemia in children. J Pediatr 72:399, 1968.

134. ———, Pinkel D: CNS radiation in children with acute lymphocytic leukemia in remission. Proc Am Assoc Cancer Res 6:22, 1965.

135. Gluckman E, Basch A, Varet B, Dreyfus B: Combination chemotherapy with cytosine arabinoside and rubidomycin in 30 cases of acute granulocytic leukemia. Cancer 31:487, 1973.

136. Goldschmidt MC, Bodey GP: Effect of chemotherapeutic agents upon microorganisms isolated from cancer patients. Antimicrob Agents Chemother 1:348, 1972.

137. Gompertz D, Brooks AP, Gaya H, Spiers ASD: Volatile fatty acids in the faeces of patients in 'germ-free' isolation. Gut 14:183, 1973.

138. Graw RG, Herzig G, Perry S, Henderson ES: Granulocyte transfusion therapy: septicemia due to Gram-negative bacteria. N Engl J Med 287:367, 1972.

139. Green RA, Dixon H: Expectancy for life in chronic lymphocytic leukemia. Blood 25:23, 1965.

140. Gunz FW, Angus HB: Leukemia and cancer in the same patient. Cancer 18:145, 1965.

141. Haddow A, Timmis GM: Myleran in chronic myeloid leukaemia. Chemical constitution and biological action. Lancet 1:207, 1953.

142. Haghbin M, Tan C, Clarkson B, Sykes M, Murphy ML: Intensive chemotherapy and

prophylactic intrathecal methotrexate in acute lymphoblastic leukemia. Proc Am Assoc Cancer Res 13:22, 1972.

143. Han T, Ezdinli EZ, Shimaoka K, Desai DV: Chlorambucil vs combined chlorambucil-corticosteroid therapy in chronic lymphocytic leukemia. Cancer 31:502, 1973.

144. _____, Stutzman L, Cohen E, Kim U: Effect of platelet transfusion on hemorrhage in patients with acute leukemia. An autopsy study. Cancer 19: 1937, 1966.

145. Harley JB, Schilling A, Glidewell O: Ineffectiveness of fluoride therapy in multiple myeloma. N Engl J Med 286:1283, 1972.

146. Hayes DM, Ellison RR: Production of remissions in blastic phase of chronic myelocytic leukemia (CML) and acute myelocytic leukemia (AML) by arabinosyl cytosine (ara-C) plus 1,3bis-(2-chloroethyl)-1-nitrosourea (BCNU). Blood 34:840, 1969.

147. Hayhoe FGJ, Quaglino D, Doll R: The Cytology and Cytochemistry of Acute Leukaemias. London, H.M. Stationery Office, 1964.

148. Heading RC, Girdwood RH, Eastwood MA: Macroglobulinaemia treated with prednisone, azathioprine, and folic acid. Br Med J 3:750, 1970.

149. Heard BE, Cooke RA: Busulphan lung. Thorax 23:187, 1968.

150. Henderson ES: Combination chemotherapy of acute lymphocytic leukemia of childhood. Cancer Res 27:2570, 1967.

151. _____: Treatment of acute leukemia. Ann Intern Med 69:628, 1968.

152. _____: Treatment of acute leukemia. Sem Hematol 6:271, 1969.

153. _____, Samaha RJ: Evidence that drugs in multiple combinations have materially advanced the treatment of human malignancies. Cancer Res 29:2272, 1969.

154. _____, Serpick A: The effect of combination drug therapy and prophylactic oral antibiotic treatment in adult acute leukemia. Clin Res 15:336, 1967.

155. _____, _____, Leventhal B, Henry P: Cytosine arabinoside infusions in adult and childhood acute myelocytic leukemia. Proc Am Assoc Cancer Res 9:29, 1968.

156. Hersh EM, Bodey GP, Nies BA, Freireich EJ: Causes of death in acute leukemia. A ten-year study of 414 patients from 1954 to 1963. J Am Med Assoc 193:105, 1965.

157. Hobbs JR: Modes of escape from therapeutic control in myelomatosis. Brit Med J 2:325, 1971.

158. Holland JF: Epidemic acute leukemia. N Engl J Med 283:1165, 1970.

159. _____, 1966. Progress in the treatment of acute leukemia. In: Dameshek W, Dutcher RM (eds.): Perspective in Leukemia. New York: Grune & Stratton, 1968.

160. _____: Therapy of acute leukemia, in Proceedings of the XIII Congress of International Society of Hematology. Munich, Lehmann, 1970, p 58.

161. _____, Glidewell O: Complementary chemotherapy in acute leukemia, in Mathé G (ed.): Advances in the Treatment of Acute (Blastic) Leukemia. New York, Springer, 1970, p 95.

162. Holt JM, Witts LJ: Splenectomy in leukaemia and the reticuloses. Q J Med 35:369, 1966.

163. Holton CP, Vietti TJ, Nora AH, Donaldson MH, Stuckey WJ, Watkins WL, Lane DM: Daunomycin and prednisone for induction of remission in advanced leukemia. N Engl J Med 280:171, 1969.

164. Hoogstraten B, Sheehe PR, Cuttner J, Cooper T, Kyle RA, Oberfield RA, Townsend SR, Harley JB, Hayes D, Costa G, Holland JF: Melphalan in multiple myeloma. Blood 30:74, 1967.

165. Howard JP, Albo V, Newton WA: Cytosine arabinoside. Results of a cooperative study in acute childhood leukemia. Cancer 21:341, 1968.

166. Huguley CM: Long-term study of chronic lymphocytic leukemia: interim report after 45 months. Cancer Chemotherapy Rep 16:241, 1962.

167. Hyman CB, Borda E, Brubaker C, Hammond D, Sturgeon P: Prednisone in childhood leukemia. Comparison of interrupted with continuous therapy. Pediatrics 24:1005, 1959.

168. _____, _____, Digumarthi G: What are normal blood values for leukemia in remission? Blood 14:369, 1959.

169. _____, Brubaker C, Sturgeon P: 6-mercaptopurine in childhood leukemia; comparison of large dose interrupted with small dose continuous therapy. Cancer Res 17:851, 1957.

170. Innes J, Rider WD: Multiple myelomatosis treated with a combination of urethane and an oral nitrogen mustard. Blood 10:252, 1955.

171. Jacquillat CL, Weil M, Boiron M: Effects de la méthode de réinduction au cours de traitement des leucémies aigués lympho-

blastiques. Nouv Rev Fr Hématol 7:677, 1967.

172. Jameson B, Gamble DR, Lynch J, Kay HEM: Five-year analysis of protective isolation. Lancet 1:1034, 1971.

173. Johnson RE: Modern approaches to the radiotherapy of lymphoma. Sem Hematol 6:357, 1969.

174. _____: Total body irradiation of chronic lymphocytic leukemia. Cancer 25:523, 1970.

175. Judson G, Jones A, Kellogg R, Buckner D, Eisel R, Perry S, Greenough W: Closed continuous-flow centrifuge. Nature 217:816, 1968.

176. Juel-Jensen BE: Symposium on the Chemotherapy of Malignancy. London, Royal Society of Medicine, 1970.

177. Kaplan HS, Smithers DW: Autoimmunity in man and homologous disease in mice in relation to the malignant lymphomas. Lancet 2:1, 1959.

178. Karon M: Preliminary report on vincristine (Oncovin) from Acute Leukemia Group B. Proc Am Assoc Cancer Res 4:33, 1963.

179. _____, et al: The role of vincristine in the treatment of childhood acute leukemia. Clin Pharmacol Ther 7:332, 1966.

180. Kaung DT, Whittington RM, Patno ME, Veterans' Administration Cancer Chemotherapy Study Group: Chemotherapy of chronic lymphocytic leukemia. Arch Intern Med 114:521, 1964.

181. Kay HEM, Knapton PJ, O'Sullivan JP, Wells DG, Harris RF, Innes EM, Stuart J, Schwartz FCM, Thompson EN: Severe neurological damage associated with methotrexate therapy. Lancet 2:542, 1971.

182. Kennedy BJ: Androgenic hormone therapy in lymphatic leukemia. JAMA 190:1130, 1964.

183. _____, Yarbro JW: Metabolic and therapeutic effects of hydroxyurea in chronic myeloid leukemia. JAMA 195:1038, 1966.

184. Khamsi F, Carstairs KC, Scott JG: Smouldering acute leukemia: A review of 21 cases. Abstract of the XIII International Congress of Hematology. Munich, Lehmann 1970, p 192.

185. Kieffer SA, Stadlan EM, D'Angio GJ: Anatomic studies of the distribution and effects of intrathecal radioactive gold. Acta Radiol 8:27, 1969.

186. Klastersky J, Cappel R, Debusscher L, Daneau D, Swings G: Use of carbenicillin and polymyxin B for therapy of gram-negative bacilli infections. Chemotherapy 16:269, 1971.

187. Krakoff IH: Use of allopurinol in preventing hyperuricemia in leukemia and lymphoma. Cancer 19:1489, 1966.

188. Krivit W, Brubaker C, Thatcher LG, Pierce M, Perrin E, Hartmann JR: Maintenance therapy in acute leukemia of childhood. Comparison of cyclic vs. sequential methods. Cancer 21:352, 1968.

189. _____, Gilchrist G, Beatty EC: The need for continued therapy after prolonged remission in acute leukemia of childhood. J Pediatr 76:138, 1970.

190. Kyle RA, Schwartz RS, Oliner HL, Dameshek W: A syndrome resembling adrenal cortical insufficiency associated with long-term busulfan (Myleran) therapy. Blood 18:497, 1961.

191. Lampkin BC, Nagao T, Mauer AM: Synchronization of the mitotic cycle in acute leukaemia. Nature 222:1274, 1969.

192. Laszlo J, Buckley CE, Amos DB: Infusion of isologous immune plasma in chronic lymphocytic leukemia. Blood 31:104, 1968.

193. Leading Article: Emergency treatment of hypercalcaemia. Lancet 2:501, 1967.

194. _____: Septic thrombophlebitis and venous cannulas. Lancet 2:406, 1970.

195. _____: Osteoporosis and fluoride therapy. Br Med J 3:660, 1970.

196. _____: Leukaemia and cytotoxic drugs. Lancet 1:70, 1971.

197. _____: Hyperviscosity syndrome. Br Med J 2:184, 1971.

198. _____: Leukaemia on myeloma. Br Med J 1:568, 1971.

199. Leidler F, Russell WO: The brain in leukemia. Arch Pathol 40:14, 1945.

200. Levi JA, Vincent PC, Gunz FW: Combination chemotherapy of adult acute nonlymphoblastic leukemia. Ann Intern Med 76:397, 1972.

201. Levine AS, Graw RG, Young RC: Management of infections in patients with leukemia and lymphoma: current concepts and experimental approaches. Sem Hematol 9:141, 1972.

202. _____: Siegel SE, Schreiber AD, Hauser J, Preisler H, Goldstein IM, Seidler F, Simon R, Perry S, Bennett JE, Henderson ES: Protected environments and prophylactic antibiotics. A prospective controlled study of their utility in the therapy of acute leukemia. N Engl J Med 288:477, 1973.

203. Lissauer: Zwei Fälle von Leucaemie. Berl Klin Wochenschr 2:403, 1865.

204. Louis J, Best WR, Limarzi LR: Effect of myleran on the blood and bone marrow in chronic granulocytic leukemia. Proc Inst Med 21:21, 1956.

205. McCredie KB, Freireich EJ: Increased granulocyte collection from normal donors with increased granulocyte recovery following transfusion. Proc Am Assoc Cancer Res 12:58, 1971.

206. McElwain TJ, Hardisty RM: Remission induction with cytosine arabinoside and L-asparaginase in acute lymphoblastic leukaemia. Br Med J 4:596, 1969.

207. McKelvey EM, Kwaan HC: Cytosine arabinoside therapy for disseminated herpes zoster in a patient with IgG pyroglobulinemia. Blood 34:706, 1969.

208. McPhedran P, Heath CW: Acute leukemia occurring during chronic lymphocytic leukemia. Blood 35:7, 1970.

209. Magnusson S, Moloney WC: Multiple myeloma. Disease-a-Month 1960, p 1.

210. Malchow H, Havemann K, Kuni H, Schmidt M: Clinical and experimental studies concerning the effect of antihuman-lymphocyte-globulin (AHLG) on chronic lymphocytic leukemia (CLL), in Proceedings of XIII Congress of the International Society of Hematology, Munich, Lehmann, 1970, p 277.

211. Martinez-Maldonado M, Yium J, Suki WN, Eknoyan G: Renal function in myeloma. J Chron Dis 24:221, 1971.

212. Mastrangelo R, Zuelzer WW, Ecklund PS, Thompson RI: Chromosomes in the spinal fluid: evidence for metastatic origin of meningeal leukemia. Blood 35:227, 1970.

213. Mathé G (ed.): Advances in the Treatment of Acute (Blastic) Leukaemias. London, Heinemann, 1970.

214. _____: Immunological approaches to the treatment of acute leukaemia. Clin Haematol 1:165, 1972.

215. _____, Amiel JL, Schwarzenberg L, Schneider M, Cattan A, Schlumberger JR, Hayat M, de Vassal F: Active immunotherapy for acute lymphoblastic leukaemia. Lancet 1:697, 1969.

216. _____, Schwarzenberg L, Mery AM, Cattan A, Schneider M, Amiel JL, Schlumberger JR, Poisson J, Wajcner G: Extensive histological and cytological survey of patients with acute leukaemia in "complete remission." Br Med J 1:640, 1966.

217. _____, _____, Schneider M, Cattan A, Schlumberger JR, Hayat M, de Vassal F: Active immunotherapy for acute lympho-

blastic leukaemia, in Proceedings of the XIII Congress of International Society of Hematology. Munich, Lehmann, 1970, p 278.

218. Mayo WJ: Mortality and end results of splenectomy. Am J Med Sci 171:313, 1926.

219. _____: Review of 500 splenectomies with special reference to mortality and end results. Ann Surg 88:409, 1928.

220. Medical Research Council: Treatment of acute leukaemia in adults: comparison of steroid therapy at high and low dosage in conjunction with 6-mercaptopurine. Br Med J 1:7, 1963.

221. _____: Treatment of acute leukaemia in adults: comparison of steroid and mercaptopurine therapy alone and in conjunction. Br Med J 1:1383, 1966.

222. _____: Chronic granulocytic leukaemia: comparison of radiotherapy and busulphan therapy. Brit Med J 1:201, 1968.

223. _____: Duration of survival of children with acute leukaemia. Report to the Medical Research Council from the Committee on Leukaemia and the Working Party of Leukaemia in Childhood. Br Med J 4:7, 1971.

224. _____: Treatment of acute lymphoblastic leukaemia. Comparison of immunotherapy (B.C.G.), intermittent methotrexate, and no therapy after a five-month intensive cytotoxic regimen (Concord Trial). Br Med J 3:189, 1971.

225. _____: Myelomatosis: comparison of melphalan and cyclophosphamide therapy. Br Med J 1:640, 1971.

226. _____: Treatment of acute lymphoblastic leukaemia: effect of "prophylactic" therapy against central nervous system leukaemia. Br Med J 2:381, 1973.

227. _____: Report on the first myelomatosis trial. 1. Analysis of presenting features of prognostic importance. Br J Haematol 24:123, 1973.

228. Meeker WR, de Perio JM, Grace JT, Stutzman L, Mittelman A: The role of splenectomy in malignant lymphoma and leukemia. Surg Clin N Am 47:1163, 1967.

229. Melhorn DK, Gross S, Fisher BJ, Newman AJ: Studies on the use of "prophylactic" intrathecal amethopterin in childhood leukemia. Blood 36:55, 1970.

230. Merigan TC, Hayes RE: Treatment of hypercalcemia in multiple myeloma. Report of two patients. Arch Intern Med 107:389, 1961.

231. Metcalf D: The nature of leukaemia: neo-

plasm or disorder of haemopoietic regulation? Med J Aust 2:739, 1971.

232. Meyers MC: Treatment of acute leukemia in adolescents and adults, in Zarafonetis CJD (ed): Proceedings of the International Conference on Leukemia-Lymphoma. Philadelphia, Lea & Febiger, 1968, p 463.

233. Miller DG: Herpes zoster and malignant lymphomas. Proc Am Assoc Cancer Res 13:21, 1972.

234. ———, Budinger JM, Karnofsky DA: A clinical and pathological study of resistance to infection in chronic lymphatic leukemia. Cancer 15:307, 1962.

235. Minot JB, Buckman TE, Isaacs R: Chronic myelogenous leukemia. Age incidence, duration and benefit derived from irradiation. J Am Med Assoc 82:1489, 1924.

236. Mittelman A, Elias EG, Wieckowska W, Jones R, Stutzman L, Grace JT: Splenectomy in patients with malignant lymphoma or chronic leukemia. Cancer Bull 22:10, 1970.

237. ———, Stutzman L, Grace JT: Splenectomy in malignant lymphoma and leukemia. Geriatrics 23:142, 1968.

238. Mitus A, Enders JF, Craig JM, Holloway A: Persistence of measles virus and depression of antibody formation in patients with giant-cell pneumonia after measles. N Engl J Med 261:882, 1959.

239. Monfardini S, Gee T, Fried J, Clarkson B: Survival in chronic myelogenous leukemia: influence of treatment and extent of disease at diagnosis. Cancer 31:492, 1973.

240. Moore EW, Thomas LB, Shaw RK, Freireich EJ: The central nervous system in acute leukemia. Arch Intern Med 105:141, 1960.

241. Mott MG, Stevenson P, Wood CBS: Methotrexate meningitis. Lancet 2:656, 1972.

242. Murphy ML: Leukemia and lymphomas in children. Pediat Clin North Am 6:611, 1959.

243. Naiman JL, Rupprecht LM, Tanyeri G, Philippidis P: Intrathecal methotrexate. Lancet 1:571, 1970.

244. Nicholls WW: Experiences with chickenpox in patients with hematologic diseases receiving cortisone. Am J Dis Child 94:219, 1957.

245. Nies BA, Creger WP: Tolerance of chemotherapy following splenectomy for leukopenia or thrombocytopenia in patients with malignant lymphomas. Cancer, 20:558, 1967.

246. ———, Thomas LB, Freireich EJ: Meningeal leukemia, a follow-up study. Cancer 18:546, 1965.

247. Nightingale D, Prankerd TAJ, Richards JDM, Thompson D: Splenectomy in anaemia. Q J Med 41:261, 1972.

248. Nissen-Meyer R, Hast H: Comparison between hematologic side effects of cyclophosphamide and nitrogen mustard. Cancer Chemother Rep 9:51, 1960.

249. Oettgen HF, Old LJ, Boyse EA, Campbell HA, Philips FS, Clarkson BD, Tallal L, Leeper RD, Schwartz MK, Kim JH: Inhibition of leukemias in man by L-asparaginase. Cancer Res 27:2619, 1967.

250. Oliner H, Schwartz R, Rubio F, Dameshek W: Interstitial pulmonary fibrosis following busulfan therapy. Am J Med 31:134, 1961.

251. Ommaya AK: Subcutaneous reservoir and pump for sterile access to ventricular cerebrospinal fluid. Lancet 2:983, 1963.

252. Osgood EE: The results of a 15-year program of treatment of chronic leukemias with titrated, regularly spaced total-body irradiation with P^{32} or x-ray, in: Proceedings of the Sixth Congress of the International Society of Hematology. New York, Grune & Stratton, 1958.

253. ———: Treatment of chronic leukemias. J Nucl Med 5:139, 1964.

255. Paolino W, Resegotti L, Rossi M, Infelise V: Treatment of acute myeloid leukaemia according to the Hammersmith protocol: Preliminary report. Br Med J 3:567, 1973.

254. Pavlovsky S, Penalver J, Eppinger-Helft M, Muriel FS, Bergna Suarez A, Vilaseca G, Pavlovsky AA, Pavlovsky A: Induction and maintenance of remission in acute leukemia. Cancer 31:273, 1973.

255. Pawelski S, Topolska R, Rechowicz K, Krzyzanowska-Woziniakowska J: Treatment of 100 cases of chronic myeloid leukemia with busulfan. Pol Med Sci History Bull 11:101, 1968.

256. Pedersen B: Karyotype profiles in chronic myelogenous leukaemia. Influence of therapy on progression of disease. Acta Pathol Microbiol Scand 67:463, 1966.

257. Petranyi G, Bobory J: Treatment of chronic myeloid leukaemia with Myelobromol (1,6-dibromo-1,6-dideoxy-D-mannitol). Ther Hung 14:136, 1966.

258. Pfisterer H, Lani K, Koczorek KH, Lamerz R, Stich W: Antilymphocyte globulin in chronic lymphocytic leukemia, in Proceedings of the Eighth Congress of the International Society of Hematology Munich, Lehmann, 1970, p 227.

259. Pinkel D: Chickenpox and leukemia. J Pediat 58:729, 1961.

260. _____: Five-year follow-up of "total therapy" of childhood lymphocytic leukemia. JAMA 216:648, 1971.

261. _____, Hernandez K, Borella L, Holton C, Aur R, Samoy G, Pratt C: Drug dosage and remission duration in childhood lymphocytic leukemia. Cancer 27:247, 1971.

262. _____, Simone J, Hustu HO, Aur RJA: Nine years' experience with "total therapy" of childhood acute lymphocytic leukemia. Pediatrics 50:246, 1972.

263. Posner JB: Reservoirs for intraventricular chemotherapy. N Engl J Med 288:212, 1973.

264. Powles R, Smith C, Kohn J, Fairley GH: Method of removing abnormal protein rapidly from patients with malignant paraproteinaemias. Br Med J 3:664, 1971.

265. Preisler HD, Goldstein IM, Henderson ES: Gastrointestinal "sterilization" in the treatment of patients with acute leukemia. Cancer 26:1076, 1970.

266. Preston FE, Ward AM: Acute renal failure in myelomatosis from intravascular coagulation. Br Med J 1:604, 1972.

267. Price RA, Johnson WW: The central nervous system in childhood leukemia: I. The arachnoid. Cancer 31:520, 1973.

268. Pusey WA: Report of cases treated with roentgen rays. JAMA 38:911, 1902.

269. Ramaran CV, Israëls MCG: Treatment of chronic myeloid leukaemia with dibromannitol. Lancet 2:125, 1969.

270. Ratcheson RA, Ommaya AK: Experience with the subcutaneous cerebrospinal-fluid reservoir. Preliminary report of 60 cases. N Engl J Med 279:1025, 1968.

271. Rheingold JJ, Kaufman R, Adelson E, Lear A: Smoldering acute leukemia. N Engl J Med 268:812, 1963.

272. Rieselbach RE, DiChiro G, Freireich EJ, Rall DP: Subarachnoid distribution of drugs after lumbar injection. N Engl J Med 267:1273, 1962.

273. Ridings GR: Radiotherapy in the leukemias. Radiol Clin North Am 6:83, 1968.

274. _____, Morse EE, Rall DP, Frei E, Freireich EJ: Intrathecal aminopterin therapy of meningeal leukemia. Arch Intern Med 111:620, 1963.

275. Ritzmann SE, Baughan MA, Levin WC: The in vivo reduction of cold agglutinin by B6-SH. Clin Res 11:34, 1963.

276. _____, Coleman SL, Levin WC: The effect of some mercaptanes upon a macrocryogelglobulin; modifications induced by cysteamine, penicillamine and penicillin. J Clin Invest 39:1320, 1960.

277. Rodriguez V, Whitecar JP, Bodey GP: Therapy of infections with the combination of carbenicillin and gentamicin. Antimicrob Agents Chemother 9:386, 1970.

278. Rosner F, Lee SL, Kagen M, Morrison AN: Intrathecal methotrexate. Lancet 1:249, 1970.

279. Rundles RW, et al: Comparison of chlorambucil and Myleran in chronic lymphocytic and granulocytic leukemia. Am J Med 27:424, 1959.

280. _____, Dillon ML, Dillon ES: Multiple myeloma. III. Effect of urethane therapy on plasma cell growth, abnormal serum protein components and Bence Jones proteinuria. J Clin Invest 29:1243, 1950.

281. Salmon SE: Immunoglobulin synthesis and tumour cell number and the natural history of multiple myeloma. Br Med J 2:321, 1971.

282. _____: Immunoglobulin synthesis and tumor kinetics of multiple myeloma. Sem Hematol 10:135, 1973.

283. Sansone G: Pathomorphosis of acute infantile leukemia treated with modern therapeutic agents: "Meningoleukemia" and "Frolich's obesity." Ann Pediatr 183:33, 1954.

284. Saunders EF, Kauder E, Mauer AM: Sequential therapy of acute leukemia in childhood. J Pediatr 70:632, 1967.

285. Scamps RA, O'Neill BJ, Newland RC: A case of multiple myeloma terminating with acute myelomonocytic leukaemia. Med J Aust 2:1129, 1971.

286. Schimpff S, Satterlee W, Young VM, Serpick A: Empiric therapy with carbenicillin and gentamicin for febrile patients with cancer and granulocytopenia. N Engl J Med 284:1061, 1971.

287. _____, Young VM, Greene WH, Ermeulen GD, Moody MR, Wiernik PH: Origin of infection in acute non-lymphocytic leukemia. Ann Intern Med 77:707, 1972.

288. Schwartz R, Dameshek W: The treatment of autoimmune hemolytic anemia with 6-mercaptopurine and thioguanine. Blood 19:483, 1962.

289. Schwarzenberg L, Mathé G, de Grouchy J, de Nava C, de Vries MJ, Amiel JL, Cattan A, Schneider M, Schlumberger JR: White blood cell transfusions. Israel J Med Sci 1:925, 1965.

290. _____, _____, Pouillart P, Weiner R, Locour J, Genin J, Schneider M, de Vassal F,

Hayat M, Amiel JL, Schlumberger JR, Jasmin C, Rosenfeld C: Hydroxyurea, leucopheresis, and splenectomy in chronic myeloid leukaemia at the problastic phase. Br Med J 1:700, 1973.

291. Seeler RA, Hahn KO: Chronic granulocytic leukemia responding to melphalan. Cancer 27:284, 1971.

292. Selawry OS: New treatment schedule with improved survival in childhood leukemia: intermittent parenteral vs. daily oral methotrexate for maintenance of induced remission. JAMA 194:75, 1965.

293. Shapiro WR, Chernik NL, Posner JB: Necrotizing encephalopathy following intraventricular instillation of methotrexate. Arch Neurol 28:96, 1973.

294. Shaw RK, Boggs DR, Silberman HR, Frei E: A study of prednisone therapy in chronic lymphocytic leukemia. Blood 17:182, 1961.

295. _____, Swzed C, Boggs DR, Fahey JL, Frei E, Morrison E, Utz JP: Infection and immunity in chronic lymphocytic leukemia. Arch Intern Med 106:467, 1960.

296. Silver RT: The treatment of chronic lymphocytic leukemia. Sem Hematol 6:344, 1969.

297. Simone JV: Use of fresh blood components during intensive combination therapy of childhood leukemia. Cancer 28:562, 1971.

298. Skipper HE: Cellular kinetics associated with 'curability' of experimental leukemia, in Dameshek W, Dutcher RM (eds.): Perspectives in Leukemia. New York, Grune & Stratton, 1968.

299. _____, Schabel FM, Wilcox WS: Experimental evaluation of anti-cancer agents. XIII. On the criteria and kinetics associated with 'curability' of experimental leukemia. Cancer Chemother Rep 35:1, 1964.

300. Snapper I, Turner LB, Moscovitz HL: Multiple Myeloma. New York, Grune & Stratton, 1953.

301. Sokal JE, Aungst CW, Grace JT: Immunotherapy of myeloid leukemia. Ann Intern Med 76:878, 1972.

302. Southam CM, Craver LF, Dargeon W, Burchenal JH: A study of the natural history of acute leukemia. Cancer 4:39, 1951.

303. Southeastern Cancer Chemotherapy Cooperative Study Group: Comparison of 6-mercaptopurine and busulfan in chronic granulocytic leukemia. Blood 21:89, 1963.

304. Speed DE, Galton DAG, Swan A: Melphalan in the treatment of myelomatosis. Br Med J 1:1664, 1964.

305. Spevak J: The prophylaxis of meningeal leukemia with intrathecal methotrexate. J Iowa Med Soc 54:238, 1964.

306. Spiers ASD: Chemotherapy of acute leukaemia. Clin Haematol 1:127, 1972.

307. _____: Cure as the aim in therapy for the acute leukaemias. Lancet 2:473, 1972.

308. _____: A multiple drug regimen for refractory acute leukaemias. Br J Haematol 23:262, 1972.

309. _____: Surgery in management of patients with leukaemia. Br Med J 3:528, 1973.

310. _____: Unpublished results.

311. _____, Baikie AG: Cytogenetic evolution and clonal proliferation in acute transformation of chronic granulocytic leukaemia. Br J Cancer 22:192, 1968.

312. _____, Booth AE: Reservoirs for intraventricular chemotherapy. Lancet 1:1263, 1973.

313. _____, Clubb JS: Meningeal involvement in acute leukaemia of adults, with a report on a patient treated by methotrexate intrathecally administered. Med J Aust 1:930, 1966.

314. _____, Firth JL: Treating the nervous system in acute leukaemia. Lancet 1:433, 1972.

315. _____, Galton DAG: Improved semilogarithmic haematological chart. Br Med J 3:458, 1970.

316. _____, Tattersall MHN, Galton DAG: Splenectomy and leucopheresis in chronic granulocytic leukaemia. Br Med J 2:610, 1973.

317. _____, Trexler PC: The use of a plastic isolator for the prevention of infection in patients with acute leukaemia. J Physiol 231:66P., 1973.

318. Spurr CL, Wilson WL, McDonald JF: Myleran in the treatment of chronic myeloid leukemia: results of treatment. Southern Med J 49:847, 1956.

319. Stavraky KM, Watson TA, White DF, Miles EM: Chronic lymphocytic leukemia and subsequent cancer in the same patient. Cancer 26:410, 1970.

320. Strumia MM, Strumia PV, Bassert D: Splenectomy in leukemia: hematologic and clinical effects on 34 patients and review of 299 published cases. Cancer Res 26:519, 1966.

321. Stuart J, Bitensky L, Chayen J: Quantitative enzyme cytochemistry of leukemic cells. J Clin Pathol 22:563, 1969.

322. _____, Simpson JS, Mann JR: Intracellular hydrogen transport systems in

acute leukaemia. Br J Haematol 19:739, 1970.

323. Sullivan MP, Haggard ME, Donaldson MH, Krall J: Comparison of the prolongation of remission in meningeal leukemia with maintenance intrathecal methotrexate (IT MTX) and intravenous bis-nitrosourea (BCNU). Proc Am Assoc Cancer Res 11:77, 1970.

324. _____, Vietti TJ, Fernbach DJ, Griffiths KM, Haddy TB, Watkins WL: Clinical investigations in the treatment of meningeal leukemia: radiation therapy regimens vs. conventional intrathecal methotrexate. Blood 34:301, 1969.

325. _____, _____, Haggard ME, Donaldson MH, Krall JM, Gehan EA: Remission maintenance therapy for meningeal leukemia: intrathecal methotrexate vs. intravenous bis-nitrosourea. Blood 38:680, 1972.

326. Sultan C, Heilmann-Goualt M, Tulliez M: Relationship between blast-cell morphology and occurrence of a syndrome of disseminated intravascular coagulation. Br J Haematol 24:255, 1973.

327. Tattersall MHN, Battersby G, Spiers ASD: Antibiotics and hypokalaemia. Lancet 1:630, 1972.

328. _____, Harrap KR: Combination chemotherapy: the antagonism of methotrexate and cytosine arabinoside. Eur J Cancer 9:229, 1973.

329. _____, Hutchinson RM, Gaya H, Spiers ASD: Empirical antibiotic therapy in febrile patients with neutropenia and malignant disease. Eur J Cancer 9:417, 1973.

330. _____, Spiers ASD, Darrell JH: Initial therapy with combination of five antibiotics in febrile patients with leukaemia and neutropenia. Lancet 1:162, 1972.

331. Thompson I, Hall TC, Moloney WC: Combination therapy of adult acute myelogenous leukemia. N Engl J Med 273:1302, 1965.

332. Till MM, Hardisty RM, Pike MC: Long survivals in acute leukaemia. Lancet 1:534, 1973.

333. Tivey H: The prognosis for survival in chronic granulocytic and lymphocytic leukemia. Am J Roentgenol 72:68, 1954.

334. _____: The natural history of untreated acute leukemia. Ann NY Acad Sci 60:322, 1954.

335. Tsirimbas AD, Pfisterer H, Hornung B, Thierfelder S, Stich W: Studies with heterologous antihuman antilymphocyte serum (ALS) as a therapy for chronic lymphocytic leukemia, in Proceedings of the XII Congress of the International Society of Hematology. New York, International Society of Hematology, 1968, p 60.

336. Ultmann JE, Hyman GA, Gellhorn A: Chlorambucil in treatment of chronic lymphocytic leukemia and certain lymphomas. JAMA 162:178, 1956.

337. Unugur A, Schulman E, Dameshek W: Treatment of chronic granulocytic leukemia with myleran. N Engl J Med 256:727, 1957.

338. Vadlamudi S, Goldin A: Influence of mitotic cycle inhibitors on the antileukemic activity of cytosine arabinoside (NSC-63878) in mice bearing leukemia L1210. Cancer Chemother Rep 55:547, 1971.

339. Venditti JM: Treatment schedule dependency of experimentally active antileukemic (L1210) drugs. Cancer Chemother Rep Pt 3, 2:35, 1971.

340. Viza DC, Bernard-Degani O, Bernard C, Harris R: Leukaemia antigens. Lancet 2:493, 1969.

341. _____, Degani O, Dausset J, Davies DAL: Lymphocyte stimulation by soluble human HL-A transplantation antigens. Nature 219:704, 1968.

342. Vogler WR, Huguley CM, Rundles RW: Comparison of methotrexate with 6-mercaptopurine-prednisone in treatment of acute leukemia in adults. Cancer 20:1221, 1967.

343. Waldenström J: Melphalan therapy in myelomatosis. Br Med J 1:859, 1964.

344. Wall RL, Conrad FG: Cyclophosphamide therapy: its use in leukemias, lymphomas and solid tumors. Arch Intern Med 108:456, 1961.

345. Wang JJ, Pratt CB: Intrathecal arabinosyl cytosine in meningeal leukemia. Cancer 25:531, 1970.

346. Watson L: Diagnosis and treatment of hypercalcaemia. Br Med J 2:150, 1972.

347. West RJ, Graham-Pole J, Hardisty RM, Pike MC: Factors in pathogenesis of central-nervous-system leukaemia. Br Med J 3:311, 1972.

348. West WO: The treatment of bone marrow failure with massive androgen therapy. Ohio State Med J 61:347, 1965.

349. Wetherley-Mein G, Cottom D: Fresh blood transfusion in leukaemia. Br J Haematol 2:25, 1956.

350. Whang-Peng J, Canellos GP, Carbone PP, Tjio JH: Clinical implications of cytogenetic variants in chronic myelocytic leukemia (CML). Blood 32:755, 1968.

351. Wheelock EF, Dingle JH: Observations on

the repeated administration of viruses to a patient with acute leukemia. A preliminary report. N Engl J Med 271:645, 1964.

352. Whitecar JP, Bodey GP, Freireich EJ: Combination chemotherapy (COAP) of adult acute leukemia. Proc Am Assoc Cancer Res 11:83, 1970.

353. Wolcott GJ, Grunnet ML, Lahey ME: Spinal subdural hematoma in a leukemic child. J Pediatr 77:1060, 1970.

354. Wolff JA, Brubaker CA, Murphy ML, Pierce MI, Severo N: Prednisone therapy of acute childhood leukemia: prognosis and duration of response in 330 treated patients. J Pediatr 70:626, 1967.

355. Zubrod CG: Present and future prospects for chemotherapy of the leukemias, in Zarafonetis CJD (ed.): Proceedings of the International Conference on Leukemia-Lymphoma. Philadelphia, Lea & Febiger, 1968, p 475.

356. Zuelzer WW: Implications of long-term survival in acute stem cell leukemia of childhood treated with composite cyclic therapy. Blood 24:477, 1964.

357. _____: Therapy of acute leukemia in childhood, in Zarafonetis CJD (ed): Proceedings of the International Conference on Leukemia-Lymphoma. Philadelphia, Lea & Febiger, 1968, p 451.

358. Zumoff B, Hart H, Hellman L: Considerations of mortality in certain chronic diseases. Ann Intern Med 64:595, 1966.

V

Epilogue

19

The Prognosis of Leukemia

Prognosis is defined in the *Shorter Oxford English Dictionary* as "a forecast of the probable course of a case of disease; also the action or act of making such a forecast." Prognosis should take account of both the immediate and long-term outlooks and should include—but often does not—a measure of the quality of survival. In this chapter an attempt is made to provide this kind of information.

It must be said at once that this is a more than usually difficult task, since both the morbidity and length of survival of leukemia and of its types are extremely variable and, save within the widest limits, unpredictable. Although the ultimate prognosis for survival is almost uniformly bad, many graduations of "badness" must be distinguished. Thus, some patients with chronic leukemia, especially the lymphocytic form, may live a relatively normal life span and die eventually from an intercurrent disease rather than from the leukemia itself. Patients with the acute disease may die within a few days from diagnosis, live for some months with or without symptoms, or, in those rare instances which restore hope to even the most pessimistic physician, survive for years in good health after only minimal treatment. Because, in general, leukemia—like life itself—terminates fatally, the "action or act" of making a prognosis for ultimate survival is not difficult. On the other hand, the much more important questions of how long, and in what health, a given patient will live once a diagnosis of leukemia has been made, never admits of an easy answer. It is clear that the physician who discusses these matters with the patient (see Chapter 20) or his relatives must be aware of the many uncertainties, as well as of those signposts in the history, and physical and hematologic findings which may indicate favorable or unfavorable aspects of the case.

DIFFICULTIES IN PROGNOSIS

Anyone reading the voluminous literature on this subject must be struck by the many contradictions; these are by no means confined to the older publications. The reasons are manifold and often unknown, but where they can be identified, they are likely to arise from one or more of the causes which follow.

Uncertainties of diagnosis. These should no longer be of importance, but formerly confusion between leukemia, "leukemoid" states, marrow aplasia, infectious mononucleosis, lymphomas, myeloproliferative disorders and other hematologic abnormalities was rife, and this must have created havoc in leukemia statistics.

Difficulties of distinguishing between types of leukemia, especially between acute and chronic. Clearly, the prognosis in a series of acute leukemias, defined as lasting less than 3 months (Committee for Clarification of Nomenclature) will differ from that of others without restrictions as to duration and defined, perhaps, according to cellular type. Even today, problems of demarcation have not been entirely overcome. Only a very individualistic classification could, for instance, have led to the statistics reviewed by Clemmesen et al.[22] from which it appeared that "acute" leukemia responded better to irradiation than to "other" treatment.

Failure to divide material into possibly meaningful subgroups, particularly according to age. Prognosis differs greatly as between children and adults, so that statistics regarding them should never be lumped together. Acute lymphocytic leukemia, whether in children or in adults, has a better prognosis than acute granulocytic leukemia, particularly with respect to therapeutic response to chemotherapy. Acute lymphocytic leukemia in children has a better prognosis than the corresponding disease in adults.

Difficulties of estimating the date of onset of leukemia. Leukemia often starts insidiously, so that patients may have difficulties in recognizing symptoms for periods which may extend back for months or even some years.[13,96] Even where symptoms such as infection or hemorrhage suddenly usher in the disease, the possibility of a much longer subclinical history is strong. Patients vary greatly in their intelligence, the ease with which they recognize symptoms as abnormal, and their sensitivity to malaise or pain. In any series, therefore, the apparent length of survival may be weighted against the less observant or the more stoical patient, and this means inevitable bias. These difficulties can only be partly overcome by measuring survival not from apparent "onset" but from time of diagnosis or first treatment; for patients see or fail to see their doctors for many reasons.

Selection of patients. This can be conscious or unconscious. Authors may select cases for inclusion in any particular series in order to bring out certain points of interest, such as the influence on prognosis of symptoms like hemorrhage or skin lesions. Naturally, such figures cannot be extrapolated to other series. Others exclude patients for various reasons such as death from ostensibly unassociated conditions. This, we believe, is an inadmissible procedure since a definite interaction of many diseases has been shown to be a fundamental law affecting the duration of life.[64] Again, patients dying soon after admission to hospital or before the beginning of treatment or surviving unusually long, are often not considered suitable for inclusion in a series. Since both very short and relatively long survivals must be expected in ultimately fatal diseases, their exclusion is bound to falsify the overall statistics. Automatic and often unrecognized selection occurs particularly in series originating from centers to which patients are referred over long distances, for here the very acute cases often fail to reach the hospital. This factor probably accounts for the striking difference between the statistics of Mangalik et al.[77] on the one hand, and those of Gunz and Burns[47] on the other; in the former about 12 percent but in the latter no less than 43 percent of all patients died within one month of admission to hospital.

The only means of obtaining really valid survival statistics for any group of patients is to resist the temptation of excluding any patients at all, however good the reason for doing so may appear at the time.

METHODS OF EXPRESSING THE PROGNOSIS

This may be done in terms of days, weeks, months, or years, either from onset or from the date of diagnosis or first treatment. The difficulties of estimating the moment of onset have already been mentioned. In a disease such as leukemia *average* or *mean* survival, with or without the standard deviation, is not a good measure of the probable survival. This is so because the survival curve is not normal but skewed to the left; in other words, numerous patients die in the early part of the period covered, whereas a comparatively small minority live very much longer than the rest (Fig. 19-1). The average in such a collection is strongly influenced by the few long-term survivors and hence is liable to overestimate the chances of survival of the rest. A better measure of the prognosis is the *median* survival time, which is the length of time which the middle patient in a series survived. The median is shorter than the average in a left, or negatively skewed, distribution. By both dividing and multiplying it by six one obtains two figures which give the approximate range of survival for 95 percent of the given population.[112,113] A more exact measure of the 95 percent confidence limits can be obtained by converting survival times into their logarithms and charting them against numbers dying, when the skewed curve is converted into a normal one[12]; 95 percent of death will turn occur in the interval, log

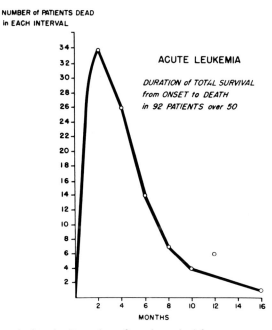

NUMBER of PATIENTS DEAD in EACH INTERVAL

ACUTE LEUKEMIA

DURATION of TOTAL SURVIVAL from ONSET to DEATH in 92 PATIENTS over 50

MONTHS

Fig. 19-1. Acute leukemia. Duration of total survival from onset to death in 92 patients over age 50.

mean plus and minus twice the standard deviation. A refinement of this method has been used by Feinleib and MacMahon.[36]

An additional difficulty in calculating median survivals in diseases like chronic leukemia is to account for those patients who are still alive at the time of review. Some authors attempt to overcome this difficulty by closing their series at a given date and counting any surviving patients among those officially "dead." The log-normal conversion method, with or without the Feinleib shortcut provides a reasonable approximation; another is the actuarial (life-table) method of Berkson and Gage,[3] as used by Green and Dixon[46] among others. Both methods give comparable results.

THE PROGNOSIS OF ACUTE LEUKEMIA

In order to assess the effect which any form of treatment may have on the course of leukemia, it is necessary to know how long the untreated patient may be expected to live. Such knowledge is relatively easily obtained in the case of acute leukemia which could not be effectively treated before 1948, when the folic acid antagonists were introduced, although symptomatic therapy was available somewhat earlier. *Untreated* series are thus those in which the form of treatment adopted, although possibly effective in relieving certain symptoms, was without any known "specific" effect on the leukemic process.

UNTREATED CASES

The untreated groups included in the following analysis were not given therapy with folic acid antagonists, antimetabolites, corticosteroids, or the more recent chemotherapeutic agents. Supportive therapy with blood transfusions or some of the earlier antibiotics was, however, frequently employed. Evidence that such treatment might by itself prolong life has not been confirmed,[9] and it will therefore be assumed that the prognosis does not differ materially in patients having various kinds of *nonspecific* supportive therapy from that of totally untreated ones.

Many large series are reported in which the survival times are either stated or can be calculated from the data provided.[16,18,25,49,84,91,92,95,98,103,105,108,118] Many of these, as well as others, were carefully analyzed by Tivey,[111] who assembled from the literature a total of 572 children and 179 adults with acute leukemia in whom the duration of the illness was reasonably well known. These patients were at first classified according to their type (lymphocytic, granulocytic, or monocytic), but no significant differences were found in the survival of the several types. The median survival in the children was 2.7 months and that in the adults 3.3 months, both from onset to death. The duration from diagnosis to death was 2.4 months in children and 1.7 months in adults, and that from onset to diagnosis was 1.2 months in children and 1.7 months in adults. The small differences between the various groups are probably not of significance, and even if they were, they would amount to only 2–3 weeks at the most.

These figures establish with reasonable certainty the life expectancy for the average patient with acute leukemia if no "specific" treatment is employed. They do not, however, give the full picture of the chances of survival. Besides the median survival figures, Tivey also estimated the range of survival of the middle two-thirds of all the patients with acute leukemia,[111] and these data are valuable in establishing the *limits* of probable survival for the majority of untreated patients. Two-thirds of children, according to them, will live between 1.0–6.9 months after the onset of their illness, and two-thirds of adults 1.0–9.8 months. It has already been pointed out that the chances for shorter survivals are greater than for more prolonged ones.

EFFECT OF TREATMENT

It is generally accepted that chemotherapy, usually combined with other measures such as transfusions and the administration of antibiotics, is capable of extending the survival of patients with acute leukemia, particularly in childhood. Figure 19-2 shows collective statistics which demonstrate a progressive improvement over successive quinquennia, compared with the baseline of untreated cases in 1940–1949. The improvement is far more pronounced in children than in adults, and is of doubtful significance at ages over 45. In children under 10 years, the median

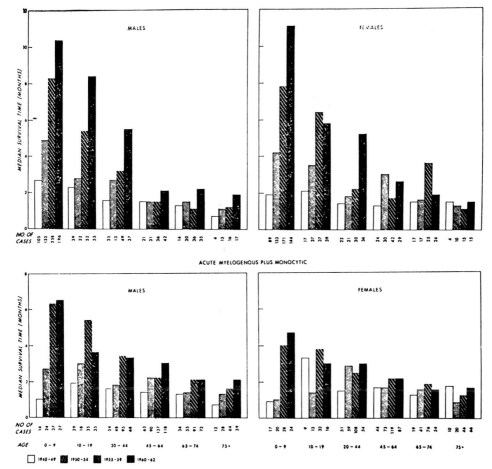

Fig. 19-2. Median survival time (months) for patients with leukemias classified as acute lymphocytic or acute (not otherwise specified), and those classified as acute myelogenous or monocytic, by age and year of diagnosis, 1940–1962. (Reproduced from Cutler, S. J., Axtell, L., and Heise, H.,[24] courtesy of the authors.)

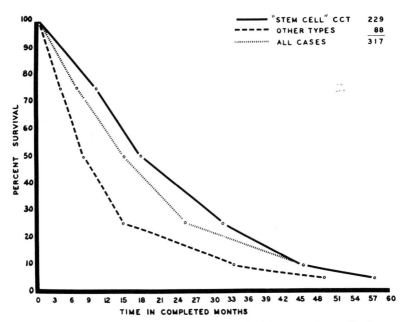

Fig. 19-3. Percentage survival for children treated with composite cyclic therapy 1955–1966. (Reproduced from Zuelzer, W. W.,[121] courtesy of the author and publishers.)

survival from diagnosis increased from about 2 to 10 months between 1940 and 1962, and more recently to 35 months.

Although distinctions between subtypes of acute leukemia are difficult (see Chapter 3), most of the published figures agree that there are appreciable differences in the response to treatment between patients with nongranular cell types ("lymphoblastic," "stem cell," "not otherwise specified," etc.) and those with predominantly myeloid or monocytoid cells ("myeloblastic," "myelomonocytic," "monocytic," etc.). Figure 19-3 shows a fivefold improvement (compared with Tivey's figures[112]) of the median survival in children with acute lymphocytic but only a threefold improvement in those with the granulocytic type. At later ages, the findings are equivocal. However, Mangalik et al.,[74] in a group of patients of all ages, found that in lymphoblastic leukemia the median survival from diagnosis increased from 3.6 months in 1947–1954[52] to 7.9 months in 1954–1957[53] and to 12.3 months in 1958–1964, while the corresponding figures for myeloblastic leukemia were 2.2, 3.4, and 5.1 months. The difference between types is also clearly seen in Fig. 19-3,[122] and it is thus apparent that both age and cell type influence the response to therapy in acute leukemia.

CHILDHOOD ACUTE LEUKEMIA

The gradual improvement in the survival of children with acute leukemia occurred *pari passu* with the introduction of new means of therapy. Thus, Farber[35] reported on 343 children treated with folic acid antagonists, ACTH, and cortisone with a median survival of 8 months; on 209 children treated additionally with 6-MP with a median survival of 11.4 months, and on a smaller number of children with improved total care and a median survival of 14.5 months. Similarly, Murphy found a

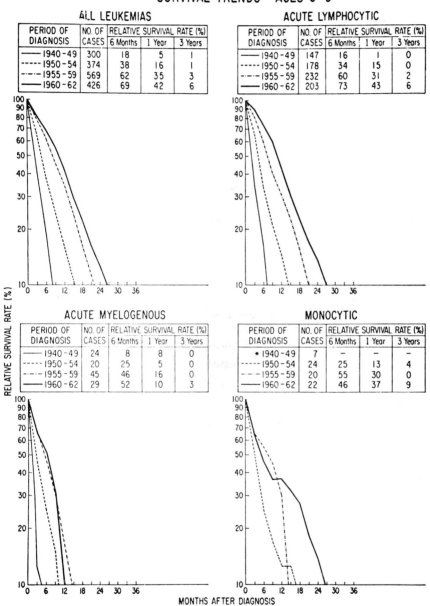

SURVIVAL TRENDS – AGES 0-9

ALL LEUKEMIAS

PERIOD OF DIAGNOSIS	NO. OF CASES	RELATIVE SURVIVAL RATE (%)		
		6 Months	1 Year	3 Years
——— 1940-49	300	18	5	1
------- 1950-54	374	38	16	1
—·—· 1955-59	569	62	35	3
——— 1960-62	426	69	42	6

ACUTE LYMPHOCYTIC

PERIOD OF DIAGNOSIS	NO. OF CASES	RELATIVE SURVIVAL RATE (%)		
		6 Months	1 Year	3 Years
——— 1940-49	147	16	1	0
------- 1950-54	178	34	15	0
—·—· 1955-59	232	60	31	2
——— 1960-62	203	73	43	6

ACUTE MYELOGENOUS

PERIOD OF DIAGNOSIS	NO. OF CASES	RELATIVE SURVIVAL RATE (%)		
		6 Months	1 Year	3 Years
——— 1940-49	24	8	8	0
------- 1950-54	20	25	5	0
—·—· 1955-59	45	46	16	0
——— 1960-62	29	52	10	3

MONOCYTIC

PERIOD OF DIAGNOSIS	NO. OF CASES	RELATIVE SURVIVAL RATE (%)		
		6 Months	1 Year	3 Years
* 1940-49	7	–	–	–
------- 1950-54	24	25	13	4
—·—· 1955-59	20	55	30	0
——— 1960-62	22	46	37	9

RELATIVE SURVIVAL RATE (%)

MONTHS AFTER DIAGNOSIS

Fig. 19-4. Survival trends for all leukemias and acute leukemia by morphologic type for ages 0-9, 1940–1962. Rates not shown for 10 cases or less. (Reproduced from Cutler, S. J., Axtell, L., and Heise, H.,[24] courtesy of the authors.)

median survival of 9.2 months in children treated with folic acid antagonists and steroids, which increased to 12.5 months when 6-MP was added,[85] and Oehme's figure for a corresponding group was 13 months.[87] Zuelzer, in a large group of children with stem cell leukemia treated with a composite cyclic or sequential therapy (steroids, folic acid antagonists, 6-MP) found a median survival of 14.2 months;[122] while Krivit et al., with the addition of vincristine to a similar regimen, obtained a median of nearly 18 months[65], and Colebatch et al., of 22–25 months.[23] These results came from leading clinics specializing in the treatment of acute childhood leukemia and probably represented the optima obtainable with the means at hand. However, elsewhere, too, corresponding improvements were taking place, as can be seen in Fig. 19-4 which was compiled from the collective results of 98 American hospitals. This shows that between 1940–1962 the 6-month survival in acute lymphocytic leukemia of children increased from 16–73 percent, the 1-year survival from 1–43 percent, and the 3-year survival from 0–6 percent, with lesser improvements in the prognosis of acute granulocytic leukemia. While much of the credit for the improved survival times must go to the new therapeutic modalities, better use of established agents, together with all those accessory means of treatment summed up as "total care" undoubtedly played their part.[23,87] It should be noted that the prognosis of children under 10 (except for those less than 1 year old) is better than that of older children or of adults with acute lymphocytic leukemia.[120]

The initial advances in the therapy of childhood leukemia were made possible by the relative ease with which remissions could be induced. With modern therapy, remissions are obtainable in 85–98 percent of cases of acute lymphocytic leukemia in children, and further improvements in the prognosis must therefore be expected, not so much from further increases in the rate of remissions as from a prolongation of their duration.

ADULT ACUTE LEUKEMIA

Whereas the prognosis of symptomatically treated acute leukemia is practically identical in children and adults (see above), treatment has much less effect in prolonging survival in the latter group. This is largely, but not solely, the result of the predominance, in adults, of the acute granulocytic type with its relatively poor remission rate. Age alone also plays a part, but the statistics are not good enough to separate the effects of the two adverse factors. Clearly, however, remissions in older adults become progressively rarer, and little save symptomatic relief can be offered to older people with acute leukemia.

In adults, as in children, the attainment of a remission is of paramount importance in the extension of life. Patients without remissions had a median survival of 4–6 months at one hospital, but if, at least, one complete remission occurred, the median became 11–13.5 months.[31,32] Corresponding figures given by Mangalik et al. for acute granulocytic leukemia were 3.0 months without and 9.5 with remissions,[74] by Wiernik and Serpick 2.8 and 11.5 months,[116] and by Levi et al. 5 and 34 weeks,[71] respectively. Gunz and Burns noted that only 6 percent of their adult patients who obtained remissions died in less than 6 months from diagnosis, while 92 percent of those failing to remit did so.[47]

However, longevity in adult acute leukemia does not depend solely on the achievement of remissions. In the first place, remissions, especially with the more recent agents such as daunorubicin, or cytosine arabinoside are often of very short duration. Second, there are a number of patients, nearly all in late-middle or old age, whose disease has a naturally slow and indolent course. This variety has been aptly described as smoldering acute leukemia[100]; examples are found in most sizeable series.[27,34,37] Such patients may live for months or years in relatively good health with nothing but symptomatic therapy, and attempts at strenuous chemotherapy may greatly worsen their condition. Statistics have shown[31,34,37] that, provided old patients survive the early part of their illness, their mean or median survival is no worse and may be better than that of much younger groups, even though they do not obtain remissions. Their disease, in a proportion of cases, appears to be biologically distinctive and comparatively benign.

LONG-TERM SURVIVAL

It has already been mentioned that the survival curve in leukemia shows a large number of early deaths but also a few patients living much longer than the rest. The median survival, though affording a satisfactory statistical parameter, does not therefore tell the full story of a patient's chances of survival. As early as 1957, Farber noted a 10 percent survival of 29.8 months in his childhood series,[35] while 10 percent of Oehme's patients lived 22 months.[87] Of Zuelzer's patients, 12.5 percent were alive 3 years or more after diagnosis,[122] and even in the combined statistics reported on by Cutler et al., 6 percent of patients under 10 had a 3-year survival rate.[24] More recently, Krivit et al. reported 16 and 27 percent of two childhood groups living 39 or more months from diagnosis,[65] while some 35 percent of Colebatch's children were alive at 30 months[23]—over 3 times the proportion found by Farber 10 years earlier.[35] More strikingly still, Jean Bernard's group has reported a 20 percent 5-year survival rate in acute lymphocytic leukemia,[60] and Pinkel a 17 percent 5-year survival rate free of leukemia.[93] Clearly, the tail of the survival curve in childhood leukemia has been lengthening, in step with the improvement of the median. A similar favorable development remains to be demonstrated in adult acute leukemia.

From very early days, instances of "cured" leukemia were also reported.[45] Although none of these are now regarded as acceptable, a considerable number of long-term survivors have been noted in the literature since the introduction of effective chemotherapy for acute leukemia in 1948. In this group are patients living 5 years or more after diagnosis, both children and adults, many of them in complete remission over periods of years. Among such reports were those by Dameshek and Mitus,[26] Fairbanks et al.,[34] Tallal,[109] Keidan,[62] Frenkel and Meyers,[38] Roath,[102] Gasser,[41] Giraud et al.,[44] and Hill et al.[56] The field was reviewed by Bernard et al.[5,6] A register of long-term survivors has been kept for some years at the Memorial Hospital, New York City, and reported on from time to time by Burchenal.[19,20] Statistics on the incidence of long-term survival are as yet unobtainable, but Burchenal estimates that a 5-year survival may occur in well under 1 percent of all cases of acute leukemia.[20]

Although long-term survivors with acute leukemia are exceedingly rare, they are of very great theoretical interest, for such patients raise the question if acute leukemia is potentially curable. Certainly, survivals of 8 years and more in good health make the distinction between long-term remission and cure seem a fine one, although very occasional relapses have been seen, even after many years of unbroken health. Careful studies have as yet produced no reasons to show why these particular individuals should have done so much better than the great majority of leukemia patients, and it is not known whether this group is merely the extreme tail of the survivors in the mortality curve, or whether it is in some respect fundamentally different.

PROGNOSIS IN INDIVIDUAL CASES

We have so far discussed the survival in groups of patients with acute leukemia. Figures obtained from statistical investigations are of some help to the physician in predicting in general terms how long the *average* patient may be expected to live; however, this is clearly of scant use in individual cases, for the range of possibilities is exceedingly wide. Thus, the doctor who tells an anxious relative that the patient in question has a 50 percent chance of living for 17 months, provided he survives the next 4 weeks, may be admired for his honesty or erudition, but hardly for his clinical acumen. The problem of supplying an exact prognosis in a given case is usually insoluble, but there are occasional signposts which may provide hints as to the immediate or more distant outlook, and may suggest, in particular, whether the case falls into the relatively favorable or unfavorable group.

As has already been stressed, age and cellular type are the most important guides, at least to the immediate prognosis. A child with acute lymphocytic leukemia has a 9:1 chance of obtaining a complete remission the first time treatment is given. If the cell type is granulocytic, the chance is reduced to about 50 percent. If the child is very young, however, the outlook is relatively poor, for infants with acute leukemia rarely live long, whatever the treatment.[95,120] In adults, worthwhile remissions occur in not more than 50 percent, except in the rarer lymphocytic or stem cell cases. The older the adult, the less the chances; but old people may do well, even without remissions. In adults, a slow onset of symptoms is often associated with a relatively long survival.[48]

Among laboratory findings, the height of the initial leukocyte count is negatively correlated with the chances for survival. In both children and adults, survival is much better when the initial leukocyte count is below 20,000 per cubic millimeter than above it.[4,28,58,103,108,122] Very high counts above 100,000 per cubic millimeter in adults carry a risk of death within a few days, usually from cerebral hemorrhage.[14,37,40,47,101]

The platelet count is of some prognostic significance, with initial counts in the normal range foreshadowing a relatively prolonged survival.[4,47] The relationship of the initial hemoglobin level to survival is more complex and less clear-cut. A possibly significant relationship has recently been reported between length of survival in childhood lymphocytic leukemia and the degree of PAS-positivity of the lymphoblasts[66]: weak PAS-positivity was correlated with short-term first remissions and survival. If confirmed, this would indicate a valuable new prognostic criterion. Similarly, Mathé and his colleagues have subdivided acute lymphocytic leukemia according to morphologic criteria and found differences in response to therapy and prognosis in the newly defined subtypes.[75] In patients with acute lymphocytic leukemia achieving complete remission, a lymphocytosis in the bone marrow appears to be associated with relatively long-term remission.[107]

THE PROGNOSIS OF CHRONIC LEUKEMIA

UNTREATED PATIENTS

For over a century it has been possible to obtain remissions in cases of chronic leukemia by means of chemotherapy,[72] and since 1902 x-irradiation has been known to exert a beneficial influence.[97,104] Taking into consideration the prolonged natural course of the disease, it is not surprising that a series of truly "untreated" patients does not exist. Admittedly, some patients with chronic leukemia are never treated; these are either individuals with extremely mild symptoms or those who were diagnosed only shortly before their death. The longer a patient survives, the greater the chance becomes that he will be treated, and, in the words of Hardin Jones,[11] the untreated series compete for cases with the treated series.[61] If any truly untreated series of chronic leukemia patients existed, it would therefore be highly selected and unsuitable for comparison with a treated series.

EFFECT OF TREATMENT

Nearly 50 years ago, Minot and his colleagues stated that neither chronic granulocytic nor chronic lymphocytic leukemia was so altered in its course by means of treatment then available that an actual extension of life could be achieved.[80,81] Since even then the majority of the untreated patients had actually received some form of therapy, Minot's conclusion can no longer be regarded as statistically tenable. It would be correct to say that his patients, as well as the controls, had had *minimal* treatment and that the results did not differ significantly regarding survival, although Minot's therapy did succeed in producing prolonged symptomatic relief.

Results similar to those of Minot appeared in numerous publications during the next 30 years, the principal therapeutic agents being various forms of ionizing radiations.[1,7,39,50,57,64,67–70,73,79,89,90,99,106,115] These and other publications were analyzed by Tivey, who calculated medians and confidence limits.[113] Among a total of 1090 patients with chronic granulocytic leukemia, he found a median survival from onset to death of 2.70 years, with a range of 2.58–2.83 years. Among 685 patients with chronic lymphocytic leukemia, the median survival was 2.77 years, with a range of 2.59–2.95 years. The figures for the two varieties of leukemia did not differ significantly, which was surprising in view of the widespread clinical impression that chronic lymphocytic leukemia tends to be a milder disease than chronic granulocytic leukemia, and that more patients with the former live longer, and sometimes very much longer. Since there are several more or less clear-cut clinical types of chronic lymphocytic leukemia with varying severities[94] (see Chapter 10), Tivey's finding of a regular overall survival curve in this disease[113] may be a coincidence rather than an accurate description of the prognosis for all cases. Several authors were unable to fit a smooth line (Fig. 19-5) when charting the survival of their patients with chronic lymphocytic leukemia[48,99]; this probably indicates heterogeneity of the material, and it seems doubtful if all cases can justifiably be grouped together for statistical purposes. It should be added that, since Tivey's figures were from onset to death,[113] the actual times which patients spent under medical observation would, in general, be much shorter. In fact, the median survival from the beginning of treatment to death was only 1.6 years for all chronic leukemias.

Even shorter median survivals were found by Feinleib and MacMahon,[36] who

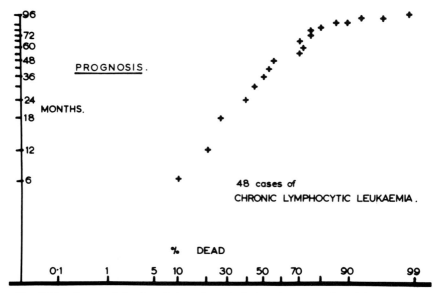

Fig. 19-5. Prognosis in chronic lymphocytic leukemia. (Reproduced from Gunz, F. W., Campbell, A. J., and Goldstein, A. M.,[48] with permission.)

collected and analyzed records of 649 white patients who had leukemia in Brooklyn during the period 1943–1952. No account was taken of treatment received. The medians from diagnosis were as follows: chronic granulocytic leukemia—males, 9.91 months; females, 11.89 months; chronic lymphocytic leukemia—males, 11.20 months; females 13.22 months; overall (both types), 11.65 months. These figures are significantly shorter than those of Tivey, and the only suggested reason for the discrepancy is dissimilarity of the material and of its selection for inclusion in the respective series.

The statistics analyzed by Tivey[113] and by Feinleib and MacMahon[36] came from a wide variety of centers, and the latest year included was 1952. Considerably better results have been published since then from individual centers, especially for chronic lymphocytic leukemia. Some of them are shown in Table 19-1.

It is unlikely that this improvement was purely the result of case selection. The more likely reason is the quality of the therapy given in units specializing in the treatment of leukemia. Although the extension of life is modest, compared with the

Table 19-1
5-Year Survival Rates for Chronic Leukemia from Diagnosis
or First Treatment

Author and Reference	5-Year Survival (%)	
	CGL	CLL
Musshoff et al.[86]	17.7	
Clark and Macdonald[21]	6.5 ± 2.6	17.9 ± 3.6
Feinleib and MacMahon[36]	5 (M) 9 (F)	8 (M) 13 (F)
Gunz et al.[48]	12.5	20.8
Green and Dixon[46]		32.8
Gerhartz[43]	10	

older figures, it nevertheless appears significant, and there seems no longer any cause for denying the efficacy of therapy in prolonging the duration of life.

Figures 19-6 and 19-7 show changes in survival in chronic leukemia according to age and period covered. These figures come from the collective statistics of 98 American and Canadian hospitals. Although details differ in the various groups, there is, in general, an improvement in survival over successive periods. This would

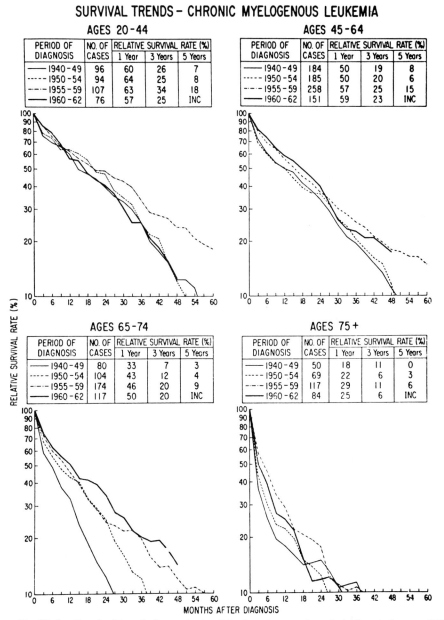

SURVIVAL TRENDS – CHRONIC MYELOGENOUS LEUKEMIA

AGES 20-44

PERIOD OF DIAGNOSIS	NO. OF CASES	RELATIVE SURVIVAL RATE (%) 1 Year	3 Years	5 Years
—— 1940-49	96	60	26	7
----- 1950-54	94	64	25	8
—··— 1955-59	107	63	34	18
—— 1960-62	76	57	25	INC

AGES 45-64

PERIOD OF DIAGNOSIS	NO. OF CASES	RELATIVE SURVIVAL RATE (%) 1 Year	3 Years	5 Years
—— 1940-49	184	50	19	8
----- 1950-54	185	50	20	6
—··— 1955-59	258	57	25	15
—— 1960-62	151	59	23	INC

AGES 65-74

PERIOD OF DIAGNOSIS	NO. OF CASES	RELATIVE SURVIVAL RATE (%) 1 Year	3 Years	5 Years
—— 1940-49	80	33	7	3
----- 1950-54	104	43	12	4
—··— 1955-59	174	46	20	9
—— 1960-62	117	50	20	INC

AGES 75+

PERIOD OF DIAGNOSIS	NO. OF CASES	RELATIVE SURVIVAL RATE (%) 1 Year	3 Years	5 Years
—— 1940-49	50	18	11	0
----- 1950-54	69	22	6	3
—··— 1955-59	117	29	11	6
—— 1960-62	84	25	6	INC

RELATIVE SURVIVAL RATE (%)

MONTHS AFTER DIAGNOSIS

Fig. 19-6. Survival trends for patients with chronic granulocytic leukemia by age, 1940–1962. (Reproduced from Cutler, S. J., Axtell, L., and Heise, H.,[24] courtesy of the authors.)

strongly suggest the effects of improved therapy. During the period under survey, chemotherapy was introduced for the treatment of chronic leukemia and replaced the use of radiotherapy in many centers. Therefore, it could be that the improvement shown in Figures 19-6 and 19-7 was at least partly due to this change, although adequately controlled trials of the comparative effects of the two modalities are not available. It is disturbing moreover, that in several of the groups the favorable trend has lately been reversed. Although this may well be a temporary check, it is

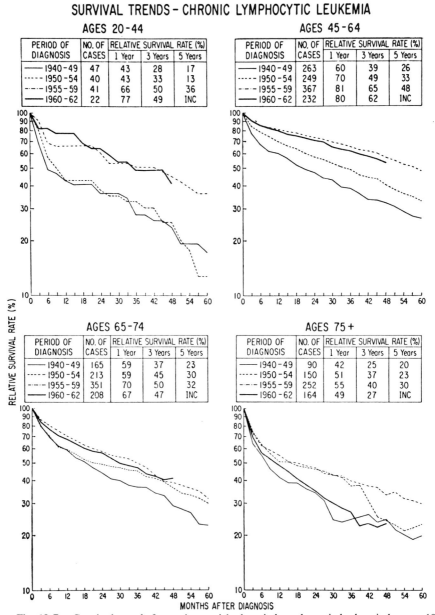

Fig. 19-7. Survival trends for patients with chronic lymphocytic leukemia by age, 1940–1962. (Reproduced from Cutler, S. J., Axtell, L., Heise, H.,[24] courtesy of the authors.)

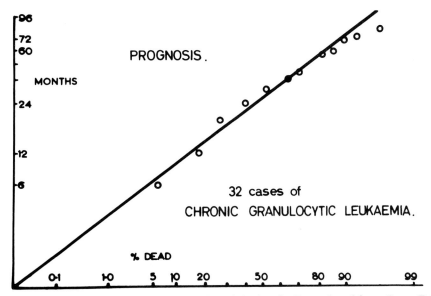

Fig. 19–8. Prognosis in chronic granulocytic leukemia. Reproduced from Gunz, F. W., Campbell, A. J., and Goldstein, A. M.,[48] with permission.)

important to search for possible causes. The question is further discussed in Chapter 18.

LONG-TERM SURVIVAL

Because of the intrinsic character of the disease, there is in chronic leukemia a far higher proportion of patients living 5 years or more than in the acute leukemias. The 5-year term is chosen because in many cancer studies 5-year survival has been equated with presumptive cure. In chronic leukemia this is certainly not the case, the survival curve being a continuous one with the number of survivors decreasing steadily year by year (when charted on log-probability paper, the survival follows a straight line in many of the published series: see Fig. 19-8). Five-year survivals for several series are shown in Table 19-2.

It is of interest that among 31 patients with chronic leukemia surviving 5 years

Table 19-2
Median Survival of Chronic Leukemia from Diagnosis
or First Treatment

Author and Reference	Median Survival (years)	
	CGL	CLL
Tivey[113]	1.65	1.70
Feinleib and MacMahon[36]	0.97	0.97
Osgood[88]	1.79	3.42
Green and Dixon[46]		3.25
Gunz et al.[48]	2.17	3.17
Musshoff et al.[86]	2.50	
Hill et al.[56]	3.38	6.46
Medical Research Council[77]	2.28 (radiotherapy)	
	3.25 (busulfan)	

who were reported by Moffitt and Lawrence,[83] half (15) were suffering from chronic granulocytic and half from chronic lymphocytic leukemia. Very long survivals in excess of 10 years occur in both types but are more common in chronic lymphocytic leukemia. Osgood reported 4.4 percent of CGL and 15.1 percent of CLL patients living 10 years or more after first treatment, an exceptionally good result.[88] Even longer survivals are reported, some in complete remission for many years. In some of these, the original diagnosis is questionable.

PROGNOSIS IN INDIVIDUAL CASES

As has been indicated, the patient with chronic lymphocytic leukemia has on average a better prognosis for survival than the one with the chronic granulocytic form. This difference extends through all age groups.[24] Young patients with chronic leukemia tend to live longer than older ones,[88] although a particularly benign form of chronic lymphocytic leukemia occurs mainly in elderly people. The prognosis is statistically slightly better in females than in males. Some workers claim that, as a general rule, those patients who have a comparatively long history before they are first seen by a physician or treated tend to live longer after treatment than those with a short history.[90] Although this is possibly true for acute leukemia, it has not been confirmed in the chronic variety.[36,113] On the other hand, it is clear that when leukemia is discovered accidentally in the absence of symptoms, considerable periods (2–5 years[117]) may elapse before symptoms are first noted. Since such patients have the same chances of survival after treatment is instituted in response to their symptoms as others who had not previously been known to have leukemia, their total survival may appear unusually prolonged.

The blood findings with which a patient first presents may be of some prognostic significance. In contrast to the acute varieties, there is no evidence that patients with low initial leukocyte counts live longer than those with leukemic levels from onset. On the contrary, it has been stated that those with initial counts below 20,000 per cubic millimeter fare substantially worse than those with higher counts.[86] This may be partly the result of diagnostic difficulties, some of the low-count cases being in reality acute rather than chronic. A low hemoglobin level at the onset or at an early stage definitely suggests short survival, especially in cases of chronic lymphocytic leukemia. In a series collected by Leavell,[69] no patients with chronic lymphocytic leukemia and with a hemoglobin of less than 30 percent survived by as much as 1 year. According to Pascucci[90] a red cell count below 3.0 million per cubic millimeter in chronic lymphocytic leukemia is of definitely bad prognostic import, and in Moffitt's and Lawrence's 16 patients with the disease, who survived for more than 5 years after diagnosis, there were only two with a red cell count of less than 4 million per cubic millimeter.[83] A marked initial thrombocytopenia is also an unfavorable sign,[90] platelet counts below 50,000 per cubic millimeter in chronic granulocytic leukemia and below 75,000 per cubic millimeter in the lymphocytic form being critical. Bleeding manifestations are unfavorable signs in the chronic leukemias, especially in the granulocytic form.[69] Skin involvement can occur early or late in chronic lymphocytic leukemia, but once it is seen in chronic granulocytic leukemia the end is very near.[42] Similarly, lymph node enlargement is a late manifestation in chronic granulocytic leukemia, and a patient first seen with it can be predicted to succumb rapidly.

SPONTANEOUS REMISSIONS IN LEUKEMIA

The prognosis of all kinds of leukemia is made a little more uncertain than has already been indicated by the possible occurrence of spontaneous remissions. These are of great rarity in the chronic forms though a few have been described in chronic lymphocytic leukemia,[51] but have been found rather more frequently in acute leukemia, although the proportion of cases in which they may be expected has been the subject of considerable argument. Furthermore, it is not altogether clear how many of the cases which have been reported were really "spontaneous," rather than being a consequence of some kind of treatment which was given at the time but held to be unimportant by the authors.[117] Most of the "spontaneous" cases tended to occur after some febrile illness or other severe strain and were preceded by a temporary marrow hypoplasia, with pancytopenic blood counts. Remissions may be complete or, more often, partial, and in some of the reported instances were of such unusually short extent that they might well have represented merely the normal fluctuations which often occur in otherwise remarkable cases of acute leukemia, aided by some optimism on the part of the medical attendant.

Spontaneous remissions have been noted in very variable proportions of the many series of cases dealing with them. Thus, no remissions were reported in one group of 152 children,[103] while in others there were 26 among 300,[30] and 12 among 83 children.[108] These figures seem inordinately high, and one wonders whether some of the patients having "remissions" actually presented full evidence for this, including bone marrow examinations. Brandberg,[16] for example, in his very full studies, discovered no single case among 140 children. It is clear, at any rate, that such remissions are much less common in adults than in children, although isolated cases have been reported in the former, some of them of remarkable length. Birge et al.[11] described the case of a 33-year-old, pregnant woman with acute stem cell leukemia, who, following eclamptic convulsions and the birth of a dead infant, had a complete remission which lasted fully 2 years before the relapse which rapidly led to her death. According to Bierman et al.,[10] who attempted to produce "spontaneous" remissions by initiating various infections in their patients, these were always preceded by a profound bone marrow hypoplasia. Should the patient survive this, a temporary regeneration of normal marrow cells may occur. This is analogous to what occurs in the course of therapy with such highly myelotoxic drugs as daunorubicin.

In one of two cases of unusually long remissions we have observed, the child developed chicken pox while taking corticosteroids. The infection was extremely severe, as it may be in these instances, and the patient was apparently close to death for several days. She then made a gradual recovery and after a prolonged convalescence, no further evidence of her previous acute leukemia was present and the patient has been completely well for at least 10 years. The adult patient developed an apparently overwhelming infection while under therapy with maximum doses of corticosteroid (1000-mg of prednisone daily). Following recovery from infection and a long convalescence, she became completely well and has remained well for 12 years. Tivey[112] thinks it probable that all such remissions are the results of an abnormal outpouring of adrenocorticosteroids in response to various stresses, such as acute infections, eclampsia, etc. The alternative explanation may be an autoimmune reaction (see Chapter 12).[2,8,15,29,54,59,82,114,119]

Quality of Survival

By this term, we mean the state of the patient's health and activity, compared to that regarded as "normal." If it were possible to assess this objectively, the results would give a better picture of the effects of therapy than would mere survival figures; for what the physician should aim at in treating leukemia, is the maximum restoration of health rather than the extension or improvement of any one statistic. This point was made by Minot who stressed that though his patients with chronic leukemia did not live longer than untreated ones, they lived much more happily and with much less invalidism.[80,81] Similar statements have been made by many others. In acute leukemia, a full remission means a full restitution to normal health; the difficulty is to express this in figures.

There are unfortunately no agreed methods of expressing the duration of "normal health" or "full remission" in the various groups of patients, and it is to be hoped that this omission can be remedied. Perhaps the closest statistical evaluation of the quality of survival can be found in Colebatch's assessment of the performance status of children treated for acute leukemia.[23] In this publication, performance class 1 means "the time spent by a child in a state of fitness for full-time attendance at school or kindergarten or for similar normal activities." Table 19-3 shows the proportion of time spent by patients in performance class 1.

The authors comment: "As would be expected, some of the short-term survivors spent much of their time unfit for school; on the other hand, 39 of the total of 86 children spent 90–100 percent of their "study period" in class 1, which is as good a performance as one commonly sees in healthy children in this age group."

In acute leukemia of adults, it has become possible only during the past few years to induce remissions with any degree of frequency, and data as to their duration and quality are still scanty. It has, in fact, been maintained that the game is not worth the candle: that the change of returning patients to anything resembling normal health, let alone a fruitful and enjoyable life, is so small that it is unjustifiable to expose them to the risks and discomforts of modern therapy. We would agree that casual therapy of acute granulocytic leukemia of adults is of doubtful value.

Table 19-3

Performance Status of Children with Acute Leukemia
Under a Comprehensive Chemotherapy Regimen

Proportion of Study Period* Spent in Class 1 (%)	Number of Patients Surviving			
	<1 Year	1 Year	2 Years	Total
60	4	3	0	7
60–79	4	7	1	12
80–89	8	15	5	28
90–94	2	7	10	19
95–100	3	14	3	20
TOTAL	21	46	19	86

Data from Colebatch, J. H. et al.[23]

*Study period does not include the first 30 days or the last 30 days before death or withdrawal from the regimen.

However, results have begun to improve in those institutions which have the specialized knowledge and facilities required for these complex therapeutic undertakings. It is now generally acknowledged that good remissions are obtainable in about half the patients seen, and that such remissions when complete allow patients to return to a normal life.[71] Although many remissions are still distressingly short, the overall arithmetic is clear enough: untreated patients, or those failing to respond to therapy may be expected to live for only 5–7 weeks, much of this time in hospital. Patients obtaining remissions have a median survival of 7–10 months of which about one quarter may be spent in hospital.[47,71] Though small, this net gain to the patient is worthwhile, especially when it is remembered that a number of remissions are prolonged. Performance status is easier to assess in adults than in children and many adults with acute granulocytic leukemia in remission have lived active, normal lives for many months. Quantitative data are, however, still too fragmentary to permit an exact evaluation of the overall prognosis in this group.

It is surely desirable to make concerted efforts to evaluate the time of optimum performance status in all groups of patients treated for leukemia, for survival figures alone give an incomplete picture of the effects of therapy and, we suspect, at times a misleading one. Only when such more meaningful statistics have been compiled, will it be possible to present an adequate account of the real prognosis of leukemia under modern therapy.

REFERENCES

1. Arendt J, Gloor W: Resultate der Röntgenbestrahlung bei chronischen Leukämien. Strahlentherapie 44:715, 1932.

2. Bassen FA, Kohn JL: Multiple spontaneous remissions in a child with acute leukemia. The occurrence of agranulocytosis and aplastic anemia in acute leukemia and their relationship to remissions. Blood 7:37, 1952.

3. Berkson I, Gage RP: Calculation of survival rates for cancer. Proc Staff Meet Mayo Clin 25:270, 1950

4. Bernard J, Boiron M, Manus A, Levy JP, Lellouch J: Factors influencing survival time in patients with acute leukemia. Natl Cancer Inst Monogr 15:359, 1964.

5. _____, Bessis M: Peut-on guêrir les leucémies? Nouv Rev Fr Hématol 5:209, 1965.

6. _____, Jacquillat C, Boiron M, Najean Y, Seligmann M, Weil M: Les très longues rémissions complètes des leucémies aiguës. Presse Méd 73:457, 1965.

7. Best WR, Limarzi LR, Poncher HG: Longevity in leucemia (abstract). J Lab Clin Med 38:789, 1951.

8. Bichel J: Temporary complete remission in acute leukemia. Case report and preliminary report of some observations on the action of pteroylglutamic acid in leukemia. Acta Haematol 3:90, 1950.

9. Bierman HR, Cohen P, McClelland JN, Shimkin MB: The effect of transfusions and antibiotics upon the duration of life in children with lymphogenous leukemia. J Pediatr 37:455, 1950.

10. _____, Crile DM, Dod KS, Kelly KH, Petrakis NL, White LP, Shimkin MB: Remissions in leukemia of childhood following acute infectious disease. Staphylococcus, varicella and feline panleukopenia. Cancer 6:591, 1953.

11. Birge RF, Jenks AL Jr, Davis SK: Spontaneous remission in acute leukemia. Report of a case complicated by eclampsia. JAMA 140:589, 1949.

12. Boag JW: Maximum likelihood estimates of the proportion of patients cured by cancer therapy. J R Stat Soc 11:15, 1949.

13. Block M: Histopathology of the preleukemic states in humans, in Proceedings of the Sixth Congress of the International Society of Hematology. New York, Grune & Stratton, 1956.

14. Boggs DR, Wintrobe MM, Cartwright GE:

The acute leukemias; analysis of 322 cases and review of the literature. Medicine 41:163, 1962.

15. Bosland HG: Acute lymphatic leukemia with remission. Minn Med 21:500, 1938.

16. Brandberg O: Studien über das klinische Bild der Leukosen und der sog. leukämoiden Reaktionen im Kindesalter. Acta Paediatr 30 (suppl 1):1, 1943.

17. Breslow N, Zandstra R: A note on the relationship between bone marrow lymphocytosis and remission duration in acute leukemia. Blood 36:246, 1970.

18. Burchenal J: In: Proceedings of the Second Conference on Folic Acid Antagonists in Leukemia Treatment. Blood 7:115, 1952.

19. Burchenal JH: Long term survival in Burkitt's tumor and in acute leukemia. Cancer Res 27:2616, 1967.

20. _____: Long-term survivors in acute leukemia, in Zarafonetis C J D (ed): Proceedings of the International Conference on Leukemia-Lymphoma. Philadelphia, Lea & Febiger, 1968, p469.

21. Clark RL, Macdonald EJ: Analysis of results of treatment of 40,000 consecutive patients at a university cancer hospital. Acta Unio Int Cancr 19:1497, 1963.

22. Clemmesen J, Sorensen BL, Hou-Jensen K: Survival of patients with leukemia. Acta Unio Int Cancr 19:1445, 1963.

23. Colebatch JH, Baikie AG, Clark ACL, Jones DL, Lee CWG, Lewis IC, Newman NM: Cyclic drug regimen for acute childhood leukaemia. Lancet 1:313, 1968.

24. Cutler SJ, Axtell L, Heise H: Ten thousand cases of leukemia: 1940–62. J Natl Cancer Inst 39:993, 1967.

25. Dale JH Jr: Leukemia in childhood. A clinical and roentgenographic study of seventy-two cases. J Pediatr 34:421, 1949.

26. Dameshek W, Mitus WJ: Seven years' remission in an adult with acute leukemia. N Engl J Med 268:870, 1963.

27. _____, Necheles TF, Finkel HE: Survival in myeloblastic leukemia of adults. N Engl J Med 275:700, 1966.

28. Darte JMM, Snelling CE, Laski B, Jackson SH, Donohue WL: ACTH and cortisone in the treatment of leukaemia in children. Can Med Assoc J 65:560, 1951.

29. Decourt J, Guillemin RAJ, Berthet G: Rechute et évolution fatale d'une leucémie aiguë après une rémission complète de trois ans et sept mois. Bull Mém Soc Méd Hôp Paris 66:47, 1950.

30. Diamond LK, Luhby AL: Pattern of "spontaneous" remissions in leukemia of childhood observed in 26 of 300 cases. Am J Med 10:238, 1951.

31. Ellison RR: Management of acute leukemia in adults. Med Clin N Am 40:743, 1956.

32. _____, Karnofsky DA, Burchenal JH: Clinical evaluation of 6-chloropurine in leukemia of adults. Blood 13:705, 1958.

33. _____, Silver RT, Engle RL Jr: Comparative study of 6-chloropurine and 6-mercaptopurine in acute leukemia in adults. Ann Intern Med 51:322, 1959.

34. Fairbanks VF, Shanbrom E, Steinfeld JL, Beutler E: Prolonged remissions in acute myelocytic leukemia in adults. JAMA 204:574, 1968.

35. Farber S: in Rebuck JW, Bethel FW, Monto RW (eds): The Leukemias. New York, Academic Press, 1959, p 623.

36. Feinleib M, MacMahon B: Variation in the duration of survival of patients with the chronic leukemias. Blood 15:332, 1960.

37. Freireich EJ, Thomas LB, Frei E III, Fritz RD, Forkner CE JR: A distinctive type of intracerebral hemorrhage associated with "blastic crisis" in patients with leukemia. Cancer 13:146, 1960.

38. Frenkel BP, Meyers MC: Acute leukemia and pregnancy. Ann Intern Med 53:656, 1960.

39. Friedell HL, Storaasli JP: The therapeutic application of radioactive phosphorus with special reference to the treatment of primary polycythemia and chronic myeloid leukemia. J Clin Invest 28:1308, 1949.

40. Fritz RD, Forkner CE Jr, Freireich EJ, Frei E III, Thomas LB: Association of fatal intracranial hemorrhage and "blastic crisis" in patients with acute leukemia. N Engl J Med 261:59, 1959.

41. Gasser C: Langdauernde Remissionen der Leukämie im Kindesalter. Med Klin 59:385, 1964.

42. Gates O: Cutaneous tumors in leukemia and lymphoma. Arch Dermatol 37:1015, 1938.

43. Gerhartz H, Eilers TH, Günther CD: Zur Symptomatik und Lebenserwartung der chronischen Myelocytenleukämien. Verh Dtsch Ges Inn Med 74:652, 1968.

44. Giraud P, Orsini A, Raybaud C, Orsini-Roubin J: Rémissions de très longue durée dans deux enfants atteints de leucose aiguë. Arch Fr Pédiatr 21:391, 1964.

45. Gloor W: Ein Fall von geheilter Myeloblasten-Leukämie. Münch Med Wochenschr 77:1096, 1930.

46. Green RA, Dixon H: Expectancy for life in lymphatic leukemia. Blood 25:23, 1965.

47. Gunz FW, Burns EW: Prognosis in acute leukaemia of adults. NZ Med J 64:555, 1965.

48. ———, Campbell AJ, Goldstein AM: The treatment of chronic leukaemia. NZ Med J 60:441,1961.

49. ———, Hough RF: Acute leukemia over the age of fifty. A study of its incidence and natural history. Blood 11:882, 1956.

50. Hamann A: External irradiation with roentgen rays and radium in the treatment of human leukemias, lymphomas, and allied disorders of the hemopoietic system. Radiology 50:378, 1948.

51. Harrison EK, Reeves RJ: The roentgen treatment of leukemia, with report of a pregnancy in a case of lymphatic leukemia. Radiology 32:284, 1939.

52. Haut A, Altman SJ, Cartwright GE, Wintrobe MM: The influence of chemotherapy on survival in acute leukemia. Blood 10:875, 1955.

53. ———, ———, Wintrobe MM, Cartwright GE: The influence of chemotherapy on survival in acute leukemia—comparison of cases treated during 1954 to 1957 with those treated during 1947 to 1954. Blood 14:828, 1959.

54. Hemmeler G, Jéquier-Doge E: Evolution atypique de la leucémie à myéloblastes, avec rémission. Schweiz Med Wochenschr 25:1239, 1944.

55. Hill JM, Khan A, Loeb E, MacLellan A, Hill NO: Probable cures in acute leukemia. Unmaintained remissions. Wadley Med Bull 1:21, 1971.

56. ———, Loeb E, Speer RJ: Colloidal zirconyl phosphate P^{32} in the treatment of chronic leukemia and lymphomas. JAMA 187:106, 1964.

57. Hoffman WJ, Craver LF: Chronic myelogenous leukemia; value of irradiation and its effect on duration of life. JAMA 97:836, 1931.

58. Huber H: Die Überlebensdauer bei Stammzellenleukämien und sie beeinflussende Faktoren—eine Austwertung von 71 Fallen. Wien Klin Wochenschr 77:388, 1965.

59. Huth EF: Die Bedeutung der sog. Spontanheilungen und Remissionen für die Therapie und Pathogenese der Leukosen und malignen Tumoren. Z Krebsforsch 58:524, 1952.

60. Jacquillat CL, Weil M, Tanzer J, Bussel A, Loisel JP, Goguel A, Schaison G, Najean Y, Goudemand M, Seligmann M, Boiron M, Bernard J: Les très longues rémissions complètes des leucémies aiguës. Presse Méd 78:253, 1970.

61. Jones HB: Demographic consideration of the cancer problem. Trans NY Acad Sci 18:298, 1956.

62. Keidan SE: Prolonged remission in acute leukaemia. Br Med J 2:1430, 1964.

63. Kienle F: Akute Hämocytoblastenleukämien mit totaler Remission und die diagnostische Bedeutung der Sternalpunktion. Dtsch Arch Klin Med 189:233, 1942.

64. Krebs C, Bichel J: Results of roentgen treatment in chronic myelogenous leukosis. Acta Radiol 28:697, 1947.

65. Krivit W, Brubaker C, Thatcher LG, Pierce M, Perrin E, Hartmann JR: Maintenance therapy in acute leukemia of childhood. Cancer 21:352, 1968.

66. Laurie JH: Duration of remissions in lymphoblastic leukaemia of childhood. Br Med J 2:95, 1968.

67. Lawrence JH, Dobson RL, Low-Beer BVA, Brown BR: Chronic myelogenous leukemia. A study of 129 cases in which treatment was with radioactive phosphorus. JAMA 136:672, 1948.

68. Lawrence JH, Low-Beer BVA, Carpender JWJ: Chronic lymphatic leukemia. A study of 100 patients treated with radioactive phosphorus. JAMA 140:585, 1949.

69. Leavell BS: Chronic leukemia. A study of incidence and factors influencing the duration of life. Am J Med Sci 196:329, 1938.

70. Leucutia T: Irradiation in lymphosarcoma, Hodgkin's disease and leukemia (a statistical analysis). Am J Med Sci 188:612, 1934.

71. Levi JA, Vincent PC, Gunz FW: Combination chemotherapy of adult acute nonlymphoblastic leukemia. Ann Intern Med 76:397, 1972.

72. Lissauer: Zwei Fälle von Leucaemie. Berl Klin Wochenschr 2:403, 1865.

73. McAlpin KR, Golden R, Edsall KS: Roentgen treatment of chronic leucemia. Am J Roentgenol Radium Ther Nucl Med 26:47, 1931.

74. Mangalik A, Boggs DR, Wintrobe MM, Cartwright GE: The influence of chemotherapy on survival in acute leukemia. III. A comparison of patients treated during 1958–1964 with those treated in two sequentially preceding periods. Blood 27:490, 1966.

75. Mathé G, Pouillart P, Sterescu M, Amiel

JL, Schwarzenberg L, Schneider M, Hayat M, de Vassal F, Jasmin C, Lafleur M: Subdivision of classical varieties of acute leukemia. Correlation with prognosis and cure expectancy. Europ J Clin Biol Res 16:554, 1971.

76. Maurice PA, Alberto P, Ferrier S, Freund M: Leucémie myélocytaire chronique: "Guérison" apparente depuis plus de 9 ans, consécutive à une hypoplasie médullaire thérapeutique. Schweiz Med Wochenschr 101:1781, 1971.

77. Medical Research Council: Chronic granulocytic leukaemia; comparison of radiotherapy and busulphan therapy. Report of the Medical Research Council's Working Party for therapeutic trials in leukaemia. Br Med J 1:201, 1968.

78. Medical Research Council (Working Party Report): Duration of survival of children with acute leukaemia. Brit Med J 4:7, 1971.

79. Medinger FG, Craver LF: Total body irradiation, with review of cases. Am J Roentgenol Radium Ther Nucl Med 48:651, 1942.

80. Minot GR, Buckman JE, Isaacs R: Chronic myelogenous leukemia. Age incidence, duration and benefit derived from irradiation. JAMA 82:1489, 1924.

81. _____, Isaacs R: Lymphatic leukemia; age incidence, duration and benefit derived from irradiation. Boston Med Surg J 191:1, 1924.

82. Moeschlin S: Subakute Paramyeloblasten-Leukämien mit mehrfachen längeren Remissionen. Dtsch Arch Klin Med 191:213, 1943.

83. Moffitt HC Jr, Lawrence JH: Chronic leukemia of long duration: with a report of 31 cases with a duration of over five years. Ann Intern Med 30:778, 1949.

84. Moody EA, Davis RW: Duration of acute leukemia in children. Review of the literature and report of a case of unusually long survival. Am J Dis Child 80:955, 1950.

85. Murphy ML: Leukemia and lymphoma in children. Pediatr Clin N Am 6:611, 1959.

86. Musshoff K, Boutis L, Obrecht P, Karsch T: Die Lebenserwartung der chronischen myeloischen Leukämie in Abhängigkeit von individuellen und krankheitsspezifischen Faktoren und der Therapie. Klin Wochenschr 47:179, 1969.

87. Oehme J, Janssen W, Hagitte C: Leukämie im Kindesalter. Stuttgart, Thieme, 1958.

88. Osgood EE: Treatment of chronic leukemias. J Nucl Med 5:139, 1964.

89. Parsons CG: Radium in treatment of leukaemia. Br J Radiol 10:573, 1937

90. Pascucci LM: Chronic leukemia: a statistical study of symptoms, duration of life and prognosis. Radiology 39:75, 1942.

91. Pierce M. Childhood leucemia J. Pediat 8:66, 1936

92. _____: in Proceedings of the Second Conference on Folic Acid Antagonists in Leukemia Treatment. Blood 7:124, 1952.

93. Pinkel D, Simone J, Hustu HO, Aur RJA: Nine years' experience with "total therapy" of childhood acute lymphocytic leukemia. Pediatrics 50:246, 1972.

94. Pisciotta AV, Hirschboeck JS: Therapeutic considerations in chronic lymphocytic leukemia. Arch Intern Med 99:334, 1957.

95. Poncher HG, Waisman HA, Richmond JB, Horak OA, Limarzi LR: Treatment of acute leukemia in children with and without folic acid antagonists. J Pediatr 41:377, 1952.

96. Propp S: Subleukemic leukemia, a common type of leukemia with emphasis on its hypoplastic form, in Proceedings of the Sixth Congress of the International Society of Hematology. New York, Grune & Stratton, 1956.

97. Pusey WA: Report of cases treated with roentgen rays. JAMA 38:911, 1902.

98. Quilligan JJ Jr: In: Proceedings of the Second Conference Folic Acid Antagonists in Leukemia Treatment. Blood 7:133, 1952.

99. Reinhard EH, Moore CV, Bierbaum OS, Moore S: Radioactive phosphorus as a therapeutic agent. A review of the literature and analysis of the results of treatment of 155 patients with various blood dyscrasias, lymphomas and other malignant neoplastic disease. J Lab Clin Med 31:107, 1946.

100. Rheingold JJ, Kaufman R, Adelson E, Lear A: Smoldering acute leukemia. N Engl J Med 268:812, 1963.

101. Rivers SL, Whittington RM, Gendel PR, Patno ME: Acute leukemia in the adult male: II. Natural history. Cancer 16:249, 1963.

102. Roath S, Israels MCG, Wilkinson JF: The acute leukaemias: A study of 580 patients. Q J Med 33:256, 1964.

103. Rodgers CL, Donohue WL, Snelling CE: Leukaemia in children. Can Med Assoc J 65:548, 1951.

104. Senn N: Case of splenomedullary leukaemia successfully treated by the use of the Roentgen ray. Med Rec NY 64:281, 1903.

105. Shimkin MB, Lucia EL, Oppermann KC, Mettier SR: Lymphocytic leukemia: an analysis of frequency, distribution and mortality at the University of California Hospital, 1913–1947. Ann Intern Med 39:1254, 1953.

106. _____, Mettier SR, Bierman HR: Myelocytic leukemia: An analysis of incidence, distribution and fatality, 1910–1948. Ann Intern Med 35:194, 1951.

107. Skeel RT, Bennett JM, Henderson ES: Bone marrow lymphocytosis in acute leukemia: a second look. Blood 35:356, 1970.

108. Southam CM, Craver LF, Dargeon HW, Burchenal JH: A study of the natural history of acute leukemia with special reference to the duration of the disease and the occurrence of remissions. Cancer 4:39, 1951.

109. Tallal L: Childhood leukemia: differing survival times by data selection. Proc Am Assoc Cancer Res 8:66, 1967.

110. Till MW, Hardisty RM, Pike MC: Long survivals in acute leukaemia. Lancet 1:534, 1973.

111. Tin Han, Sokal JE: Spontaneous remission of leukemic lymphoproliferative disease. Cancer 27:586, 1971.

112. Tivey H: The natural history of untreated acute leukemia. Ann NY Acad Sci 60:322, 1954.

113. _____: The prognosis for survival in chronic granulocytic and lymphocytic leukemia. Am J Roentgenol Radium Ther Nucl Med 72:68, 1954.

114. Wagner A: Remission einer akuten lymphatischen Leukämie durch komplizierende Eiterung. Klin Wochenschr 7:266, 1928.

115. Watt WL: Leukaemia and deep x-ray therapy. Guy's Hosp Rep 86:175, 1936.

116. Wiernik PH, Serpick AA: A randomized clinical trial of daunorubicin and a combination of prednisone, vincristine, 6-mercaptopurine and methotrexate in adult acute nonlymphocytic leukemia. Cancer Res 32:2023, 1972.

117. Wintrobe MM, Hasenbush LL: Chronic leukemia. The early phase of chronic leukemia, the results of treatment and the effects of complicating infections; a study of eighty-six adults. Arch Intern Med 64:701, 1939.

118. Wollstein M: Leukemia in young children. Am J Dis Child 44:661, 1932.

119. Young LE, Platzer RF, Lawrence JS: Unusual anemia associated with chronic myeloid leukemia. Acta Haematol 5:345, 1951.

120. Zippin C, Cutler SJ, Reeves WJ Jr, Lum D: Variation in survival among patients with acute lymphocytic leukemia. Blood 37:59, 1971.

121. Zuelzer WW: Implications of long-term survival in acute stem cell leukemia of childhood treated with composite cyclic therapy. Blood 24:477, 1964.

122. _____: Therapy of acute leukemia in childhood, in Zarafonetis CJD (ed): Proceedings of the International Conference on Leukemia-Lymphoma. Philadelphia, Lea & Febiger, 1968, p 451.

20

What Should One Tell the Patient?

'And what does the doctor say?' asked Mary.

'Oh! Much what all doctors say: he puts a fence on this side and a fence on that, for fear he should be caught tripping in his judgment. One moment he does not think there is much hope—but while there is life there is hope; th'next he says he should think she might recover partial, but her age is again her.'—From E. C. Gaskell, *Mary Barton* (Everyman's Library Edition, p 189)

Until recently, doctors almost universally withheld from patients with leukemia all knowledge of their disease, usually under the impression that it would be bad for the patient's morale to realize that he had an incurable disease. We believe that there are grave objections to this practice and that, in the great majority of cases, patients, as well as their relatives, should be taken into the doctor's full confidence, advised of the correct diagnosis, and encouraged to cooperate in the treatment to the best of their ability. We have personally followed this policy for many years and though there must be differences arising from the opinions and emotions of individual physicians, certain principles seem to us to be generally tenable in our communications with patients, and these will be explained in this brief chapter. There are at least five strong arguments in favor of a candid approach to the patient and each will be discussed in turn.

Leukemia is better known to the public by name than many much more common diseases. More than half our patients have already decided on the diagnosis themselves, their suspicions having been aroused by blood tests which were followed by prompt referral to a hematologist. Further blood and bone marrow tests, perhaps with subsequent transfusions, rapidly convince the patient that he has a serious blood disorder, and leukemia, the subject of so much sensational publicity in books, magazines, radio, television, and motion pictures, is by far the best-known blood disease. A patient who finds himself in a ward with several other patients who have leukemia is almost certain to conclude that he, too, has leukemia, even if he has an altogether different complaint. Thus, difficulties may even arise when patients have to be convinced that they do *not* have leukemia. Clearly, most patients with leukemia are not reassured in any way if their diagnosis is withheld.

The patient who diagnoses his own leukemia almost certainly attaches the worst possible interpretation to the concept. "Leukemia" is nearly always thought to be acute, for the existence of the chronic forms seems relatively little known. One of our patients with chronic lymphocytic leukemia spent an agonizing 48 hours after becoming aware that he had leukemia, because his mother had died from the acute disease and he expected, like her, to live no more than a week or two and to die a distressing death. Only after lengthy further explanation was he finally persuaded that he had a relatively mild complaint which needed little treatment and was unlikely to shorten his life materially.

The longer the disease lasts, the less likely is it that its nature can be concealed. This is especially so in acute leukemia entering remission, with its need for continuing complex maintenance therapy. It is preferable that the patient be given truthful and accurate information from his doctor instead of obtaining it in roundabout ways, in which case it will probably be inaccurate and unnecessarily frightening.

To tell nothing or a deliberate lie about his illness to the patient is felt by many to be morally wrong, for of all those concerned, he has the clearest right to know the truth. Moreover, such deceptions are usually self-defeating, for as the disease progresses, its nature becomes more obvious. The patient may then justifiably lose all trust and confidence in his medical attendants, and even in the friends and relatives around him: he may eventually have to face his final illness among people from whom he has become estranged; a predicament very movingly described by Tolstoy:

"What tormented Ivan Ilyich most was the pretence, the lie . . . that he was merely ill and not dying, and the pretence made him wretched: it tormented him that they refused to admit what they knew and he knew to be a fact, but persisted in lying to him concerning his terrible condition, and wanted him and forced him to be a party to the lie: this lying which would only degrade the awful, solemn act of his death."* We believe that, practical considerations apart, it is morally indefensible to withhold from a patient the information that he has leukemia, for such a paternalistic attitude detracts from the patient's own human dignity.

Modern treatments for leukemia are often highly demanding on the patient's stamina and can only be tolerated when he is willing to cooperate fully. It is unreasonable to expect him to do so without adequate explanations, and, indeed, we have found it difficult to establish relations of confidence with patients who were uncertain of their diagnosis—such patients often distrust their physician, question his judgment, fail to follow instructions, or default in treatment. Once the diagnosis has been given, explained and discussed, there are no barriers between patient and doctor and all can work together in the attempts to conquer the disease.

The disclosure of the diagnosis can often be of great help to the patient's mental stability. The suspicion that he has leukemia may produce profound anxiety and depression which may not be expressed, either because the patient is afraid to ask or because he seeks to spare the doctor the distressing task of having to tell him the truth. A frank discussion may greatly ease the mind in such a situation, as shown in the following letter from one of our patients:

During the first phase I was in ill health and was subjected to numerous tests.

*From Leo Tolstoy *The Death of Ivan Ilyich,* trans. Rosemary Edmonds (Baltimore, Md.: Penguin Classics, 1971) pp. 142–143.

At this stage I suffered severely mentally with the fear that this blood disorder could be leukemia. It was this fear that prompted me to ask the doctor directly if my disease was in fact leukemia. The second phase covers the period following an affirmative answer. The news was upsetting, but not the shock one would expect. A little time settled me down and I am extremely grateful that I do know of the disease I suffer because the fear of the possibility was worse in all respects than the actual knowledge.

We do not tell the diagnosis to those we consider unable to understand a reasonable explanation. This includes small children and some senile or intellectually subnormal patients. All other patients are told, not excluding those thought to be "unstable" or "neurotic" whose symptoms are often the reflection of worry about their possible diagnosis and who may, in our experience, become much more stable and cooperative once their condition has been fully explained to them. Relatives sometimes want to shield the patient from a knowledge of his disease, especially in the case of adolescents or young adults, but it is usually possible to dissuade them from this course. Such relatives tend to underestimate the patient's resilience and find to their surprise that the reaction to the diagnosis is better than they had feared.

What then should patients be told, and at what particular moment? This has to be decided for each individual, and both content and timing of the information are of great importance. In general, we tell each patient as much as he can understand about his disease and its treatment. One of the first things to explain is the nature of the common leukemias and their responsiveness to treatment. The truth about the median survival in well-treated cases of the chronic leukemias and acute leukemias in childhood is usually much better than the patient or his relatives had previously believed. Even in acute leukemias in adults, the outlook is now significantly better than it was even a few years ago, and here a varnish of optimism may be applied to the less encouraging picture, at least initially. The word *leukemia* is specifically mentioned, but only when the diagnosis has been thoroughly established. It is a word evocative of fear in most people, but its gradual introduction and reiteration produces eventual familiarity and, with it, a reduction in its highly emotional overtones.

The timing of communication is important, especially in the acute leukemias. It is desirable to get to know the patient and form a relationship with him before discussing the diagnosis. Adult patients and parents should not be told lies at any stage, but there is no need to volunteer the information at once that leukemia is included in the differential diagnosis. The relatively uncommon patient who asks for his diagnosis point-blank should be told at once, provided the answer can be definite. In most other instances, not too much should be told at one time. The simplest facts are given first. Anything more may be imperfectly understood, depending on intelligence, previous suspicion of the diagnosis, and the emotional impact of its confirmation.

When the patient has been told the basic facts, he may then be given a copy of one of the booklets especially written for this purpose (for example, *Leukaemia and Its Treatment: The Disease Explained,* prepared by Clinical Haematology Unit, Kanematsu Memorial Institute, Sydney Hospital, Sydney, New South Wales, 2000, Australia). At subsequent interviews a more detailed account of the situation may be given and questions invited and answered. The treatment to be followed, its likely discomforts and probable benefits, are outlined in some detail, with the emphasis on optimism. Prognosis is discussed in general terms. In the chronic leukemias, we have often found it valuable to put this in perspective by comparing leukemia with a more familiar disease such as myocardial infarction or chronic nephritis which is less evocative of fear but may have a poorer outlook than many chronic leukemias. We explain to such patients that they will need continuing supervision and treatment, but that there is every chance of their being able to pursue normal lives in good health for at least some years. Elderly patients with chronic lymphocytic leukemia can often be assured that the disease needs no treatment and probably will not harm them, but that a blood count, perhaps twice a year, is a useful precaution.

Even in acute leukemia, a general attitude of hope is justifiable. This is best created by modest reference to recent improvements in treatment—very modest in older adults but much more optimistic in acute lymphocytic leukemia of children. Mention may be made of the probability of further improvements arising in the lifetime of the patient. We do not generally use the term *cure,* but in selected patients the possibility of cure need no longer be categorically dismissed. The examples of other patients with relatively long remissions may also be quoted and a reassurance be given about the international dissemination of knowledge about the leukemias, together with a caution against accounts of leukemia to be found in obsolete medical books or in the popular press. Indeed, a general word of warning against false hopes and false prophets is advisable.

Many of the questions patients ask are basically requests for reassurance: reassurance against the fear that nothing done—or left undone—in the past, by patients or relatives, can have determined the appearance of the disease; reassurance about the absence of familial risk (the most common single question we have encountered is, Will my children be affected?); reassurance, above all, against the nagging suspicion that something dreadful is being concealed from them. Patients commonly fear not being told more than they fear bad news itself, but once they have acquired confidence in the integrity of those looking after them, they will readily accept their explanations, even if these cannot always be as definite as they would like. Outlining the plan of the proposed therapy is often comforting to the patient, for this shows that much can and will be done for him.

We invariably give an implicit or actual reassurance that patients and relatives will have a continuing ready access to the physician in the future, either for further counseling or to answer specific questions. We aim at creating a relationship of mutual trust, and in this context we emphasize that treatment will mean a team effort, and that both the patient and his next of kin belong to the team and will remain part of it. A corollary to this approach is an assurance that if things are not going well, the complete team will understand the situation and will take appropriate steps to change and, if possible, improve it. This conveys to the patient the message that he will not be deserted, even when death is imminent, a point whose psychologic importance can scarcely be overemphasized.

Where teamwork is necessary, as in the treatment of the leukemias, it is often helpful for the patient to have an especially close relationship with one physician. Where such a relationship is accepted, even tacitly, the possibility of his or her absence at times critical to the patient, should be faced. It is often helpful to introduce a second physician to whom special responsibility will fall, so that a second, even if subsidiary, special relationship may develop. If this precaution is not taken, even the patient who is not especially dependent may be unhappy when his or her particular physician is unavoidably absent.

In the lifetime of the patient with leukemia, death and the preterminal state, while not to be denied, should hardly be mentioned. The general attitude should be one of hopeful optimism. This attitude is best inculcated by close attention to all the details of management, with the implication that it is all worthwhile. When we approach a patient with leukemia, we endeavour to treat the whole man or woman, and not only the blood or marrow. For this are needed sympathy, frankness, and reassurance as well as technical knowledge; and we have found few patients who have not responded favorably to this combination. Finally, one aspect of communication should be considered, even after the patient's death. It is often helpful to offer to see the relatives, if they wish it, a few weeks after death. This is especially helpful for the parents of young children, whether or not they may still harbor fears about the patient's siblings. Even the relatives of adult patients may welcome this opportunity, since they often have to be reassured that they themselves fulfilled all their responsibilities to the deceased, even to the end. This offer of a postmortem interview is, of course, a feature of complete medical care and it should not be restricted to the relatives of patients with leukemia.

REFERENCES

1. Binger CM, Ablin AR, Feuerstein RC, Kushner JH, Zoger S, Mikkelsen C: Childhood leukemia. Emotional impact on patient and family. N Engl J Med 280:414, 1969.

2. Evans AE: If a child must die. . . . N Engl J Med 278:138, 1968.

3. Farber S: Management of the acute leukemia patient and family. CA 15:14, 1965.

4. Hinton J: Dying. Ringwood, Victoria, Penguin Books, 1967.

5. Kübler-Ross E, Wessler S, Avioli LV: On death and dying. JAMA 221:174, 1972.

6. Lewis IC: Leukaemia in childhood: Its effects on the family. Aust Paediat J 3:244, 1967.

21

Recent Advances

In this chapter we cite briefly some findings which were published while our manuscript was being prepared for the printer and which appeared to us to be of outstanding importance. They are arranged in the order of the relevant chapters.

CLASSIFICATION

Two major reports on a total of 61 cases[17,29] describe the characteristics of hairy cell leukemia which is identical with Bouroncle's "leukemic reticulo-endo-theliosis" (q.v.). This is a rare leukemia, accounting for less than 3 percent of acute leukemias. It has a subacute course, neutropenia, often massive splenomegaly, and the characteristic "hairy cells" which belong to the lymphocytic series and are mostly B-cells.[18] Cytochemical studies show these B-cells to have a specific tartrate-resistant acid-phosphatase iso-enzyme.

Hairy cell leukemia is not considered either by that name or by any of its synonyms in a recent critical review of the histiocytic disorders[20], embracing all the recognized neoplasms of histiocytes or macrophages, including all forms of monocytic leukemia. This review accepts both the recognized types of monocytic leukemia as being variants of a single form, in contrast to our clearer separation of acute myelomonocytic leukemia from the rare acute monocytic form.

The status of eosinophilic leukemia is further confounded by a description of two cases of acute lymphocytic leukemia with marked eosinophilia at presentation. Indirect cytogenetic evidence is provided to support the contention that the eosino-philia was a reactive and not a neoplastic process. In both cases there were elec-trocardiographic changes and skin manifestations which could not be attributed to thrombocytopenia.[78] Another little known aspect of acute leukemia may be related to treatment and is likely to be seen often as more radical regimens are increasingly used in the treatment of acute leukemia.[77] These changes are hematologic features of moderate anemia, thrombocytosis, and neutropenia with monocytosis but without leukopenia. It commonly occurs 14 days after the last chemotherapy and is

readily misinterpreted as evidence of relapse, or the superimposition of a granulocytic leukemia on the already recognized acute lymphocytic leukemia.

No convincing explanation has yet emerged from either studies of cell kinetics
or theories about the multistage induction of leukemia to account for the latent period of leukemias. Experiments with transplantable murine leukemias[39] suggest that
both the latent period and the emergence or nonemergence of leukemia depend on
interaction between tumor cells and host. The host factors probably involve physiologic mechanisms as well as immunologic responses.

Children with acute lymphocytic leukemia are of greater birth weight than their
nonleukemic sibs.[88] This puzzling association suggestive of prenatal determination
of childhood acute leukemia cannot be explained by either maternal age or the
child's birth rank in the sibship.

ETIOLOGY

Radiation

A further large and well-studied group of patients who were subjected to
internal irradiation has been shown to have a greatly increased incidence of leukemia
as well as of other blood dyscrasias, mostly termed aplastic anemia, but also
probably atypical leukemias.[21] These individuals, all Portuguese, were exposed to
systemic injections of radiothorium, mainly for cerebral angiography, during the
years 1930 to 1955. Among 988 who could be traced, there were 12 leukemias (all
acute or chronic granulocytic) and 11 other blood dyscrasias. The leukemia incidence was estimated to be at least 12–16 times higher than in controls. This was a
considerably greater excess than that among the irradiated spondylitics in Britain.
However, the most remarkable difference was that, whereas the peak leukemia incidence in all previously reported series of patients receiving external radiation occurred some 6 years after exposure, the latent period in those given radiothorium
was about three times longer, with a peak 20 years after exposure. The reasons for
this difference are not clear, but the special characteristics and distribution of the
alpha radiation emitted are probably important. It is also noteworthy that the effect
of radiothorium should have been so different from that of radium which, as mentioned in Chapter 5, was not found to be leukemogenic when ingested or injected in
large doses.

New approaches have been made to the problem of the increased incidence of
leukemia in young children exposed to preconception or intrauterine irradiation.
When children with leukemia and a history of irradiation were arranged in groups,
according to previous experience of infections or allergies, it was found that those
with allergic diseases (asthma or urticaria) as well as radiation histories had the
highest leukemia incidence; those with bacterial diseases (pneumonia, whooping
cough, dysentery) and radiation a somewhat lower one; those with virus diseases
(measles, varicella) and radiation, lower again; and those with radiation alone, the
lowest incidence[11,62] It is suggested that children, especially those under 4, with histories of allergies and, to a lesser extent, of infections, are especially susceptible to
radiation exposure and that doses of radiation innocuous to most children may be
leukemogenic in the susceptible groups. In this connection it may be significant that
a preliminary report[26] suggesting a higher leukemia incidence in the children of

mothers who had influenza during pregnancy has now been confirmed, at least for maternal influenza of the so called Asian type.[38] Conceivably the offspring of such mothers may form another susceptible group. On the other hand, a recent prospective survey has shown that black children, in contrast to white ones, do not have an increased leukemia incidence following intrauterine irradiation, probably because of a genuine difference in susceptibility.[23]

In 61 cases of leukemia amongst atomic bomb survivors at Hiroshima and Nagasaki, autopsy findings have been compared with those in a control series without unusual radiation exposure.[52] On pathologic features no case of leukemia could be recognized as radiation induced or otherwise differentiated from cases without unusual radiation exposure. Recently, with accurate measurements of the radiation dose received by survivors now available, an excess of malignant lymphoma and myeloma has been shown in those who received 100 rad or more at Hiroshima.[64] No such effect has been found in the survivors at Nagasaki: this difference may be due to difference in the bombs dropped on the two cities, or to difference in the irradiated populations.

Viruses

Rapid progress has been made in biochemical and immunologic studies of oncogenic viruses and their constituents. The discovery of the DNA polymerase of RNA tumor viruses (oncornaviruses), the so-called *reverse transcriptase,* has been energetically followed up, and evidence has accumulated which shows that reverse transcriptase of the viral type is present in some human leukemic cells.[73] At first there was some confusion when it was found that normal lymphocytes contain at least two major DNA polymerases capable of some DNA-RNA synthetic functions. Since then, it has been shown that there are definite and reproducible differences in the activities of the DNA polymerases of normal tissues and the reverse transcriptase of RNA viruses.[31] Several groups of investigators[7,31,41] have found that the reverse transcriptase in leukemic and some other neoplastic cells closely resembles that of known oncornaviruses (Rauscher virus, avian myeloblastosis virus). It has also been shown[84] that the activity of the transcriptase can be inhibited by certain rifamycin derivatives.

The present theory of the life cycle of RNA viruses, as first postulated by Temin,[44] is as follows: the virus, having entered a susceptible cell, uses its reverse transcriptase to produce a DNA "provirus" from its RNA template. This becomes integrated with the cellular DNA but at a later stage is transcribed again to viral RNA and, with the acquisition of a protein coat, becomes new infectious oncornavirus. In this cycle, the viral reverse transcriptase plays an essential part, and the discovery of this enzyme in a tissue is now regarded as an unmistakable "footprint" of the virus. If this reasoning is accepted, there now appears to be definite, though indirect, evidence that RNA viruses closely resembling animal oncornaviruses are present in some human leukemic cells. Some investigators have found them only in blasts from acute leukemias,[31] others also in chronic leukemic cells.[48] It should, however, be clearly understood that even though such viruses may indeed be present and active, no proof exists as yet that they are directly concerned in the process of human leukemogenesis; nor is their relationship to other etiologic factors understood.

New and rather simple techniques have been discovered which make it possible to demonstrate the presence of feline leukemia virus (FeLV) in infected cats. By means of these tests it has been shown that, contrary to the situation in experimental mice, transmission of cat lymphoma is *horizontal* and not vertical, and that this common leukemia-like neoplasm is thus truly an infectious disease.[40] A carrier state has been found to occur in some apparently normal cats. Transmission is by saliva, urine, and possibly, blood transferred by blood-sucking insects. However, no evidence has been obtained that FeLV is transmissible to man, although it may be able to grow in vitro in human tissues.

SIMIAN LEUKEMIA VIRUSES

A second herpesvirus, H. ateles, has been isolated from spider monkeys and shown to be leukemogenic in marmosets and owl monkeys.[55] It appeared possible that in the host marmosets, the virus could be propagated horizontally.[43] Similarly, H. saimiri, isolated from squirrel monkeys, was highly leukemogenic when injected into marmosets,[91] but this virus did not spread to cage mates. The fact that two DNA herpesviruses isolated from primates have now been found to be leukemogenic raises afresh the possibility that other herpesviruses, including the EB virus in man, may be oncogenic. Obviously there is urgent need for further studies in this field.

It has been shown for both children[10] and adults[9] that twice as many patients with acute leukemia as matched controls had had contact with a sick cat. For adults with acute leukemia there was even stronger evidence of association with sick canaries and parakeets, but in neither children nor adults was any similar link found between acute leukemia and sick dogs. Although these associations suggest that in some cases of acute leukemia a virus or viruses harbored by sick animals may play a part in the etiology, other investigators, working on similar lines, failed to find any correlation between animal and human leukemias in the same households, as discussed in Chapter 5. An excess of cases of childhood leukemia was found in a group of children whose mothers had chickenpox in pregnancy.[1]

CYTOCHEMISTRY

The importance of the myeloperoxidase of neutrophil polymorphs in the defense against certain bacterial and fungal infections has been stressed, and it was shown that this enzyme is absent from the neutrophils of a high proportion of patients with acute granulocytic leukemia, especially the myeloblastic type.[16] The lack of bactericidal power of such cells may account in part for the susceptibility to serious infections found in patients with acute leukemia. The inability of leukocytes in acute granulocytic leukemia to ingest and kill *Candida albicans* may be especially important.[36]

CHROMOSOMES

The long-standing question whether the Ph[1] chromosome originates by deletion or translocation has been settled by the use of fluorescence and Giemsa banding techniques. Rowley[69] found that in patients with chronic granulocytic leukemia there was a consistent "extra" piece of chromatin attached to one of the C group chromosomes (usually No. 9), and that this corresponded in size to the piece "missing" from the Ph[1] chromosome. Clearly therefore the Ph[1] abnormality resulted from a translocation and not a deletion. This unexpected finding is of much interest, for it signifies for the first time that in the history of cellular development— including conversion of normal to leukemic cells—the *position* within the genome of some pieces of genetic information can be of the greatest importance.

While the discovery that the Ph[1] stems from a translocation is so far the most important result in the leukemia field of the introduction of the new "banding" techniques, considerable work has also been done with these techniques on acute leukemic cells in efforts to show chromosome abnormalities not revealed in conventional cytogenetic preparations. Early findings[57] suggest that in some acute leukemias there may indeed be abnormalities of banding patterns, but because of difficulties in the reproducibility of these techniques, there is need for more confirmatory studies.

More recent studies have shown the acquisition of an additional C group chromosome in myelofibrosis with myeloid metaplasia,[22,47] polycythemia vera, and thrombocythemia.[70] Similar acquisitions have been observed in Ph[1]-positive cases of chronic granulocytic leukemia at metamorphosis.[69] The C group chromosomes acquired in these various conditions have been identified as Nos. 8, 9, and 10.

An important case report[15] concerns a patient who was accidentally found to have a Ph[1] positive clone in his marrow 5 years before he developed symptoms and signs of a rapidly fatal leukemia. During this 5-year period the clone grew from 22 percent—with a normal differential count—to 90 percent, with 46 percent blasts in the marrow and 64,000 blood leukocytes. Treatment with oral hydroxyurea produced a short remission, but the marrow Ph[1] count rose to 100 percent. Three months later a relapse occurred, and after therapy for acute granulocytic leukemia the patient died 11 months later. During this period a 47XY hyperdiploid cell line appeared while the patient became refractory to treatment. This case was interpreted as an example of two cell lines—a normal one and a second carrying the Ph[1]— coexisting for years in a "preleukemic" condition, with a subsequent abortive phase of chronic granulocytic leukemia which in turn led to metamorphosis and the acquisition of aneuploidy. It appears likely that this was an example of events which occurred also in other published cases of chronic granulocytic leukemia with a rapid metamorphosis, including cases of so-called Ph[1]-positive acute granulocytic leukemia. Tantalizing questions arise from this case report: what might have happened if energetic chemotherapy had been given while the Ph[1]-positive clone was relatively small? Could this patient have been "cured" before the onset of symptoms? And, generally, does this signify curability of chronic granulocytic leukemia if it can be diagnosed early enough?

There has been a continued accumulation of evidence, understandably provided by studies of single cases, for the clonal origin of chronic granulocytic leukemia. In one case the evidence arose in a female heterozygote for glucose-6-phosphate-dehydrogenase deficiency.[5] In another case, acquired sex chromosome mosaicism of the 45, XO, Ph[1]/46, XY, Ph[1] type in bone marrow enabled the clonal origin of new cell lines at metamorphosis to be deduced.[60]

CELL KINETICS

Recent studies have shown that monocytes, rather than neutrophils, are responsible for the stimulatory effect of blood leukocytes on the growth of marrow colonies in culture.[34,37,72] Alveolar macrophages have also been shown to be stimulatory.[35] In the mouse, the release of colony stimulating factor from monocytes in vitro can be increased by the addition of endotoxin or polyinosinic-polycytidylic acid to the medium, a phenomenon which corresponds to the increased level of serum CSF seen in mice given endotoxin in vivo.[68]

The nature of the colony-forming cell in bone marrow has been investigated further. There is conflicting evidence as to whether it is capable of adhering[37] or not adhering[56] to glass surfaces. Isolation of colony-forming cells from normal blood using a density gradient technique has been reported.[71] With the use of a short-term suspension culture technique and cytogenetic methods, it was confirmed that leukemic cells could proliferate in such cultures and required a conditioned medium containing a substance released by leukemic blast cells.[4]

Among the many reports of studies of colony-forming cells in human leukemia is one[58] suggesting that this technique may have a place in the control of treatment. In both acute and chronic granulocytic leukemia, remission was accompanied by a return to normal of several features of the colony-forming cells derived from peripheral blood or bone marrow. Extension and confirmation of these results will be eagerly awaited.

CLINICAL FEATURES

Dramatic developments in this field are now unlikely, except as regards modification of clinical features by treatment or the appearance of new features as a concomitant of longer survival. The most important of the latter is, of course, neurologic involvement in acute leukemia, especially in children. By reason of its frequency, importance as a cause of morbidity, and bad prognostic import, interest continues in its occurrence, clinical features, diagnosis, prevention, and treatment. Further evidence is now available of the value of the cytocentrifuge in the diagnosis of meningeal leukemia, and in monitoring its treatment.[25] Where clinical features are lacking and atypical cells in the cerebrospinal fluid are few, cytochemical methods may be applied to cytocentrifuge preparations (see Chapter 18). Sudan Black B, peroxidase, and the periodic-acid-Schiff reaction (PAS) have all been used in this way. The finding of PAS positive lymphoblasts, and especially their persistence after treatment, has been found to have grave prognostic significance.[27]

Another concomitant of longer survival in acute leukemia in childhood is the leukemic ileocecal syndrome. The syndrome includes inflammation, perforation, and necrosis in the ileocecal region of the gastrointestinal tract, including the appendix. It seems to depend on previously silent leukemic infiltration, followed by inflammation or therapeutically induced necrosis of the leukemic tissue.[74]

Chloromas and other manifestations of extramyeloid leukemia continue to arouse new interest, possibly because they are more often seen at relapse after long remission, or because of the challenge they provide to planned eradication of all leukemic cells. In one study[61] the importance of demonstrating myeloperoxidase activity is emphasized, as is involvement of the ovary, epidural, and perineural structures. Involvement of the iris in acute leukemia is not related to survival, has characteristic clinical features, and is usually bilateral; it may occur in children and in adults.[44] Bone pains are more frequent in children with acute leukemia than in adults, and usually occur in long bones. Back pain is less common, but when it does occur, it may be associated with vertebral collapse.[63] Pain is relieved when remission of the leukemia is induced, but usually without radiologic evidence of improvement in the bone lesions.

There have now been several case reports of patients with acute leukemia presenting with lactic acidosis. This serious complication, which is nevertheless amenable to treatment, is of uncertain pathogenesis.[87]

Cytomegalovirus infection is common in children with acute leukemia.[19] Although it is usually a late event attributable to naturally occurring and iatrogenic immunosuppression, it may also occur early in the disease. In early cases it appears to be clinically silent and to be transmitted by blood transfusion.

MYELOPROLIFERATIVE DISORDERS

A review originating from the Mayo Clinic[75] has shown that acute granulocytic leukemia, either myeloblastic or myelomonocytic, is a not uncommon terminal event in "idiopathic" MMM. Eight of 165 patients (4.8 percent) with MMM arising *de novo* died from acute granulocytic leukemia. In addition, 5 of 29 patients (17.2 percent) with MMM following polycythemia vera died from acute leukemia. No significant role could be attributed to therapy in the evolution of idiopathic MMM to acute leukemia. These statistics reinforce the concept of a group of myeloproliferative disorders which comprises both chronic and acute varieties, with frequent transitions between them. The same interpretation may be placed upon a report[79] of two patients with chronic granulocytic leukemia who developed metamorphosis characterized by large numbers of bizarre megaloblastoid erythroblasts, a picture resembling that in the Di Guglielmo syndrome.

LYMPHOPROLIFERATIVE DISORDERS

Further work in many laboratories has confirmed the fact that chronic lymphocytic leukemia and the lymphomas can in many instances be reclassified according to their origin from B- or T-cells. In the great majority of cases, CLL lymphocytes are predominantly B-cells, usually abnormal ones with reduced quantities of surface-bound immunoglobulins (SIg). In some cases nonimmunoglobulin-bearing B-cells may seemingly predominate.[54] Solid B-cell lymphomas carry much more SIg.[3,67] T-cell forms of chronic lymphocytic leukemia[50,81] and of solid lymphomas[76] have been seen in a minority of cases,[90] while the Sézary syndrome is now clearly recognized as having its origin from T-cells.[8,12,53] Dissociated loss of T-cell characteristics by the lymphocytes in Sézary's syndrome has been invoked to account for cases in which these cells do not respond to PHA.[45] By methods not used in earlier studies both B- and T-cell markers have now been found on individual human peripheral blood lymphocytes.[24] Although most lymphocytes can be assigned to one or other category, the existence of a subpopulation of cells with characteristics of both must complicate attempts to identify as B- or T-cells the lymphocytes of the leukemias and malignant lymphomas.[54]

Some improvement in prognosis of mycosis fungoides following total skin irradiation with 2.5 MeV electrons has been reported. In one series[5] '0 percent of patients were in remission 3–14 years after a single treatment and some of these may be cured.

In two patients with chronic lymphocytic leukemia, the disease was shown to undergo an acute blast cell crisis with blasts which had B-cell characteristics which, in one case, were identical with those of the original CLL lymphocytes.[13] It thus seemed likely that the leukemic cells found during the acute and chronic phases of the disease had originated from the same clone. Another important case report[28] concerns a woman with chronic lymphocytic leukemia who carried the constitutional chromosomal abnormality Gp-(Ch[1]). After treatment with chlorambucil over 8 years, she developed an acute leukemia with plasma cell characteristics and increased IgM levels. The nature of the terminal disease is open to several interpretations, including the possible role of the constitutional chromosomal aberration and the patient's previous treatment in its development.

The new methods for classifying the lymphoproliferative disorders—including the use of the scanning electron microscope[51,65]—may be particularly useful in showing connections and transitions between the various members of the group.

PARAPROTEINEMIAS

Gamma heavy chain disease has been reviewed and attention drawn to its occurrence in young adults, as well as in older patients.[6] Bone lesions and hypercalcemia may be less unusual in this rare condition than was formerly thought.

TREATMENT

Preliminary reports have appeared of the use of 5-azacytidine[46] and adriamycin[80] in the treatment of acute leukemia in children. Adriamycin (see Chapter 18) seems to be an effective agent for remission induction in both acute lymphocytic and acute granulocytic leukemia in children: 5-azacytidine is more effective against acute granulocytic leukemia. These early trials were of each drug used alone. Their place in combined drug regimens has yet to be explored and may be very much more important than when used alone. Neocarzinostatin is an antitumor antibiotic first used in the treatment of solid tumors several years ago. The first report of its use in acute leukemia has appeared only recently.[42] Used alone in both children and adults, it produced complete remission in 7 of 14 patients. Reports of further experience are awaited with interest.

Leukapheresis in chronic granulocytic leukemia was first described several years ago,[14,59] not as a primarily therapeutic procedure, but as a means of obtaining large numbers of granulocytes for infusion into neutropenic recipients. It has now been reported to produce symptomatic improvement and regression of splenomegaly and hepatomegaly when used in the chronic phase of the disease.[85] It had, if anything, a deleterious effect on hemoglobin levels and some patients required transfusion with packed red cells. It would appear that metamorphosis is not delayed or prevented by leukapheresis, but other possible benefits have not yet been fully explored. It has been suggested that the place of leukapheresis may lie in the prevention or treatment of the accumulative stage of the chronic phase, which follows one of cyclic leukocytosis with spontaneous return of leukocyte levels to base-line values.[32]

Both the recent papers on relatively large series of cases of leukemic reticuloendotheliosis ("hairy cell leukemia")[18,29] are in agreement on the value of splenectomy in this condition. In addition, Catovsky et al.[18] found adrenal corticosteroids to be effective.

In a preliminary report of the British Medical Research Council Working Party for Childhood Leukemia,[89] optimal therapy for overt meningeal leukemia is described. This at present appears to be 2,400 rad to the cranial vault, 1,000 rad to the spinal axis, and at least six intrathecal injections of methotrexate in a dose of 10 mg. per sq. m. at weekly intervals.

In a small series of cases of both chronic lymphocytic leukemia and myelofibrosis[66] oxymetholone has been shown to increase hemoglobin levels, decrease transfusion needs, and improve platelet levels. The patients thus treated were all of the difficult group previously found to be refractory to antineoplastic chemotherapy.

The ability of patients with leukemias to produce interferon is reduced, and interferon levels are likely to influence the ability to recover from serious viral infections. There is evidence that such infections in children with acute leukemia may be prevented by intramuscular injection of human leukocytic interferon.[2] Any antileukemic effect of the interferon is at present uncertain.

PROGNOSIS

The increasing number of patients with *acute leukemia,* especially children between 1 and 10 years of age, who survive for long periods has brought with it a continuing discussion on the possibility of cures, and, more practically, on the likelihood of relapses in long-term survivors. A study from Britain[83] has provided evidence on the latter question. Among 100 patients with acute leukemia who survived at least 4 years after diagnosis—only 11 of them more than 15 years old and the majority females—there was a 25 percent annual death rate during the fifth and sixth years, and one of 6 percent thereafter: no patient died after the tenth year. The most important prognostic sign in this group was the occurrence of relapses before the fifth year. Among the patients who had been in continuous remission from first treatment, 70 percent appeared likely to survive indefinitely, whereas only 17 percent of those with one or more relapses in the first 4 years had a similarly favorable prognosis. Clearly, therefore, the longer the first remission, the greater the chance of long survival. Although these authors took 4 years as their initial cut-off point, it could well be that 3 or even fewer years without relapse might have a similar significance.

In a recent study of 1024 cases of childhood acute leukemia from 1958 through 1970, the prognostic importance of age, race, cytologic type of leukemia, the leukocyte count at diagnosis, initial platelet count, and the extent of extramyeloid disease have all been confirmed.[33] In this multicenter cooperative study, the patient's sex, the hemoglobin level at diagnosis, and the proportion of blast cells in the initial bone marrow sample were of no prognostic significance. In contrast, an earlier report[49] of the prognostic value of enumeration of PAS positive blasts in marrow in acute lymphocytic leukemia in childhood has recently been confirmed.[86] Of a group of children treated by a cyclic regimen, none with less than 35 percent PAS-positive blast cells in marrow at diagnosis survived beyond the median: most of those with more than 35 percent survived longer.

A retrospective study of 839 patients with *chronic lymphocytic leukemia*[92] revealed an overall 5-year survival rate of 34 percent which, when adjusted for expected mortality from other causes (relative survival rate), rose to 44 percent: 50 percent for females and 41 percent for males. The rate declined with increasing age at diagnosis. Although minor prognostic differences were found in groups with differing clinical and hematologic manifestations and different forms of therapy, the major differentials attributed to sex and age persisted even after adjustments for other variables had been made. An unexpected finding was that in both sexes the best survivals occurred in individuals with initial leukocyte counts between 25,000 and 49,000 per cu.mm. Although it was not known what accounted for this finding, it should be said that our own experience tends to confirm it. These results, which originated from the combined results of a large group of hospitals, probably form the best existing baseline with which survival in other series can be compared.

REFERENCES

1. Adelstein AM, Donovan JW: Malignant disease in children whose mothers had chicken-pox, mumps or rubella in pregnancy. Br Med J 4:629, 1972.

2. Ahstrom L, Dohlwitz A, Strander H, Carlström G, Cantell K: Interferon in acute leukaemia in children. Lancet 1:166, 1974.

3. Aisenberg AC, Bloch KR: Immunoglobulins on the surface of neoplastic lymphocytes. N Engl J Med 287:272, 1972.

4. Aye MT, Till JE, McCullough EA: Growth of leukemic cells in culture. Blood 40:806, 1972.

5. Barr RD, Fialkow PJ: Clonal origin of chronic myelocytic leukemia. N Engl J Med 289:307, 1973.

6. Bloch KJ, Lee L, Mills JA, Haber E: Gamma heavy chain disease—an expanding clinical and laboratory spectrum. Am J Med 55:61, 1973.

7. Bowen JM, Allen PT, East JL, Maruyama K, Newton WA, Georgiades J, Priori ES, Dmochowski L: Molecular probes in studies of the relationship of viruses to human neoplasia. Am J Clin Path 60:88, 1973.

8. Broome JD, Zucker-Franklin D, Weiner MS, Brianco C, Nussenzweig V: Leukemic cells with membrane properties of thymus derived (T) lymphocytes in a case of Sézary's syndrome: morphologic and immunologic studies. Clin Immunol Immunopathol 1:319, 1973.

9. Bross IDJ, Bertell R, Gibson R: Pets and adult leukemia. Am J Public Health 62: 1520, 1972.

10. _____, Gibson R: Cats and childhood leukemia. J Med 1:180, 1970.

11. _____, Natarajan N: Leukemia from low-level radiation. N Engl J Med 287:107, 1972.

12. Brouet J-C, Flandrin G, Seligmann M: Indications of the thymus-derived nature of the proliferating cells in six patients with Sézary's syndrome. N Engl J Med 289:341, 1973.

13. _____, Preud'homme J-L, Seligmann M, Bernard J: Blast cells with monoclonal surface immunoglobulin in two cases of acute blast crisis supervening on chronic lymphocytic leukaemia. Br Med J 4:23, 1973.

14. Buckner D, Graw RG, Eisel RJ, Henderson ES, Perry S: Leukapheresis by continuous flow centrifugation (CFC) in patients with

chronic myelocytic leukemia (CML). Blood 33:353, 1969.

15. Canellos GP, Whang-Peng J: Philadelphia-chromosome-positive preleukaemic state. Lancet 2:1227, 1972.

16. Catovsky D, Galton DAG, Robinson J: Myeloperoxidase-deficient neutrophils in acute myeloid leukaemia. Scand J Haematol 9:142, 1972.

17. ———, Pettit JE, Galetto J, Okos A, Galton DAG: The B-lymphocyte nature of the hairy cell of leukaemic reticuloendotheliosis. Br J Haematol 26:21, 1974.

18. ———, ———, Galton DAG, Spiers ASD, Harrison CV: Leukaemic reticuloendotheliosis ("Hairy" cell leukaemia): a distinct clinico-pathological entity. Br J Haematol 26:1, 1974.

19. Caul EO, Dickinson VA, Roome AP, Mott MG, Stevenson PA: Cytomegalovirus infections in leukaemic children. Int J Cancer 10:213, 1972.

20. Cline MJ, Golde DW: A review and re-evaluation of the histiocytic disorders. Am J Med 55:49, 1973.

21. da Silva Horta J, Abbatt JD, Cayolla da Motta L, Tavares H: Leukaemia, malignancies and other late effects following administration of thorotrast. Z Krebsforsch 77:202, 1972.

22. Davidson WM, Knight LA: Acquired trisomy 9. Lancet 1:390, 1973.

23. Diamond EL, Schmerler H, Lilienfeld AM: The relationship of intra-uterine radiation to subsequent mortality and development of leukemia in children. A prospective study. Am J Epidemiol 97:283, 1973.

24. Dickler HB, Adkinson NF, Terry WD: Evidence for individual human peripheral blood lymphocytes bearing both B- and T-cell markers. Nature 247:213, 1974.

25. Drewinko B, Sullivan MP, Martin T: Use of the cytocentrifuge in the diagnosis of meningeal leukemia. Cancer 31:1331, 1973.

26. Fedrick J, Alberman ED: Reported influenza in pregnancy and subsequent cancer in the child. Br Med J 2:485, 1972.

27. Feldges AJ: Diagnosis of meningeal leukemia in acute childhood lymphocytic leukemia with periodic acid-Schiff reaction of cytocentrifuged liquor. Acta Haematol 49:154, 1973.

28. Fitzgerald PH, Rastrick JM, Hamer JW: Acute plasma cell leukaemia following chronic lymphocytic leukaemia: Transformation or two separate diseases? Br J Haematol 25:171, 1973.

29. Flandrin G, Daniel MT, Fourcade M,

Chelloul N: Leucémie à "tricholeucocytes" (Hairy cell leukaemia), étude clinique et cytologique de 55 observations. Nouv Rev Fr Hématol 13:609, 1973.

30. Fuks ZY, Bagshaw MA, Farber EM: Prognostic signs and the management of mycosis fungoides. Cancer 32:1385, 1973.

31. Gallo RC: Summary of recent observations on the molecular biology of RNA tumor viruses and attempts at application to human leukemia. Am J Clin Pathol 60:80, 1973.

32. Gatti RA, Robinson WA, Deinard AS, Nesbit M, McCullough JJ, Ballow M, Good RA: Cyclic leukocytosis in chronic myelogenous leukemia: new perspectives on pathogenesis and therapy. Blood 41:771, 1973.

33. George SL, Fernbach DJ, Vietti TJ, Sullivan MP, Lane DM, Haggard ME, Berry DH, Lonsdale D, Komp D: Factors influencing survival in pediatric acute leukemia: the SWCCSG experience, 1958–1970. Cancer 32:1542, 1973.

34. Golde DW, Cline MJ: Identification of the colony-stimulating cell in human peripheral blood. J Clin Invest 51:2981, 1972.

35. ———, Finlay TN, Cline MJ: Production of colony-stimulating factor by human macrophages. Lancet 2:1397, 1972.

36. Goldman JM, Th'ng KH: Phagocytic function of leucocytes from patients with acute myeloid and chronic granulocytic leukaemia. Br J Haematol 25, 299, 1973.

37. Granström M, Gahrton G: Colony-forming and colony-stimulating cells in normal human peripheral blood. Exp Cell Res 80:372, 1973.

38. Hakulinen T, Hovi L, Karkinen-Jääskeläinen M, Penttinen K, Saxén L: Association between influenza during pregnancy and childhood leukaemia. Br Med J 4:265, 1973.

39. Haran-Ghera N: Relationship between tumour cell and host in chemical leukaemogenesis. Nature New Biol., 246:84, 1973.

40. Hardy WD Jr, Old LJ, Hess PW, Essex M, Cotter S: Horizontal transmission of feline leukaemia virus. Nature 244:266, 1973.

41. Hehlmann R, Baxt W, Kufe D, Spiegelman S: Molecular evidence for a viral etiology of human leukemias, lymphomas, and sarcomas. Am J Clin Pathol 60:65, 1973.

42. Hiraki K, Kamimura O, Takahashi I, Nagao T, Kitajima K, Irino S: Neocarzinostatin: une approche nouvelle dans la chimiothérapie des leucémies aiguës. Nouv Rev Fr Hématol 13:29, 1973.

43. Hunt RD, Melendez LV, Garcia FG, Trum BF: Pathologic features of *herpesvirus ateles*

lymphoma in cotton-topped marmosets *(Saguinus oedipus)*. J Natl Cancer Inst 49:1631, 1972.

44. Johnston SS, Ware CF: Iris involvement in leukaemia. Br J Ophthalmal 57:320, 1973.

45. Kalden JR, Peter HH, Odriozola J, Richter W, Richter R: Sézary syndrome. Lancet 1:688, 1974.

46. Karon M, Sieger L, Leimbrocks S, Finklestein JZ, Nesbit ME, Swaney JJ: 5-azacytidine: a new active agent for the treatment of acute leukemia. Blood 42:359, 1973.

47. Knight LA, Davidson WM, Cuddigan BJ: Acquired trisomy 9. Lancet 1:688, 1974.

48. Kufe DW, Spiegelman S: Molecular probing for a viral etiology of human leukemias and lymphomas, including Burkitt's disease. Wadley Med Bull 3:83, 1973.

49. Laurie HC: Duration of remissions in lymphoblastic leukaemia of childhood. Br Med J 2:95, 1968.

50. Lille I, Desplaces A, Meeus L, Saracino RT, Brouet J-C: Thymus-derived proliferating lymphocytes in chronic lymphocytic leukaemia. Lancet 2:263, 1973.

51. Lin PS, Cooper AG, Wortis HH: Scanning electron microscopy of human T-cell and B-cell rosettes. N Engl J Med 289:548, 1973.

52. Liu PI, Ishimaru T, McGregor DH, Yamamoto T, Steer A: Autopsy study of leukemia in atomic bomb survivors. Hiroshima-Nagasaki, 1949–1969. Cancer 31:1315, 1973.

53. Lutzner MA, Emerit I, Durepaire T, Flandrin G, Grupper Ch, Pruniéras M: Cytogenetic, cytophotometric, and ultrastructural study of large cerebriform cells of the Sézary syndrome and description of a small-cell variant. J Natl Cancer Inst 50:1145, 1973.

54. McLaughlin H, Wetherley-Mein G, Pitcher C, Hobbs JR: Non-immunoglobulin bearing 'B' lymphocytes in chronic lymphatic leukaemia? Br J Haematol 25:7, 1973.

55. Melendez LV, Hunt RD, King NW, Barahona HH, Daniel MD, Fraser CEO, Garcia FG: *Herpesvirus ateles*. A new lymphoma virus of monkeys. Nature New Biol 235:182, 1972.

56. Messner HA, Till JE, McCullough EA: Interacting cell populations affecting granulopoietic colony formation by normal and leukemic human marrow cells. Blood 42:701, 1973.

57. Milligan WJ, Garson OM: Giemsa banding of "normal" leukaemic chromosomes: a preliminary report. Pathology 6:143, 1974.

58. Moore MAS, Williams N, Metcalf D: *In vitro* colony formation by normal and leukemic human hematopoietic cells: characterization of the colony-forming cells. J Natl Cancer Inst 50:603, 1973.

59. Morse EE, Freireich EJ, Carbone PP, Bronson W, Frei E: The transfusion of leukocytes from donors with chronic myelocytic leukemia to patients with leukopenia. Transfusion 6:182, 1966.

60. Motomura S, Ogi K, Horie M: Monoclonal origin of acute transformation of chronic myelogenous leukemia. Acta Haematol 49:300, 1973.

61. Muss HB, Moloney WC: Chloroma and other myeloblastic tumors. Blood 42:721, 1973.

62. Natarajan N, Bross IDJ: Preconception radiation and leukaemia. J Med 4:276, 1973.

63. Newman AJ, Melhorn DK: Vertebral compression in childhood leukemia. Am J Dis Child 125:863, 1973.

64. Nishiyama H, Anderson RE, Ishimaru T, Ishida K, Ii Y, Okabe N: The incidence of malignant lymphoma and multiple myeloma in Hiroshima and Nagasaki atomic bomb survivors, 1945–65. Cancer 32:1301, 1973.

65. Polliack A, Lampen N, Clarkson BD, De Harven E, Bentwich Z, Siegal FP, Kunkel HG: Identification of human B and T lymphocytes by scanning electron microscopy. J Exp Med 138:607, 1973.

66. Presant CA, Safdar SH: Oxymetholone in myelofibrosis and chronic lymphocytic leukemia. Arch Intern Med 132:175, 1973.

67. Preud'homme JL, Seligmann M: Surface-bound immunoglobulins as a cell marker in human lymphoproliferative diseases. Blood 40:777, 1972.

68. Quesenberry P, Morley A, Stohlman F Jr, Rickard K, Howard D, Smith M: Effect of endotoxin on granulopoiesis and colony-stimulating factor. N Engl J Med 286:227, 1972.

69. Rowley JD: A new consistent chromosome abnormality in chronic myelogenous leukaemia identified by quinacrine fluorescence and Giemsa staining. Nature 243:290, 1973.

70. ———: Acquired trisomy 9. Lancet 2:390, 1973.

71. Rubin SH, Cowan DH: Assay of granulopoietic progenitor cells in human peripheral blood. Exp Hematol 1:127, 1973.

72. Ruscetti FW, Chervenick PA: Release of colony-stimulating factor from monocytes by endotoxin and polyinosinic-polycytidylic acid. J Lab Clin Med 83:64, 1974.

73. Sarngadharan MG, Sarin PS, Reitz MS,

Gallo RC: Reverse transcriptase activity of human acute leukaemic cells: purification of the enzyme, response to AMV 705 RNA, and characterization of the DNA product. Nature New Biol 240:67, 1972.

74. Sherman NJ, Woolley MM: The ileocecal syndrome in acute childhood leukemia. Arch Surg 107:39, 1973.

75. Silverstein MN, Brown AL, Linman JW: Idiopathic myeloid metaplasia. Its evolution into acute leukemia. Arch Intern Med 132:709, 1973.

76. Smith JL, Barker CR, Clein GP, Collins RD: Characterization of malignant mediastinal lymphoid neoplasm (Sternberg sarcoma) as thymic in origin. Lancet 1:74, 1973.

77. Spiers ASD: Blood abnormalities during leukaemia treatment. Lancet 1:674, 1974.

78. Spitzer G, Garson OM, Lymphoblastic leukemia with marked eosinophilia: a report of two cases. Blood 42:377, 1973.

79. Srodes CH, Hyde EH, Boggs DR: Autonomous erythropoiesis during erythroblastic crisis of chronic myelocytic leukemia. J Clin Invest 52:512, 1973.

80. Starling KA, Berry DH, Britton HA, Humphrey GB, Vats T, Ragab AH: Adriamycin for induction of remission in acute leukemia in children. Blood 42:1015, 1973.

81. Sumiya M, Mizoguchi H, Kosaka K, Miura Y, Takaku F, Yata J: Chronic lymphocytic leukaemia of T-cell origin? Lancet 2:910, 1973.

82. Temin HM: The protovirus hypothesis: speculations on the significance of RNA-directed DNA synthesis for normal de-velopment and for carcinogenesis. J Natl Cancer Inst 46:iii, 1971.

83. Till MM, Hardisty RM, Pike MC: Long survivals in acute leukaemia. Lancet 1:534, 1973.

84. Ting RC, Yang SS, Gallo RC: Reverse transcriptase RNA tumour virus transformation and derivatives of rifamycin SV. Nature New Biol 236:163, 1972

85. Vallejos CS, McCredie KB, Brittin GM, Freireich EJ: Biological effects of repeated leukapheresis of patients with chronic myelogenous leukemia. Blood 42:925, 1973.

86. Vowells MR, Willoughby MLN: Cyclic chemotherapy in acute lymphoblastic leukaemia of childhood. 5-year survivals. Arch Dis Child 48:436, 1973.

87. Wainer RA, Wiernik PH, Thompson WL: Metabolic and therapeutic studies of a patient with acute leukemia and severe lactic acidosis of prolonged duration. Am J Med 55:255, 1973.

88. Wertelecki W, Mantel N: Increased birth weight in leukemia. Pediatr Res 7:132, 1973.

89. Willoughby MLN: Treatment for overt meningeal leukaemia. Lancet 1:363, 1974.

90. Wilson JD, Hurdle AD: Surface immunoglobulins on lymphocytes in chronic lymphocytic leukaemia and lymphosarcoma. Br J Haematol 24:563, 1973.

91. Wolfe LG, Falk LA, Deinhardt F: Oncogenicity of herpesvirus saimiri in marmoset monkeys. J Natl Cancer Inst 47:1145, 1971.

92. Zippin C, Cutler SJ, Reeves WJ Jr, Lum D: Survival in chronic lymphocytic leukemia. Blood 42:367, 1973.

Index

817

        a
4   b
5   c
6   d
7   e
8   f
9   g
0   h
1   i
8   2   j